MEDIEVAL PERIOD (5TH TO 15TH CENTURY)

Characteristics. Breakdown of social conditions due to wars, plagues, migrations. Life was unpredictable, precarious, and anxiety-ridden. Contributions made by the Greeks and Romans were offset by a regression to primitive treatments and beliefs. General hospitals were established as well as Bedlam, a hospital for the mentally ill. Patients would go into the streets and beg if they were well enough; if not, they were chained, treated inhumanely, and exhibited to the general public.

Treatments. Exorcisms by priests, harsh primitive methods; banishment of mentally ill to fend for themselves.

Therapists. Sorcerers, priests.

Nursing. Although society was chaotic, nursing developed roots, purpose, direction, and leadership as the profession moved into the missions and monasteries. Nuns and monks did much of the work of the nurse. In the village of Gheel, housewives took the mentally ill into their homes, accepted them as foster family members, and treated them kindly.

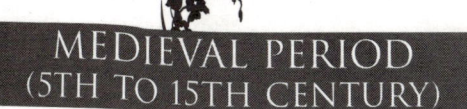

RENAISSANCE (16TH CENTURY)

Characteristics. The beginning of modern science and the age of enlightenment, during which the basis for modern clinical descriptions of mental illness was established. Many contradictions concerning mental illness. Ruthless witch-hunting and persecution of mentally ill continued. All human frailties were viewed as works of the devil. At the same time, the humane movement was underway with deep sympathy for the unfortunate and the sick.

Treatments. Harsh punishments, along with rebirth of clinical observation and humane treatment.

Therapists. Sorcerers. **Juhann Weyer**, known as father of modern psychiatry, viewed "possession" as mental illness. **Paracelsus** was the first to refer to unconscious motivation as a contributor to mental illness.

Nursing. Men and women delivered nursing care to those with varying health needs, across the age continuum. Nurses became more educated and continued to treat the patient physically, as well as psychosocially.

Contemporary Psychiatric–Mental Health Nursing

The Brain-Behavior Connection

Contemporary Psychiatric–Mental Health Nursing

The Brain-Behavior Connection

Carol A. Glod, RN, CS, PhD
Assistant Professor
Northeastern University College of Nursing
Lecturer
Department of Psychiatry
Harvard Medical School
Boston, Massachusetts

Bipolar and Psychotic Disorders Program
McLean Hospital
Belmont, Massachusetts

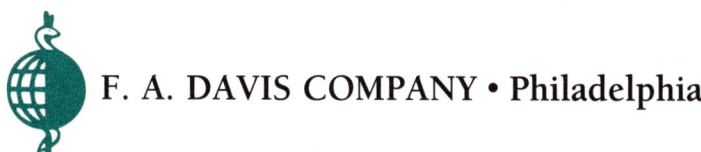

F. A. DAVIS COMPANY • Philadelphia

F. A. Davis Company
1915 Arch Street
Philadelphia, PA 19103

Copyright © 1998 by F. A. Davis Company. All rights reserved. This book is protected by copyright. No part of it may be reproduced, stored in a retrieval system, or transmitted in any form or by any means, electronic, mechanical, photocopying, recording, or otherwise, without written permission from the publisher.

Printed in the United States of America

Last digit indicates print number: 10 9 8 7 6 5 4 3 2 1

Acquisitions Editor: Joanne Patzek DaCunha, RN, MSN
Developmental Editor: Melanie Freely
Production Editors: Michael Schnee, Nancee Morelli
Cover Designer: Louis J. Forgione
Cover Artwork: Susan Miyamoto

As new scientific information becomes available through basic and clinical research, recommended treatments and drug therapies undergo changes. The authors and publisher have done everything possible to make this book accurate, up to date, and in accord with accepted standards at the time of publication. The authors, editors, and publisher are not responsible for errors or omissions or for consequences from application of the book, and make no warranty, expressed or implied, in regard to the contents of the book. Any practice described in this book should be applied by the reader in accordance with professional standards of care used in regard to the unique circumstances that may apply in each situation. The reader is advised always to check product information (package inserts) for changes and new information regarding dose and contraindications before administering any drug. Caution is especially urged when using new or infrequently ordered drugs.

Library of Congress Cataloging in Publication Data

Contemporary psychiatric–mental health nursing : the brain-behavior
  connection / [edited by] Carol A. Glod.
      p.   cm.
    Includes bibliographical references and index.
    ISBN 0-8036-0293-6 (alk. paper)
    1. Psychiatric nursing.   2. Community health nursing.   I. Glod,
Carol A., 1958– .
    [DNLM: 1. Psychiatric Nursing.   2. Community Health Nursing.   WY
160 C761 1998]
RC440.C585 1998
610.73′68—dc21
DNLM/DLC
for Library of Congress   97-46122
                                                            CIP

Authorization to photocopy items for internal or personal use, or the internal or personal use of specific clients, is granted by F. A. Davis Company for users registered with the Copyright Clearance Center (CCC) Transactional Reporting Service, provided that the fee of $.10 per copy is paid directly to CCC, 222 Rosewood Drive, Salem, MA 01923. For those organizations that have been granted a photocopy license by CCC, a separate system of payment has been arranged. The fee code for users of the Transactional Reporting Service is: 8036-0293 / 98 0 + $.10.

Dedication

To my parents.

To my mother, Jennie, a beautiful, vibrant woman struck by postpartum depression after my birth, who first taught me about the pain and suffering that mental illness causes and how it steals away the person you once were. Her ongoing struggles with mental illness have helped me become a better educator and human being and have shown me how health professionals and society can either help or harm individuals who suffer from psychiatric conditions.

To my father, Bill, a generous, caring, and devoted father. He provided the nurturing that shaped me into who I am today; he showed me how to overcome fear and muster the courage to face unbearable pain; he taught me to understand and accept others' behaviors and problems by recognizing the inherent goodness in their souls; and he instilled in me the belief that I could do anything I really wanted.

Preface

Carol A. Glod, RN, CS, PhD

I didn't set out to be a psychiatric nurse. I was raised during the feminist movement; new doors were opening and I could be anything that I wanted. With more options than my mother and her generation, I wasn't limited to traditional careers like teaching or nursing.

I began college as a biology major. But one summer, while doing cancer research, I realized that I was becoming bored with biochemistry. I longed for someone to talk to. It was then that I switched my major to nursing.

All nurses use a number of interpersonal and psychiatric nursing skills to help clients cope with their medical problems. Psychiatric nurses have a unique role: They promote the psychological health of individuals, families, and communities and help people deal with grief, crisis, or developmental difficulties. They also care for those with intractable illnesses such as schizophrenia, depression, and posttraumatic stress disorder. How they do that is part of what this book is about.

For years, experts believed that inadequate parenting and mothers who gave "mixed messages" contributed to mental illness. Then Congress declared the 1990s "The Decade of the Brain," sparking a biological revolution. Research dollars were dedicated to discovering biological and genetic markers and abnormalities in brain functioning and structure. Researchers found that like neurological conditions, psychiatric disorders may result from problems in the brain. This emphasis on the biological basis of psychiatric disorders led to new medications (psychopharmacology) and the treatment of psychiatric disorders with these agents (pharmacotherapy). Although some individuals have been helped dramatically, others continue to have intermittent or chronic mental health problems.

Psychobiology describes the interplay between biological and genetic makeup and life experience. Psychobiologists look at the synergism between the workings of the mind, the so-called psyche, and biology, particularly the structural and functional aspects of the brain. This framework has been refined into a new theoretical position that is called developmental or neural plasticity. It says that the brain, an organ that continues to develop well into adolescence, is shaped by both physical and psychological experiences that account for disturbances in thinking, emotions, and behavior.

We still know little about the actual psychological and biological causes of psychiatric disorders. What is clear, however, is that they affect people's abilities to work, function, and relate to others. For psychiatric nurses, the challenge is to understand and balance the latest psychological and neurobiological developments. Just as important is the nurse's ability to recognize how illness affects the client's ability to attend school or work or remain connected to others in healthy, satisfying relationships. For example, knowing that schizophrenia can be inherited or that it is caused by some abnormality in the brain does little to help individuals or their families cope with the havoc the disease causes. For some clients, medications will control their symptoms, allowing them to live a more satisfying life in the community and pursue some of their interests. But, for others, medication may have little effect or have difficult and uncomfortable side effects.

Today, clients may be treated briefly in the hospital, but they receive the majority of psychiatric care in the community. Psychiatric nurses are trained at homeless shelters, community-based day programs, crisis centers, psychiatric home care agencies, and other community settings. This book explores community-based psychiatric nursing treatment based on the program offered at Northeastern University's Center for Community Health, Education, and Research (CCHERS—pronounced "cheers"). The program uses a comprehensive holistic model of care that is designed to be responsive to the needs of individuals, families, and the community. Every clinical course, including psychiatric nursing, is focused on providing health care in the community, where most treatment actually takes place. Students begin their nursing training in community health centers, which target vulnerable and underserved populations.

The first unit of this book discusses the theories that are the foundation for linking, or bridging, brain and behavior. It also focuses on the legal and ethical issues in the care of persons with psychiatric problems. In addition, assessing physical and psychological functioning, planning care, and effective therapeutic communication are addressed. The delivery of care in various settings, particularly the community, is emphasized.

Unit Two explores healthy psychological development. The classic theories from Piaget and Erikson are presented, as well as newer ones on the psychology of women. A comprehensive chapter on neuroanatomy and neurophysiology provides a basis for understanding the pathophysiology of psychiatric conditions and treatment. **Included is an eight-page color insert that illustrates the structural and functional aspects of the healthy and the unhealthy brain.**

Treatment of psychiatric problems ranges from medications to somatic therapies to many different types of psychotherapy, including so-called talk therapy. The third unit begins with an in-depth overview of the major classes of psychiatric medications. This section also reviews the latest advances in each of the major forms of psychotherapy, including cognitive-behavior therapy (CBT). Finally, the latest information on some controversial biological treatments, such as electroconvulsive therapy (ECT), psychosurgery, and phototherapy (light therapy) are discussed.

The fourth unit of this text details the nursing care of clients with major psychiatric disorders, generally following the *Diagnostic and Statistical Manual of Mental Disorders, Fourth Edition (DSM-IV)*. DSM-IV represents how all disciplines categorize psychiatric conditions. Each chapter contains the essential information on diagnostic criteria and descriptions of the illness. Clinical vignettes illustrate the clients' and their families' experiences with psychiatric illness. Clinical management tips and care plans help outline effective interventions. The latest treatments based on available research are presented along with research notes—descriptions of specific nursing and interdisciplinary research studies. For psychiatric nursing to move into the 21st century, we must learn and continually study why we do what we do and what works the best. The focus of caring for the client is also based on the continuum of psychiatric nursing care, from crisis centers to inpatient units to the community, where the bulk of treatment occurs. Contemporary psychiatric nursing means caring for clients and their families in the community, and with helping them mobilize community resources.

Nurses have a primary role in caring for vulnerable groups with community-based problems. Many of these clients do not have one disorder, but suffer from many psychiatric, medical, emotional, financial, and social problems. They present a special challenge to care providers in nonpsychiatric settings.

Unit Five addresses those conditions that cut across nursing specialities: abuse, violence, incarceration, grief, AIDS, severe and persistent psychiatric illness, and homelessness.

The book ends with a chapter on future trends that discusses how the present health care environment has affected treatment for those with mental disorders. The challenges and opportunities for psychiatric nurses in what is expected to be a time of continuing change are explored.

On the cover and throughout this book are contributions from the National Alliance for Research on Schizophrenia and Depression (NARSAD) Artworks. NARSAD Artworks provides art by and on behalf of mentally ill persons to promote their employment and recovery and to reduce the stigma associated with psychiatric disorders. NARSAD raises money that directly supports ongoing research of major mental illnesses. I am a beneficiary of their work. My NARSAD Young Investigator Award supports my research on sleep and activity disturbances in adolescents with depression and posttraumatic stress disorder. I am thankful for the direct support NARSAD has provided to my research career and feel privileged to be able to include such creative works of art in this text.

It is an exciting time for psychiatric research. New discoveries and technological advances point to the neurosciences as the foundation for understanding psychiatric disorders. The challenge, however, is to maintain a focus on the individual and the nurse-client relationship balanced against new knowledge about pathophysiology. Psychobiology and research in developmental plasticity of the brain offers important insights into the causes of mental illness and the care of those suffering from it.

Acknowledgments

I am indebted to many people for helping the ideas in this book come together. First, I thank the many patients whom I have worked with over the years, who have shared their experiences with me and allowed me to learn about their illnesses and reactions along with them. Second, each of the contributors, nurses, psychiatrists, psychologists, and students generously gave their time, energy, and insight to provide the "latest and greatest" information. Writing has many rewards, yet also many challenges. I thank them for all of their hard work and patience as their chapters were revised and finessed into final form. Third, this book would not have been possible without the dedication and wisdom of the staff at F. A. Davis, particularly Joanne DaCunha, MSN, and Melanie Freely. They, too, generously gave their encouragement, advice, and time to help produce each chapter. We met as author and editors, but we have become good friends. Finally, this book would not have been begun or completed without the great deal of help that I received from my friends and colleagues:

Nicole Phillips, who was always willing to call a contributor or chase down an article;

Nancy Torkewitz, who was always there when I needed her;

Kate Detwiler, whose direct and honest remarks kept me on track ("you know this book is really making you irritable; I won't take it personally");

Pamela and Alex Campbell, who encouraged me along the way;

Dr. Barbara Wolfe, for supporting me in the ups and downs;

Dr. Geoffrey McEnany, for keeping me laughing;

and my mentors, Drs. Carol Hartman and Marty Teicher.

C.A.G.

Contributors

Susan L. Andersen, PhD
Instructor of Psychiatry
Harvard Medical School/McLean Hospital
Belmont, Massachusetts

Billie Barringer, BSN, MA, RNC, CNS
Associate Professor
Northeast Louisiana University
Monroe, Louisiana

Anne Bateman, RN, CS, EdD
Assistant Professor
College of Nursing
Northeastern University
Boston, Massachusetts

Thröstur Björgvinsson, MA
Psychology Intern
Psychology Department
McLean Hospital
Belmont, Massachusetts
Clinical Fellow
Department of Psychiatry
Harvard Medical School
Boston, Massachusetts

Pamela D. Campbell, BS/OTR, MS/CIS
Director of Training Services
Technology Resource Group
Wayland, Massachusetts
Associate Professor
Boston University
Boston, Massachusetts

Doreen Cawley, RN, MS, CS, ARNP
Outpatient Therapist/Nurse Practitioner
The Hitchcock Clinic—Behavioral Health
Nashua, New Hampshire

Margery Chisholm, RN, EdD, CS, ABPP
Associate Professor
Northeastern University
Lecturer
Harvard Medical School
Boston, Massachusetts

Patricia Dahme, MSN, ARNP, CS
Psychiatric Nurse Practitioner
Clinical Nurse Specialist
Private Practice
Concord, New Hampshire

Debra Ann Danforth, MS, ARNP
Adult Nurse Practitioner
University of South Florida
Tampa, Florida

Nicole Duane, RN, MSc
Graduate Student
College of Nursing
Northeastern University
Boston, Massachusetts

Linda M. Gorman, RN, MN, CS, OCN, CRNH
Clinical Nurse Specialist
Cedars Sinai Medical Center
Los Angeles, California

Barbara A. Jones, RN, DNSc
Associate Professor
School of Nursing
Gwynedd-Mercy College
Gwynedd Valley, Pennsylvania

Karen Hogan King, RN, MS, CS, PC
Psychiatric Clinical Nurse Specialist
McLean Hospital
Belmont, Massachusetts

Philip Levendusky, PhD, FAClinP
Vice President, Network Development
Chairman, Psychology Department
Director of Clinical Training
McLean Hospital
Belmont, Massachusetts
Assistant Professor of Psychiatry
Department of Psychiatry
Harvard Medical School
Boston, Massachusetts

Suzanne Levy, RN, PhD
Nurse Psychotherapist
West Chester Psychiatric Associates
West Chester, Pennsylvania

Cindy A. Peternelj-Taylor, RN, MSc
Associate Professor
College of Nursing
University of Saskatchewan
Saskatoon, Saskatchewan

Sonja Stone Peterson, RN, EdD
Professor
University of Massachusetts
North Dartmouth, Massachusetts

Shari Petronis-Gibson, MSW, LSW
Administrative Director of Psychiatry
Abington Memorial Hospital
Abington, Pennsylvania

Ann Polcari, RN, CS, PhDc
Doctoral Student
School of Nursing
Boston College
Boston, Massachusetts
Research Associate
Developmental Biopsychiatry Research Program
McLean Hospital
Belmont, Massachusetts

Gail Schober, MS, RN, CS, CNA
Nurse Manager
Hebrew Rehabilitation Center for the Aged
Boston, Massachusetts

Roberta Schweitzer, RN, CS, PhD
Assistant Professor
Orvis School of Nursing
University of Nevada—Reno
Reno, Nevada

Joyce Dagnal Shields, RN, MS, CS, CGP
Private Practice
Individual, Couples, and Group Psychotherapy
Associate in Nursing
McLean Hospital
Cochair, Conference Committee
Northeastern Society for Group Psychotherapy
Belmont, Massachusetts
Cofounder
Aftercare Resource Associates
Arlington, Massachusetts

Anne L. Silva, RN, MS, CS
Private Practice
Individual, Family, and Group Psychotherapy
Cofounder
Aftercare Resource Associates
Arlington, Massachusetts

George Byron Smith, RNC, MSN, CCM
Mental Health Case Manager and Consultant
Columbia Home Care
Clearwater, Florida
Visiting Instructor and Adjunct Faculty
University of South Florida
Tampa, Florida

Stephanie Stockard Spelic, MSN, RN, CS, CPC, LMHP
Assistant Professor
Psychiatric–Mental Health Nursing
School of Nursing
Creighton University
Omaha, Nebraska

Nancy Valentine, RN, MPH, PhD, FAAN
Chief Consultant
Nursing Strategic Health Care Group
Department of Veteran Affairs
Washington, D.C.

Gail Wangerin, RN, PhD
Director of Program Development
Arbour Counseling Services
Lawrence, Massachusetts

Barbara E. Wolfe, RN, CS, PhD
Clinical Nurse Specialist
Department of Psychiatry
Beth Israel Deconess Hospital
Assistant Professor of Psychiatry
Harvard Medical School
Boston, Massachusetts

Consultants

Naomi Ballard, RN, MA, MS, CNRN
Associate Professor
Oregon Health Sciences University
Portland, Oregon

Cecilia R. Barron, RN, PhD
Associate Professor
University of Nebraska Medical Center
Omaha, Nebraska

George Blake, RPh
Practice Manager
Eastern Medical Associates
Blue Bell, Pennsylvania

Judy Bourrand, BSN, MSN
Assistant Professor of Nursing
Samford University
Birmingham, Alabama

Marcia Cohen, MS, RN, CS, CGP
Adjunct Clinical Instructor
Columbia University Medical Center
Columbia, New York

Barbara Crosson, RN, MSN
Assistant Professor
Valdosta State University
Valdosta, Georgia

Edward J. Edwards, RN, MSN, EdD, CHES
Assistant Professor
Indiana University of Pennsylvania
Indiana, Pennsylvania

Karen Espeland, CCDN, RN, MSN
Associate Professor
Medical Center One
Bismarck, North Dakota

Amy Govoni, CS, RN, MSN
Assistant Professor
Cleveland State University
Cleveland, Ohio

Connie S. Heflin, MSN
Associate Professor
Paducah Community College
Paducah, Kentucky

Mildred Hogstel, RN, C, PhD
Emeritus Professor of Nursing
Texas Christian University
Fort Worth, Texas

Julia F. Houfek, RN, PhD
Assistant Professor
University of Nebraska Medical Center
Omaha, Nebraska

David Keller, RN, MS
Professor
Brigham Young University
Provo, Utah

Alice R. Kempe, MEd, MSN, PhD
Associate Professor
Ursuline College
Pepper Pike, Ohio

Judy Kendall, RN, PMHNP, PhD
Associate Professor
Oregon Health Sciences University
Portland, Oregon

Dianne Kinzel, RN, MN
Lecturer
Intercollegiate Center for Nursing
    Education
Spokane, Washington

Doris K. Kowalski, RN, MA
Professor
Carl Sanburg College
Galesburg, Illinois

Judy A. Malone, RN, PhD
Associate Professor
Ball State University
Muncie, Indiana

Judith Matana, RN, MS
Instructor
Somerville Hospital
Somerville, Massachusetts

Joan Q. McDevitt, RN, BSN, MSN, EdD
Professor
Gwynedd-Mercy College
Gwynedd Valley, Pennsylvania

Daryl Minicucci, RN, MSN, PhDc
Assistant Professor
Rochester University
Rochester, New York

Linda Nance Marks, RN, EdD
Associate Professor
University of Texas
Arlington, Texas

Ann Parkinson, RN, MS
Assistant Professor
University of Utah
Salt Lake City, Utah

Dawn Margaret Scheick, RN, MN, CS
Associate Professor
Alderson Broaddus College
Phillipi, West Virginia

Marcia Shannon, RN, MSN
Assistant Professor
Saginaw Valley State University
University Center, Michigan

Margaret P. Shepard, RN, PhD
Professor
University of Rochester
Rochester, New York

Janet Teets, RN
Assistant Professor
Miami University
Hamilton, Ohio

Susan M. Weeks, RN, MS
Professor
Texas Christian University
Fort Worth, Texas

Kathleen Spor Wilson, BSN, MSN, PhD
Professor
Houston Community College
Houston, Texas

NARSAD Artworks artists whose works are reproduced on Unit and Chapter opening pages:

Unit 1	Susan Miyamoto	Chapter 17	Chris Humphrey
Chapter 1	Chris Humphrey	Chapter 18	Aranda Michaels
Chapter 2	Chris Humphrey	Chapter 19	Carol Schum
Chapter 3	Ruth McDowell	Chapter 20	Karen Avery
		Chapter 21	Aranda Michaels
Unit 2	Ruth McDowell	Chapter 22	Chris Humphrey
Chapter 4	Aranda Michaels	Chapter 23	Aranda Michaels
Chapter 5	Aranda Michaels	Chapter 24	Connie Witt English
		Chapter 25	Louise Dickinson Miller
Unit 3	Aranda Michaels	Chapter 26	Aranda Michaels
Chapter 6	Carol Schum	Chapter 27	Louise Dickinson Miller
Chapter 7	Aranda Michaels	Chapter 28	Debbie Specht
Chapter 8	LaRue Alegria		
Chapter 9	Annick Hollister	Unit 5	Ruth McDowell
Chapter 10	Aranda Michaels	Chapter 29	Chris Humphrey
Chapter 11	Louise Dickinson Miller	Chapter 30	Ralph Kay
Chapter 12	John Christy	Chapter 31	Ruth McDowell
Chapter 13	John Christy	Chapter 32	John Christy
Chapter 14	David England	Chapter 33	Aranda Michaels
		Chapter 34	Chris Humphrey
Unit 4	William Nguyen		
Chapter 15	Bijan Naderi	Unit 6	Susan Miyamoto
Chapter 16	Aranda Michaels	Chapter 35	Eclare' Hannifen

Brief Contents

UNIT ONE
Introduction to Psychiatric Nursing 1

CHAPTER 1
Contemporary Psychiatric–Mental Health Nursing 2

CHAPTER 2
The Nursing Process in Psychiatric–Mental Health Nursing 24

CHAPTER 3
Therapeutic Relationship and Effective Communication 46

UNIT TWO
Etiologic Theories of Mental Illness 63

CHAPTER 4
Developmental and Psychological Theories of Mental Illness 64

CHAPTER 5
The Biological Basis of Mental Illness 73

UNIT THREE
Treatment and Therapies 91

CHAPTER 6
Psychopharmacology 92

CHAPTER 7
Cognitive-Behavior Therapy 129

CHAPTER 8
Crisis Intervention 142

CHAPTER 9
Group Therapy and Therapeutic Groups 157

CHAPTER 10
Family Therapy 177

CHAPTER 11
Sexual Therapy 194

CHAPTER 12
Reminiscence Therapy 201

CHAPTER 13
Milieu Therapy 212

CHAPTER 14
Electroconvulsive Therapy and Other Biological Therapies 219

UNIT FOUR
Psychiatric Disorders 231

CHAPTER 15
Delirium, Dementia, Amnestic, and Other Cognitive Disorders 232

CHAPTER 16
Mental Illness due to a General Medical Condition ... 260

CHAPTER 17
Substance-related Disorders 275

CHAPTER 18
Schizophrenia and Other Psychotic Disorders 305

CHAPTER 19
Mood Disorders 341

CHAPTER 20
Anxiety Disorders 377

CHAPTER 21
Somatoform Disorders 401

CHAPTER 22
Posttraumatic and Dissociative Disorders 426

CHAPTER 23
Sexual and Gender Identity Disorders 444

CHAPTER 24
Eating Disorders 460

CHAPTER 25
Sleep Disorders..................................... 478

CHAPTER 26
Adjustment Disorders 499

CHAPTER 27
Personality Disorders............................. 509

CHAPTER 28
Attention-Deficit/Hyperactivity Disorder 529

UNIT FIVE
Problems in the Community 551

CHAPTER 29
Prolonged Mental Illness: Clients and Their Families in the Community 552

CHAPTER 30
The Faces of Homelessness........................... 574

CHAPTER 31
Victims of Abuse 589

CHAPTER 32
Persons Living with HIV Disease and AIDS 604

CHAPTER 33
Care of Individuals in Correctional Facilities.......... 620

CHAPTER 34
Grieving... 634

UNIT SIX
Future Challenges to Delivering Care to the Mentally Ill 641

CHAPTER 35
Future Trends.. 642

Detailed Contents

UNIT ONE
Introduction to Psychiatric Nursing 1

CHAPTER 1
Contemporary Psychiatric–Mental Health Nursing 2
INFLUENCE OF CONCEPTUAL MODELS OF NURSING ON PSYCHIATRIC–MENTAL HEALTH NURSING, 4
  Contemporary Mental Health Care, 4
  Historical Aspects, 6
  Mental Health Care in the Community, 6
DEFINING AND CLASSIFYING MENTAL ILLNESS, 9
  Definition of Mental Illness, 9
  Influence of Culture, Spirituality, and Environment, 10
  Diagnostic and Statistical Manual of Mental Disorders, Fourth Edition, 13
ROLES OF THE PSYCHIATRIC–MENTAL HEALTH NURSE IN CONTEMPORARY MENTAL HEALTH CARE, 15
  Role of the Generalist, 15
  Role of the Specialist, 16
  Primary Care Nurse, 16
  Psychiatric Nurse as Collaborative Member of the Interdisciplinary Team, 16
  Role in Mental Health Promotion, 17
  Nurse Case Manager, 17
  Director or Manager of the Therapeutic Milieu, 17
  Psychiatric Consultation–Liaison Nurse, 18
  Nurse Psychotherapist, 18
  Nurse Psychopharmacologist, 19
LEGAL AND ETHICAL ISSUES, 19
  Confidentiality, 19
  Admission to a Psychiatric Inpatient Facility, 20
  Discharge from a Psychiatric Inpatient Facility, 20
  Duty to Warn, 20
  Rights of Individuals Who Receive Psychiatric Care, 20
  Informed Consent and the Right to Refuse Treatment, 21
  Seclusion and Restraint, 21
  Advocate for Clients, 21

CHAPTER 2
The Nursing Process in Psychiatric–Mental Health Nursing 24
ASSESSMENT, 25
  Before the Assessment, 25
  During the Assessment, 26
  After the Assessment, 40

PLANNING CARE, 42
  Establishing Priority, 42
  Setting Long-term Goals, 42
  Setting Short-term Goals, 42
  Designing Interventions, 42
  Implementation, 42
  Evaluation, 43
  The Collaborative Plan of Care, 44

CHAPTER 3
Therapeutic Relationship and Effective Communication 46
DEFINING THE THERAPEUTIC RELATIONSHIP, 47
  Differences between Social and Therapeutic Relationships, 47
  Boundaries of the Therapeutic Nurse-Client Relationship, 48
  Phases of the Therapeutic Relationship, 50
  Guidelines for Conducting the Therapeutic Relationship, 51
UNDERSTANDING THE COMMUNICATION PROCESS, 52
  Levels of Communication, 52
  Elements of Communication, 53
PERFORMING THERAPEUTIC COMMUNICATION, 54
  Objectivity, 54
  Active Listening, 54
  Types of Communication in Psychiatric Nursing, 54
  Techniques of Therapeutic Communication, 55
  Barriers to Therapeutic Communication, 55

UNIT TWO
Etiologic Theories of Mental Illness 63

CHAPTER 4
Developmental and Psychological Theories of Mental Illness 64
THE PSYCHOANALYTIC THEORIES OF DEVELOPMENT, 65
  Freud's Psychosexual Theory, 65
  Ego Psychology, 65
  Object Relations Theory, 66
ERIKSON'S LIFE CYCLE THEORY, 66
PIAGET'S COGNITIVE THEORY OF DEVELOPMENT, 67

xix

INTERPERSONAL THEORIES OF DEVELOPMENT, 67
  Client-centered Therapy, 67
  Behavioral Theories, 68
THE EMERGENCE OF A NEW PSYCHOLOGY OF WOMEN, 68
DEVELOPMENTAL PROBLEMS OF CHILDHOOD, 70
DEVELOPMENTAL PROBLEMS OF ADULTHOOD, 71
REDISCOVERY OF THE EFFECTS OF TRAUMA ON DEVELOPMENT, 71
DEVELOPMENT AND AGING, 71

CHAPTER 5
The Biological Basis of Mental Illness 73
NEUROANATOMY, 75
  Membranes, 76
  Convoluted Surfaces, 76
  Two Hemispheres, 76
  Cortex, 76
  Frontal Cortex, 78
  Limbic System, 78
  Basal Ganglia, 78
  Diencephalon, 79
BASIC PROPERTIES OF NEUROTRANSMISSION, 79
  Structure and Activity of a Neuron, 79
  Synthesis and Storage, 80
  Release, 80
  Response, 80
  Inactivation, 81
SPECIFIC NEUROTRANSMITTERS, 81
  Biogenic Amines, 81
  Cholinergics, 83
  Neuropeptides, 83
  Amino Acids, 84
TOOLS OF THE TRADE, 85
GENETICS AND HEREDITY, 85
CIRCADIAN RHYTHMS AND MENTAL ILLNESS, 86
PSYCHONEUROIMMUNOLOGY, 87
  HPA Axis Functioning, 87
  Immune Function and Mental Illness, 88

UNIT THREE
Treatment and Therapies 91

CHAPTER 6
Psychopharmacology 92
NEUROPHARMACOLOGY, 93
PHARMACOKINETICS AND PHARMACODYNAMICS, 94
  Cultural and Gender Factors, 94
  Pregnancy and Lactation, 94
ANTIDEPRESSANTS, 95
  General Information, 95
  Tricyclic Antidepressants, 96
  Monoamine Oxidase Inhibitors (MAOIs), 99
  Selective Serotonin Reuptake Inhibitors (SSRIs), 101
  Novel Antidepressant Medications, 104
  Nursing Considerations, 105
MOOD STABILIZERS, 107
  General Information, 107
  Lithium Carbonate, 107
  Carbamazepine, 109
  Valproic Acid, 110
  Nursing Considerations, 110
ANTIPSYCHOTIC MEDICATIONS (NEUROLEPTICS), 112
  General Information, 112
  Nursing Considerations, 118
ANXIOLYTICS AND SEDATIVE-HYPNOTICS, 120
  General Information, 120
  Benzodiazepines, 121
  Buspirone, 123
  Nursing Considerations, 123
PSYCHOSTIMULANTS, 124
  General Information, 124
SYNOPSIS OF CURRENT RESEARCH, 126
AREAS FOR FUTURE RESEARCH, 127

CHAPTER 7
Cognitive-Behavior Therapy 129
PURPOSE OF COGNITIVE-BEHAVIOR THERAPY, 131
THE NURSE'S ROLE, 131
BEHAVIORAL THEORIES, 132
  Conditioning, 132
BEHAVIORAL ASSESSMENT AND OUTCOME MEASUREMENT, 133
COGNITIVE-BEHAVIOR THERAPY, 134
BEHAVIOR THERAPY PROCEDURES, 135
  Relaxation Exercises, 135
  Biofeedback, 135
  Systematic Desensitization, 136
  Token Economies, 137
  Shaping, 137
  Extinction and Punishment, 137
  Modeling, 138
  Exposure-Response Prevention, 138
  Social Skills Training, 138
  Assertiveness Training, 138
EXPECTED OUTCOMES, 138
SYNOPSIS OF CURRENT RESEARCH, 139
AREAS FOR FUTURE RESEARCH, 139

CHAPTER 8
Crisis Intervention 142
THE PURPOSE OF CRISIS INTERVENTION, 143
  The Nurse's Role, 143
  Historical Evolution, 143
CRISIS DEFINED, 143
  Characteristics of a Crisis, 144
  Developmental Phases in a Crisis Situation, 145
  Types of Crises, 146
CRISIS INTERVENTION AND THE NURSING PROCESS, 149
  Assessment, 149
  Diagnosis, 151
  Planning and Implementing Interventions, 151

Evaluation of the Nursing Process and Expected Outcomes, 154
Coping with Crisis Work, 154
IMPLICATIONS FOR EDUCATION AND RESEARCH, 154
AREAS FOR FUTURE RESEARCH, 155

CHAPTER 9
Group Therapy and Therapeutic Groups 157
DEFINING GROUP THERAPY, 159
PURPOSE OF GROUP THERAPY, 160
Therapeutic Factors, 160
CREATION OF THE GROUP, 162
GROUP PURPOSE AND GOALS, 162
The Nurse's Role, 163
Membership Selection, 166
Group Environment, 166
Client Preparation for Group, 168
GROUP INTERVENTION STRATEGIES, 169
Observing for Defensive Maneuvers, 169
Fostering Connections to Other Members, 169
Being Empathetic and Supportive, 170
Being Curious about Group Behavior, 170
Balancing Group-as-a-Whole Interpretations with Individual Interpretations, 170
STAGES OF GROUP DEVELOPMENT, 170
Initial Phase, 170
The Responsive Phase, 171
The Focused Phase, 172
The Termination Phase, 173
EXPECTED OUTCOMES, 173
THE ROLE OF THE NURSE IN GROUP THERAPY, 174
Educational Preparation, 174
Supervision, 174
Type of Group Leadership, 174
Leadership Styles, 175
AREAS FOR FUTURE RESEARCH, 175

CHAPTER 10
Family Therapy 177
PURPOSE OF FAMILY THERAPY, 179
THE NURSE'S ROLE, 179
ASSESSING THE FAMILY SYSTEM, 180
Genogram, 181
Structural Mapping, 181
Family Assessment Guide, 182
NURSING AND PSYCHIATRIC DIAGNOSES, 185
FAMILY THERAPY APPROACHES, 185
Multigenerational Theories and Therapies, 186
Structural and Systemic Family Therapy, 189
EXPECTED OUTCOMES, 190
SYNOPSIS OF CURRENT RESEARCH, 191
AREAS FOR FUTURE RESEARCH, 191

CHAPTER 11
Sexual Therapy 194
PURPOSE OF SEXUAL THERAPY, 195
NURSE'S ROLE, 195
Assessment of Sexual Functioning, 195
Referral for Sexual Therapy, 196

SEXUAL THERAPY, 196
Types of Sexual Therapy, 197
EXPECTED OUTCOMES, 198
SYNOPSIS OF CURRENT RESEARCH, 199
AREAS FOR FUTURE RESEARCH, 199

CHAPTER 12
Reminiscence Therapy 201
TYPES OF REMINISCENCE, 203
Simple Reminiscence, 203
Informative Reminiscence, 203
Life Review, 203
Oral History and Autobiography, 204
DEFINITION OF REMINISCENCE THERAPY, 204
PURPOSES OF REMINISCENCE THERAPY, 204
NURSE'S ROLE IN REMINISCENCE THERAPY, 205
INTERVENTION STRATEGIES, 207
EXPECTED OUTCOMES, 208
AREAS FOR FUTURE RESEARCH, 209

CHAPTER 13
Milieu Therapy 212
PURPOSE OF MILIEU THERAPY, 213
FUNCTIONS OF THE MILIEU, 213
Containment, 214
Support, 214
Structure, 214
Involvement, 214
Validation, 214
NURSE'S ROLE AS MILIEU MANAGER, 215
EXPECTED OUTCOMES, 216
AREAS FOR FUTURE RESEARCH, 216

CHAPTER 14
Electroconvulsive Therapy and Other Biological Therapies 219
TYPES OF BIOLOGICAL THERAPIES, 221
Electroconvulsive Therapy (ECT), 221
Psychosurgery, 224
Phototherapy, 225
Sleep Deprivation Therapy, 228
SYNOPSIS OF CURRENT RESEARCH, 228
AREAS FOR FUTURE RESEARCH, 229

UNIT FOUR
Psychiatric Disorders 231

CHAPTER 15
Delirium, Dementia, Amnestic, and Other Cognitive Disorders 232
NORMATIVE AGING AND COGNITION, 233
DELIRIUM, 234
Definition, 234
Characteristic Behaviors, 234
Culture, Age, and Gender Features, 235
Etiology, 235
Prognosis, 235
Assessment, 235
Interventions for Hospitalized Clients, 235
Expected Outcomes, 237

DEMENTIA, 239
    Definition, 239
    Characteristic Behaviors, 241
    Diagnostic Aids, 245
    Culture, Age, and Gender Features, 245
    Etiology, 246
    Prognosis, 249
    Assessment, 249
    Planning Care, 249
    Interventions for Clients in the Community, 250
    Client and Family Education, 254
    Expected Outcomes, 254
    Differential Diagnosis, 254
AMNESTIC DISORDERS, 255
    Definition, 255
    Characteristic Behaviors, 255
    Diagnostic Aids, 256
    Culture, Age, and Gender Features, 256
    Etiology, 256
    Prognosis, 256
    Planning Care, 256
    Interventions for Clients in the Community, 256
    Expected Outcomes, 256
SYNOPSIS OF CURRENT RESEARCH, 256
AREAS FOR FUTURE RESEARCH, 257

CHAPTER 16
Mental Illness due to a General Medical Condition... 260

COMMON MENTAL ILLNESSES DUE TO GENERAL MEDICAL CONDITIONS, 261
    Characteristic Behaviors, 261
    Culture, Age, and Gender Features, 264
    Etiology, 265
    Prognosis, 268
    Planning Care, 268
    Interventions for Hospitalized Clients, 268
    Intervention for Clients in the Community, 271
    Expected Outcomes, 271
    Differential Diagnosis, 271
CRITICAL CARE UNIT PSYCHOSIS, 272
    Characteristic Behaviors, 272
    Culture, Age, and Gender Features, 272
    Etiology, 272
    Prognosis, 272
    Interventions for Hospitalized Clients, 272
    Expected Outcomes, 273
    Differential Diagnosis, 273
SYNOPSIS OF CURRENT RESEARCH, 273
AREAS FOR FUTURE RESEARCH, 273

CHAPTER 17
Substance-related Disorders... 275

DEFINITION, 277
CHARACTERISTIC BEHAVIORS, 278
    Substance Abuse, 278
    Alcohol Abuse, 281
    Substance Dependence, 282
    Enabling, 282
    Intoxication and Withdrawal, 282
CULTURE, AGE, AND GENDER FEATURES, 284
    Culture, 284
    Age, 285
    Gender, 285
ETIOLOGY, 285
    Biological Theories, 285
    Imaging Studies, 286
    Genetic Theories, 286
    Behavioral Theories, 286
PROGNOSIS, 287
ASSESSMENT, 288
    Short Alcohol and Drug History, 289
    Screening Tools, 289
    Family and Significant Others, 290
    Physical Findings and Mental Status Examination, 290
    Laboratory Findings, 290
PLANNING CARE, 291
INTERVENTIONS FOR HOSPITALIZED CLIENTS, 292
    Acute Intoxication, 292
    Acute Withdrawal, 292
INTERVENTIONS FOR CLIENTS IN THE COMMUNITY, 295
    Brief Interventions, 295
    Cognitive-Behavior Therapy, 295
    Long-Term Substance Dependence, 297
    Family Interventions, 298
    Pharmacologic Treatments, 299
    Alcohol Dependence, 300
    Benzodiazepines and Sedative-Hypnotic Withdrawal, 300
    Opioids, 300
    Stimulant Withdrawal, 301
    Nicotine Withdrawal, 301
EXPECTED OUTCOMES, 301
DIFFERENTIAL DIAGNOSIS, 301
    Medical Disorders, 301
    Mood Disorders, 301
    Psychotic Disorders, 301
    Anxiety Disorders, 301
    Personality Disorders, 301
    Attention-Deficit/Hyperactivity Disorder (ADHD), 302
COMMON NURSING DIAGNOSES, 302
AREAS FOR FUTURE RESEARCH, 302

CHAPTER 18
Schizophrenia and Other Psychotic Disorders 305

SCHIZOPHRENIA, 308
    Characteristic Behaviors, 308
    Culture, Age, and Gender Features, 313
    Etiology, 313
    Prognosis, 317
OTHER PSYCHOTIC DISORDERS, 317
    Schizophreniform Disorder, 319
    Schizoaffective Disorder, 319
    Delusional Disorder, 319
    Brief Psychotic Disorder, 319
    Assessing Acute Episodes of Illness, 319
    Assessing the Prodromal Phase of Schizophrenia in the Community, 325
    Planning Care, 327
    Interventions for Hospitalized Clients, 327
    Interventions for Clients in the Community, 330
    Client and Family Education, 335
    Differential Diagnosis, 336
    Expected Outcomes, 337

Common Nursing Diagnoses, 337
Synopsis of Current Research, 337
Areas for Future Research, 337

CHAPTER 19
Mood Disorders *341*

MAJOR DEPRESSION, 345
Definition, 345
Characteristic Behaviors, 345
Culture, Age, and Gender Features, 348
Etiology, 350
Prognosis, 353
Assessment, 353
Planning Care, 353
Interventions for Hospitalized Clients, 357
Interventions for Clients in the Community, 357
Expected Outcomes, 362

BIPOLAR DISORDER, 363
Characteristic Behaviors, 363
Culture, Age, and Gender Features, 365
Etiology, 366
Prognosis, 368
Planning Care, 368
Interventions for Hospitalized Clients, 368
Interventions for Clients in the Community, 368
Client and Family Education, 371
Expected Outcomes, 372

DIFFERENTIAL DIAGNOSIS, 373

COMMON NURSING DIAGNOSES, 374

SYNOPSIS OF CURRENT RESEARCH, 374

AREAS FOR FUTURE RESEARCH, 375

CHAPTER 20
Anxiety Disorders *377*

GENERALIZED ANXIETY DISORDER, 380
Characteristic Behaviors, 380
Culture, Age, and Gender Features, 381
Etiology, 381
Prognosis, 381
Interventions for Hospitalized Clients, 381
Interventions for Clients in the Community, 382

PANIC DISORDER WITH OR WITHOUT AGORAPHOBIA, 382
Characteristic Behaviors, 382
Culture, Age, and Gender Features, 384
Etiology, 384
Prognosis, 386
Interventions for Clients in the Community, 386

PHOBIAS, 387
Characteristic Behaviors, 387
Culture, Age, and Gender Features, 389
Etiology, 389
Interventions for Clients in the Community, 389

OBSESSIVE-COMPULSIVE DISORDER (OCD), 389
Characteristic Behaviors, 389
Diagnostic Aids, 392
Culture, Age, and Gender Features, 392
Etiology, 393
Prognosis, 393
Interventions for Hospitalized Clients, 393
Interventions for Clients in the Community, 393

DIFFERENTIAL DIAGNOSIS, 396

EXPECTED OUTCOMES, 397

COMMON NURSING DIAGNOSES, 397

SYNOPSIS OF CURRENT RESEARCH, 398

AREAS FOR FUTURE RESEARCH, 398

CHAPTER 21
Somatoform Disorders *401*

SOMATIZATION, 403
Definition, 403
Characteristic Behaviors, 404
Culture, Age, and Gender Features, 404
Etiology, 404
Prognosis, 408
Assessment, 408
Planning Care, 409
Interventions for Hospitalized Clients, 409
Interventions for Clients in the Community, 409
Expected Outcomes, 410
Differential Diagnosis, 410

UNDIFFERENTIATED SOMATOFORM DISORDER, 411

CONVERSION DISORDER, 411
Characteristic Behaviors, 411
Culture, Age, and Gender Features, 411
Etiology, 411
Assessment, 412
Planning Care, 412
Interventions for Hospitalized Clients, 412
Interventions for Clients in the Community, 413
Expected Outcomes, 413

PAIN DISORDER, 413
Characteristic Behaviors, 413
Etiology, 413
Assessment, 415
Planning Care, 415
Interventions for Hospitalized Clients, 415
Interventions for Clients in the Community, 415
Expected Outcomes, 415

HYPOCHONDRIASIS, 416
Characteristic Behaviors, 416
Culture, Age, and Gender Features, 417
Etiology, 417
Prognosis, 418
Assessment, 418
Planning Care, 419
Interventions for Clients in the Community, 419
Expected Outcomes, 420

BODY DYSMORPHIC DISORDER, 421
Characteristic Behaviors, 421
Culture, Age, and Gender Features, 421
Etiology, 421
Assessment, 422
Planning Care, 422
Interventions for Clients in the Community, 422
Expected Outcomes, 422

SOMATOFORM DISORDER NOT OTHERWISE SPECIFIED (NOS), 422
Expected Outcomes, 423

COMMON NURSING DIAGNOSES, 423

SYNOPSIS OF CURRENT RESEARCH, 423

AREAS FOR FUTURE RESEARCH, 424

CHAPTER 22
Posttraumatic and Dissociative Disorders 426

- POSTTRAUMATIC STRESS DISORDER (PTSD), 428
  - Characteristic Behaviors, 428
- DISSOCIATIVE DISORDERS, 428
  - Characteristic Behaviors, 428
- RISK FACTORS, 431
- PREVALENCE, 433
- CULTURE, AGE, AND GENDER FEATURES, 433
- ETIOLOGY, 434
- PROGNOSIS, 435
- PLANNING CARE, 435
- INTERVENTIONS FOR HOSPITALIZED CLIENTS, 436
- INTERVENTIONS FOR CLIENTS IN THE COMMUNITY, 436
- CLIENT AND FAMILY EDUCATION, 440
- EXPECTED OUTCOMES, 440
- DIFFERENTIAL DIAGNOSIS, 440
- COMMON NURSING DIAGNOSES, 441
- SYNOPSIS OF CURRENT RESEARCH, 441
- AREAS FOR FUTURE RESEARCH, 441

CHAPTER 23
Sexual and Gender Identity Disorders................. 444

- NORMAL SEXUAL FUNCTIONING IN MEN AND WOMEN, 445
- SEXUAL DYSFUNCTIONS, 446
  - Characteristic Behaviors, 446
  - Culture, Age, and Gender Features, 449
  - Etiology, 450
  - Prognosis, 451
  - Planning Care, 451
  - Interventions for Clients in the Community, 451
- GENDER IDENTITY DISORDER, 453
  - Characteristic Behaviors, 453
  - Culture, Age, and Gender Features, 453
  - Etiology, 453
  - Prognosis, 454
  - Interventions for Clients in the Community, 454
- PARAPHILIAS, 454
  - Characteristic Behaviors, 454
  - Culture, Age, and Gender Features, 456
  - Etiology, 456
  - Prognosis, 456
  - Interventions for Clients in the Community, 456
- CLIENT AND FAMILY EDUCATION, 457
- EXPECTED OUTCOMES, 457
- COMMON NURSING DIAGNOSES, 457
- SYNOPSIS OF CURRENT RESEARCH, 457
- AREAS FOR FUTURE RESEARCH, 457

CHAPTER 24
Eating Disorders 460

- CHARACTERISTIC BEHAVIORS, 463
- CULTURE, AGE, AND GENDER FEATURES, 463
  - Culture, 463
  - Age and Gender, 463
- ETIOLOGY, 463
  - Neurobiological Factors, 464
  - Genetic Factors, 465
- PROGNOSIS, 465
- ASSESSMENT, 465
  - Anorexia Nervosa, 467
  - Bulimia Nervosa, 467
- PLANNING CARE, 468
  - How to Determine an Effective Treatment Strategy, 468
  - When to Refer, 469
- INTERVENTIONS FOR HOSPITALIZED CLIENTS, 469
  - Effective Communication Strategies, 469
  - Milieu Therapy, 470
  - Cognitive-Behavior Approaches, 470
  - Behavior and Interpersonal Therapies, 470
  - Pharmacologic Treatments, 471
- INTERVENTIONS FOR CLIENTS IN THE COMMUNITY, 471
- EXPECTED OUTCOMES, 471
- DIFFERENTIAL DIAGNOSIS, 472
  - Anorexia Nervosa, 472
  - Bulimia Nervosa, 472
  - Comorbidity, 472
- COMMON NURSING DIAGNOSES, 472
- AREAS FOR FUTURE RESEARCH, 473

CHAPTER 25
Sleep Disorders.. 478

- NORMAL SLEEP-WAKE PATTERNS, 479
  - Culture, Age, and Gender Features, 481
- PRIMARY INSOMNIA, 485
  - Characteristic Behaviors, 485
  - Etiology, 485
- PRIMARY HYPERSOMNIA, 486
  - Characteristic Behaviors, 486
  - Etiology, 486
- BREATHING-RELATED SLEEP DISORDERS, 486
  - Characteristic Behaviors, 486
  - Etiology, 486
- NARCOLEPSY, 486
  - Characteristic Behaviors, 486
  - Etiology, 487
- CIRCADIAN RHYTHM SLEEP DISORDER, 487
  - Characteristic Behaviors, 487
  - Etiology, 487
- DYSSOMNIA NOT OTHERWISE SPECIFIED (NOS), 487
  - Characteristic Behaviors, 487
- PARASOMNIAS, 487
  - Characteristic Behaviors, 487
  - Etiology, 488
- SLEEP DISORDERS DUE TO MEDICAL AND PSYCHIATRIC DISORDERS, 488
- PROGNOSIS, 488
- PLANNING CARE, 488
- INTERVENTIONS FOR HOSPITALIZED CLIENTS, 488

Detailed Contents **XXV**

INTERVENTIONS FOR CLIENTS IN THE COMMUNITY, 490
CLIENT AND FAMILY EDUCATION, 494
EXPECTED OUTCOMES, 494
DIFFERENTIAL DIAGNOSIS, 495
COMMON NURSING DIAGNOSES, 496
SYNOPSIS OF CURRENT RESEARCH, 496
AREAS FOR FUTURE RESEARCH, 497

CHAPTER 26
Adjustment Disorders 499

CHARACTERISTIC BEHAVIORS, 501
   Beginning Symptoms, 501
CULTURE, AGE, AND GENDER FEATURES, 503
ETIOLOGY, 503
   Stress-Adaptation Theories, 503
   Neuropharmacologic Theories, 503
PROGNOSIS, 503
PLANNING CARE, 503
INTERVENTIONS FOR CLIENTS IN THE COMMUNITY, 504
   Interventions for Chronic Adjustment Disorders, 505
   Cognitive-Behavior Therapy, 505
   Pharmacologic Interventions, 506
CLIENT AND FAMILY EDUCATION, 506
EXPECTED OUTCOMES, 506
DIFFERENTIAL DIAGNOSIS, 506
   Mood Disorders, 506
   Posttraumatic Stress Disorder (PTSD) and Acute Stress Disorder, 506
   Bereavement, 507
COMMON NURSING DIAGNOSES, 507
SYNOPSIS OF CURRENT RESEARCH, 507
AREAS FOR FUTURE RESEARCH, 507

CHAPTER 27
Personality Disorders................................ 509

CLUSTER A PERSONALITY DISORDERS, 511
   Characteristic Behaviors, 511
   Culture, Age, and Gender Features, 514
   Etiology, 514
   Prognosis, 515
   Planning Care, 515
   Interventions for Hospitalized Clients, 515
   Interventions for Clients in the Community, 515
CLUSTER B PERSONALITY DISORDERS, 517
   Characteristic Behaviors, 517
   Culture, Age, and Gender Features, 518
   Etiology, 519
   Prognosis, 520
   Interventions for Hospitalized Clients, 520
   Interventions for Clients in the Community, 521
CLUSTER C PERSONALITY DISORDERS, 523
   Characteristic Behaviors, 523
   Culture, Age, and Gender Features, 524
   Etiology, 525
   Prognosis, 525
   Interventions for Clients in the Community, 525
EXPECTED OUTCOMES, 525

DIFFERENTIAL DIAGNOSIS, 525
COMMON NURSING DIAGNOSES, 526
CLIENT AND FAMILY EDUCATION, 526
SYNOPSIS OF CURRENT RESEARCH, 526
AREAS FOR FUTURE RESEARCH, 527

CHAPTER 28
Attention-Deficit/Hyperactivity Disorder 529

CHARACTERISTIC BEHAVIORS, 531
   Children, 531
   Adolescents, 533
   Adults, 533
CULTURE, AGE, AND GENDER FEATURES, 533
   Culture, 533
   Age, 534
   Gender, 534
ETIOLOGY, 535
   Genetics, 535
   Brain Development, 536
   Brain Function and Structure, 536
   Neurotransmitters in ADHD, 536
ASSESSMENT, 537
   Clinical Assessment Interview, 537
   Assessment Instruments, 538
PLANNING CARE, 539
   Role of the Nurse as Resource, 540
   Role of the Nurse as Teacher, 540
   Role of the Nurse as Leader, 540
   Role of the Nurse as Surrogate, 540
   Role of the Nurse as Counselor, 541
INTERVENTIONS FOR HOSPITALIZED CLIENTS, 541
INTERVENTIONS FOR CLIENTS IN THE COMMUNITY, 541
   Cognitive-Behavior Interventions, 542
   Psychopharmacologic Interventions, 542
EXPECTED OUTCOMES, 544
DIFFERENTIAL DIAGNOSIS, 544
   Mood, 544
   Learning, 545
   Traumatic Experiences, 545
   Conduct and Oppositional Behaviors, 546
   Mental Retardation, 546
   Pervasive Developmental Disorders, 546
   Tic Disorders, 547
   Anxiety, 547
   Psychotic Disorder, 547
SYNOPSIS OF CURRENT RESEARCH, 547
AREAS FOR FUTURE RESEARCH, 547

UNIT FIVE
Problems in the Community 551

CHAPTER 29
Prolonged Mental Illness: Clients and Their Families in the Community 552

CHARACTERISTICS OF PROLONGED MENTAL ILLNESS, 553
CONCEPT OF RECOVERY AND NURSING CONSIDERATIONS, 553
IMPACT OF PROLONGED MENTAL ILLNESS, 554

PROGNOSIS, 554
HISTORICAL PERSPECTIVES, 554
   Managed Costs and Rationed Care, 554
   Nursing Process within a Systems Context, 556
OPEN SYSTEMS MODEL WITHIN THE COMMUNITY, 556
   Assessment and Data Collection, 556
   Dilemmas Experienced by Individuals with PMI: Nursing Diagnoses, Outcomes, and Intervention Strategies, 560
   Environments and Support Systems, 561
MODELS OF TREATMENT AND REHABILITATION, 567
   Case Management, 567
   Continuous Treatment Teams, 568
   Residential Care, 568
   Psychosocial Rehabilitation Programs, 569
EVALUATING OUTCOMES, 571
AREAS FOR FUTURE RESEARCH, 571

CHAPTER 30
The Faces of Homelessness 574

DEFINING HOMELESSNESS, 575
HISTORICAL PERSPECTIVES AND RELATED ISSUES, 576
   Deinstitutionalization and Homelessness, 576
   Economic and Public Policy Factors, 577
HOMELESS SUBGROUPS AND PSYCHIATRIC–MENTAL HEALTH CONCERNS, 577
   The Homeless Experience and Psychiatric–Mental Health Issues, 578
   Vulnerable Homeless Subgroups, 578
CONCEPTUAL MODELS: THE PROCESS OF BECOMING HOMELESS, 581
   Social Distress Theory and Homelessness, 581
   Individual Styles of Coping with Social Distress, 582
   Model of the Homelessness Process, 582
PSYCHIATRIC–MENTAL HEALTH NURSING AND THE HOMELESS, 583
   Historical Background, 583
   Theoretical Basis for Nursing Practice, 583
   Psychiatric–Mental Health Nursing Intervention Strategies, 584
   Advocacy Role for the Homeless, 584

CHAPTER 31
Victims of Abuse 589

PREVALENCE, 591
TYPES OF ABUSE, 592
   Physical Abuse, 592
   Sexual Abuse, 592
   Psychological Abuse, 593
   Economic Abuse, 593
DISCLOSURE AND SUBSTANTIATION OF ABUSE, 593
COMPONENTS OF ABUSE, 593
   Perpetrator, 593
   Violence in the Home, 593
   Violence in the Environment, 594
   Survivor, 594
TRAUMA RESPONSES, 594

ASSESSMENT OF ABUSE, 595
   Indicators, 595
   Abuse-related Symptoms, 596
KEY PRINCIPLES OF TREATMENT, 598
   Maintain Safety, 598
   Empower the Individual, 598
   Report by Mandated Laws, 598
   Minimize Intrusiveness, 599
   Keep No Secrets, 599
   Identify Symptom Clusters, 599
   Know Your Level of Expertise, 600
   Do Not Pathologize, 600
   Do Not Reinforce Perceptions of Shame or Vulnerability, 600
   Be Aware of Possible Cognitive Distortions, 600
TREATMENT OF ABUSE VICTIMS, 600
   Individual Psychotherapy, 601
   Group Psychotherapy, 601
   Family, Couples, and Sex Therapy, 601
   Pharmacologic Treatment, 601
   Potential Countertransference, 602

CHAPTER 32
Persons Living with HIV Disease and AIDS 604

MODE OF TRANSMISSION, 606
EPIDEMIOLOGY, 606
   A Mother's Story, 607
   Personal Awareness, 608
CLINICAL MANIFESTATION AND THE SPECTRUM OF HIV DISEASES, 608
   Early Stage, 608
   Middle Stage, 609
   Late Stage, 610
NEUROPSYCHIATRIC TESTING, 610
NEUROPSYCHOLOGICAL COMPLICATIONS, 611
OTHER PSYCHIATRIC DISORDERS, 613
PATIENT CARE, 614
   Assessment, 615
   Nursing Diagnosis, 615
   Planning and Therapeutics, 616
   Hope for a Future: Protease Inhibitors, 616
VULNERABLE POPULATIONS, 617
   The Severely and Persistently Mentally Ill, 617
   Women, 617
   Substance Abusers, 618
AREAS FOR FUTURE RESEARCH, 618

CHAPTER 33
Care of Individuals in Correctional Facilities 620

CHARACTERISTICS OF THE CLIENT POPULATION, 621
   The Mentally Ill Offender, 621
   Gender Issues, 622
   Cultural Issues, 622
CONFLICTING CONVICTIONS: CUSTODY AND CARING, 623
THE CONTEXT OF NURSING CARE IN CORRECTIONAL FACILITIES, 624
   Nurse-Client Relationship, 624
   Treatment Setting, 627

Professional Role Definition, 629
Societal Norms, 630

AREAS FOR FUTURE RESEARCH, 631

CHAPTER 34
Grieving 634

CHARACTERISTICS OF THE GRIEVING PROCESS, 635

TYPES OF GRIEVING EXPERIENCED BY CLIENTS, 636

THE CONTEXT OF NURSING CARE IN THE GRIEVING PROCESS, 637
The Nurse-Client Relationship, 637
Assisting Clients in the Grieving Process, 637

UNIT SIX
Future Challenges to Delivering Care to the Mentally Ill 641

CHAPTER 35
Future Trends 642

THE PRESENT AND FUTURE OF PSYCHIATRIC–MENTAL HEALTH CARE: MANAGED CARE, 643
The Fee-for-Service Delivery System, 643
The Managed Care Delivery System, 644

THE EFFECTS OF MANAGED CARE ON PSYCHIATRIC–MENTAL HEALTH CARE DELIVERY, 645

OPPORTUNITIES FOR PSYCHIATRIC NURSES, 645
Roles for the Psychiatric-Generalist Nurse, 646
Roles for the Psychiatric Clinical Nurse Specialist (CNS), 647

CHALLENGES FOR FUTURE PSYCHIATRIC NURSES, 647

APPENDIX 1
DSM-IV Classification 651

APPENDIX 2
A Patient's Bill of Rights 660

APPENDIX 3
Tips for Psychiatric Home Visits 662

APPENDIX 4
Psychopharmacology Guidelines 664

APPENDIX 5
Comparison of the Major Features of Alzheimer's Disease, Parkinson's Disease, Acquired Immunodeficiency Syndrome—Dementia Complex 668

APPENDIX 6
Selected Resources 670

Glossary 673

Index 683

UNIT One
Introduction to Psychiatric Nursing

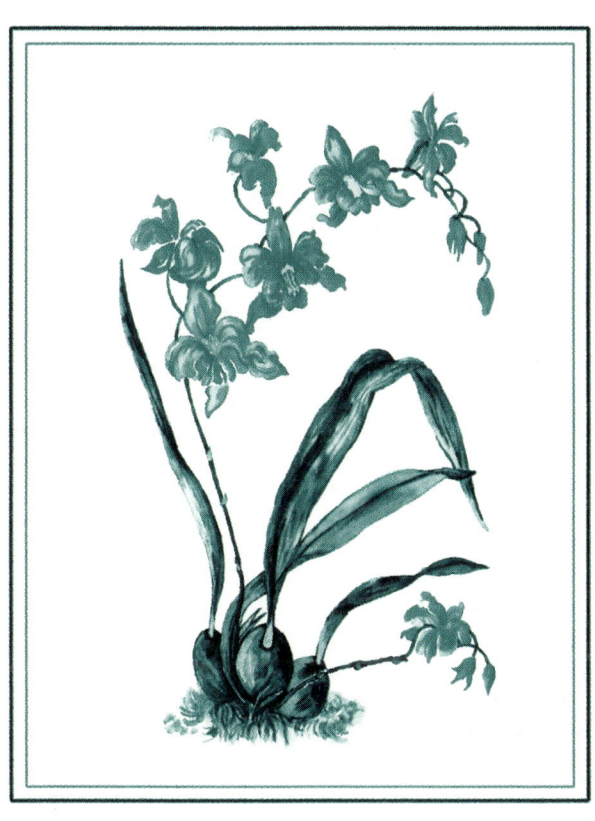

CHAPTER 1
Contemporary Psychiatric–Mental Health Nursing

CHAPTER 2
The Nursing Process in Psychiatric–Mental Health Nursing

CHAPTER 3
Therapeutic Relationship and Effective Communication

CHAPTER 1

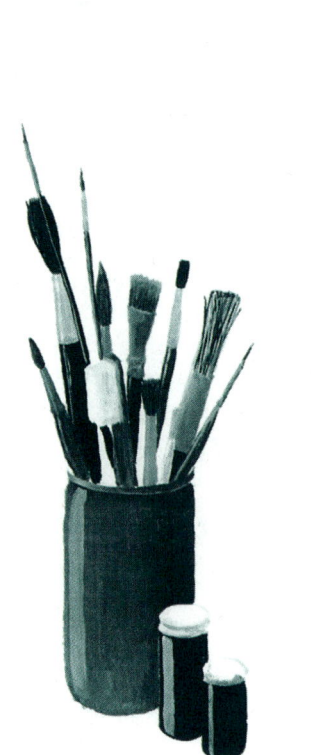

CHAPTER OUTLINE

Influence of Conceptual Models of Nursing on Psychiatric–Mental Health Nursing
Contemporary Mental Health Care
Historical Aspects
Mental Health Care in the Community

Defining and Classifying Mental Illness
Definition of Mental Illness
Influence of Culture, Spirituality, and Environment
Diagnostic and Statistical Manual of Mental Disorders, Fourth Edition

Roles of the Psychiatric–Mental Health Nurse in Contemporary Mental Health Care
Role of the Generalist
Role of the Specialist
Primary Care Nurse
Psychiatric Nurse as Collaborative Member of the Interdisciplinary Team
Role in Mental Health Promotion
Nurse Case Manager
Director or Manager of the Therapeutic Milieu
Psychiatric Consultation–Liaison Nurse
Nurse Psychotherapist
Nurse Psychopharmacologist

Legal and Ethical Issues
Confidentiality
Admission to a Psychiatric Inpatient Facility
Discharge from a Psychiatric Inpatient Facility
Duty to Warn
Rights of Individuals Who Receive Psychiatric Care
Informed Consent and the Right to Refuse Treatment
Seclusion and Restraint
Advocate for Clients

Carol A. Glod, RN, CS, PhD
Billie Barringer, MA, BSN, RNC, CNS

Contemporary Psychiatric–Mental Health Nursing

LEARNING OBJECTIVES

After completing this chapter, the reader should be able to:
- Define current views of mental health and mental illness.
- Discuss the roles of the psychiatric nurse in contemporary mental health care.
- Outline the history of mental illness treatment from primitive times to the present.
- Explain the role of the neurosciences and psychopharmacology in psychiatric nursing care.
- Describe the legal and ethical issues in psychiatric nursing.
- Explain the classification system used in *Diagnostic and Statistical Manual of Mental Disorders, Fourth Edition (DSM-IV)*, its benefits, and its drawbacks.

KEY TERMS

client advocacy
clients' rights
commitment
confidentiality
culture
developmental plasticity
Diagnostic and Statistical Manual of Mental Disorders, Fourth Edition (DSM-IV)
environment
mental health
mental illness
primary mental health care
primary prevention
psychiatric clinical nurse specialist (CNS)
psychiatric–mental health generalist nurse
psychiatric–mental health nursing
psychobiology
secondary prevention
tertiary prevention

A 15-year-old girl sits in the hospital room of her dying father. He's been diagnosed with untreatable cancer and has slipped into a coma. The nurse walks into the room and tells the teenager that her father, despite the coma, can probably hear her. Even though no one has overtly said so, the girl knows her father is dying. On the one hand, she hopes that his pain will end. On the other hand, she cannot imagine losing the most important person in her life. As she talks about her mixed feelings, the nurse listens.

A few minutes later, the girl's father is dead. Her mother, overtaken with grief and shock, sits at the nursing station, staring off into space. As the girl cries by herself, the nurse comes over to her and holds and comforts her. They walk arm in arm down the hallway, while other nurses tend to her father's postmortem care. The girl can't imagine what will happen to her now.

The actions of the nurse in this example reflect the essence of psychiatric nursing. Whether helping a person deal with grief, crisis, or developmental difficulties, or caring for those with intractable and persistent mental illnesses such as schizophrenia and posttraumatic stress disorder, psychiatric nurses promote the psychological health of individuals, families, and communities. Some nurses are drawn to the specialty because of their own life experiences; others find that people with psychiatric problems present an interesting challenge. That is partly what this book is about: the myriad factors that are thought to account for reactions to crisis, the devastation of depression, the bizarre and disordered thoughts of schizophrenia, the frenetic pace of hyperactive children, and the severe regression of dementia. However, explaining the complex relationship between the components that lead to, promote, and foster the development of these psychiatric problems sometimes creates more questions than answers. Part of the challenge of psychiatric nursing is devising effective interventions and making a difference in the lives of people who suffer from these devastating disorders.

Psychiatric–mental health nursing, a subspecialty of nursing, emphasizes use of the nursing process with clients who have unmet psychiatric or psychosocial needs. The ANA, in its *Statement on Psychiatric–Mental Health Clinical Nursing Practice*, defines psychiatric nursing as a "specialized area . . . employing theories of human behavior as its science and purposeful use of self as its art."[1] It focuses on human aspects and responses to illness and is therefore part and parcel of all areas of nursing.

INFLUENCE OF CONCEPTUAL MODELS OF NURSING ON PSYCHIATRIC–MENTAL HEALTH NURSING

According to the work of Hildegard Peplau,[2] psychiatric–mental health nursing is accomplished through a counseling role, the nurse-client relationship, and therapeutic communication skills. Nurses use a holistic approach, considering biological, genetic, developmental, environmental, social, cultural, spiritual, physical, and emotional aspects of the client. They build on the strengths of individuals, while remaining aware of their deficits.[3]

Many nurse leaders have influenced this definition and the practice of psychiatric nursing through their theories of nursing, health, person, and environment. Table 1–1 lists their conceptualizations of nursing.[4]

CONTEMPORARY MENTAL HEALTH CARE

Psychiatric disorders were once thought to rise from some disruption in early life experiences. For example, "schizophrenigenic mothers" gave "mixed messages" that caused their children to become schizophrenic, and harsh, rigid toilet training led to unrelenting thoughts and behaviors like repeated hand washing and to obsessive-compulsive disorder. Given these etiologies, it was thought that reflecting on one's own childhood could unravel what "caused" an arrest in psychological development. Deciphering the impact of childhood experiences was the process used

TABLE 1–1. Nursing Theorists

Name	Nursing	Person	Health	Environment
Calista Roy	The knowledge that provides the analysis and action related to the care of the ill or potentially ill person. Roy's model emphasizes assessment and intervention, which are carried out as part of the nursing process.	A biopsychosocial, open system, constantly adapting to a changing environment.	A process that results from successful adaptation.	Conditions, circumstances, and influences surrounding and affecting the development of a person or group.
Martha Rogers	A learned profession characterized by promoting health and by caring for and rehabilitating the infirm and disabled. Nursing activities include promoting "symphonic" interaction between the environment and man.	An energy field characterized by pattern and organization, and manifesting characteristics and behaviors that are greater than the sum of its parts.	Defined by cultures and individuals to denote behaviors that are of high or low value.	An energy field that encompasses all that is not within any given human field; for example, those things that are external to the individual.
Dorothea Orem	A service whose aim is to promote self-care actions to overcome limitations. Nurses make their own judgments as to the need for nursing.	A unified whole, functioning biologically, symbolically, and socially.	Integration of the individual, his or her parts, and modes of functioning (physical, psychological, social).	A subcomponent of the person that with the other components comprise an integrated system related to self-care.
Hildegard Peplau	A significant, therapeutic interpersonal process. It functions cooperatively with other human processes that make health possible for individuals in communities. Nursing is an educational instrument, a maturing force that aims to promote forward movement in the direction of creative, constructive, productive, personal and community living.* Nursing is driven by goal-oriented, interpersonal processes.	A biological, physical, and psychological self-system with emphasis on the psychological.	The state, characterized by a manageable level of anxiety, that facilitates forward movement of personality and other human processes.	A person's significant others.

*Mariner-Tomey, A: American Nursing Theorists and Their Work. Mosby, St. Louis, 1994.

to understand and change a lifetime of unhappiness and depression.

A new wave of theories of causation then emerged: Biological and genetic factors accounted for the symptoms of psychiatric illness. People were manic-depressive, not because of poor parenting or other difficulties in childhood, but because their genes were shuffled into a life of severe mood swings. "Chemical imbalances," similar to the insulin deficiencies in diabetes, caused the psyche to be odd, bizarre, depressed, compulsive, or otherwise disrupted. If these imbalances could be corrected—that is, if the client took the right pill or combination of pills—the brain's chemistry could be altered and psychiatric symptoms reversed.

Not surprisingly, neither of these extreme positions fully explains the complexity of the brain and the mind; it is more likely that psychiatric disorders result from some combination of the two theories. **Psychobiology**, the melding of biology with the workings of the mind, describes the interplay between one's inherent biological and genetic makeup and one's life experiences. This thinking has been refined into a new theoretical position, "developmental plasticity." Simply stated, **developmental plasticity**, or neural plasticity, is the capacity for experience to alter the brain's structure and function, particularly during the first decade or so of life.

Each person is born with a certain biological substrate, a brain. The brain is like a lump of clay, made up of all kinds of interconnecting parts that govern movement, feelings, thoughts, and behaviors. More important, this lump of clay is molded by our physical and psychological experiences well into adolescence. The interplay of the brain and experience shapes who we are; it also accounts for disturbances in thinking, emotions, and behavior. The inherent makeup of the brain is the foundation upon which experiences help or hinder psychological and emotional development. The nature of experiences during pregnancy, infancy, and childhood shapes the brain's structure and functioning, which in turn affect relationships, personality, and behavior. In this model, other people do not directly "cause" psychiatric problems, but poor nutrition, emotional neglect, exposure to drugs, physical abuse and head trauma, and major losses can impede the development of the brain. Exposure to drugs or viruses during pregnancy may lead to the expression of symptoms that arise later in childhood as the brain continues its development. As a result of these negative experiences, the pathways, synaptic connections, and even the structure of the brain may fail to develop fully or may change in shape or function.

Because the brain continues to develop throughout childhood, positive and negative experiences shape its final form, which in turn affects mental health or psychiatric problems. Experiences that occur during certain sensitive periods in infancy and childhood potentially alter brain structure and functioning, thereby changing behavior. For instance, children exposed to classical music in utero have been shown to have higher intelligence quotients. Conversely, children exposed to substance, alcohol, or nicotine abuse during pregnancy have higher rates of hyperactivity and inattention.

Language development needs to be stimulated in childhood because the areas of the brain responsible for language development become less plastic during adolescence. Children under age 10 can learn a language more quickly and with less of a foreign accent than can older children. Other factors also affect language acquisition. Children with head trauma that affects the brain's language centers can use other parts of their brains that are not generally associated with language.

One of the most extreme examples of developmental plasticity is the effect of sexual and physical abuse. Children subjected to ongoing abuse early in childhood have less-developed brains, particularly the left side.[5] The consequences of abuse impede the different connections in the left hemisphere and lead to psychiatric symptoms such as depression, memory problems, impulsivity, and difficulty in relationships.

Rapid discoveries and technological advances have recently promoted neuroscience as the foundation for understanding psychiatric disorders. More knowledge about the structure and function of the brain has led to further research about the relationship between behavior and cellular and molecular processes. These advances have included knowledge about the heritability of psychiatric illness and about genetic markers that can identify affected individuals. The development of magnetic resonance imaging (MRI), magnetic resonance spectroscopy, and positron emission tomography has enabled the identification of physiological and structural brain changes. Imaging studies now allow researchers to study the living brain to better understand psychiatric disorders. The refinement of diagnostic categories has allowed practitioners to relate observable biological changes to psychiatric illnesses. Some authors who believe that environmental influences alone shape individual development have suggested that psychiatric nursing should remain skeptical about polarized views that claim that biology is the cause of psychiatric illness.[6] Others suggest that psychiatric nursing demands a paradigm shift to these new approaches.[7,8] The challenge is to maintain a focus on the individual and the nurse-client relationship to balance new understanding about the expression of psychiatric behaviors. Psychobiology and research in the developmental plasticity of the brain offer important opportunities to understand the underlying themes that can promote more effective nursing care of the individual.

Progress in neuroscience and its relationship to psychiatric disorders moved slowly until the twentieth century. The last 35 to 40 years have witnessed a revolution in the understanding of the brain and how it functions. According to the National Institute of Mental Health, in fact, 90% of what is known about the brain has been discovered in the past 10 years. Developments in this arena were slow in part because of the enormous complexity of the brain, with its more than 100 billion interconnected neurons and brain cells.[9] Furthermore, refined technology that allows close scrutiny of the brain has evolved only recently. The result has been an explosion of knowledge that has reshaped our understanding of psychiatric disorders and led to another revolution in the care and treatment of the mentally ill.

Some of the major achievements in the past decades include effective psychopharmacologic medications, knowledge about degenerative brain diseases such as Alzheimer's and Parkinson's diseases, the use of MRI to delineate the relationship between brain lesions and specific behavioral deficits, discoveries about the ongoing development of the brain into adolescence, and the application of molecular biology to investigate the heritability of psychiatric disorders. Critics charge that this medicalization of psychiatry shifts the emphasis away from the individual client, and they urge nurses to preserve the focus on interpersonal relationships.[6] Advocates of incorporating neuroscientific insights suggest that an overreliance on interpretation and disruption in relationships is impeding the true discovery of abnormal brain functioning. In fact, McEnany[8] claims that ignoring new biological evidence defies reason and logic. Instead of maintaining polarized views, psychiatric nursing can build on the strengths of both the psychological and neuroscientific biological perspectives to reach a new synergistic position: one that uses psychoneurobiological principles to guide practice, education, and research. The philosophy that the mind affects brain functioning and that brain structure and function affect the mind is inherent in many of the existing psychological or psychiatric models. The time is now for nursing models to embrace past accomplishments and traditions while simultaneously applying the burgeoning information about the neurosciences.

HISTORICAL ASPECTS

Over the years, attitudes toward mental health and the care of those with mental illness have undergone revolutionary changes and have continually shaped and influenced the practice of all mental health disciplines. The following example describes a young woman who could have presented for help at any point in history.

A 20-year-old postpartum woman abusing illicit substances is found running naked through the streets, shouting obscenities. When strangers approach her, she is initially suspicious and withdrawn and mumbles unintelligible words to herself. She frequently screams out and shakes a clenched fist for no apparent reason. If touched, she quickly runs away, claiming that rape was attempted. Without adequate attention, however, she will succumb to the cold and vile conditions of living on the street.

Historically, how would this woman have been treated, and what conditions would have supported the restoration of her physical and mental health? Prior to the twentieth century, people believed that such behaviors resulted from satanic possession, tropical climates, tea, menopause, masturbation, or other social, moral, or personal excesses.

In the mid-nineteenth century, practitioners would say she had "idiocy" (insanity), the only "diagnosis" available. Few treatments were effective, and most treatments were cruel and inhumane. The police would probably have taken her to a "madhouse," a private boarding house without any legal or therapeutic guidelines to govern her care, but only if she had had money. They might instead have taken her to an "almshouse," the precursor to an asylum. Almshouses had notoriously deplorable conditions: bare, filthy cells where individuals were confined to straitjackets. The woman would probably have been locked in a room, attic, or outhouse, or tied to a chair or bed and been forced to take noxious, unproven concoctions.

At the end of the nineteenth century, private and public psychiatric hospitals began, although they provided largely custodial care.

Her family might have taken her to a psychiatric institution that emphasized the need for pleasant surroundings. Recent graduates trained by Linda Richards at the McLean Hospital Training School, the first educationally prepared nurses in the country, might have given her nursing care. Their attitude toward her would have been respectful and compassionate. The institution would have discouraged physical and mechanical restraint. The woman would have filled her days with structured activities. The beginning of milieu treatment, with consistent schedules and planned activities, would have dominated her care. Nurses would have encouraged her to participate in outdoor activities such as horseback riding, golfing, and gardening.

The 1950s saw the advent of new medications that revolutionized the treatment of psychiatric disorders and dramatically reduced the number of hospitalized clients.

The woman would probably have been hospitalized at a public psychiatric facility. Treatment with chlorpromazine (Thorazine), an antipsychotic medication used to reduce and eliminate hallucinations and bizarre thoughts, would have calmed her agitation. Nurses would have restrained her if her behavior remained aggressive, not as a punishment but as a means of containing her behavior. She also would have met with a psychiatrist for individual psychotherapy, three to five times each week for 1 hour. Based on principles of psychoanalysis, the psychotherapist would have targeted an understanding of how past childhood experiences such as difficulties in the mother-child relationship or problems with toilet training led to her mental health problems. After her behavior "normalized," she might have been discharged, but only after years of hospitalization.

MENTAL HEALTH CARE IN THE COMMUNITY

In the 1960s, the community mental health movement first emerged. In the words of President Kennedy, the goal of community mental health care was to replace "the cold mercy of custodial isolation with the open warmth of community concern and capability."[10] This model shifted the emphasis of mental health care from hospitals to community mental health centers, and from "patients" to "clients." Although deinstitutionalization in America failed to produce the intended results, mental health care today emphasizes community-based or community-linked care, partly because of economic pressures and managed care. Using grants and government funds, public and private agencies attempt to facilitate and maintain the care of individuals living in home or homelike settings, including foster homes, group homes, congregate living facilities, apartment complexes, or supervised living facilities designed for special populations. Box 1–1 describes an innovative program for community-based nursing practice.

Today, the woman described previously might be treated briefly in the hospital, but she would receive most of her care in the community. Psychiatric nurses and other mental health professionals might engage her in treatment at a homeless shelter, in a community-based hospital program, or in a crisis center or emergency room.

Ann, a psychiatric nurse working in the nursing clinic of a homeless shelter, first met Sally after her brief hospitalization and discharge to the shelter. The hospital staff had learned little about her. Ann used kind words and simple phrases such as "we'd like to help" to begin the therapeutic relationship with Sally. She helped her get suitable clothes and toiletries. Sally seemed thankful and began to trust Ann. A treatment team that included Ann, a social worker, and the consulting psychiatrist from the shelter met to discuss a plan of care. The discussion centered on how best to understand the client and develop the most effective interventions in the community. Sally, whose diagnosis was tentatively given as schizophrenia, undifferentiated type, had major self-care deficits and appeared to be abusing both drugs and alcohol. To work with her effectively, Ann wanted to obtain a detailed history and gather more information to assess her level of current functioning. Sally was extremely resistant to treatment but began to make an important connection with Ann. Ann decided to foster the relationship and engage her in her own treatment. Ann understood that Sally's symptoms might be worsened by the alcohol and drugs, or that she might be "self-medicating" the symptoms to get some relief from internal "voices." Ann's short-term goal was to build the relationship and complete a psychiatric history; the long-term goal was to help Sally become sober and begin a medication trial.

Psychiatric nurses provide community-based care to people with mental illness. The goal is consistent with the aim of tertiary prevention: to reduce the severity of a mental health problem and to help the person live at the highest functional capacity possible. Special knowledge and tech-

---

Box 1–1. Outline of Clinical Activities for Psychiatric Nursing Students

Site Homeless shelter for women with substance abuse problems and their children

Theme of Clinical Assignment Mental health promotion with mothers

Design of Experience Contact time is 2–3 hours for 10 weeks

Objectives:

For clients:
1. Identify mental health-care concerns and choose assistance
2. Identify parenting concerns and choose assistance

For student:
1. Employ and develop interviewing skills
2. Assess actual and potential mental and physical health problems of adult clients
3. Assess actual and potential mental and physical health problems of children
4. Apply interventions and referrals as indicated

Implementation:

- Students work with women to assess their individual and group health-care needs, with an emphasis on mental health needs.
- Students develop an individual relationship with one family group within the shelter. By talking with the women, students learn some of the factors that led to their clients' present situations.
- Students continue to assess the needs of the families as well as their individual clients and develop appropriate responses.
- Students learn from the mothers and teach them information specific to their needs, such as parenting skills, and information about sexual abuse, acquired immunodeficiency syndrome (AIDS), safe sex, and hygiene. Students use written materials and videotapes, and develop posters to assist teaching.
- Students help clients locate and secure appropriate referrals.
- Students develop group workshops on substance abuse, parenting, and other topics specific to their clients.

Hints for Success:
- Clients may react initially with indifference and hostility toward students. Do not take it as a personal insult, but see it as a learned response to prior events.
- The relationship often takes time to develop; be patient, persistent, and consistent.
- Clients may be similar to students; some are highly educated, have jobs, and may be familiar individuals.
- Students should talk about reactions and feelings to the situation with the clinical instructor and in clinical group conferences.

Source: Adapted from Matteson, PS (ed): Teaching Nursing in the Neighborhoods: The Northeastern University Model. Copyright © 1995, Springer Publishing Company, Inc., New York 10012, used by permission.

niques are required, namely, creation of a professional space within the home, observation, insight into the client's and family's problems, independent practice, and the ability to make referrals. Box 1–2 lists an experience of psychiatric nursing students working in a community-based shelter for children and their mothers recovering from substance abuse.

Today, psychiatric nurses also integrate psychobiological theories of mental illness and advances in psychopharmacology in their practices. The ANA developed the *Psychopharmacology Guidelines for Psychiatric Mental Health Nurses*[11] to help nurses direct medication teaching, administration, management, and maintenance; integrate psychopharmacology with other treatment modalities; and foster interdisciplinary collaboration. These guidelines clearly state that "psychiatric nurses must continuously integrate the neurosciences, particularly psychopharmacology, into practice."[11] The guidelines clearly delineate the scope of practice in three broad content areas: neuroscience, psychopharmacology, and clinical management, which includes physical, neuropsychiatric, psychosocial, and psychopharmacologic assessment; diagnosis; and treatment. Table 1–2 presents a synopsis; the complete guidelines can be found in Appendix 4.

> A few days after Sally arrived at the shelter, her behavior became so disruptive that she began accosting and pushing other residents; she was physically restrained. The shelter staff sent her to the city hospital emergency room for further psychiatric evaluation. Hospital staff physically examined Sally and gave her a drug screen; Sally was anemic, had low potassium levels, and tested negative for street drugs. Shortly after admission to the hospital's brief treatment unit, she appeared suspicious and talked to herself. The nurses and psychiatrist tried to give her haloperidol (Haldol), an antipsychotic medication, but she refused it. She also refused to attend the groups on the unit but did agree to meet with Ann. Sally slowly told Ann her history, including a previous psychiatric hospitalization for depression and a suicide attempt; she also revealed a recent head injury. The staff sent Sally to the MRI center for a brain scan, which ruled out specific neuroanatomic problems secondary to the head trauma. Sally also told Ann that she had been attending a community college and working part-time delivering pizzas. While working late one night, she had intercourse, became pregnant, and miscarried several weeks later.

The evaluation and history suggested that Sally might be suffering from major depression, with postpartum onset and psychotic features. A variety of factors including the unplanned pregnancy, the miscarriage, and chemical imbalances probably caused the depression, which then worsened in the months after the miscarriage.

Box 1–2. Community-Based Nursing Education: A Model for Learning, Teaching, and Research

CCHERS (pronounced cheers), the Center for Community Health Education, Research, and Service, is an integrated program that stresses community-based nursing and medical education. It is based on the idea that traditional acute health-care settings have not effectively prepared nurses for competent and comfortable service to community-based populations. CCHERS stresses the philosophy that most treatment of illness, including emotional and psychiatric disorders, occurs in the community rather than in acute medical centers, and thus education should be based in the person's natural setting. As part of their education, nursing and medical students are assigned to one of 12 neighborhood health centers for all of their clinical experiences. Neighborhood health centers, founded in the late 1960s, "provide comprehensive health-care services that are geographically, linguistically, and culturally accessible to community members," particularly the underserved. Nursing students learn to provide psychiatric–mental health care, health education, outreach, and counseling services to individuals, families, and the community. The goal is to provide students with the "knowledge, attitudes, and practice skills of community caregiving." Each clinical nursing course in the 4-year program contains a clinical experience at the health center to meet the student's educational requirements and the health-care needs of the community. Students learn to assess and treat clients with acute and chronic psychiatric problems, including:

- Developing psychiatric communication and interviewing techniques
- Contributing to taking a psychiatric history
- Performing a mental status examination
- Integrating physical and psychiatric assessment skills
- Collaborating with an interdisciplinary psychiatric and primary care team
- Developing community workshops and educational programs on depression, alcohol abuse, and other conditions
- Becoming familiar with the effects of living conditions and the environment on mental health problems
- Understanding and referring clients to available community resources
- Assisting in school screenings for psychiatric problems such as attention deficit hyperactivity disorder and depression
- Presenting classroom topics on health issues such as adolescent suicide
- Conducting community or school surveys of health concerns
- Learning the criteria for a psychiatric evaluation to assess children at high risk for psychiatric–mental health problems
- Understanding community-based day treatment of clients with chronic and persistent mental illnesses, dementia, and AIDS
- Applying an understanding of developmental stages to psychiatric nursing care

- Conducting screenings for depression in supermarkets and shopping centers

Placements include:
- Client advocacy in a court clinic for battered women
- Day care centers for children and their mothers with alcohol and substance abuse
- Day treatment centers focusing on special populations with chronic mental illness, AIDS, and Alzheimer's disease
- Medication clinics based in community mental health centers
- Senior housing projects

This program's community-based philosophy prepares nurses for the changing job market. The shortage of hospital-based positions has increased the need for well-prepared community mental health nurses in places such as community health centers, home health agencies, nursing homes, and housing projects. The clinical experiences of CCHERS allow students to explore these different agencies, equip them with essential community-based skills, help them make important connections with community-based staff, and provide unique experiences that distinguish them from other new graduates.

Source: Adapted from Matteson, PS (ed): Teaching Nursing in the Neighborhoods: The Northeastern University Model. Springer, New York, 1995; and the CCHERS Student Guide, Northeastern University College of Nursing

---

TABLE 1–2. Psychopharmacology Guidelines

I Neurosciences
Commensurate with level of practice, the psychiatric–mental health nurse integrates current knowledge from the neurosciences to understand etiologic models, diagnostic issues, and treatment strategies for psychiatric illness.

II Psychopharmacology
The psychiatric–mental health nurse involved in the care of clients who have been prescribed psychopharmacologic agents demonstrates knowledge of psychopharmacologic principles—including pharmacokinetics, pharmacodynamics, drug classification, intended and unintended effects, and related nursing implications.

III Clinical Management
The psychiatric–mental health nurse applies principles from the neurosciences and psychopharmacology to provide safe and effective management of clients being treated with psychopharmacologic agents. Clinical management includes assessment, diagnosis, and treatment considerations.

Source: From American Nurses' Association: Psychopharmacology guidelines for psychiatric mental health nurses. In Psychiatric Mental Health Nursing Psychopharmacology Project. ANA, Washington, DC, 1994, pp 41–42, with permission.

After a few days, the hospital discharged Sally, and she went back to live in the homeless shelter. Now that a relationship had been built, Ann wanted to help Sally improve her nutritional status. She also encouraged her to take medications. Antidepressants might reduce her depression and restore the balance of affected neurotransmitters such as serotonin. Antipsychotic medications could reduce or eliminate the hallucinations and false ideas Sally experienced. Ann tried to learn more about Sally's family and hoped to involve them in her treatment. Once stabilized physically and mentally, Sally might be able to live in a residential setting such as a halfway house and begin to work a few hours each week at a volunteer job.

DEFINING AND CLASSIFYING MENTAL ILLNESS

DEFINITION OF MENTAL ILLNESS

There are many different ways to conceptualize mental health and illness. Freud defined **mental health** as the ability to work and to love; the ANA defines mental health as a state of well-being in which individuals function well in society and are generally satisfied with their lives.[1] The result is socially acceptable behavior and the ability to respond productively and appropriately in the environment. **Mental illness** is a disturbance in an individual's thinking, emotions, behaviors, and physiology. Mental illness implies some disruption in "mental" as opposed to physical processes; however, clinicians increasingly recognize that there is substantial overlap between physical and psychiatric conditions and that each one affects the other in complex ways, leading to problems with behavior, relationships with people, and the ability to function in the environment. For example, when a client has a thought disorder, behavior may be socially inappropriate because of problems in thinking and problem solving. Likewise, people suffering from the profound sadness of depression have problems concentrating and creating thoughts, and their behavior slows to the point of stupor in some cases. In both instances, individuals are unable to interact socially with others and the environment.

One formal definition of mental illness or a psychiatric disorder is as follows:

A clinically significant behavioral or psychological syndrome or pattern that occurs in an individual and that is associated with present distress (e.g., a painful symptom) or disability (i.e., impairment in one or more important areas of functioning), or with a significantly increased risk of suffering death, pain, disability, or an important loss of freedom. In addition, this syndrome or pattern must not be merely an expectable and culturally sanctioned response to a particular event, for example the death of a loved one. Whatever its original cause, it must currently be considered a manifestation of a behavioral, psychological, or biological dysfunction in the individual.[12]

How many people have a mental disorder or substance abuse/dependence?

The National Comorbidity Survey estimates that approximately 52 million people, age 15 to 54, had some type of alcohol, drug abuse, or mental health (ADM) disorder within the past year. Of these, an estimated 20 million had substance abuse/dependence and 40 million had some type of mental disorder. An estimated 8 million people (4.5% of the 15- to 54-year-olds) had both a mental disorder and substance abuse/dependence within the past year. Overall, 30% of the population had at least one ADM disorder in the past year, and the severity of their disorder varied.

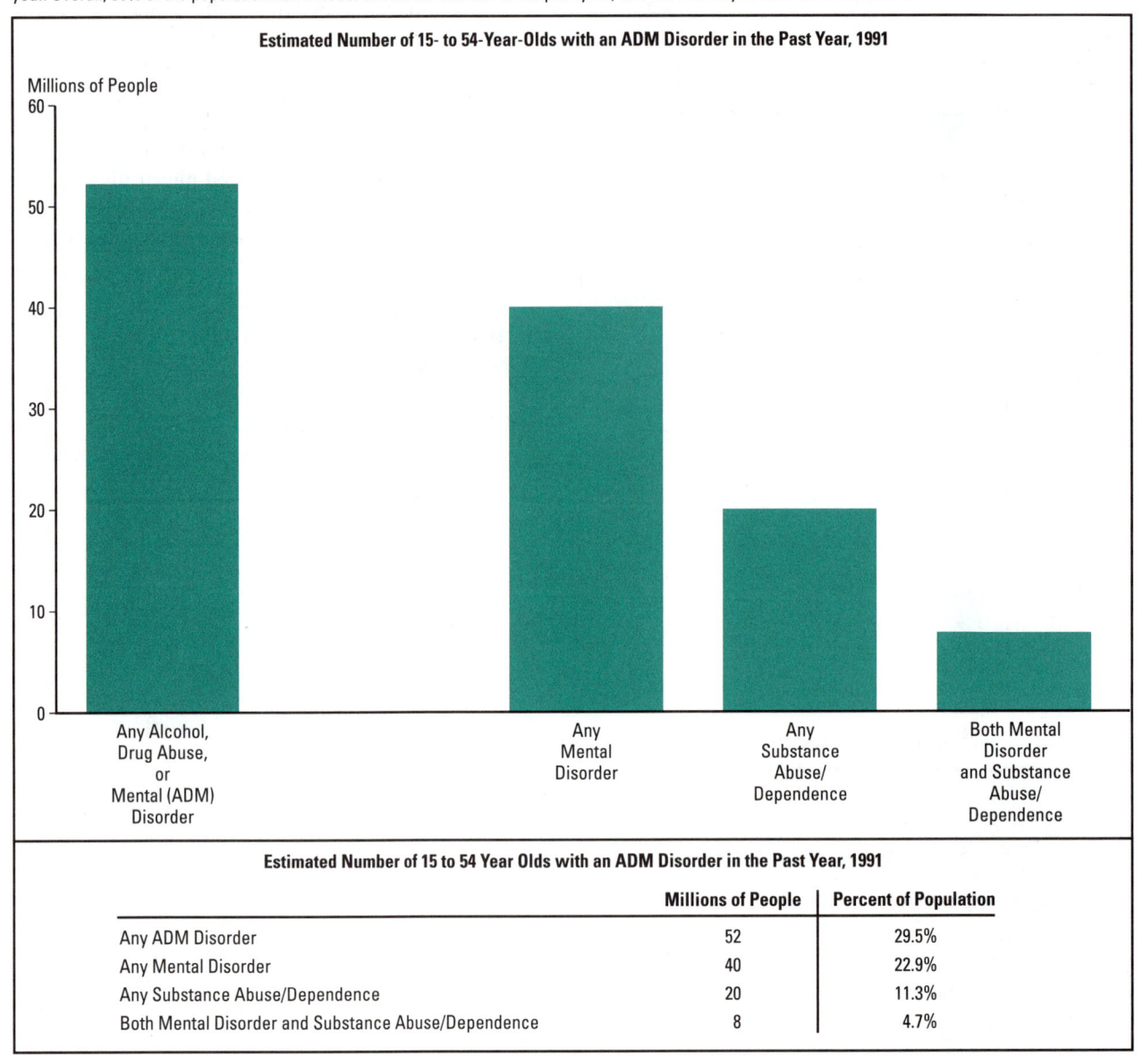

Estimated Number of 15- to 54-Year-Olds with an ADM Disorder in the Past Year, 1991

Millions of People:
- Any Alcohol, Drug Abuse, or Mental (ADM) Disorder: ~52
- Any Mental Disorder: ~40
- Any Substance Abuse/Dependence: ~20
- Both Mental Disorder and Substance Abuse/Dependence: ~8

Estimated Number of 15 to 54 Year Olds with an ADM Disorder in the Past Year, 1991

	Millions of People	Percent of Population
Any ADM Disorder	52	29.5%
Any Mental Disorder	40	22.9%
Any Substance Abuse/Dependence	20	11.3%
Both Mental Disorder and Substance Abuse/Dependence	8	4.7%

Source notes: Kessler et al. (1994): Lifetime and 12-Month Prevalence of DSM-III-R Psychiatric Disorders in the U.S., Archives of General Psychiatry, 51:8-19 and unpublished data from the survey. These estimates are from the National Comorbidity Survey (NCS). The survey was based on interviews administered to a probability sample of the non-institutionalized U.S. civilian population. The NCS sample consisted of 8,098 respondents, age 15-54 years. This survey was conducted from September 1990 to February 1992. DSM-III-R criteria were used as the basis for assessing disorders in the general population. The "substance abuse disorder" category includes drug or alcohol *dependence or abuse*. Any ADM disorder includes the following categories of disorders: affective, anxiety, substance abuse/dependence, non-affective psychosis, and antisocial personality.

Figure 1–1. Percentages of Americans with a mental disorder or substance abuse/dependence. (Rouse, B. A. [ed]: Substance Abuse and Mental Health Statistics Source Book. DHHS Publication No. [SMA] 95-3064, Washington, DC: Superintendent of Documents, U.S. Government Printing Office, 1995, p. 33.)

As seen in Figure 1–1, 52 million people, or about 30% of the young adult population has had a psychiatric disorder in the past year. Figure 1–2 shows how these disorders affect individuals' ability to work and be productive and how they are associated with increased health-care costs and crime.

INFLUENCE OF CULTURE, SPIRITUALITY, AND ENVIRONMENT

Culture, spirituality, and environment may influence mental health or illness. Understanding and respect for the client's culture, religious beliefs and practices, and environment are

What is the cost of alcohol, drug abuse, and mental health disorders to our nation?

Alcohol, drug abuse, and mental health (ADM) disorders are costly in terms of health, productivity, and crime. The total costs of ADM disorders in 1990 are estimated at $314 billion. The greatest portion of these costs comes from the loss of productivity due to injury or illness ($108 billion or 34%). About $81 billion, or 26% of costs, is due to health-care costs, which include the treatment of ADM disorders and their medical consequences. About $68 billion (22%) is due to crime, criminal justice costs, and property damage.

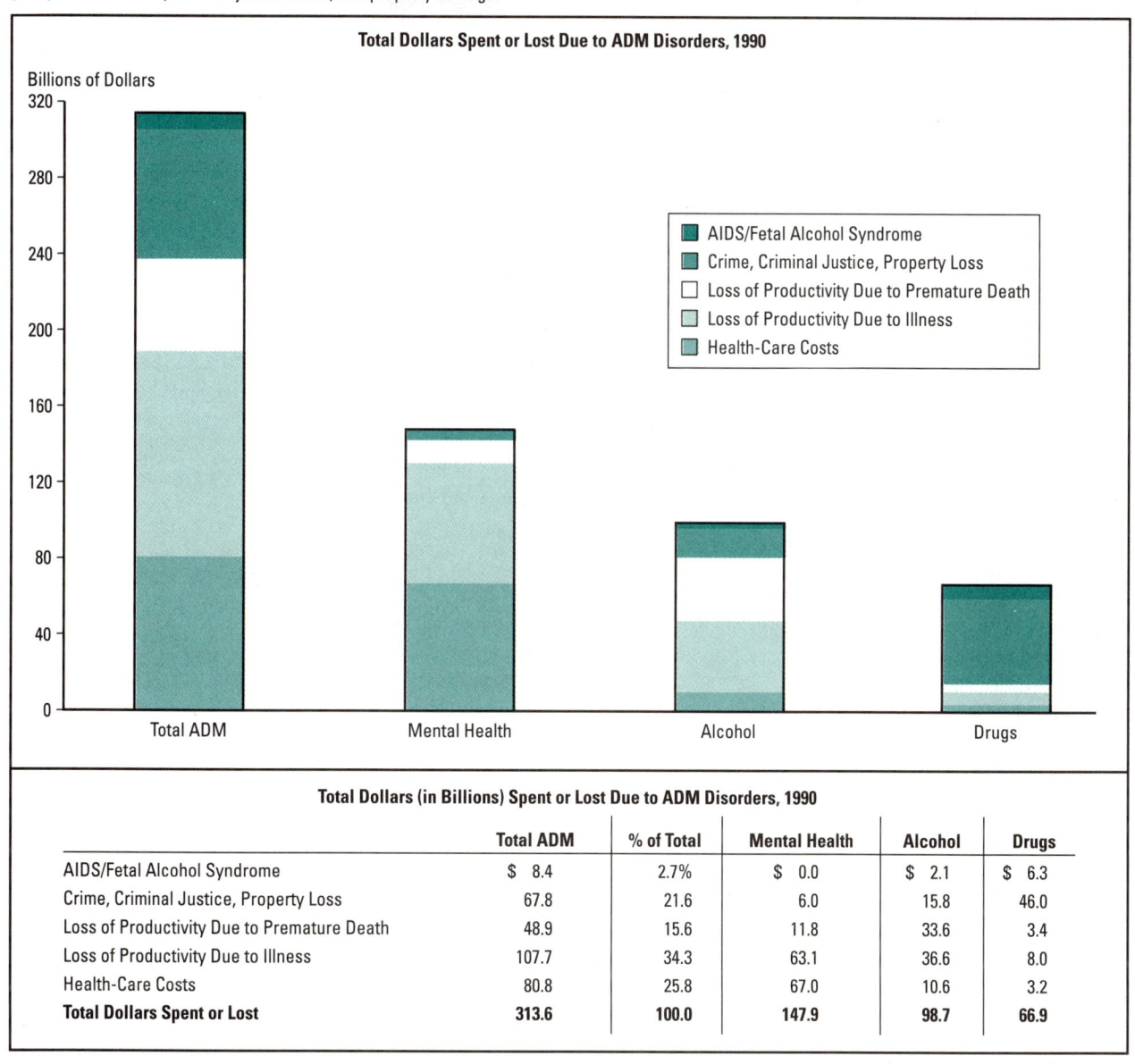

Total Dollars (in Billions) Spent or Lost Due to ADM Disorders, 1990

	Total ADM	% of Total	Mental Health	Alcohol	Drugs
AIDS/Fetal Alcohol Syndrome	$ 8.4	2.7%	$ 0.0	$ 2.1	$ 6.3
Crime, Criminal Justice, Property Loss	67.8	21.6	6.0	15.8	46.0
Loss of Productivity Due to Premature Death	48.9	15.6	11.8	33.6	3.4
Loss of Productivity Due to Illness	107.7	34.3	63.1	36.6	8.0
Health-Care Costs	80.8	25.8	67.0	10.6	3.2
Total Dollars Spent or Lost	**313.6**	**100.0**	**147.9**	**98.7**	**66.9**

Source notes: Rice DP & Miller LS (1992): Costs of Mental Illness, In: Hu Teh-Wei, Rupp A, eds. *Advances in Health Economics and Health Services Research: Research In the Economics of Mental Health, Vol 14*. Costs of substance abuse In: Robert Wood Johnson Foundation (1993); *Substance Abuse: The Nation's Number One Health Problem: Key Indicators for Policy*. Above estimates are projections from basic conceptual and analytic work done under contract with the Alcohol, Drug Abuse and Mental Health Administration and presented in Rice DP, Kelman S, Miller LS, Dunmeyer S (1990): *The Economic Costs of Alcohol and Drug Abuse, and Mental Illness: 1985*, DHHS Publication No. (ADM) 90-1964. Subsequent analysis of the alcohol data by Miller TR and Blincoe LJ (in Incidence and Cost of Alcohol-Involved Crashes in the United States, *Accident Analysis and Prevention*, 26(5):583-591, 1994) estimated the total dollars spent or lost due to alcohol to be $116.5 billion.

Figure 1–2. The cost of alcohol, drug abuse, and mental health disorders in the United States. (Rouse, B. A. [ed]: Substance Abuse and Mental Health Statistics Source Book. DHHS Publication No. [SMA] 95-3064, Washington, DC: Superintendent of Documents, U.S. Government Printing Office, 1995, p. 3.)

an important part of psychiatric nursing care. Griffith and Gonzolaz[13] define **culture** as an abstract concept that describes the way of life of a particular group of people who live together. Culture encompasses shared patterns of beliefs, feelings, and knowledge that guide behavior. For example, some cultures view mental illness as a punishment for moral transgressions. Therefore, shame may be a major symptom of mental illness in that group. In other cultures, people may

TABLE 1-3. DSM-IV Classification

If criteria are currently met, one of the following severity specifiers may be noted after the diagnosis: Mild, Moderate, Severe.

If criteria are no longer met, one of the following specifiers may be noted: In Partial Remission, In Full Remission, Prior History.

Disorders Usually First Diagnosed in Infancy, Childhood, or Adolescence
Mental Retardation
Learning Disorders
Motor Skills Disorder
Communication Disorders
Pervasive Developmental Disorders
Attention-deficit and Disruptive Behavior Disorders
Feeding and Eating Disorders of Infancy or Early Childhood
Tic Disorders
Elimination Disorders
Other Disorders of Infancy, Childhood, or Adolescence

Delirium, Dementia, and Amnestic and Other Cognitive Disorders
Delirium
Dementia
Amnestic Disorders
Other Cognitive Disorders

Mental Disorders Due to a General Medical Condition Not Elsewhere Classified

Substance-related Disorders
Alcohol-related Disorders
Amphetamine (or Amphetamine-like)–related Disorders
Caffeine-related Disorders
Cannabis-related Disorders
Cocaine-related Disorders
Hallucinogen-related Disorders
Inhalant-related Disorders
Nicotine-related Disorders
Opioid-related Disorders
Phencyclidine (or Phencyclidine-like)–related Disorders
Sedative-, Hypnotic-, or Anxiolytic-related Disorders
Polysubstance-related Disorder
Other (or Unknown) Substance-related Disorders

Schizophrenia and Other Psychotic Disorders

Mood Disorders
Depressive Disorders
Bipolar Disorders

Anxiety Disorders

Somatoform Disorders

Factitious Disorders

Sexual and Gender Identity Disorders
Sexual Dysfunctions
Paraphilias
Gender Identity Disorders

Eating Disorders

Sleep Disorders
Primary Sleep Disorders
Sleep Disorders Related to Another Mental Disorder
Other Sleep Disorders

Impulse-Control Disorders Not Elsewhere Classified

Adjustment Disorders

Personality Disorders

Other Conditions That May Be a Focus of Clinical Attention
Psychological Factors Affecting Medical Condition
Medication-induced Movement Disorders
Other Medication-induced Disorder
Relational Problems
Problems Related to Abuse or Neglect
Additional Conditions That May Be a Focus of Clinical Attention

Additional Codes

Multiaxial System
   Axis I: Clinical Disorders, Other Conditions That May Be a Focus of Clinical Attention
   Axis II: Personality Disorders, Mental Retardation
   Axis III: General Medical Conditions
   Axis IV: Psychosocial and Environmental Problems
   Axis V: Global Assessment of Functioning

Source: Reprinted with permission from the Diagnostic and Statistical Manual of Mental Disorders, Fourth Edition. Copyright 1994 American Psychiatric Association.

---

scatter salt to dispel evil spirits or bring clergy or a folk healer into the treatment process. Social status, income, education, and social advantage influence perceptions that people have regarding treatment of mental illness and can inhibit or shape responses. For these reasons, the ethnic and cultural backgrounds of all persons entering the treatment process are important.

Spirituality is a deeply personal inner experience that both integrates and transcends the physical, emotional, and social aspects of mental health as it influences thoughts, feelings, and behaviors. Individuals may draw their spirituality from religion, nature, or a higher power. In treatment, it is useful to identify people's spiritual orientation and values. Clients may bring talismans (consecrated religious articles), amulets, or other items they believe possess magical or spiritual powers into treatment settings. Native Americans may have a "medicine bag," which contains items for healing purposes; Roman Catholic clients may have a crucifix to which they affix great importance for their convalescence. Some behaviors that would be interpreted as psychotic in treatment settings, such as hearing voices, may be seen in certain religious groups as evidence of divine intervention.

Environment refers to physical circumstances that surround the client. Examples include temperature, air, presence of infection, natural disaster, sensory overload or deprivation, or exposure to toxic substances. Social factors in the environment also affect mental health or illness. Consider work pressures, competition, sexual harassment, neighborhood crime, and living conditions. Some forms of mental illness are situational, and changing the physical or social aspects of the environment results in improvement.

> In her work with Ann, Sally revealed her Irish heritage, Catholic upbringing, and the importance of children in her family. Her first pregnancy, the result of a chance sexual encounter, was a terrible burden. She felt she could not share this experience with her family because "they wouldn't understand." She considered an abortion, but felt it was "against her religion," even though she did not consider herself religious. Sally also talked about the importance of having children in the future. Now, suffering the effects of the pregnancy and miscarriage, Sally was ambivalent about reconnecting with her family and the church.

DIAGNOSTIC AND STATISTICAL MANUAL OF MENTAL DISORDERS, FOURTH EDITION

All mental health disciplines use the *DSM-IV*,[12] a classification system for the diagnosis of psychiatric illness. It is a taxonomy that has three purposes:
- to provide a standardized nomenclature and language for all mental health professionals
- to present defining characteristics that differentiate specific conditions
- to assist in the identification of the underlying cause of a disorder

Specific diagnostic criteria are outlined for every category based on the phenomena observed in clinical experience and empirical research. Table 1–3 lists the major categories of disorders currently included in *DSM-IV*. All categories are listed in Appendix 1.

A multiaxial classification scheme allows for the interrelation of biological, psychological, and social aspects of an individual's condition.
- Axis I cites a client's major psychiatric disorder; for example, major depression. Each condition has certain key features listed.

TABLE 1–4. Axis IV: Psychosocial and Environmental Problems

AXIS IV
Psychosocial and Environmental Problems
Problems with primary support group
Problems related to the social environment
Educational problems
Occupational problems
Housing problems
Economic problems
Problems with access to health-care services
Problems related to interaction with the legal system/crime
Other psychosocial and environmental problems

Source: Reprinted with permission from the Diagnostic and Statistical Manual of Mental Disorders, Fourth Edition. Copyright 1994 American Psychiatric Association.

- Axis II consists of the personality disorders and mental retardation; for example, borderline personality (see Chapter 27 for a discussion of borderline personality disorder).
- Axis III reflects the client's medical conditions that are potentially relevant to understanding the individual's circumstances. Medical conditions that complicate the client's diagnosis or treatment, yet are not responsible for the cause of the psychiatric illness, would also be coded on Axis III.
- Axis IV provides a checklist of negative life events, environmental difficulties, housing needs, stressors, inadequate social supports, and other problems that describe the personal circumstances (Table 1–4).
- Axis V presents a Global Assessment of Functioning (GAF) that rates the overall psychological functioning of the client on a scale of 0 to 100. The GAF summarizes the clinician's assessment of the present psychological, social, and occupational ability to function.[1] Table 1–5 lists the GAF.

> The treatment team reevaluated Sally's provisional diagnosis after Ann further assessed the nature and course of her symptoms. Using the classification system based on *DSM-IV*, Sally had the following diagnoses:
>
> Axis I: Major Depressive Disorder, Recurrent, Severe with Postpartum Onset; Alcohol Abuse (Provisional); Acute Stress Disorder (Provisional)
> Axis II: None
> Axis III: Anemia, Hypokalemia, Complications of Pregnancy and the Puerperium
> Axis IV: Miscarriage, Homelessness, Unemployment
> Axis V: GAF = 30 (current)

TABLE 1–5. Axis V: Global Assessment of Function

AXIS V
Global Assessment of Functioning Scale
Consider psychological, social, and occupational functioning on a hypothetical continuum of mental health–illness. Do not include impairment in functioning due to physical (or environmental) limitations.

Code	(Note: Use intermediate codes when appropriate, e.g., 45, 68, 72.)
100 | 91	**Superior functioning in a wide range of activities, life's problems never seem to get out of hand, is sought out by others because of his or her many positive qualities. No symptoms.**
90 | 81	**Absent or minimal symptoms** (e.g., mild anxiety before an exam), **good functioning in all areas, interested and involved in a wide range of activities, socially effective, generally satisfied with life, no more than everyday problems or concerns** (e.g., an occasional argument with family members).
80 | 71	**If symptoms are present, they are transient and expectable reactions to psychosocial stressors** (e.g., difficulty concentrating after family argument); **no more than slight impairment in social, occupational, or school functioning** (e.g., temporarily falling behind in schoolwork).
70 | 61	**Some mild symptoms** (e.g., depressed mood and mild insomnia) **OR some difficulty in social, occupational, or school functioning** (e.g., occasional truancy, or theft within the household), **but generally functioning pretty well, has some meaningful interpersonal relationships.**
60 | 51	**Moderate symptoms** (e.g., flat affect and circumstantial speech, occasional panic attacks) **OR moderate difficulty in social, occupational, or school functioning** (e.g., few friends, conflicts with peers or co-workers).
50 | 41	**Serious symptoms** (e.g., suicidal ideation, severe obsessional rituals, frequent shoplifting) **OR any serious impairment in social, occupational, or school functioning** (e.g., no friends, unable to keep a job).
40 | 31	**Some impairment in reality testing or communication** (e.g., speech is at times illogical, obscure, or irrelevant) **OR major impairment in several areas, such as work or school, family relations, judgment, thinking, or mood** (e.g., depressed man avoids friends, neglects family, and is unable to work; child frequently beats up younger children, is defiant at home, and is failing at school).
30 | 21	**Behavior is considerably influenced by delusions or hallucinations OR serious impairment in communication or judgment** (e.g., sometimes incoherent, acts grossly inappropriately, suicidal preoccupation) **OR inability to function in almost all areas** (e.g., stays in bed all day; no job, home, or friends).
20 | 11	**Some danger of hurting self or others** (e.g., suicide attempts without clear expectation of death; frequently violent; manic excitement) **OR occasionally fails to maintain minimal personal hygiene** (e.g., smears feces) **OR gross impairment in communication** (e.g., largely incoherent or mute).
10 | 1	**Persistent danger of severely hurting self or others** (e.g., recurrent violence) **OR persistent inability to maintain minimal personal hygiene OR serious suicidal act with clear expectation of death.**
0	Inadequate information.

The rating of overall psychological functioning on a scale of 0–100 was operationalized by Luborsky in the Health-Sickness Rating Scale (Luborsky L: "Clinicians' Judgments of Mental Health." *Archives of General Psychiatry* 7:407–417, 1962). Spitzer and colleagues developed a revision of the Health-Sickness Rating Scale called the Global Assessment Scale (GAS) (Endicott J, Spitzer RL, Fleiss JL, Cohen J: "The Global Assessment Scale: A Procedure for Measuring Overall Severity of Psychiatric Disturbance." *Archives of General Psychiatry* 33:766–771, 1976). A modified version of the GAS was included in *DSM-III-R* as the Global Assessment of Functioning (GAF) Scale.

Source: Reprinted with permission from the Diagnostic and Statistical Manual of Mental Disorders, Fourth Edition. Copyright 1994 American Psychiatric Association.

ROLES OF THE PSYCHIATRIC–MENTAL HEALTH NURSE IN CONTEMPORARY MENTAL HEALTH CARE

Trends and issues in the U.S. health-care system currently affect the roles of the psychiatric–mental health nurse. Although psychiatric nurses have traditionally worked on inpatient psychiatric units, they have continued to expand their role into the community. Those working with hospitalized clients once had a broad span of time for developing the nurse-client relationship; however, they must now contend with a reduced length of stay and less time for helping clients with their emotional needs. Community-based treatment allows more time to develop a therapeutic relationship, participate in the "real-life" context of the client's illness, and share responsibility for health-care decisions.

The funding of health care impacts on psychiatric nursing, not only by dictating the length and type of a client's treatment but also by mandating increased efficiency, accountability, and meticulous justification for both inpatient and outpatient therapy. The documentation of the client's treatment process demands the attention and energy of the nurse and often competes with time spent with the client.

Because of the reduced length of inpatient stays, rarely are the client's long-term goals attained during hospitalization. Instead, they become part of an aftercare or continuing-care plan based in the client's home and community. Numerous opportunities exist for the psychiatric–mental health nurse in this rehabilitation process.

There are essentially two levels of psychiatric–mental health nurses: the generalist and the specialist. The scope and roles of both are guided by nurse practice acts and by standards of care and professional performance developed by the ANA.[1] Table 1–6 lists the ANA standards of care.

ROLE OF THE GENERALIST

The **psychiatric–mental health generalist nurse** is a licensed RN with an aptitude for and demonstrated expertise in psychiatric–mental health practice. Generalists deliver **primary mental health care**, care that includes comprehensive and continuous services for the prevention of mental illness and maintenance of mental health, as well as the diagnosis and treatment of psychiatric disorders, their consequences, and rehabilitation.[14] Primary mental health care incorporates both physical and mental health care.[14] Generalists exercise a holistic approach to practice and perform psychiatric nursing in prevention programs, community and day treatment centers, psychiatric rehabilitation facilities, homeless shelters, and many other settings. Those with a bachelor's degree are eligible to take a specialized certification examination from the ANA. Table 1–7 lists the

TABLE 1–6. ANA Standards of Care and Standards of Professional Performance

Standard I Assessment
The psychiatric–mental health nurse collects client health data.

Standard II Diagnosis
The psychiatric–mental health nurse analyzes the assessment data in determining diagnoses.

Standard III Outcome Identification
The psychiatric–mental health nurse identifies expected outcomes individualized to the client.

Standard IV Planning
The psychiatric–mental health nurse develops a plan of care that prescribes interventions to attain expected outcomes.

Standard V Implementation
The psychiatric–mental health nurse implements the interventions identified in the plan of care.

Standard VI Evaluation
The psychiatric–mental health nurse evaluates the client's progress in attaining expected outcomes.

Source: Adapted from American Nurses' Association: A Statement on Psychiatric–Mental Health Clinical Nursing Practice and Standards of Psychiatric–Mental Health Clinical Nursing Practices. American Nurses' Association, Washington, DC, 1994.

TABLE 1–7. Major Responsibilities of the Psychiatric–Mental Health Nurse Generalist

- Advocacy
- Knowledge of personality development
- Knowledge of group dynamics
- Knowledge of theories of mental illness
- Use of psychosocial principles
- Understanding of behavior patterns
- Therapeutic communication
- Ability to create, maintain, and terminate a therapeutic nurse-client relationship
- Promotion of health, physical and mental
- Health maintenance
- Health screening
- Crisis intervention
- Counseling
- Understanding of relationship of theories and methods on nursing care
- Home visits
- Medication management
- Understanding of theories of treatment for mental illness
- Somatic and other psychobiological interventions
- Teaching client self-care
- Membership in professional organizations
- Health teaching
- Milieu therapy
- Case management
- Research-based practice interventions

major functions of the generalist. Box 1–3 describes an innovative role for psychiatric nurse generalists.

ROLE OF THE SPECIALIST

In contrast to the generalist, the **psychiatric clinical nurse specialist (CNS)** holds a master's degree in psychiatric–mental health nursing, does supervised postgraduate hours of direct clinical practice, and successfully passes the ANA certification examination as a psychiatric CNS, in either child or adult psychiatric nursing. The CNS is an advanced practice nurse who demonstrates depth and breadth of knowledge, competence, and skill in the practice of psychiatric–mental health nursing.[1] Table 1–8 lists the major roles of the psychiatric CNS.

Recent trends have witnessed the emergence of the role of the psychiatric nurse practitioner (NP). Substantial disagreement and ambiguity exist around this term. For example, is this an expanded CNS role that encompasses increased knowledge and experience in pathophysiology and pharmacology, or is this an NP role with expanded training in psychotherapeutic and psychopharmacologic modalities? Because there is no defined consistent curriculum for the psychiatric NP or any current ANA certification standards or examination, the nature and scope of this role remain ambiguous and controversial. Talley and Caverly[15] offer a proposal for expanding the role of the psychiatric CNS in primary mental health-care services. Their model extends biological and therapeutic management of psychopharmacology, expands the role of differential diagnosis of medical problems, and emphasizes prevention, coordination of care, education, and assessment of health risks associated with mental health and treatment.

TABLE 1–8. Major Responsibilities of the Psychiatric–Mental Health Nurse Specialist

- Individual, group, and family therapy
- Prescriptive authority
- High degree of proficiency in interpersonal skills and nursing process
- Leadership
- Advancement of nursing theory
- Nursing research
- Clinical supervision
- Consultation
- Education of staff and trainees
- Expert witness testimony
- Leadership in professional organizations
- Peer review
- Research-based practice interventions

Box 1–3. A Unique Role for Psychiatric Nursing in the Community: The Sexual Assault Nurse Examiner

The Sexual Assault Nurse Examiner (SANE) is a nurse with specialized training in the assessment and treatment of women who have been physically or sexually assaulted.[1] The SANE program focuses on the medical, social, psychological, cultural, and legal implications of this type of trauma. It emphasizes providing sensitive and competent care during the victim's initial contact with the health-care system to facilitate recovery and promote effective coping. The idea stemmed from the need to develop a cadre of specialized staff to ensure that legally admissible evidence would be collected from rape victims. Although being a psychiatric nurse is not a requirement for joining this cadre of nurses, much of the training is based on principles of psychiatric–mental health care. In fact, prior to instituting this program, nurses cared primarily for the physical needs of the victim of an assault. Originally, women's health practitioners and outpatient clinic nurses comprised most SANEs. Since emergency room (ER) nurses are usually the first to treat a traumatized individual, today many nurse examiners are based in or provide "on call" services to the ER. This unique program, which has expanded to include physicians and other health-care professionals in its training, assists victims in the emotional aftermath of severe trauma, while simultaneously obtaining forensic evidence. In fact, most SANEs are expected to testify about the victim and report on evidence from the assault. This unique role promotes client advocacy and victim recovery, along with public safety and community advocacy.

1. Lenehan, G: Sexual assault nurse examiners: A SANE way to care for rape victims. Journal of Emergency Nursing 17:1, 1991.

PRIMARY CARE NURSE

Recent trends have shown that primary care psychiatric nursing is effective in delivering care in inpatient settings. This modality shifts from a task-oriented perspective to client-centered nursing in which a primary nurse is responsible for applying the nursing process to an assigned client.[1] Research on the initiation of this model finds that more individual and accountable care results, nurses develop a more positive attitude toward the nursing process, and clients are more self-sufficient and independent.[17]

PSYCHIATRIC NURSE AS COLLABORATIVE MEMBER OF THE INTERDISCIPLINARY TEAM

Regardless of practice at the generalist or specialist level, the psychiatric nurse is responsible for being a collaborative member of the mental health treatment team. Collaboration implies a commitment to common goals, with shared responsibility for the outcome of care. It also implies helping to facilitate the mental health of the client, family, or community within the context of the treatment team. Nurses bring their own specialized knowledge to the treatment process, thereby enhancing information about the client's assessment, treatment needs, and progress. Saur and Ford[16] describe seven characteristics of effective collaboration: trust, respect, commitment, cooperation, coordination, communication, and flexibility.

ROLE IN MENTAL HEALTH PROMOTION

Psychiatric nurses have a role in all levels of health promotion. **Primary prevention** of mental health problems means avoiding the development of psychiatric conditions, whereas **secondary prevention** enables people to regain previous functioning and to prevent further problems, once an illness has been identified. **Tertiary prevention** focuses on the prevention or reversal of the consequences of illness and may include rehabilitative interventions. Table 1–9 lists functions of the nurse at each level.

NURSE CASE MANAGER

Case management has been a key role for psychiatric nursing for decades. It arose in response to the need to coordinate services for clients during the time of deinstitutionalization.[1] Now, in response to decreased length of hospital stays and cost-containment measures, there is an increased need for case management to integrate the client's entire health-care needs. Table 1–10 lists characteristics of the role of the nurse case manager.

TABLE 1–9. Functions of the Psychiatric–Mental Health Nurse in the Levels of Prevention

Primary—fostering mental health
- Identifying high-risk groups
- Teaching parenting classes
- Teaching stress management
- Conducting support groups for those who have medical problems
- Counseling about everyday stressors and problems
- Promoting growth and development across the life span
- Counseling on mental health problems
- Providing anticipatory guidance

Secondary–treating illness
- Screening and identifying mental illness in its early form to prevent disabling consequences
- Making referrals
- Conducting individual, group, and family psychotherapy
- Intervening in crises
- Applying brief psychotherapy techniques
- Administering and managing medication
- Managing therapeutic milieu
- Assisting with electroconvulsive therapy

Tertiary—rehabilitating
- Referring clients to step-down programs, halfway houses, psychiatric home health agencies, and psychiatric rehabilitation centers
- Continuing health teaching
- Providing case management

TABLE 1–10. Role of the Psychiatric–Mental Health Nurse as Case Manager

- Anticipation and prevention of crises
- Medication maintenance
- Maintenance of regular medical and dental needs
- Psychosocial rehabilitation
- Prevention of hospitalization and maintenance of community living
- Enhancement of quality of life
- Help with problems of living
- Money management
- Client advocacy
- Integrated care planning
- Facilitation of application for public assistance programs
- Brokerage and negotiation with agencies to provide services to client
- Early identification and intervention for worsening of symptoms
- Treatment planning jointly with client
- Administrative support of long-term clients
- Facilitation of access to services
- Provision of a full array of mental-health services, including individually tailored treatment and flexible program offerings
- Coordination of agencies that serve the client
- Recognition of cultural factors that affect treatment

Sources: Adapted from Sledge, WH, et al. Case management in psychiatry: An analysis of tasks. Am J Psychiatry 152:1259, 1995. American Nurses Association: Nursing Case Management. American Nurses Association, Kansas City, 1988. Stetler, C: Case management plans. In Zander, K, Etheridge, M, and Bower, K (eds): Nursing Case Management: Blueprints for Transformation. New England Medical Center Hosptials, Boston.

DIRECTOR OR MANAGER OF THE THERAPEUTIC MILIEU

Some agencies employ nurses as program directors or nurse managers of a treatment unit such as an inpatient hospital unit, a day treatment center, or a specialized community-based program, for example, an Alzheimer's treatment center. Four broad areas of expertise are needed.

First, specialized leadership skills should include the ability to provide clear and consistent direction, with a visionary perspective. Leadership also implies the promotion and protection of the values of the program, conflict resolution skills, and communication ability. Effective milieu leaders convey ethical integrity and focus on the needs and rights of clients.

Second, the manager keeps the therapeutic milieu running smoothly: scheduling staff, determining appropriateness of

> **RESEARCH NOTE**
>
> Baradell, JG: Clinical outcomes and satisfaction of patients of clinical nurse specialists in psychiatric–mental health nursing. Arch Psychiatr Nurs 9:240–250, 1995.
>
> **Findings.** The purpose of the study was to examine clinical outcomes and satisfaction of clients of psychiatric CNSs. A total of 100 individuals (45%) responded to a series of questionnaires designed to measure mood, quality of life, and client satisfaction with care provided by six clinical specialists. The respondents rated significant improvement in symptoms of anxiety, depression, anger, confusion, fatigue, and vigor. With psychotherapy provided by the CNS, clients' reports of their quality of life indicated greater improvement in all three domains (family, social, and job functioning) after receiving therapy. Overall, the clients were satisfied with the care they received, and 97% responded that therapy had helped at least somewhat. Nearly all respondents reported that the clinical specialist listened to their needs and understood them. This study is the first to systematically evaluate the effectiveness and satisfaction of clinical specialist–delivered psychotherapy to a large group of individuals with psychiatric conditions.
>
> **Application to Practice.** The psychiatric CNS is a cost-effective independent provider of mental health services who should have a major role in new health-care delivery systems. Although other skills such as prescriptive authority were not evaluated in this study, the evolving responsibilities of the CNS place them in key positions to provide comprehensive and effective mental health care. The psychiatric CNS can help identify, assess, and treat major psychiatric disorders as well as help patients and family cope with stress, loss, and family issues. As independent clinicians, they provide primary psychiatric–mental health care.

client admission, co-leading groups, teaching, providing clinical supervision, role modeling, and making timely decisions.

Third, the manager derives and modifies mental health policies to implement the organization's mission in the changing health-care market. As part of this function, the administrator is partially responsible for cost control and quality assessment and improvement.

Fourth, the nurse as milieu manager uses psychotherapeutic principles to understand the behavior of other staff and self and thus promote effective professional work relationships.

PSYCHIATRIC CONSULTATION–LIAISON NURSE

The role of the consultation-liaison (CL) nurse has generally been based in the hospital setting, but now the psychiatric CL nurse also works in home care. In this role, the nurse provides expert psychotherapeutic interventions to clients, staff of medical and surgical units, or other nurses working in home care. A hallmark of this activity is an understanding of human behavior and the expert ability to construct an appropriate plan of action quickly.

- The psychiatric CL nurse may talk with a particularly difficult client and recommend a course of action or consult with nursing staff about clinical dilemmas. For example, oncology nurses may request training to help clients cope with the diagnosis of cancer and with staff responses to this process.
- CL nurses may assist with staff issues, such as concerns about substance abuse among employees.
- The CL has a primary prevention role of anticipating mental health needs of clients and staff, thereby preventing unnecessary transfers to psychiatric units or escalations of unhealthy behaviors.
- CLs facilitate increased sensitivity of the nursing staff to mental health needs, decreased nurse-client conflicts, and provision of additional emotional and educational support to staff.

Psychiatric CNSs are beginning to provide consultation in unique settings, including industry, school nursing, home health-care agencies, nursing homes, burn units, and intensive care units.[18–20] In industry, psychiatric nurse consultants assist with communication problems, role clarification, and interpersonal and group dynamics. They design and implement employee-based stress management, wellness, behavioral change such as weight loss, and substance abuse programs. On burn units, psychiatric nurse consultants have helped nurses to assess and intervene in the psychosocial needs of the client and family and helped reduce the stress of nursing staff caring for these clients. In intensive care units, CL nurses provide support and direction to clients who require cessation of life-sustaining treatment. Consultation to home health-care agencies and nursing homes involves interventions similar to the traditional hospital-based CL role but also includes leading support groups for staff, clients, or families and recommending medication changes.

Unfortunately, with the current emphasis on cost reduction and reduced lengths of stay, less time is allotted for dealing with emotional needs, and many clients do not get the benefit of liaison nursing services in the hospital. Also, this role may be difficult to fund because insurance companies generally do not reimburse for it.

NURSE PSYCHOTHERAPIST

The one-to-one therapeutic relationship is key to psychiatric nursing practice. With advanced practice comes the opportunity to build on these skills and develop independent practice as a psychotherapist. Different from counseling abilities, psychotherapy implies a defined agreement between nurse and client to address and treat psychological issues in an intensive manner.

Today, providing individual, group, and family therapy is an integral role of the psychiatric CNS. In a recent study, 73% of psychiatric CNSs indicated they use individual psychotherapy and spend 35% of their practice in this modality.[21] As psychotherapists, nurses at the advanced practice level are engaged in either independent private practices or as equal partners in group or clinical settings. Many states allow direct insurance reimbursement for these services. The underlying theoretical framework for therapy may be based on both nursing and psychological models. These models may include cognitive-behavior theory, brief or short-term therapy models, supportive therapy, systems theory, psychoanalytic theory, and so forth. In the child subspecialty, play therapy with toys, games, and stories facilitates treatment of young clients.

One emerging role in the current health-care system is the nurse who provides brief psychotherapy. Shires and Tappan[22] describe several aspects of the CNS as brief psychotherapist:

- the combination of advanced assessment skills
- the knowledge of community resources
- the focus on health, developmental, group, and crisis skills
- the ability to set clear, distinct short-term goals

NURSE PSYCHOPHARMACOLOGIST

One of the newest roles is nurse psychopharmacologist—the psychiatric CNS with prescriptive authority. Although physicians traditionally prescribe, advanced practice nurses such as psychiatric CNSs and NPs also have this privilege. Prescriptive practice is defined as:

> The ability of the nurse in advanced practice to prescribe or authorize (through cosignature) or recommend a drug, controlled or uncontrolled, device or therapy independently based on nursing assessment or the delegation of medical acts or as conditioned by a protocol or collaborative arrangement or as authorized by exemption from nurse or medical practice act (for state employees) to a patient who is under the direct care of the nurse.[23]

As part of this role, the nurse psychopharmacologist is charged with obtaining a complete physical and psychological assessment of the individual: psychiatric diagnosis, review of medical history, assessment of past and present medications, and referral for a physical examination and other necessary procedures. Then the nurse psychopharmacologist initiates a joint plan of care with the client, which may include psychopharmacology as one aspect of the overall treatment plan. The nurse would then start, monitor, and adjust the medication, determine whether a partial or full clinical response is evident, and monitor and manage side effects. Because psychiatric nurse generalists have long been the individuals who administer and help monitor the response to medication, the CNS is in a prime position to use expanded knowledge in initiating medication and assessing the client's response.

The parameters of prescriptive authority vary considerably from state to state.[24] Three states currently permit the psychiatric CNS to write prescriptions without any limitation or supervision, whereas most require some level of physician involvement: direct supervision, written contracts that describe the prescribing practice, cosignature of prescriptions, or detailed medication protocols that outline exact procedures for medication monitoring. Regardless of whether the nurse actually writes the prescription, medication management is becoming an integral part of the psychiatric CNS role.

There is little research on the role of the psychiatric CNS as psychopharmacologist. However, studies of other advanced practice nurses, such as NPs and certified nurse midwives, have demonstrated their ability to use prescriptive authority effectively.[25] In fact, some studies have found that nurse prescribers are less likely to aggressively initiate medication than their physician counterparts and more likely to obtain further assessment data or suggest nonpharmacologic interventions such as diet and exercise. The cost-effectiveness of care delivered by nurse prescribers is an added advantage.

LEGAL AND ETHICAL ISSUES

From the beginning, psychiatric nurses have played a major role in the moral treatment of individuals with mental health problems. Moral treatment means conveying respect and tolerance for clients regardless of social, ethnic, economic, or personal situations. Promoting humane care and environmental conditions that facilitate recovery rather than disease are important values that the specialty continues to hold.

Another obligation is the nurse's assumption of responsibility for his or her actions, decisions, and competence. Psychiatric nurses, as professionals, are charged with maintaining high standards of personal and professional accountability to ensure high-quality care and to champion the rights of psychiatric clients. Guidance for the moral, legal, and ethical components emanates from three important sources: The ANA *Standards of Psychiatric–Mental Health Practice*, the ANA *Code of Ethics for Nurses* (Table 1–11), and state and federal laws that govern the care and treatment of the mentally ill.

CONFIDENTIALITY

Psychiatric nurses are bound by ethical principles to maintain **confidentiality** unless prior consent is given. Protecting the identity and rights of the individual who is receiving psychiatric care is essential in developing a trusting relationship. Only when clients are in danger of harming themselves or others can confidentiality be violated. In the hospital, clients are told who has access to their records and must give their written permission for others, including insurers, to review their files. With technological developments that promote computerized medical records, the challenge is to protect clients from others' unauthorized access to their records.

TABLE 1-11. American Nurses' Association Code of Ethics for Nurses

1. The nurse provides services with respect for human dignity and the uniqueness of the client unrestricted by considerations of social or economic status, personal attributes, or the nature of health problems.
2. The nurse safeguards the client's right to privacy by judiciously protecting information of a confidential nature.
3. The nurse acts to safeguard the client and the public when health care and safety are affected by the incompetent, unethical, or illegal practice of any person.
4. The nurse assumes responsibility and accountability for individual nursing judgments and actions.
5. The nurse maintains competence in nursing.
6. The nurse exercises informed judgment and uses individual competence and qualifications as criteria in seeking consultations, accepting responsibilities, and delegating nursing activities to others.
7. The nurse participates in activities that contribute to the ongoing development of the profession's body of knowledge.
8. The nurse participates in the profession's efforts to implement and improve standards of nursing.
9. The nurse participates in the profession's efforts to establish and maintain conditions of employment conducive to high-quality nursing care.
10. The nurse participates in the profession's effort to protect the public from misinformation and misrepresentation and to maintain the integrity of nursing.
11. The nurse collaborates with members of the health profession and other citizens in promoting community and national efforts to meet the health needs of the public.

Source: From American Nurses' Association: Code of Ethics for Nurses, American Nurses' Association, Washington, DC, 1985, with permission.

For example, in a recent criminal case, a custodian accessed admission lists of a hospital with home phone numbers of young women and began to harass them. In another case, confidential information about a famous individual was leaked to the press by a hospital staff worker. These represent not only a breach of trust and confidentiality but also a potentially dangerous situation for the client.

ADMISSION TO A PSYCHIATRIC INPATIENT FACILITY

All states have laws that govern commitment of clients to mental health facilities. Generally, an individual with a psychiatric disorder severe enough to warrant hospitalization enters voluntarily. Unfortunately, a person sometimes does not recognize the need for intense treatment, is too afraid or suspicious to enter the hospital, or is too impaired by the current psychiatric behavior to make an adequate judgment. In these circumstances, involuntary hospitalization, or **commitment**, may be considered. In all states, there are two main reasons for psychiatric hospitalization. First, the individual is a severe danger or poses a threat of harm to himself or herself or to someone else. This includes suicidal or homicidal threats or actions. Second, the individual is unable to care for himself or herself or provide for basic needs. In either case, the situation is potentially dangerous, and mental health professionals are mandated to act to protect the client. In some states, other criteria exist for involuntary commitment. Nurses should become familiar with the mental health laws of their states to protect themselves and their **clients' rights.**

DISCHARGE FROM A PSYCHIATRIC INPATIENT FACILITY

Ideally, clients are released from the hospital when they have received sufficient care to promote recovery and sustain treatment in the community. However, some individuals with psychiatric illness feel that they do not require hospitalization, largely because of denial or lack of insight, and press for early discharge. Also, pressures of managed care lead to the possibility of premature discharge. In either case, careful assessment of the client's ability to reside in the community and receive adequate treatment must be made. If the client disagrees with the clinical decision of the treatment team to continue hospitalization, several options are available in most states.

Nurses should understand the mental health laws of their states and follow procedures governing discharge. They should protect the client's rights to call an attorney. And, if a nonvoluntary commitment is imminent, the nurse can lend support by explaining the legal ramifications to the client, showing sensitivity, and acknowledging the client's feelings of anger, lack of power, or consternation.

DUTY TO WARN

In the Tarasoff case, a psychotherapist was held liable for failing to warn the client's intended victim of harm when the client was released from care. Although no one can truly foresee the possibility of a crime, the law requires therapists and physicians to warn the potential victim of a client's violent act and to notify the authorities. Individuals who receive care and then directly threaten to harm another need to be carefully assessed. The client's right to confidentiality is overridden by the need to protect another individual from severe and dangerous consequences.

RIGHTS OF INDIVIDUALS WHO RECEIVE PSYCHIATRIC CARE

Clients' rights include those cited in the U.S. Constitution, basic rights of all patients, and special rights of the mentally ill, which are found in some of the state mental health laws (see Appendix 2). The nurse is ethically responsible to understand and to respect these rights. If for any reason a client's right is limited, the nurse must understand the reasons why and how to proceed. This problem then becomes part of the client's treatment plan. For example, a client who has been fired begins harassing the employer and making threats from the hospital telephone. The treatment team feels this way of dealing with feelings is unsafe and unproductive. Therefore, "ineffective management of anger" becomes a problem in the client's treatment plan. The client's goal is to learn to replace aggression with assertiveness. In the intervention, the client agrees to ban telephone calls to the employer and seeks to express angry feelings in therapy instead.

INFORMED CONSENT AND THE RIGHT TO REFUSE TREATMENT

One of the major rights of an individual is to be adequately informed about mental health care and treatment (informed consent). The right is founded in part on an ethical and legal precedent, the right of self-determination. Simply put, every individual has the right to determine what will or will not be done to his or her body. It is also based on the notion that any health-care provider is obligated to disclose the nature of the condition, risks, alternatives, and consequences of care, and the results of receiving no treatment.

Psychiatric nurses have a key role in **client advocacy**, that is, promoting and defending clients' rights and ensuring that informed consent takes place. The goal is to promote the individual's independence and ability to make decisions based on knowing and understanding the process, which implies that the client has received a reasonable amount of information to make a decision about treatment and has voluntarily and freely agreed to it. A prerequisite for informed consent is that the individual is an adult who is competent. Competency includes the ability to understand the proposed treatment choice, make a treatment decision, and verbally or nonverbally communicate that choice. The exceptions to obtaining informed consent are emergency situations, incompetency, a client's waiver of the right, and therapeutic privilege, an infrequent case where disclosure of risks and alternatives might have a deleterious effect on the client.

One of the most difficult issues today is understanding the right to refuse treatment. Individuals with psychiatric illnesses are increasingly afforded more freedom in choosing not to engage in treatment. Sometimes, however, these decisions are counter to the clinical judgment of the clinician recommending care. For example, an individual who is experiencing severe paranoia and hearing voices (auditory hallucinations) can refuse to take medication known to alleviate these symptoms in the absence of any emergency or danger.

TABLE 1–12. Indications for the Use of Seclusion or Restraint

- To prevent self-destructive behavior
- To prevent harm to others
- To prevent serious disruption to treatment environment
- To control serious agitation and behavioral escalation
- If appropriate, at the client's request
- To decrease stimulation (seclusion only)

Source: Adapted from Tardiff, K: Violence. In Hales, RE, Yudofsky, SC, and Talbott, JA (eds): Textbook of Psychiatry. American Psychiatric Press, Washington, DC, 1994, p 1278, with permission.

SECLUSION AND RESTRAINT

Nurses are confronted daily with the need to use a variety of management techniques, including restraint and seclusion. The major uses of these interventions are to prevent further escalation of dangerous behavior and to maintain the safety of the client, other individuals, and the hospital environment. Table 1–12 lists behaviors that justify seclusion or restraint.

Seclusion refers to the removal of the client from the usual treatment setting into a safe, empty room specifically designed with a locked door. However, in some states, depriving a client of interaction with others through room restriction or "time out" procedures also constitutes seclusion.

Restraint may take several forms. Mechanical restraints include leather cuffs, cloths, or poseys used to tie the person to a bed or chair. Chemical restraints are medications usually administered intramuscularly to control acute behavior. Restricting a client's movement by using "geri-chairs," four-point side rails, or a wheelchair positioned into the wall so that the client cannot move are also forms of restraint.

Seclusion and restraint are never used as punishment. The American Psychiatric Association's Task Force on Seclusion and Restraint[26] has devised specific guidelines (Table 1–13). Every treatment setting should have a similar policy for the use of these procedures, and all staff should be educated in their proper use consistent with state laws.

ADVOCATE FOR CLIENTS

One of the major ethical components of psychiatric nursing is to protect clients from misrepresentation and abuse. Championing the clients' rights, protecting them from exploitation, and devising individual interventions to promote health constitute the advocate's role. Nowhere is this advocacy needed more than in promoting psychiatric conditions as illnesses, similar to medical disorders, rather than as personal weaknesses or "craziness." The advocate role includes influencing public policy and the passage of laws in favor of the mentally ill. Box 1–4 describes how a psychiatric nurse

TABLE 1–13. Guidelines for the Use of Seclusion or Restraint

- Do not use to punish client or solely for convenience of staff or other clients.
- Take medical and psychiatric status of client into consideration (e.g., drug overdose, medical disease, self-mutilation).
- Follow institution's written guidelines.
- Make sure adequate staff (minimum of four) is present for implementation.
- Once decision is made, give client seconds to voluntarily comply and walk to seclusion room.
- If client does not comply, have each staff member grab a limb and bring client to ground.
- Apply restraint devices or carry client to seclusion.
- Search client for dangerous objects (belts, pins, watches), and remove shoes.
- Have physician examine client within 1 to 3 hours.
- Contact physician for subsequent episodes; physician may elect to not see client.
- Have physician observe client every 12 hours.
- Have staff outside the unit review clients in seclusion or restraint continuously over 72 hours.
- Observe client every 15 minutes at a minimum.
- Examine and reevaluate the client at least every 2 hours.
- Provide meals (without utensils) and fluids, allow toileting, and monitor vital signs at appropriate times and with caution.
- Loosen four-point restraints every 15 minutes.
- Continuously evaluate the outcome of seclusion or restraint on client's behavior.
- Gradually release client from seclusion or restraint.
- Document in detail in the medical record or in a log each decision, observation, measurement, medication administered, and nursing care given.
- "Debrief" (discuss the seclusion or restraint) with client after each episode.

Source: Adapted from Tardiff, K: Violence. In Hales, RE, Yudofsky, SC, and Talbott, JA (eds): Textbook of Psychiatry. American Psychiatric Press, Washington, DC, 1994, p 1279, with permission.

Box 1–4. Teaming Up to Provide Intensive Psychiatric Treatment in the Community

White and Shields,[1] a psychiatrist and psychiatric clinical nurse specialist, were confronted with clients with severe and persistent psychiatric conditions that required intensive and often long-term treatment. Each client's "outpatient" insurance benefits totaled only about $500 per year, allowing only six to nine individual therapy or medication follow-up sessions. However, the insurance company would and did pay for several acute hospitalizations for many clients that totaled hundreds of thousands of dollars. These clinicians found that these clients were hospitalized frequently and received little follow-up care, which increased the need for expensive inpatient care. White and Shields proposed to restructure the nature of the reimbursement system and "prove" to the insurance company that this would be a successful strategy for everyone. In fact, the plan could also save the company money. With that in mind, these clinicians were able to successfully manage the first conversion of benefits for a psychiatric client: The reimbursement for inpatient services was "converted" to an extensive outpatient management program, which included daily phone calls, halfway house living, emergency visits, medication, and frequent counseling. The goal was to maintain the individual in the community by providing a network of necessary services, thereby minimizing or avoiding hospitalization. In this model, psychiatric nurses provide more than case management; they are actively involved in daily treatment with their clients. The essence of this model, conversion of benefits, has been a prototype for many other services for clients with psychiatric and medical conditions such as clients with AIDS or conditions leading to workers' compensation.

1. White, K, and Shields, J: Conversion of inpatient mental health benefits to outpatient benefits. Hosp Community Psychiatry 42:570, 1991.

and psychiatrist teamed up to advocate and provide mental health care for their clients in the community.

CASE STUDY

Mrs. Damon is a 50-year-old woman who is referred to the home health agency for follow-up and treatment of major depression. She is a widow, lives alone, and has no friends or social supports other than her two sons, who live in distant cities. She is unable to function in any of her usual roles because of her depression. The psychiatric diagnosis is complicated by Mrs. Damon's chronic pain from a previous automobile accident and her diabetes. Her sons voice frustration at their mother's unwillingness to care for herself. They describe her as "clinging, needy, and attention seeking." In fact, Mrs. Damon's dependency is so profound that nursing home placement is an option. Major stressors in the client's life include the death of her husband 1 year ago, her inability to maintain her present living arrangements, and her physical problems. Her diagnosis follows:

Axis I: Major Depressive Disorder, Recurrent, Severe Without Psychotic Features
Axis II: Dependent Personality Disorder
Axis III: Chronic pain, diabetes mellitus
Axis IV: Problems with primary support group
Axis V: GAF = 41

CRITICAL THINKING QUESTIONS

1. From examining the GAF in Table 1–5, is "41" a fair score for Mrs. Damon? Explain.
2. Cite the factors in the case study that support the Axis IV diagnosis: Problems with primary support group. Refer to Table 4–3. Develop a nursing diagnosis for Mrs. Damon from the information you have on the medical axes.

KEY POINTS

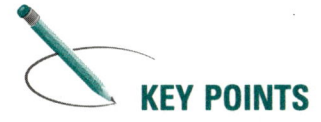

- Mental health is a state of well-being in which individuals function well in society and are generally satisfied with their lives in the context of their culture and environment.
- Mental illness is a significant behavioral or psychological problem that leads to distress and impaired functioning.
- The history of psychiatric nursing began during primitive times when intuitive, caring, and compassionate women of the society ministered to the sick. The profession has evolved into one that treats the whole person and emphasizes the neuroscientific and psychosocial aspects.
- According to Peplau, psychiatric–mental health nursing is accomplished through a counseling role, the nurse-client relationship, and therapeutic communication skills. The discipline uses a holistic approach; considers biological, genetic, developmental, environmental, social, cultural, spiritual, physical, and emotional implications; and builds on the strengths of the individual, while remaining aware of deficits.
- Experiences during pregnancy, infancy, and childhood shape the brain's structure and functioning, which in turn affect relationships, personality, behavior, and the potential for psychiatric problems.
- Rapid discoveries and technological advances have recently promoted neuroscience as the foundation for understanding psychiatric disorders.
- Contemporary mental health is characterized by increased knowledge and technology, use of the *DSM-IV* for classifying mental illness, and community-based care.
- Mental health care today emphasizes community-based or community-linked care, partly because of economic pressures and managed care.
- Mental illness is now recognized as a medical condition with distinct etiologies.
- Psychiatric nursing is challenged with incorporating new understanding of the neuroscientific and medical aspects of mental wellness into practice while retaining the traditional roles of the nurse.
- Psychiatric nursing is practiced at all levels of prevention: primary, secondary, and tertiary.
- There are essentially two areas of practice: generalist and clinical specialist. Both have clearly identified roles.
- Psychiatric nurses are guided by legal and ethical requirements and aim always to protect the client's rights.

REFERENCES

1. American Nurses' Association: A Statement on Psychiatric–Mental Health Clinical Nursing Practice and Standards of Psychiatric–Mental Health Clinical Nursing Practice. ANA, Washington, DC, 1994.
2. Peplau, HE: Interpersonal Relationships in Nursing: A Conceptual Frame of Reference for Psychodynamic Nursing. GP Putnam's Sons, New York, 1952.
3. Beeber, LS: The one-to-one relationship in psychiatric nursing: The next generation. In Anderson, CA (ed): Psychiatric Nursing 1974 to 1994: A Report on the State of the Art. Ohio State University, Columbus, 1995, pp. 9–36.
4. Marriner-Tomey, A: American Nursing Theorists and Their Work. Mosby, St. Louis, 1994.
5. Teicher, MH: Preliminary evidence for abnormal cortical development in physically and sexually abused children using EEG coherence and MRI. Ann NY Acad Sci, 1977.
6. Peplau, HE: Some unresolved issues in the era of biopsychosocial nursing. Journal of the American Psychiatric Nurses Association 1:92, 1995.
7. Hayes, A: Psychiatric nursing: What does biology have to do with it? Arch Psychiatr Nurs 9:216, 1995.
8. McEnany, GW: Psychobiology and psychiatric nursing: A philosophical matrix. Arch Psychiatr Nurs 5:255, 1991.
9. Judd, LL, and Murphy, DC: Neuroscience past to present. In Broadwell, RD (ed): Neuroscience, Memory, and Language, Vol 1. Library of Congress, Washington, DC, 1995, p 25.
10. Sutton, SB: Crossroads in Psychiatry: A History of the McLean Hospital. American Psychiatric Press, Washington, DC, 1986.
11. American Nurses' Association: Psychopharmacology guidelines for psychiatric mental health nurses. In Psychiatric Mental Health Nursing Psychopharmacology Project. ANA, Washington, DC, 1994, pp 41–45.
12. American Psychiatric Association: Diagnostic and Statistical Manual of Mental Disorders, fourth edition. American Psychiatric Association, Washington, DC, 1994.
13. Griffith, EEH, and Gonzolaz, CA: Essentials of Culture Psychiatry. In (eds): p 1379.
14. Haber, J, and Billings, C: Primary mental health care: A model for psychiatric-mental health nursing. Journal of the American Psychiatric Nurses Association 1:154, 1995.
15. Talley, S, and Caverly, S: Advanced-practice psychiatric nursing and health care reform. Hospital Community Psychiatry 45:545, 1994.
16. Saur, C, and Ford, S: Quality, cost-effective psychiatric treatment: A CNS-MD collaborative practice model. Arch Psychiatr Nurs 9:332, 1995.
17. Armitage, P, Champney-Smith, J, and Andrew, K: Primary nursing and the role of the nurse preceptor in changing long-term mental health care: An evaluation. J Adv Nurs 16:413, 1991.
18. Newton, L, and Wilson, KG: Consultee satisfaction with a psychiatric consultation–liaison nursing service. Arch Psychiatr Nurs 4:264, 1990.
19. Stickney, SK, and Hall, RCW: The role of the nurse on a consultation-liaison team. Psychosomatics 22:224, 1981.
20. Hart, CA: The role of psychiatric consultation–liaison nurses in ethical decisions to remove life-sustaining treatment. Arch Psychiatr Nurs 4:370, 1990.
21. Betrus, PA, and Hoffman, A: Psychiatric–mental health nursing: Career characteristics, professional activities, and client attributes of members of the ANA Council of Psychiatric Nurses. Issues Mental Health Nursing 13:39, 1992.
22. Shires, B, and Tappan, T: The clinical nurse specialist as brief psychotherapist. Perspectives Psychiatr Care 28:15, 1992.
23. Carson, WY: Prescriptive practice in the 1990s: A crazy quilt of overregulation. Unpublished manuscript, p 1.
24. Talley, S, and Brooke, PS: Prescriptive authority for psychiatric clinical specialists: Framing the issues. Arch Psychiatr Nurs 6:71, 1992.
25. Safriet, B: Health care dollars and regulatory sense: The role of advanced practice nursing. Yale J Regulation 9:417, 1992.
26. Tardiff, K (ed): The Psychiatric Uses of Seclusion and Restraint. American Psychiatric Press, Washington, DC, 1984.

CHAPTER 2

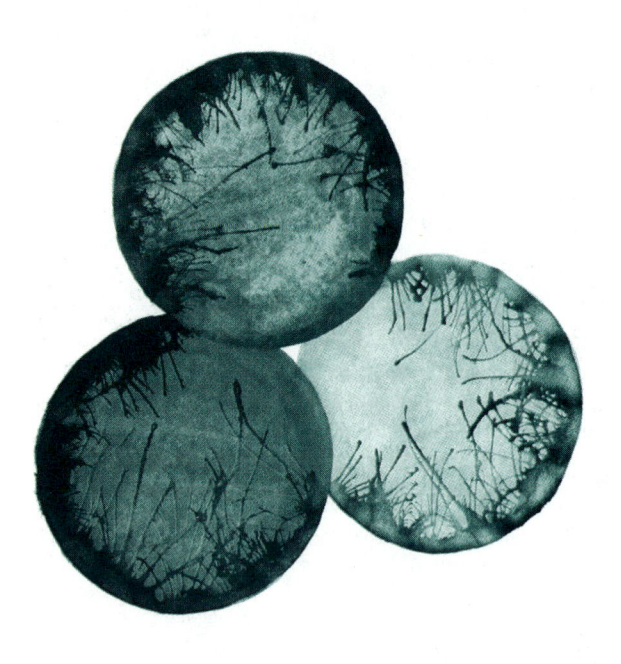

CHAPTER OUTLINE

Assessment
   Before the Assessment
   During the Assessment
   After the Assessment
Planning Care
   Establishing Priority
   Setting Long-term Goals
   Setting Short-term Goals
   Designing Interventions
Implementation
Evaluation
The Collaborative Plan of Care

LEARNING OBJECTIVES

After completing this chapter, the reader should be able to:

- Perform a Mental Status Examination.
- Identify major components of the nursing assessment process.
- Discuss common biases and prejudices that may affect the nursing process.
- Explain the role of specific types of testing beyond the nursing assessment.
- Construct a plan of care for the client with a psychiatric problem.
- State the importance of reevaluation against an initial baseline.

KEY TERMS

affect	delusions
ambivalence	dysphoric
blunted	euphoric
cognition	flat
confabulation	hallucinations
countertransference	inappropriate
culture	insight

Pamela Campbell, MS, OTR
Billie Barringer, MA, BSN, RNC, CNS

The Nursing Process in Psychiatric–Mental Health Nursing

lability
Mental Status Examination
mood
obsession
orientation
outcomes
phobia
signs
symptoms
transference

In all settings in which nursing takes place, the method used for delivering individualized, quality nursing care is the *nursing process*. The process is never static. As problems are solved, new ones emerge. The nursing process is two-way; that is, it involves the nurse and client, the family, or a group in an interpersonal interaction. Each affects the other and is influenced by factors within the situation. Applying the nursing process demands intellectual, interactional, and technical skills, plus a well-defined relationship with the multidisciplinary team. According to the North American Nursing Diagnosis Association's (NANDA) *Standards of Psychiatric and Mental Health Nursing Practice*,[1] six standards guide nurses in using the nursing process:

Standard I: (Re-)Assessment
Standard II: Nursing Diagnosis
Standard III: Outcome Identification
Standard IV: Planning
Standard V: Implementation
Standard VI: Evaluation

Figure 2–1 shows the cyclic relationship of the six steps to each other.

ASSESSMENT

On initially encountering the psychiatric client, the nurse performs a holistic assessment and applies the **Mental Status Examination (MSE)** to elicit information about the client, the environment, and behaviors and beliefs indicative of pathology. The nurse is usually the first member of the treatment team to interact with the client, and the nurse's assessment becomes the basis for initiating the treatment plan, also called a *collaborative plan of care*. Any family member, friend, police officer, or social worker who accompanies the client can supply information from his or her perspective to explain the client's situation.

BEFORE THE ASSESSMENT

A nurse must establish rapport and trust before the client can be comfortable discussing problems. Therefore, the attention given to arranging an environment in which the client feels comfortable and secure must be meticulous.

- Make sure the client has privacy to encourage uninhibited discussion and ensure confidentiality.
- Obtain appropriate releases for information. If family or friends are present, ask for the client's consent to include them in the interview.
- Make sure the client signs a voluntary commitment form if inpatient hospitalization is requested. Admission

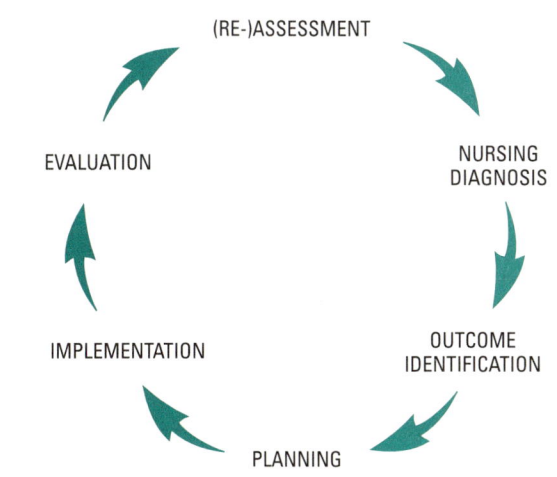

Figure 2–1. NANDA Six Step Assessment Process. Initial Assessment components of the ANA Psychiatric Standard of Care.

to community-based nursing facilities likewise requires the client's consent.
- Allow plenty of time to conduct the interview to avoid appearing rushed or hurried.
- Convey concern, interest, and empathy toward the client.
- Examine the way your own feelings and behavior influence the client. Your own anxiety could prevent your hearing the client or cause you to talk too much, display nervous habits, fail to sit down with the client, or misperceive the client's problem.
- Give the client necessary information about the purpose of the interview and about yourself, such as your affiliation or credentials. Inform the client that you will record information in a nursing history form and that the client may read the notations if desired. This approach establishes honesty, puts the client at ease, and starts the bonding process. See Figure 2–2 for a nursing history form.
- Search for existing medical records. Obtain written permission from the client before requesting records from other institutions or clinics and before discussing the client with other caregivers. For home visits, study the client's discharge summary and other information available from previous records.

DURING THE ASSESSMENT

The contents and style of the assessment will reflect the treatment setting, the types of clients encountered, the available resources, and the perceived need of the client. Older clients

Identifying Data

Name

Address

Date (always ask the client to state the date.)

Work and home telephone numbers

Date of birth

Marital status

Employer or profession

Emergency contact/legal guardian

Physical Assessment

- Allergies
- Current medication, the schedule of administration, and time of last dose
- Recent surgeries and/or major illnesses
- Chronic conditions
- Respiration (rate, cough, wheezing, asthma history)
- Pulse (strong, weak, rapid, slow)
- Skin tone and condition (pale, flushed, cyanotic, moist, cold, presence of cuts or other self-inflicted injuries, bruises, scars, tattoos)
- Date of last physical and the name and telephone of primary care physician
- Use of stimulants, alcohol, cigarettes, drugs (amount, duration, and time of last use)
- Anomalies of gait, any asymmetrical conditions (coordination)

Figure 2–2. Example of Nursing History for the Holistic Assessment. Reprinted with permission from Folstein, MF, Folstein, SE, McHugh, PR: Mini mental state exam: A practical method for grading the cognitive state of patients for the clinician. J Psychiatr Res 12:189–198, 1975.

- Nutritional status, special diets, recent weight loss or gain, appetite

- Ability to perform activities of daily living

- Sleep (normal, changes, duration, disturbances)

- Physical impairment, pain (duration, treatment)

- Elimination (constipation, diarrhea, colostomy, incontinence), or (urinary frequency, pain, burning, bleeding, retention)

- Sexual function (sexually active or not, sexual orientation, numbers of children, dysfunction, date of last menstrual period)

- Substance abuse history (type of drug, route of administration, length of addictive episode, history of withdrawal symptoms)

Psychological Assessment

Problem statement (in client's own words)

- Onset, or start. Simply ask the client, "When did this problem begin?"

- Duration refers to the length of time the problem has existed. Ask the client, "How long have you been bothered by this problem?"

- The precipitating event is the most recent occurrence, which made the client decide to seek treatment. Ask, "What happened during the past few days that made you decide to seek treatment?"

- Coping mechanisms are those conscious and unconscious mechanisms a client enlists to deal with a problem. Ask, "What have you done about the problem?" Coping may be effective or ineffective.

- Insight and motivation for change. Insight refers to the client's own understanding about the problem. Motivation refers to the client's willingness to participate in therapy and to cope differently. Questions such as, "What can be done about your problem?" Or, "Who will have to change?" will assist in evaluating these aspects.

Personality Development

Life-cycle history and current stresses associated with present developmental stage

Past Experience with Mental Illness

(prior hospitalization, counseling)

Figure 2–2. (Continued)

Assessing Suicide

- Does the client have a plan?
- How specific is the plan?
- How lethal is the method?
- Is the method available?

Violence Potential

- History of frequent arrests, fights, or assaults
- History of impulsive behavior
- History of reckless disregard for others or self

Sociological Aspects

- Marital status
- Current living arrangements
- Family members, along with history of family illnesses and chemical dependence
- Community support systems and relationships
- Occupational history
- Educational history (highest degree attained, problems at school, problems with learning)
- Spiritual and/or religious affiliations (include spiritual or religious factors that may influence treatment)
- Sexual orientation and reproductive history (children, pregnancies, sexual difficulties, AIDS risk)
- Coping style of the family
- Culture (include cultural practices that should be observed during treatment)
- Spiritual

Strengths

- Methods of successful coping during previous difficulty

Figure 2–2. (Continued)

may be unable to tolerate a lengthy initial session, and the nurse may need to see them more than once. Young clients require care in the wording of questions and may need specialized assessments that include more nonverbal interaction. The nurse may need to see clients with attention disorders or confusion more than once before the "initial" contact is concluded. The level of the client's wellness, the availability of family members, and the nurse's own ability to establish rapport influence the success of the initial interview.

Identifying Information

The assessment begins with the collection of identifying information, not only to provide needed data about the client but also to allow the nurse to begin testing the client's orientation, memory, level of consciousness, and self-esteem. See Figure 2–2 for an example of identifying information.

Performing the Physical Assessment

The client frequently receives a complete physical as part of the intake process, regardless of setting. If a physical is not routinely part of the treatment setting, the nurse is responsible for conducting a physical assessment appropriate to the circumstances. The focus of the physical examination should be to isolate any physical factors that influence the current clinical picture and to identify physical problems that should be addressed.

Assessing physical well-being is important because mental illness affects physiological processes, such as sleep, appetite, and energy level. Clients who are suffering psychiatric problems complain of a variety of physical complaints that need to be dealt with during therapy. Some physical illnesses that overlap with psychiatric illnesses include peptic ulcers, certain dermatologic disorders, and asthma. Recording these problems and assessing their acuity provide for continuity of care.

Then again, physical illness influences one's mental well-being. Consider a client who has chronic pain and is depressed as a result. Some types of physical problems assume priority and need to be dealt with first, for example, lithium toxicity resulting from an acute episode of diarrhea.

Most people are more comfortable discussing their physical problems than their mental illness. Assessment of the client's physiological well-being is a tangible way of conveying concern and caring, provides a time span during which rapport and bonding occur, and facilitates the assessment of the psychosocial aspects. See Figure 2–2 for specifics.

Asking for the Problem Statement

The "problem" is the client's statement of the reason for admission. Document it in the client's own words. The problem is defined by determining the following:

- Onset. Simply ask, "When did this problem begin?"
- Duration. Ask, "How long have you been bothered by this problem?"
- Precipitating event. Ask, "What happened during the past few days that made you decide to seek treatment?"
- Coping mechanisms. Ask, "What have you done about the problem?" Coping may be effective or ineffective.
- **Insight.** Those who are willing to take responsibility for the problem generally have more insight than those who blame others or rationalize their problem.
- Motivation. Questions such as "What can be done about your problem?" or "Who will have to change?" assist in evaluating the client's willingness to participate in therapy and to cope differently.
- Functioning. It is also helpful to talk with the client about life stress and pressures, which are often related to current problems. Many practitioners collect a developmental history and track the client's behavior throughout the life span as a way of identifying problems and premorbid functioning.

Determining Life Cycle Developments

An individual passes through phases of the life cycle beginning with prenatal development and ending with death. Each phase opens new horizons, provides new areas to explore, requires developmental task mastery, and demands acquisition of new skills and abilities. This phasic nature of the life cycle is based on the individual's maturation, cognitive development, expectations set by society, and roles modeled by the family.

Often, clients do not accomplish even the most basic tasks of psychosocial development (such as the development of trust). Conflicts and pressures of previous unmet developmental stages spill over into the present and make attainment of new development requirements difficult. Whether or not a developmental history is taken, explore the stress and pressures associated with the client's current developmental stage and success with task attainment.

Performing the MSE

During the interview with the client, the nurse simultaneously applies the MSE (Figure 2–3), which is an assessment of the way the mind is working. A complete MSE provides opportunities for observation of the client's response to a variety of simple tests of cognitive functioning. Responses provide a comprehensive baseline for initial assessment, and continued monitoring of areas of dysfunction becomes a measure of progress and an indicator of prognosis. Nurses should be familiar with the components of the MSE and may routinely administer it in their setting. Many facilities use the Mini–Mental State Examination (MMSE) developed by Folstein for a short but complete assessment (Figure 2–4).

Melrose-Wakefield Hospital
Admission Assessment for Psychiatric Services

Patient: LEE M.   INTAKE: 11/09/96
Dr. WATSON

Room #: O.P.C.

Current Mental Status Evaluation:

APPEARANCE: Well Groomed___ Disheveled ✓ Bizarre___ Inappropriate___ Poor Hygiene ✓
Comments: DIRTY FINGERNAILS, HAIR

ATTITUDE: Cooperative ✓ Guarded___ Suspicious___ Uncooperative___ Belligerent___ Confused___
Hostile___ Defensive___ Attentive___ Seductive___ Entitled___ Apathetic ✓
Comments: _____

MOTOR ACTIVITY: Calm ✓ Agitated___ Hyperactive___ Hypomotoric___ Tremors/Tics___ Muscle Spasm___
Comments: _____

AFFECT: Appropriate___ Labile___ Expansive___ Constricted___ Blunted___ Flat ✓
Comments: _____

MOOD: Euthymic___ Depressed ✓ Anxious___ Euphoric___ Hostile___ Irritable___
Panicky___ Fearful___ Overwhelmed___ Angry___
Comments: _____

SPEECH: Normal___ Delayed___ Soft ✓ Loud___ Slurred___ Monotonous___ Excessive___ Pressured___
Perseverating___ Incoherent___ Hesitant ✓ Goal Directed___ Stuttering___
Comments: FREQUENT SIGHING

FACIAL EXPRESSION: Appropriate___ Staring___ Masked___ Threatening___ Distorted___ Asymmetrical___ Other___
Comments: SAD

EYE CONTACT: Direct___ Glaring___ Fixed___ Indirect___ Darting___ Avoidant ✓ Vacuous___
Comments: _____

THOUGHT PROCESS: Intact___ Circumstantial___ Loosening of Associations___ Tangential___ Blocking___
Indecisive___ Flight of Ideas___ Concrete___ Vague/Abstract ✓ Confabulation___
Perseveration___ Neologisms/Clang___ Rumination/Obsession___ Echolalia___
Comments: _____

THOUGHT CONTENT: *Hallucinations:* Not Present ✓ Present: Auditory___ Visual___ Olfactory___ Tactile___
Gustatory___ Denies___
Delusions: Not Present ✓ Present: Persecutory___ Being Controlled___ Grandiose___
Thought Insertion/Deletion___ Bizarre___ Somatic___ Denies___
Comments: _____

SUICIDAL IDEATION: Denies ✓ Vague/Passive___ With Plan___ With Impulse___ With Means to Act___
Comments: (Hx) MAY HAVE PLAN — HAS SAVED 3 MONTHS OF MEDS   NO ATTEMPTS KNOWN

HOMOCIDAL IDEATION: Denies ✓ Vague/Passive___ With Plan___ With Impulse___ With Means to Act___
Comments: (Hx) NO HISTORY

ORIENTATION: Fully Oriented ✓ Disoriented: Always___ Sometimes___ Time___ Place___ Person___
Comments: _____

MEMORY: Intact ✓ Impaired: Immediate___ Recent___ Remote___ Amnesia: Partial___ Global___
Comment: _____

COGNITIVE FUNCTION: General Knowledge Intact: Yes ✓ No___ Serial Sevens Intact: Yes___ No___
Simple Calculations Intact: Yes ✓ No___
Comments: SLOW ANSWERS — NEEDED PROMPTING

ABSTRACTION: Proverb Interpretation Intact ✓ Impaired: Concrete___ Idiosyncratic___
Comment: _____

JUDGEMENT: Intact ✓ Impaired: Minimal___ Moderate___ Severe___
Comment: _____

INSIGHT: Intact___ Impaired: Minimal___ Moderate ✓ Severe___
Comment: DENIES ILLNESS

Psychiatric Nursing Assessment Completed by: J. M. Lenning   Date: 11/9/96   Time: 2:25 p.m.

Figure 2–3. A sample MSE. (Courtesy of Melrose-Wakefield Hospital, Melrose, MA.)

Instructions for Administration of Mini–Mental State Exam

Orientation

1. Ask for the date. Then ask specifically for part omitted, e.g., "Can you also tell me what season it is?" One point for each correct.
2. Ask in turn, "Can you tell me the name of this hospital?" (town, county, etc.). One point for each correct.

Registration

Ask the patient if you may test his memory. Then say the names of 3 unrelated objects, clearly and slowly, about 1 second for each. After you have said all 3, ask him to repeat them. This first repetition determines his score (0–3) but keep saying them until he can repeat all 3, up to 6 trials. If he does not eventually learn all 3, recall cannot be meaningfully tested.

Attention and Calculation

Ask the patient to begin with 100 and count backwards by 7. Stop after 5 subtractions (93, 86, 79, 72, 65). Score the total number of correct answers.

If the patient cannot or will not perform this task, ask him to spell the word "world" backwards. The score is the number of letters in correct order, e.g., dlrow=5, dlorw=3.

Recall

Ask the patient if he can recall the 3 words you previously asked him to remember. Score 0–3.

Language

Naming: Show the patient a wrist watch and ask him what it is. Repeat for pencil. Score 0–2.

Repetition: Ask the patient to repeat the sentence after you. Allow only one trial. Score 0 or 1.

3-Stage command: Give the patient a piece of plain blank paper and repeat the command. Score 1 point for each part correctly executed.

Reading: On a blank piece of paper print the sentence "Close your eyes," in letters large enough for the patient to see clearly. Ask him to read it and do what it says. Score 1 point only if he actually closes his eyes.

Writing: Give the patient a blank piece of paper and ask him to write a sentence for you. Do not dictate a sentence; it is to be written spontaneously. It must contain a subject and verb and be sensible. Correct grammar and punctuation are not necessary.

Coding: On a clean piece of paper, draw intersecting pentagons, each side about 1 in., and ask him to copy it exactly as it is. All 10 angles must be present and 2 must intersect to score 1 point. Tremor and rotation are ignored.

Estimate the patient's level of sensorium along a continuum, from alert on the left to coma on the right.

Figure 2–4. Mini–Mental State Examination (MMSE). (Reprinted with permission from Folstein, MF, Folstein, SE, McHugh, PR: Mini mental state exam: A practical method for grading the cognitive state of patients for the clinician. J Psychiatr Res 12:189–198, 1975.)

Maximum Score	Score	
		Orientation
5	( )	What is the (year) (season) (date) (day) (month)?
5	( )	Where are we (state) (county) (town) (hospital) (floor)?
		Registration (Memory)
3	( )	Name three objects: Give 1 second to say each. Then ask the client to repeat all three after you have said them. Give 1 point for each correct answer. Then repeat them until the client learns all three. Count trials and record.
		Attention and Calculation
5	( )	Serial sevens. Give 1 point for each correct. Stop after five answers. Alternately spell "world" backwards.
		Recall
3	( )	Ask for three objects repeated above. Give 1 point for each correct.

Maximum Score	Score	
		Language
9	( )	Name a pencil and watch when pointed to. (2 points) Repeat the following: "No ifs, ands, or buts." (1 point) Follow a three-stage command: "Take a paper in your right hand, fold it in half, and put it on the floor." (3 points) Read and obey the following: "Close your eyes." (1 point) Write a sentence. (1 point) Copy design. (1 point)

Total Score _____

The maximum score is 30 points; a score below 24 probably indicates clinically significant cognitive impairment.

Figure 2–4. (Continued)

Others have developed their own short version of an MSE. Box 2–1 outlines the components of the MSE.

Appearance, Behavior, and Attitude. Appearance describes the physical characteristics of the client. The following areas are observed and noted, if significant:
- Apparent age
- Cleanliness (hygiene)
- Appropriateness and manner of dress (appropriate for season, setting, age; indicative of financial hardship)
- Eye contact
- Posture

Box 2-1. Components of the MSE

- Appearance, behavior, and attitude
- Attention
- Orientation
- Language function and characteristics of speech
- General intellectual evaluation and memory
- Cortical and cognitive functions
- Mood and affect—emotional state
- Thought content—preoccupations and experiences
- Insight

- Gait and use of any aids
- Facial expression

Table 2–1 contains examples of subtle cultural differences that may influence this often subjective aspect of the MSE.

Attention. Attention is the ability to focus and concentrate. Identify attention problems early, because difficulties in this area may affect the rest of the examination. Attention disorders may stem from psychiatric conditions such as anxiety, depression, or the intrusion of unwanted thoughts. Organic deterioration, as seen in senile dementia, in brain damage, or as a result of toxic conditions such as lead poisoning or metabolic disorders, may affect attention. Children and some adults may be inattentive and easily distracted because of attention deficit hyperactivity disorder. Notice whether the client seems to hear your questions. Does the client have difficulty answering? Is the client preoccupied with other thoughts? Is the client able to spell the words *heart* or *watch* backwards?

Children's attention may be tested by microcomputers that present the client with a series of precisely timed tests requiring that the child attend and respond. Testing continues until the client fails or a satisfactory level of attention has been demonstrated. Such automated testing has the advantage of administering and assessing the test results in precisely the same manner each time and is very useful when used periodically to chart progress.

Orientation. Orientation refers to the client's awareness of person, place, and time. If clients correctly identify all three and understand the circumstances surrounding the need for treatment, they are oriented "times 4." Clients who do not know answers to time and date questions should be pressed to guess or estimate. The response under pressure should be noted.

Language Function and Characteristics of Speech. Language function includes both written and spoken language. Speech is easily assessed and usually evaluated before writing. Clients who speak a different language may exhibit difficulties that are not related to a psychiatric condition. Similarly, clients with a history of stroke or brain damage may exhibit speech difficulties. An initial assessment of speech is usually obtained early in the interview as the client responds to the first questions. Speech is evaluated as follows:

- Volume (loud or soft)
- Presence of accent
- Hesitancy, stuttering, stammering
- Fluency, rate, quantity. *Fluency* is the flow of speech, with pauses and breaks. *Rate* refers to slow, fast, or normal. Rate may fluctuate with topic of discussion, which should be noted. Quantity, or amount of verbiage, may also vary with content.
- Coherence. Note any tendency to illogical thinking, vagueness, or loose associations (jumping from topic to topic). Incoherent speech may be characterized by quickly straying from the topic to unrelated material or may be as extreme as to consist only of a word salad of unrelated or invented words (*neologisms*.) Table 2–2 lists a variety of thought processes and speech dysfunctions.
- Naming and word finding. The ability to correctly name articles can be tested by pointing to objects and asking the client to supply the name of each item. The following categories are available in most settings and can be used:
  ○ Body parts: eye, leg, arm, hand, fingernail, ear
  ○ Clothing: shirt, shoe, sock, earring, belt
  ○ Objects: pen, pencil, chair, coin, lamp
  ○ Parts of objects: watchband, pencil eraser, light bulb

The client with no impairment should correctly identify all items. Any difficulty is worthy of further exploration. To

TABLE 2–1. Critical Questions to Identify Cultural and Common Biases

Even subtle value differences between the nurse and the client can influence the nurse's judgment of the client's presentation. The nurse is responsible for identifying any potential biases and minimizing the impact of cultural bias on assessments. The following questions are designed to raise awareness of areas of potential bias:

- If the client is illiterate (as an estimated 20–30 million American adults are), will the assessments used measure the client's mental state without bias?
- Different cultures accept differing amounts of "personal space" between conversants. Is this client shrinking from contact? Is another client "aggressive" in taking the nurse's space?
- Not all cultures are accepting of direct eye contact. Is the client evasive? Is he or she "boldly staring" at the nurse?
- Hygiene standards may differ between the nurse and the client. Should "poor hygiene" be regarded in this instance as an indication of psychosis or depression?
- Is the dress or speech of the client appropriate for his or her culture, age group, socioeconomic level, or lifestyle? Is the client "flamboyant," "bizarre," or "verbally abusive"?

Some common prejudices and biases have been identified:

- **Ageism:** Belief that a person of one age is superior to another.
- **Ethnocentrism:** Belief that one's own culture is superior to others.
- **Heterosexism:** Belief that everyone should be of a heterosexual orientation and that heterosexual behavior is best, normal, and superior to all others. May be accompanied by homophobia.
- **Homophobia:** Morbid fear of those who support a homosexual lifestyle, often characterized by fear of inadvertent contact, ridicule, and derision.
- **Racism:** Belief that one race is superior to another.
- **Sexism:** Belief that members of one sex are superior to the other.
- **Xenophobia:** A morbid fear of strangers and those who are not a member of one's own ethnic group.

TABLE 2–2. Thought-Process Descriptions and Speech Dysfunctions

- **Circumstantial:** Thought and speech are excessive and include unnecessary detail that is usually irrelevant to answering a question.
- **Flight of ideas:** Overproductive speech characterized by rapid shifting from one topic to another. Includes fragmented ideas. May include punning, rhyming, clang associations (based on similar sounds), and may demonstrate distractibility as well.
- **Loose associations:** Lack of a logical relationship between thoughts and ideas. Renders speech and thought inexact, vague, and unfocused.
- **Mutism:** Valid assessment only when no response is given even though the client appears alert and aware of the environment.
- **Neologisms:** New words or words created by the client. Words may be a blend of other words.
- **Perseveration:** Repetition of sounds, words, or phrases, despite efforts to create a new response. Not the same as stammering or stuttering. May be observed with motor activity as well. Can be tested with actions by asking the client to alternately turn palm up and then palm down. After several repetitions, the pattern is changed to palm up, palm down, make a fist, and repeat. Client is unable to repeat new pattern.
- **Tangential:** Similar to circumstantial but the person never returns to the central point and never answers the original question.
- **Thought blocking:** Sudden stoppage in train of thought or in the midst of a sentence.
- **Word salad:** Series of words that seem totally unrelated.

mask inability, the client may launch into an elaborate description of how the object is used or a visual description of the item: "It is round, clear, it seems to be a cover of some kind. It might be made of glass. . . ." The client is describing a watch crystal, although he or she is unable to recall the correct name of the item.

General Intellectual Evaluation and Memory. Typically, three general types of memory are tested:

- *Short-term memory* means recall after only a few minutes. To test for this, cover your name pin and ask the client to state your name.
- *General recall* is the ability to retain and recall the information needed to conduct one's daily life, such as the location of one's eyeglasses or medications. The client's ability to discuss precipitating events is a good indicator of general recall.
- *Long-term memory* is the ability to recall with accuracy over days, months, or years. Questions, which should be independently verifiable from family or medical records, may include "Where did you grow up?" or "How many children do you have?" Recognize that some clients, particularly those with memory problems, may fabricate responses to cover memory lapses; this is called **confabulation**.

Cortical and Cognitive Functions. Cortical and cognitive functions, also referred to as higher functions, are evaluated and include the following:

- Assessment of the general fund of knowledge, which is the facts and information a client commands. Educational background, culture, and age are closely related to it. The nurse assesses fund of knowledge by listening to the content of the client's talking, by noticing vocabulary, and by exploring educational background. The client's need for teaching and the method the nurse will use for instruction are based on this element of mental status.
- Calculation ability. The client's ability to perform mathematical operations also gives an assessment of cortical functioning. Use "serial 7s," asking the client to subtract 7 from 100; 7 from 93; and so forth, to evaluate **cognition**.
- Concept formation. The nurse evaluates the client's ability to think in concepts, or to conceptualize. Mental illness often affects this ability, and the client responds literally. Knowing this alerts the nurse to respond to the client at that level, be specific, and avoid generalizations.
- Judgment. The client's ability to understand a situation and to react to it logically is judgment. It can be assessed by listening to the client's reports of past and present coping and can be directly tested by asking the client to describe what he or she would do, for example, after discovering a stamped, addressed envelope on the street. Knowing about a client's ability to use good judgment directs the nurse in establishing realistic goals and plans.
- Evaluation of the sequencing of normal activities such as dressing and grooming. Clients with sequencing difficulties may forget to remove their clothing before showering or be unable to perform a simple sequence such as removing the pen cap before attempting to write. Sequencing information is often not obtained in the formal MSE but may be available through observations obtained by nurses in inpatient settings or during other parts of the initial interview.

Mood and Affect—Emotional State. Mood refers to emotions and feelings generally related to the emotions. **Affect** is the term used to characterize behaviors that convey a mood or an emotion. Affect may be described as heightened, **flat, inappropriate,** restricted, bland, **blunted, euphoric, dysphoric,** or bright (see glossary for definitions). A rapid change in emotions is called **lability**. It is important to compare the exhibited affect with the circumstances and to judge whether it is appropriate. The nurse's ability to empathize will help determine the appropriateness of a client's feelings to the situation.

Thought Content—Preoccupations and Experiences. Thought content is what the client seems to want to talk about the most. It should be organized and coherent. By asking questions, the nurse provides an opportunity for the client to reveal impaired thought. Questions are most effective if they cannot be answered with a simple "yes" or "no." For example, say, "Tell me about what has been happening in your life the past few days." Insight is the ability to understand one's own character and the inner meaning of one's behavior.

Specific questions may establish the existence of preoccupations and unusual experiences: "Do you hear or see things that others do not see or hear?" In other cases, unusual thought content such as **delusions, hallucinations, obsessions,** and **phobias** may be blatantly expressed. Table 2–3 lists descriptions of common impairments to thought patterns and open-ended questions that may be used to elicit such information.

Noting Medication Side Effects

Clients with previous histories of mental illness may be receiving medication such as neuroleptics or antipsychotics. These medications, such as dopamine, affect neurotransmitters, improve thought processes, and potentially cause numerous side effects. Nurses need to be able to recognize the symptoms of untoward reactions to antipsychotics and should watch for and document them during the assessment. The prevalence of these behaviors and movements in chronic psychiatric populations may even mistakenly be assumed to be part of the psychotic syndrome being observed. Because many clients come into psychiatric treatment because of medication problems, medication compliance and follow-up are major activities of the community-based psychiatric nurse (see Chapter 6).

Assessing Suicidal Potential

In the general population, an average of 12 per 100,000 individuals commit suicide. In the psychiatric population, the incidence can be as high as 370 per 100,000 with as many as 6% occurring in the psychiatric inpatient setting.[2] These figures underscore the importance of assessing suicidal potential and of periodic reassessment during treatment. In the general population, the average suicide victim is an elderly, depressed man with access to firearms. Recent studies[2] reveal that in psychiatric settings, hanging is the most common method, and the age of the victim is between

TABLE 2–3. Impaired Thought Patterns

- **Compulsion:** Repetitive act performed through some inner drive that produces anxiety if not indulged. Common acts are hand washing, touching of specific objects, and ritualistically performing common tasks in a specific and unvarying order, such as dressing.
- **Delusion:** Client may describe persistent untrue beliefs unsupported by social reality.
- **Delusion of alien control:** Belief that one's feelings, thoughts, or behaviors are being directed by others. Suggested questions: Have you ever felt that your feelings or thoughts were controlled by others? Have you ever done anything against your will?
- **Delusion of grandeur:** Belief that one possesses great strength, unreal wealth, unusual powers, sexual potency, or even that one is a deity. Suggested questions: Do you have any unusual powers or godlike qualities? Are you physically stronger than most people?
- **Delusion of a paranoid nature:** Excessive or irrational suspiciousness and distrustfulness of others, characterized by belief that others are "out to get them" or are spying on them. Suggested questions: Are others watching you? Are you the subject of surveillance?
- **Delusion of reference or persecution:** Belief that one is the subject of scrutiny or undue attention. Suggested questions: Do you ever feel that people are watching you? Do you often feel you are the center of attention?
- **Delusion of thought broadcasting:** Belief that thoughts are being aired to the outside world (others hear the client's thoughts). Suggested questions: Can others hear your thoughts?
- **Delusion of thought insertion:** Belief that thoughts are being placed in one's mind. Suggested questions: Has anyone ever placed thoughts in your mind?
- **Hallucination:** False sensation such as seeing objects or people that no one else can see, hearing voices, smelling unusual odors, or experiencing the sensation of being touched. Hallucinations can involve any of the five senses. Clients may express depersonalization, such as being changed or feeling unreal.
- **Hypochondriasis:** Somatic overconcern with and morbid attention to details of body functioning.
- **Magical thinking:** Belief that thinking or wishing equates with doing. Often accompanied by an unrealistic association between cause and effect.
- **Nihilistic delusion:** Belief that nothing exists, that everything is lost, or that body parts are missing. Suggested questions: Have you ever experienced the feeling that everything is gone and no longer exists? Have you ever felt part of your body is missing?
- **Obsession:** Persistent thought often regarded by the client as absurd and meaningless, but which cannot be ignored.
- **Phobia:** Unreasonable fear of common situations or objects. Phobias may be expressed for flying, open spaces, heights, closed spaces, crowds, or subways. Fear is unreasonable if it prevents one from completing tasks or attending appointments, or significantly interferes with conducting normal activities of daily living.
- **Somatic delusion:** Unfounded belief that one has cancer or other disfiguring, terminal disease. Suggested questions: Do you have any illnesses that your doctor doesn't recognize or believe?

> **RESEARCH NOTE**
>
> Dawes, SS, et al: Center for Technology in Government (1995) Supporting Psychiatric Assessment in Emergency Rooms. Available at www.ctg.albany.edu/projects/projmain.htm
>
> **Findings:** In 1995, the Center for Technology in Government sponsored a research project to identify a model for conducting psychiatric assessments in emergency rooms (ER). They sought to develop a decision model that identified key indicators influencing the decision to hospitalize an ER client. Their second objective was to characterize the decision process through the development of software that would present the decision process in question form and present a usable score.
>
> The decision model identified the following 10 key indicators that provide the most important information for a psychiatric assessment:
> - Danger to self
> - Danger to others
> - Mental health status
> - Functional impairment
> - Substance abuse
> - Environmental factors
> - Client and family preferences
> - Availability of services
> - Medical conditions
> - Potential to benefit from treatment
>
> One item of interest in this research is the use of an expert panel of practitioners, consumers of emergency psychiatric services, families of consumers, and officers of the American Association of Emergency Psychiatry. In the process of achieving consensus, the group identified specific factors in each area of the psychiatric assessment that were considered "essential."
>
> The prototype system was developed in Microsoft's Windows environment, written in MS Visual Basic, with questions that develop descriptive profiles for a client in each of the ten categories listed previously. Seventy-three questions are available, although the program's branching may not result in all questions needing to be answered. The prototype is also able to accommodate situations in which only partial information is available. It is designed to be used by ER personnel either during or after the interview.
>
> The prototype was field tested at Westchester Medical Center, Valhalla, NY. Although practitioners felt the full set of questions was too long and complex to be routinely administered in an ER setting, they agreed that the target areas were valid and that the scoring was especially useful in identifying disparities between the clinician's "gut reactions" and the scores. Such disparity prompted the clinicians to explore the reasons for the difference and to seek further information or a consultation from a colleague. The highly structured interview process was seen to be a valuable training tool. Further information on this research can be found through the Internet server at the Center for Technology in Government.
>
> **Application to Practice:** An inappropriate decision to admit or discharge a psychiatric client from the ER setting can result in serious consequences. An individual who is inappropriately admitted is involved in a serious, disruptive, often stigmatizing event, and is deprived of liberty. An average length of stay of 17 days incurs a cost of $10,000, and if inappropriate, is a misuse of resources. The inappropriate admission of a client may deprive a truly needy client of access to that hospital bed. If a client who should be admitted is not admitted, they may engage in inappropriate or violent behavior and will not receive the care they need. Psychiatric nurses play an important role in helping to assess acutely ill individuals in the ER and in the community. This research assists nurses to better evaluate clients and make appropriate decisions about the need for treatment.

30 and 50 years. A higher proportion of inpatient suicides are women. Symptomatology should always have priority over demographic information for assessing suicidal clients.

Several factors predispose a client to suicide: biological predisposition, cultural beliefs, family history, environment exposure, and situational stressors.[1] Ambivalence is a key element. **Ambivalence** is the experience of having opposing feelings or behaviors about a situation and is accompanied by indecision. It increases the importance of initial and ongoing assessment because clients may move between suicidal and nonsuicidal states.

Clients usually give clues that they are suicidal to their family, friends, or to the examining nurse. These clues are indicative of *suicidal ideation*.
- The client may offer verbal clues such as "I wish I could go to sleep and never wake up," or "I wish I were dead."
- The client may plan a suicidal act, such as saving pills, purchasing a handgun, concocting a poison to drink, giving possessions away, or disposing of treasured items.
- The client might exhibit a change in affect. Clients who were formerly depressed may paradoxically appear calmer and happier after making the decision to end their lives.
- The client might make small, superficial attempts, such as reckless action with disregard for safety (speeding tickets), frequent nicks with a razor, or combining drugs and drinking.

If suicidal ideation is present, the nurse determines if the client has a definite *plan*. Suicide plans should be evaluated in terms of their specificity (time, place, and means), the availability of the means described (drugs, guns), and the lethality of the measures described. The most lethal measures are gunshot and hanging. See Table 2–4 for questions to consider regarding suicidal risk.

TABLE 2–4. Questions to Consider Regarding Potentially Suicidal Clients

- Does the client threaten to commit suicide?
- Does the client describe a plan for committing suicide?
- How realistic is the plan? Are the means available to the client?
- Is there a time frame for the suicide? Is it near?
- Has the client attempted suicide in the past? How serious was the attempt? Does the current plan include any elements of the previous attempt?

Clients are most at risk of suicide at two times: when they are moving into a psychiatric illness and when they approach wellness. At both of these points, the client has the energy to carry out suicidal plans together with the ability to cognitively execute a plan. External stressors such as financial or job changes, divorce, and family problems may trigger a resurgence of symptoms at other times during treatment.

Assessing Violence Potential

To assess violence potential, ask, "Is this client a danger to others?" Be sure to ascertain the interventions needed and to protect others, both inside and outside the treatment facility.

The incidence of violence among the mentally ill is the same as that in the general population. Ask and listen carefully to the client's answers to identify whether a client is at risk for violence toward others. Those who report their anger, hallucinations, and delusions in a highly agitated manner may be likely to harm others as a result of the specific pathology.

Another way to assess violence is to ask the client's family. They can supply relevant data about the client, based on their unique understanding. See Table 2–5 for specific questions.

Assessing Family and Sociological Aspects

Because health is influenced by the interaction between the client, family, and environment, an assessment of sociological variables should be made. Determine whether the family

TABLE 2–5. Questions to Consider Regarding Potentially Violent Clients

- Does the client threaten to harm? Is it physical harm, harm to property, or psychological harm?
- Does the client threaten serious harm such as murder or assault?
- How likely is it that the harmful act will occur? Is the client capable of carrying out this threat?
- Is there a time frame for the act? Is it near?
- Has the client engaged in violent behavior in the past? Does the threatened violence repeat any of those elements (i.e., same harm, same target)?

functions effectively as a support system for the client. Interaction among family members is reciprocal. When any member is in distress, others are affected, and family therapy may be needed. The family is also an important aspect of aftercare that may need teaching, support, and encouragement.

Assess the client's ability to function in the major family roles, such as parent, breadwinner, sibling, spouse, manager, and so forth. Mental illness often prevents the client from functioning.

Healthy individuals and families who participate in their community achieve support and social rewards that can affect mental health. The assessment of community support systems includes those to which the client turns when help is needed, as well as the availability of agencies and support groups.

A family's ability to problem solve is an insight into its strengths. Some families have few resources for dealing with crises and are prone to periods of intense disruption. An assessment of strengths helps the nurse predict the family's ability to overcome adversity. Examples of strengths include health, financial security, education, and ability to communicate support, caring, and respect.

Work history, income, and success or failure are related both to self-esteem and to relationship needs. The nurse assesses what the client thinks about his or her job, relationship with superiors, and job-related pressures.

Some **cultures** experience a much higher incidence of certain disorders than others. Words and behaviors of clients that are understood in their culture may be misinterpreted as psychotic when judged out of context. Specific syndromes that occur within certain groups have been identified. Table 2–6 gives examples of culture-bound syndromes as described in the appendix of the *Diagnostic and Statistical Manual of Mental Disorders (DSM-IV)*.[3]

Assess the client's spiritual needs. The spiritual dimension of a person's life is that part that adds a zest for living, an enjoyment of the beauty in the world, a philosophy of life, an understanding of one's own purpose, and the ability to lead an enriched existence. Ask the following questions for assessing the spiritual domain:

- "What kinds of things add meaning to your life?"
- "What do you see as your life's purpose?"
- "What do you enjoy doing?"
- "What is your religion?"
- "What religious practices of yours should I respect as your nurse?"

Determining Strengths

Discovering client talents, strengths, and assets promotes his or her self-esteem and helps the nurse formulate goals and plans with the client. Ask clients for a list of their strengths. If they are unable to list any, ask them to describe how they have handled difficult situations in the past. No matter how handicapped a client may be, there are always abilities that can be emphasized.

TABLE 2–6. Examples of Culture-bound Syndromes

Anorexia, bulimia

North Americans

Bizarre eating patterns, distorted body image, and severe caloric restriction illustrate anorexia, a disorder almost exclusively seen in females. Bulimia can include food binging and purging.

Ataque de nervios

North and South Americans, particularly Latin Americans, and Latin Mediterraneans

Symptoms include uncontrollable shouting, attacks of crying, trembling, heat rising into the head, and verbal or physical aggression. Frequently occurs as a result of a stressful family event (death of a relative, divorce from a spouse, or witnessing an accident involving a family member). Amnesia may occur during the attack; otherwise functioning rapidly returns. Distinguished from *DSM-IV* panic disorder by the precipitating event and the lack of hallmark symptoms of fear or apprehension.

Bilis and colera (also referred to as *muina*)

Latin Americans

Strongly experienced anger or rage that disturbs core body balances. Symptoms may include acute nervous tension, headache, trembling, screaming, stomach disturbances, and in severe cases, loss of consciousness.

Falling out, blacking out

African-Americans, Bahamians, and Haitians throughout North America

Characterized by sudden collapse, often preceded by feelings of dizziness or "swimming" in the head. Loss of voluntary movement and vision, although hearing is unaffected.

General somatic syndromes: brain fag, nervios, shenjing shuairuo (China), shin-byung (Korea)

Asians, Africans (brain fag), Latin Americans, and Latin Mediterraneans (nervios)

All are characterized by low mental and physical energy, poor sleep, and vague somatic complaints such as headaches and other pains. Shenjing shuairuo may include irritability and excitability, as well as sexual dysfunction. Shin-byung may include spirit possession. Brain fag is characterized by difficulties in concentrating, remembering, and thinking, and may be described as fatigue from "too much thinking." Brain fag was initially used to describe a condition experienced by high school or university students responding to the challenge of schooling. Nervios (called *nevra* among the Greeks) includes a range of symptoms including headache, "brain aches," irritability, stomach upsets, and dizziness, in addition to the other symptoms mentioned previously.

Ghost sickness

Native American

Includes a preoccupation with death and the deceased and is sometimes associated with witchcraft. Symptoms include bad dreams, weakness, generalized fear, loss of appetite, fainting, dizziness, hallucinations, loss of consciousness, and a sensation of suffocation.

Mal de ojo

Mediterranean and Spanish cultures

Translates as "evil eye." Children are usually victims, and symptoms include fitful sleep, crying, diarrhea, vomiting, and fever. Women may also have the condition.

Pibloktoq, chakore, grisi siknis, or frenzy witchcraft

Arctic natives, Ngawbere tribe of Panama, Miskito tribe of Nicaragua, and Navajos

An initial lethargy, depression, anxiety, followed by a brief (30-minute) episode of agitation, violence, purposeless running, and other irrational or dangerous acts. This is followed by exhaustion, sleep, or coma for up to 12 hours, and then amnesia for the incident.

Spirit possession

Asians and Africans

Brief, reversible episodes of dissociation with client behaving as though possessed by a spirit or deity, followed by amnesia for episode.

Susto ("fright" or "soul loss")

Latin Americans

Also referred to as *espanto, pasmo, tripa ida, perdida del alma,* or *chibih*. An illness attributed to a frightening event that causes the soul to leave the body. May appear days to years after the fright is experienced. Symptoms include appetite disturbance, sleep disorder, bad dreams, feelings of sadness, and lack of motivation. Somatic complaints such as headaches, muscle aches, stomachache, and diarrhea may occur.

Witchcraft, rootwork, or voodoo

Southern African-Americans and Caribbean societies (rootwork) and Latinos (mal puestro or brujeria)

A set of cultural interpretations that ascribe illness to hexing, witchcraft, sorcery, or the evil influence of another person. Symptoms may include generalized anxiety and gastrointestinal complaints (nausea, vomiting, diarrhea), weakness, dizziness, fear of being poisoned, and sometime fear of being killed. "Roots," "spells," or "hexes" can be "put" on other persons, causing the problems.

See Appendix I of the *DSM-IV* for more information.

Source: Adapted from the Diagnostic and Statistical Manual of Mental Disorders, Fourth Edition. Copyright 1994 American Psychiatric Association.

TABLE 2–7. NANDA Nursing Diagnoses through 12th NANDA Conference

NANDA DIAGNOSES, 1995–1996	
Activity Intolerance	Incontinence, functional
Activity Intolerance, risk for	Incontinence, reflex
Adaptive Capacity: intracranial, decreased	Incontinence, stress
Adjustment, impaired	Incontinence, total
Airway Clearance, ineffective	Incontinence, urge
Anxiety	Infant Behavior, disorganized
Aspiration, risk for	Infant Behavior, disorganized, risk for
Body Image Disturbance	Infant Behavior, organized, potential for enhanced
Body Temperature, altered, risk for	Infant Feeding Pattern, ineffective
Bowel Incontinence	Infection, risk for
Breastfeeding, effective	Injury, risk for
Breastfeeding, ineffective	Knowledge Deficit (specify)
Breastfeeding, interrupted	Loneliness, risk for
Breathing Pattern, ineffective	Memory, impaired
Cardiac Output, decreased	Noncompliance (specify)
Caregiver Role Strain	Nutrition: altered, less than body requirements
Caregiver Role Strain, risk for	Nutrition: altered, more than body requirements
Communication, impaired verbal	Nutrition: altered, risk for more than body requirements
Community Coping, potential for enhanced	Oral Mucous Membrane, altered
Community Coping, ineffective	Pain
Confusion, acute	Pain, chronic
Confusion, chronic	Parental Role Conflict
Constipation	Parent/Infant/Child Attachment, altered, risk for
Constipation, colonic	Parenting, altered
Constipation, perceived	Parenting, altered, risk for
Coping, defensive	Perioperative Positioning Injury, risk for
Coping, individual, ineffective	Peripheral Neurovascular Dysfunction, risk for
Decisional Conflict (specify)	Personal Identity Disturbance
Denial, ineffective	Physical Mobility, impaired
Diarrhea	Poisoning, risk for
Disuse Syndrome, risk for	Post-Trauma Response
Diversional Activity Deficit	Powerlessness
Dysreflexia	Protection, altered
Energy Field Disturbance	Rape-Trauma Syndrome
Environmental Interpretation Syndrome, impaired	Rape-Trauma Syndrome: compound reaction
Family Coping: ineffective, compromised	Rape-Trauma Syndrome: silent reaction
Family Coping: ineffective, disabling	Relocation Stress Syndrome
Family Coping: potential for growth	Role Performance, altered
Family Process, altered: alcoholism	Self Care Deficit, feeding, bathing/hygiene, dressing/grooming, toileting
Family Processes, altered	
Fatigue	Self Esteem, chronic low
Fear	Self Esteem disturbance
Fluid Volume Deficit	Self Esteem, situational low
Fluid Volume Deficit, risk for	Self-Mutilation, risk for
Fluid Volume Excess	Sensory/Perceptual Alterations (specify): visual, auditory, kinesthetic, gustatory, tactile, olfactory
Gas Exchange, impaired	
Grieving, anticipatory	Sexual Dysfunction
Grieving, dysfunctional	Sexuality Patterns, altered
Growth and Development, altered	Skin Integrity, impaired
Health Maintenance, altered	Skin Integrity, impaired: risk for
Health-Seeking Behaviors (specify)	Sleep Pattern Disturbance
Home Maintenance Management, impaired	Social Interaction, impaired
Hopelessness	Social Isolation
Hyperthermia	Spiritual Distress (distress of the human spirit)
Hypothermia	Spiritual Well-Being, potential for enhanced

Continued on following page

TABLE 2–7. NANDA Nursing Diagnoses through 12th NANDA Conference (Continued)

NANDA DIAGNOSES, 1995–1996	
Spontaneous Ventilation, inability to sustain	Tissue Integrity, impaired
Suffocation, risk for	Tissue Perfusion, altered (specify): cerebral, cardiopulmonary, renal, gastrointestinal, peripheral
Swallowing, impaired	
Therapeutic Regimen: community, ineffective management	Trauma, risk for
Therapeutic Regimen: families, ineffective management	Unilateral Neglect
Therapeutic Regimen: (individuals) effective management	Urinary Elimination, altered
Therapeutic Regimen (individuals) ineffective management	Urinary Retention
Thermoregulation, ineffective	Ventilatory Weaning Response, dysfunctional (DVWR)
Thought Processes, altered	Violence, risk for, directed at self/others

Source: Permission from North American Nursing Diagnosis Association (1994): NANDA Nursing Diagnoses: Definitions and Classifications 1995–1996. Philadelphia: NANDA. Copyright 1994 by the North American Nursing Diagnosis Association.

Responding to the Interview

What takes place between the nurse and the client in the interview is a crucial part of assessment. The nurse develops feelings toward the client during the interaction that may interfere with the approach if not recognized.

> A client told a nurse about the way his alcoholism contributed to the breakup of his marriage, his financial ruin, and the alienation of his two children. The nurse later told a colleague, "I feel so sorry for him." The nurse recognized her feelings and resisted the urge to notify the client's children and to ask them to visit their father. Instead, she suggested that the client contact his children and begin reconciliation. This type of intervention facilitated what the client needed most—to assume independence and assertive behavior.

Understanding the concepts of **transference** and **countertransference** allowed the nurse to take a more positive and respectful approach. Transference occurs when the client unconsciously attributes feelings and behavioral predispositions, formed toward a significant other earlier in life, to the nurse. In the example cited previously, the client could have "hooked" the nurse, as he had manipulated his own family, into becoming a "caretaker."

Countertransference occurs when the nurse develops feelings toward the client in return. In the example, although the nurse felt sorry, she recognized her feelings and avoided becoming the rescuer that the client was in the habit of finding.

AFTER THE ASSESSMENT

Following the assessment, thank the client and compliment his or her ability as a historian. Then share with the client your perception of the major problems and ask for verification. Using the list of nursing diagnoses, decide with the client where to begin work.

Making a Nursing Diagnosis

After collecting assessment data, the next step is to analyze the data and make relevant nursing diagnoses. NANDA defines a nursing diagnosis as a clinical judgment about individual, family, or community responses to actual and potential health problems and life processes. Although *DSM-IV* diagnoses guide the clinician in the treatment approach, NANDA diagnoses provide the basis for selecting nursing interventions to achieve outcomes for which the nurse is accountable[1] (Table 2–7). The nursing diagnosis changes with accumulation of new data about the client. An advantage to using nursing diagnoses is that the common language facilitates a uniform standard of care among nurses.

Testing and Evaluating beyond the Initial Assessment

Other members of the mental health team perform their own specific assessments. Nurses refer to others' assessments to

TABLE 2–8. Mental-Health Team Assessments

Psychological Testing
Those measurements that assess aspects of cognition such as intellect, personality, mood, or thought content.

Intelligence Tests. Used to diagnose mental retardation.
- **Wechsler Adult Intelligence Scale—Revised (WAIS-R):** Measures IQ.
- **Wechsler Intelligence Scale for Children (WISC):** Measures IQ of those ages 5 to 15.
- **Wechsler Preschool and Primary Scale of Intelligence (WPPSI):** Standardized for children ages 4–6½.

Personality Tests. Projective tests that allow the client to use the process of projection in interpreting and assigning meaning to stimuli.
- **Draw-A-Person:** Tests body image.

Continued on following page

understand the client. They should know about the procedures and importance of each study to provide teaching and to obtain *informed consent*. See Table 2–8 for an overview of tests. Box 2–2 lists available rating scales for further psychiatric evaluation and monitoring.

TABLE 2–8. Mental-Health Team Assessments (Continued)

- **Thematic Apperception Test (TAT):** Presents the client with pictures from which a story is constructed. Useful in determining underlying personality dynamics.
- **Rorschach:** Ten inkblots used as a basis for eliciting associations.

Neuropsychological Testing. Seeks to establish any neurological basis for responses and behaviors. Useful in establishing presence of learning disabilities and attention deficit disorders in children and adults.

Laboratory Testing

Assesses physical or biological basis of illness.

Brain Imaging Tools.

- **Positron Emission Tomography (PET) scan:** Identifies cortical and subcortical brain functions along a continuum from "cool" to "hot." Uses the principle that blood flow is increased in the more active areas of the brain to provide needed oxygen and nutrients. A blue image indicates a metabolically cool, or low-activity area; yellow to red indicates high, or hot, metabolic areas. Useful in determining presence of tumors, multiple sclerosis, strokes, trauma, Alzheimer's disease, or other illnesses.
- **Computed Tomography (CT) scan:** Uses radiation (x-ray) to create a series of computer images, or "sections," of the brain. Useful in identifying brain structures and in diagnosis and monitoring of conditions such as stroke and tumors.
- **Magnetic Resonance Imaging (MRI):** Uses radiofrequency signals to create detailed images of cerebral anatomy. Delineates white and gray matter.
- **Single Photon Emission Computed Tomography (SPECT):** Uses tracer isotopes such as xenon or iodine to visualize and measure density of neuroreceptors.
- **Electroencephalogram (EEG):** Measures electrical activity patterns of the brain by use of leads connected to surface electrodes on the scalp and nasopharyngeal area. Useful in diagnosing seizure disorders.
- **Polysomnography (Sleep EEG):** An EEG performed during sleep.
- **Brain Electrical Activity Map (BEAM):** Computerized maps of brain.

Pharmacologic Challenge Testing

Involves the administration of psychotropic substances, followed by laboratory testing. Used to provoke a measurable physiological response. Assists in understanding biobehavioral relationships observed in psychiatric nursing. Outcome measurements include behaviors such as mood or sleep patterns, neuroendocrine parameters (cortisol levels), and other physiological measures (basal temperature).

Genetic Testing

Useful in identifying inherited gene characteristics.

- **Restriction Fragment Length Polymorphisms (RELPs):** Uses restriction enzymes to cut a DNA strand at sites where the enzyme recognizes a specific coding sequence. The fragment length has been shown to be inherited, and transmitted through families.

Box 2–2. Available Psychiatric Rating Scales Used in Assessment and Monitoring

General Psychiatric
- Assessment of Coping Strategies
- Clinical Global Impression (CGI)
- Global Assessment Scale (GAS)
- National Institute of Mental Health Global Consensus Rating Scales
- Symptom Checklist-90 (SCL-90)
- Assessment of Suicidality Potentiality

Affective Disorders
- Center for Epidemiologic Studies Depression Scale (CES-D)
- Geriatric Depression Scale (GDS)
- Hamilton Depression Scale (HAM-D)
- Manic-State Scale

Anxiety Disorders
- Dissociative Experience Scale
- Hamilton Rating Scale for Anxiety (HAM-A)
- Maudsley Obsessional Compulsive Inventory
- Yale-Brown Obsessive-Compulsive Scale (Y-BOCS)

Child and Adolescent
- Behavior Problems Checklist
- Brief Psychiatric Rating Scale for Children
- Children's Global Assessment Scale (CGAS)
- Conner's Parent Rating Scale
- Yale-Brown Obsessive-Compulsive Scale (Y-BOCS-C) for Children

Eating Disorders
- Body Attitudes Test
- Diagnostic Survey for Eating Disorders (DSED)
- Eating Habits Checklist
- Eating Disorders Inventory (EDI)

Organic Mental Disorders
- Alzheimer's Disease Rating Scale (ADRS)
- Blessed Dementia Scale
- Cornell Scale for Depression in Dementia
- Memory and Behavior Problem Checklist

Psychotic Disorders
- Scale for Assessment of Negative Symptoms (SANS)
- Brief psychiatric rating scale (BPRS)
- Life Skills Profile: Schizophrenia (LSP)

Substance Use Disorders
- Addiction Severity Index (ASI)
- Brief Drug Abuse Screen Test (B-DAST)

PLANNING CARE

In psychiatric nursing, as well as in other areas of nursing, the care plan is the blueprint the nurse develops for delivering goal-oriented intervention. The plan also assists in communicating to health-care team members and provides a measure of quality assurance that the client's needs are being addressed. The plan consists of prioritized nursing diagnoses; expected **outcomes**, which are derived from the long-term and short-term goals; designated interventions; and evaluation. The plan, along with the assessment, is documented carefully[4] in the client's record (Box 2–3).

ESTABLISHING PRIORITY

After the nursing diagnoses are written, the nurse considers which one to initiate first. The nurse uses judgment, relies on knowledge of basic human needs, and consults with the client in assigning priorities.

SETTING LONG-TERM GOALS

Although long-term goals may be the result of the sustained performance of short-term goals, by definition they cannot be attained in the short term. For example, the short-term goal of selecting appropriate foods each day to meet caloric needs contributes to a long-term goal of reaching a desired weight by discharge. Furthermore, many long-term goals continue into aftercare and into long-term treatment, where other health-care team members may continue to address and monitor them.

The nurse involves the client and family in constructing the long-term goals. To build individual and family self-esteem, the nurse writes realistic and attainable goals that are specific and give direction.

SETTING SHORT-TERM GOALS

Short-term goals are those small steps toward achieving a long-term goal. They are stated as client or family behaviors; for example, the client will express anxiety as it occurs, rather than keep the feeling suppressed. Short-term goals should be realistic and achievable; measurable, observable, and behavioral; client-centered; time-limited; and established mutually with the client and family. Short-term goals serve as motivators for the client because the satisfaction of reaching a short-term goal produces a desire to continue on toward maximum functioning.

After the goals have been established, the nurse sets *outcome criteria* against which nursing interventions are evaluated. Outcomes should be attainable, measurable, and realistic. A decrease in the number of self-mutilating behaviors is a measurable outcome; a less measurable outcome is a better self-image.

DESIGNING INTERVENTIONS

After establishing goals, the nurse, client, and family begin a list of all the possible alternatives for achieving goals. The nurse's ability to design interventions is based on knowledge of the psychiatric nursing specialty and clinical expertise. However, room for creativeness is abundant.

The nurse and client designate responsible parties for each intervention; for example, "The *nurse* will instruct the client in use of the self-rating scale." However, much of the work of psychotherapy is done by the client or the family, and they should also be designated as implementors when appropriate.

IMPLEMENTATION

The implementation phase begins when the care plan is put into action. Interventions specified on the plan are tested

---

Box 2–3. The Computerized Patient Record (CPR)

The computer is now part of the data collection process and the person's medical record, regardless of setting. The use of computers for direct client care has been developing since 1990. Computerized systems have several advantages. Unlike the paper record that "anyone" can see and have access to, computerized records can limit access. For example, employees of the accounting department can only access billing information, not full-text descriptions of intimate and personal client encounters.

Computerized systems also allow nurses to quickly search relevant information, regardless of its location in the medical record. Bulky physical charts make it sometimes impossible to examine, recall, and locate information scattered throughout the record or spread among several sections. Horizontal coverage refers to the ability to view the information chronologically, from oldest to newest. Vertical coverage is the ability to view all current services such as medicine, pharmacy, physical therapy, and others. Easy identification of information promotes data collection to document outcomes of care.

These systems also can continually move the most recent client data to the "front of the chart." For example, new material can be flagged for nurses or others to examine, similar to putting information on the top of the chart. The major difference is that the computerized record can flag several new pieces, while only one sheet could be first in the old system.

Although they are not perfect, computers have great promise of changing the way psychiatric nursing care is provided, documented, and assessed. Future trends include client rating scales, where clients telephone an automated system and report their symptoms; psychopharmacology programs that automatically identify and warn nurses of drug interactions and contraindications; and videos "on-line" that show problems such as tardive dyskinesia to help identify treatment-emergent issues.

RESEARCH NOTE

Griffith, EEH, and Gonzalez, CA: Essentials of cultural psychiatry. In Hales, RE, Yudofsky, SC, Talbott, JA (eds): Textbook of Psychiatry. American Psychiatric Press, Washington, DC, 1994, pp. 1379–1404.

Findings: The International Pilot Study on Schizophrenia (IPSS) involved 1202 clients from nine countries: Columbia, Czechoslovakia, Denmark, India, Nigeria, Taiwan, the Soviet Union, Great Britain, and the United States. The study focused on symptoms and signs. **Symptoms** are the subjective descriptions by the client of pathological phenomena such as hallucinations. **Signs** are an observable manifestation of a pathological condition, observed by the nurse rather than merely reported by the patient. Examples are weeping or flattened affect. Certain symptoms reported by the clients in the study, such as hallucinations and delusions, displayed the greatest interrater reliability. In contrast, reports by the evaluators of signs such as estimates of affect were below acceptable reliability ranges. Assessment of premorbid level of functioning displayed the greatest variability when assessed by a rater whose culture differed from that of the client. This study dramatically illustrates the care that must be taken to assess clients whose cultural background differs from the caregiver's. The inter-rater reliability in cross-cultural diagnosis of the IPPS is summarized in the following table.

Application to Practice: Across the nine countries, the IPSS found the greatest similarity of symptoms among clients who were diagnosed with depression. The similar symptoms were depressed mood, gloomy thoughts, hopelessness, early-morning waking, delusions of self-depreciation, and sleep problems. Reliability between raters evaluating symptoms is unacceptable, however, when the diagnostic information becomes more subjective. Only symptoms reported by the client, such as hallucinations and delusions, could be reliably identified by those outside the culture of the client. Even external observations frequently identified as "objective," such as flatness or incongruity of affect, cannot be reliably reported between cultures.

Summary of IPSS Interrater Reliability Findings

Diagnostic Information	How Obtained	Reliability
Symptoms (e.g., hallucinations, delusions)	Client report	Acceptable
Signs (e.g., flatness of affect, incongruity of affect)	Observation	Unacceptable
Historical data (e.g., work history, social relationships)	Cross-culture exchange	Least acceptable

---

according to their success or failure in ameliorating the client's problem.

In psychiatric nursing, implementation is carried out mainly through the nurse-client relationship (see Chapter 3.) In this interpersonal interaction, the client is in need of experiences the nurse is able to provide. A basic ingredient is a firm belief in the worth and dignity of every human being and a commitment to the idea that every person has an innate capacity for self-help. Of equal importance is the nurse's understanding of the self. Implementation is the use of intellectual, interpersonal, and technical skills.

Interpersonal skills are a major tool for effecting behavioral change in the client. The nurse exerts a powerful influence on the client just by being accepting, interested, and concerned and conveying warmth, respect, and honesty.

Although the nurse's role of "doing" for the client is emphasized to a lesser degree in psychiatric nursing, many clients require assistance with bathing, eating, or toileting. Many are dependent to the degree that the nurse gives much supervision.

Individuals, families, and groups depend on the psychiatric nurse for *teaching*. The nurse may supply information, such as facts about medication, or teach by example and behavior. For instance, if a client does not trust others, the nurse teaches trust by maintaining a predictable approach and being consistently accepting.

The *leadership* role is significant during implementation. The nurse takes the initiative in establishing the nurse-client relationship, in leading groups, and in working with families.

The major role of the psychiatric nurse is *counselor*. A counselor is a facilitator who aids the client in identifying problems, reporting difficulties, expressing feelings, and finding solutions. The nurse uses communication skills in assisting the client to report events, feelings, or changes that need to be made. (Other interpersonal techniques required of a good counselor are discussed in Chapter 3.)

EVALUATION

The outcome of activities identified in the planning phase is assessed during evaluation. Evaluation begins and ends with the client's goals and consists of comparing new data collected about the client's progress and treatment response with the goals. If goals were not attained, the nurse asks, "Why not?" (Box 2–4).

Box 2–4. Evaluating Goals

- Was the nursing diagnosis correct?
- Were the goals realistic?
- Was the intervention appropriate and successful?
- Were the expected outcomes attained?
- Have new problems emerged?
- What else should be done?

Evaluation results in reassessment, replanning, trying out different solutions, and reevaluation. It is a cycle that continues for the length of the nurse's contact with the client.

Because the nursing process is two-way, the nurse should examine his or her own behavior. The following questions, all common pitfalls, should be explored.

- Is your approach to the client effective?
- Are you allowing your own needs and feelings to interfere with the relationship?
- Are your communication techniques effective?
- Have you pressured the client or made demands?
- Are you demonstrating acceptance or forcing your own values and judgments on the client?

THE COLLABORATIVE PLAN OF CARE

Treatment team membership depends on the setting. Typically, a psychiatric team consists of a nurse, a social worker, an occupational and a recreational therapist, and the client's physician. A psychologist may conduct psychological or neuropsychological testing, if needed. The psychiatric nurse is responsible for communicating assessment, plans, and results to other members of the team and may identify interventions to be performed jointly. The nurse may refer appropriate clients for further testing or for assessment and treatment by another caregiver. Successful collaboration requires assertiveness by the nurse, coupled with respect for the opinions of others. The nurse is frequently the only team member, with the exception of the physician, who has trained in both physical and psychiatric practice.

CASE STUDY

Lee M., a 68-year-old widower, visits the psychiatric clinic of a community-based mental health center on the advice of his internist after telling him during an appointment that he has "no will to live" and revealing that he hasn't been taking a prescribed antidepressant but is instead "saving" the pills. His married daughter, Evelyn, accompanies him.

Interviewed separately, Evelyn freely admits she has been very concerned about her father's mental health since the death of her mother 14 months ago. Approximately 6 months ago, Lee's closest friend unexpectedly died. Evelyn works a full-time, demanding job that often involves overtime. She lives an hour away from her father's home and visits approximately once a week. Evelyn's older brother, Fred, lives in Arizona and visits annually. Evelyn telephones her father frequently during the week.

Lee, when initially interviewed, states he has come to the center because he's been " a little depressed lately." He denies any suicidal ideas or plans for suicide. When questioned about his daily routine, he states he has no difficulties. Lee describes an active schedule that includes church activities, shopping, and walking in the neighborhood.

When asked about her father's mood and recent behavior, Evelyn describes frequently arriving for a weekend visit to find her father still in pajamas at lunchtime and often with unkempt hair. She suspects her father is not bathing daily and has noticed that he is not cleaning his house on a regular basis. Evelyn relates that when she has asked her father why he isn't dressed, he replies, "I don't have any energy to do that. Besides, I'm not going to be doing anything or going out." Over the past few months, Lee has spontaneously said to Evelyn, "I wish I would just die" and "I have no reason to go on living." Evelyn suspects her father is eating inadequately, and his internist has confirmed a weight loss of 15 pounds during the past 4 months. When asked about her father's activities, Evelyn relates that he has stopped church activities and shopping since the death of his friend. The friend had accompanied Lee and done all the driving. Evelyn doubts that her father has been walking regularly because it was an evening ritual that he and his wife completed each night.

Evelyn explains that she had become concerned during her last visit and contacted her father's physician when she found three full bottles of antidepressants in the bathroom cabinet. When she asked her father why he hadn't been taking the antidepressants, he stated he felt they were not helping him. (See sample MSE, Fig. 2–3.)

CRITICAL THINKING QUESTIONS

1. What factors in the suicide assessment does this client appear to have?
2. What are the objective signs of illness that Lee is displaying?
3. What are the subjective symptoms reported by the client?
4. What aspects of a complete assessment have been addressed by the case study?
5. What additional questions should be asked?
6. What testing would be helpful in establishing a diagnosis?
7. Describe some possible short-term and long-term goals.
8. Describe an objective outcome that could be tracked to indicate improvement.

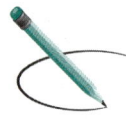

KEY POINTS

- Psychiatric nursing assessments are holistic, even though the emphasis is on unmet psychological needs.
- Before conducting an assessment, arrange for comfort and privacy, convey concern and empathy, ensure confidentiality, and examine your own feelings about the client and interaction.
- Use the interview as the vehicle for collecting data for the nursing assessment.
- Apply the MSE simultaneously with the interview.
- The MSE is the method for determining the way a client's mind is working.
- Following assessment, diagnose those problems the client has that can be managed by nurses. Use NANDA terminology.
- Cooperatively establish goals and outcomes with the client and family.
- The client and family will perform many of the interven-

tions in psychiatric nursing with encouragement and support from you, the nurse.
- The roles you will use during implementation include those of counselor, teacher, leader, and manager; the role of the counselor is emphasized.
- Evaluation is continuous throughout the nursing process. Begin and end evaluation with the client's goals.
- Remember that part of the evaluation includes self-examination.

REFERENCES

1. North American Nursing Diagnosis Association: Nursing Diagnosis Definitions and Classification 1995–1996, NANDA, Philadelphia, 1994.
2. Cardell, R, and Horton-Deutsch, S: A Model or Assessment of Inpatient Suicide Potential. Arch Psychiatr Nurs 6:366, 1994.
3. American Psychiatric Association: Diagnostic and Statistical Manual of Mental Disorders, ed 4. American Psychiatric Press, Washington, D.C., 1994, pp 843–849.
4. Blue Cross and Blue Shield Association: Medical Record Keeping Guidelines. Blue Cross and Blue Shield of Massachusetts, Boston, MA, 1995.

CHAPTER 3

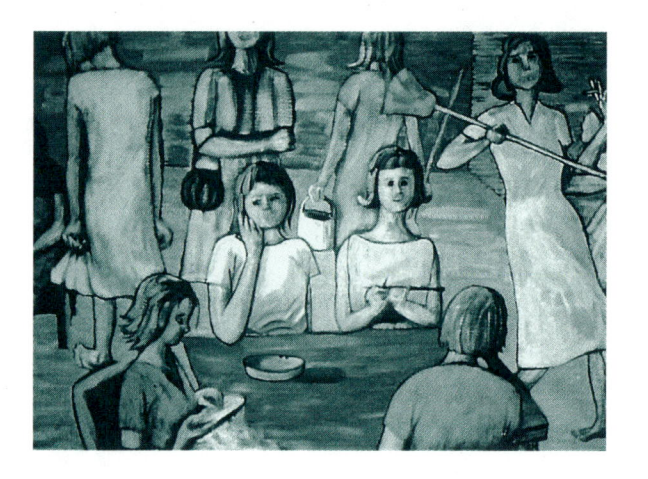

CHAPTER OUTLINE

Defining the Therapeutic Relationship
- *Differences between Social and Therapeutic Relationships*
- *Boundaries of the Therapeutic Nurse-Client Relationship*
- *Phases of the Therapeutic Relationship*
- *Guidelines for Conducting the Therapeutic Relationship*

Understanding the Communication Process
- *Levels of Communication*
- *Elements of Communication*

Performing Therapeutic Communication
- *Objectivity*
- *Active Listening*
- *Types of Communication in Psychiatric Nursing*
- *Techniques of Therapeutic Communication*
- *Barriers to Therapeutic Communication*

LEARNING OBJECTIVES

After completing this chapter, the reader should be able to:

- Explain the nature and scope of the nurse-client therapeutic relationship.
- Differentiate social and therapeutic relationships.
- Compare and contrast the stages of the therapeutic relationship.
- Identify potential boundary crossings and boundary violations that threaten the therapeutic relationship.
- Apply guidelines for developing and maintaining a therapeutic relationship.
- Demonstrate the use of effective communication skills.
- Identify roadblocks to therapeutic communication.
- Describe principles and guidelines for therapeutic communication.
- Discuss the way communication with groups differs from nurse-client interaction.

Billie Barringer, MA, BSN, RNC, CNS
Carol A. Glod, RN, CS, PhD

Therapeutic Relationship and Effective Communication

KEY TERMS

active listening
boundary
empathy
helpful communication techniques
nonverbal communication
orientation phase
self-disclosure
termination phase
therapeutic relationship
working phase

DEFINING THE THERAPEUTIC RELATIONSHIP

The essence of psychiatric nursing is the **therapeutic relationship**. The one-to-one therapeutic relationship is defined as the systematic interaction of a psychiatric nurse and an individual client for the purpose of providing psychiatric–mental health care.[1] This definition can be expanded to groups, families, and communities. Six important dimensions comprise the therapeutic relationship: genuineness, **empathy**, unconditional positive regard, communication patterns, trust, and caring. Each of these factors plays a major role in the development and sustenance of the psychiatric nurse–client relationship. Table 3–1 defines these elements.

DIFFERENCES BETWEEN SOCIAL AND THERAPEUTIC RELATIONSHIPS

Social relationships exist for the reciprocal pleasure of both individuals. People often choose their friends on the basis of personal needs for satisfaction and fun. Conversely, in the nurse-client relationship, the nurse is in a professional role that exists for the client's benefit. The goal is to care for the client and to assist in **self-disclosure**. Often this activity is not "pleasurable"; however, it is challenging and requires work for both the nurse and the client.

Social relationships are characterized by "friendship alliances," whereas the "therapeutic alliance" is the emotional bond that develops between the nurse and the client. Without the therapeutic alliance, clients cannot be expected to reveal their innermost thoughts, feelings, or fears.

Social interactions are based on codes of social conduct that are culturally tailored. In social relationships, a person has a choice about continuing or ending the interaction if behavior breeches social codes. In the therapeutic relationship, the client must be accepted, regardless of socially unacceptable behavior, cultural differences, illness, race, or other factors. For example, if you have dinner with a friend who uses bad table manners, you have the option of never accepting another dinner date with that person. If your client exhibits bad manners during mealtimes, however, you accept the behavior, avoid criticism, and use tactful suggestions to produce socially acceptable behavior.

Social relationships usually do not possess as much integrity as the nurse-client interaction. The therapeutic relationship is bound by professional ethics not to harm, exploit, or take advantage of the client. The nurse respects the client's confidentiality. No appointments are made that cannot be kept. No false reassurance is given. The client participates in decisions involving care and gives an informed consent. The nurse uses an open and honest approach consistently throughout the relationship.

In a social relationship, problems, issues, experiences, and feelings are shared. In the therapeutic relationship, the personal life and issues of the nurse do not become the focus. Rather, the client's problems, family dynamics, daily fluctuations, and emotions are the main concerns for the nurse. Only in certain situations, and under supervision, does the nurse share experiences with the client.

A nursing student who worked in a health clinic serving minority single mothers and their children participated in group therapy. Many of the women were poor, in abusive relationships, and at risk for being battered. After forming an alliance with the group, the student requested advice from the instructor about sharing previous experience with family violence. An

TABLE 3–1. Elements of the Therapeutic Nurse-Client Relationship

Genuineness
The ability of the nurse to be honest, open, and sincere. Genuineness is demonstrated by congruence between the nurse's verbal and nonverbal behavior.

Empathy
The ability to understand the situation from the client's point of view without losing objectivity in the process. Empathy is a characteristic inherent in everyone, although some are better able to empathize than others. The nurse can make a conscious effort to use empathy as a way of building the nurse–client relationship and thereby retrain the self in the use of empathic understanding of the client and others.

Unconditional Positive Regard
The ability to accept the client exactly as he or she is. The nurse uses this concept by being consistently respectful and nonjudgmental and by avoiding criticism, both verbally and through attitude.

Communication Patterns
Planned communication through the deliberate use of helpful communication skills and through avoidance of communication roadblocks and barriers. The nurse studies, applies, and evaluates communication skills and techniques constantly throughout the nurse-client relationship. The aim of interaction is to assist the client to vent concerns, problem solve, and express feelings.

Trust
The client's belief that the nurse will behave predictably and competently and will respect his or her needs. Trust provides the basis for progress during future encounters. It is the very basis of the relationship and produces comfort rather than anxiety during the interaction.

Caring
The level of emotional involvement between the nurse and the client. Caring provides the client with knowledge that the nurse is willing to help.

---

advantage of disclosing this information was the chance of building better rapport with group members; a danger was that the student would be satisfying her own needs by discussing her issues rather than those of the group. The student shared her experience and became a role model for the other women. The personal resources she contributed helped the others deal with their own episodes of violence.

This example demonstrates the way sharing personal experiences can have a profound effect on others' ability to cope and to change. It also indicates another requirement of the therapeutic relationship: supervision. Working with clients with psychiatric problems can cause the nurse to lose objectivity or to misinterpret communication. Supervision from an objective "outsider" helps keep the interaction in perspective.

Communication in social relationships consists of chit-chat. In the therapeutic relationship, communication is planned. The nurse acquires, applies, and studies the way communication skills are used in the interaction.

Social relationships are intuitive. Friends interact without wondering about the way their performance influences the other. Nurses, however, consciously study their own behavior with clients and evaluate its effect on the interaction. Often the process recording is used as a way for the nurse to gain self-understanding and growth.

> A nurse whose husband was dying visited a client who had recently returned home from inhospital treatment for schizophrenia and tuberculosis. When the nurse studied a process recording made of the session, it was apparent that each time the client mentioned his concerns about dying, the nurse abruptly changed focus. The nurse realized that the client's concern about death was forcing her to face her own anxieties about her husband. Only after studying her approach was she able to help the client with his needs.

Inherent in developing self-understanding is discovering beliefs and biases about individuals who have mental illness. Preconceived ideas can seriously hamper effective nursing care. Table 3–2 describes some questions nurses can ask themselves to determine personal biases and to promote the therapeutic relationship.

BOUNDARIES OF THE THERAPEUTIC NURSE-CLIENT RELATIONSHIP

Boundaries are typically thought of as lines of demarcation. The term **boundary** in psychiatric settings refers to the "line" between a therapeutic and nontherapeutic relationship. Every encounter with a psychiatric client is a therapeutic relationship, and boundaries establish the nature and scope of the interactions. Boundaries serve to protect the client from practices that are beyond the typical standard of care. Nursing conduct that extends beyond usual standards of safe and ethical practice is termed "boundary crossing" or "boundary violation."[2] These boundary crossings may be viewed as nontherapeutic or therapeutic depending on the intent, conduct, and rationale for the behavior.

Is meeting a client for lunch a boundary crossing? This situation is beyond the standard level of care delivered by a psychiatric nurse. However, in psychiatric home care, nurses may develop a treatment plan that includes encouraging a very isolated or anxious client to socialize and adapt to activities outside the home. In this case, the deviation from the normal intervention clearly supports therapeutic objectives in the overall plan of care. By contrast, if the *nurse* weekly met the client for lunch to avoid eating alone, this social engagement would constitute a boundary crossing. Ques-

TABLE 3–2. Ways to Explore Reactions to Clients' Behaviors

If the client *scares* you, ask yourself the following questions:
- What observable behaviors suggest violent or disruptive behaviors?
- Have you experienced directly any past violent or near-violent behaviors?
- Are others experiencing similar fears?
- Could your lack of experience with this client be contributing to your concerns?
- Is the individual's speech or communication pattern a barrier to understanding the behavior?
- Is the ethnic or cultural background a factor that may lead you to misinterpret behavior?
- Has the individual displayed threats or actual harm to others or self?

If the client *offends* or *outrages* you, ask yourself the following questions:
- What are the observable behaviors and statements?
- Is there some factor that biases you against this person?
- Is the client resisting or rejecting help that you believe is needed?
- What are your beliefs about respectful interpersonal relationships?
- How does the client react to other staff and clients?
- Are you reacting with anger and hurt?
- Could the client be angry and hurt, yet is disguising it as offensive behaviors?
- Is the client arousing your own fears and insecurities?
- Are you concerned that the client doesn't like you?

---

tionable behavior should be discussed in detail with a supervisor and expert colleagues to determine if the plan is consistent with an appropriate level of care.

Guidelines for Establishing Boundaries

The following guidelines apply to nurses and nursing students engaged in psychiatric–mental health practice, regardless of setting. They are intended to promote the development of a safe and ethical therapeutic relationship.

Defining the Parameters of the Relationship. On the initial contact, the nurse informs the client of name, affiliation, purpose of the interaction, confidentiality, and date of termination of the relationship. For example, a nursing student might say, "My name is Susan Smith. I am a nursing student from the university, and I will be doing a clinical practice here on Wednesdays until October 15th. I would like to meet with you each week and discuss your concerns. Everything you say will be confidential." If the client agrees, a contract is obtained for the interaction; for example, "Let's meet between 8 and 9 AM in the interview room." This approach defines the nature of the therapeutic relationship as a professional, goal-oriented, business encounter.

Avoiding Physical Contact. In psychiatric nursing, physical contact is avoided. An initial handshake is appropriate, but other physical contact is limited to basic nursing care such as taking vital signs, giving injections, providing nursing care, and applying restraints. The client may misunderstand or take out of context any behaviors that go beyond these measures, usually because of distortions of reality, confusion, sexual identity issues, or a history of sexual abuse by primary caretakers. Therefore, hugs, kisses, back rubs, holding hands, and putting an arm around a client are not the usual standard of care. These gestures carry the potential for extreme conscious and unconscious reactions and thus are viewed as "boundary crossings" in therapeutic relationships. Their use is guided by careful prior thought and review with the supervisor and other colleagues.

The client may use physical contact as a way of testing the nurse for acceptance. When this happens, the nurse must set limits without rejecting the client.

A client said to a nurse, "I am going to kiss you." The nurse, although alarmed, understood the underlying meaning of the client's act and was able to refocus with the reply, "You must be feeling lonely." The two then sat down and discussed the client's needs.

Maintaining Confidentiality. Confidentiality is essential for establishing and maintaining a therapeutic relationship. (See Chapter 1 for a discussion of confidentiality.) Disclosing information about the client to other people (except to the clinical instructor and staff) without written consent constitutes a boundary crossing.

Avoiding Self-Disclosure. The nurse usually does not disclose personal information, such as marital status, address, age, religious background, or other private information. Doing so goes beyond the boundaries of the therapeutic relationship. However, the nurse would appear cold and aloof by not responding if a client asked some personal questions. The best way to place the interaction back on course is to reply, "Yes, I am married. And you?" From there, the nurse refocuses on the client.

Accepting Gifts. Gifts are a common social means of showing gratitude. However, other motivations for giving the nurse a present are possible. Often, the client feels it is "the thing to do." Despite financial hardship, the client feels obligated to thank the nurse with a gift. In other cases, the gift is a way of continuing the relationship past its termination point. Refuse expensive gifts or those of an intimate or sexual nature. Accept gifts that the client makes for you during the course of the relationship. Depending on the motivation, some ways of dealing with gifts are to say, "You do not need to give me a gift to make me stay and talk to you. I will be here for our session anyway." Or, at termination time, the nurse might say, "I cannot accept this gift, but I will always remember you and our time together."

The nurse does not generally give presents or cards to the client. However, exceptions occur. For example, a psychiatric nurse who is engaged in an ongoing relationship with a client may send a sympathy card to acknowledge a parent's death, or a nurse may give to a client a paperback book explaining psychotropic medication. In this context, gifts are shared as part of the treatment plan and not as a social pleasure for the nurse.

Avoid other economic transactions with the client and family. Examples include accepting special favors, frequenting a client's place of business, exchanging services, or purchasing items from the client. Ideally, these boundaries continue after discharge and hinder the development of a business, social, or romantic liaison.

Addressing the Client. While it might feel comfortable to address clients by their first names, call adults by their surnames, until told otherwise, to convey respect and place the relationship on a professional plane. Conversely, the nurse gives first and last names to clients and allows them to choose how to respond. Regardless of choice, the aim is for the client to feel comfortable addressing the nurse.

Managing Social Relationships or Encounters. It may be impossible to avoid social encounters with clients in restaurants or stores. When these accidental encounters occur, allow the client to acknowledge you first, because confidentiality extends even after the therapeutic relationship ends. Unless carefully outlined in the nursing care plan, avoid meeting the client in social settings and situations. For example, a nurse would not ask a client to go shopping to avoid going alone. However, if the nurse was making a home visit to a socially isolated client, they might meet at a shopping mall. The goal would be to decrease social isolation and encourage the client to interact more in the future, which is consistent with the overall treatment plan.

Guidelines for Boundaries with Children

Many of the same boundaries exist for a therapeutic relationship with children and adolescents, although some leeway is possible. Children with psychiatric disorders have a right to confidentiality; however, their parents have the ultimate responsibility, and therefore the family is an active part of the therapeutic relationship. Parents and legal guardians have the right to information that the nurse obtains from and about their child. The family (not the child) must give written authorization before any data are shared. Physical contact with younger children is generally allowed, primarily in the form of touch or hugs, yet the circumstances are still carefully considered. The interaction between nurse and client may take place in more informal settings, for instance, on the floor of an interview room or bedroom. The therapeutic relationship is enhanced through toys, games, art, and play. More latitude is generally allowed for self-disclosure and exchange of gifts, pictures, and food. Each of these activities can be a specific nursing intervention to establish and maintain the therapeutic relationship, keeping in mind the developmental level of the child.

Decision Making about Boundaries in Therapeutic Relationships

The previously suggested boundaries apply to all therapeutic relationships; however, clinical judgment and individual client needs determine the exact implementation. While many of the parameters may seem distinct, the nurse holds the responsibility for evaluating the standard of care and deciding when deviating is appropriate. Novice nurses are challenged to begin to understand and adhere to these guidelines, although expert nurses may be in a better position to mold nursing practice by using strategies that go beyond the usual standards. Nonetheless, nursing care must remain within acceptable and safe conduct and support therapeutic objectives.

PHASES OF THE THERAPEUTIC RELATIONSHIP

Hildegard Peplau[3] describes four stages of relationship development. They are fluid, and individuals pass back and forth throughout each stage depending on the situation. Together, the psychiatric nurse and client embark through this process on a journey toward mental health.

Preinteraction Phase

In the first stage, the nurse prepares for initial contact. During the preinteraction stage, the nurse makes assessments and gathers data from all available sources.

Another key aspect of preinteraction is self-assessment or countertransference, the process by which the nurse unconsciously projects feelings, thoughts, and wishes from the past that interfere with treatment. As a result, the client's feelings and behaviors can become obscured by the nurse's own experiences. Self-understanding requires the nurse to examine feelings and to make them conscious and readily apparent. An honest and open appraisal produces growth, an important outcome of the nurse-client interaction.

Orientation Phase

In the **orientation phase**, clients begin to learn about their behaviors and need for assistance. The nurse continues to assess, to identify strengths and weaknesses, to construct nursing diagnoses, and to design an individual plan of care with the client.

The orientation phase is uncomfortable because the nurse and client are strangers and they lack trust. Therefore, establishing the therapeutic alliance comprises a major part of orientation (Box 3–1).

Working Phase

Progress in the therapeutic nurse-client relationship occurs during the **working phase**. The working phase aims to help the clients maintain or reestablish their best possible level of functioning based on their behaviors, personality, ability,

Box 3–1. Tips for Trust

- Be honest, open, sincere.
- Ensure confidentiality.
- Introduce yourself, giving name, affiliation, purpose, and termination date.
- Be consistent.
- Avoid pressuring or probing the client during assessment.
- Obtain an understanding of the problem from the client's frame of reference.
- Be respectful.
- Treat the client with the same courtesy you would accord any other stranger until trust is established.

and life circumstances. Together, the nurse and client problem solve and evaluate progress in goal attainment. Much can be accomplished because the client knows the nurse better and trusts more (Box 3–2).

Termination Phase

The **termination phase** may be the most difficult. Ideally, termination occurs when the client has reached the goals for treatment. However, time constraints and pressures of managed care may promote early discharge. The therapeutic relationship may also be terminated when the nurse or student leaves the clinical setting.

After termination is initiated, the nurse and client should address several issues.

- They review the course of treatment, progress, and unresolved areas.
- They examine feelings associated with termination such as sadness, rejection, abandonment, anger, or emotions from past unresolved losses. The nurse allows adequate time for recognition and exploration of these feelings and, with forethought and supervision, also may share feelings about saying goodbye.

Termination can be an especially growth-promoting process. Clients can use the termination phase to develop increased confidence and independence, along with the capacity to deal with loss (Box 3–3).

GUIDELINES FOR CONDUCTING THE THERAPEUTIC RELATIONSHIP

When interacting with the client, the nurse should keep several guidelines in mind. This knowledge helps the nurse to understand the client, provide unconditional positive regard, and interact effectively. These guides are also referred to as *interpersonal skills*.

- Identify behavior that is expressive of emotional needs and recognize the meaning it serves for the client. The individual expresses emotional needs through behavior. For example, a client who is fearful and nontrusting might say, "Go away and leave me alone." The nurse who understands the client's behavior would say, "All right, I will leave; but I will be back." Not understanding the client's emotional needs could cause the nurse to respond personally, feel hurt, and possibly withdraw from future interaction.
- Allow the client to express a wide range of feelings without fear of retaliation. Feelings are categorized under the broad headings of "mad," "glad," "sad," or "scared." Feelings are neither right nor wrong. They are like breathing; they are a necessary accompaniment of living. In mental illness, feelings are often dissociated or repressed; however, they continue to influence behavior. One aim of psychiatric treatment is to uncover

Box 3–2. Tips for Intervening

- Use interventions that build on the client's strengths and foster the therapeutic relationship.
- Reinforce healthy behaviors.
- Provide encouragement and reassurance.
- Teach needed concepts or information.
- Use confrontation when the client is ready.
- Assist the client to restructure thinking, i.e., to think positively.
- Set limits as needed.
- Use problem-solving interventions to help the client make changes in relationships, lifestyle, and occupational functioning.
- Use role play as a way of helping the client test actual or potential situations.
- Model responsible, positive behavior for the client.
- Use evocative techniques, such as art and literature, to facilitate expression of feelings.

Box 3–3. Tips for Terminating

- Inform the client about the termination date on the first contact.
- Inoculate the client emotionally throughout the relationship with reminders of termination day.
- Provide the opportunity to discuss termination before it occurs.
- Consider cutting down on the amount of time spent with the client prior to terminating.
- Involve other health team members with the client prior to leaving.
- Make referrals.
- Allow time for expression of feelings.
- Avoid seeking out new problems; rather, review progress.
- Indicate confidence in the client.

> **RESEARCH NOTE**
>
> Beeber, LS: The one-to-one relationship in psychiatric nursing: The next generation. In Anderson, C (ed): Psychiatric Nursing 1946 to 1994: A Report on the State of the Art. Ohio State University, Columbus, OH, 1995.
>
> **Findings:** In this study, specific interventions are developed within the one-to-one therapeutic relationship to assist individuals with depression and anxiety. This model, based on the theoretical notions of Peplau and Sullivan, emphasizes an empathetic link with the client. The nurse then engages the depressed client through a specific sequence of interventions designed to change past patterns of interpersonal relating. First, the nurse develops an empathetic connection that elicits the need for tenderness in the client. In response, the client begins to distance from and withhold connection to the nurse. These behaviors are hypothesized to be based on past patterns of associating the need for tenderness with anxiety and avoidance. The nurse then sets limits on these distancing defenses, and remains neutral, not reacting with anger.
>
> **Application to Practice:** This approach promotes the ongoing connection with the client without impeding the giving of tenderness. Simultaneously, the client is encouraged to relate emerging anxious feelings. The results show that clients with depression are able to express their emotions. Their need for tenderness is validated as well. This set of interventions provides a specific framework to foster the nurse's provision of tenderness with the client's need for tenderness, to alleviate the depression in the context of a therapeutic relationship.

uncomfortable emotions, examine them, and determine their meaning for the client. To do this, the nurse must be accepting.

- Whenever possible, find ways of promoting the client's self-esteem. Focus on strengths. Avoid criticism by words or attitudes that undermine the client's morale. Praise the client for accomplishments. Include the client in the plan of care. Encourage the client to set realistic goals in an incremental way by beginning with small steps and increasing the difficulty with progress. Promote decision making, and involve the client in activities at which he or she can succeed.
- Give attention and recognition to the client on each contact. Nurses have structured encounters with clients through the nurse-client relationship contract. Many contacts, however, are unplanned, spontaneous meetings. Regardless of the brevity of these contacts, the nurse can make them therapeutic by giving undivided attention to the client. Also, some clients ask for attention and recognition through such ways as refusing to participate, making demands, or resisting. Rather than ignoring them, the best approach is to respond to the process. Often, the client's demanding behavior stops, once attention and recognition are given.

A client who was a resident of a convalescent home wandered the halls, wringing her hands, and saying, "I want to go home. I want out of here." Because the staff ignored her, her protests escalated to the point where she threatened to hit the staff with her walking cane. The nurse approached the client, helped her make a telephone call to her family, and took her outside on the patio. After a few minutes of sitting with the client, the nurse was able to resume her work, and the client sat peacefully in the courtyard, watching the birds and looking at the autumn leaves.

- Provide for the client's need to feel secure. Because many clients do not trust others, they feel anxious and afraid. The nurse helps the client to be more trusting by using a consistent approach, offering reassurance, and adhering to the boundaries that define the relationship.
- Convey understanding. The ability to empathize helps the nurse understand the client's situation, but communicating on the client's level of understanding is also important. Children require a different approach than adults. Educated and uneducated clients have different levels of comprehension. Because the thought process becomes concrete due to impaired concept formation, mental illness sometimes influences a client's level of understanding. Different cultural groups use language differently. In each of these instances, your approach is modified to gain and to convey understanding.
- Consider the client's readiness before requiring change. Evaluate the level of health prior to making certain therapeutic demands. Otherwise, you may unwittingly cause the client to fail. Careful assessment and evaluation help in determining readiness.
- Learn and use therapeutic communication skills.

UNDERSTANDING THE COMMUNICATION PROCESS

In nursing, communication is the tool for establishing the nurse-patient relationship. According to Reusch[4], communication includes "all of the procedures by which one mind may affect another." Therefore, verbal and nonverbal behavior, the arts and literature, and literally all aspects of being constitute communication.

LEVELS OF COMMUNICATION

There are four levels of communication, and each builds upon the next.

Intrapersonal Level

Individuals think or talk to themselves as they communicate. They generate messages through their own private thoughts and from responding to internal and external stimuli. As they receive messages from others or from the surroundings, they also talk to themselves as they organize, interpret, and assign meaning to input. Miscommunication often occurs because of differences in perceiving. Also, too much "self talk" results in an inability to give full attention to the client, and lack of understanding results.

Interpersonal Level

Interpersonal communication occurs between two people, and each party communicates intrapersonally at the same time. Face-to-face encounters, telephone conversations, letter writing, and computer transactions are all examples of interpersonal communication. In nursing, this form of communication is basic to establishing the interpersonal relationship.

Small Group Communication

When three or more people engage in face-to-face or other types of encounters, there is communication among a group. Each party continues to communicate intrapersonally and interpersonally, as well as with the group; therefore, communication is more complex. The events that take place during small group interaction and the development of cliques or subgroups are called *group dynamics*.

Nurses constantly deal with structured and unstructured groups. Examples include group therapy, family interaction, treatment team meetings, committees within the setting, and staff meetings.

Organizational Communication

Organizational communication occurs when small groups within the agency meet together to establish and reach common goals. This type of communication is inherent to the management role of the nurse and involves formal channels, such as organizational charts, lines of command, and policy manuals.

ELEMENTS OF COMMUNICATION

The Sender

Communication starts when a person has an idea and sends out a message to others, verbally, nonverbally, or through the arts. Messages are generated by internal stimulation, such as hunger, and by external factors, such as what one hears.

The Message

The message is the stimulation produced by the sender and directed toward a receiver.

Verbal Messages. The messages are expressed through language or writing and are embellished by *paraverbal* cues like tone of voice, pitch, speed, inflections, loudness or softness, and the way words are spoken. These characteristics add to the meaning of the verbal message and often influence the listener more than the actual message.

Nonverbal Messages. These are the unspoken messages people give that are often more reliable than verbal content. Table 3–3 cites examples of nonverbal communication.

The Channel

The channel is the medium through which messages are transmitted.

The Visual Channel. Communication occurs by seeing and observing people and events. However, when meaning is assigned to the visual event, *perception* occurs.

The Auditory Channel. Communication occurs through hearing, the reception of an auditory stimulus. More important than hearing is listening, which involves understanding the underlying messages and feelings associated with an auditory experience.

The Kinesthetic Channel. The nurse communicates whenever touch is used. *Procedural touch* occurs during nursing procedures and techniques. *Caring touch*, which is used much more by psychiatric nurses, conveys emotional support.

The Receiver

This person intercepts the message through hearing and mental abilities. Messages must be interpreted when they are noticed, and the ability to think is crucial. Often, mental illness interferes with thinking. Anxiety restricts the perceptual field, so that one hears less, sees less, and feels less. Also, too much "self-talk" will influence a person's communication with others.

TABLE 3–3. Types of Nonverbal Communication

- Facial expressions communicate happiness, sadness, fear, and anger.
- Eyes, eyebrows, and eyelids show interest, concern, sadness, alarm, shyness, pleasure, displeasure, excitement, and flirtation.
- Posture indicates tenseness, relaxation, and positive or negative self-concept.
- Gestures add a dimension to communication; consider a shrug of the shoulders, tapping of the feet, or a wave of the hand.
- Artifact messages enhance or hinder the spoken words. Consider use of clothing, jewelry, hair style, and grooming.
- Invasion of personal space produces anxiety.
- Lips smile, pout, snarl, or quiver to communicate feelings.
- Jaws clamp shut to indicate unwillingness to talk.

Feedback

Once a receiver gains awareness of the sender's message, feedback is provided. The function of feedback is to alert the sender to the receiver's perception of the message. Then the sender can adjust the message strategy to communicate more effectively.

Time and Space

Communication occurs within the context of time and space. The time of day influences communication. For example, information given to a client at 3:00 AM may not be remembered as well as information provided at 3:00 PM when the client is awake. Likewise, noise in the environment, heat or cold, light, and the presence or absence of fresh air all influence the communication process.

PERFORMING THERAPEUTIC COMMUNICATION

Therapeutic communication is helping a client with needs, concerns, and problems. It is the medium for establishing the nurse-client relationship and for using the nursing process. According to Peplau,[3] therapeutic communication focuses on the reactions of the client to illness and health problems. Similarly, Carl Rogers[5] states that therapeutic communication is client-centered and exists for the purpose of the client's self-expression. Besides use of elements for creating a therapeutic alliance, the nurse must be objective and an active listener to communicate therapeutically (Box 3–4).

OBJECTIVITY

To be an active listener, the nurse must become "selfless"; that is, personal biases, prejudices, feelings, anxieties, and other baggage are put aside during the interaction, allowing the nurse to pay attention to the client and to be unencumbered by personal complications that might interfere with listening.

ACTIVE LISTENING

Being an active listener includes hearing the client, interpreting the language, noticing nonverbal and paraverbal enhancements, and identifying underlying feelings. Through analyzing and validating the conversation, the nurse gains a better understanding of the client. The nurse also suspends judgment, listens between the lines, empathizes, notes discrepancies between facts and feelings, and uses communication techniques. According to Kemper,[6] therapeutic listening includes maintaining eye contact and an attentive posture; staying within conversational distance; responding with facial expressions, touch, gestures, and encouragement;

Box 3–4. Tips for Therapeutic Communication

- Provide privacy. Find a place for your interview where others cannot overhear the client. This also ensures confidentiality.
- Sit in comfortable chairs. Regulate the temperature. Make the client comfortable.
- Establish yourself as an interested, concerned nurse.
- Be aware of your own feelings and their effect on your behavior as well as on the session itself.
- Let the client start the interview. Talk about present issues and concerns. Give timely interjections and prompting after the client begins.
- Avoid the use of a direct approach. Allow the client time to get ready to discuss painful issues.
- Avoid using statements that sound final. Instead, use comments and techniques that have prompting qualities. For example, "You were saying . . . " or "Tell me about. . . . "
- Use minimal verbal activity. The client gets the opportunity to say more when the interviewer says less. Even during health teaching, give the client the chance to ask questions, to provide information, and to dominate the session.
- Use techniques that encourage the client to be spontaneous. The client will reveal more about problems and issues with spontaneity.
- Allow the client to express feelings. Talking for the sake of talking is not interviewing. Only when the client is addressing issues and revealing feelings does therapy really occur.
- Explore issues and areas that are emotionally laden. Watch body language, listen to vocal characteristics, be aware of things left unsaid, and notice the way communication changes with the topic of discussion. All of this will help you identify emotionally charged areas.
- Listen to the client and focus on verbal, nonverbal, written, or artifact clues. By responding to clues, the nurse avoids asking extraneous questions and requesting information about unexpressed issues.

---

asking relevant questions; and interpreting and summarizing key points by using specific words spoken by the client. As a result of the nurse's approach, the client gains the opportunity to self-disclose more freely and to problem solve. **Active listening** also enhances the client's self-esteem.

TYPES OF COMMUNICATION IN PSYCHIATRIC NURSING

Assessment Interview

Because the purpose of the assessment interview is fact-finding, the nurse has more liberty in the use of direct questioning techniques. A direct questioning technique is used within the context of the nursing process for establishing baseline data and for constructing a nursing care plan; therefore, it is therapeutic. However, facilitative communication skills may be employed throughout the assessment to allow the client to vent concerns.

Counseling

Counseling is the medium the psychiatric nurse uses to help clients solve problems. The nurse assumes a counselor's role and uses techniques to encourage the client to self-disclose. Discussing problems and feelings brings relief to the client, and the logical consequence is behavioral change for improved relationships with others.

Group Interaction

The nurse works with families and groups of clients and continues to identify problems, problem solve, and use group discussion as a means of self-disclosure. Communication is more difficult because more people are involved. Subgroups form and further complicate the communication process. Nevertheless, the psychiatric nurse serves as a catalyst, observes group dynamics, and promotes the work and growth of groups. Table 3–4 illustrates differences between interpersonal and small-group communication.

Communication with the Treatment Team

A treatment-team meeting includes all mental health disciplines, the client, and the family for establishing treatment plans, reviewing progress, and arranging or maintaining community-based care. Usually a leader and a recorder are appointed at each meeting. The nurse shares in this leadership at the designated time and uses group communication skills to promote the work and productivity of the team. Maintaining the focus is a major task for the group facilitator. The recorder documents the client's progress toward the short-term goals and the plans for revision.

TECHNIQUES OF THERAPEUTIC COMMUNICATION

During interaction with the client, the nurse deliberately uses **helpful communication techniques** that encourage self-disclosure. To avoid pressuring or probing the client, a nondirective approach, based on work by Hays and Larson,[7] is recommended (Box 3–5).

Process recordings are effective techniques to reflect on and analyze therapeutic communications. Table 3–5 shows a portion of a process recording. Each recording usually has five columns: the client's communication, the student nurse's communication, the student nurse's thoughts and feelings, an analysis, and a critique. After an interaction with a client that lasts about 10 to 15 minutes, the student writes down the entire conversation, noting both verbal and **nonverbal communication**. Next, the student reflects on any thoughts or feelings that arose during the therapeutic interaction. With the help of textbooks and other readings, the student analyzes the communication and notes patterns and interpretations. Finally, the student evaluates the entire interaction to improve her or his communication techniques with this client and others.

BARRIERS TO THERAPEUTIC COMMUNICATION

Several common obstacles interfere with effective communication. Although these **communication roadblocks** inter-

TABLE 3–4. Differences between Interpersonal and Group Communication

Interpersonal	Group
• One sender, one receiver, both engaging in self-talk	• Numerous senders and receivers, each engaging in self-talk
• Facilitative communication techniques used in one-to-one interaction	• Facilitative communication techniques used with the group
• Influenced by dynamics of nurse-client relationship (creating, maintaining, and terminating)	• Requires knowledge of theoretical framework to guide both interventions and interpretations (examples: transactional analysis, Gestalt theory, existential theory, group dynamics, family therapy, and interpersonal communication. The approach selected will influence the kind and amount of communication used by the leader.)
• Requires understanding of nurse-client relationship theory, communication theory, and a basis of approach (such as Peplau[3])	
• May be done by the generalist nurse	• Communication influenced by group dynamics
• Identification of problems and problem solving done by client with help from nurse.	• May be done by the generalist nurse in certain instances (e.g., educational groups); nurse clinical specialist, with greater depth of understanding of group process, handles group and family therapy
• Nurse is major support for client during interaction	
• Logical outcome of one-to-one communication is development of the nurse-client relationship	• Identification of problems and problem solving done by group with help from leader
	• Group is major support for clients during interaction
	• Logical outcome is group cohesiveness and group productivity

56 Introduction to Psychiatric Nursing

TABLE 3–5. Partial Process Recording of a Therapeutic Interaction between a Student Nurse and Client in a Psychiatric Day Program for Elders

The client was sitting in a chair by herself when the student approached her. Before beginning the interaction, the student had read her chart, and understood that one of the client's major issues was a possible cerebrovascular accident (CVA). She had been prescribed "pills" for her condition, which apparently she did not take consistently. The purpose of the interaction was to further assess the patient's health status.

Patient (verbal & nonverbal)	Nurse (verbal & nonverbal)	Nurse's thoughts & feelings	Analysis	Critique
[Mrs. S. is standing near the table. She smiles as I approach her.]	"Hi. My name is Frances, one of the nursing students. Would you have a few minutes for me to ask some questions about your health? [I approach her at the table, looking directly into her eyes.]	I had just finished reading Mrs. S.'s chart, and another client pointed Mrs. S. out. I was wondering to myself, "How's this going to go?"	This is the beginning or orientation phase. Giving the person a choice about participating allows her control, to increase self-esteem, trust.	This approach was effective, because I explained the purpose of the interview and clarified my role to give her an overview.
	[I return her smile.]	She appeared younger than her stated age, and looked physically fit.	According to my reading, most older people remain healthy and active in later life.	
"Me? I have no health problems. But, you can ask me anything you like [laughing]."	"Thank you, this won't take long. How would you describe your health?"	Because she had keys, I did not want to delay her.	Setting a clear time frame for interview to increase understanding.	This clarified some of the expectations for the interview.
[Mrs. S.'s hair is well kept, she is dressed appropriately in a jogging suit, and is holding a set of keys.] "It's perfect. Well, up to about 2 months ago."	"What changed?" [Sympathetic tone.]	I wondered why she said that, and what had changed lately. It might be a recent loss, emergent health problem, financial problem, or change in mental health status.	This is an open-ended question to encourage a broad response.	

"I may have taken a little spell, or stroke." [She rubs her left arm.] "That's what we think."	"You and your doctor?"	A more effective question would have been to use an open-ended approach: "Who's we?"
"No. I haven't seen her yet."		
"My side felt strange, and this side [points to left] seemed limp. Since then, I don't want to do as much."	"What makes you think you had a stroke?"	If she had a stroke, I don't notice any obvious residual effect. I wonder if she recovered. A CVA often results in some physical consequences. She seems to be downplaying or minimizing it.
"I went into the hospital for a few days, but the hardest part was leaving home."	"That must have been very hard for you."	The relationship appears to be developing more. She appears to trust me, and is opening up somewhat.
	"Leaving home?" [Making good eye contact]	
"Yes, my daughter, you know she works a lot and has her own family to deal with." [Looks sad and looks down toward the floor.]		One of the consequences of CVA can be depression.
	"Hmmm."	I'm wondering if she has had a major adjustment or if there may be a more severe problem like major depression going on. I'm not sure exactly what to say here. Oh no—I made her sad. There are several ways to proceed here, and I'm also hoping to think a little about what to do. Empathy and silence can be used to effectively establish rapport and build trust.

Therapeutic Relationship and Effective Communication   **57**

Box 3-5. Tips for the Nondirective Approach

Techniques That Allow the Client to Begin the Conversation

- Offering self. The nurse is available physically and emotionally and communicates a willingness to help. Example: "I'll sit with you awhile."
- Giving broad openings. The nurse makes statements that indicate the client should begin. Example: "What would you like to discuss today?"
- Silence. The nurse remains quiet and allows the client the opportunity to direct the session. Example: The nurse waits for the client to begin or to continue talking.
- General leads. The nurse allows the client to direct the discussion by indicating interest in what comes next. Examples: "And then . . . " or "Go on."

Techniques That Have a Prompting Quality

- Open-ended statements. The nurse uses incomplete sentences to prompt the client. Example: "You were saying. . . . " Minimal verbal activity. The nurse monitors and controls the amount of verbiage so that the client will say more. Examples: "Oh," "Yes . . . ," or simply acknowledging the client as he or she speaks.
- Reflection. The nurse repeats the client's last words to prompt. Example: The client says, "I'm upset." The nurse responds, "upset. . . . "
- Restatement. The nurse repeats the client's major theme to gain a better perception of the problem. Example: The client says, "I did not sleep at all last night." The nurse says, "You are having difficulty sleeping."
- Encouraging a description of perception. The nurse asks for a description of a situation from the client's point of view. Example: "How do you see your situation at this point?" or "What do you think about . . . ?"

Techniques Used for Responding to Verbal or Nonverbal Leads, Clues, or Signals from the Client

- Exploring. The nurse directs the client to a specific component of the session for a more thorough discussion. Example: "I would like to backtrack to what you said about. . . . "
- Recognition. The nurse points out behaviors of the client. Example: "I notice that you became upset when. . . . " Or, "I notice that you have a photograph of your husband."
- Focusing. The nurse focuses on topics that need further elaboration. Examples: "You mentioned that you have a problem with. . . . " And "You say you're anxious."
- Direct questions. The nurse uses comments that elicit specific information about issues and problems the client brings into the session. Examples: Any number of questions beginning with "Who, what, where, when, and how." These questions are directed toward the specific topic at hand and serve to further define it.
- Verbalizing the implied. The nurse makes the client's communication more explicit by putting ideas and concepts into concrete terms. Example: The client says,

Box 3-5. Tips for the Nondirective Approach (Continued)

"Nobody ever comes to see me. I might as well be nonexistent." The nurse replies, "You must feel very lonely."
- Seeking clarification. The nurse alerts the client about misunderstood communication. Example: "I'm not sure I follow you" or "Explain what you meant by. . . . "

Techniques That Focus on the Client's Feelings

- Asking for thoughts. The nurse asks for thoughts about problems and concerns. Example: "What do you think about . . . ?"
- Decoding or translating into feelings. The nurse uncovers the true meaning behind the client's words. Example: "How much is this bottle of hand lotion costing me, nurse?" The nurse responds, "You're worried about your medical bill?"
- Encouraging evaluation. The nurse encourages the client to consider people or events from his or her frame of reference. Example: The client says, "I am going home today." The nurse responds, "What do you think about going home today?"

Techniques That Convey Recognition to the Client

- Recognition. The nurse voices awareness of a change or a personal effort by a client. Example: "I notice that you participated in group today."
- Observation. The nurse voices awareness of the client's behavioral or affective characteristics. Example: "You seem tense today."
- Suggesting collaboration. The nurse offers support to the client as the client faces and solves problems. Example: "Perhaps you and I can work together to decide on your goals for treatment."

Techniques That Promote Thinking

- Voicing doubt. The nurse challenges the client's beliefs by not reinforcing perceptions. Examples: "Really?" or "Oh?"
- Presenting reality. The nurse objectively points out reality for the client, without arguing with or reinforcing the client's beliefs. Example: "I know you think there are worms in your food, but I do not see any."
- Encouraging formulation of a plan of action. The nurse encourages the client to consider ways of dealing with problems. Example: "What could you do about your loneliness?"

fere with the exchange of ideas, most of them can be overcome.

Language

The most prominent communication barrier is language. Many clients speak English as a second language, and a smaller proportion are hearing impaired or deaf. These groups present nursing with the greatest challenge. Some agencies have interpreters available to translate important information. Keeping a foreign language dictionary handy might help. Many clinicians learn sign language to communicate with the hearing-impaired client.

Cultural Considerations

Specific cultural considerations can provide important insight into effective communication. For example, as a result of political, religious, or ethnic persecution or to obtain better economic or educational opportunities, individuals have left their countries of origin. Aside from the relocation and resettlement processes, immigrants often do not have adequate health insurance and may be reluctant to seek care. Lack of knowledge about treatment options and backgrounds of exploitation or torture also contribute to treatment resistance. Distrust of government and differing philosophies about health and illness may further promote alienation from health-care providers. As a result, many immigrants are fearful of communicating to others about their intimate physical and mental health needs.

Different cultures use language differently. For example, medical personnel have a jargon of their own. Clients may not understand "PET scan" or "borderline." Therefore, dispensing with hospital jargon is one way of overcoming this type of cultural barrier.

Age and Development Level

Age differences may pose communication problems. With aging can come loss of hearing, eyesight, or cognition. In addition, the elderly hold values that may be different than those of younger people. Children do not think abstractly, and reaching their level of understanding requires a more concrete approach. In both cases, relating on the clients' level is necessary for understanding.

Level of Health

An individual with depression may speak little because of the level of illness, and initiating and maintaining communication may be difficult. Those with mania may have unusual speech patterns, so the nurse may need to set limits. The client who has paranoia may be suspicious and difficult to bond with, whereas clients who are delirious need simple, short sentences repeated to them to communicate.

Knowledge Level

Communication is affected by the amount and kinds of facts the client has at hand. The nurse assesses the client's fund of knowledge and educational background at the time of admission. The knowledge level will dictate both teaching needs and the method of instruction. The nurse also speaks in words that are commensurate with the client's level of understanding.

Time

Counseling takes time, and the need to hurry blocks communication. Therefore, plan to interview when neither you nor the patient is pressured. Hectic times to avoid include changes of shift, visitations, doctors' rounds, or when other appointments are pending.

Daydreaming or Self-talk

People speak at a rate of 125 to 150 words a minute.[9] However, they have the ability to listen to 800 words per minute. Therefore, as the client talks, the nurse's mind may wander. Be sure to constantly attend to what the client says, to control personal thoughts, and to stay alert.

The Nurse's or Client's Feelings

Whenever the nurse or client becomes anxious, communication changes. Talking about or listening to disturbing experiences or information is uncomfortable. Therefore, be aware of anxiety in the interview and deal with it directly, both in self and in the client.

Unhelpful Communication Techniques

Nurses overcome responses that halt communication by being aware of the approach. Most of these responses consist of statements that change the focus, finalize the interview, or result in the client's feeling inadequate, threatened, or confused. Table 3–6 provides a list of communication techniques to avoid.

CASE STUDY

Juanita Hernandez, a 35-year-old Spanish immigrant, is admitted to the psychiatric hospital because she has become increasingly noncommunicative and fearful of others. According to the family, Juanita's problem began 4 weeks ago, following an unexpected encounter with an uncle who had abused her sexually when she was age 6. Following this encounter, Juanita began withdrawing, locking herself in the house, and refusing to open the door. She stopped functioning in most of her usual roles of cooking, cleaning the house, bathing, and grooming herself.

Juanita expressed concern that neighbors were plotting to set fire to her house. On the day of admission, she had loaded a shotgun and fired it out into the yard at an invisible intruder. The police investigated and notified Juanita's husband at work. He initiated commitment proceedings on the basis that Juanita is dangerous to others and is "gravely disabled."

At the hospital, Juanita continues to be fearful and suspicious of others. The nurse notes that Juanita speaks a few words of English but has difficulty expressing herself. She speaks with a thick accent and searches for words to describe her problem. The client sits alone, watching the movements of others. She

TABLE 3–6. Communication Techniques to Avoid

- **Reassurance.** A comment that indicates to the client that feelings are unwarranted. Example: "Everything will be fine. Don't worry."
- **"Why" questions.** Questions beginning with "why" that intimidate by probing or posing questions the client is unable to answer. Example: "Why do you feel that way?"
- **"Do You" questions.** Questions that arrange a "yes–no" and give the client hints about how to respond. Example: Nurse, "Do you want soup for lunch?" Client, "Yes, I want soup for lunch."
- **Agreeing.** Indicating that the client is correct before fully evaluating the facts. Example: "I agree with you" or "That's good."
- **Disagreeing.** A comment that criticizes the client and indicates disapproval. Example: "I do not think you should have done that."
- **Focusing on the self rather than the client.** A comment that allows the nurse to share experiences or feelings. Example: "I know you are angry. I get angry easily, too."
- **Defending.** A comment that explains the nurse's or other's actions. Example: "I did not mean to upset you. I was only trying to help."
- **Premature discussion.** Comments that introduce data into the interview and are not based on clues given by the client. Example: "Let's discuss your problem with your husband." (The client has not indicated a need to discuss this subject.)
- **Challenging.** A comment that stems from the nurse's belief that confronting the client will result in better perception of reality. Example: "You are not the Virgin Mary" or "If those voices were real, why can't I hear them, too?"
- **Belittling the client's feelings.** A comment that indicates the client's problem is not important. Example: "I would not worry" or "You should not feel that way."
- **Giving advice.** A comment that problem solves for the client. Example: "I think you should . . ."
- **Minimizing the problem.** A comment that indicates disrespect for the seriousness of the client's problem and conveys false reassurance. Example: "Maybe everything will be all right" or "That's not so bad."
- **Magical knowing.** Indicating understanding when not enough facts have been obtained. Example: "I see" or "I understand."
- **Global statements.** Use of vague terminology. Example: Nurse, "How are you today?" Client, "Fine." Nurse, "Good."
- **Troublesome pronouns.** Use of pronouns when the reference person has not been mentioned. Example: Client, "Nurse, he told me I could go outside." (The nurse does not know who "he" is.)

retreats to her room whenever she can and refuses to interact with anyone. When the nurse approaches her, Juanita says loudly, "Go away." Feeling rejected, the nurse leaves.

CRITICAL THINKING QUESTIONS

1. What could the nurse do to overcome the language barrier?
2. What could the nurse do to make Juanita less fearful?
3. What should the nurse do when the client says, "Go away"?
4. Why should the nurse examine her own feelings about Juanita?

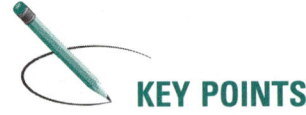

KEY POINTS

- The therapeutic relationship is the systematic interaction of a psychiatric nurse and a client for the purpose of providing psychiatric–mental health care.
- Dimensions of the therapeutic relationship include genuineness, empathy, unconditional positive regard, communication patterns, trust, and caring.
- Social and therapeutic relationships are distinctly different.
- A boundary is a line of demarcation between a therapeutic and a social relationship and serves to protect the client from practices that are beyond the typical standard of care.
- Clinical judgment and the client's needs direct the nurse in establishing boundaries.
- There are four phases of the nurse-client relationship—preorientation, orientation, working, and termination—and each has its own characteristics.
- There are four levels of communication, and each level builds upon the next: intrapersonal, interpersonal, group, and organizational.
- Elements of a model of communication include sender, receiver, message, channel, feedback, self-talk, and the time and place context.
- Specific types of communication used in psychiatric nursing include assessment interview, counseling interview, group communication, and communication with the treatment team.
- Nondirective communication techniques may be used in encouraging self-disclosure by the client.
- Several roadblocks may interfere with communication, but ultimately they produce challenges that the nurse can overcome.

REFERENCES

1. Beeber, LS: The one-to-one relationship in psychiatric nursing: The next generation. In Anderson, C (ed): Psychiatric Nursing 1946 to 1994: A Report on the State of the Art. Ohio State University, Columbus, OH, 1995.
2. Guthiel, T, and Gabbard, G: The concept of boundaries in clinical practice: Theoretical and risk-management dimensions. Am J Psychiatry 150: 188, 1993.
3. Peplau, H: Interpersonal Relationships in Nursing: A Conceptual Frame

of Reference for Psychodynamic Nursing. GP Putnam's Sons, New York, 1952.
4. Reusch, J: Therapeutic Communication. WW Norton, New York, 1961.
5. Rogers, C: Client-centered Therapy. Houghton Mifflin, Boston, 1951.
6. Kemper, BJ: Therapeutic listening: Developing the concept. Psychosoc Nurs Ment Health Serv 30:21, 1992.
7. Hays, J, and Larson, K: Interacting with Patients. Macmillan Publishing Company, Indianapolis, IN, 1963.
8. Gaw, AC: Culture, Ethnicity, and Mental Illness. American Psychiatric Press, Washington, DC, 1993.
9. Communication Research Associates: Communicate. Kendall/Hunt Publishing Company, Dubuque, IA, 1990.

UNIT Two
Etiologic Theories of Mental Illness

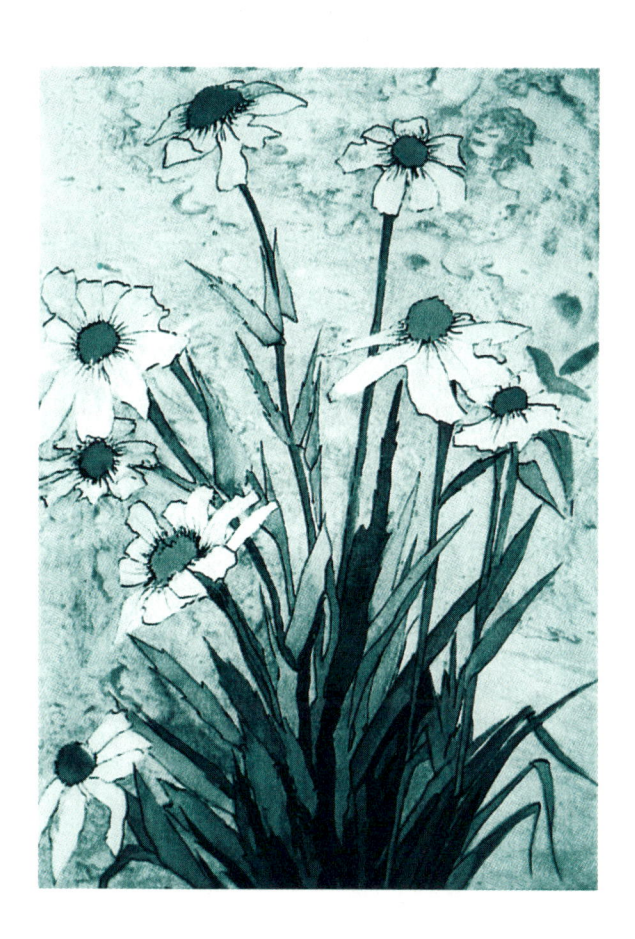

CHAPTER 4
Developmental and Psychological Theories of Mental Illness

CHAPTER 5
The Biological Basis of Mental Illness

CHAPTER 4

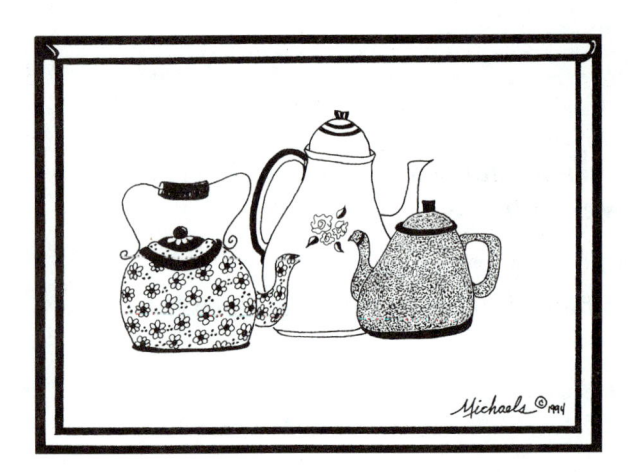

CHAPTER OUTLINE

The Psychoanalytic Theories of Development
  Freud's Psychosexual Theory
  Ego Psychology
  Object Relations Theory
Erikson's Life Cycle Theory
Piaget's Cognitive Theory of Development
Interpersonal Theories of Development
  Client-centered Therapy
  Behavioral Theories
The Emergence of a New Psychology of Women
Developmental Problems of Childhood
Developmental Problems of Adulthood
Rediscovery of the Effects of Trauma on Development
Development and Aging

LEARNING OBJECTIVES

After completing this chapter, the reader should be able to:
- List the key stages of psychological development.
- Distinguish between the different theories of normal psychological development.
- Identify developmental hypotheses about the emergence of psychopathology.
- Differentiate the major psychological theories of development.
- Understand emerging theories about women's development and distinguish them from traditional developmental theories.

KEY TERMS

conscious
defense mechanisms
development
object relations

psychosocial stages
self-in-relation theory
unconscious

Carol A. Glod, RN, CS, PhD

Developmental and Psychological Theories of Mental Illness

Developmental theories provide a basis for understanding the process of normal **development** and how psychopathology emerges. Each theory provides a framework for relating life history and past circumstances to the child's ability to function, form healthy relationships, and develop ways of understanding the world. Recent discoveries at the cellular level suggest that environment has a major impact on the developing central nervous system. Just as muscles grow and are strengthened with use, experience, and nutrition, so, too, environmental factors can foster or stress the developing brain.

Traditional views of psychological development range from the psychoanalytic theories of Sigmund Freud and Erik Erikson to the interpersonal ones of Harry Stack Sullivan and Carl Rogers. Developmental theories propose that individuals evolve through increasing levels of separation, mastery, and independence. Sigmund Freud first articulated the idea that the first 5 years of childhood have a tremendous impact on both normal and pathological development.[1] Several feminist psychologists have recently challenged existing theories and propose that traditional developmental views fail to adequately describe and reflect women's development.[2,3] Each of these theories suggests how normal and abnormal psychological development occurs.

THE PSYCHOANALYTIC THEORIES OF DEVELOPMENT

FREUD'S PSYCHOSEXUAL THEORY

Freudian theory proposes that innate sexual impulses, largely taboo and hidden from awareness, play an essential role in the psychological development of infants and children.[1] *Repression*, a key defense mechanism, serves to hide and modify early sexual thoughts from conscious awareness. Children are thought to progress through four stages of psychosexual development: the oral, anal, phallic (Oedipal), and latency stages. In Freudian theory, psychopathology emerges when problems arise during the transitions. Difficulties arise in two major ways. First, *fixation*, an arrest or interruption in the progress of psychosexual development, can occur at a particular stage. Second, the individual can "regress" to an earlier stage of development. *Regression* is a symbolic or functional return to an earlier way of acting or thinking.[4] Along with these difficulties in development come certain **defense mechanisms**, ways of protecting (defending) the self against uncomfortable urges and anxieties (Table 4–1). Anxiety arises and becomes known to the awareness (the "conscious") when repression fails. This anxiety signals an impending dangerous situation to the individual, and uncomfortable thoughts, previously hidden in the unconscious, are now forced into conscious awareness.

According to Freud's psychoanalytic theory, two major parts of the mind exist: the conscious and the unconscious. The **conscious** mind represents thoughts that are accessible to the individual, whereas the **unconscious** mind contains unwanted and uncomfortable thoughts hidden from awareness. This theory also contains the structural functions of the *id, ego,* and *superego.* The id represents the individual's innate drives and desires. Instinctual drives such as anger, aggression, and sexual impulses, considered essential to this model, are kept hidden from consciousness by defense mechanisms (see Table 4–1). The superego is thought to reflect morality and internalized parental concepts of acceptable behavior and thoughts. Ego (here, not meaning selfishness) is the integration of perception, memory, and defense mechanisms used to resolve conflict and promote psychological functioning. The ego serves to balance the instinctual drives of the id with the stringent rules and taboo behavior imposed by the superego and reality.

EGO PSYCHOLOGY

Other psychoanalytic developmental models grew out of Freud's original theories. Ego psychology, based largely on the work of Margaret Mahler,[5] emphasizes separation-individuation; the infant starts out totally dependent upon the caretaker (usually the mother) and then psychologically builds the various ego strengths necessary for separation. The child moves through various stages to develop indepen-

TABLE 4–1. Common Defense Mechanisms

Denial. Intensely avoiding unwanted or disturbing feelings or information. Common in substance and alcohol abuse.

Identification. Taking on qualities of other individuals.

Projection. Displacing an unacceptable feeling or thought onto an external source or individual. Common in paranoid clients.

Projective Identification. A form of projection in which the unacceptable feeling or thought is pinned on and assumed by another individual, who identifies with the projected feeling or thought.

Reaction Formation. Changing a feeling into its opposite to avoid the true feeling.

Regression. Returning to earlier levels of developmental functioning or ways of behaving.

Repression. A means of "forgetting" or keeping unwanted feelings, memories, and drives from consciousness so that they remain out of awareness. Common in sexual abuse survivors.

Reversal. Acting out or feeling the opposite of an impulsive wish.

Splitting. Seeing the world and individuals as "good" or "bad," "black" or "white."

Sublimation. Channeling uncomfortable feelings, memories, and drives into healthy and creative outlets.

Undoing. A way of dissolving feelings and actions by means of actions that negate or cancel out previous, uncomfortable ones; reversing a previous behavior.

---

dence. The infant moves from a state totally dependent on the mother (*autism*) to a normal state of enmeshment (*symbiosis*) and begins to differentiate at age 6 to 10 months, a time when the child begins to discover the world on his or her own. During *rapprochement* (10 to 16 months), Mahler's subphase of separation-individuation, the child displays temper tantrums, whininess, moodiness, and severe reactions to separation. Initially the child searches for the mother when separated, seeking to reconnect with her visually and physically, and then progresses to feeling more comfortable and tolerant of the separation. According to this model, the child is usually ambivalent at first, wanting to be with the caretaker, while simultaneously wanting to be separate. At this point, the child develops a sense of omnipotence, an all-powerful feeling or sense of greatness. At 2 to 3 years of age, the child develops a sense that the mother or caretaker is a separate and distinct individual, an "object." This heralds the arrival of *object constancy,* the ability to view others as separate individuals in the world. Along with this view comes the ability to distinguish and integrate "good" and "bad" aspects in a given individual or relationship. The stability of the mother-child relationship is thought to help establish her as a distinct "object" and to differentiate the child's sense of self as an autonomous, discrete entity, able to engage in flexible interpersonal relationships. The goal of psychotherapy is to help the ego overcome developmental obstacles that occur early in life, often during toddlerhood, to establish increasing levels of independence.

OBJECT RELATIONS THEORY

Object relations theory is partly based on the work of Sigmund Freud's daughter, Anna Freud. Key concepts in this model include the "good-enough mother," transitional objects, and projective identification. Winnicott[6] conceptualizes the "good-enough mother" as the caretaker who is not perfect but provides for the child's basic needs in a sufficient manner, without overly frustrating or gratifying the infant. Winnicott[6] proposes that a mother who is unable to adequately address the child's needs will foster development of a "false self" that protects the "true self" (manifested by children who can "be themselves" in the presence of their mother). *Transitional objects* serve to link the child and mother and, later in life, connect any two people, particularly in the face of separations.[6] Examples include blankets or toys that children (even adults!) keep to soothe transitions and difficult times and help them deal with isolation and separation. *Projective identification* is the unconscious projection of uncomfortable or painful feelings such as anger to another individual in order to avoid and disconnect from them.

ERIKSON'S LIFE CYCLE THEORY

Unlike other developmental theories, Eriksonian[7] theory proposes eight sequential phases of development from infancy to older adulthood. As seen in Table 4–2, each phase of normal development requires that the individual accomplish age-appropriate developmental tasks. According to this theory of **psychosocial stages**, the infant first learns to trust others for basic needs. The child then progresses through a series of distinct phases to develop autonomy, initiative, and industry. During the teenage years, identity formation is solidified. The task of young adulthood is to develop intimate relationships, whereas the task of adulthood is *generativity,* productive and creative work and loving relationships. In the last stage, old age, the individual develops a sense of integrity, accepting a sense of being complete. In Erikson's theory, individuals who fail to master a particular stage of development can return to a developmental task and relearn it.

Erikson was also one of the first developmental theorists to suggest that the interaction between caretaker and child is essential to healthy psychological growth. He proposes that although the parent raises the child, the child influences the parent:[7]

> Babies control and bring up their families as much as they are controlled by them; in fact, we may say that the family brings up the baby by being brought up by him. Whatever reaction patterns are given biologically and whatever schedule is pre-

TABLE 4–2. Erikson's Stages of Psychological Development

Stage	Task
Trust vs. mistrust	Viewing the universe as reliable and relationships as stable and available.
Autonomy vs. shame & doubt	Understanding control over one's body and thinking. Understanding disappointment in others and self.
Initiative vs. guilt	Genital issues predominate.
Industry vs. inferiority	Dealing with latency, school, and relationships outside the family.
Identity vs. role confusion	Clarifying personal identity, and depersonifying internal representations.
Intimacy vs. isolation	Rediscovering attachment and mature bonding.
Generativity vs. stagnation	Being creative, productive, and carrying out parental responsibilities.
Integrity vs. despair	Feeling a sense of completeness, based on an integrated philosophy of one's unique life.

determined developmentally must be considered to be a series of potentialities for changing patterns of mutual regulation. (p. 69)

PIAGET'S COGNITIVE THEORY OF DEVELOPMENT

Piaget's[8] major interest was to understand how children evolve ways of knowing and how they develop right and wrong answers. In Piaget's theory, infants innately possess both fixed and flexible reflexes that enable them to develop abstract intelligent behavior. Children move through four general periods of cognitive development. Infants begin in the sensory-motor stage, where feelings and actions are inseparable. At first, actions such as sucking and touching are innate. By the end of this stage, children begin to understand how their behavior affects the world; they are involved in a set of trial-and-error actions. For instance, if they reach for a toy, they will be able to hold onto it. Next, in the preoperational stage, children can maintain stable and consistent images and are able to create a representational world. They are able to fantasize and symbolically represent objects and feelings. During the operational stage, from ages 7 to 14 years, children devise rules to govern behavior, and trial and error is replaced by the ability to problem solve. In the last stage of formal operations, developing adolescents use reasoning and abstract conceptualizations to help guide future actions. In this stage they accomplish the ability to "walk in another's shoes" and can use deductive logic.

INTERPERSONAL THEORIES OF DEVELOPMENT

Harry Stack Sullivan[9] reframed developmental theory to stress the role of interpersonal relationships in shaping development. In Sullivan's theory, healthy development is based on repeated experiences between parents and children that lead to the development of a good "me self" and a bad "me self." During infancy, both good and bad self-representations are evident. In this stage, children develop a sense of sequential time in which things are causally related. To Sullivan, anxiety results from any threats to interpersonal security; that is, identity develops in the context of secure, consistent relationships.[9] In the next stage, childhood, children begin to develop interpersonal relationships with peers, language skills, and gender identity. In the juvenile stage, children expand their interactions to social, group, and societal relationships. The fourth stage, preadolescence, marks the formation of a "chum" relationship with a same-sex peer. Healthy development consists of the ability to form a meaningful nondependent relationship. Next, early adolescence heralds the development of sexuality and gender identity. Late adolescence is characterized by beginning to assume adult responsibility. Last, adulthood contains these interpersonal themes that continue to emerge in new relationships. Overall, these stages represent processes by which the individual's identity develops in the context of relationships. Because personality is shaped by previous relationships, difficulties in development are then seen as manifestations of disordered interpersonal relationships. Table 4–3 contrasts the stages of development proposed by Sullivan with those outlined by Freud and Erikson.

CLIENT-CENTERED THERAPY

Carl Rogers's[10] development of client-centered therapy marked a major shift in theories about interpersonal development. Rogers's theories are considered to be humanistic, based more on an existential philosophy of life, and in sharp contrast to the deterministic views of the developmental theories and the mechanistic ones of behaviorism. One of his major contributions was to provide a better understanding of the treatment of psychological problems. Rogers emphasized the subjective, personal, and experiential aspects of human existence and individuals' suffering. The first school of therapy designed in the United States, Rogerian therapy or client-centered therapy is a flexible approach based on an "open and accepting attitude" by the therapist. In this model, clients are viewed as active participants who take responsibility for their situation and voluntarily seek help. Specific therapeutic techniques are replaced by accurate, empathic understanding.[10] His theory stressed genuineness, warmth, empathy, and unconditional positive regard for the individ-

TABLE 4-3. Comparison of Developmental Theories of Personality

Period	Psychoanalytic Theories — Freud	Psychoanalytic Theories — Erikson	Interpersonal Theories — Sullivan
Infancy 0–12 months	Oral	Trust vs. mistrust	Infancy
Toddler 12–36 months	Anal	Autonomy vs. shame & doubt	Childhood
Preschool 3–5 years	Phallic Oedipal	Initiative vs. guilt	Childhood
School-age 5–12 years	Latency	Industry vs. inferiority	Juvenile Preadolescence
Adolescence 12–18 years		Identity vs. role confusion	Early adolescence / Late adolescence
Early Adulthood 18–25 years		Intimacy vs. isolation	Adulthood
Adulthood 26–65 years		Generativity vs. stagnation	
Older Adulthood > 65 years		Integrity vs. despair	

ual. According to Rogers, personal growth and the ability to change unhealthy ways of relating are facilitated by exhibiting openness in the relationship rather than by the removed objectivity of psychoanalytic and behavioral theories. As a result, self-disclosure on the part of the therapist plays a role in therapy based on Rogerian principles. While many of these principles are important to develop therapeutic nurse-client relationships, Rogers's theory was a radical idea initially:

> I have said that constructive personality growth and changes come about only when the client perceives and experiences a certain psychological climate in the [therapeutic] relationship. The conditions that constitute this climate do not consist of knowledge, intellectual training, orientation in some school of thought, or techniques. They are feelings or attitudes that must be experienced by the counselor and perceived by the client, if they are to be effective.[11]

BEHAVIORAL THEORIES

In contrast to the emphasis on drives, instincts, conflict, separation, and other concepts in the developmental models, behavioral theorists propose that human behavior, like that of animals, derives from behavioral principles and aversive childhood experiences. Based on observations of performance and behavior, this model is a radical departure from previous theories about how the mind works. Deriving in part from Pavlov's work in the classical conditioning of dogs, behavior theory suggests that internal responses can be changed by modifying behavior. In classical conditioning, a once-neutral stimulus becomes associated with a response, after "learning" to relate the two. In his classic experiments, Pavlov's dogs began to salivate after they "learned" to associate a bell (the neutral stimulus) with food.[12] In humans, individuals are influenced by the effect of their behaviors, and these action responses also reflect that learning. Behavior can be shaped by introducing certain stimuli that act as "reinforcers." The basis of behavioral therapy is designing strategies to help individuals unlearn problematic behaviors and substitute healthier ones.

Watson[13] is credited with defining "behaviorism," the study of only experimental and observational techniques rather than the introspection of earlier psychoanalytic models. Using "little Albert," a child without any fear of rats, as an experiment, Watson showed that the child could learn to fear rats through a series of conditioned behaviors. The rat was presented to the child, along with repeated, loud, and distressing noises. "Little Albert" learned to associate the two stimuli with fear and then, when presented with the rat alone, reacted fearfully as a result of his "conditioning." These principles are the basis for understanding the development of psychopathology. For instance, phobias or specific fears (e.g., of heights, dogs, public speaking, crowds, germs) can be learned through the tenets of conditioning and can also be unlearned through a series of specific "counterconditioning" techniques.

Skinner[14] extends Pavlovian theories to human behavior, paving the way for the development of behavior therapies. In Skinner's theory, environmental consequences of behavior determine which actions are weakened or strengthened during development. In this model, positive and negative reinforcers, those events that increase or decrease the likelihood that a given action will result, shape behavior. Thoughts and perceptions are no different from physical responses and obey the principles of stimulus, response, reinforcement, and conditioning. In this model, therapy for disturbed behaviors and psychiatric symptoms is not related to unearthing an underlying "cause" but is accomplished simply through introducing variables to shape and teach healthier behaviors. Skinner's view of problematic behaviors is quite simple: "the variables to be considered in dealing with a probability of response are simply the response itself and the independent variables of which it is a function"[14] (p. 374).

THE EMERGENCE OF A NEW PSYCHOLOGY OF WOMEN

Several psychologists at the Stone Center at Wellesley College in conjunction with others at Harvard University have

> **RESEARCH NOTE**
>
> **Williams, LM: Recall of childhood trauma: A prospective study of women's memories of child sexual abuse. Journal of Consulting and Clinical Psychology 62:1167–1176, 1994.**
>
> **Findings:** Researchers interviewed 129 adult women with previously documented histories of sexual victimization during childhood. The interviewers asked women detailed questions about their abuse histories to determine the actual rate of forgetting the traumatic events. This investigation was undertaken because recent reports have raised serious questions about the accuracy of retrospective accounts of abuse, which has led to a debate about the validity of repressed traumatic memories and the processes by which they are recovered.
>
> More than one-third (38%) of the women interviewed failed to report sexual abuse in childhood, despite clear documentation of the event in their medical records. Although some participants may have chosen to conceal the abuse that occurred a decade or more earlier, additional questions revealed that withholding of information was probably not intentional. The researchers determined that the participants did not censor their answers because of having to talk about multiple incidents of abuse. Similarly, alcohol and substance abuse was not a factor, and the use of force during the event was not associated with poor recall. From the original records of the abuse, these investigators found that, when physical evidence of genital trauma was present, more than half of the women failed to remember the abuse. Those abused at a younger age and by someone closely related were more likely to forget the traumatic events in adulthood. However, some individuals who were abused before age 3 were able to remember their abuse. Developmental theories have proposed that infant abuse before age 3 cannot be remembered because of the child's lack of capacity for language. The present study fails to support these notions.
>
> **Application to Practice:** Overall, these results suggest that forgetting documented traumatic events in childhood happens often. Having a history of previous abuse does not appear to affect whether women remember the event. Even though, during a nursing or psychiatric assessment, an individual denies the presence of early trauma, one cannot be sure that the client was not, in fact, subjected to abuse. It is possible that very young children who were abused by someone close to them are more likely to forget these incidents. These data suggest that substantial numbers of abused women may not present for psychiatric treatment but may present to health-care clinics and other professionals without remembering their trauma history. Therefore, nurses should be open and sensitive to the possibility that clients may have suffered childhood abuse, even if they deny it.

begun to develop a new paradigm for understanding women's development. In part because of ideas that emerged from the feminist movement, the developmental psychology of women proposes a distinct and novel theory for understanding how female children grow and develop. In sharp contrast to developmental theories that stress the formation of an autonomous, self-sufficient, "separate self," attained though mastery of sequential crises or stages, the psychology of women emphasizes the development of a self inseparable from dynamic interactions. In this model, the idea of "self" and "separation-individuation" are not synonymous with female development and may not be appropriate for male development either. The major tenet of the psychology of women is that development is based on maintaining a relationship with key individuals. Sometimes referred to as the **self-in-relation** theory, this idea is gaining increasing support and evidence for its validity.

Whereas Sullivan hypothesized that interpersonal relationships are key to female development, the psychologists based at the Stone Center suggest a more complex relational dynamic. In infancy, the child is actively paying attention to and responding to the caretaker. In this way, development is based more on the relatedness to another individual rather than on a loss of part of oneself. Self-esteem emerges when the individual feels a part of relationships and takes care of those relationships, themes that emerge early in life. In early childhood, a more complex sense of self develops in response to more complex relationships with others.[2] Also, during that time healthy development is characterized by increasing caring and relatedness between the child and the caretaker. In adolescence, a conflict ensues but, unlike the traditional notions of puberty, this model proposes that the sense of self is in conflict with the need to remain connected in the relationship. The conflict is between the teenage girl's own desires and the needs and desires of the relationship. For instance, girls learn that their sexuality is wrong, bad, evil, dirty, and shameful, putting their own needs in conflict with the interpersonal needs of the "other" (the boy) in a relationship. Miller[2] suggests that in adolescence, girls "shut down," whereas boys "open up."

Although many of these ideas are still under development, this concept of female development challenges previously held beliefs. The goal of treatment for women who experience psychological difficulties is not for them to develop more separateness or independence, but to value themselves and their uniquely feminine perceptions and desires, while finding others who will relate to them in that same manner.[2] This theory suggests that women more than men want to talk about relationships, yet according to the psychoanalytic models, such desires may be viewed as dependency. It also

> Levant and Pollack, prompted partly by the feminist critiques of women's psychological development, challenge some of the traditional views of men's development. A central component of classic theories is that healthy development results in a separate autonomous self, achieved by the child's disconnection with the mother. The authors suggest that the development of male autonomy needs to be balanced with the need to feel intimate and understood by others. Shame and fear may prevent some men from acknowledging these needs and desires because of child-rearing biases that teach boys to be strong and invulnerable. This fear may lead to the male child's suppression of loving and connected feelings to females and other males. Levant and Pollack suggest that men are "not self-sufficient loners who care for no one else. They are frightened searchers, looking to connect but very unsure of what safety net they need should the connection go awry." The authors propose that male children's separation from others may lead to difficulties in relationships later in life. For instance, men may be less capable of displaying empathy and intimacy. In this new model, typical male traits such as aggression and autonomy can remain valuable, but not to the exclusion of connection to others.
>
> **Source**: From Levant, RF, and Pollack, WS: A New Psychology of Men. New York, Basic Books, 1995.

implies that the goal for women is not to develop more independence (and hence less dependence) but to be engaged in relationships. This framework suggests that women strive to really comprehend other people, understand another's feelings, and contribute to the well-being of others. Carol Gilligan,[3] in her studies of girls, proposes that women's sense of self and morality revolves around the responsibility for, care of, and inclusion of other individuals. Overall, in this model, the female child's capacity for healthy development is based on engagement with others, mutuality, empathic relating, and "relational growth."

DEVELOPMENTAL PROBLEMS OF CHILDHOOD

Developmental theories provide a mechanism for examining problems in physical, neurological, sensory-motor, cognitive, and affective development in childhood. Developmental delays may occur in any of these areas. Infants who are unable to turn over by themselves at age 4 months or sit by age 6 months may evidence these delays. By 10 months, children can usually grasp objects in both hands, and by the time they reach their first birthday, they have usually mastered standing and walking. Also at this time, the infant can attend selectively to specific individuals. Between 10 and 16 months, children are continuing to develop motor skills, moving around, and exploring their environments, with comfortable separation from the major caretaker evident by age 3. Because motor and cognitive behaviors are influenced by the environment, healthy child-rearing factors such as adequate nutrition, nurturing behaviors, healthy interaction, and time for play, feeding, and sleep need to be assessed. Developmental language delays may present as early as the first year of life, when the child begins to produce sounds and to attend selectively to sound and visual stimuli in the environment. Language then develops rapidly, and abnormalities may be found in 2-year-olds who are unable to use single words to communicate. If the 3-year-old child is unable to speak three- to six-word phrases, developmental delays are evident.

Similarly, 3-year-old children can be expected to use language to communicate their needs and investigate the world that surrounds them. They are "social beings." Children who are unable to behave in limited social situations, cooperate with rules, take turns, share playthings, or participate in fantasy play may be experiencing other psychological problems. Again, normal developmental task achievement provides the framework for assessing difficulties or delays in each domain. However, temporary lags that can resolve over time may occur in an individual child.

In middle childhood, developmental shifts continue. Relationships outside the family—for example, with peers and teachers—expand, and children develop a relationship with a "best friend." Social withdrawal or inhibition of these relationships may reflect anxiety or depressive disorders. Although 6-year-old children can be very emotional and display angry outbursts, sustained irritability may be a sign that a more serious problem, such as depression, is emerging. Because earlier developmental theories proposed that latency-aged children are incapable of abstract reasoning, it was thought that depression did not occur in young children. Current views suggest that depression with adult characteristics can arise in middle childhood. School phobias and separation anxiety may be most prominent at the beginning of middle childhood as the child develops more social relationships and enters school.

Adolescence marks a time of major turmoil, accompanying physical, social, and affective growth. Distinguishing between "normal" behaviors and moods and signs of greater difficulties can be difficult for even experienced nurses. Several themes tend to characterize developmental progress during puberty. Although teenagers are striving for and gaining independence, they remain ambivalent about their dependence on parents, teachers, and other authority figures. This ambivalence represents a normal developmental struggle to separate from family and develop and pursue individual goals. During this time, experimentation with drugs, sexuality, and challenging rules generally occurs. However, defiant behavior and more severe actions, such as stealing, truancy, starting fights, or consistent lying, may signal the development of a psychiatric disorder, for example, substance abuse, conduct disorder, or oppositional defiant disorder.

Adolescents can also be expected to join peer groups and identify with friends through dress, hairstyle, and language. The development of identity, including sexual identity and role, should occur at this time. Although teenagers tend to be attracted to groups, they have a simultaneous need for privacy, which should be distinguished from ongoing lack of interactions with others or extreme social withdrawal, which may reflect the emergence of depression or schizophrenia. Mood shifts can be common during this phase of development; however, in the extreme, combined with changes in sleep, appetite, and energy, these mood swings may reflect the beginning of bipolar mood disorder.

DEVELOPMENTAL PROBLEMS OF ADULTHOOD

Developmental theories have contributed to the outdated classifications of neuroses and psychoses. For instance, hysterical neurosis was presumed to result from repression of unwanted sexual drives and urges. Despite emerging evidence for biological and genetic bases for disorders, some personality disorders are still thought to arise from key developmental difficulties. The most notable are borderline personality and narcissistic personality, both characterized by severe disturbances in the ability to relate interpersonally. In fact, their diagnostic criteria are partly based on deficits in developmental phases.

In borderline personality disorder, developmental theories focus on concepts of object constancy and splitting. Instead of developing *object constancy,* people lack the ability to "hold onto" and internalize the image of the mother (or other significant relationships) in her absence. In essence, the individual views others as "out of sight, out of mind." Instead of developing a consistent, cohesive sense of self and others, the individual with borderline personality disorder uses *splitting* to divide the world into "good" or "bad" parts. One of the key features of this disorder is the tendency to use the defense mechanism of splitting to an extreme degree. Individuals are either idealized or devalued. The ability to tolerate ambivalence—the notions that good and bad are contained in the same object or that good and bad feelings exist in themselves—is problematic. As a result of these developmental impairments, severe conflicts arise in relationships, and images of the good self and bad self fail to be integrated. Severe shifts in mood and anger also result.

Narcissistic personality disorder arises from the infant's concern with the self and with being in love with himself or herself. In healthy development, the child becomes less self-absorbed, less omnipotent, and more able to love others for who they are. Narcissism implies an arrest or regression to this stage in which others are viewed as "love objects." These objects are actually narcissistic ties to maintain the individual's sense of self-esteem. Instead of developing a healthy ego, individuals depend on others to define their sense of self and their very being.

REDISCOVERY OF THE EFFECTS OF TRAUMA ON DEVELOPMENT

Early developmental theorists largely ignored the important role of severe psychological trauma on the developing self. However, several theorists, including Janet,[15] observed that acute and chronic forms of trauma were associated with psychological difficulty and could lead to disturbances in personality development. Although the effects of severe trauma secondary to combat experiences, physical and sexual abuse, and natural disasters have been well described (see Chapter 22), the effects of trauma upon development have only recently been rediscovered; the *repetition of trauma* is an emerging theme. For instance, a woman who was sexually abused in childhood marries a man who repeatedly batters her and her child. The early traumatic experience during childhood continues to be reenacted during adulthood in intimate relationships.

The connection between trauma and dissociation is also gaining widespread attention. Dissociation can range from feelings of unreality or detachment to the actual fragmentation of personality as seen in dissociative identity disorder, such as the well-publicized case of "Sybil." Dissociation can also be conceptualized as a combination of repression and denial used to protect the developing self from intolerable and unbearable situations. The child who is subjected to repeated acts of severe abuse "dissociates" from the experience, blocking out awareness of the traumatic event, emotions about it, and memories of it, which interferes with normal development. Although some question the validity of "repressed memories," recent studies have shown that severe documented episodes of abuse were forgotten (i.e., repressed) by about one-third of adult women (see Research Note).

DEVELOPMENT AND AGING

Until the nineteenth century, human life expectancy remained fairly constant, but since the 1960s, it has increased. With longer lifespan comes increased risk for physical deterioration and certain psychiatric conditions. However, the majority of healthy older adults continue to remain active and healthy, and a major nursing role is to carefully distinguish between "normal" signs of aging and changes related to specific disease processes. Age affects hearing, vision, renal function, systolic blood pressure, bone density, pulmonary function, glucose tolerance, immune function, sympathetic nervous system activity, performance speed, and certain cognitive parameters. Although some minor memory loss occurs with aging, signs of memory disruption usually signal the beginning of more disabling conditions such as dementia. Similarly, other cognitive abilities such as language, spatial or temporal orientation, judgment, and abstract thought remain intact in later life, whereas impairment in these areas is evidence of more serious problems such as dementia. Memory impairment occurs in about 5% of elderly individuals living within the community, with a higher prevalence among nursing home residents.

In later life, adults face a series of losses, including a decline in physical abilities, retirement, death of friends and spouses, and increased potential for isolation. Suicide risk increases with lack of social and emotional ties, loneliness, and bereavement; older widowed men are at highest risk for suicide. Nurses evaluating older adults should allow patients extra time because of visual, hearing, and functional impairments. Focus on what the client can do, relative to what they should be able to do or on what they want to do. A complete review of systems, medications, and functional ability may uncover reversible factors that are contributing to impairment. The major task is to help elderly individuals maintain the highest levels of functioning and to promote their mental and physical health status.

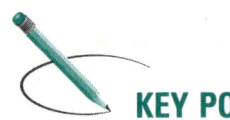

KEY POINTS

- Development theories propose that individuals evolve through stages consisting of increasing levels of separation, mastery, and independence.
- Freudian theory proposes that children progress through four stages of psychosexual development: oral, anal, phallic (Oedipal), and latency.
- Erikson's life cycle theory proposes eight sequential phases of development from infancy to old age.
- Object relations theory and ego psychology focus on the child's emotional relationship with the major caretaker, the so-called object.
- Piaget's theory of cognitive development suggests that children progress through four general periods of intellectual development: sensory-motor, preoperational, concrete operational, and formal operational.
- Harry Stack Sullivan reframed development theory to stress the role of interpersonal relationships.
- Carl Rogers's theories are considered humanistic and based on an existential philosophy of life. According to Rogers, personal growth and the ability to change unhealthy ways of relating are facilitated by the therapist exhibiting an openness in the therapeutic relationship rather than the removed objectivity of psychoanalytic and behavioral theories.
- Behavioral theories suggest that internal responses can be changed by modifying behavior.
- A new paradigm for understanding women's development, the "self-in-relation" theory, suggests that women's development is based on maintaining close relationships with key individuals instead of forming an autonomous "separate self."
- The recent rediscovery of the effects of early childhood experiences suggests that sexual and physical abuse severely affect development, leading to dissociation and a tendency to reenact abusive relationships repeatedly in adulthood.
- Developmental theories provide a mechanism for examining problems in physical, neurological, sensory-motor, cognitive, and affective development throughout the lifespan of the individual.

REFERENCES

1. Freud, S: Inhibitions, symptoms and anxiety. In Strachey, J (ed, trans): The Standard Edition of the Complete Psychological Works of Sigmund Freud, Vol 18. Hogarth Press, London, 1959, pp. 1–64.
2. Miller, JB: The development of women's sense of self. In Jordan, JV, et al (eds): Women's Growth in Connection. Guilford Press, New York, 1991, pp. 11–26.
3. Gilligan, C: In a Different Voice: Psychological Theory and Women's Development. Harvard University Press, Cambridge, MA, 1982.
4. Shapiro, T, and Hertzig, ME: Normal child and adolescent development. In Hales, R, Yudofsky, SC, and Talbott, JA (eds): Textbook of Psychiatry, ed 2. American Psychiatric Press, Washington, DC, 1994, pp. 105–142.
5. Mahler, MS, Pine, F, and Bergman, A: The Psychological Birth of the Human Infant: Symbiosis and Individuation. Basic Books, New York, 1975.
6. Winnicott, DW: The Maturational Processes and the Facilitating Environment. Hogarth/Institute of Psycho-Analysis, London, 1965.
7. Erikson, E: Childhood and Society, ed 2, rev. WW Norton & Co. Inc, New York, 1963.
8. Piaget, J: Origins of Intelligence in Children, trans. Cook, M. International Universities Press, New York, 1952.
9. Sullivan, HS: The Interpersonal Theory of Psychiatry. WW Norton & Co Inc, New York, 1953.
10. Rogers, CR: Client-Centered Therapy. Houghton Mifflin, Boston, 1951.
11. Rogers, CR: The interpersonal relationship: The core of guidance. Harv Educ Rev 416, 1962.
12. Pavlov, IP: Conditioned Reflexes: An Investigation of the Physiological Activity of the Cerebral Cortex. Oxford University Press Inc, New York, 1927.
13. Watson, J: Psychology from the Standpoint of a Behaviorist. JB Lippincott Co., Philadelphia, PA, 1919.
14. Skinner, BF: Science and Human Behavior. Macmillan, New York, 1953.
15. Janet, P: The Mental State of Hystericals. Alcan, Paris, 1911.

CHAPTER 5

The Biological Basis of Mental Illness

CHAPTER 5

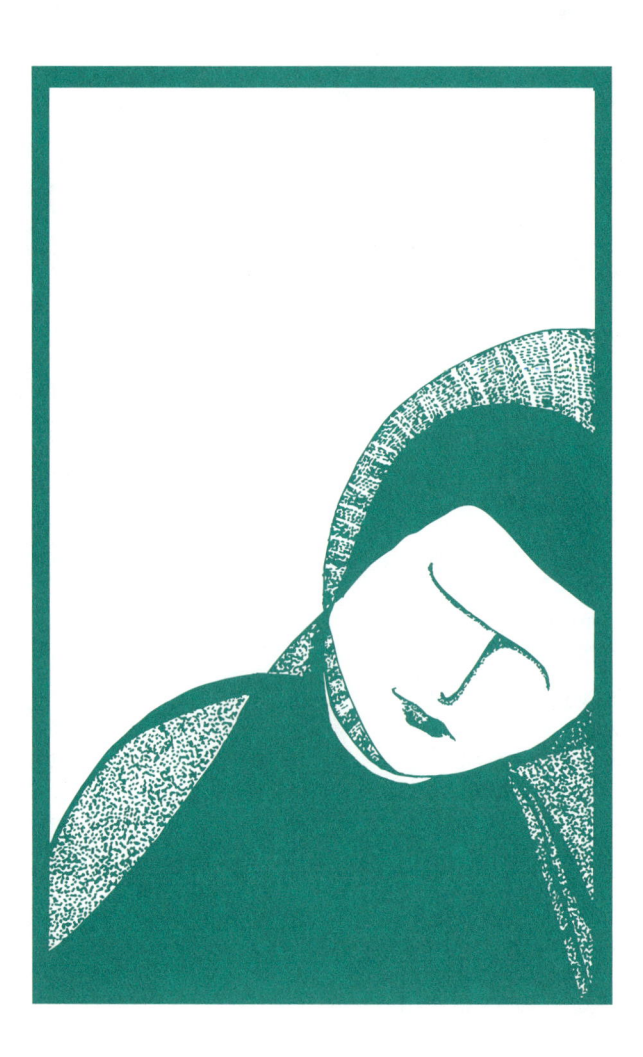

CHAPTER OUTLINE

Neuroanatomy
 Membranes
 Convoluted Surface
 Two Hemispheres
 Cortex
 Frontal Cortex
 Limbic System
 Basal Ganglia
 Diencephalon
Basic Properties of Neurotransmission
 Structure and Activity of a Neuron
 Synthesis and Storage
 Release
 Response
 Inactivation
Specific Neurotransmitters
 Biogenic Amines
 Cholinergics
 Neuropeptides
 Amino Acids
Tools of the Trade
Genetics and Heredity
Circadian Rhythms and Mental Illness
Psychoneuroimmunology
 HPA Axis Functioning
 Immune Function and Mental Illness

Susan L. Anderson, PhD

The Biological Basis of Mental Illness

LEARNING OBJECTIVES

After completing this chapter, the reader should be able to:

- List major structures of the brain and their relationship to mood, activity, and other physiological and psychological factors.
- Explain the relationship between the brain, its chemistry, and psychiatric illness.
- Discuss relationships between stress, immune system functioning, and psychiatric illness.
- Identify the basic structures of a neuron and describe the process of neurotransmission as it relates to treatment of mental illness.
- Understand the advantages and disadvantages of the various neuroimaging techniques.

KEY TERMS

catecholamines
corpus callosum
dendrite
dura mater
hemispheres
indolamines
myelin
neurotransmitters
receptor
reuptake
synapse
ventricles

Terry B. is a 40-year-old man who first started showing unusual behavior in his teens. As a child he was somewhat quiet and withdrawn but excelled in school and demonstrated high intelligence. In adolescence he began to hear "God's voice" telling him he had unique powers. Although he was accepted to a prestigious college, he failed to complete his first semester. He sat for hours staring out of his window, concocted bizarre outlines for required college papers, and began to "see" people following him. As his behavior became more bizarre, he stopped attending class and failed to follow through on assignments. One night, he paraded through the campus naked, screaming unintelligible remarks. He was examined in the school infirmary and transferred to a psychiatric unit for further evaluation and care.

Terry's parents described their ordeal as terrifying because the professionals "criticized" them for his difficulties. Adding to their feelings of guilt, a social worker initially told them that Terry was schizophrenic, that there was little hope for recovery, and that his early childhood experiences were responsible for his symptoms. His mother remembers feeling that she "caused" his problems.

In later years, with the help of psychiatric nurses and other mental health professionals, she found out that schizophrenia may be caused by certain biological or brain abnormalities and tends to be inherited in families. Terry's parents joined a support group, the National Alliance for the Mentally Ill (NAMI), and learned more about their son's illness. In addition to defining schizophrenia as a "brain disorder" rather than the result of parenting deficits, this group provided the information and support they needed to cope with their son's debilitating disorder. They were also able to join national efforts to promote a better understanding of schizophrenia as a disease with a biological basis.

Men ought to know that from the brain, and from the brain only, arise our pleasures, joys, laughter, and jests, as well as our sorrows, pains, griefs, and fears. Through it, in particular, we think, see, hear. . . .

—HIPPOCRATES

Since Congress declared the years 1990 to 2000 as "The Decade of the Brain," psychiatric nurses have been exposed to increasing amounts of information about the brain. To use the panoply of drug therapies to treat mental illness and the brain-imaging techniques that offer new insights into brain dysfunction during the course of the illness, nurses should have a basic understanding of the various brain regions and their specific chemical messengers to clarify how their function or dysfunction results in mental illness. With this knowledge, psychiatric nurses can help to educate and treat their clients and improve their overall quality of life.

NEUROANATOMY

The brain (shown in the color figures) is composed of many different smaller systems (Figure 5–1). These systems inter-

76 Etiologic Theories of Mental Illness

connect to form complicated networks that allow us to perform sophisticated actions or think abstractly. Because the expression of who we are is a culmination of many different brain areas interacting to affect behavior, emotion, and cognition,[1] damage to any single part of the brain has significant effects on our quality of life.[2]

MEMBRANES

The brain is encased in the skull to protect it from damage and is further protected within a layer of durable membranes. These membranes are known collectively as the *meninges*, the inflammation of which is *meningitis*. The outer membrane, the **dura mater**, a leatherlike covering, is the thickest. Beneath the dura are the thinner protective membranes, the *arachnoid* and *pia mater*. The arachnoid matter is named because it resembles a spider's web; the innermost layer, the pia mater, is soft and very thin.

The brain has another major form of defense, *the blood-brain barrier*. Proteins and other molecules circulating in blood vessels cannot leave the blood and enter the brain tissue. The blood-brain barrier, a significant obstacle for a number of drugs, is discussed in Chapter 6. Blood traveling through the brain carries oxygen and nutrients such as glucose and dietary amino acids. A second fluid, *cerebrospinal fluid (CSF)*, is found within hollow cavities of the brain, called **ventricles**, and around the outside of the brain between the dura mater and the skull. CSF acts as a shock absorber and permits some nutrient exchange. It also circulates into the spinal column and is the fluid collected by a lumbar puncture (a spinal tap) to evaluate the chemicals in the brain.

CONVOLUTED SURFACE

The human brain is convoluted to provide a maximum surface area, more than 2.5 ft^2, which increases our capacity to store information. The "grooves" are called *sulci* (the singular form is *sulcus*), and the "bumps" are referred to as *gyri* (singular, *gyrus*). The main sulcus that divides the brain is the midsagittal fissure, and the lateral fissure subdivides the hemispheres. Loss of this convoluted structure (and thus loss of information) is apparent in different disease states.

TWO HEMISPHERES

The brain is divided into two **hemispheres** and, except for the pineal gland, all of the cortical lobes and definitive structures are found in both hemispheres. The two lobes are interconnected by a number of pathways, especially the **corpus callosum**. This pathway is sometimes surgically cut to prevent seizures on one side of the brain from spreading to the opposite side, which has led to the interesting discovery of hemispheric dominance. The Nobel prize–winning work of Roger Sperry that began in the 1950s led to the concept of *hemispheric laterality*. The left hemisphere is dominant for "more scientific functions"—that is, language, complex voluntary movement, reading, writing, and mathematical tasks. Associated with the "conscious self," this side is involved in decision making. In contrast, the right hemisphere is more "artistic" and specializes in nonlanguage-based tasks, including visual, tactile, and auditory pattern recognition, intuition, and sense of direction. Furthermore, the left hemisphere controls the right side of the body, whereas the right hemisphere controls the left side.

CORTEX

The cortex, the most complex structure in the brain, is composed of six distinct layers of different cell types (Figure 5–2). Overall, the cortex is the area of higher-level thinking and is intimately involved in the qualities that make us human, including our ability to use language and think abstractly. The cortex forms associations by integrating information that it receives from sensory stimuli (sight, hearing, smell, taste, and touch) and motor stimuli (body position) with memories and past patterns of behavior to evaluate a situation and decide on an output.

The cortex can be divided into many subregions, based on a number of functions. The most basic divisions are the frontal, parietal, occipital, and temporal lobes (Figure 5–3). From the 1940 to 1970, neurosurgeon Wilder Penfield and others mapped brain structure and function by repeatedly stimulating electrically a specific area of the cortex in awake clients. Instead of pain, which the brain itself cannot feel, clients reported detailed hallucinatory sights and sounds.

Brain

Systems:	Cerebrum	Diencephalon	Basal Ganglia	Limbic System	Brain Stem	Cerebellum
Function:	Higher-level thought	Integration; modulation	Motor	Emotions	Vital life functions	Muscle synergy
Brain Regions:	Frontal Parietal Occipital Temporal	Thalamus Hypothalamus Pineal Gland	Caudate Putamen Globus Pallidus	Hippocampus Amygdala Fornix	Midbrain Pons Medulla Oblongata Reticular Formation	

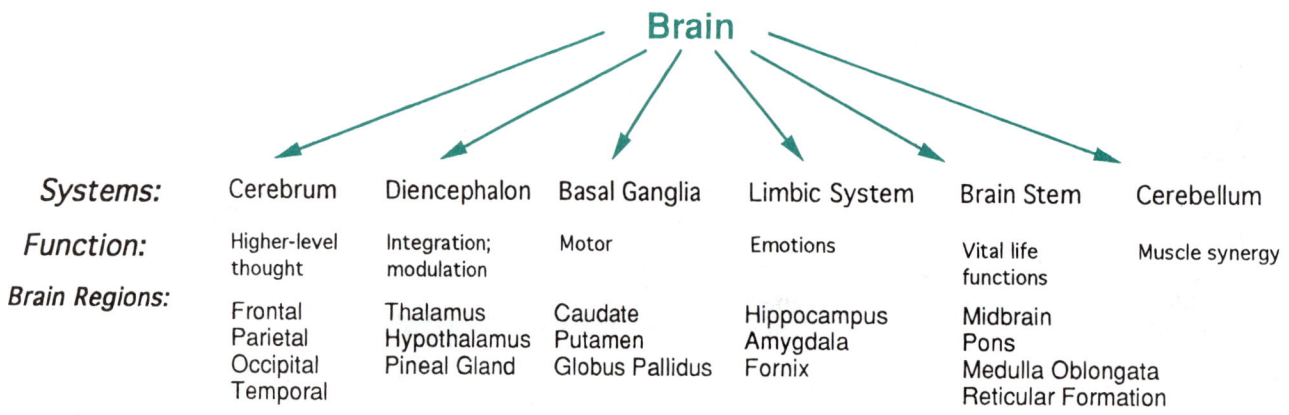

Figure 5–1. Diagram illustrating the division of the brain into smaller systems that are composed of individual brain areas.

1. Molecular layer
2. External granular layer
3. Pyramidal cell layer
4. Internal granular layer
5. Ganglionic layer
6. Polymorphonuclear cells

Golgi-Stained   Nissl-Stained

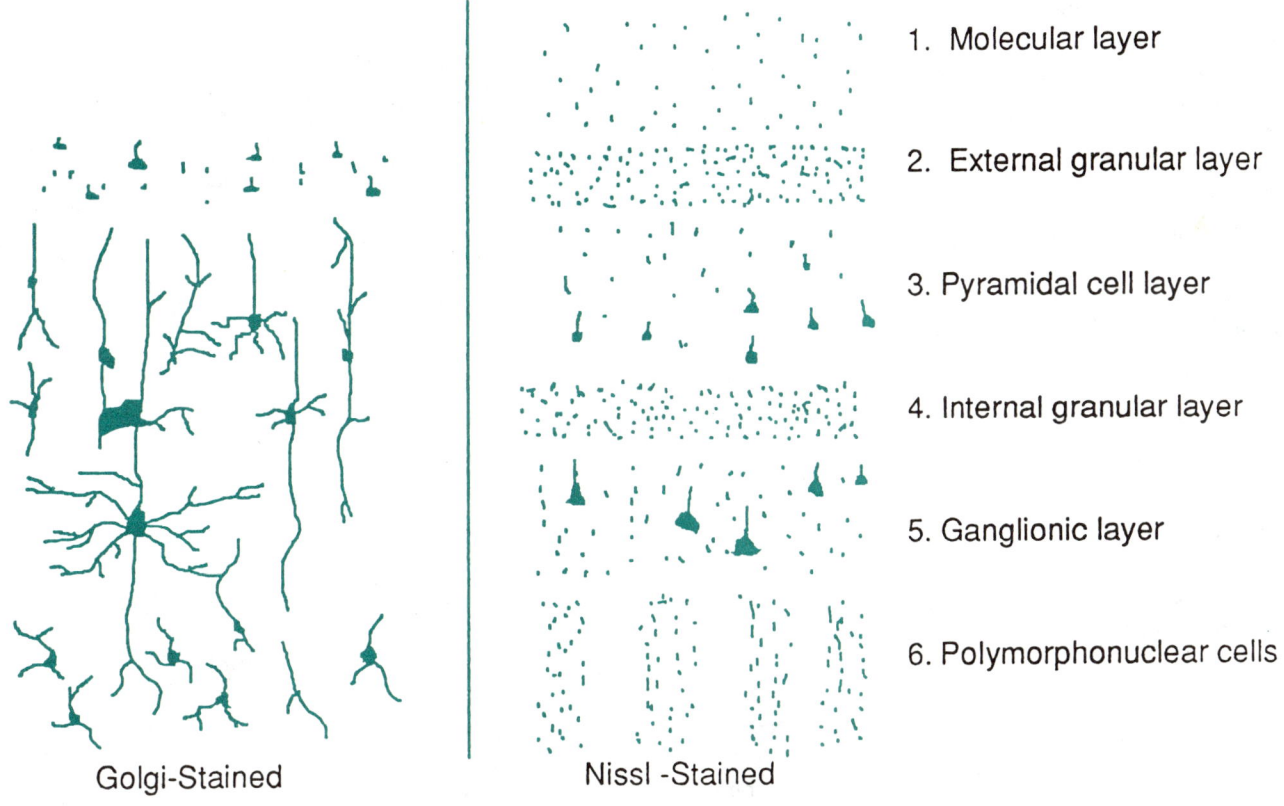

Figure 5–2. Schematic of the six different layers of cells in the cortex (specifically, the primary visual cortex). Two different methods of staining the tissue were used to show different parts of the neuron. A golgi stain illustrates a whole neuron but stains fewer than 1 in a 1000 neurons. To better estimate how many neurons are in an area, a Nissl stain, which stains everything, is used. Adapted from D'Armond, SJ, Fusco, MM, and Dewey, MM: Structure of the Human Brain: A Photographic Atlas. New York: Oxford University Press, 1974.

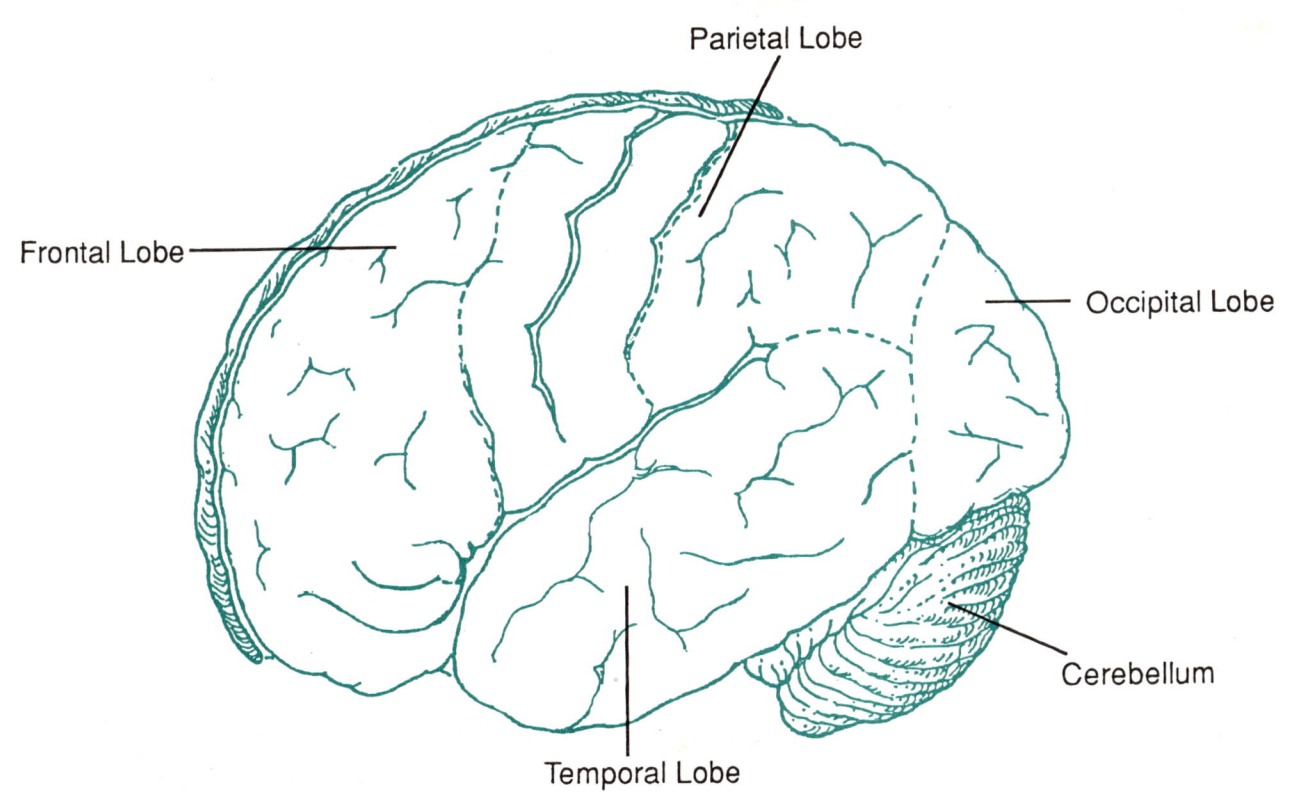

Figure 5–3. The four major divisions of the cortex: frontal, parietal, occipital, and temporal lobes.

For example, a young client of Penfield reported, "I think I heard a mother calling her little boy somewhere. It seemed to be something that happened years ago . . . in the neighborhood where I lived." Sensory input from all body regions is mapped onto very specific regions in the brain (Figure 5–4). Areas of the body that have greater sensitivity, such as the lips and hands, are mapped to a larger proportion of the cortex. This map is known as a *homunculus* (the "little man"). Motor pathways are mapped similarly.

FRONTAL CORTEX

The frontal cortex is the most highly integrated brain area and the last to mature in the mammalian brain. Input from all areas of the brain travels to the cortex, which integrates information about body position, memories, arousal states, and emotions. This combined information helps regulate arousal, focuses our attention, and allows us to make decisions before actions.

The case of Phineas Gage in the early 1900s demonstrates the importance of the frontal cortex. A railroad tie accidentally struck him and damaged his frontal lobes. After this event, he was reported to be uncharacteristically undependable, inattentive, and impulsive. In the 1950s, frontal lobotomies were performed to reduce clients' inappropriate social behavior, but this surgery also deprived them of their human qualities and capabilities. Abnormalities in the frontal cortex play a role in a number of mental illnesses, including schizophrenia, attention deficit hyperactivity disorder (ADHD), and various dementias, sometimes referred to as "frontal dementias" because clients' affect is noticeably blunt.

The remaining three lobes are known as "association areas" because they integrate sensory and motor information. The parietal and the temporal lobes help individuals focus on environmental events. In addition to their higher-level processing of integrated information, the lobes receive specialized information. Specifically, the parietal lobe receives and integrates information about taste and touch, the temporal lobe integrates smell and hearing, and the occipital lobe is involved in the perception of visual input. Because of its proximity to a set of brain areas known collectively as the *limbic system*, the temporal lobe plays a role in memory and emotional functioning. The occipital lobe receives information from the eyes indirectly and recreates the whole image, which aids in depth perception. The occipital lobe is also responsible for the "stars" people see when they bump their heads, owing to the stimulation of the visual pathways. Alterations in the occipital lobe have been observed in individuals with schizophrenia, although these changes may be secondary to the primary disorder.

LIMBIC SYSTEM

The limbic system, located under the cortex, is composed of the hippocampus, amygdala, and fornix. The limbic system controls emotion, memory, and learning and mediates feelings of aggression, sexual impulses, and submissive behaviors. Disturbances in the limbic system have been implicated in a number of mental illnesses. Damage to the hippocampus greatly reduces a person's ability to learn new information. Because the hippocampus is the site where new information is consolidated into memories, its loss is most apparent in individuals with Alzheimer's disease (see Chapter 15). One of the characteristic indices of neuronal destruction in this area is the presence of plaques and tangles in the brains of people with Alzheimer's disease. The amygdala mediates fear and aggression; studies in animals show that damage to the amygdala results in fearlessness and plays a role in aggressive behaviors. The loss of this tissue in chronic alcoholics who have Korsakoff's syndrome prevents the formation of new memories. The fornix is a neuronal pathway between the hippocampus and the hypothalamus.

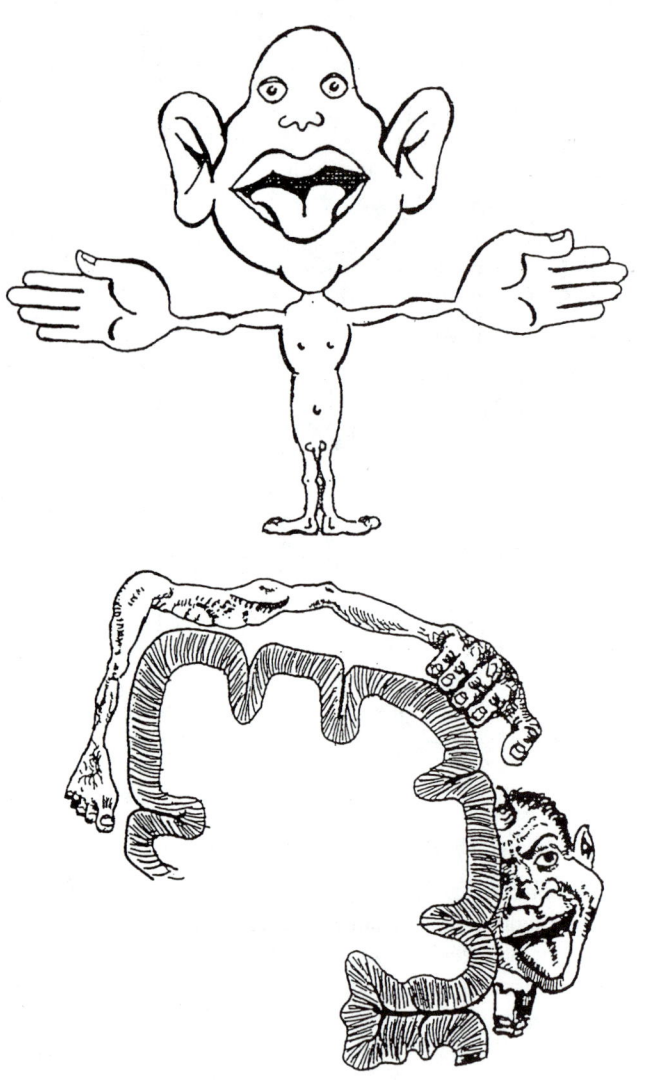

Figure 5–4. A homunculus of the human brain. Also known as the "little man," the size of various structures represents the cortical area devoted to the processing of sensory and motor information. (Artwork by Dr. M. Didier, McLean Hospital.)

BASAL GANGLIA

The basal ganglia initiates and controls activity, muscle tone, posture, and muscle movements and works primarily to inhibit motor movements. The specific regions of this system are the caudate, putamen, and the globus pallidus. This system is also known as the *extrapyramidal system*. Before movement occurs, the basal ganglia receives and integrates information from lower regions of the brain, such as the thalamus and the substantia nigra, as well as higher regions, such as the cerebral cortex.

Among the diseases associated with the basal ganglia is obsessive-compulsive disorder (OCD). It is also related to some of the major motor tics and other motor side effects such as extrapyramidal symptoms due to antipsychotic medications (see Chapter 6). Dysfunction of this system is mainly associated with motion-based diseases, although dementia is an unfortunate accompaniment in the final stages. The loss of a specific part of the basal ganglia, the substantia nigra, occurs in Parkinson's disease, in which approximately 90% of these neurons have degenerated before muscular rigidity is apparent.

Huntington's disease is more dramatic. Several brain areas atrophy and the ventricles widen as a result of the missing tissue. Although clients at risk can be identified from genetic markers found in DNA, given the debilitating course of the illness, both physically and mentally, few family members at risk have chosen genetic analysis in order to know their fate.

DIENCEPHALON

The thalamus, hypothalamus, and pineal gland comprise the diencephalon. The thalamus serves as a large relay center through which all sensory information passes en route to various cortical areas. The thalamus is divided into more than 20 regions, and information is integrated and segregated before reaching its destination. Recent research on individuals with schizophrenia suggests that dysfunction in the thalamus may mediate difficulties in integrating information, possibly playing a role in thought disorder.

Located below the thalamus, the hypothalamus is the control center for endocrine, somatic, and autonomic functions. Hormones from the hypothalamus are released into the bloodstream, and these chemicals modulate feeding, drinking, salt balance, sexual activity, body temperature, cardiac function, and feelings of fear and rage. For instance, the hypothalamus partially mediates aggression associated with steroid use.

Once described as the "seed of the soul" by Descartes, the pineal gland is the only unpaired structure in the brain. It secretes melatonin, a hormone that affects the sleep-wake cycle, and has the largest concentration of serotonin. The pineal gland, melatonin, and circadian rhythms are discussed later in this chapter.

BASIC PROPERTIES OF NEUROTRANSMISSION

STRUCTURE AND ACTIVITY OF A NEURON

In *neurotransmission*, information transfers between brain regions through neurons,[3] which "talk" to each other in one of two ways. The first form of communication is electrical, via a process known as an *action potential* (Figure 5–5). An action potential is the exchange of an electrical charge across

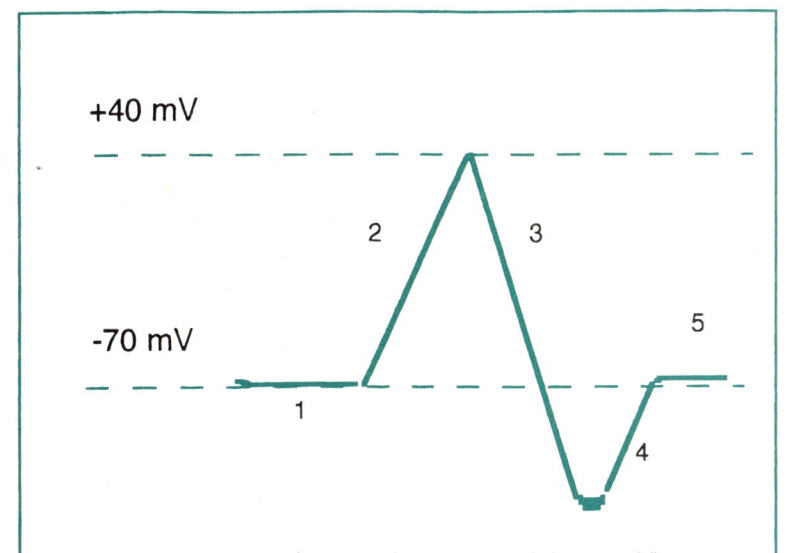

1. Neuron is at resting membrane potential (-70 mV).
2. Electrical charge causes Na+ channels to open, causing the membrane to become ++ charged (+40 MV).
3. K+ ions leave neuron to reestablish negative potential.
4. Na+ and K+ return to normal concentrations across the membrane.
5. Resting membrane potential is reestablished.

Figure 5–5. A schematic of an action potential.

TABLE 5–1. General Neurochemical Effects and Treatments

Neurotransmitter System	Receptor Subtypes	Disease	Example Drug	Mechanism
Dopamine	D_1, D_2, D_3, D_4, and D_5	Schizophrenia	Haloperidol	D_2 antagonist
		ADHD	Methylphenidate	Indirect agonist
Norepinephrine	α_1 (A, B, C, D)	Posttraumatic stress disorder	Clonidine	α_2 antagonist
	α_2 (A, B, C, D)			
	β_1; β_2			
Serotonin	$5\text{-}HT_{1(A,B,C,D,F,P,R,S)}$	Depression	Fluoxetine	Uptake blocker
	$5\text{-}HT_{2(A,B,C,F)}$		Sertraline	
	$5\text{-}HT_3$, $5\text{-}HT_4$, $5\text{-}HT_{(A,B)}$			
	$5\text{-}HT_6$, $5\text{-}HT_7$			
Acetylcholine	M_1, M_2, M_3, M_4, M_5	Alzheimer's disease	Tacrine	Cholinesterase inhibitor
	N (6 α and 3 β subtypes)			
GABA	GABA-A and GABA-B	Anxiety disorders	Diazepam	GABA-A antagonist
Mixed neurotransmitter pharmacotherapy	D_4 and $5\text{-}HT_2$	Schizophrenia	Risperidone	D_4 antagonist
			Clozapine	$5\text{-}HT_2$ antagonist

the membrane of a neuron, allowing information to travel from one part of the neuron to its end. The transfer of information between neurons occurs in a series of steps. First, chemical messengers from the previous neuron arrive at a receptive area, the **dendrite**, of the next neuron. The chemical information is either excitatory, inhibitory, or a combination of excitatory and inhibitory. After the dendrite is stimulated, the information travels to the cell body. If the sum of all of the information is sufficiently excitatory, an action potential is initiated. The neuron then becomes positively charged, a process referred to as *depolarization*, and the action potential, in the form of electrical energy, travels down the axon to the nerve terminal. Information generally flows from the cell body to the terminal region in one direction, with few exceptions.

The speed at which the message reaches the nerve terminal depends on the degree of myelination of the nerve. **Myelin** is a fatty substance that wraps around neurons and works to increase the speed of information exchange by allowing the information to skip over parts of the neuron. Because myelin is a white substance, axons with myelin are called *white matter*, whereas cell bodies, dendrites, and some axons without myelin are called *gray matter*. Myelination increases as the brain develops and is lost with dementia.

The second method of conveying information from one neuron to the next is by chemical messengers, called **neurotransmitters**. When the action potential reaches the nerve terminal, neurotransmitters are released into the synapse. A **synapse** is the 15- to 20-nanometer space between a neuron terminal and the dendrite of the next neuron. Table 15–1 summarizes the role of neurotransmitters in specific psychiatric disorders.

SYNTHESIS AND STORAGE

Most neurotransmitters are synthesized and stored in the terminal region of the neuron. They are often synthesized from chemicals in our diets. For instance, tryptophan, which is found in relatively high levels in cheese, turkey, and red wine, is used in the synthesis of serotonin. Tryptophan used to be available commercially as a home remedy for sleeping problems; however, a contaminated batch that produced life-threatening illness led to its removal from the marketplace.

Before their release into the synapse, neurotransmitters are stored in membranous sacs called *vesicles*. This kind of "packaging" protects them from being destroyed by enzymes and gives them a chance to work. Researchers found by accident that the drug reserpine triggers depression. Reserpine also affects the storage of neurotransmitters; this discovery led to studies on the relationship between depression and drug effects on neurotransmitters.

RELEASE

Neurotransmitters are released from the nerve terminal following electrical stimulation (an action potential) from the cell body. To release a neurotransmitter, the membrane of the vesicle fuses to the membrane and dumps its contents into the synapse. It was once believed that one neuron was associated with one neurotransmitter for communication across a synapse. With technological advances in detecting chemicals, Dale's law has been refuted; we now know that neurochemicals within a synapse work together to produce an effect. For instance, one chemical may have an effect that lasts only seconds, whereas a second chemical's effect may last from several hours to several days.

RESPONSE

In order to transmit information, a neurotransmitter binds to a **receptor**, which is a unique protein found in the membrane of the neuron. The analogy of a lock and key describes this relationship; the lock is the receptor, and the key is the neurotransmitter. A receptor can be located either postsynaptically, on the next neuron it excites or inhibits, or presynaptically, on the neuron that released the transmitter modulating the activity of that neuron. More than 10 kinds of receptors can be activated by a single neurotransmitter (see Table 5–1). Whether the message is excitatory or inhibitory depends on the receptor. Using the techniques of molecular genetics, researchers have identified the majority of receptors, although the functions of many of them remain unknown. As discussed in Chapter 6, different psychotropic medications are aimed at individual subtypes of receptors to produce a specific effect. However, not all medications are precise in their effects; they can inadvertently cause unwanted side effects by activating other receptors or other neurotransmitter systems.

After the receptor is bound, the action of the first message, the neurotransmitter, is converted into action by a "second messenger." Second-messenger systems are complicated; however, basically, the effects of a single neurotransmitter are amplified through the subsequent activation of multiple systems. Different kinds of receptors are linked to different chemical second-messenger systems. Examples of second messengers are calcium, G-proteins, cyclic adenosine monophosphate (cyclic AMP), and arachidonic acid. The effects of second messengers last longer than those of neurotransmitters, and thus the process is described as "neuromodulatory." For instance, lithium, which is used to treat bipolar disorder, is believed to modulate the specific second-messenger system of G-proteins.

INACTIVATION

The exchange of information across a synapse needs to be tightly controlled so that the rapid transfer of information is not dulled by extra "noise" in the form of excess neurotransmitter. This noise is similar to fuzzy reception on a radio that makes it difficult to hear a song. For this reason, the nervous system controls the level of noise by efficient removal of a neurotransmitter from the synapse in a matter of milliseconds (0.001 second) after it has been released. Inactivation occurs by two main methods: breakdown by enzymes, primarily monoamine oxidase (MAO), or return of the neurotransmitter back into the neuron by a process known as **reuptake**.

Mechanisms of inactivation are targeted by various antidepressants such as tricyclic antidepressants (TCAs), MAO inhibitors (MAOIs), or selective serotonin reuptake inhibitors (SSRIs). These antidepressants acutely increase levels of the neurotransmitter in the synapse. As the main mechanism of inactivation, most neurotransmitters use reuptake by means of a special protein molecule. Other neurotransmitters, like acetylcholine, depend on specific enzymes for inactivation. Although these enzymes degrade the neurotransmitter into smaller proteins (metabolites), the metabolites themselves can participate in neural transmission. For instance, the major metabolite of fluoxetine, norfluoxetine, is active for many hours after the drug is degraded. Because inactivation is so efficient, levels of metabolites can be measured in the CSF more easily than the transmitter itself. Measuring metabolites of these neurotransmitters is imprecise; diet, movement, stress, and other factors can affect the results. Only a small fraction of metabolites are derived from the brain, and the rest come from the rest of the body.

SPECIFIC NEUROTRANSMITTERS

Four major types of neurotransmitters in the brain are involved in psychiatric illness: biogenic amines, cholinergics, neuropeptides, and amino acids.

BIOGENIC AMINES

The biogenic amines consist of the monoamines and histamine. Based on their chemical structure, the monoamines are subdivided into **catecholamines**, which include dopamine, norepinephrine, and epinephrine, and the **indolamines**, serotonin and melatonin. The monoamines have received the most attention in the study and treatment of psychiatric disorders. Specific drugs, developed with knowledge of the different chemical structures of neurotransmitters, "fool" the brain into thinking they are the transmitters themselves.

Dopamine

Dopamine receptors are classified into two main families, D_1 and D_2. The D_1-receptor family contains two subtypes, D_1 and D_5, and has stimulatory properties on second-messenger systems. The D_1-receptor family does not appear to be involved in mental illness. In contrast, the D_2-receptor family contains D_2, D_3, and D_4 subtypes, is inhibitory, and is the target of a number of pharmacotherapies, including antipsychotic medications. For instance, the atypical antipsychotic clozapine is believed to work at the D_4 receptor.

Dopamine is an inhibitory neurotransmitter found in discrete systems. Three major projection systems—the *mesolimbic, nigrostriatal,* and *mesocortical*—send neurons from the midbrain (*meso*), where the cell bodies are located, to forebrain structures, where dopamine is released. Increased levels of dopamine in the mesolimbic system are involved in the pleasurable feelings of reward, such as that felt from cocaine, as well as increased locomotion similar to amphetamine effects; therefore, this system has been implicated in drug addiction.

The nigrostriatal system sends projections from the substantia nigra to the caudate nucleus and the putamen. An increase of dopaminergic activity in the nigrostriatal system is associated with motor tics, such as those found in Tourette's disorder. In contrast, a deficit of dopamine in the nigrostriatal system is associated with retarded locomotion or the inhibition of the initiation of a motor task. The importance of dopamine is readily observed in clients who are medicated with neuroleptics, which decrease the availability of dopamine in the nigrostriatal system and produce the shuffling gait and slow motion seen in such clients.

The mesocortical system includes dopamine neurons traveling to the cortex, cingulate, and entorhinal cortex. This system is exquisitely sensitive to stress, has a high level of electrical activity, lacks an important self-regulatory system, and does not show compensatory changes to long-term treatment with antipsychotic medications. Because this area demonstrates unique characteristics not found in the other two major projection systems, researchers connect it with a number of mental illnesses, especially schizophrenia. Initially it was believed that schizophrenia resulted from excess dopamine activity. Based partly on the action of new antipsychotic medications, researchers now believe that dysregulation in the serotonin system is also involved. A dysregulation model suggests that dopamine systems are no longer in a state of homeostasis, resulting in decreased activity in the mesocortical system and hyperactivity in the nigrostriatal region.

The synthesis of dopamine involves the conversion of tyrosine, one of the essential amino acids, to L-dopa by the enzyme tyrosine hydroxylase. L-aromatic amino acid decarboxylase acts on L-dopa to form dopamine. Most of the dopamine in the synapse is inactivated by reuptake, and the rest is degraded into its metabolites, dihydroxyphenylacetic acid (DOPAC) and homovanillic acid (HVA). HVA is measured in CSF as an indicator of dopamine function in the brain. Extensive research on HVA levels in the CSF or blood levels in clients with schizophrenia has yielded equivocal results.

Norepinephrine

Norepinephrine has two main receptor subtypes, α and β. Many different forms of norepinephrine receptors are found in the brain and body. To date, at least two forms of the β-receptor and five forms of the α-receptor subtypes have been identified. Beta receptors may sound familiar because they are implicated in various cardiac disorders and in the pharmacologic treatment of hypertension. These implications are important for understanding the side effects of some psychotropic agents.

Norepinephrine and its derivative, epinephrine, are also known as noradrenaline and adrenaline, respectively. Norepinephrine is the most prevalent neurotransmitter in the nervous system. Its cell bodies are located in the small hindbrain area of the locus caeruleus. Noradrenergic neurons are projected throughout the brain in a major package of neurons called the *medial forebrain bundle*. These projections, which include five separate systems, are sent to the neocortex, hippocampus, thalamus, olfactory system, brain-stem nuclei, and the cerebellum. Projections also travel to the amygdala and the septum. A third projection system innervates the hypothalamus and modulates melatonin secretion, which is involved in the day-night cycle.

Given this anatomical localization, it should not be too surprising that norepinephrine plays a role in the regulation of awareness of the external environment, attention, learning, memory, and arousal, and has been implicated in mood disorders. Research with laboratory animals shows that excess norepinephrine increases startle reactions and aggression, and thus norepinephrine has been implicated in generalized anxiety disorder, panic disorder, and posttraumatic stress disorder (PTSD). In contrast, a deficit of norepinephrine may affect memory loss, social withdrawal caused by decreased awareness of and interest in the environment, depression, and ADHD.

Synthesis of norepinephrine follows the same pathway as that of dopamine, and dopamine β-hydroxylase converts dopamine to norepinephrine. Conversion of norepinephrine to epinephrine occurs by an enzyme, phenylethanolamine-N-methyl transferase (PNMT). Norepinephrine is then metabolized into two metabolites, namely, 3-methoxy-4-hydroxyphenylglycol (MHPG) and 3-methoxy-4-hydroxymandelic acid (VMA). Urinary MHPG levels can be detected and have been measured in clients with mood disorders, such as major depression, but with equivocal results. Norepinephrine is mainly inactivated by reuptake and is degraded by MAO and COMT.

Epinephrine has limited distribution in the brain. Epinephrine controls the fight-or-flight response in the peripheral nervous system that arouses people when they are threatened.

Serotonin

Serotonin is believed to have an impact on mood and psychotic disorders.[4] Like dopamine, this neurotransmitter has

---

RESEARCH NOTE

Pearlson, GD, et al: In vivo D_2 dopamine receptor density in psychotic and nonpsychotic patients with bipolar disorder. Arch Gen Psychiatr 52:471–477, 1995.

Findings: Previous work has shown that dopamine D_2 receptors are elevated in the brains of individuals with schizophrenia. Whether this elevation in receptor density reflects the biological nature of schizophrenia specifically or is related to the psychotic state of the patient is not known. This study examined the density of dopamine D_2 receptors in patients with bipolar disorder with psychosis (n = 7), bipolar disorder without psychosis (n = 7), schizophrenia (n = 10), and controls (n = 12) with PET to address this hypothesis.

Application to Practice: The results of this study show that elevated D_2-receptor density correlates with the severity of psychotic symptoms (assessed by the Present State Examination) but not with the severity of mood symptoms. These results suggest that the D_2 receptor plays a role in affective disorders with psychosis, and that the reported elevation in D_2 receptors in schizophrenia is not unique to this form of mental illness.

been the subject of a tremendous amount of research on the etiology and maintenance of mental illness. Serotonin is found in the periphery, and only 1 to 2% of all serotonin is actually in the brain, with the greatest concentration in the pineal gland. Serotonin neurons send projections from the cell bodies in the raphe nucleus in the hindbrain to the entire brain: Serotonin neurons project into the neocortex, hippocampus, thalamus, and cerebellum. Synthesis of serotonin requires dietary tryptophan and its conversion to an intermediate compound. Serotonin has at least 14 receptor subtypes and is inactivated primarily by reuptake. Degradation by MAO produces serotonin's main metabolite, 5-hydroxyindoleacetic acid (5-HIAA), or serotonin may be converted to melatonin.

The structural similarity of serotonin to the hallucinogen D-lysergic acid diethylamide (LSD) prompted researchers to hypothesize that serotonin is a factor in psychosis. Low levels of serotonin have been implicated in depression, aggression, violent suicide attempts, risk taking, and impulsivity. Thus, the relationship between serotonin and depression, mania, borderline personality disorder, and some cases of schizophrenia should not be unexpected. In contrast, excess serotonin leads to the opposite symptoms, that is, behavioral inhibition, fearfulness, and harm avoidance and is implicated in anxiety disorders such as generalized anxiety disorder, phobias, and obsessive-compulsive disorder.

Changes in blood levels of serotonin, serotonin uptake into blood platelets, or receptor density may prove to be a biological marker that clinicians can use to monitor the course and severity of depression in the future.

Histamine

Histamine is predominantly found in mast cells in the blood and has limited distribution in the brain. Involved primarily in allergic responses in the periphery, its role in the central nervous system remains elusive. Histamine has three receptor subtypes, H_1, H_2, and H_3. The drowsiness and hunger caused by antihistamines results from the blockade of stimulatory H_1 receptors in the hypothalamus. H_2 receptors have inhibitory effects in the neocortex and the hippocampus, although their specific action is not known with certainty. To date, histamine is not believed to play a role in mental illness.

CHOLINERGICS

Acetylcholine

At the turn of the century, acetylcholine was one of the first neurotransmitters to be described because of its stimulatory action on motor neurons in the periphery; it does not appear to share characteristics with the other transmitters. Acetylcholine is localized primarily in the hippocampus, amygdala, caudate and putamen, nucleus accumbens, cortex, thalamus, and the brain stem. Like serotonin, whose formation depends on the availability of tyrosine from the diet, the formation of acetylcholine depends on the dietary intake of its precursor, choline, from red meat and many different vegetables. Choline is transported into the neuron, converted into acetylcholine with the enzymes acetyl-CoA and choline acetylase, and packaged into vesicles. Acetylcholine is degraded rapidly by acetylcholinesterase, and the choline byproduct is reused.

Acetylcholine has two main receptor subtypes, nicotinic and muscarinic. Nicotine, found in tobacco, has at least 10 possible receptor subtypes and is stimulatory through its actions on ion channels. Activity at nicotine receptors has been shown to improve learning and memory performance. In contrast, activity at muscarinic receptors, caused when acetylcholine binds, is associated with memory dysfunction and some of the adverse side effects, such as dry mouth, found in antipsychotic drug use. At least five subtypes of muscarinic receptors exist. Activation of muscarinic receptors can be either stimulatory or inhibitory, depending on the second-messenger system.

The role of acetylcholine in the brain is to mediate cognitive function either directly or, by modulating another neurotransmitter system, indirectly. One of the most profound characteristics of Alzheimer's disease is the loss of cholinergic neurons in the hippocampus and entorhinal cortex. Clients with this disease are more sensitive to the memory-impairing effects of cholinergic blockade. The treatment of choice for Alzheimer's disease is cholinesterase inhibitors that increase the amount of available acetylcholine in the synapse.

NEUROPEPTIDES

Neuropeptides represent the newest class of neurotransmitters; already more than 50 peptides, chains of amino acids that range in size from 2 to more than 40 amino acids, have been identified. Initially, researchers thought these chemicals were involved in various endocrine functions and were released from the hypothalamus and transported into the anterior pituitary. The first neuropeptides to be isolated were releasing hormones, including thyrotropin-releasing hormone (TRH), gonadotropin-releasing hormone (GnRH), somatostatin, and adrenocorticotropic hormone (ACTH); they have primarily endocrine functions. The neuropeptides that have captured the interest of psychiatric researchers include the opiate-like peptides (endorphins and enkephalins), neurotensin, vasoactive intestinal peptide (VIP), cholecystokinin (CCK), and substance P. Neurotensin is found in high concentrations in the limbic regions of the hypothalamus, amygdala, septum, and nucleus accumbens; VIP and CCK are concentrated in the cortex and the hippocampus.

The unique characteristic of the neuropeptides is their presence in the same neuron with the major monoaminergic neurotransmitters, a situation known as *co-localization*. Table 5–2 provides a summary of some of the neuropeptides and their locations in the brain. Neuropeptides are primarily

TABLE 5–2. Neuropeptides

Neuropeptide	Co-Localized Neurotransmitter	Location	Associated Illness	Change
Cholecystokinin (CCK)	Acetylcholine	Ventrotegmental area	Anxiety	Increase
	Dopamine	Hypothalamus		
	Vasopressin	Cortex		
	GABA	Caudate and putamen		
		Hippocampus and amygdala		
Corticotropin-releasing factor (CRF)		Cortex	Depression	Increase
		Hypothalamus and pituitary	Alzheimer's disease	Decrease
		Hippocampus and amygdala	Parkinson's disease	Decrease
Neurotensin	Dopamine	Hypothalamus	Schizophrenia	Decrease
	CCK	Substantia nigra	Parkinson's disease	Decrease
		VTA		
		Hippocampus, amygdala	Alzheimer's disease	Decrease
		Nucleus accumbens		
NPY	Epinephrine	Brain stem	Depression	Decrease
	Norepinephrine	Brain stem	Anxiety	Increase
Opioids	Dopamine	Hippocampus	Drug addiction	Increase
		Locus caeruleus	Anorexia nervosa	Increase
			Autism	Increase
Somatostatin	GABA	Cortex, hippocampus	Parkinson's disease	Decrease
	Norepinephrine	Peripheral nervous system	Alzheimer's disease	Decrease
			Depression	Decrease
Substance P	Acetylcholine	Brain stem		
	Serotonin	Medulla		

inactivated by enzymatic degradation, diffusion away from the synapse, or reuptake.

AMINO ACIDS

Amino acids may be divided into two classes: excitatory and inhibitory. The excitatory amino acids include aspartic acid, glutamic acid, cysteic acid and homocysteic acid. With the exception of glutamate, information on the relationship between these excitatory neurotransmitters and psychiatric illness is sparse. The inhibitory neurotransmitters include γ-aminobutyric acid (GABA), glycine, taurine, and β-alanine. GABA, the subject of much research, has been implicated in schizophrenia, epilepsy, senile dementia, and anxiety disorders.[5]

The excitatory amino acids, especially glutamate, are important in neuropathology because of their toxic nature when levels are too high. Glutamate has three main classes of complex receptors that are named for the kinds of compounds that activate them: N-methyl-D-aspartic acid (NMDA), kainate/quisqualate, and α-amino-3-hydroxy-5-methyl-lisoxazole-4-propionic acid (AMPA). The NMDA-receptor complex modulates a calcium and sodium ion channel and has multiple binding sites for compounds like phencyclidine (PCP), glutamate, and glycine. This receptor subtype is believed to play a role in brain development, especially in learning.

The food additive monosodium glutamate (MSG) produces dizziness and headaches in some individuals who are sensitive to its effects. Glutamate has been shown to destroy neurons in the immature brains of laboratory animals and has been implicated in neurodegenerative disorders, including Alzheimer's disease. At the cellular level, glutamate has been linked as the causative agent in brain damage produced by hypoglycemia, sustained epileptic seizures, hypoxia and ischemia, and even central nervous system trauma. Experimental research is currently investigating the effects of calcium channel or specific glutamatergic-receptor blockers to prevent this excitotoxic cascade of events.

GABA is the major inhibitory neurotransmitter in the brain. Its highest concentrations are in the globus pallidus and the substantia nigra; smaller amounts have been found in the cortex, thalamus, caudate, and cerebellum. It acts as an intermediary, modulating the other neurotransmitter systems rather than providing a stimulus itself. GABA is derived from glutamate and is degraded by GABA transaminase (GABA-T) to γ-hydroxybutyrate (GHB), which is present in bodily fluids. Elevated levels of GHB have been associated with both motor and mental retardation.

GABA has two receptor subtypes, A and B. The type A GABA receptor has been extensively characterized and is quite complex. Once activated, this receptor has inhibitory effects on neurotransmission by modulating a chloride ion channel. It has specific binding sites for pharmacologic

The Normal Brain

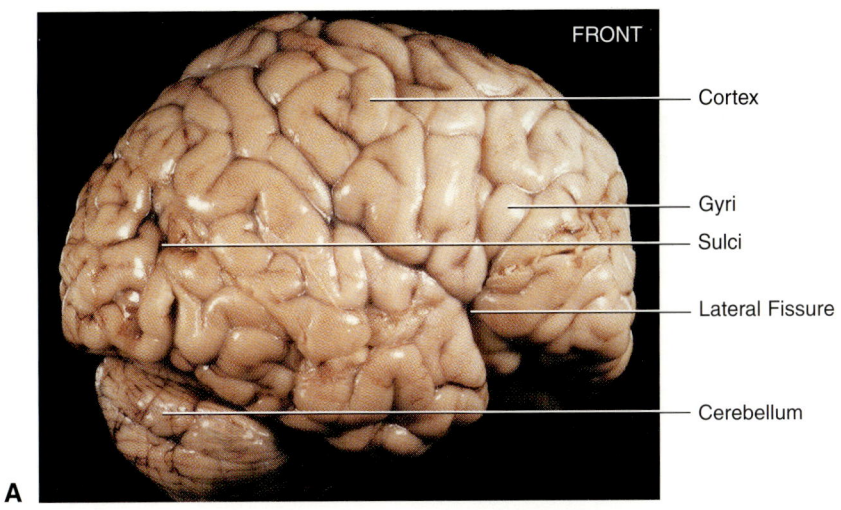

A

- Cortex
- Gyri
- Sulci
- Lateral Fissure
- Cerebellum

The cortex is the area of higher level thinking. Coordination is controlled by the cerebellum. Note the convoluted surface area. It increases the surface of the brain to more than 2.5 square feet. The bumps are referred to as gyri, the grooves are called sulci. A deep sulcus is known as a fissure.

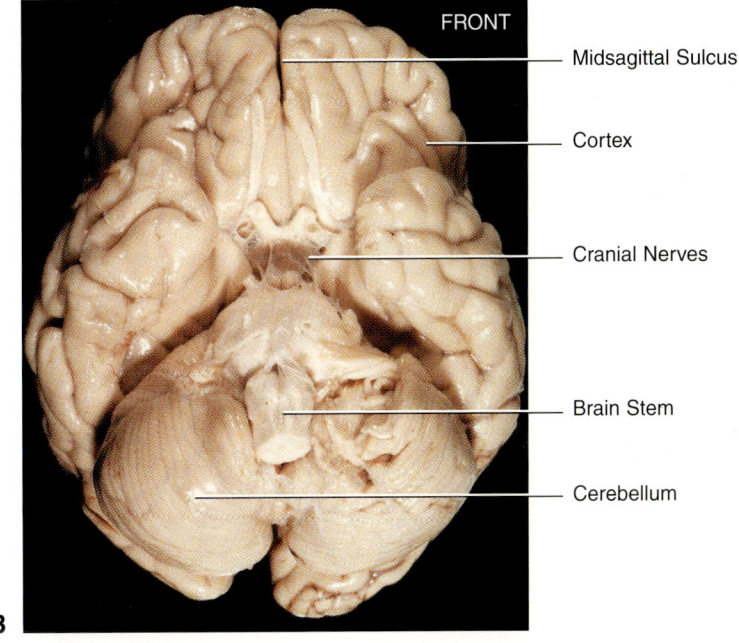

B

- Midsagittal Sulcus
- Cortex
- Cranial Nerves
- Brain Stem
- Cerebellum

From the ventral view, the cortex and the cerebellum are visible, as well as the beginning of the brain stem and some of the cranial nerves. The brain is divided into two hemispheres by the midsaggital sulcus.

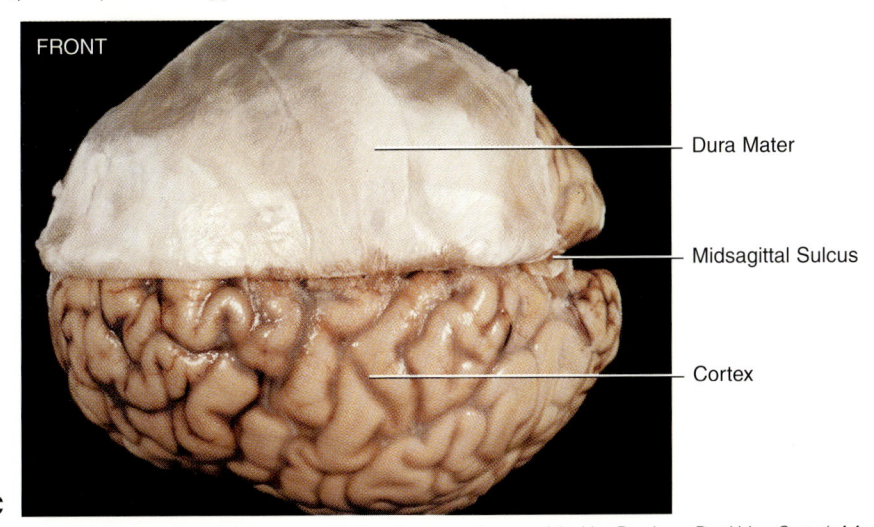

C

- Dura Mater
- Midsagittal Sulcus
- Cortex

A dorsal view reveals the dura mater, the thick covering of the cortex. *Color photographs provided by Dr. Jean Paul Von Sattel, Massachusetts General Hospital.*

Map of Normal Brain Function

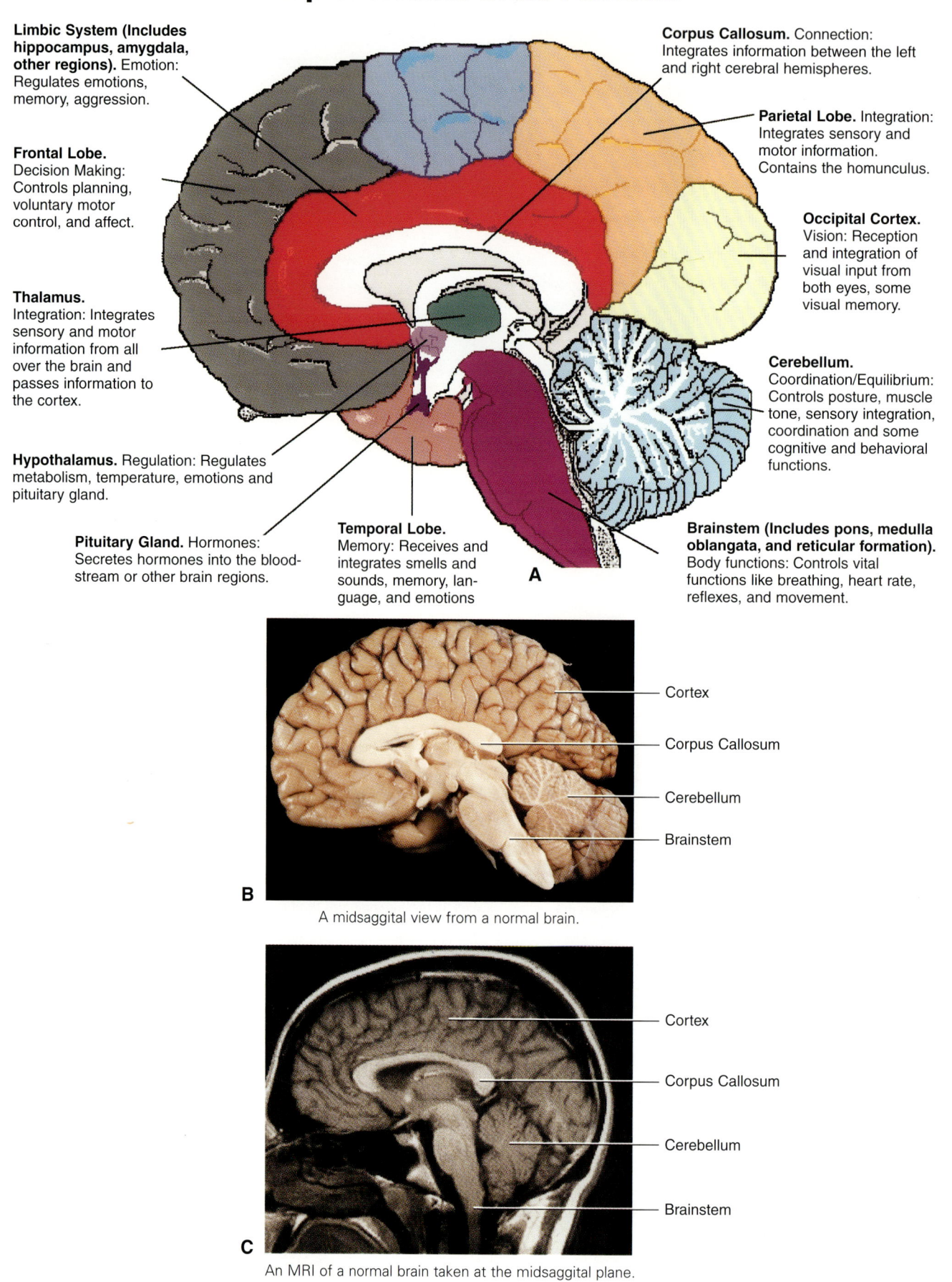

Limbic System (Includes hippocampus, amygdala, other regions). Emotion: Regulates emotions, memory, aggression.

Frontal Lobe. Decision Making: Controls planning, voluntary motor control, and affect.

Thalamus. Integration: Integrates sensory and motor information from all over the brain and passes information to the cortex.

Hypothalamus. Regulation: Regulates metabolism, temperature, emotions and pituitary gland.

Pituitary Gland. Hormones: Secretes hormones into the bloodstream or other brain regions.

Corpus Callosum. Connection: Integrates information between the left and right cerebral hemispheres.

Parietal Lobe. Integration: Integrates sensory and motor information. Contains the homunculus.

Occipital Cortex. Vision: Reception and integration of visual input from both eyes, some visual memory.

Cerebellum. Coordination/Equilibrium: Controls posture, muscle tone, sensory integration, coordination and some cognitive and behavioral functions.

Temporal Lobe. Memory: Receives and integrates smells and sounds, memory, language, and emotions.

Brainstem (Includes pons, medulla oblangata, and reticular formation). Body functions: Controls vital functions like breathing, heart rate, reflexes, and movement.

A

B — A midsaggital view from a normal brain.
- Cortex
- Corpus Callosum
- Cerebellum
- Brainstem

C — An MRI of a normal brain taken at the midsaggital plane.
- Cortex
- Corpus Callosum
- Cerebellum
- Brainstem

The Ventricular System

A

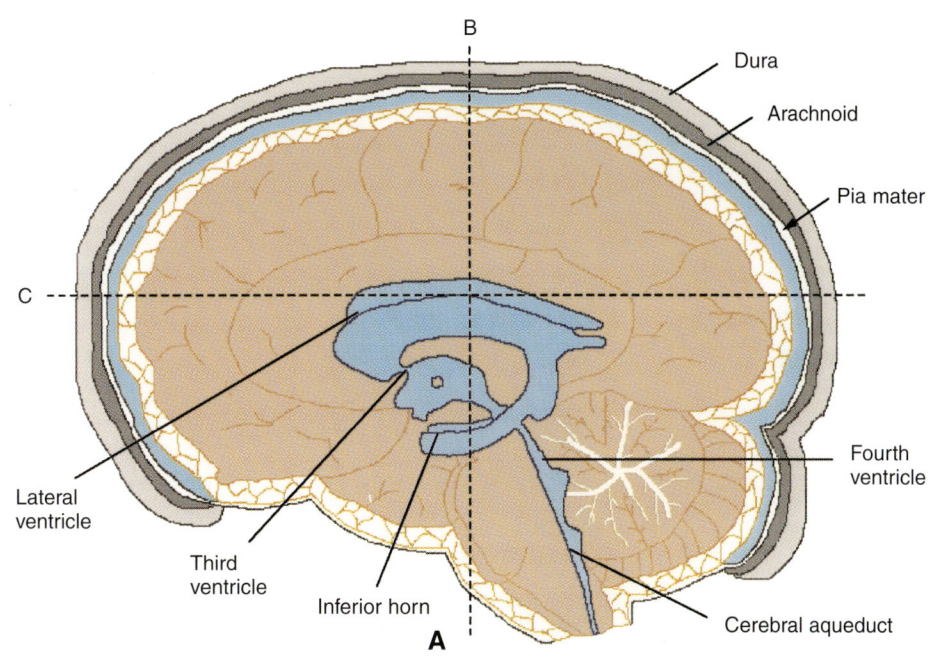

Cerebrospinal fluid (shown in blue) diffuses around the brain, in the ventricles, and down the spinal column. It provides bouyancy for the brain, acting as a shock absorber. CSF also permits some nutrient exchange and drains unwanted substances away from the brain. The lines show the plane of section for B and C.

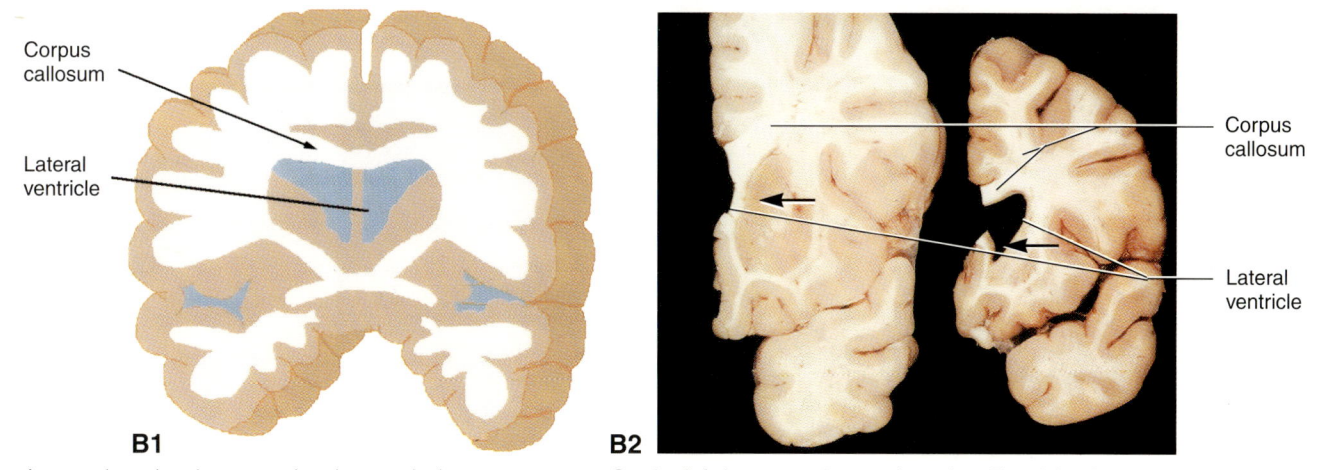

B1

A coronal section demonstrating the ventricular system.

B2

On the left is a normal coronal section. The right shows a section from a patient with Huntington's disease. Note the enlarged ventricles, the result of atrophying of the caudate nucleus (as indicated by the arrows).

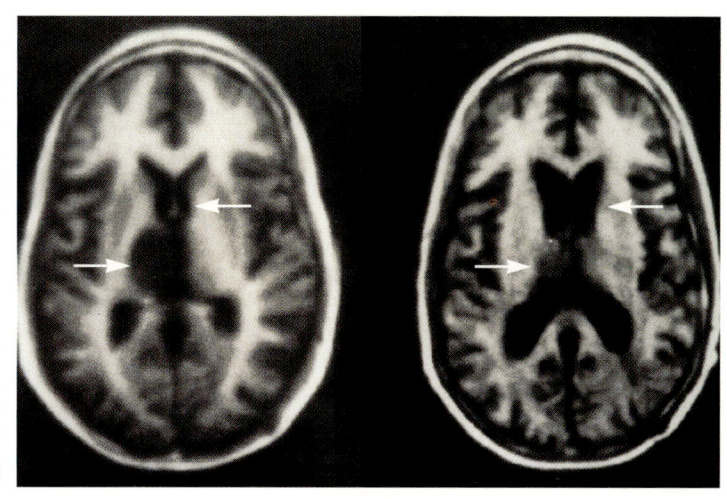

C

A horizontal section taken with a CT scanner. The left scan is a control, the right scan shows the enlarged ventricles of a patient with schizophrenia.

The Limbic System

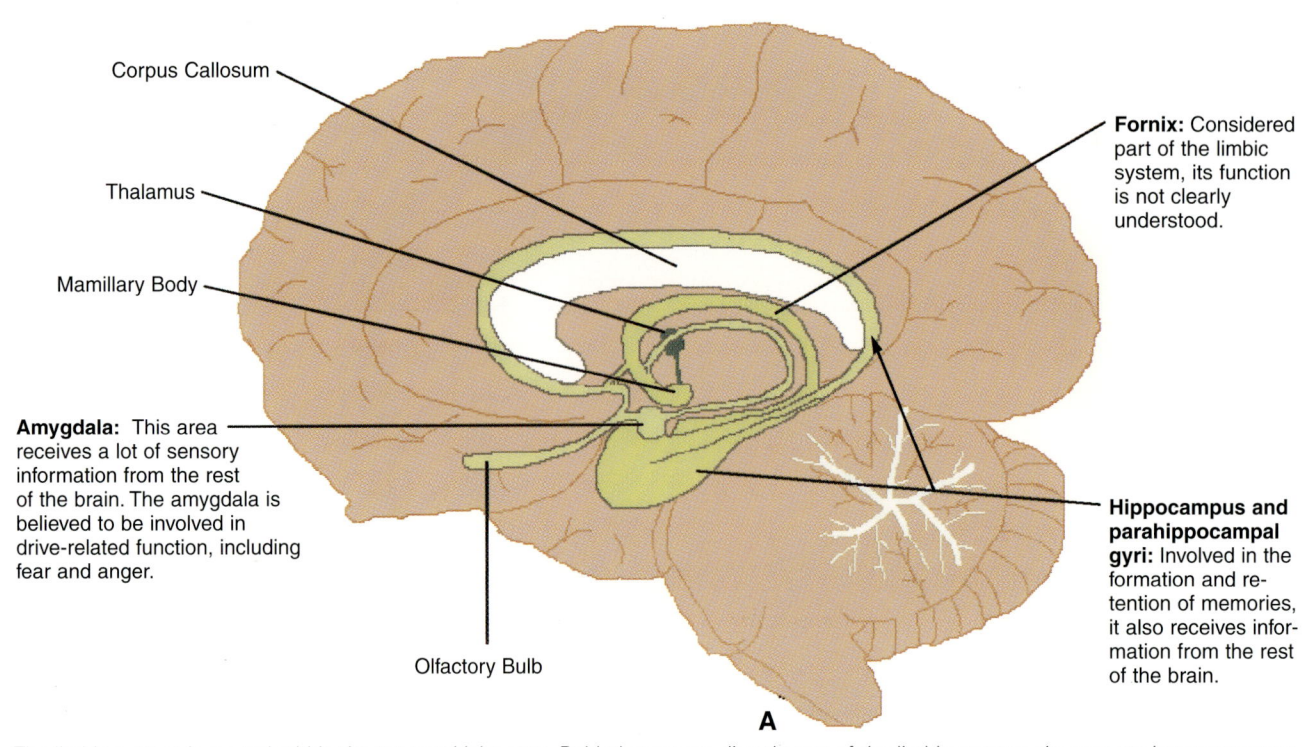

A

- Corpus Callosum
- Thalamus
- Mamillary Body
- **Amygdala:** This area receives a lot of sensory information from the rest of the brain. The amygdala is believed to be involved in drive-related function, including fear and anger.
- Olfactory Bulb
- **Fornix:** Considered part of the limbic system, its function is not clearly understood.
- **Hippocampus and parahippocampal gyri:** Involved in the formation and retention of memories, it also receives information from the rest of the brain.

The limbic system is nested within the temporal lobe area. Bolded areas are directly part of the limbic system; the rest are important areas involved in the limbic system's elaborate circuitry with other brain regions.

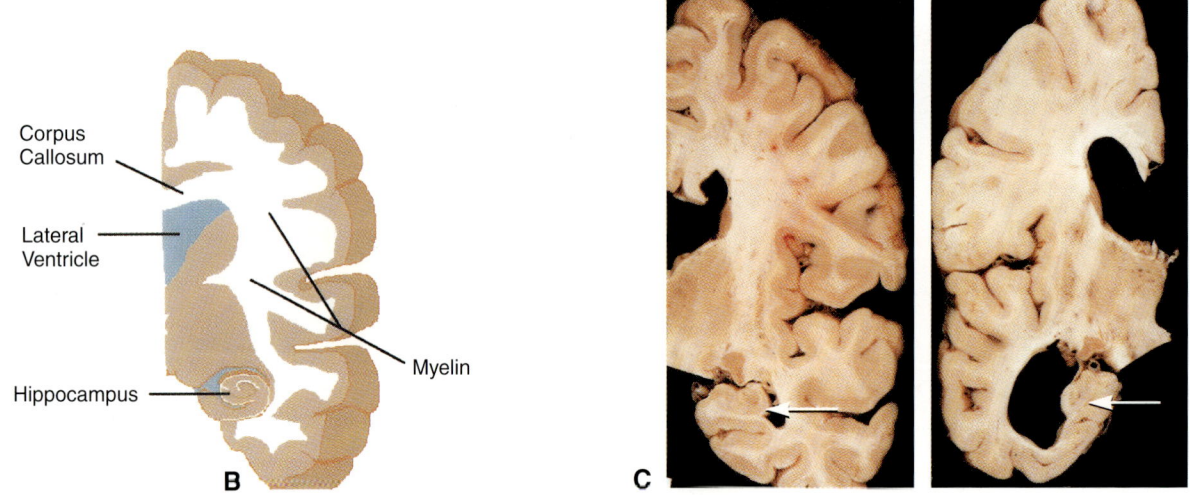

B

- Corpus Callosum
- Lateral Ventricle
- Myelin
- Hippocampus

Coronal section showing the hippocampus. Hippocampus comes from Latin for seahorse, which can be seen in its cytoarchitecture.

C

Coronal section demonstrating the profound loss of the hippocampus (shown by the arrows) due to Alzheimer's disease. Normal brain is on the left, while the Alzheimer's brain is pictured on the right.

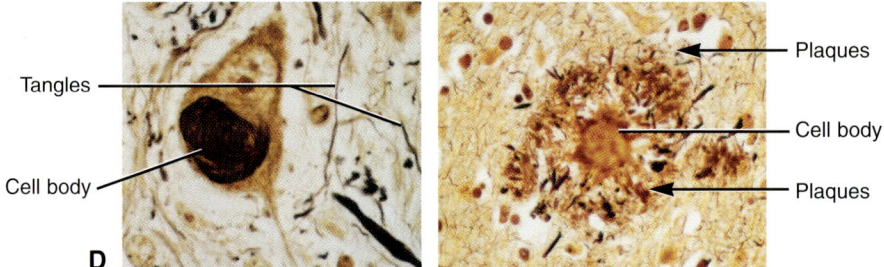

D

- Tangles
- Cell body
- Plaques
- Cell body
- Plaques

Tangles and plaques (right, all the extra matter surrounding the cell body) that characterize Alzheimer's disease. Their presence is used as a post-mortem diagnostic criteria for the disease.

Parts of a Neuron

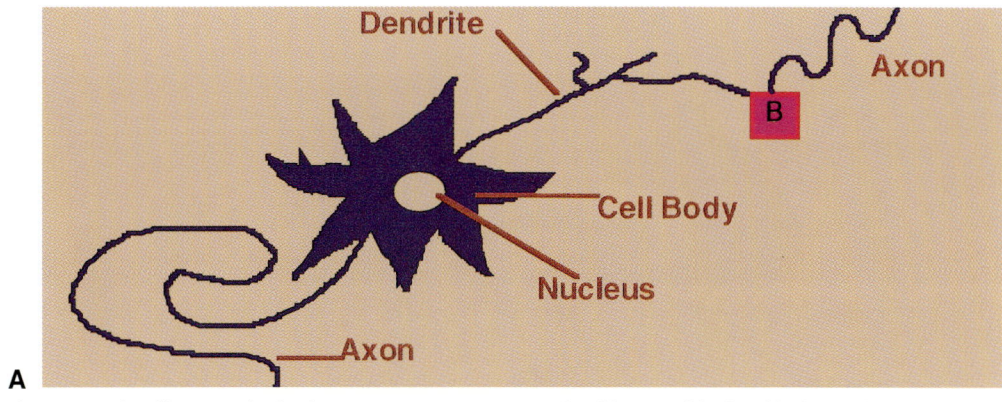

A

A schematic of a neuron that illustrates its basic components: an axon, a dendrite, a cell body with the nucleus (the site of DNA production), and nerve terminal and a synapse. (shown enlarged below)

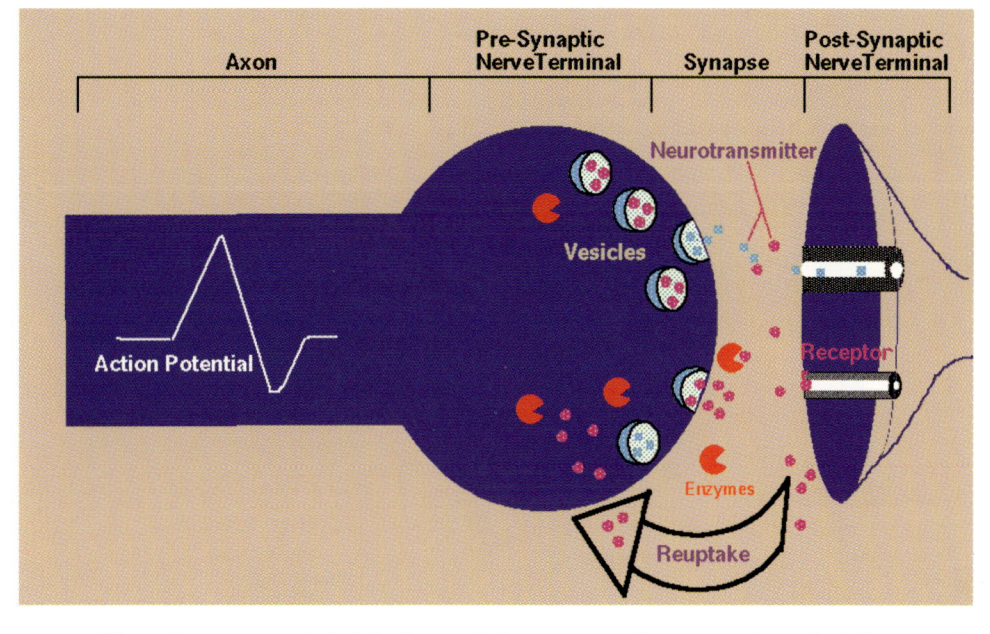

B

A schematic of a synapse. The major components include the terminal, synapse, and post-synaptic terminal. Drugs work at the level of the synapse, depending on their mechansim of action. Drugs can directly bind receptors, inhibit enzymes or reuptake, or reduce action potentials.

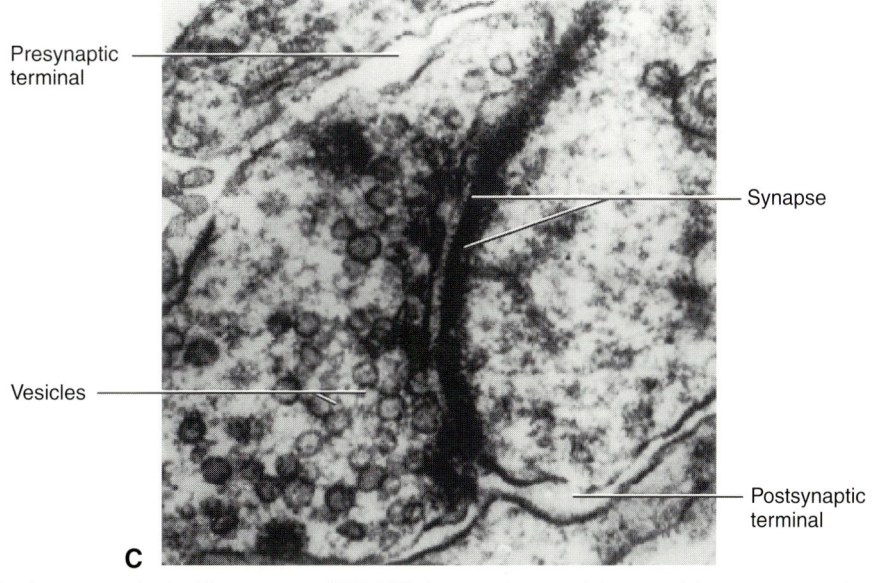

C

An electron micrograph of a synapse in the hippocampus (X55,000). Arrows show vesicles containing neurotransmitters and the membranes of the pre- and postsynaptic neuron. *Courtesy of C. Santefemio, McLean Hospital.*

The Role of Neurotransmitters

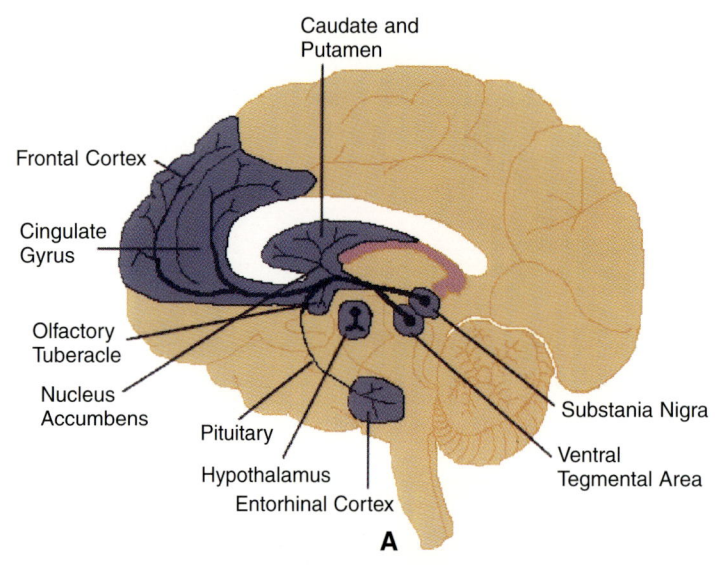

A

The Dopamine System: This system (shown in blue) serves a modulatory role on the other monaminergic systems. Its dysfunction has been implicated in a number of disorders, including schizophrenia and ADHD.

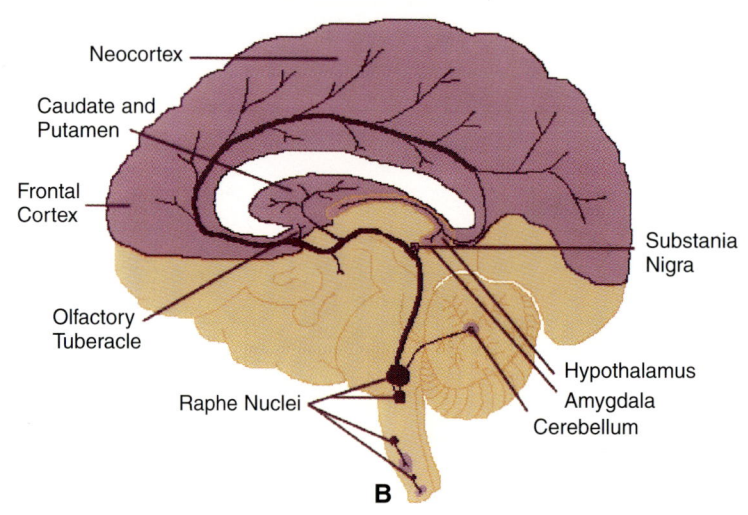

B

The Serotonin System: This system (shown in purple) plays a prominent role in psychiatric illness. Serotonin has been implicated in affective disorders more often than the dopamine system.

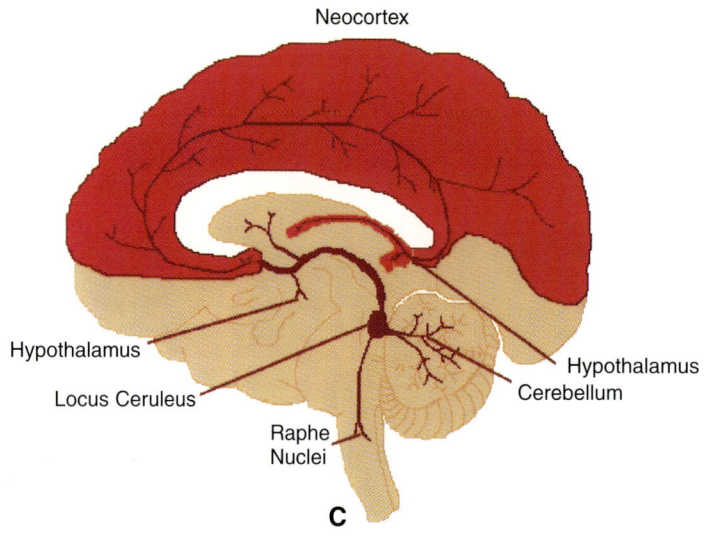

C

The Noradrenergic System: This system (in red) is involved in fight or flight responses and controls levels of arousal. Dysfunction of this system has not been as strongly implicated in psychiatric illness as the dopamine or serotonin systems. However, blockade of norepinephrine receptors is common pharmacotherapy for depression.

Imaging Technique

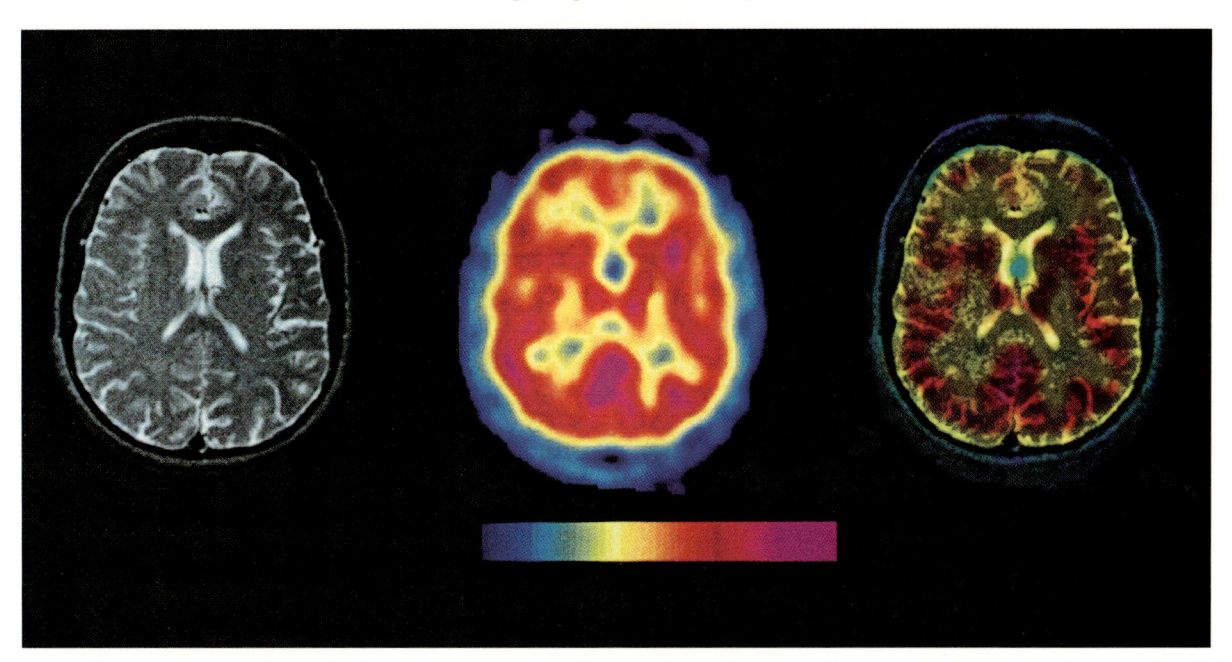

Different profiles generated by the available imaging techniques. The far left is a CT scan, which uses X-rays. The middle image is a SPECT scan, a technique that involves the injection of a radioactive tracer to light up the brain. The degree of activation is indicated by the color strip below this image with pink representing more activity than blue. The image on the right is a combined image, which provides both anatomical and functional resolution. *Courtesy of Dr. B. Cohen, McLean Hospital.*

The Extrapyramidal System

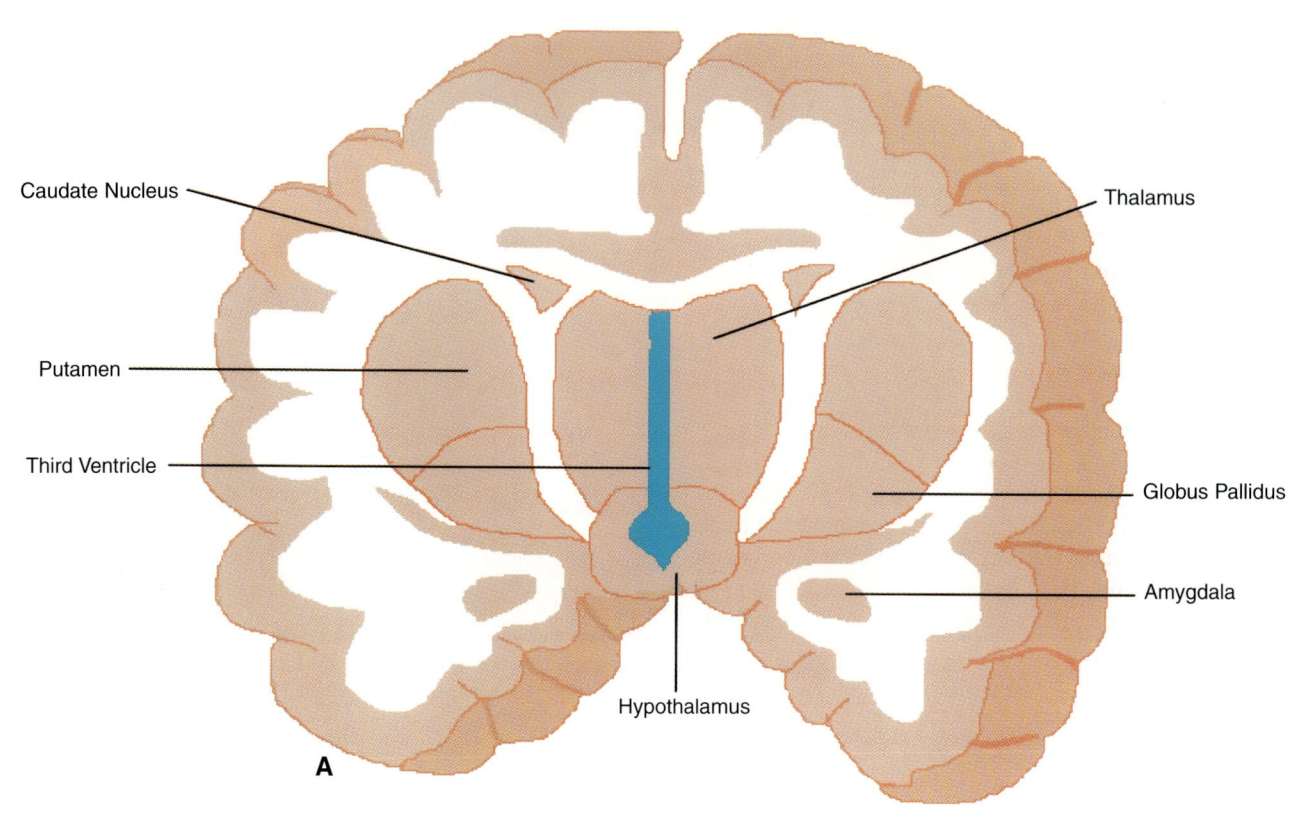

A

Schematic of the basal ganglia. The main structures that compose this system are the caudate nucleus, the putamen, and the globus pallidus. These areas send and receive information from the cortex and the main relay station, the thalamus, and are involved in the switching gears from one thought to another. Dysfunction of these areas causes one to "get stuck" and is associated with obsessive-compulsive disorder and some of the unwanted side effects of chronic neuroleptic treatment.

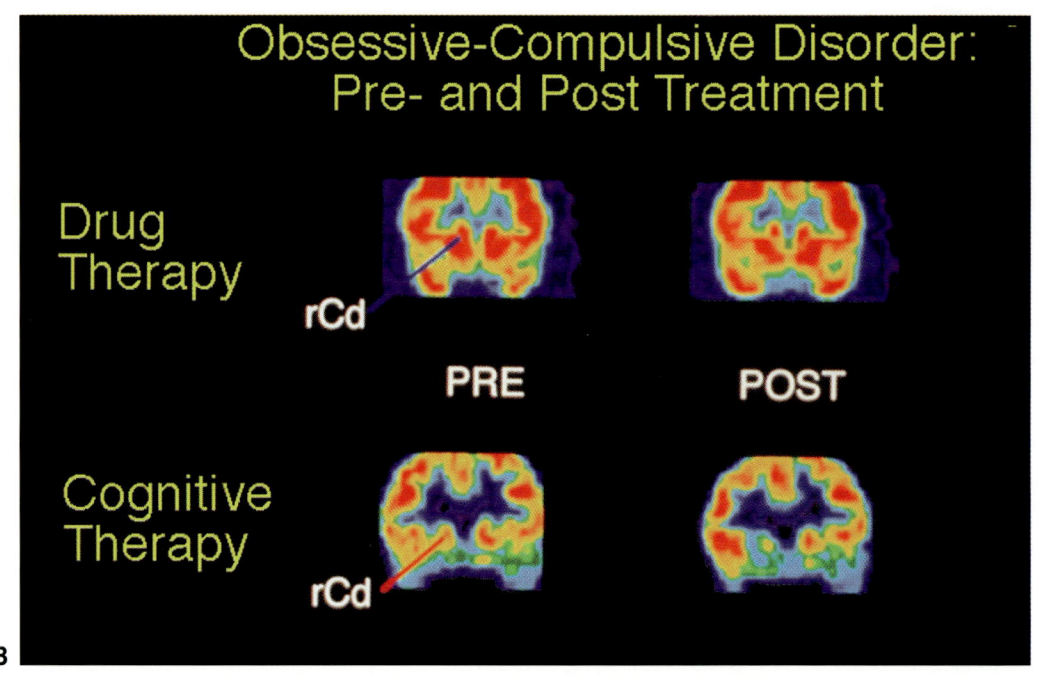

B

Shown are PET scans of the brains of two patients with obsessive-compulsive disorder (OCD) pre- and post-treatment. Red indicates the most activity, yellow intermediate, and blue little activity. The top scans are from a patient who took medication (a selective serotonin reuptake inhibitor, SSRI). The bottom scans are from a patient who underwent cognitive therapy. Both treatments decreased the activity of the caudate nucleus (rCD) (the more anterior section is shown here). *Scans were provided by Jeffry M. Schwartz, M.D., UCLA School of Medicine, copyright of the American Medical Association, Arch. Gen. Psychiatry, 53:109-113, 1996.*

agents used to treat mental illness, including benzodiazepines often used to treat anxiety and seizure disorders. Anxiolytics and anticonvulsants that target this receptor subtype and are discussed in Chapter 6.

TOOLS OF THE TRADE

The tools used to study mental illness are wide-ranging. Until recently, most of what was known about the biological changes of mental illness was based on surgery or postmortem assays. In some cases, specific brain changes are readily noticeable, such as in end-stage Alzheimer's disease. In other diseases, such as schizophrenia and depression, the changes are molecular, and researchers study small pieces of brain tissue for alterations in chemical levels. These studies are complicated, partly because of the limited amount of tissue available. Also, factors like chronic drug treatment during the client's lifetime, the circumstance of death such as drowning or suicide, a time delay in obtaining the brain tissue, and tissue preservation can influence the findings. With neuroimaging and chemical analysis of bodily fluids, researchers are trying to identify biological markers in the living client to track the course of mental illness. The main purpose is early detection for early intervention, with the ultimate goal of prevention.

The field of neuroimaging (Table 5–3) has advanced rapidly in the past 20 years. It is relatively noninvasive and can be used to identify gross anatomical deficits in the living client. The structural images from computed tomography (CT) and magnetic resonance imaging (MRI) are used to rule out treatable conditions such as cerebral vascular accidents (CVAs), tumors, and hydrocephalus when the client presents with alterations in personality. Data from CT and MRI have detected enlarged ventricles in schizophrenia, corroborating results from postmortem studies. The more advanced imaging techniques of positron-emission tomography (PET), single photon emission computed tomography (SPECT), and some MRIs can provide limited information on functional—namely, physiological—changes in the brain, through the use of a radioactive tracer to study blood-flow patterns, energy and glucose metabolism, and drug localization. Based on different patterns of blood flow, energy use, or drug distribution, dementias such as Alzheimer's disease can be better identified.

Although neuroimaging techniques are promising, they have a number of limitations. The first is the number of times the client can have a brain scan. Multiple CTs and MRIs can be generated in the same individual, in contrast to PET or SPECT, where the use of radioactivity limits the number of times a scan can be performed. Second, imaging services are not always found in smaller hospitals because the cost and maintenance of the machines are prohibitive. Third, imaging takes place in narrow chambers that make many individuals claustrophobic and unable to remain still for the length of time required; most are given a sedative to make the experience tolerable. Finally, these techniques currently lack the sophistication to detect subtler differences such as those believed to occur at the network and chemical levels in disorders like schizophrenia.

Chemical analysis of body fluids is another tool that is available to study psychiatric disorders in living clients. Research compares blood, urine, saliva, and CSF levels of neurotransmitters and their metabolites in clients with a specific diagnosis and normal controls, as well as changes in DNA levels to find genetic markers. These studies have yielded exciting findings, which are discussed in other chapters in more detail.

GENETICS AND HEREDITY

The goal of the Human Genome Project is to identify all of the human DNA and what it encodes. Among the interesting results of this project is the identification of two genes for Alzheimer's disease on chromosomes 14 and 21.

Genes are located on chromosomes; each person has 23 pairs, for a total of 46. One set of 23 comes from the mother and the other set from the father at the time of conception. Genes are composed of pairs of nucleic acids in specific sequences that contain an enormous amount of coding information. This information serves as a "blueprint" for biological processes. The mechanism of decoding the DNA is complex (Figure 5–6). First, DNA, a double-stranded mol-

TABLE 5–3. Neuroimaging Techniques

Neuroimaging Method	Imaging Procedure	Clinical Utility	Estimated Cost ($)	Disadvantages	Duration
Computed tomography (CT)	Serial x-rays through brain	Structural	700–900	Low resolution / Radiation exposure	20 min
Magnetic resonance imaging (MRI)	Radio waves from brain detected by magnet	Structural / Some functional	1100–1300	Moderate resolution	35–45 min
Positron-emission tomography (PET)	Radioactive tracer	Functional	1500–2000	Radioactivity exposure	2–3 hrs
Single photon emission computed tomography (SPECT)	Radioactive tracer	Functional	700–800	Radioactivity exposure	1–2 hrs

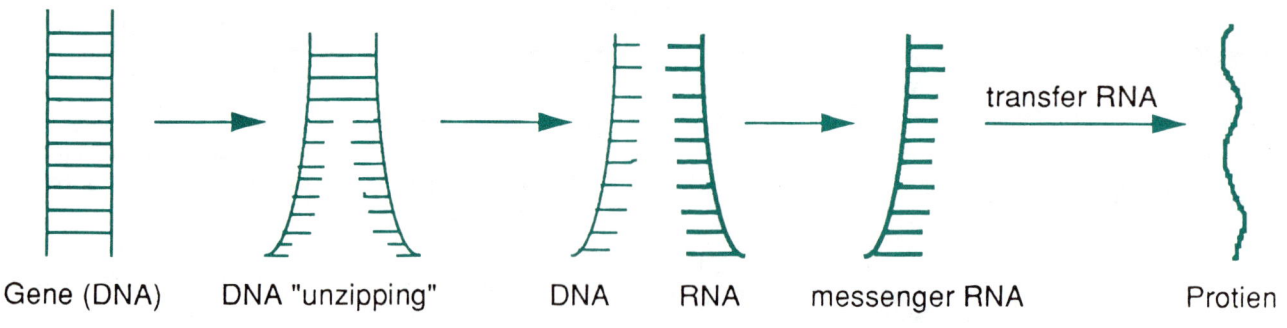

Gene (DNA)　　DNA "unzipping"　　DNA　　RNA　　messenger RNA　　Protien

Figure 5–6. Synthesis of protein from DNA. The double-stranded DNA molecule divides into two pieces ("unzips"), and one strand serves as a template for the formation of messenger RNA. Protein is then made from this blueprint of mRNA.

ecule, divides in half for replication. Second, the DNA is "read" by another molecule, ribonucleic acid (RNA). Through different RNA molecules, specifically transfer RNA (tRNA) and messenger RNA (mRNA), the sequence for a given protein is deciphered. The mRNA is then used in the construction of a new protein molecule, and the body uses this and other molecules as building blocks.

Although a good portion of brain structure and function is dictated by genes and DNA, there is room for errors in the process of construction. For example, Down syndrome involves an extra replication of chromosome 21, resulting in three copies instead of the normal two. Hence, Down syndrome is also known as *trisomy 21*. For the most part, however, the relationship between genes and psychiatric illness is not clear, and the classic issue of nature versus nurture plays itself out. If it is in the genes to develop a psychiatric illness, why does illness not manifest itself in all children of diagnosed psychiatric clients? To that end, a number of studies support observations that mental illness is not transmitted by typical Mendelian genetics.

Researchers can determine the probabilities of inheritance of a gene by examining twins with a given disorder. In monozygotic (identical) twins, the genes are the same; dizygotic (fraternal) twins share only 50% of their genes. In both cases, the twins share approximately the same in utero environment as well as many aspects of their environment during postnatal development. An example of how twin studies work is prevalence of dyslexia. Research suggests that if one twin has the illness, there is a 90% chance that the second monozygotic twin will have dyslexia (known as a 90% *concordance rate*). In contrast, only 30% of dizygotic twins will show the learning disorder between sets of twins. However, not all disorders have such a high genetic disposition. Concordance rates of schizophrenia in monozygotic twins are only 50%, suggesting that the relationship between environment and genetics is more complicated. Other etiologic factors in schizophrenia include the season of birth, viral infection, and obstetric complications.

The second type of commonly used genetic study is an adoption study, in which one sibling is removed from a given environment at the time of adoption. This type of study allows researchers to compare the effects of the 50% of genes that all siblings share. Results from adoptive studies are not as conclusive as twin studies, and more effort has been expended on the collection of genetic information from monozygotic twins than any other type of genetic study.

A third form of genetic studies, family studies, determines how common a trait is among family members. Researchers examine the frequency of appearance of a mental illness in parents, offspring, and distant relatives through the use of pedigrees. This information is then compared to the frequency in the general population, and genetic probabilities are calculated. From this information, researchers look for a specific genetic marker for the disease in the population with a high frequency of occurrence of the illness. In this manner, Nancy Wexler discovered a genetic basis for Huntington's disease. By studying the frequency of Huntington's disease in a village of fewer than 1000 individuals in Venezuela, she was able to examine enough DNA that contained a high frequency of the mutant gene to determine that it was causing the disease.

CIRCADIAN RHYTHMS AND MENTAL ILLNESS

Eating, drinking, sleeping, body temperature, and menstruation are all subject to cyclic variation.[6] Although these patterns can be manipulated by the environment to some extent, they are greatly influenced by our internal pacemakers. For instance, some individuals are "night owls," preferring to stay up late at night, whereas others are "larks," rising early in the morning. The amount of light in the environment at bedtime or awakening influences how long and when we sleep; however, most people fare better if they stick to the schedule dictated by their own bodies.

The term *biological rhythms* is used to describe these cyclical fluctuations in physiological functioning. Depending on their length of time, different biological rhythms have different names. A *circadian rhythm* refers to a period of ap-

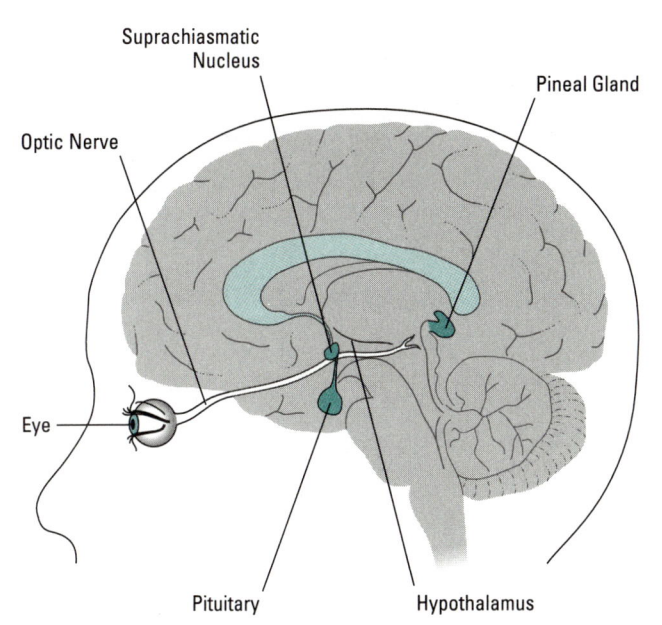

Figure 5–7. Pathway showing how light information travels through the retina of the eye to the suprachiasmatic nucleus and the pineal gland.

proximately 24 hours and is most observable in our patterns of rest and activity. *Infradian rhythms*, such as the menstrual cycle, are fluctuations that last longer than a day. Parts of our sleep cycle are examples of *ultradian rhythms, those that are shorter than a day.* Alterations in the light and dark cycle and social cues are important in regulating circadian rhythms.

Circadian rhythms influence our rest and activity cycle, body temperature, blood pressure, and hormone secretions. All of these physiological changes, in turn, greatly influence our moods, fertility, and even susceptibility to illness.

The mechanism by which light influences circadian rhythms has been well studied. Specifically, light enters the eye and stimulates a set of nerves that stimulate an area of the hypothalamus in the diencephalon (Figure 5–7). (The hypothalamus is the region where eating, drinking, sexual activity, cardiac function, and fear responses are mediated through the release of hormones.) Located within the hypothalamus is a specific set of neurons, the suprachiasmatic nucleus (SCN), which, in turn, controls many brain regions involved in circadian rhythms. Evidence for the role of the SCN in circadian rhythms comes from animal studies, in which a lesion in the SCN disrupts the rhythmicity of activity, sleep and wake cycles, corticosteroid secretion, temperature, drinking, and the synthesis of melatonin. Melatonin, a metabolite of serotonin, is released from the pineal gland in response to changes in light. Light also influences body temperature, which decreases at night. The brain modulates the circadian rhythm of activity, melatonin, body temperature, and other physiological processes. Given the cyclical nature of melatonin and serotonin, it should not be surprising that clients with depression often complain of a change in sleeping patterns.

The desynchronization of infradian rhythms is most readily observed in seasonal affective disorder (SAD). The seasonal nature of this depression parallels the shortening of the days during fall and winter. Many of these individuals respond favorably to bright light treatment, or phototherapy. In clients affected by SAD, the symptoms disappear by springtime, when the amount of daylight increases, and return during the fall.

PSYCHONEUROIMMUNOLOGY

Practitioners, pathologists, and researchers are beginning to understand how psychiatric functioning can alter the course of infectious disease and vice versa. The emerging field of psychoneuroimmunology looks at the links between how a person feels emotionally and the functioning of the immune system and how both factors alter central nervous system function.[7,8] By understanding this relationship, psychiatric nurses can intervene during the course of stress-related or stress-susceptible mental illnesses.

The function of the immune system is to distinguish "self" from "nonself." The mechanism by which psychosocial stressors influence the immune function is primarily mediated by the hypothalamic-pituitary-adrenal (HPA) axis via the glucocorticoids. Most of what is known involves the interaction of the HPA axis with depression or PTSD.

HPA AXIS FUNCTIONING

Since the pioneering work of Hans Selye, who brought the effects of stress to the forefront, nurses have taken an important clinical and theoretical interest in the relationship between stress and illness. Leading the way, Callista Roy extended existing theories to develop a framework for nursing based on stress and adaptation. Psychiatric researchers have developed theories based on the observed effects of stress, stress hormones such as corticosteroids, and HPA dysregulation in certain disorders. Activation of the "stress system" and its many interconnections with the locus caeruleus, prefrontal cortex, hippocampus, and amygdala sets the level of emotional and physical arousal, resulting in a person's ability to respond intellectually and physically.

When faced with physical or psychological stress, neurotransmitters activate the hypothalamus to release corticotropin-releasing factor (CRF), which causes the release of adrenocorticotropic hormone (ACTH) from the pituitary gland. ACTH is released into the bloodstream and travels to the adrenal cortex, where it stimulates the release of the corticosteroids, including cortisol. This cascade is shown in Figure 5–8. As major stress hormones, cortisol and other corticosteroids affect this cascade through negative feedback; excess cortisol binds to glucocorticoid receptors in the brain

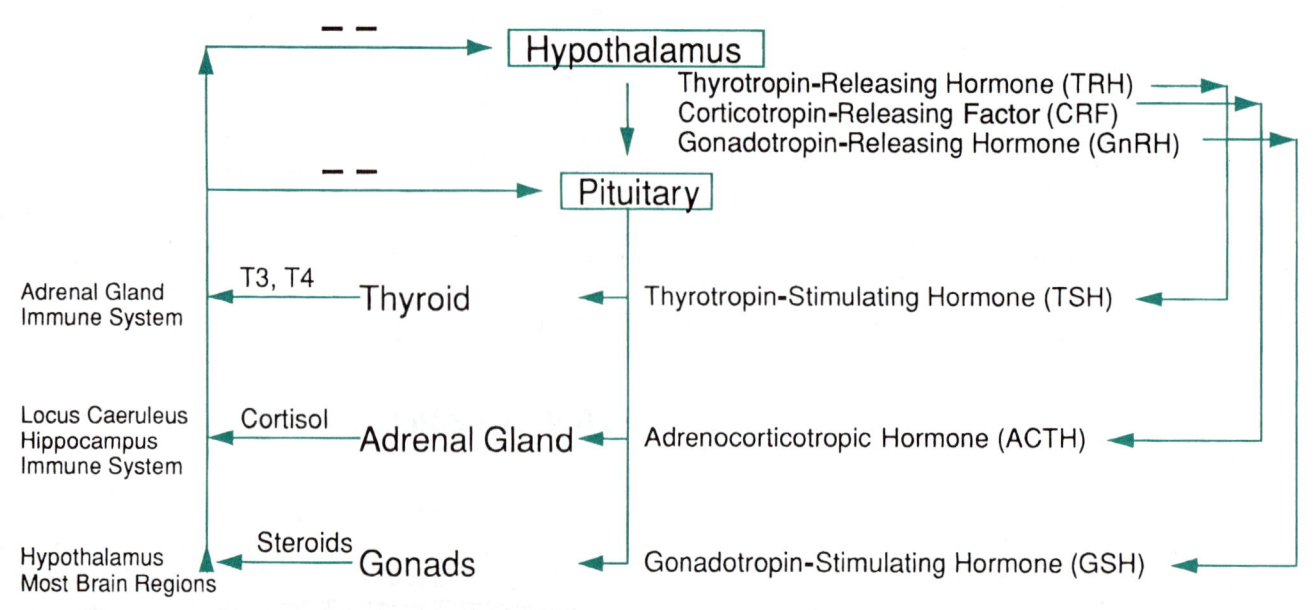

Figure 5–8. Schematic of the hypothalamic-pituitary-adrenal axis. Diagram illustrates the network of negative feedback systems involved in the regulation of stress-related hormones.

and shuts off the release of CRF. This system can fail in depressed or traumatized individuals, resulting in an abnormal stress response.

At every step, these neuroendocrine effects produce the stress response in the nervous system. For instance, CRF stimulates the locus caeruleus to release norepinephrine, which increases blood pressure and body temperature. As the individual is repeatedly exposed to the stressor, the individual's response either diminishes or increases each time, depending on the perception of the stress. In preclinical (animal) and clinical (human) studies of this system, the HPA axis was implicated in major depression and in some anxiety disorders, particularly PTSD. In general, exposure to acute stress results in overactivation of the HPA axis, with increased release of glucocorticoids, whereas chronic stress or repeated exposure to the same stressor leads to an attenuation of the adrenal cortical stress response.

In studies of adults with depression, increased cortisol levels (cortisolemia) and continued cortisol release are apparent when stimulated in a specific challenge study, the dexamethasone suppression test (DST) (see Chapter 19). The explanation for the DST changes is that the feedback to the HPA axis fails to occur in some depressed individuals, and thus cortisol release continues. Unlike many medical conditions that have few to no biological markers for screening, identification, or diagnosis, DST is a possible marker for depression. If the results are consistently replicated, these investigations may lead to a clinical test to measure cortisol, aiding in the diagnosis and treatment of depression.

IMMUNE FUNCTION AND MENTAL ILLNESS

Stress greatly influences psychological functioning and the exacerbation of symptoms in psychiatric clients. Stress can also impact how the immune system functions; it is a powerful psychological influence on the body's overall functioning. The emerging field of psychoimmunology is dedicated to elucidating the mechanisms of this process.

Through the use of various molecules, including lymphocytes, T-helper cells, natural killer cells, and macrophages, the body attacks and destroys anything that is foreign. These foreign molecules, known as *antigens*, can be bacterial or viral in nature (see the following discussion on Jakob-Creutzfeldt disease). Various stressors suppress immune function, rendering the individual more susceptible to illness. Among these stressors are physical and sexual abuse, sleep deprivation, and death of a family member. For instance, depression is associated with a suppression of natural killer cells, lymphocytes, and T-helper cells. Antibody titers are also increased, indicating poor immune function, in students during examination time and in individuals with depression.

Both the autonomic nervous system and the neuroendocrine system, via the pituitary gland, mediate the response with the immune system.[7] These effects are mediated primarily by the HPA axis via glucocorticoids. Lesions of the hypothalamus lead to a decrease in T and B lymphocytes. Stress and immune system interactions are also mediated by catecholamines, endogenous opioids, and pituitary hormones. In fact, some lymphocytes, macrophages, and granulocytes have receptors for some of these neurotransmitters.

The relationship between immune function and the nervous system is to protect the individual; that is, if a person is injured or ill, it is important to modulate behavioral responses appropriately. For a list of stress-related factors that influence immune functioning, see Table 5–4.

Another aspect of immune functioning that can influence nervous system functioning is autoimmune disease, in which

TABLE 5–4. Stress and Immune Function

Important Factors	Duration
Stress-related factors	Degree and duration of stress
	Ability to effectively cope with stressor
Immune system–related factors	Degree and duration of immunogenic activation
	Dependent on which specific immune system is activated
	Environmental factors
	Individual factors (e.g., sex, age, nutritional state)

Source: Adapted from Ader, R, Cohen, N, and Felten, D: Psychoneuroimmunology: Interactions between the nervous system and the immune system. Lancet 345:99–103, 1995.

the body fails to recognize itself as "self." An example of an autoimmune disease is multiple sclerosis, which attacks myelin and impairs the nervous system by slowing down or destroying nerve pathways. Narcolepsy (uncontrollable drowsiness) may be another autoimmune disorder.

Finally, from a different perspective on immune dysfunction and the nervous system, very few bacteria or viruses can directly attack the brain because of the protective blood-brain barrier. One theory of obsessive-compulsive disorder posits that antibodies produced during repeated exposure to strep throat in genetically vulnerable individuals attack the basal ganglia, thereby producing obsessive-compulsive–like symptoms. Other illnesses that can pass through this barrier are rabies and acquired immunodeficiency syndrome (AIDS), presumably because these diseases break down the barrier itself. A disorder that is much rarer but has captured public interest is Jakob-Creutzfeldt disease, also known as "mad cow disease" or scrapie in animals. A "slow virus" was first blamed for this disease. However, mad cow disease is produced by a protein, not a virus, that has eluded scientists for years. This abnormal protein has been transmitted to humans through consumption of infected meat from cows or sheep. The symptoms can remain dormant for decades and then, within months, the disease can produce rapid mental deterioration and death. The anatomical effect of this virus in the brain is literally to produce holes in neurons, dramatically reducing their functioning.

SEX DIFFERENCES IN BRAIN HEMISPHERES

The brain is a lateralized structure and, interestingly, there are sex differences in how the brain reacts to the outside world. PET scans have shown that the resting metabolism of the brain is higher in the more primitive areas of the brain associated with motion and action in males. Metabolism in female brains is higher in more language-based areas, although these areas tend to be smaller in men than in women. One possible implication is that whereas men are more likely to act on their thoughts and feelings, women are more likely to want to talk about them first.

Clinically, differences in brain metabolism have been observed between men and women during periods of sadness. Blood flow into the limbic system of women is eight times higher than that in the men, even though both sexes rate their sadness equally. These results may help explain why the prevalence of depression is twofold higher in women.

KEY POINTS

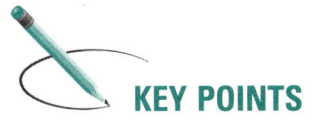

- Many different brain areas interact to affect behavior, emotion, and cognition.
- The blood-brain barrier protects the brain. It can prevent medications, proteins, and other molecules circulating in blood vessels from leaving the blood and entering brain tissue.
- The brain is divided into two hemispheres. Except for the pineal gland, all of the different cortical lobes and definitive structures are found in each hemisphere. The major pathway connecting the two hemispheres is the corpus callosum.
- *Hemispheric laterality* refers to specialized functioning in different sides of the brain. The left hemisphere is dominant for "more scientific functions" such as language, complex voluntary movement, reading, writing, and mathematical tasks, whereas the right hemisphere is more "artistic," specializing in nonlanguage-based tasks, including visual, tactile, and auditory pattern recognition; intuition; and sense of direction.
- The cortex is the area of higher-level thinking and is intimately involved in the qualities that make us human, including our ability to use language and think abstractly.
- Abnormalities in the frontal cortex play a role in a number of mental illnesses, including schizophrenia, attention-deficit hyperactivity disorder (ADHD), and various dementias.
- The limbic system, composed of the hippocampus, amygdala, and the fornix, is involved in emotion, memory, and learning and mediates feelings of aggression, sexual impulses, and submissive behaviors.
- The basal ganglia initiates and controls activity, muscle tone, posture, and muscle movements and works primarily to inhibit motor movements. It is associated with Tourette's disease, Parkinson's disease, and Huntington's disease.
- The thalamus, hypothalamus, and pineal gland comprise the diencephalon.

- The pineal gland secretes melatonin, a hormone that regulates the sleep and wake cycle, and has the largest concentration of serotonin.
- Information transfer between brain regions occurs through neurons. Neurons "talk" to each other through neurotransmission.
- Four major types of neurotransmitters in the brain are involved in psychiatric illness: biogenic amines, cholinergics, neuropeptides, and amino acids.
- Neuroimaging techniques are currently used to study brain abnormalities. CT and MRI are neuroimaging techniques that may identify gross anatomical changes in the brain. PET, SPECT, and some MRI scans may provide limited information about functional, that is, physiological changes.

REFERENCES

1. Fischbach, GS: Mind and brain. Scientific American, September, 48–57, 1992.
2. Gershon, ES, and Rieder, RO: Major disorders of mind and brain. Scientific American, September, 127–133, 1992.
3. Cooper, J, Bloom, F, and Roth, RH: The Biological Basis of Neuropharmacology. Oxford University Press, New York, 1996.
4. Goodwin, FK, and Redfield-Jamson, K: Manic Depressive Illness. Oxford University Press, New York, 1990.
5. Olney, JW: Excitatory amino acids and neuropsychiatric disorders. Biological Psychiatry 26:505–525, 1989.
6. Wever, R: The Circadian System of Man. Springer Verlag, New York, 1979.
7. Ader, R, Cohen, N, and Felten, D: Psychoneuroimmunology: Interactions between the nervous system and the immune system. Lancet 345: 99–103, 1995.
8. Chrousos, G, and Gold, PW: Concepts of stress and stress system disorders: Overview of physical and behavioral homeostasis. JAMA 267: 1244–1252, 1985.

UNIT THREE

Treatment and Therapies

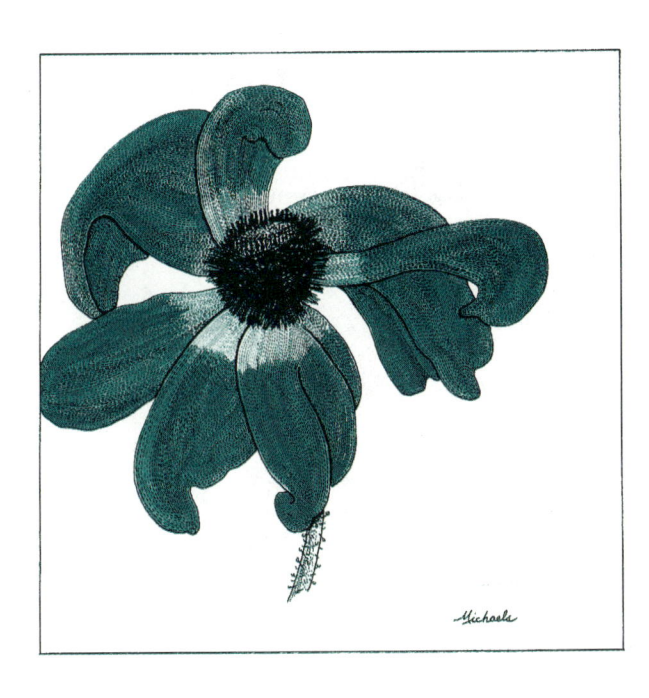

CHAPTER 6
Psychopharmacology

CHAPTER 7
Cognitive-Behavior Therapy

CHAPTER 8
Crisis Intervention

CHAPTER 9
Group Therapy and Therapeutic Groups

CHAPTER 10
Family Therapy

CHAPTER 11
Sexual Therapy

CHAPTER 12
Reminiscence Therapy

CHAPTER 13
Milieu Therapy

CHAPTER 14
Electroconvulsive Therapy and Other Biological Therapies

CHAPTER 6

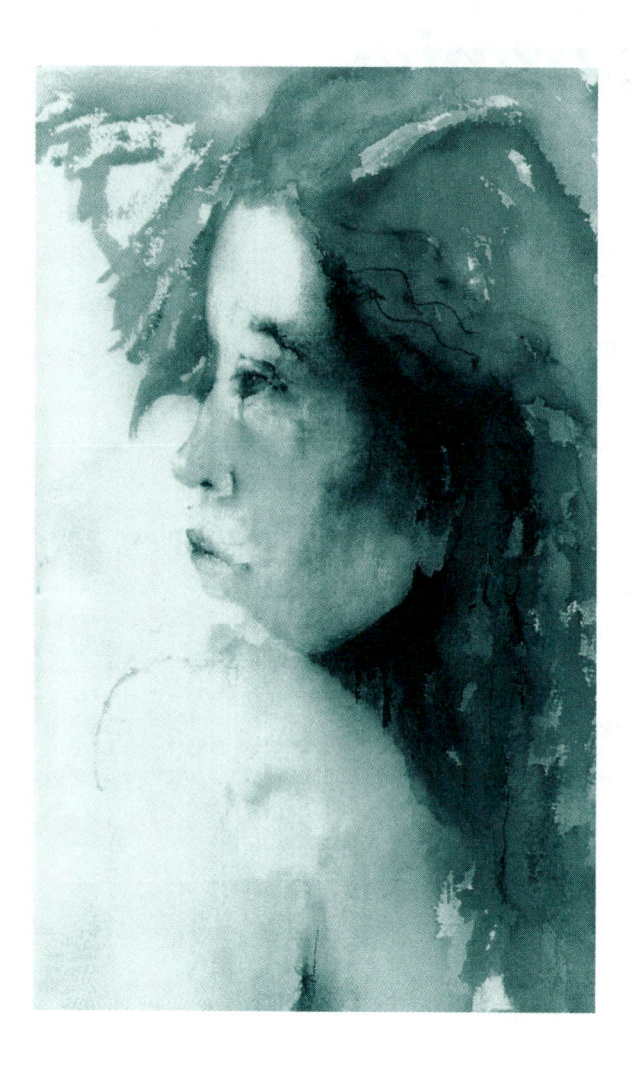

CHAPTER OUTLINE

Neuropharmacology
Pharmacokinetics and Pharmacodynamics
  Cultural and Gender Factors
  Pregnancy and Lactation
Antidepressants
  General Information
  Tricyclic Antidepressants
  Monoamine Oxidase Inhibitors (MAOIs)
  Selective Serotonin Reuptake Inhibitors (SSRIs)
  Novel Antidepressant Medications
  Nursing Considerations
Mood Stabilizers
  General Information
  Lithium Carbonate
  Carbamazepine
  Valproic Acid
  Nursing Considerations
Antipsychotic Medications (Neuroleptics)
  General Information
  Nursing Considerations
Anxiolytics and Sedative-Hypnotics
  General Information
  Benzodiazepines
  Buspirone
  Nursing Considerations
Psychostimulants
  General Information
Synopsis of Current Research
Areas for Future Research

Carol A. Glod, RN, CS, PhD
Suzanne Levy, RN, PhD

Psychopharmacology

LEARNING OBJECTIVES

After completing this chapter, the reader should be able to:

- Understand the indications, dosage, contraindications, and adverse reactions of antidepressants, anxiolytics, mood stabilizers, antipsychotics, and psychostimulants.
- Differentiate between common and uncommon side effects of the major psychopharmacologic agents.
- Describe the proposed mechanism of action of the psychotropic medications.
- Teach patients about positive outcomes anticipated with psychopharmacotherapy, as well as potential adverse reactions and management strategies.
- Distinguish between symptoms of a disorder and side effects that emerge during the course of treatment.
- Devise a medication teaching plan based on the individual's beliefs, intelligence, culture, and age.

KEY TERMS

akathisia
anxiolytics
dystonias
extrapyramidal syndrome (EPS)
mood stabilizers
neuroleptic malignant syndrome (NMS)
pharmacodynamics
pharmacokinetics
psychopharmacotherapy
reuptake
selective serotonin reuptake inhibitors (SSRIs)
tardive dyskinesia (TD)

Psychopharmacotherapy, also called *pharmacotherapy*, is the treatment of psychiatric disorders with psychotropic medications, those drugs that affect the central nervous system (CNS) and reduce or eliminate the symptoms of psychiatric disorders. Researchers have made significant advances in the understanding of the biological basis of psychiatric disorders. An outgrowth of this research has been many new medications to aid in treatment of these disorders. Pharmacotherapy offers safe and effective treatment and is aimed at helping individuals resume their previous level of functioning with improved quality of life. Before pharmacologic treatment is initiated, a diagnostic evaluation is necessary to assess past history of symptoms or illnesses, current physical and mental status, current medications, drug and alcohol abuse, family history of any psychiatric disorders, and target symptoms. The selection of a particular pharmacologic agent depends on the nature of the person's behavior and symptoms, past history, past response to medication, family members' responses to treatment, and concurrent disorders.

The following sections detail the key aspects of treatment with major classes of psychotropic medications (agents used to treat psychiatric disorders). Antidepressants, mood stabilizers, antipsychotics, benzodiazepines and sedative-hypnotics, and psychostimulants represent the major pharmacotherapeutic options. The doses, indications, pharmacokinetics, mechanisms of action, contraindications and precautions, adverse reactions, and clinically significant interactions are an important part of the nurse's knowledge base. In particular, common, occasional, and potentially dangerous side effects are noted here.

NEUROPHARMACOLOGY

How do the psychopharmacologic agents work? Most of the medications have their effects at the neuronal synapse, producing changes in neurotransmitter release and the receptors they bind to. Table 6–1 lists the possible effects linked with specific receptor blockade. Each class of psychopharmacologic medications is briefly discussed; however, their specific effects are detailed as mechanisms of action within each section.

Researchers hypothesize that most antidepressants work by blocking the reuptake of neurotransmitters, specifically, serotonin and norepinephrine. **Reuptake** is the process of neurotransmitter inactivation by which the neurotransmitter is reabsorbed into the presynaptic neuron from which it had been released. Blocking the reuptake process allows more serotonin and norepinephrine to be available for neuronal transmission. Blockade of norepinephrine and serotonin may also result in undesirable side effects (see Table 6–1). Some antidepressants also block receptor sites that are unrelated to their mechanisms of action. These include α-adrenergic, histaminergic, and muscarinic cholinergic receptors. Blocking these receptors is associated with the development of certain side effects (see Figure 6–1).

Mood stabilizers may exert their main effects by inhibiting a process called *kindling*. They act to diminish repetitive

TABLE 6–1. Neuropharmacologic Effects on Neurotransmitters

NE reuptake blockade	Alleviation of depression Tachycardia, sexual dysfunction
SE reuptake blockade	Alleviation of depression, anxiety, obsessive-compulsive disorder Nausea, headache, nervousness, akathisia, sexual dysfunction, tremor
DA reuptake blockade	Alleviation of psychosis; possible antidepressant properties Behavioral activation; aggravation of psychosis
5-HT_2 blockade	Alleviation of depression, psychosis
Muscarinic-cholinergic blockade	Dry mouth, constipation, blurred vision, urinary hesitancy, sinus tachycardia, memory dysfunction
α_1-adrenergic blockade	Orthostatic hypotension, dizziness, reflex tachycardia
α_2-adrenergic blockade	Priapism, potentiation of antihypertensives
Histaminergic blockade	Sedation, weight gain, drowsiness, hypotension, potentiation of CNS depressants

mood cycles by making each episode less likely to appear or worsen. Antipsychotic medications block dopamine receptors, and some affect muscarinic cholinergic, histaminergic, and α-adrenergic receptors. The "atypical" antipsychotics block a specific serotonin receptor. Benzodiazepines facilitate the transmission of the inhibitory neurotransmitter γ-aminobutyric acid (GABA). The psychostimulants work by increasing norepinephrine, serotonin, and dopamine release.

Although each psychotropic medication affects neurotransmission, the specific drugs within each class have varying neuronal effects. Their exact mechanisms of action are unknown. Many of the neuronal effects occur acutely; however, the therapeutic effects may take weeks for some medications such as antidepressants and antipsychotics. Acute alterations in neuronal function do not fully explain how these medications work. Long-term neuropharmacologic reactions to increased norepinephrine and serotonin levels relate more to their mechanisms of action. Recent research suggests that the therapeutic effects are related to the nervous system's adaptation to increased levels of neurotransmitters (see Research Note).[1] These adaptive changes result from a homeostatic mechanism, much like a thermostat, that regulates the cell and maintains equilibrium.

PHARMACOKINETICS AND PHARMACODYNAMICS

Pharmacodynamics refers to the clinical effects of the drug, both positive and negative, on the individual. A positive effect could be relief from depressive symptoms. A negative effect could be dry mouth or constipation. **Pharmacokinetics** refers to drug movement within the body, that is, absorption, distribution, metabolism, and half-life. *Half-life* refers to the amount of time it takes for half of the drug to be removed from the bloodstream. Little relationship exists between half-life and onset of clinical effectiveness, but half-life is a useful concept because a medication's onset of effect, dosage schedule, and duration of action may be related to this parameter. Multiple daily dosing may be necessary with medications that have short half-lives. Longer half-lives imply more time to reach steady-state drug levels and more time for removal from the system. On average, it will take about five half-lives for a medication to be completely eliminated from the system in a healthy individual after a steady state has been reached.

Metabolism is the process by which medications are eliminated from the body. Because of the liver's size, high blood flow volume, and concentration of isoenzymes that metabolize drugs, one of the most common routes is hepatic metabolism. Some psychotropic medications inhibit major groups of liver enzymes, the cytochrome P-450 isoenzymes, needed to break down many prescription and over-the-counter drugs. When used together, these drugs are not metabolized effectively and may remain in the bloodstream longer, leading to possible toxicity. Nurses need to be aware of all medications a client is taking that may affect response to psychotropic medications.

Medications also vary in their protein binding. Those agents that are highly bound to plasma protein will displace other drugs from protein binding and elevate their plasma levels.

CULTURAL AND GENDER FACTORS

Ethnicity, race, and gender may play a role in pharmacokinetics. Recent research has described differential responses to psychotropic medications in individuals from different races. Compared with whites and African Americans, Asians have increased sensitivity to alcohol, antipsychotics, antidepressants, and benzodiazepines, and they require lower dosages. African Americans, on the other hand, may develop quicker antidepressant responses because they have higher plasma levels of tricyclic antidepressants. Because lithium metabolism is less efficient, African Americans need lower daily lithium doses. Very little is known about the effects of gender on drug metabolism. Some preliminary evidence suggests that women may respond better to serotonin reuptake inhibitors than to tricyclic antidepressants. Future research may determine more precise information on the relationship between psychopharmacology and the variables of race and gender.

PREGNANCY AND LACTATION

Psychotropic medications may be passed on to the developing fetus and are secreted in breast milk. Treatment during the first trimester of pregnancy poses the greatest risk to the

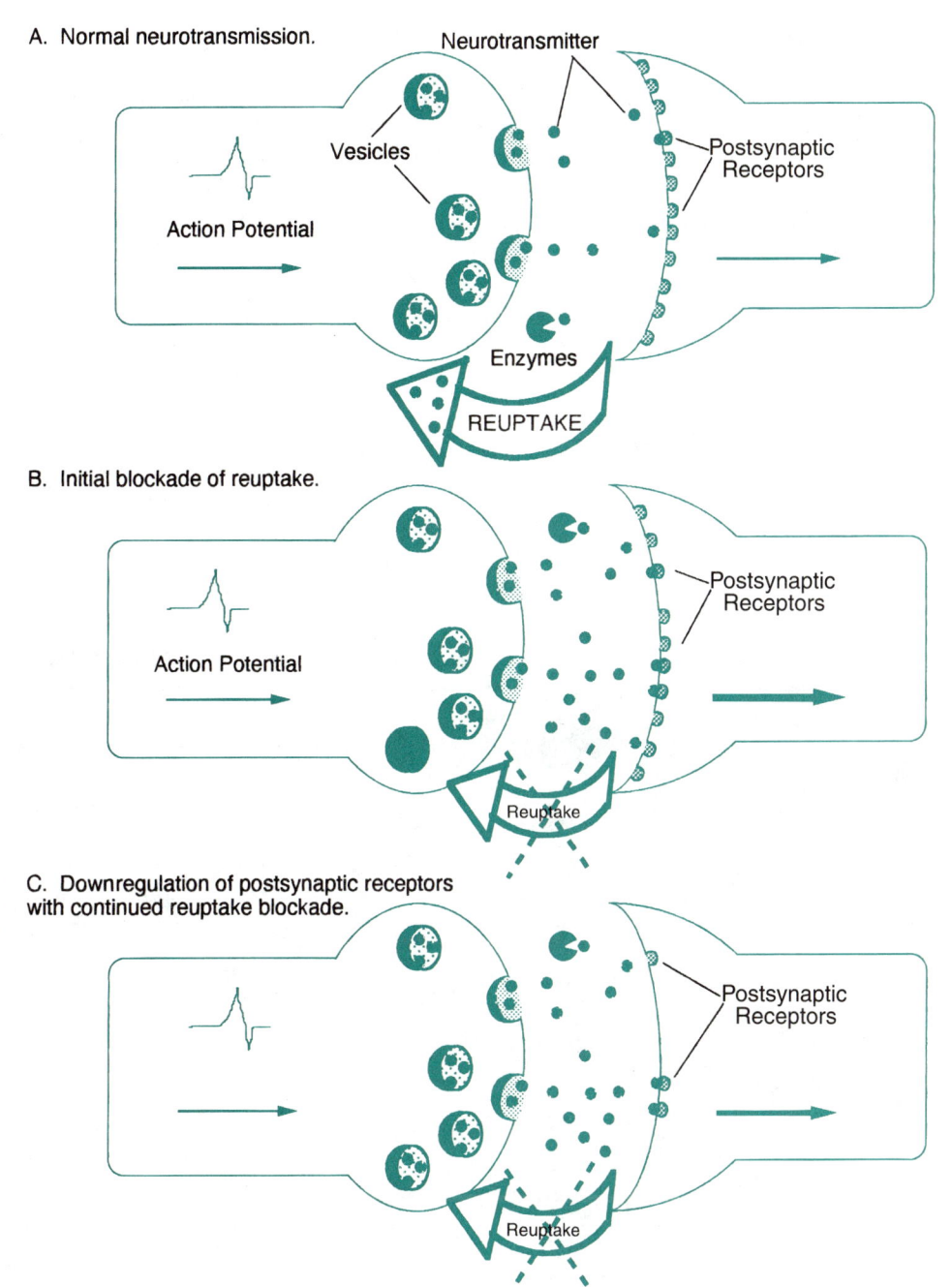

Figure 6-1: The effects of a reuptake blocker on neurotransmission. The arrows indicate the strength of the response, both presynaptically and postsynaptically. (A) Shows normal neurotransmission. (B) The acute effects of reuptake blockade. Neurotransmitter levels increase in the synapse, and the output of the postsynaptic neuron is much stronger. (C) During the course of chronic treatment, the postsynaptic receptors downregulate (decrease in number) and the response moderates. (Courtesy of Susan L. Andersen, PhD, McLean Hospital.)

developing fetus. Some medications complicate the third trimester and parturition. However, an untreated psychiatric disorder also poses substantial prenatal risk. To determine whether to institute or maintain pharmacotherapy during pregnancy, prescribing physicians and nurses carefully weigh the benefits of medication versus the risks to the fetus.

ANTIDEPRESSANTS

GENERAL INFORMATION

Since their introduction in the 1950s, antidepressant medications have provided countless individuals with undeniable relief. However, some clients receive only a partial response. Despite drug studies demonstrating antidepressant efficacy in 65 to 80% of clients, the placebo response rate in some depression studies is as high as 40%, and even higher in studies of childhood depression. The onset of action for antidepressants in the treatment of depression is usually at least 2 to 4 weeks. Overall, all antidepressants are equally effective in treating the symptoms of major depression. Expanding uses of some antidepressants include anxiety, eating disorders, pain disorders, and smoking cessation. Side effects may occur with any of these agents despite recent efforts to develop drugs with different or less bothersome side effects. Nonetheless, for the treatment of acute depressive symptomatology, antidepressants are clearly indicated, and some individuals respond favorably.

The first classes of antidepressants introduced were the tricyclic antidepressants and monoamine oxidase inhibitors (MAOIs). These agents have been used for more than 40 years. In the last decade, new agents have proliferated. **Selective serotonin reuptake inhibitors (SSRIs)** were developed as a unique class of antidepressants, without the bothersome side effects of tricyclic antidepressants. Next, several other miscellaneous antidepressant medications became available. The currently available antidepressants and their dosages, half-lives, and major side effects are listed in Table 6–2.

TRICYCLIC ANTIDEPRESSANTS

Indications

Tricyclic antidepressants (TCAs) are indicated for the treatment of major depression, the depressed phase of bipolar disorder, and dysthymia. Some of the tricyclic antidepressants are specifically indicated for certain conditions including chronic pain syndrome, panic disorder, obsessive-compulsive disorder (OCD), borderline personality disorder, attention deficit hyperactivity disorder (ADHD), bulimia, migraine headaches, peptic ulcer, fibromyalgia, and nocturnal enuresis in children.

Pharmacokinetics

TCAs are rapidly and well absorbed after oral administration. Oral doses are administered in either divided or once-daily doses depending on the particular agent's half-life. TCAs with activating action are taken in the morning, whereas those with sedative effects are taken at bedtime. TCAs are lipophilic, strongly bound to plasma protein and tissues, and not removed effectively by hemodialysis after overdose.

When absorbed, these medications are widely distributed

TABLE 6–2. Common Antidepressant Medications, Elimination Half-Lives, Dosages, and Relative Side Effects

	Dose/Day	Half-Life (hrs)‡	Anticholinergic	Anxiety/ Agitation	Insomnia	Sedation	GI Distress
Tricyclic Antidepressants							
Amitriptyline (Elavil)	75–300	10–46	****	*	*	***	*
Amoxapine (Ascendin)	75–300	8	****	*	***	***	*
Clomipramine (Anafranil)	75–250	17–28	****	*	*	****	*
Desipramine (Norpramin)	75–300	12–76	**	***	*	*	*
Doxepin (Sinequan)	75–300	8–36	***	*	*	***	*
Imipramine (Tofranil)	75–300	4–34	***	***	*	***	**
Nortriptyline (Pamelor)	50–200	13–88	**	*	*	*	*
Protriptyline (Vivactil)	20–60	54–124	****	***	**	*	*
Trimipramine (Surmontil)	75–300	7–30	****	*	*	****	*
Monoamine Oxidase Inhibitors†							
Phenelzine (Nardil)	30–90	2	**	*	****	***	*
Tranylcypromine (Parnate)	20–60	2	**	***	****	**	*
Selegiline (Eldepryl)§	5–10	2–21	*	*	**	*	***
Selective Serotonin Reuptake Inhibitors							
Fluvoxamine (Luvox)	50–300	15–22	*	**	***	***	***
Fluoxetine (Prozac)	10–80	24–518	*	***	***	**	***
Paroxetine (Paxil)	10–50	3–20	*	***	***	**	***
Sertraline (Zoloft)	50–200	24–66	*	***	***	**	***
Novel Antidepressants							
Trazodone (Desyrel)	150–450	4–9	*	**	*	****	*
Bupropion (Wellbutrin)††	150–450	10–14	*	***	**	*	*
Venlafaxine (Effexor)	150–375	5–16	*	***	**	*	***
Nefazodone (Serzone)	200–500	5	*	*	*	***	***
Mirtazapine (Remeron)	20–35	20–40	*	*	*	****	*

* = very low, ** = low, *** = moderate, **** = high
†Isocarboxazid (Marplan) is no longer available.
‡Elimination half-life includes parent drug and active metabolites.
§Indicated for the treatment of Parkinson's disease.
††Also available in a sustained-release formulation. Teicher, MH, Glod, CA, and Cole, JO: Antidepressant drugs and the emergence of suicidal tendencies. Drug Safety 8:186, 1993.
Source: Adapted from Physician's Desk Reference, 1996, and Teicher et al, 1993.

and excreted in the urine. The major route of metabolism of most antidepressants is by the liver. The tricyclic compounds imipramine and amitriptyline yield active metabolites, desipramine and nortriptyline. The elimination half-lives of TCAs range from 20 to 126 hours (decreased in the elderly); with ordinary clinical doses, most of the drug should be eliminated 1 week after discontinuing treatment (except with protriptyline.

TCAs are distributed across the placenta to the developing fetus. Similarly, TCAs and their metabolites may be passed on to infants during lactation.

Therapeutic Blood Levels and Monitoring. TCAs are the only antidepressants with established therapeutic plasma levels, although reliable data exist only on imipramine, nortriptyline, and possibly desipramine. Blood levels are monitored for dosage titration, to determine whether the drug is being metabolized, and with prescription of high dosages. For imipramine and desipramine, a linear relationship exists between dose and drug responsiveness. Thus, with increased dose comes increased effectiveness. For imipramine, blood levels above 220 ng/mL are generally associated with clinical response. With nortriptyline, a different relationship exists: that of the "therapeutic window." Clinical improvement is associated with blood levels between 50 and 200 ng/mL. Blood levels below or above the therapeutic window usually provide poor response.

Mechanism of Action

TCAs have broad-spectrum neuronal effects. They block the reuptake of neurotransmitters such as norepinephrine and serotonin into the presynaptic neuron (Figure 6–2). Some TCAs such as desipramine more selectively block norepinephrine, others such as amitriptyline block serotonin, whereas others affect both systems. Reuptake blockade allows more available neurotransmitter in the synaptic cleft. Increased availability means that more of the substance can be transmitted across the cleft to connect with postsynaptic receptors. Next, the neurotransmitter disperses to different parts of the brain. These effects all occur acutely, hours or days after antidepressant administration. Acute administration of antidepressants produces little in the way of therapeutic benefit. However, acute administration of TCAs leads to blockade of muscarinic cholinergic, histaminergic, and α-adrenergic receptors (Figure 6–2). Blocking these receptors is associated with the development of substantial side effects and does not contribute to antidepressant efficacy.

Increased levels of neurotransmitters occur after the first doses of antidepressants; however, the positive clinical effects may take weeks. Long-term neuropharmacologic reactions relate more to understanding how they work. For example, in response to the outpouring of norepinephrine, β-adrenergic receptors downregulate (decrease in number: Figure 6–1). This decrease corresponds to the second phase of medication effects. These adaptive responses are the result of a homeostatic mechanism, much like a thermostat, that regulates the cell and maintains equilibrium. Recent theories suggest that the nervous system's adaptation to increased neurotransmitters produces therapeutic responsiveness.[1]

Contraindications and Precautions

TCAs lower seizure threshold, and the risk of developing a seizure is about 1 to 2 in 1000 individuals. Therefore, TCAs should be used cautiously in clients with known seizure disorders. Of the TCAs, clomipramine has the greatest effect on lowering seizure threshold.

TCAs have known cardiac effects and are contraindicated in clients with underlying conduction disturbances. Avoid TCAs in clients with bifascicular block, left bundle branch block, or a prolonged QT interval.[1]

Use TCAs cautiously in clients with prostatic hypertrophy, urinary retention, and narrow-angle glaucoma because of the drug's enhanced anticholinergic effects.

Warn patients to avoid alcohol during antidepressant treatment, as it may worsen symptoms or potentiate the effect of medication. Excess sedation may result, along with impairment in motor and cognitive performance. Because the primary route of elimination appears to be hepatic metabolism to inactive metabolites excreted by the kidney, use these agents cautiously in clients with liver and renal disease. Known hypersensitivity to a TCA also contraindicates treatment.

Safe use during pregnancy has not been established for the majority of antidepressant agents. Congenital malformations during administration of some TCAs have been reported, but studies fail to demonstrate a causal effect. A recent study found that the risk of miscarriages was 12% for women treated with TCAs and 14% with SSRIs, compared with 6% for those who were exposed to nonteratogenic medications.[2] TCAs can also be passed on in breast milk and are used cautiously during lactation (see Research Note: Antidepressant treatment during breast-feeding). They may be prescribed during pregnancy after an in-depth, risk-benefit analysis is completed.

Adverse Reactions

Common Effects. Because TCAs block muscarinic cholinergic receptors, clients develop anticholinergic side effects such as dry mouth, constipation, urinary hesitancy, drying of nasal passages, and blurred vision. Other common side effects include sedation, weight gain, orthostatic hypotension, and tachycardia (see Table 6–2). If the dose is increased too rapidly, these side effects become more problematic. Amitriptyline is one of the most potent anticholinergic agents, whereas desipramine has fewer anticholinergic effects (see Table 6–2). Tolerance may develop to anticholinergic effects; however, clients usually experience these reactions as unpleasant and uncomfortable.

Because of these uncomfortable effects, clients may not regularly take their medication or may discontinue it alto-

Tricyclic Antidepressants

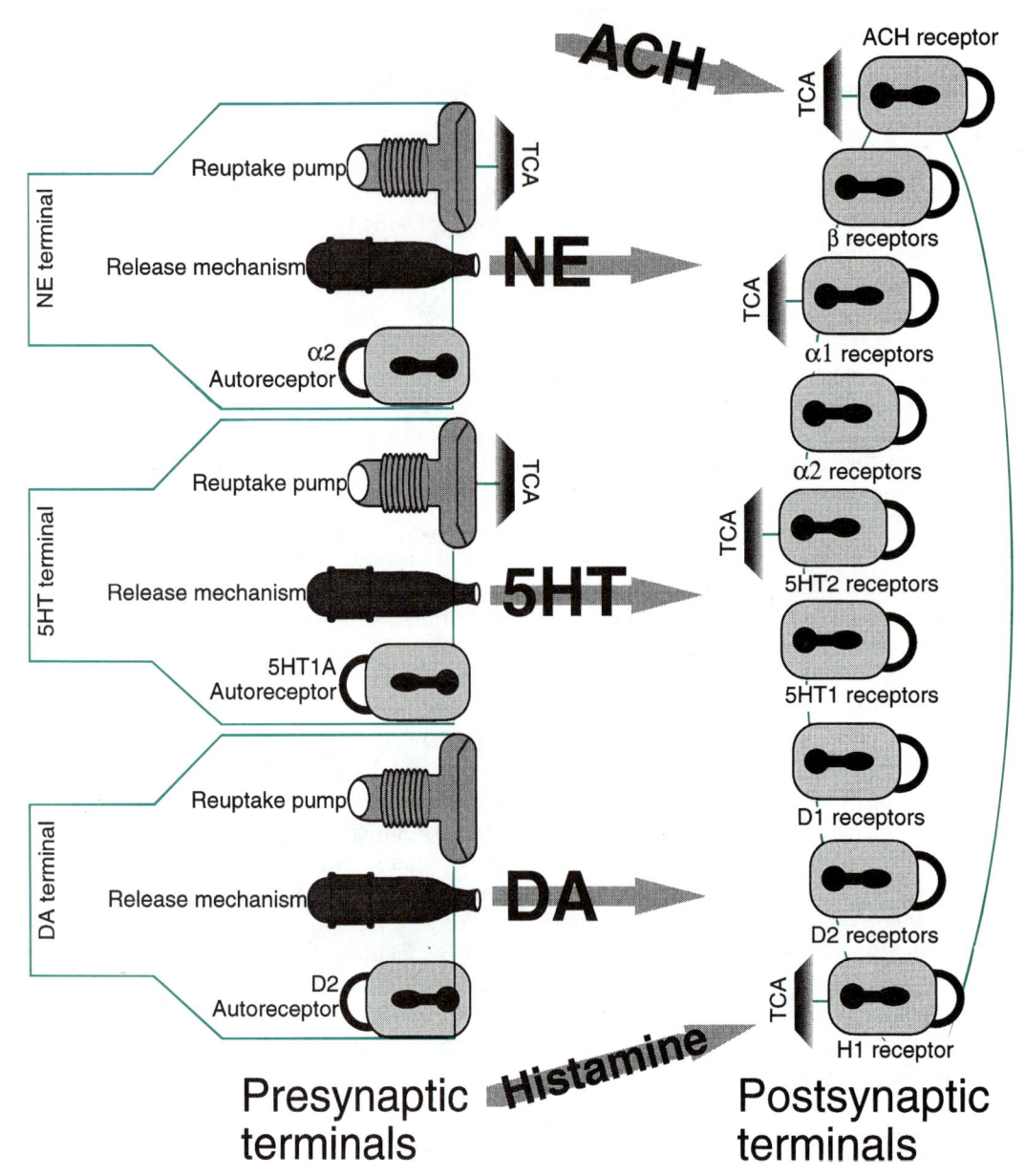

Figure 6–2: The neuropharmacological action of tricyclic antidepressants (TCAs). TCAs block the reuptake pumps of norepinephrine (*Top Left*) and serotonin, also known as 5-hydroxytryptamine (5-HT; *Middle Left*). These actions may explain some of their antidepressant effects. Tricyclics also block several postsynaptic receptors, like a key fits into a lock; these actions are unrelated to their antidepressant effects and are shown on the right side of the figure. TCAs block acetylcholine (ACH), alpha (α), and histaminic (H$_2$) receptors, leading to anticholinergic, cardiac, and sedative effects, respectively. (Courtesy of Martin H. Teicher, MD, PhD, McLean Hospital.)

gether. An important component of the nurse's role is to regularly assess anticholinergic and other effects and teach ways to manage them. Dry mouth can be relieved by rinsing the mouth with water (drinking fluids rarely helps), and increased fiber and laxatives may be necessary for constipation. Regularly assess clients with impaired memory or reality testing for the development of severe constipation.

TCAs block histaminergic receptors, leading to even more uncomfortable effects such as sedation and weight gain. Each TCA differs in its potential for inducing sedation. Amitriptyline, clomipramine, trimipramine, and doxepin have the most potent effects. Adjusting dosage or dosing schedule does not usually minimize sedation. If the client's symptom presentation is more agitated and insomniac, a more sedating agent may prove beneficial and more easily tolerated. Weight gain is a long-term consequence, most likely due to increased appetite and carbohydrate cravings. Some individuals have gained 10 to 20 lb during the first 6 months of treatment. Although weight gain can be minimized by dieting, many clients are unable to control their appetites. Although these side effects also contribute to potential noncompliance, nurses can encourage their continued use while educating the client about coping strategies such as dose timing, diet plans, or a possible medication change.

Cardiac effects, including orthostatic hypotension and tachycardia, result from tricyclic blockade of α_1-adrenergic receptors. *Orthostatic hypotension* is a drop in blood pressure secondary to a change in position. Clients may complain of feeling dizzy or being off balance. Orthostatic changes can lead to dizziness and falls and, in elderly clients, to secondary consequences such as bone fractures. Tachycardia, with increases of 15 to 20 beats per minute, is another common side effect of TCAs. Obtain and regularly monitor a baseline blood pressure and pulse during treatment (daily for inpatients, bimonthly for outpatients), especially during dosage adjustment or for individuals with preexisting hypotension. Take blood pressure measurements while the client sits and then immediately when the client stands to determine if an orthostatic change results. To minimize these effects, instruct clients to rise carefully when changing positions, for example, when first arising in the morning. Severe hypotension or tachycardia requires drug discontinuation.

Occasional Effects. At times, clients develop difficulty with sexual function during treatment with a TCA. Blocking reuptake of norepinephrine or serotonin may account for the development of sexual difficulties. Clients often fail to spontaneously report sexual dysfunction or even recognize it as a possible adverse reaction. Sexual dysfunction may respond to adding amantadine, yohimbine, or cyproheptadine. Dose reduction of TCAs seems to have little effect.

Uncommon but Potentially Serious Effects. TCAs are also associated with uncommon but potentially serious adverse reactions. The most potentially dangerous consequences are cardiac effects. TCAs slow impulse conduction and may precipitate bundle branch block or complete heart block. Sudden cardiac death is a rare but possible effect during treatment with these agents. Cardiac death has been reported in several prepubertal children taking tricyclic medications, most likely because of slowing of cardiac conduction; however, a clear causal relationship has not been established. These deaths occurred with children who took desipramine.

Until recently, researchers widely assumed that TCAs adversely affected left ventricular function (LVF); however, research reports indicate that it is infrequent.[3] Similarly, while TCAs were initially contraindicated in clients with preexisting arrhythmias, imipramine and nortriptyline (and perhaps other TCAs) have significant antiarrhythmic effects against premature ventricular contractions.[3]

TCAs may induce mania in clients with known bipolar disorder or in clients with no underlying manic history. Many clients will not recognize manic symptoms in the beginning; therefore, it is important for nurses to assess the client for these behaviors. If mania occurs, immediate pharmacologic intervention is necessary. The interventions will depend on the severity and duration of the manic symptoms, the client's history, and past response to other agents. Dose reduction or discontinuation is generally the first step. Treatment with antimanic agents (neuroleptics or lithium) is often initiated.

Clinically Significant Interactions

TCAs should not be used in combination with monoamine oxidase inhibitors (MAOIs—see the following). Additive anticholinergic effects arise in combination with certain antipsychotic medications. Blood levels of tricyclics may be increased when used in combination with cimetidine (Tagamet), neuroleptics, stimulants, calcium channel blockers, or SSRIs. TCAs may also affect other drugs and lead to a variety of complications. Tricyclics combined with antiarrhythmic drugs lead to cardiac toxicity secondary to prolonged cardiac conduction. TCAs also decrease the antihypertensive effects of clonidine, methyldopa, and guanethidine. Conversely, tricyclics may increase the effects of warfarin. Some anticonvulsants (for example, carbamazepine) decrease TCA levels, whereas others (for instance, valproic acid) increase levels. TCAs increase levels of carbamazepine because of inhibition of metabolism. Because of their sedating and hypotensive effects, use TCAs cautiously with any medication that also possesses these characteristics.

MONOAMINE OXIDASE INHIBITORS (MAOIs)

Indications

MAOIs are indicated for the treatment of major depression, atypical depression, the depressed phase of bipolar disorder, dysthymia, panic disorder, bulimia, and borderline personality disorder. Less commonly, MAOIs may be used for the treatment of OCD, narcolepsy, posttraumatic stress disorder (PTSD), social phobia, and chronic pain syndrome. Overall, this class of antidepressants is reserved for treatment-resistant depression (episodes of depression that have failed to respond to other antidepressant medication trials), because of their potential for severe interactions and the need for dietary restrictions (see the following). Selegiline (Eldepryl), another MAOI, is used to treat Parkinson's disease.

Pharmacokinetics

MAOIs are rapidly absorbed from the gastrointestinal tract, widely distributed, and given in divided doses. These medications are relatively lipophilic, although at low pH levels they are highly soluble. The major route of metabolism is by the liver, although the metabolism of MAOIs is not well understood. MAOIs are distributed across the placenta to the developing fetus and are passed on to infants during lactation.

Mechanism of Action

MAOIs inhibit the action of two isoenzymes, monoamine oxidase A (MAO-A) and monoamine oxidase B (MAO-B), present in the CNS that metabolize neurotransmitters (serotonin, norepinephrine, and dopamine). The two MAOIs currently approved for the treatment of depression affect both isoenzymes, whereas selegiline is selective for MAO-B at lower doses. Two agents that selectively inhibit the MAO-A enzyme, moclobemide and brofaromine, are currently being studied for the treatment of depression.

Normally, the enzyme monoamine oxidase (MAO) degrades norepinephrine and serotonin in the presynaptic neuron. MAOIs inhibit the enzyme MAO. However, inhibition of these enzymes halts the degradation and leads to increased availability of neurotransmitters. The end result is that more norepinephrine and serotonin are released for dispersion postsynaptically and to the rest of the brain.

Contraindications and Precautions

Avoid MAOIs in clients with known seizure disorders and in pregnant or lactating women, and use them cautiously in individuals with liver and renal disease. Warn clients to avoid alcohol.

Adverse Reactions

Common Effects. The most common side effects of the MAOIs are daytime sedation, insomnia, weight gain, dry mouth, orthostatic hypotension (dizziness), peripheral edema, and sexual dysfunction. Daytime sedation may be so severe that individuals fall asleep during work or while driving. MAOI-induced sedation and insomnia are difficult to treat, and switching the time of administration offers little relief. Insomnia may be treated with trazodone. If the client's insomnia is severe, the nurse may need to change to a different class of antidepressant. Manage peripheral edema by suggesting that the client use elastic support stockings or increase salt in the diet. At times a salt-retaining steroid may be necessary.

Occasional Effects. Less common effects may include myoclonic jerks (muscle spasms of the legs). These reactions may be treated with either cyproheptadine or with pyridoxine hydrochloride therapy (vitamin B_6).

Uncommon but Potentially Serious Effects. MAOIs selectively pose a dangerous and potentially life-threatening situation: hypertensive crisis. It occurs most frequently when the MAOI is taken with a substance containing tyramine or a restricted medication such as meperidine (Table 6–3). Tyramine, an amino acid, is normally degraded by MAO in the intestine. With MAOI use, tyramine is not degraded. Ingestion of this substance leads to a massive outpouring of norepinephrine that cannot be metabolized, leading to symptoms of a hypertensive crisis. Clients experience sudden onset of severe headache that may be accompanied by neck stiffness, nausea, sweating, or palpitations. Blood pressure increases abruptly, usually within minutes of ingesting the substance. This rise in blood pressure may lead to hyperpyrexia (increased body temperature) and potentially to stroke, coma, or death. Although rarely clients may ingest tyramine-containing foods without any ill effects, instruct clients to follow the restrictions very carefully.

Other uncommon but potentially dangerous adverse reactions include mania, peripheral neuropathy, and paresthesia. To treat these problems, the MAOI is decreased or discontinued altogether, depending on the severity of symptoms. A deficiency in pyridoxine may lead to the de-

TABLE 6–3. Dietary and Medication Restrictions for Individuals Taking Monoamine Oxidase Inhibitors

Foods to Be Definitely Avoided
All cheeses (with the exception of cottage, cream, ricotta, American)
Broad bean pods, or fava beans
Marmite or veg-o-mite (hydrogenated yeast products)
Beer, red wine*
Sauerkraut*
Soy sauce*
Smoked or pickled fish*
Sausage, pepperoni, salami, bologna, mortadella*
Foods to Be Avoided in Large Quantities or after Freshness Has Expired
Other alcoholic beverages
Ripe avocados, bananas, banana bread
Sour cream
Yogurt
Liver
Medications to Be Avoided
Asthma tablets or inhalers
Weight-reduction aids
Products with dextromethorphan, ephedrine, phenylephrine, phenylpropanolamine
Selective serotonin reuptake inhibitors
Clomipramine
Buspirone
Venlafaxine
Nefazodone
L-dopa
Meperidine
Amphetamines, cocaine

*Small amounts may be tolerated in some individuals under certain conditions.

Source: Adapted from the McLean Hospital Department of Dietetics MAOI Diet

> **RESEARCH NOTE**
>
> Rothschild, AJ: Selective serotonin reuptake inhibitor–induced sexual dysfunction: Efficacy of a drug holiday. Am J Psychiatry 152: 1514–1516, 1995.
>
> **Findings:** In this study, the author devised and tested a strategy to help clients with sexual dysfunction. Because decreased sex drive and difficulty achieving an erection or orgasm is a common side effect of SSRI therapy, brief weekend drug holidays were used to try to improve sexual functioning. In addition, this research explored whether the skipped doses were associated with a relapse of depressive symptoms.
>
> Thirty men and women who were taking paroxetine, sertraline, or fluoxetine participated. Different rates of improvement of sexual functioning were apparent. Fifty percent of the clients taking paroxetine or sertraline reported return of sexual functioning after the medication was discontinued for the weekend. Sexual dysfunction returned when the medication was restarted. In contrast, those who took fluoxetine experienced little to no benefit from the drug holiday. None of the subjects in the entire sample reported that their depressive symptoms returned.
>
> **Application to Practice:** The results of this investigation suggest that SSRI-induced sexual dysfunction can be treated successfully with weekend drug holidays, if the client is taking either paroxetine or sertraline. This may provide a very practical alternative that avoids the addition of another medication to treat sexual dysfunction. It appears that because fluoxetine has a longer half-life, brief medication-free periods are ineffective. Based on this preliminary evidence, psychiatric nurses can suggest that clients "skip" doses of paroxetine or sertraline as a method of treating sexual dysfunction.

velopment of peripheral neuropathy, which responds to pyridoxine therapy.

Clinically Significant Interactions

Many prescription and over-the-counter medications contain ingredients that cause hypertensive reactions when taken along with MAOIs. Table 6–3 lists foods and medications that are contraindicated. Because meperidine and other narcotics can produce a syndrome characterized by hypertension, hyperpyrexia, and coma, pain medications such as meperidine must also be avoided. Aspirin, acetaminophen (Tylenol), and ibuprofen (Advil, Motrin) are *not* restricted and may also be taken concomitantly.

Because of the potential adverse reaction of MAOIs with other medications, therapy with new antidepressants must be started after all of the interacting substances have been eliminated from the body. The combination of MAOIs and SSRIs (for example, fluoxetine) causes a serotonergic syndrome characterized by agitation, confusion, myoclonus, hypertension, tremor, diarrhea, and hypomania.[4] Do not start SSRI therapy until the MAOI has been discontinued for at least 2 weeks. Do not start MAOI therapy until 5 to 6 weeks after discontinuing fluoxetine, and 2 weeks after treatment with other SSRIs. Buspirone and clomipramine, other medications that strongly affect serotonin, lead to a serotonin syndrome when taken along with MAOIs. Their use is also contraindicated.

SELECTIVE SEROTONIN REUPTAKE INHIBITORS (SSRIs)

Indications

The SSRIs are indicated for the treatment of major depression, the depressed phase of bipolar disorder, dysthymia, OCD, panic disorder, and bulimia. Studies are currently underway to assess their effectiveness in borderline personality disorder, premenstrual syndrome, chronic fatigue, smoking cessation, and alcoholism.

Pharmacokinetics

Substantial variability exists in pharmacokinetic properties between the currently available SSRIs. Fluoxetine has the longest half-life, whereas the remaining three SSRIs have half-lives of less than 24 hours (see Table 6–2). As a result, these medications are usually administered in once-daily doses. Fluoxetine and sertraline each have active metabolites with elimination half-lives of 7 to 15 days and 66 hours, respectively. On the other hand, paroxetine and fluvoxamine have metabolites with little or no activity. Although a longer half-life (of the parent drug and metabolites) may provide greater protection against noncompliance, it poses a greater risk for drug-drug interactions. For example, following discontinuation of fluoxetine, a 5- to 6-week washout period is necessary before an MAOI is initiated.

All of the SSRIs are extensively bound to plasma protein, although fluvoxamine has the least effect. They are distributed across the placenta to the developing fetus and are passed on to infants during lactation. The SSRIs inhibit the activity of cytochrome P-450 isoenzymes in the liver. These isoenzymes are needed to metabolize many prescription and over-the-counter medications. Without adjusting doses for these drugs, blood levels can increase and lead to toxicity. The SSRIs have differential effects on cytochrome P-450 isoenzymes, thereby affecting levels of certain classes of medication. For example, fluoxetine increases levels of TCAs, whereas fluvoxamine augments levels of some benzodiazepines (see Table 6–4).

Mechanism of Action

The SSRIs block the reuptake of serotonin into the presynaptic neuron (Figure 6–3). Reuptake blockade occurs

TABLE 6-4. Effect of Newer Antidepressants on Cytochrome P-450 Isoenzymes and Potential Interactions

	Cytochrome P-450 Isoenzyme			
	IA$_2$	IIC	IID$_6$	IIIA$_4$
Antidepressant	Fluvoxamine	Fluvoxamine Fluoxetine	Fluoxetine Paroxetine[†] Sertraline	Fluvoxamine Nefazodone
Medications Affected*	Theophylline Warfarin	Diazepam Imipramine	Desipramine, Other triclyclics Cimetidine Propranolol Haloperidol Risperidone Phenytoin Mirtazapine Cold preparations	Alprazolam Triazolam Terfenadine Astemizole Erythromycin Nifedipine

*Blocking the particular enzyme inhibits metabolism, leads to interactions, and may lead to increased levels of these agents when both are administered.
[†]May have minimal effects.

acutely, and, in response, serotonin is increased in the synaptic cleft. After several days or weeks, receptors located on presynaptic serotonin neurons (autoreceptors) desensitize—a homeostatic neuronal response secondary to increased serotonin. These chronic adaptive reactions probably account for the therapeutic effectiveness of these drugs.

Contraindications and Precautions

Avoid giving SSRIs to clients with known seizure disorders, and use them cautiously in clients with liver and renal disease and in pregnant or lactating women. Instruct clients to avoid alcohol during SSRI therapy.

Adverse Reactions

Common Effects. Enhancing serotonin transmission leads to several common side effects, including agitation, anxiety, akathisia, nausea, insomnia, and sexual dysfunction. Clients may complain of feeling nervous, anxious, or "hyper," have "caffeine-like" effects, or actually experience a form of motor restlessness in which they need to pace or move their legs (**akathisia**). Administration of low-dose beta-blockers such as propranolol or benzodiazepines is necessary to treat akathisia. Clients can minimize nausea by taking the medication with food. Sleep disruption is a common side effect and does not correspond to the timing of medication administration. Thus, clients report insomnia even when the SSRI is taken early in the morning. Insomnia often requires treatment with either a sedative-hypnotic agent or low-dose trazodone.

One of the most troubling side effects is sexual dysfunction. Overlooked in the initial research studies, the incidence of sexual dysfunction may be a high as 33%. Clients experience diminished sex drive or difficulty achieving orgasm or an erection. Often, individuals fail to report these effects either because of embarrassment or lack of knowledge. Because of its effect on medication compliance, ask if any sexual dysfunction is present. Although sexual dysfunction may respond to the addition of amantadine, yohimbine, or cyproheptadine, some individuals do not receive relief. Switching to another antidepressant that does not lead to sexual dysfunction, such as bupropion or nefazodone can be helpful. Finally, for the shorter-acting SSRIs, "drug holidays"—that is, weekends without medication—may treat sexual dysfunction successfully (see Research Note).

Occasional Effects. Less commonly, the SSRIs may cause sedation, sweating, diarrhea, hand tremor, and headache, due to enhanced serotonin neurotransmission. Sedating effects may arise only after high dosages are administered. If moderate or severe sedation emerges, the client will need to switch to another antidepressant. Similarly, excessive sweating is difficult to manage and may require drug discontinuation. Diarrhea can be treated with antidiarrheal agents, and headache, with acetaminophen, aspirin, or ibuprofen.

Uncommon but Potentially Serious Effects. Uncommon but potentially dangerous side effects include seizures, mania, and the induction of severe hostility or suicidal ideation. Recently, the development of obsessive suicidal ideation was described in clients taking fluoxetine.[5] The onset of these effects may occur days to weeks after initiation of the drug and are characterized by intrusive, ruminatory urges or violent images to hurt or mutilate oneself. This side effect appears to be serious but relatively rare. After the antidepressant has been discontinued, the effects generally subside. Some researchers have suggested that suicidal ideation may emerge or intensify because the underlying depression

Selective Serotonin Reuptake Inhibitor

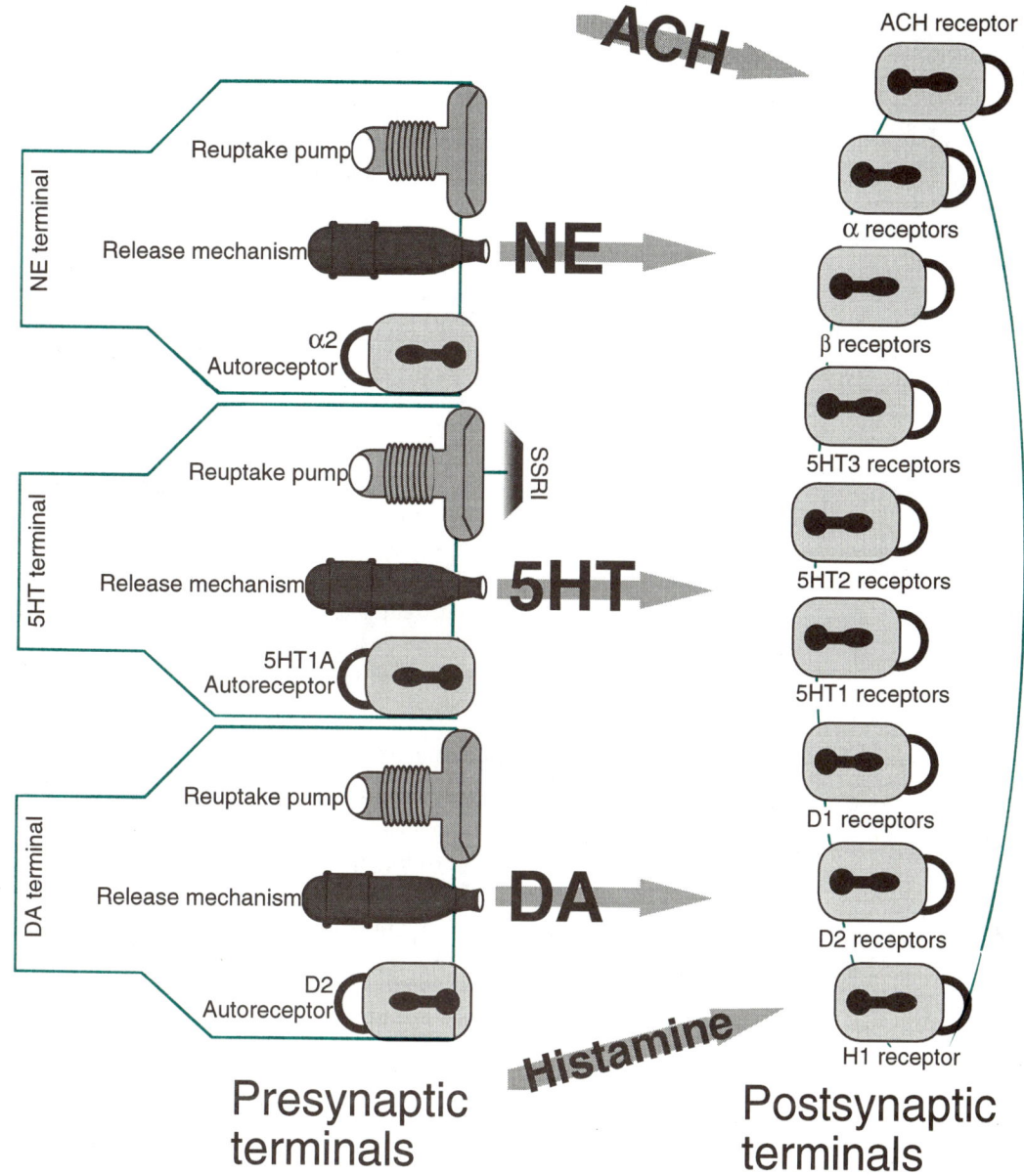

Figure 6–3: The action of selective serotonin reuptake inhibitors (SSRIs). Unlike the tricyclic antidepressants, SSRIs exert antidepressant effects by blocking the reuptake of serotonin (5-hydroxytryptamine [5-HT]; *Middle Left*). Since they do not block any of the postsynaptic receptors, SSRIs fail to cause the uncomfortable side effects associated with the TCAs. (Courtesy of Martin H. Teicher, MD, PhD, McLean Hospital.)

is worsening, rather than as a result of medication use. If severe suicidal ideation arises, drug discontinuation is usually necessary, and hospitalization should be considered. SSRIs are discontinued if seizures or mania results.

Clinically Significant Interactions

Of the SSRIs, fluoxetine and paroxetine appear to have the greatest effects on the P-450 IID$_6$ isoenzyme and have been associated with increasing certain medications to toxic levels (see Table 6–4). SSRIs used in combination with TCAs are not contraindicated; however, take careful precautions. The addition of an SSRI generally leads to a marked elevation of TCA levels and exacerbation of anticholinergic effects.

SSRIs do not appear to potentiate the effects of alcohol.[6] Concomitant MAOI–SSRI therapy leads to the development of a central serotonin syndrome. The SSRIs may increase antiarrhythmic, anticonvulsant, anticoagulant, antipsychotic, oral hypoglycemic, and lithium levels. Cimetidine may inhibit metabolism of SSRIs, thereby increasing their

WHO ARE WE REALLY?

> Do medications change personality? Is society entering a phase of "cosmetic pharmacology," using drugs to enhance our personalities?
>
> Peter Kramer first raised many of these questions in a book called *Listening to Prozac*. In it, he outlines how people without major psychiatric disorders describe their revolutionary response to fluoxetine (Prozac); how it altered their lives and seemingly changed their personalities. He suggests that antidepressant medications can significantly change who we are.
>
> My first meeting with Prozac had been heightened for me by the uncommon qualities of the patient who responded to the drug. I found it astonishing that a pill could do in a matter of days what psychiatrists hope, and often fail, to accomplish by other means over a course of years: to restore a person robbed of it in childhood the capacity to play. Yes, there remained a disquieting element to this restoration.... Charisma, courage, character, social competency—Prozac seemed to say that these and other concepts would need to be reexamined, that our sense of what is constant in the self and what is mutable, what is necessary and what contingent, would need, like our sense of the fable of transformation, to be revised.*
>
> Robert Aranow and other clinicians have noticed that antidepressants may be "mood enhancers": medications that brighten the periodic down days of people who are not clinically depressed, without causing the "highs" of illicit drugs such as cocaine. Antidepressants may promote energy and optimism. However, what are the risks of prescribing these medications to those without depression? These and many other ethical questions remain unanswered.
>
> ---
> *Kramer, P. Listening to Prozac: A Psychiatrist Explores Anti-Depressant Drugs and the Remaking of the Self. Viking Penguin, New York, 1994, p. 21.

levels. Because of the possibility of cardiac effects, use risperidone cautiously with the SSRIs.

NOVEL ANTIDEPRESSANT MEDICATIONS

Several other new antidepressants do not fit into any particular class. They include nefazodone, trazodone, bupropion SR, venlafaxine, and mirtazapine.

Indications

These agents are indicated for the treatment of major depression, the depressed phase of bipolar disorder, and dysthymia. Studies are currently underway to assess the effectiveness of venlafaxine in treatment-resistant depression, ADHD, and panic disorder. Trazodone is indicated for the treatment of sleep disturbances, particularly insomnia induced by other antidepressants. Bupropion effectively treats ADHD and bupropion SR is effective as a treatment for smoking cessation, marketed under the trade name Ziban.

Pharmacokinetics

All of the novel compounds have relatively short half-lives and on average require twice-daily dosing. Trazodone and venlafaxine have active metabolites. They are rapidly absorbed after oral administration, metabolized in the liver, and excreted in urine. All of the miscellaneous antidepressants are distributed across the placenta to the developing fetus and are secreted in breast milk.

Mechanism of Action

Both nefazodone and trazodone block the serotonin 5-HT$_2$ receptor; however, nefazodone has greater effects on serotonin reuptake inhibition than trazodone. Venlafaxine, like TCAs, blocks both serotonin and norepinephrine reuptake but does not block cholinergic, histaminergic, or α_1-adrenergic receptors. Bupropion and bupropion SR are potent dopamine reuptake inhibitors that, with long-term administration, increase levels of norepinephrine. Mirtazapine increases the release of norepinephrine and serotonin.

Contraindications and Precautions

Avoid giving any of the miscellaneous antidepressants during pregnancy and lactation and in individuals with liver and kidney disease.

Bupropion is contraindicated in clients with seizure disorders or bulimia and should be used cautiously if head trauma is present. Bupropion is associated with a rare risk of seizures, approximately 4 in 1000. However, the sustained-release form of bupropion has a seizure rate similar to most antidepressants. The exact reason for the induction of seizures was never discovered; however, seizure history, eating disorders, and, possibly, head trauma are risk factors. Use cautiously the remaining agents in individuals with seizures.

Venlafaxine has been reported to be associated with dose-dependent increases in blood pressure (BP). About 2% of individuals experience increased BP at doses greater than 100 mg. Because clinically significant increases in diastolic BP of greater than 15 mm Hg have been observed in 5.5% of clients who receive doses above 200 mg, it is used cautiously for individuals with hypertension and cardiovascular disease.

Adverse Reactions

Common Effects. Nefazodone, trazodone, and mirtazapine commonly cause sedation. Trazodone can be given all at bedtime; however, nefazodone requires twice-daily dosing because of its shorter half-life. Gradual dose titration mini-

> **RESEARCH NOTE**
>
> Wisner, KL, Perel, JM, and Findling, RL: Antidepressant treatment during breast-feeding. Am J Psychiatry 153: 1132–1137, 1996.
>
> **Findings:** Postpartum psychiatric disorders are common; postpartum depression occurs in the 3 months following childbirth and affects up to 15% of women. Because most women choose to breast-feed their infants and few exact guidelines are available for medication prescription for lactating mothers, this article reviews the risks and benefits of antidepressant treatment.
>
> Fifteen studies that systematically investigated antidepressants during the postpartum period revealed that sertraline and several tricyclic antidepressants including amitriptyline, nortriptyline, desipramine, clomipramine, and doxepin fail to exert significant adverse effects on the infant. These antidepressants also do not increase antidepressant levels in the children. In contrast, colic and increased blood levels have been reported in breast-fed infants whose mothers took fluoxetine. Respiratory depression occurred in babies whose mothers were treated with doxepin. Longer-term effects are more difficult to understand because of the lack of studies; the data to date suggest that no documented developmental delays are evident in 9- to 36-month-old infants of antidepressant-treated mothers.
>
> **Application to Practice:** Breast-feeding offers babies decreased risk of illness and infections, improved digestion, and lowered risk of mortality; new mothers benefit from decreased cost and may reduce their risk of breast cancer as well. In the past, women who needed antidepressant treatment were told to avoid or discontinue lactation. This review suggests that sertraline and some of the TCAs appear relatively safe; the mother can continue to breast-feed and receive antidepressants. The decision to use medications should be based on the potential risks of failure to treat the mother's depression pharmacologically versus the unknown future risks to the child. Parents should be told that the long-term effects are unknown. The findings from this article need to be discussed with both parents before medications are started.

mizes the sedating effects. If severe, sedation requires drug discontinuation and alternate antidepressant treatment. Both nefazodone and trazodone also commonly produce headache, which can be managed by giving acetaminophen or administering the medication with food. Nefazodone can lead to nausea and dry mouth.

Bupropion and venlafaxine may lead to decreased appetite, nausea, agitation, and insomnia. Venlafaxine may also produce dizziness, sweating, anxiety, or sedation. The side effect profile of venlafaxine is similar to that of SSRIs because of its effects on serotonin reuptake inhibition. Mirtazapine commonly causes dizziness, increased appetite, and weight gain.

Occasional Effects. Bupropion and nefazodone lead to sexual dysfunction much less frequently than the SSRIs. Because venlafaxine may lead to elevations in BP, baseline and regular BP monitoring is necessary to detect clinically significant changes.

Uncommon but Potentially Serious Effects. An important, although uncommon, side effect of trazodone in males is *priapism* (sustained erection). Priapism requires immediate drug discontinuation and immediate evaluation in the emergency room or by a urologist. Seizures are possible with any of the miscellaneous antidepressants, and the regular formulation of bupropion poses a slightly higher risk.

Three clients have developed severe blood disorders, agranulocytosis, and neutropenia while being treated with mirtazapine. Further research is needed to determine how common this reaction is.

Clinically Significant Interactions

Nefazodone affects the cytochrome P-450 IIIA$_4$ isoenzyme and may increase levels of some benzodiazepines, terfenadine, astemizole, and potentially digoxin (see Table 6–4). Reduced doses of alprazolam or triazolam are necessary when combined with nefazodone. Terfenadine and astemizole are contraindicated because of the potential for serious cardiac complications, including QT prolongation.

Trazodone can potentiate the effects of other CNS depressants, leading to increased drowsiness and sedation. Avoid the coadministration of trazodone and CNS depressants or alcohol. In combination, trazodone reduces clonidine's antihypertensive effects. Serotonergic syndrome can occur with trazodone and buspirone.

Venlafaxine, in combination with cimetidine, may increase BP in individuals with preexisting hypertension. It has minimal effects on the cytochrome P-450 IID$_6$ isoenzyme system. Therefore, only minor elevations of drugs metabolized by this process can be expected, but further research is necessary. Venlafaxine should be not be combined with MAOIs (because of possible serotonergic syndrome).

Bupropion should not be administered with an MAOI. In combination with L-dopa, bupropion can lead to hallucinations, confusion, and dyskinesia and therefore should be avoided. Because of the potential for lowering seizure threshold, cautious use of bupropion and an SSRI is necessary.

NURSING CONSIDERATIONS

Nurses have an important role in educating clients about their disorders and the medications used to treat debilitating psychiatric disorders. To treat depression, antidepressants may take 2 to 6 weeks to take effect. Educate clients about this "lag time," and monitor them carefully for any potential response or worsening of depressive symptoms. It is important to know the client's baseline behaviors prior to pharmacotherapy to establish response and to distinguish between depressive symptoms and side effects. Generally, new behaviors and reactions during the course of antidepressant therapy can be attributed to the medication.

All antidepressants are associated with side effects, even the more specific agents that do not block muscarinic cholinergic, histaminergic, and α-adrenergic receptors, such as SSRIs and novel antidepressants. By and large, side effects worsen with dose escalation. Educate clients about common and uncommon effects and potentially dangerous reactions. Some individuals experience few side effects or develop tolerance to them. Assess the severity of side effects and help the individual to manage the reactions (Table 6–5). Teach clients that drug discontinuation is usually necessary for serious side effects and that an alternative antidepressant treatment must be started.

Many of the newer agents are metabolized through liver enzymes (Table 6–4). Although some drug-drug interactions are known, further research is necessary to determine other potential interactions. Caution clients about potential reactions when certain prescription and over-the-counter medications are combined with antidepressants, such as hypertensive crisis during MAOI treatment and toxicity with commonly used medications and SSRIs.

Suicide remains a major risk for individuals on antidepressants. Clients can successfully overdose with a week's supply of TCAs or MAOIs. The SSRIs and most newer antidepressants are less toxic in overdose and have a wider safety margin. However, in combination with other drugs or alcohol, they still can produce serious reactions or death. Regularly assess suicidal potential prior to and during antidepressant therapy.

CASE STUDY

Kathleen is a 32-year-old woman, married, with two young children. She reports feeling sad with decreased interest and pleasure in activities she once enjoyed. Her ability to concentrate, especially on reading, is greatly reduced. She has lost 15 lb in the past month. Kathleen awakens nearly every night and has difficulty returning to sleep. Kathleen reports also having felt this way about 2 years ago. She reports that her mother was "moody" and would become tearful and withdrawn periodically throughout Kathleen's childhood. Kathleen was evaluated by a psychiatric clinical nurse specialist, diagnosed with major depressive disorder, recurrent episode, and started on sertraline daily.

The nurse helps Kathleen understand the diagnosis of depression. She explains that depression results from a combination of factors, including a chemical imbalance of the neurotransmitters in the brain. The medication that has been prescribed is an SSRI that specifically works by balancing the brain's serotonin. The rebalancing is expected to relieve Kathleen's symptoms of depression. She tells Kathleen that the medication needs to be taken every day, even though a positive response could take several weeks. Some people may respond much more rapidly, beginning to feel some relief after a week, she adds. Kathleen experiences a slight headache, nausea, and restlessness. These side effects are mild and she is encouraged to continue to take the medication along with food to minimize nausea. The clinical nurse specialist prescribes a low dose of

TABLE 6–5. Treatment of Common Medication-induced Side Effects

GI disturbance	
Nausea	Decrease dose; administer with meals
Vomiting	Hold or decrease dose; if severe, switch to another agent
Diarrhea	Decrease dose; use antidiarrheal agents
Constipation	Decrease dose; use laxative; increase fiber
Dry mouth	Sugar-free candy; rinsing mouth with water; if severe, switch agent
Orthostatic hypotension	Monitor carefully; if severe, switch agent
Dizziness	Instruct client to rise carefully during position changes
Weight gain	Diet and exercise
Edema	Decrease dose; carefully add diuretic
Sedation	Decrease dose; switch to another agent
Lethargy and fatigue	Decrease dose; switch to another agent
Neurological	
Tremor	Decrease dose; give low-dose beta-blocker
Vision disturbance	Decrease dose; prescribe ophthalmologic consultation
Ataxia	Decrease dose; if severe, switch agent
Headache	Acetaminophen; assess for interaction if taking MAOI
Rash	Dermatologic consultation; assess for hematologic dysfunction (blood counts)
Increased LFTs	Monitor carefully; may require drug discontinuation
Agranulocytosis	If WBC <3000, discontinue drug
Sexual dysfunction	
Impotence, anorgasmia	Amantadine (if due to increased prolactin); yohimbine
Decreased libido	Cyproheptadine; switch to another agent
Priapism	Discontinue medication; urology consultation

propranolol to treat the restlessness. Kathleen denies having any symptoms of sexual dysfunction or insomnia.

Because many clients discontinue medications after their symptoms are relieved, the nurse tells her about the importance of taking the medication consistently. A 9- to 12-month course is necessary for the treatment of a first episode. Longer-term treatment may be recommended with recurrent episodes. She warns Kathleen to avoid alcohol. The nurse remains available to educate and support the client's family, who can facilitate compliance with treatment.

MOOD STABILIZERS

GENERAL INFORMATION

Mood stabilizers are used to treat the cycles of bipolar disorder. These agents prevent recurrent episodes of mania and depression, maintain and balance the individual's level of functioning, and decrease the severity and frequency of manic and depressed mood states. One goal of pharmacotherapy is *euthymia*, stable moods without depression or euphoria. Mood stabilizers also quell the overexcitement, euphoria, and insomnia characteristic of *acute* manic episodes. Lithium carbonate is the oldest and most established mood stabilizer. Others include two widely used anticonvulsants, valproic acid (also known as divalproex [Depakote]) and carbamazepine (Tegretol). In general, therapeutic effects occur 7 to 10 days after initiation.

LITHIUM CARBONATE

Lithium is available in several different oral formulations, each equally effective. Lithium citrate syrup, the liquid preparation, is used for individuals who have difficulty swallowing pills or who are noncompliant. Lithium carbonate also comes in pills, capsules, and a sustained-release form.

Indications

Lithium is indicated for the treatment of acute manic episodes, the prevention of bipolar disorder and cluster or migraine headaches, and augmentation of antidepressant treatment. Some research data suggest that it may be effective for schizophrenia, schizoaffective disorder, prevention of major depression, and severe aggression.

Pharmacokinetics

Lithium, given orally, absorbs readily through the GI tract. Sustained-release forms are 60 to 90% absorbed and have a higher likelihood of causing lower GI effects. The half-life is approximately 24 hours, and lithium is metabolized by the kidneys. Lithium crosses the placenta to the developing fetus and is secreted in breast milk.

Blood Level Monitoring. For lithium to be effective, adequate serum levels need to be maintained. Generally, dosing strategies are determined by measuring blood levels. Measure plasma levels 12 hours after the last dose is taken for optimal usefulness. Lithium levels of 0.8 to 1.2 mEq/L are considered therapeutic. Measuring blood levels also helps detect toxicity. During the start of treatment, obtain levels two to three times per week and then once every month to several months when the client is stabilized. As seen in Tables 6–6 and 6–7, several factors can affect the accuracy and reliability of plasma lithium concentration, leading to lower (nontherapeutic) or higher (possibly toxic) levels. Levels above 1.5 mEq/L are potentially dangerous. Poor concentration, mental status changes, coarse tremors, drowsiness, loss of appetite, severe nausea or vomiting, diarrhea, lethargy, ataxia, or confusion may indicate toxicity, which may progress to severe coma, convulsions, renal failure, or death. If toxicity occurs, hold the lithium, and monitor blood levels every several hours until levels decrease. Lithium can then be restarted at a lower dose to obtain levels in the therapeutic range.

Mechanism of Action

Lithium's mechanism of action is poorly understood. It normalizes the reuptake of certain neurotransmitters such as serotonin, norepinephrine, dopamine, and acetylcholine. It also reduces the release of norepinephrine through competition with calcium. Unlike most psychotropic medications, lithium does not produce its effects within neuronal synapses. Instead, it produces its effects intracellularly, affecting certain enzyme subsystems such as cyclic adenosine monophosphates (cAMP) and phosphatidylinositol biphosphate (PIP$_2$). These processes in turn alter calcium-mediated intracellular functions to release calcium, affecting many other cellular processes.

Contraindications and Precautions

Lithium carbonate is contraindicated in individuals with known hypersensitivity or renal, hepatic, or cardiovascular disease. It should not be used during pregnancy or lactation. Because the ability to excrete lithium decreases with age, it

TABLE 6–6. **Conditions That May Affect Serum Lithium Levels**

Increased Lithium Levels	*Decreased Lithium Levels*
• Increased dose	• Missed doses
• Drug interactions	• Drug interactions
• Diets, salt deficiency	• Timing of blood test
• Renal disease	
• Dehydration	
• Excessive sweating	
• Severe diarrhea	
• Physical illness	
• Timing of blood test	
• Severe vomiting	
• Pregnancy	

TABLE 6–7. Significant Interactions between Mood Stabilizers and Other Medications

Medications that increase lithium levels
- Anesthetics
- Angiotensin-converting enzyme inhibitors
- Nonsteroidal anti-inflammatory medications
- Tetracycline
- Thiazide diuretics

Medications that decrease lithium levels
- Acetazolamide
- Aminophylline
- Mannitol
- Sodium bicarbonate
- Osmotic diuretics
- Xanthines

Medications that increase carbamazepine levels
- Erythromycin
- Cimetidine
- Propoxyphene
- Isoniazid
- Calcium channel blockers
- Verapamil
- Fluoxetine, possibly other SSRIs

Medications that decrease carbamazepine levels
- Divalproex
- Phenytoin
- Phenobarbitol

Carbamazepine may decrease levels of
- Oral contraceptives
- Warfarin
- Theophylline
- Antipsychotics
- Divalproex
- Anticoagulants
- Doxycycline

Interactions with divalproex
- Potentiates the effects of alcohol
- Aspirn, warfarin—prolonged bleeding time
- Aspirin may increase levels of divalproex
- Decreased levels of carbamazepine

should be used cautiously with elderly clients. Warn clients to avoid alcohol.

Administration of lithium during the first trimester of pregnancy increases the risk of a cardiac defect, Ebstein's anomaly, in the infant. One study found that the risk of serious congenital anomalies was two to six times greater for infants whose mothers took lithium during pregnancy.[7] Women are also at greater risk for toxicity when treated with lithium during the third trimester, because of fluid changes. If taken postpartum, lithium passes in breast milk to the infant at about half the level of that in the mother. Childbirth can increase the risk of bipolar cycling, so benefits of treatment versus risks of nontreatment need to be considered.

Adverse Reactions

Common Effects. Common side effects of lithium therapy include nausea, anorexia, and diarrhea. Individuals also frequently experience polydipsia (increased thirst), polyuria (increased urination), weight gain, fatigue, lethargy, and hand tremor. These symptoms usually emerge during dose titration and are dose-related; as the dose is increased, side effects worsen. When they emerge later in treatment, these adverse reactions may reflect toxicity. Use the strategies listed in Table 6–5 to manage side effects. Using slow-release preparations or taking the medication with food minimizes GI distress. However, diarrhea may be more common with slow-release preparations. Increased thirst and urination can be very bothersome and lead to nocturia. Several strategies can minimize these effects: lowering (but maintaining) a therapeutic dose, taking all of the lithium at bedtime, or adding potassium-sparing diuretics. Diuretics paradoxically decrease urine outputs.

Weight gain, fatigue and lethargy, and hand tremor may occur and are the most difficult to manage. Although dieting and exercise can help mitigate increased weight, these efforts may be futile. Continued fatigue and lethargy often lead to noncompliance. Switching to another mood stabilizer may be more beneficial. Some clients, particularly those who work with their hands, find that hand tremor impedes their performance. Others find it embarrassing and a physical reminder that they are taking medication. Tremor often responds to the administration of low doses of propranolol (Inderal). Worsening of these neurologic-like symptoms may represent signs of lithium toxicity.

Occasional Effects. Less commonly, lithium may lead to vomiting, abdominal pain, edema, cognitive dulling, and dermatologic reactions such as rash, acne, psoriasis, and hair loss. Some of these effects will respond to dose reduction, but edema of the face or lower extremities usually resolves over time. Skin and hair reactions require consultation with a dermatologist, additional treatments, or drug discontinuation.

Five percent of individuals will develop hypothyroidism and another 3% will have a nontoxic goiter. Obtain baseline and regular thyroid function tests. The client may show signs of fatigue, lethargy, or appetite change suggestive of hypothyroidism. Synthetic thyroid medication, for example, levothyroxine sodium (T_4), is necessary to treat lithium-induced hypothyroidism.

Uncommon but Potentially Serious Effects. Uncommon but potentially dangerous reactions include nephrogenic diabetes insipidus or cardiac toxicity. Lithium therapy is the most common cause of nephrogenic diabetes insipidus and requires referral to a urologist. Diuretic therapy usually treats the condition.

The client's ECG may show benign flattening or inversion of T waves. Sinus and ventricular arrhythmias may develop, particularly in individuals with preexisting cardiac disease. Individuals may complain of dizziness, palpitations, or syncope, which reflect these abnormalities. Assess clients carefully for any cardiac-related reactions. These side effects require immediate attention and discontinuation of lithium treatment.

One of the most serious concerns is the development of lithium toxicity. At levels of 1.5 to 2.0 mEq/L, toxic side effects emerge. The initial treatment is to discontinue lithium therapy. Levels in excess of 2 mEq/L require symptomatic treatment: first, restore fluid and electrolyte balance. Alkaline diuresis or dialysis may be necessary to restore renal function. If convulsions occur, short-acting barbiturates may be used. Monitor individuals intensively for renal or cardiac failure and seizures. Death has occurred when levels exceed 4 mEq/L.

Clinically Significant Interactions

Nurses should assess clinically significant interactions (Table 6–7). Because of the risk of severe toxicity, many medications can increase lithium to toxic levels. Other agents can reduce lithium levels, which negates its therapeutic effectiveness, and lithium may affect serum concentrations of other medications.

CARBAMAZEPINE

Indications

Carbamazepine is indicated for the treatment of acute mania, prevention of bipolar disorder, temporal lobe (partial complex) and limbic seizures, and chronic pain disorders such as trigeminal neuralgia and neuropathic pain. It appears to be more effective than lithium in certain subtypes of bipolar disorder, for example, rapid-cycling or dysphoric mania. Less commonly, carbamazepine may be used for schizoaffective disorder, episodic dyscontrol, and posttraumatic stress disorder.

Pharmacokinetics

Carbamazepine is more slowly absorbed, with a half-life of 15 to 30 hours initially (8 to 15 hours, maintenance). It is metabolized by the liver and inhibits the metabolism of medications that are metabolized by the cytochrome P-450 isoenzymes (see Clinically Significant Interactions section, following). Carbamazepine crosses the placenta to the developing fetus and is passed on to infants during lactation.

Therapeutic levels are approximately 6 to 12 mEq/L; however, no exact therapeutic range has been established. Nonetheless, obtain carbamazepine levels to monitor for toxicity, and obtain levels at baseline and regular intervals.

Mechanism of Action

Carbamazepine affects sodium and calcium channels and this decreases the release of neurotransmitters. A recent concept, *kindling,* explains the development of bipolar disorder and the effectiveness of carbamazepine. Borrowed from the treatment of seizure disorders, kindling refers to repeated subthreshold stimuli that build and eventually culminate in a seizure. Similarly, bipolar disorder may start with minor episodes that lead to the development of the full condition. Researchers theorize that mood stabilizers quell episodes of mania and depression and prevent recurrence by inhibiting the kindling process. Less frequent and severe mood states result. Like water on a fire, these medications may extinguish the phases of bipolar disorder, impeding the recurring cycles.

Contraindications and Precautions

Carbamazepine is contraindicated in clients with hepatic or cardiovascular disease, blood dyscrasias, or known hypersensitivity. Avoid giving carbamazepine during pregnancy and lactation. A higher rate of craniofacial defects, finger hypoplasia, and developmental delays has been associated with prenatal treatment. It is secreted in breast milk at 60% of the mother's plasma level. Instruct the client to avoid alcohol.

Adverse Reactions

Common Effects. The most common effects include sedation, drowsiness, rash, and neurological reactions, such as dizziness, clumsiness, ataxia, and double or blurred vision. Each of these reactions can lead to significant disruption in daily functioning and task performance. For example, driving, studying, and concentrating may be impeded. These reactions are dose-related and are the result of rapid escalation of dose or high serum levels. They can be managed successfully by slow initiation of carbamazepine therapy or dose reduction.

Up to 20% of clients on carbamazepine therapy develop a rash. If urticaria and pruritic skin reactions result, discontinue the drug. Rarely, clients develop a fatal rash secondary to Stevens-Johnson syndrome.

Occasional Effects. Carbamazepine therapy can decrease sodium secondary to its antidiuretic properties. Benign minor elevations in liver function tests have also been reported. Monitor clients both at baseline and regular intervals for electrolyte levels and liver function to detect these reactions. Nausea and vomiting may develop transiently and respond to gradual dose titration or dose reduction.

Uncommon but Potentially Serious Effects. The most dangerous effect is the development of bone marrow depression. Carbamazepine can lead to serious and irreversible reduction of white and red blood cells and platelet count (for example, agranulocytosis and aplastic anemia). Clients may display fever, sore throat, pallor, petechiae, or easy bruising and should report these effects immediately. Nurses should also carefully observe individuals for these signs of hematologic toxicity. Baseline and regular monitoring of complete blood cell (CBC) counts is necessary. Discontinue the drug if a white blood cell count drops below 3000 or a neutrophil count drops below 1500.

Carbamazepine therapy is also associated with sinus bradycardia and heart block. Assess clients for cardiac complaints and slowing of the heart rate. If present, discontinue the drug.

Clinically Significant Interactions

As with any medication, there are potential interactions between carbamazepine and many other agents (see Table 6–7). Because severe toxicity may result, assess important clinically significant interactions. Medications that decrease carbamazepine levels reduce its therapeutic efficacy and lead to breakthrough symptoms. Carbamazepine used in combination with either an anticonvulsant or a neuroleptic may lead to neurotoxicity.

VALPROIC ACID

Indications

Valproic acid, also known as divalproex, is indicated for treatment of acute mania, prevention of bipolar disorder, and simple or complex absence seizures. It appears to be more effective than lithium in certain subtypes of bipolar disorder, such as the rapid-cycling and dysphoric mania subtypes. Less commonly, valproic acid may be used for schizoaffective disorder and episodes of behavioral dyscontrol.

Pharmacokinetics

Valproic acid is available in several different preparations including Depakene and Depakote, the enteric-coated form. Divalproex, comprised of valproic acid and sodium valproate, is more commonly used. It is more slowly absorbed than valproic acid, with a half-life of about 8 hours. Valproic acid is 80 to 95% protein bound and is metabolized by the liver. It crosses the blood-brain barrier and is secreted in breast milk. Therapeutic levels are usually 50 to 150 mcg/mL; however, no exact therapeutic range has been established. Nonetheless, obtain levels to monitor for toxicity and at baseline and regular intervals. Valproic acid is distributed across the placenta and is secreted in breast milk.

Valproic acid inhibits the metabolism of medications that are metabolized by the cytochrome P-450 isoenzymes (see Clinically Significant Interactions, following).

Mechanism of Action

The exact action of valproic acid is unknown. This agent increases levels of the inhibitory neurotransmitter γ-aminobutyric acid (GABA). However, its therapeutic actions, like those of carbamazepine, are more likely related to inhibiting kindling of mood episodes.

Adverse Reactions

Common Effects. Valproic acid commonly leads to nausea, heartburn, anorexia, sedation, hand tremor, and weight gain. Most of these effects worsen during dose titration and diminish with ongoing treatment. GI side effects can be minimized by taking the medication with food or by using the enteric-coated formulation. Sedation can be helped by shifting the dose to bedtime. Hand tremor responds to treatment with low-dose propranolol. Because weight gain can be substantial, it can lead to noncompliance; dieting and exercise are the best management strategies.

Occasional Effects. Less commonly, valproic acid leads to ataxia, dysarthria, and reversible changes in blood count (thrombocytopenia). These uncomfortable effects require dose reduction or switching to another mood stabilizer.

Uncommon but Potentially Serious Effects. The most serious potential consequence of valproic acid therapy is increased liver function tests (LFTs) and hepatic failure. Monitor clients for signs of liver toxicity: severe anorexia, weight loss, vomiting, lethargy, jaundice, and edema. Although several deaths have resulted from liver damage, the majority were infants who were treated with multiple anticonvulsants. Overall, the risk for adults treated with valproic acid alone is minimal.

Platelet dysfunction and pancreatitis have been reported during valproic acid therapy. Baseline and regular monitoring of platelet counts and pancreatic enzymes is also necessary. If severe abnormalities in hepatic or pancreatic enzymes or platelets emerge, discontinue the drug.

Avoid using valproic acid during pregancy and lactation. Prenatal exposure may lead to increased risk of spina bifida (1.2% risk) and neural tube defects (1.5% risk). Valproic acid levels in breast milk have been reported to be 1 to 10% of the mother's serum concentration.

Clinically Significant Interactions

Valproic acid may increase levels of the SSRIs, other anticonvulsants, and other medications metabolized by the liver (see Table 6–7). Because it is highly protein-bound, it increases levels of other highly protein-bound agents such as aspirin and warfarin, or valproic acid may be displaced by these medications, leading to valproic acid toxicity. Conversely, drugs that induce liver enzymes can lead to decreased valproic acid levels.

NURSING CONSIDERATIONS

One of the key aspects of effective nursing care is to assess and monitor side effects related to the mood stabilizers. Weight gain, associated with each of these agents, may lead to missed doses as well as dose reduction and discontinuation. The underlying condition worsens and breakthrough symptoms can then readily result. Anticipate potential adverse reactions and help clients manage their response. Instruct clients to try appropriate interventions to deal with the emergence of any uncomfortable side effects. If side effects are severe, a change to a different mood stabilizer can be suggested. As advocates for clients, nurses are in a key position to help them weigh the advantages of long-term continued compliance over the discomfort of any potential short-term adverse reactions.

Side effects need to be distinguished from worsening episodes of the underlying disorder. For example, signs of lethargy, appetite disturbance, and weight gain may reflect an impending depressive episode or lithium-induced hypothyroidism. Cognitive dulling may represent an adverse reaction or a sign of depression. When effects develop shortly after initiation of a mood stabilizer, they are more likely to reflect an adverse reaction; a complaint that coincides with a group of other moods and behaviors implies the presence of undiagnosed mania or depression. Help clients sort out when complaints represent side effects and when they indicate worsening of the underlying disorder.

Teach clients to avoid alcohol and illicit substances because of the potential for dangerous interactions. In addition, substance abuse is associated with higher rates of medication noncompliance. Educate clients on the need for medication monitoring to ensure therapeutic blood levels and for potential hematologic and hepatic abnormalities. Review the signs and symptoms of hematologic and liver dysfunction with the client and family.

CASE STUDY

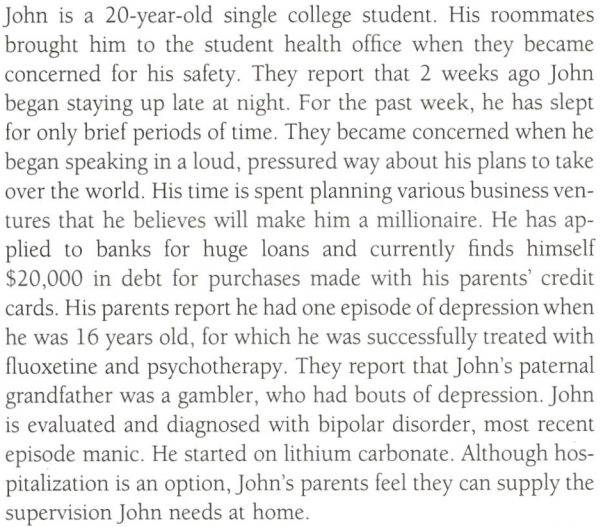

John is a 20-year-old single college student. His roommates brought him to the student health office when they became concerned for his safety. They report that 2 weeks ago John began staying up late at night. For the past week, he has slept for only brief periods of time. They became concerned when he began speaking in a loud, pressured way about his plans to take over the world. His time is spent planning various business ventures that he believes will make him a millionaire. He has applied to banks for huge loans and currently finds himself $20,000 in debt for purchases made with his parents' credit cards. His parents report he had one episode of depression when he was 16 years old, for which he was successfully treated with fluoxetine and psychotherapy. They report that John's paternal grandfather was a gambler, who had bouts of depression. John is evaluated and diagnosed with bipolar disorder, most recent episode manic. He started on lithium carbonate. Although hospitalization is an option, John's parents feel they can supply the supervision John needs at home.

The first goal for the nurse is to ensure that John and his family understand the diagnosis of bipolar disorder. They should be aware that this disorder is believed to have a genetic and biological component. Because the course of the disease is often recurrent, both John and his parents need to understand the importance of treatment compliance. A positive, trusting relationship between the nurse and the client is essential. Family involvement is important in ensuring compliance, especially because John may be reluctant to initiate or maintain treatment while manic.

The nurse needs to educate John and his family about regularly monitoring lithium levels during the course of treatment, with the first level drawn after a few days on the medication. The lithium dose will be adjusted depending on the lithium level in the blood. John will also have baseline kidney and thyroid function tests done before beginning the drug and then at intervals of 6 to 12 months after treatment has begun. The nurse should teach John and his family about possible early side effects, including nausea and diarrhea. Nausea can be ameliorated by taking the lithium with a meal. Diarrhea usually responds to antidiarrheal medications. There may be increased frequency of

RESEARCH NOTE

Hyman, SE, and Nestler, EJ: Initiation and adaptation: A paradigm for understanding psychotropic drug action. Am J Psychiatry 153:151–162, 1996.

Findings: In this theoretical paper, the authors try to answer the complicated question, how do psychotropic medications work? They focus on the mechanism of action of several classes of agents, particularly antidepressants. Initially, antidepressants block the reuptake of norepinephrine, serotonin, or both into the presynaptic neuron. The net result is an increase in neurotransmitters. These effects all occur acutely, hours or days after antidepressant administration. Acute administration produces little in the way of behavioral change, but does lead to side effects. However, because antidepressants have a protracted onset of action, acute alterations in neuronal function are probably inappropriate to their mechanism of action. Instead, they propose an alternate hypothesis: long-term neuropharmacologic reactions to increased norepinephrine and serotonin are more relevant to understanding mechanism of action. With this recognition, antidepressant action is distinguished between "acute" and "chronic" effects. These researchers suggest that the nervous system's adaptation to increased neurotransmitters produces therapeutic responsiveness. The long-term response, more relevant to understanding how antidepressants work, is to decrease and then balance neurotransmission. They propose that it is these adaptive reactions that are crucial to understanding the mechanism of action.

Application to Practice: The acute effects of antidepressant treatment, increased norepinephrine or serotonin, are probably an oversimplification. These are the initial effects. The long-term effects are for the neuron to balance the neurotransmission of norepinephrine and serotonin. Therefore, when clients ask about how these drugs work, the answer becomes very complicated. Education can include how the drugs initially affect neurotransmitters, but the real answer lies in their long-term adaptive response.

urination, weight gain, or fine tremors of the hand. Urinary frequency is usually a minor effect and requires further evaluation only if the client complains of excessive thirst along with increased need to urinate. This could signal diabetes insipidus and requires immediate attention. Weight gain may be addressed by stressing the importance of diet and exercise. Fine tremors are usually not troublesome.

The nurse's role is vitally important in providing education and support to clients and their families. Offer hope that treatment will be successful in stabilizing the client's mood and limiting the potentially devastating effects of untreated bipolar disorder.

ANTIPSYCHOTIC MEDICATIONS (NEUROLEPTICS)

GENERAL INFORMATION

Since their discovery in the 1950s, antipsychotic medications have revolutionized the care of individuals with major psychiatric disorders. Initially observed to have a calming effect when used as an adjunct to anesthesia, the antipsychotic agents treat a range of major psychiatric disorders. However, they also have the potential for severe short- and long-term side effects; they are referred to as neuroleptics because of their capacity to induce neurological-type adverse reactions. Used for both adults and children, these medications have allowed many individuals to live more natural lives without the confinement of long-term hospitalization. The onset of therapeutic effect often takes weeks or months. These medications are classified as either "typical" or "atypical" antipsychotics. Typical antipsychotics are equally effective. Recent development of drugs that preferentially affect certain symptoms of schizophrenia has heralded the second major wave in the treatment of psychotic disorders. Clozapine, olanzapine, quetiapine (Seroquel), sertindole, and possibly risperidone represent "atypical" antipsychotic medications because they usually produce few to no extrapyramidal side effects. Quetiapine and sertindole are scheduled for release on to the U.S. market in 1997 but were not FDA approved at the time of publication.

Antipsychotic medications can be classified into low, moderate, and high potencies. Potency refers to relative dosage strengths that are necessary to achieve maximal effect. Low-potency agents reflect larger doses, while high-potency medications indicate lower doses. Relative potency may indicate differential side effects; for instance, low-potency antipsychotic therapy is associated with more anticholinergic, sedating, and cardiac reactions. Table 6–8 lists the typ-

TABLE 6–8. Comparison of Typical Antipsychotic Medications

Drug Name Generic/Trade	Potency 1 mg = x mg CPZ*	Sedation	Hypotension	Anticholinergic	EPS	Seizure
Low-potency agents						
Chlorpromazine (Thorazine)	1	++++	++++	+++	++	++++
Thioridazine (Mellaril)	1.1	++++	++++	++++	++	++
Mesoridazine (Serentil)	1.8	++++	++++	++++	+++	++
Chlorprothixene (Taractan)	2.3	++†	++++	++++	++	+++
Moderate-potency agents						
Loxapine (Loxitane)	8	+++	+++	+++	+++	++++
Molindone (Moban)	11	+++	++	+++	++	++
Perphenazine (Trilafon)	11	++	++	++	++++	+++
High-potency agents						
Thiothixene (Navane)	19	++	++	++	++++	+++
Trifluoperazine (Stelazine)	36	++	++	++	++++	++
Haloperidol (Haldol)	63	++	++	++	++++	+++
Pimozide (Orap)	67	++	++	++	++++	++
Fluphenazine (Prolixin)	83	++	++	++	++++	++

*CPZ = Chlorpromazine. Potency estimates vary significantly and are only approximate indicators to determine equivalent dose. Typical doses are from 300–600 mg or equivalent of chlorpromazine. EPS = Extrapyramidal symptoms. + = very low, ++ = low, +++ = moderate, ++++ = high.
†Sedating initially, then becomes activating with continuous use.
Note: Risperidone is associated with little to no EPS in daily doses less than 6 mg in adults.
Source: Adapted from Teicher, MH, and Glod, CA: Neuroleptic drugs: Indications and guidelines for their rational use in children and adolescents. J Child Adolesc Psychopharmacol 1:33, 1990.

TABLE 6–9. Comparison of Atypical Antipsychotic Medications and Haloperidol

Generic Name Trade Name	Clozapine Clozaril	Risperidone Risperdal	Olanzapine Zyprexa	Sertindole Serlect	Quetiapine[†] Seroquel	Haloperidol Haldol
Dose*						
Initial dose	25–50	1–2	5–10	4	50	2–5
Common dose	300–600	6–8	10–15	12–20	300	6–8
Maximum dose	900	12	20	24	500	20
Common Side Effects						
EPS	+	++	+	+	+	++++
Anticholinergic	++++	+	++	+	++	++
Sedation	++++	++	+++	+	+++	++
Hypotension	++++	++	+	+	+	+
Seizure	++++	+	+	+	+	+
Weight gain	++++	++	++	++	++	++
Treatment Effect						
Positive symptoms	marked	marked	marked	marked	marked	marked
Negative symptoms	marked	moderate	marked	marked	moderate	mild

*In mg
[†] FDA approved doses not established at time of publication.
Note: Risperidone is associated with little to no EPS in daily doses < 6 mg in adults. + = very low, ++ = low, +++ = moderate, ++++ = high.
Source: Adapted from the Physician's Desk Reference, 1997; Teicher, MH, and Glod, CA: Neuroleptic drugs: Indications and guidelines for their rational use in children and adolescents. J Child Adolesc Psychopharmacol 1:33, 1990; and Cosey, DE: Seroquel (Quetiapine): Preclinical and clinical findings of a new atypical antipsychotic. Experimental Opinions Investigational Drugs 5:939–957, 1996.

ical antipsychotic agents, dosage, and differential side effect profiles. Table 6–9 lists the major characteristics of the atypical agents.

Indications

Antipsychotic medications are indicated for the treatment of schizophrenia, schizoaffective disorder, acute psychotic states (including drug-induced psychosis), mania (while awaiting the effects of a mood stabilizer), psychotic depression (in combination with an antidepressant), pervasive developmental disorder, severe nausea and vomiting, and intractable hiccups. Less commonly, they may be used for severe agitation and aggression, preoperative sedation, borderline personality disorder, and ADHD in children. One antipsychotic, pimozide, is used mainly for movement disorders such as Tourette's disorder.

Pharmacokinetics

Following oral administration, the antipsychotic medications are well absorbed into the GI tract and metabolized by the liver. Food or antacids can decrease their absorption. Liquid formulations are more reliably and rapidly absorbed. The average half-life for most agents taken orally is 18 to 40 hours. Fluphenazine and haloperidol are also available in long-acting decanoate preparations, which possess a half-life of approximately 2 weeks. Smoking leads to decreased plasma neuroleptic levels because of induction of metabolism.

Antipsychotic medications are highly protein-bound and lipophilic. Therapeutic blood levels have not been established. These medications are also passed on prenatally to the developing fetus and are secreted in breast milk.

Mechanism of Action

Typical Antipsychotics. Although a great deal has been learned about the antipsychotic medications, their effects are varied and not fully understood. Typical antipsychotic medications have their primary effects on dopamine. As seen in Figure 6–4, they block a specific dopamine (D_2) receptor located on the postsynaptic neuron that transiently increases levels of dopamine. With ongoing treatment, dopamine levels are reduced.

These agents affect two areas of the brain: the striatal (nigrostriatal) and limbic (mesocorticolimbic) dopamine systems. Affecting the striatal region produces extrapyramidal side effects; acting upon dopamine in the limbic system probably explains the reduction in psychotic symptoms.

Atypical Antipsychotics. One of the newer atypical neu-

Haloperidol - typical antipsychotic

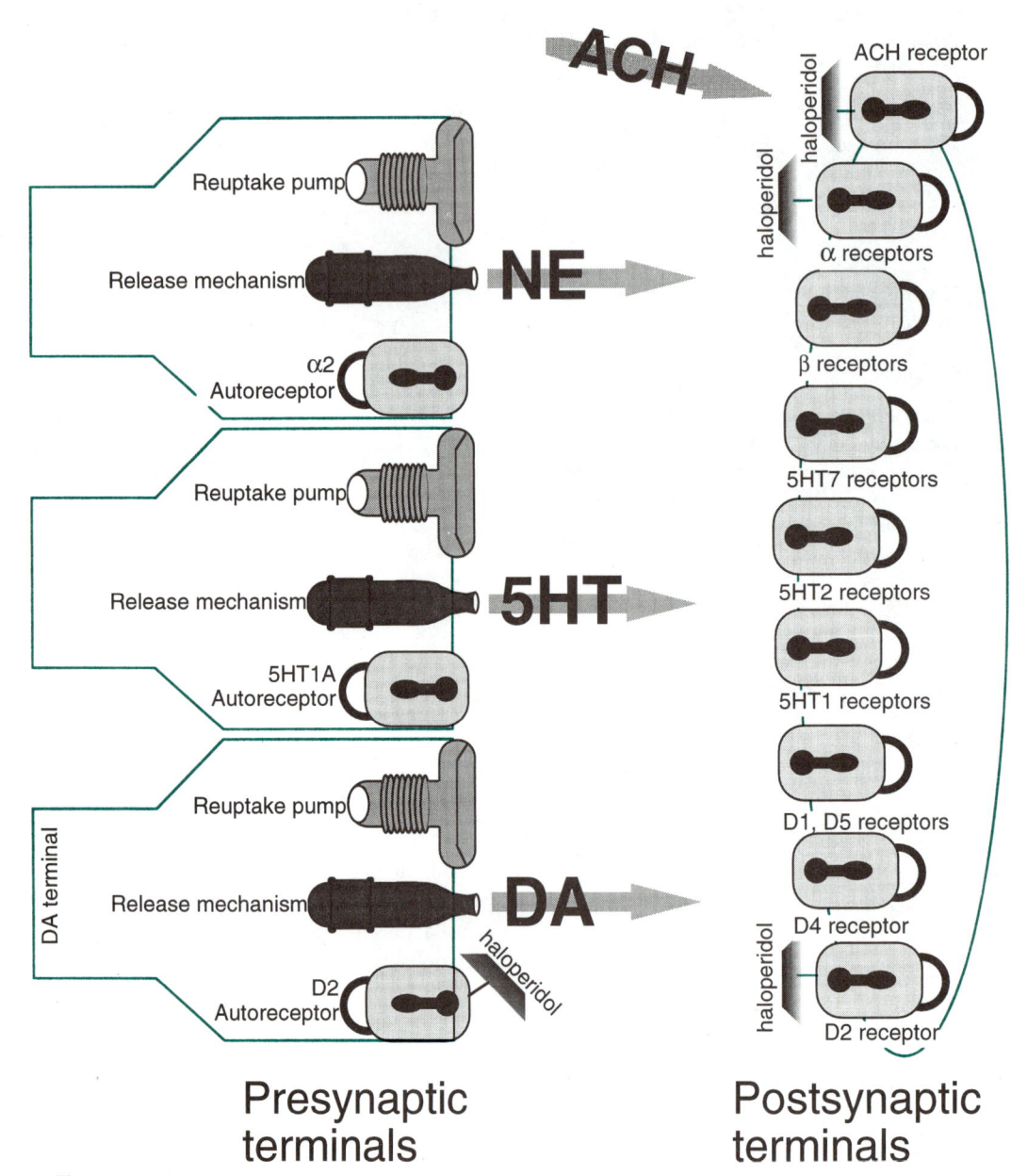

Presynaptic terminals | **Postsynaptic terminals**

Figure 6–4: The mechanism of action of a typical antipsychotic such as haloperidol. Haloperidol blocks the dopamine (D_2) receptors postsynaptically, and presynaptically, known as the D_2 autoreceptor. These actions were once thought to explain their antipsychotic effects. Typical antipsychotic medications also block several postsynaptic receptors, like a key fits into a lock; these actions are unrelated to their antipsychotic effects and are shown on the right side of the figure. Haloperidol blocks acetylcholine (ACH) and alpha (α) receptors leading to anticholinergic and cardiac effects, respectively. (Courtesy of Martin H. Teicher, MD, PhD, McLean Hospital.)

roleptic agents, clozapine, is a weak dopamine D_2 receptor–blocker and a potent D_4 blocker. As seen in Figure 6–5, clozapine and the other atypical agents block a specific serotonin receptor (5-HT_2). These unique effects may explain greater efficacy of these drugs; however, because they act on a wide range of receptors, it is difficult to argue that any one effect is responsible for therapeutic effectiveness (see Sidebar).

Atypical antipsychotics produce changes only in the mesocorticolimbic system. By acting on the limbic system, psychotic symptoms are treated without the development of extrapyramidal side effects.

Clozapine - atypical antipsychotic

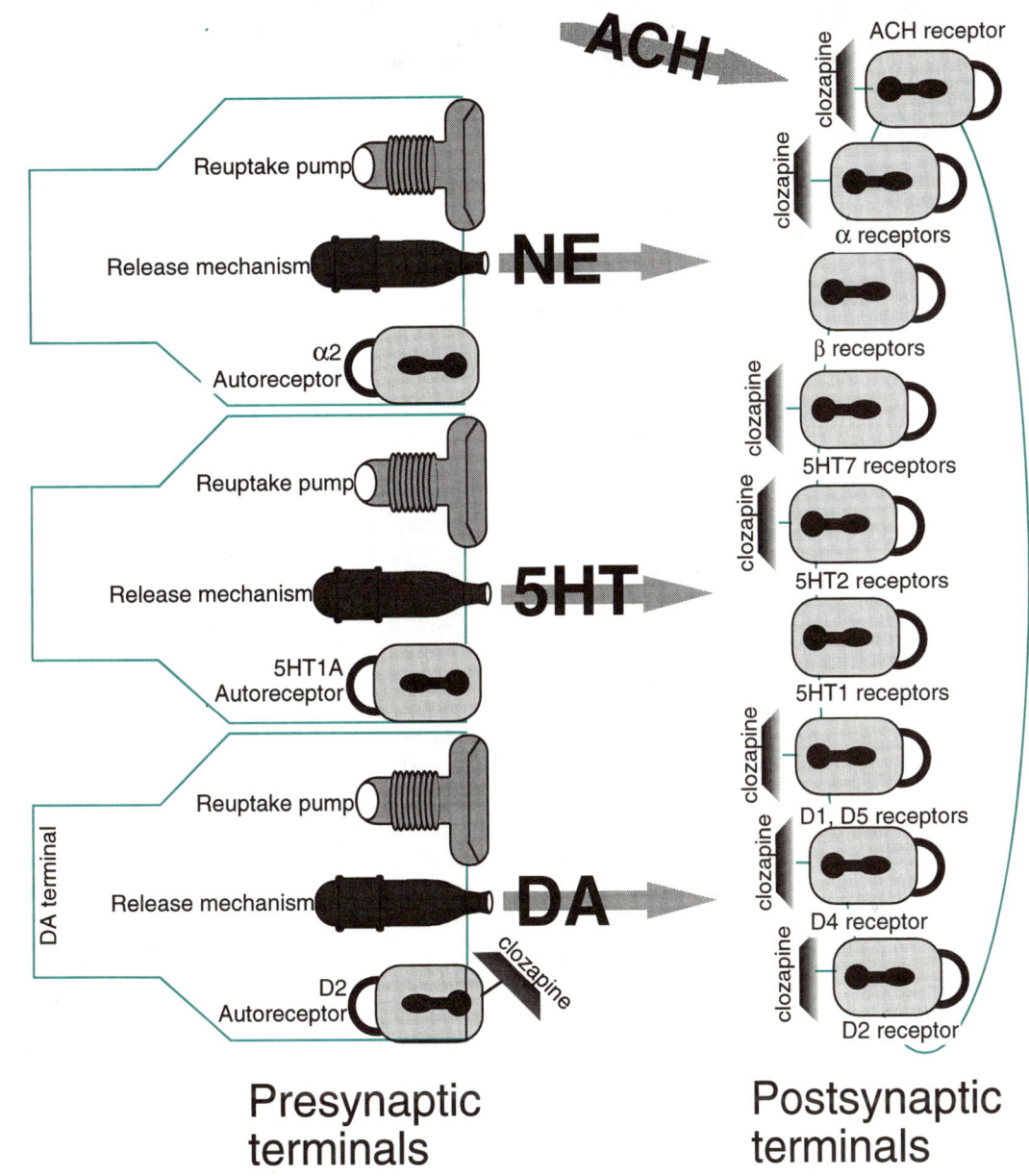

Figure 6–5: The effects of clozapine, an atypical antipsychotic, on neurotransmitters. Clozapine may exert its unique antipsychotic properties because of its effects on blocking dopamine receptors (D_1, D_5, D_4, and D_2; *Lower Right*) and serotonin receptors (5-HT_2, 5-HT_7; *Middle Right*). Clozapine also blocks the dopamine D_2 autoreceptor located on the presynaptic neuron (*Bottom Left*). Side effects of clozapine such as anticholinergic and cardiac effects are best explained by its effects on acetylcholine (ACH) and alpha (α) receptors (*Top Right*). (Courtesy of Martin H. Teicher, MD, PhD, McLean Hospital.)

Contraindications and Precautions

Avoid antipsychotic medications in comatose clients and in individuals with agranulocytosis (especially clozapine), circulatory collapse, narrow-angle glaucoma, poorly controlled seizure disorders, and neuroleptic malignant syndrome (NMS). Use antipsychotic medications cautiously in hepatic or renal insufficiency, cardiac arrhythmias, or tardive dyskinesia.

Very few data are available on the use of antipsychotics during pregnancy and lactation; ideally they are avoided. Chlorpromazine, the most widely studied of the antipsychotics, has not been associated with any clear problems

ATYPICAL ANTIPSYCHOTIC MEDICATIONS

- Medications that treat the so-called positive symptoms of schizophrenia, such as hallucinations and paranoia, and negative symptoms, such as lack of motivation, blunted emotions, and social withdrawal.
- Those that reduce or eliminate problems in attention and processing of information.
- Medications that cause few or no extrapyramidal motor side effects.
- Those that cause little or no tardive dyskinesia.
- Those that fail to cause increases in prolactin levels.

when given to clients during the first two trimesters. Administration of chlorpromazine during the third trimester has been associated with neonatal jaundice and extrapyramidal syndrome (EPS) (see the following). Similarly, an infant exposed to antipsychotic medication during lactation can also display EPS.

Adverse Reactions, Typical Antipsychotics

Common Effects. The development of common side effects depends on the medication's relative potency (see Tables 6–8 and 6–9). Antipsychotic medications can lead to weight gain and cognitive blunting. Low-potency typical antipsychotic medications are associated with a higher likelihood of anticholinergic effects, sedation, and orthostatic hypotension. Moderate-potency agents have mixed effects, whereas high-potency agents are usually related to the development of **extrapyramidal syndrome** (EPS). EPS consists of three possible reactions: akathisia, parkinsonian symptoms, and dystonia. Each of these side effects can be very uncomfortable and fail to remit without intervention.

Akathisia is an uncomfortable sense of motor restlessness or desire to pace or move the legs. Individuals may describe it as the inability to sit still, "wanting to jump out of my skin," or an internal sense of itchiness. Akathisia has been associated with increased potential for aggression. Clients may not readily recognize this very uncomfortable side effect. Similarly, nurses might mistake the restlessness and agitation for worsening psychosis rather than as akathisia. In this scenario, the nurse might observe increased agitation and give a "prn" dose of neuroleptic, worsening the akathisia. Instead, the nurse should suspect akathisia even if the client does not complain about it and it is distinguished from agitation. Akathisia can be successfully treated with either low-dose benzodiazepines or beta-blockers such as propranolol. It may also respond to dose reduction or a switch to an atypical antipsychotic.

Parkinsonian symptoms include behaviors observed in Parkinson's disease: shuffling gait, masked facies, drooling, tremor, stiff posture, and muscle rigidity. Clients may not recognize these side effects, but nurses should be aware of their development. Parkinsonian symptoms are treated by dose reduction, the addition of an anticholinergic agent (Table 6–10), or switching to an atypical agent.

Occasional Effects. Antipsychotic medications can lead to rash or sunburn on exposure to the sun (photosensitivity). Oftentimes clients are unaware of these effects until they burn severely. The most effective treatment is to avoid outdoor exposure or wear protective sunblock. Because antipsychotic medications can raise prolactin levels, irregular menses, galactorrhea, or impotence may emerge. One neuroleptic, thioridazine, also has the potential to cause retrograde ejaculation. Because clients frequently fail to reveal sexual side effects, question them about such problems to prevent noncompliance. Dose reduction, addition of amantadine, or switching to another antipsychotic agent is necessary to treat sexual dysfunction.

Uncommon but Potentially Serious Effects. One of the extrapyramidal symptoms, **dystonias**, can be very frightening. These are generally muscle spasms of the jaw, tongue, neck, or eyes. Dystonic reactions usually occur early in treatment with high-potency, typical agents such as haloperidol. Young men or muscular individuals may be more at risk. These reactions can be a very frightening and surprising side effect. If the dystonic reaction involves the larynx, severe respiratory distress or death may result. Ideally, clients take both a neuroleptic and an anticholinergic agent to prevent the development of a dystonia. However, anticholinergic medications can lead to dry mouth, constipation, blurred vision, and, in very high doses, toxic psychosis. Therefore, some clients will not receive prophylactic treatment with an antipsychotic agent, particularly if they are on a low-potency neuroleptic (associated with less EPS). If a dystonic reaction emerges acutely, intramuscular anticholinergic agents are administered initially, followed by daily oral doses.

Neuroleptic malignant syndrome (NMS) is a serious idiosyncratic reaction characterized by severe catatonia, parkinsonian rigidity, fever, changes in blood pressure or mental status, irregular pulse, tachycardia, sweating, and elevated creatine kinase and myoglobin, secondary to muscle breakdown. Not all symptoms may be present, and the diagnosis

TABLE 6–10. Medications Used to Treat Extrapyramidal Symptoms

Medication	Dose
Benztropine (Cogentin)	0.5–2 mg bid
Biperiden (Akineton)	0.5 mg–2 mg bid
Diphenhydramine (Benadryl)	25–50 mg tid
Trihexyphenidyl (Artane)	1–3 mg bid
Clonidine (Catapres)*	0.05 mg bid–qid
Lorazepam (Ativan)*	0.5–2 mg bid
Propranolol (Inderal)*	10–30 mg tid

*Indicated for the treatment of akathisia.

may be difficult. It is more likely in the first 2 weeks after initiation of treatment or after an increased dose, but NMS may occur at any point in the treatment. Although it can result from any neuroleptic, high-potency agents pose the greatest risk. The progression of NMS can be rapid, and death may result from cardiac, respiratory, or renal failure. Discontinue the neuroleptic, and provide supportive measures such as cooling blankets, adequate hydration, and frequent monitoring of side effects. Dantrolene or bromocriptine may also be prescribed to relieve the rigidity and catatonia.

Severe cardiac effects can also occur during antipsychotic therapy. Pimozide, thioridazine, and mesoridazine slow cardiac conduction and may lead to heart block and ventricular tachycardia. Obtain baseline and regular pulse and blood pressure on all clients who take neuroleptics. Because of the increased risk of cardiac abnormalities, baseline and regular ECG monitoring is essential for individuals treated with pimozide and high doses of clozapine.

All antipsychotic medications lower the seizure threshold. Chlorpromazine and loxapine pose a greater risk. High doses of thioridazine have been associated with pigmentary retinopathy.

Tardive dyskinesia (TD), a severe reaction, refers to the late onset (tardive) of abnormal movements (dyskinesia). It is generally associated with long-term use of antipsychotics. Clients experience involuntary movements of the mouth, tongue, and face. In more severe cases, TD may involve the fingers, arms, trunk, and respiratory muscles, and the drug must be discontinued. Increasing age and female gender are known risk factors. Emerging evidence suggests that the presence of an affective disorder may pose an additional risk. Clozapine therapy is associated with much less risk of TD, and switching to it may help diminish or even treat the condition. Although TD has no known treatment, drug discontinuation may minimize the movements over time.

Adverse Reactions, Atypical Antipsychotics

Common Effects. Weight gain is a common reaction, particularly with clozapine. The side effects of clozapine are similar to the low-potency, typical antipsychotic agents and include anticholinergic effects, weight gain, sedation, and orthostatic hypotension, as well as transient increases in body temperature. Sertindole, quetiapine, and olanzapine were developed to have fewer side effects. The most common side effects of sertindole are nasal congestion and one specific type of sexual dysfunction, decreased ejaculatory volume. Twenty percent of men treated with sertindole have decreased ejaculatory volume that usually resolves. Side effects of quetiapine include sedation, sleepiness, and mild, transient, and reversible increases in liver enzymes. Olanzapine may lead to sedation, particularly during the first 1 to 2 weeks of treatment. Other common side effects include agitation and nervousness.

> **LESSONS LEARNED FROM CLOZAPINE**
>
> Clozapine ushered in a new wave of treatment, particularly for those with schizophrenia because of its unique properties, which led to the introduction of several other atypical antipsychotics and the ongoing development of other agents. How does understanding the mechanism of action of clozapine further the search for more effective antipsychotic medications? Three major hypotheses exist about how clozapine works. First, it selectively affects the limbic system, an area of the brain that appears to be disturbed in schizophrenia. Unlike the typical antipsychotics, it does not affect the striatal region, responsible for movement disorders such as EPS. Second, clozapine affects both dopamine and serotonin systems, as well as other neurotransmitters such as norepinephrine, glutamate, acetylcholine, and certain neuropeptides. This theory suggests that the combined effects, particularly on dopamine and serotonin, are responsible for the effectiveness of what are now called "$D_2/5\text{-}HT_2$ antagonists." Third, clozapine selectively binds to specific dopamine receptors, the D_1 and D_4 receptors. This theory proposes that clozapine balances dopamine-receptor binding affinities. Whatever the exact mechanism of action, clozapine and the new generation of antipsychotics continue to offer hope for clients and their families.

Occasional Effects. Clozapine may cause enuresis and increased salivation during the night. Clozapine is also associated with tachycardia.

Sertindole can lead to a mild increase in the Q_T interval on the ECG similar to typical antipsychotics.

Clozapine, olanzapine, sertindole, and risperidone (in daily doses less than 6 mg) are not likely to cause EPS, but rarely it may occur.

Uncommon but Potentially Serious Effects. Agranulocytosis is a serious complication of clozapine therapy that affects about 1% of all clients. Weekly white blood cell counts (WBC) are necessary to detect agranulocytosis. Individuals are given a 1-week supply of clozapine after their WBC count has been screened. Signs of infection may also signal agranulocytosis. Despite adequate monitoring, several deaths have occurred. The mechanism of agranulocytosis is unknown. The risk increases with age and when clozapine is combined with other medications that reduce WBCs. If it occurs, the medication is discontinued immediately.

The risk of seizures is low, except with clozapine. Higher doses of clozapine are associated with higher risk.

NMS and TD rarely occur in clients treated with clozapine. The frequency of occurrence of NMS and TD on risperidone, olanzapine, quetiapine, and sertindole has not been fully established because of their relative lack of extensive use.

Clinically Significant Interactions

The most important interactions are listed in Table 6–11. Combined with other medications, neuroleptics may worsen side effects such as sedation and extrapyramidal and anticholinergic effects. Anticonvulsants reduce clearance and decrease neuroleptic plasma levels. Lithium and antipsychotic therapy can lead to neurotoxicity. Clozapine, while providing many potential benefits, cannot be combined with medications such as carbamazepine that lead to hematologic effects. In combination with an SSRI, clozapine levels increase.

TABLE 6–11. Drug Interactions with Antipsychotic Medications

Antipsychotics may increase effects of:
- Alcohol, barbiturates
- Antidepressants
- Anticholinergic agents
- Phenytoin
- Beta-blockers
- Tetracylcine, other antibiotics
- Thiazide diuretics
- Antihypertensives
- Surgical muscle relaxants
- Quinidine

Antipsychotics may reduce effects of:
- Lithium
- Anticonvulsants, barbiturates
- Antibiotics
- Guanethidine
- L-dopa, methyldopa
- Hypoglycemic agents

Medications that may increase antipsychotic effects include:
- Antidepressants
- Beta-blockers
- Barbiturates
- Methyldopa

Medications that may reduce the effectiveness of antipsychotics include:
- Lithium
- Cimetidine
- Antidiarrheal agents
- Antacids
- Anticholinergic agents

Source: Adapted from Teicher & Glod, 1990

*CPZ = Chlorpromazine. Potency estimates vary significantly and are only approximate indicators to determine equivalent dose. Typical doses are from 300–600 mg or equivalent of chlorpromazine. EPS = Extrapyramidal symptoms. + = very low, ++ = low, +++ = moderate, ++++ = high.

†Sedating initially, then becomes activating with continuous use.

Note: Risperidone is associated with little to no EPS in daily doses less than 6 mg in adults.

Source: Adapted from Teicher, MH, and Glod, CA: Neuroleptic drugs: Indications and guidelines for their rational use in children and adolescents. J Child Adolesc Psychopharmacol 1:33, 1990.

Concomitant clozapine and clonazepam therapy has resulted in sedation, severe dizziness, delirium, and respiratory arrest.

NURSING CONSIDERATIONS

A major role for psychiatric nurses is to evaluate the individual's response to antipsychotic medications. Because of their protracted onset of action, psychotic symptoms take time to diminish. The tendency may be to escalate the dose to manage continued symptoms. In most situations, high doses fail to treat the condition. Instead, side effects increase dramatically. Adults usually require daily doses equivalent to 300 to 600 mg of chlorpromazine.

Uncomfortable side effects emerge early and should be distinguished from antipsychotic effects. The nurse should regularly monitor key target symptoms and adverse reactions. For example, sedation may lead to slowed behaviors, which is different from lessening of psychotic thoughts. Side effects frequently lead to noncompliance, and clients need to be encouraged to continue pharmacotherapy. Simple, concrete instructions are the most useful.

Carefully monitor acute and serious reactions. For example, the frightening effects of a dystonic reaction can lead to increased paranoia, fear, and noncompliance. Clients may not notice signs of infection that signal a drop in WBC count. Early intervention with potentially dangerous side effects is essential. For all individuals who receive antipsychotic medications, baseline and regular assessment for TD is necessary. Psychiatric nurses have a key role in assessing this side effect. It is most commonly evaluated by completing the *Abnormal Involuntary Movement Scale (AIMS*; Table 6–12). This instrument is used to systematically observe, assess, and document facial, oral, extremity, and truncal movements. The severity of any movement is coded from minimal to severe. At a minimum, complete the AIMS at baseline and every 6 months, and record it in the individual's medical record.

As advocates for individuals with major psychiatric disorders, nurses can suggest that a trial of an atypical neuroleptic be initiated when poor response or uncomfortable side effects are present. Teach clients and families the benefits of these medications; they are less likely to cause EPS and may be superior in treating certain symptoms such as the "negative" symptoms of schizophrenia. However, many of the atypical agents are expensive, and clozapine requires close monitoring. Help families request an atypical antipsychotic when their family member has not responded to typical antipsychotics, when uncomfortable side effects emerge, or if ongoing negative symptoms such as apathy and social withdrawal prevail. Support the family in their efforts to ensure compliance. Atypical agents hold the hope for enhanced therapeutic efficacy; explain that potential benefits are possible, whereas dramatic effects are unlikely. For instance, treatment with clozapine may improve clients' quality of life and allow them a greater degree of independence. It may mean that the individual can live in a structured living situation, tolerate part-time work, or have less frequent hospitalizations.

TABLE 6–12. AIMS

DEPARTMENT OF HEALTH AND HUMAN SERVICES PUBLIC HEALTH SERVICE ALCOHOL DRUG ABUSE AND MENTAL HEALTH ADMINISTRATION NATIONAL INSTITUTE OF MENTAL HEALTH ABNORMAL INVOLUNTARY MOVEMENT SCALE (AIMS)	STUDY	PATIENT	PERIOD	RATER	HOSPITAL
	PATIENT'S NAME					
	RATER					
	DATE					

INSTRUCTIONS: Complete Examination Procedure (next page) before making ratings
MOVEMENT RATINGS: Rate highest severity observed. Rate movements that occur upon activation one *less* than those observed spontaneously.

Code 0 = None
1 = Minimal, may be extreme normal
2 = Mild
3 = Moderate
4 = Severe

		(Circle One)
FACIAL AND ORAL MOVEMENTS:	1. Muscles of Facial Expression e.g., movements of forehead, eyebrows, periorbital area, cheeks; include frowning, blinking, smiling, grimacing	0 1 2 3 4
	2. Lips and Perioral Area e.g., puckering, pouting, smacking	0 1 2 3 4
	3. Jaw e.g., biting, clenching, chewing, mouth opening, lateral movement	0 1 2 3 4
	4. Tongue Rate only increase in movement both in and out of mouth, NOT inability to sustain movement	0 1 2 3 4
EXTREMITY MOVEMENTS:	5. Upper *(arms, wrists, hands, fingers)* Include choreic movements (i.e., rapid, objectively purposeless, irregular, spontaneous), athetoid movements (i.e., slow, irregular, complex, serpentine). Do NOT include tremor (i.e., repetitive, regular, rhythmic)	0 1 2 3 4
	6. Lower *(legs, knees, ankles, toes)* e.g., lateral knee movement, foot tapping, heel dropping, foot squirming, inversion and eversion of foot	0 1 2 3 4
TRUNK MOVEMENTS:	7. Neck, shoulders, hips e.g., rocking, twisting, squirming, pelvic gyrations	0 1 2 3 4
GLOBAL JUDGMENTS:	8. Severity of abnormal movements	None, normal 0 Minimal 1 Mild 2 Total ____ Moderate 3 Severe 4
	9. Incapacitation due to abnormal movements	None, normal 0 Minimal 1 Mild 2 Moderate 3 Severe 4
	10. Patient's awareness of abnormal movements Rate only patient's report	No awareness 0 Aware, no distress 1 Aware, mild distress 2 Aware, moderate distress 3 Aware, severe distress 4

Continued on following page

TABLE 6–12. AIMS (Continued)

DENTAL STATUS:	11. Current problems with teeth and/or dentures	No 0 / Yes 1
	12. Does patient usually wear dentures?	No 0 / Yes 1
EXAMINATION PROCEDURE:	Either before or after completing the Examination Procedure observe the patient unobtrusively, at rest (e.g., in waiting room) The chair to be used in this examination should be a hard, firm one without arms.	

1. Ask patient whether there is anything in his/her mouth (i.e., gum, candy, etc.) and if there is, to remove it.
2. Ask patient about the *current* condition of his/her teeth. Ask patient if he/she wears dentures. Do teeth or dentures bother patient *now*?
3. Ask patient whether he/she notices any movements in mouth, face, hands, or feet. If yes, ask to describe and to what extent they *currently* bother patient or interfere with his/her activities.
4. Have patient sit in chair with hands on knees, legs slightly apart, and feet flat on floor. (Look at entire body for movements while in this position.)
5. Ask patient to sit with hands hanging unsupported. If male, between legs, if female and wearing a dress, hanging over knees. (Observe hands and other body areas.)
6. Ask patient to open mouth. (Observe tongue at rest within mouth.) Do this twice.
7. Ask patient to protrude tongue. (Observe abnormalities of tongue movement.) Do this twice.
8. Ask patient to tap thumb, with each finger, as rapidly as possible for 10–15 seconds; separately with right hand, then with left hand. (Observe facial and leg movements.)
9. Flex and extend patient's left and right arms (one at a time). (Note any rigidity and rate on DOTES.)
10. Ask patient to stand up. (Observe in profile. Observe all body areas again, hips included.)
11. Ask patient to extend both arms outstretched in front with palms down. (Observe trunk, legs, and mouth.)
12. Have patient walk a few paces, turn, and walk back to chair. (Observe hands and gait.) Do this twice.

CASE STUDY

Joseph is an 18-year-old high school student. He is described as a loner, usually shy and quiet around peers. He has been an excellent student prior to the past semester. His parents report that he began failing subjects and became more withdrawn at home. They have recently noticed him talking to himself and acting in a secretive manner. His appearance is uncharacteristically disheveled. On evaluation, Joseph reports hearing voices telling him he is "bad" and he believes that "aliens are coming" who will "punish" him. He reports spending time in his room to protect himself from the "invaders." His parents report that a grandfather, uncle, and two cousins have had similar symptoms. Joseph is given a battery of blood and other diagnostic tests to rule out other causes for his psychosis. These tests are negative. Although a definite diagnosis of paranoid schizophrenia cannot positively be made without additional data about the course of the symptoms over time, a working diagnosis of schizophrenia is reasonable. Joseph is started on risperidone for treatment of his psychotic symptoms.

The nurse needs to be sure the client and his family understand that schizophrenia is believed to be the result of a genetic and biological defect that causes brain abnormalities, not faulty parenting. The nurse can support the family while they learn how to best support Joseph. Medication can control the delusions and hallucinations, although it cannot cure the disease. The nurse educates the parents and Joseph about the possible side effects of the medication: parkinsonian side effects (tremor, rigidity, and shuffling gait) or akathisia (restlessness), particularly when the dose is above 6 mg. These effects usually occur after a few weeks of treatment and respond to additional medications. Education about dystonic reactions is important. An anticholinergic medication will probably be prescribed in addition to the antipsychotic to avoid the development of this side effect. If Joseph responds well to the antipsychotic and long-term treatment is indicated, then Joseph and his parents need to be taught about TD, a rare side effect of long-term treatment. The nurse should also educate them about the rare, but life-threatening complication, NMS. Any severe rigidity, difficulty breathing, high fever, or sweating indicates the need for emergency treatment at a hospital. The nurse should assess Joseph for any side effects at each contact. Although the antipsychotic medications have potential side effects, the nurse can explain to the family and client that schizophrenia is a serious disease and that untreated psychosis has severe repercussions for the person and the family. The nurse's role as educator and supporter for the client and the family is integral because compliance with treatment is essential.

ANXIOLYTICS AND SEDATIVE-HYPNOTICS

GENERAL INTRODUCTION

When anxiety becomes severe and diagnosable as a discrete disorder, treatment with **anxiolytics** may be necessary. Similarly, persistent insomnia may require temporary treatment with a sedative-hypnotic. Unlike many of the other medications used to treat major psychiatric disorders, anxiolytics and sedative-hypnotics are generally well tolerated and work acutely to reverse symptoms. However, they carry potential for abuse and dependence. The major class of anxiolytics is benzodiazepines. A unique nonbenzodiazepine, buspirone, is also available to treat anxiety. Several specific benzodiazepines are sedative/hypnotics. One sedative-hypnotic, zolpidem, is chemically unrelated to the benzodiazepines. Because it acts similarly on neuronal receptors, produces similar side effects, and is pharmacologically related, however, it is included under the benzodiazepines. Table 6–13 lists the medications and dosages commonly used to treat anxiety and insomnia.

BENZODIAZEPINES

Indications

Benzodiazepines are indicated for the treatment of panic disorder with or without agoraphobia, generalized anxiety disorder, temporary relief of situational anxiety, management of acute alcohol withdrawal, preoperative sedation, seizures, temporary relief of insomnia, and short-term treatment of acute mania. Less commonly, they are used for the acute treatment of aggression, OCD, schizophrenia, and akathisia.

Pharmacokinetics

Benzodiazepines are rapidly absorbed through the GI tract after oral administration, widely distributed, and metabolized by the liver. Intramuscular absorption of benzodiazepines may be slow and inconsistent. Benzodiazepines differ in several ways: dosage strength, onset of action, and elimination half-life (see Table 6–13). Dosage strength is the amount of medication necessary to effectively treat symptoms. Onset of action reflects how rapidly benzodiazepines produce sedating and anxiolytic effects. The more rapid the onset of action, the greater the sedating and anxiolytic properties. Elimination half-life refers to the amount of time required for the drug and its active metabolites to be eliminated from the body. With repeated administration, benzodiazepines with longer half-lives have a greater duration of action.

Benzodiazepines are highly lipid soluble. As a result, they get into the brain quickly to produce anxiolytic and sedating effects. Age, smoking, liver dysfunction, and other medica-

TABLE 6–13. Characteristics of Anxiolytic and Sedative-Hypnotic Medications

Anxiolytics	Dose/Day	Onset after Oral Dose	Elimination Half-Life*
Benzodiazepines			
Alprazolam (Xanax)	0.75–6	Intermediate	6–20
Chlordiazepoxide (Librium)	15–100	Intermediate	30–100
Clonazepam (Klonopin)	1–4	Intermediate	18–50
Clorazepate (Tranxene)	7.5–30	Rapid	30–100
Diazepam (Valium)	5–40	Rapid	30–100
Halazepam (Paxipam)	60–160	Intermediate–slow	30–100
Lorazepam (Ativan)	2–6	Intermediate	10–20
Oxazepam (Serax)	30–120	Intermediate–slow	8–12
Prazepam (Centrax)	10–60	Slow	30–100
Nonbenzodiazepines			
Buspirone	15–60	Slow	2–11
Sedative-Hypnotics			
Benzodiazepines			
Flurazepam (Dalmane)	15–60	Rapid–intermediate	50–160
Quazepam (Doral)	7.5–30	Rapid–intermediate	50–160
Temazepam (Restoril)	10–30	Intermediate	8–20
Triazolam (Halcion)	0.25–0.5	Intermediate	1.5–5
Nonbenzodiazepines			
Zolpidem (Ambien)	5–10	Rapid	2–3

*Half-life in hours, includes all active metabolites. The elderly tend to have longer half-lives than those listed above.

Source: Adapted from Arana, Hyman, and Rosenbaum: Handbook of Psychiatric Drug Therapy, ed. 3. Boston: Little, Brown, 1995, and the Physicians' Desk Reference, 1997.

tions can influence their distribution and elimination. Benzodiazepines freely cross the placenta and are secreted in breast milk.

Mechanism of Action

Benzodiazepines are hypothesized to exert some of their main effects through an inhibitory neurotransmitter, GABA, which acts like a natural anxiety reducer. Benzodiazepines facilitate the transmission of GABA by binding to GABA-A receptors and opening chloride ion channels. Benzodiazepines also decrease serotonin turnover and decrease the activity of serotonergic neurons.[8]

Contraindications and Precautions

Benzodiazepines are contraindicated for individuals with known hypersensitivity, sleep apnea, narrow-angle glaucoma, shock, coma, and alcohol or substance abuse. They should not be combined with alcohol or other CNS depressants because of the risk of severe sedation and respiratory depression. Because the primary route of elimination appears to be hepatic metabolism to inactive metabolites excreted by the kidney, use these agents cautiously in clients with liver and renal disease.

Few research data exist on the use of benzodiazepines during pregnancy and lactation, and therefore they should be avoided. Early reports suggested that diazepam caused cleft lip and palate; however, recent research fails to support this association. Benzodiazepines may be associated with decreased fetal and infant growth or CNS dysfunction. If these medications are administered late in the third trimester, newborns experience benzodiazepine withdrawal and floppy infant syndrome.

Adverse Reactions

Common Effects. Benzodiazepines can cause sedation, fatigue, reduced motor coordination, impaired memory, and cognitive dysfunction. Sedation and fatigue usually resolve with repeated administration and respond to dose reduction. Impaired motor coordination, memory, and cognition may result in difficulty performing tasks or driving, remembering new information, and concentrating. Warn clients that these effects can develop. Short-acting high-potency agents such as triazolam are associated with greater memory impairment. Switching to a longer-acting low-potency agent may reduce difficulty with memory. If severe motor or cognitive problems result, use should be tapered and finally discontinued.

Zolpidem commonly leads to sedation, nausea, diarrhea, headache, and dizziness. Dose reduction or discontinuation manages these effects successfully.

Occasional Effects. Less commonly, benzodiazepines may cause nausea, headache, or dizziness. Reducing the dose usually alleviates these effects.

Uncommon but Potentially Serious Effects. Rapid discontinuation of benzodiazepines and zolpidem can produce withdrawal symptoms of insomnia, agitation, anxiety, sweating, irritability, and nausea 1 to 2 days after short-acting benzodiazepines are stopped or 5 to 10 days after discontinuation of long-acting agents. Severe reactions include seizures, coma, and psychosis. Withdrawal is more common after prolonged regular administration, when steady-state levels have been achieved. Instruct clients not to discontinue medication abruptly or miss doses, and educate them about the possible untoward reactions. Withdrawal is treated by restarting the benzodiazepine. Clients who are tapered too quickly can also experience withdrawal symptoms.

Rebound symptoms occur when the benzodiazepine "wears off," usually several hours after the last dose is taken. Alprazolam, because of its short half-life, may pose the most risk for interdose rebound symptoms. Clients notice reemergence of their anxiety or insomnia. They then begin to "clock-watch": Symptoms of anxiety occur between doses, and they watch the clock to decide when to take their next dose. Switching to a longer-acting agent such as clonazepam is the most common intervention.

Benzodiazepines also carry the potential for abuse and dependence. Although the majority of individuals do not abuse them, some clients may repeatedly escalate the dose to achieve the same desired effects, usually a "high." Increasing the dose usually reflects addictive behavior or dependency and should signal the potential for dangerous consequences. Careful tapering for discontinuation of benzodiazepine therapy is necessary.

Respiratory depression is a major risk, particularly with parenteral administration and high doses. Monitor the respiratory rate in clients who receive high doses or who have compromised respiratory ability.

Paradoxical behaviors may also result. Agitation, loss of control, rage reactions, or aggressive behaviors signal the need for immediate intervention. Treatment consists of careful drug discontinuation or switching to another agent such as oxazepam, which is less likely to induce these reactions.

Clinically Significant Interactions

The most serious interaction occurs with coadministration of a benzodiazepine or zolpidem with alcohol, TCAs, antihistamines, or other CNS depressants. This mixture can lead to severe impairment in motor and cognitive abilities, respiratory depression, or death. Benzodiazepines lower alcohol tolerance and may produce alcohol intoxication or enhance the effects of other CNS drugs.

Several medications have the potential to increase benzodiazepine levels: cimetidine, disulfiram, erythromycin, estrogens, nefazodone, and the SSRIs (particularly fluoxetine and fluvoxamine). Conversely, certain anticonvulsants, such as carbamazepine, phenobarbital, and phenytoin decrease benzodiazepine effects. Antacids interfere with absorption of benzodiazepines. To minimize this effect, tell clients to take benzodiazepines prior to antacids.

BUSPIRONE

Indications

Buspirone (BuSpar) is indicated for the treatment of generalized anxiety disorder. Emerging uses include the treatment of aggression in some individuals with organic brain conditions or developmental delays and treatment of children with disruptive aggressive behaviors.

Pharmacokinetics

Buspirone is completely absorbed into the GI tract after oral administration and is metabolized by the liver. It has a half-life of 2 to 11 hours.

Mechanism of Action

Unlike benzodiazepines and zolpidem, this agent does not affect GABA receptors. Its primary mechanism of action is on serotonin receptors. Buspirone partially acts on the 5-HT$_{1A}$ autoreceptor. The result is to send a signal back to the presynaptic neuron to release less serotonin. Decreased serotonin is thought to have anxiolytic actions.

Contraindications and Precautions

Because the primary route of elimination is hepatic metabolism, buspirone is used cautiously in clients with liver disease. Few research data exist on use during pregnancy and lactation; therefore, it should be avoided.

Because buspirone is not a benzodiazepine, no cross-tolerance with benzodiazepines is possible. Therefore, buspirone is not used in alcohol or benzodiazepine withdrawal. Buspirone has a protracted onset of action and therefore cannot be used in emergency situations or for rapid relief of anxiety.

Adverse Reactions

Common Effects. Headache and restlessness are the most common side effects. Headache can be treated with acetaminophen, ibuprofen, or aspirin. The restlessness is similar to akathisia and can be observed as motor restlessness. It is treated by dose reduction or low-dose beta-blockers.

Occasional Effects. Less common effects include dizziness and stomach upset. These effects may subside with ongoing administration or respond to dose reduction.

Uncommon but Potentially Serious Effects. Buspirone has only one known serious effect to date. Rare cases of mania have been reported. Drug discontinuation is usually necessary.

Clinically Significant Interactions

Buspirone in combination with MAOIs leads to the development of a serotonergic syndrome. Agitation, confusion, myoclonus, hypertension, tremor, and death may result.

NURSING CONSIDERATIONS

Although benzodiazepines carry the potential for abuse, they are highly beneficial for individuals diagnosed with anxiety disorders. Most clients do not abuse their medication; however, those with a history of alcohol or substance abuse are at greatest risk.

Once taken regularly, benzodiazepines reach steady-state concentrations and can lead to physical dependence. If discontinued abruptly, symptoms of withdrawl may result. Clients should be instructed to take each dose as directed and avoid any missed doses. Sudden medication discontinuation commonly leads to insomnia, agitation, anxiety, sweating, irritability, and nausea; more severe reactions such as seizures, coma, and psychosis are possible. The onset of withdrawal is similar to half-life, and symptoms are more likely with shorter-acting agents. As a result, careful weaning of the medication is necessary. Detailed tapering schedules are available for each of the benzodiazepines to prevent and minimize withdrawal effects. For example, alprazolam is tapered by about 0.25 mg every week. Another strategy is to switch the client from a short-acting to a longer acting benzodiazepine (for example, from alprazolam to clonazepam) and then taper the medication.

Clients should be educated about the properties of sedative-hypnotic agents. These medications are indicated for the short-term relief of insomnia and should not be prescribed for long periods (that is, several weeks or months). Sedative-hypnotics treat insomnia successfully, rapidly, and with little "hangover" effect because they tend to wear off quickly. However, insomnia is often a symptom associated with other conditions and may not always be recognized as part of an underlying disorder. Nurses should carefully assess whether an undiagnosed disorder is present. Several sleep disorders have insomnia as their primary complaint, as do many psychiatric illnesses, for example, depression, mania, and PTSD. Thus, if the undiagnosed condition is ignored, the insomnia generally persists, and sedative-hypnotics fail to provide adequate treatment.

Because buspirone does not have the properties of benzodiazepines, psychiatric nurses can suggest it as a possible alternative for the treatment of anxiety. However, clients need to be aware that it is effective only for generalized anxiety disorder and is ineffective for other disorders such as panic disorder. Buspirone has a protracted onset of action, and no immediate effects are seen. Instruct clients that anxiolytic effects may take 2 to 4 weeks. While awaiting positive effects, individuals are at high risk for missed doses or drug discontinuation. A major role for the nurse is to encourage

ARE PSYCHOSTIMULANT MEDICATIONS BEING OVERPRESCRIBED?

Methylphenidate, an amphetamine, paradoxically quells hyperactivity and focuses the attention of both children and adults with ADHD. Early reports suggested that use of this medication has sextupled in the last 5 years. More recent research suggests that methylphenidate use has doubled or tripled. Why is it being prescribed more? Although the answer is not certain, several possibilities exist. First, children are probably taking the medication longer than before. Most children do not "outgrow" ADHD and continue to need medication. Second, more adults are recognizing that they have ADHD, which was not diagnosed during their childhood, and are being prescribed stimulant medications to treat their restlessness and inattention. Third, ADHD is recognized as having several subtypes, including a predominantly inattentive type that can also be helped pharmacologically. Fourth, although unproven, some people have suggested that methylphenidate is being given to children who are active rather than those diagnosed with ADHD. Fifth, other clinicians think that society influences decisions about beginning medication, and that some people are looking for a "quick fix." Whatever the answer, more children and adults are probably receiving pharmacotherapy. The bottom line is that if medication adequately treats hyperactivity and inattention, the benefits, that is, improved quality of life, ability to attend to school and work, and relating better to others, outweigh the risks.

compliance and to remind the client that the drug's effect may take several weeks.

CASE STUDY

Caroline is a 35-year-old married woman. She presents to the emergency room with chest pain, rapid heart rate, sweating, nausea, and shaking and reports feeling as if she is going to die. This is her third visit to the emergency room in the past 2 months for similar symptoms. Cardiac and other medical difficulties, including substance abuse, have been ruled out. She reports that since her first attack, she has been afraid and worried about another attack. She has been significantly altering her activities in an attempt to ward off further episodes. Caroline is evaluated, diagnosed with panic disorder, and started on alprazolam.

The nurse can help Caroline understand that her symptoms are partly biological in origin, with her fear subsequently contributing a psychological component. The nurse should reassure Caroline that anxiety disorders are common and respond well to treatment. Given that Caroline does not have a history of substance abuse, a benzodiazepine is an appropriate choice of medication. She is told to take the drug as prescribed and not increase it without consulting the prescribing clinician. She should also be told to use caution when driving, at least initially, because the drug can cause sedation. She should avoid alcohol. The nurse also tells the client not to stop the drug abruptly because this can lead to withdrawal symptoms (nervousness, headache, decreased appetite, or decreased energy). The nurse can offer support by explaining that the symptoms are anxiety-based and not a reflection of an underlying cardiac or other medical disease.

PSYCHOSTIMULANTS

GENERAL INFORMATION

Methylphenidate, dextroamphetamine, pemoline, and a mixture of amphetamine formulations constitute the class of medications called psychostimulants. They are called stimulants because of their propensity to induce CNS stimulation. Their use dates back to the 1930s, when psychiatrists began administering stimulant medication to hospitalized children with behavior problems. Children who were very active initially were calmed by the medication, whereas those who were shy became more active. Since that time, many studies have demonstrated their effectiveness in treating a wide range of symptoms from depression to overactivity. Despite these benefits, stimulants carry a high risk of abuse. Common stimulant medications, dosages, and half-lives are found in Table 6–14.

Indications

Psychostimulants are used to treat ADHD in children and adults and narcolepsy. Emerging evidence suggests that they may be useful for treatment-resistant depression and geriatric depression.

Pharmacokinetics

These medications are well absorbed after oral administration. With the exception of pemoline, the psychostimulants

TABLE 6–14. Available Stimulants, Half-Life, and Dose

Generic (Trade) Name	Half-life (hrs)	Dose (mg/kg)	Dosage range
Methylphenidate (Ritalin)	2–3[†]	0.3–1.5	10–60 mg
Dextroamphetamine (Dexedrine)*	3–6	0.3–1.5	5–40
Pemoline (Cylert)	9–14	0.5–3.0	18.75–112.5

*Approved for children as young as age 3 years.
[†]2-6 hours for the sustained-release preparation.

have short half-lives, requiring frequent daily dosing (see Table 6–14). Because of its longer half-life, pemoline can be administered once daily; however, onset of its therapeutic effects may take weeks. It also has less potential for abuse. Methylphenidate is metabolized by the liver, whereas dextroamphetamine and pemoline are metabolized partially by the liver and excreted partly unchanged in urine.

Mechanism of Action

Psychostimulants act directly on neuronal synapses to increase the release of norepinephrine, serotonin, and dopamine. Because they also block the reuptake of norepinephrine and dopamine, they further increase levels of these neurotransmitters. Increased dopaminergic neurotransmission is probably responsible for their euphoric effects, whereas enhanced noradrenergic neurotransmission explains their CNS-stimulating effects. How psychostimulants work to paradoxically quell the hyperactive and impulsive behaviors of ADHD is not known.

Contraindications and Precautions

Avoid psychostimulants in clients with substance abuse, seizure disorders, or liver disease and in pregnant or lactating women. Use them cautiously in individuals with renal disease, hypertension, or other cardiac disorders such as tachyarrhythmias. Stimulants may worsen abnormal motor and vocal tics in clients with movement disorders such as Tourette's disorder. Warn clients to avoid alcohol.

Adverse Reactions

Common Effects. Appetite loss, insomnia, agitation, and irritable or dysphoric mood are the most common side effects. Originally prescribed as appetite suppressants, psychostimulants reduce appetite, sometimes resulting in unwanted weight loss. For example, children may experience stimulant-induced appetite suppression and fail to maintain their weight. In this case, the medication is reduced in dosage or discontinued, or another medication is substituted. Insomnia may be lessened by taking the medication earlier in the day; but if insomnia persists, drug discontinuation or switching to another class of medication may be necessary. Agitation is best treated with dose reduction.

Shifts in mood, resulting in grouchy, irritable, or depressed mood states, can occur with psychostimulants. Dose reduction may help these effects; however, drug discontinuation is usually necessary.

Occasional Effects. Headache, mild abdominal pain, and increases in blood pressure have been reported with psychostimulants. Over-the-counter analgesics can effectively treat headaches, which usually subside with ongoing treatment. Mild abdominal pain responds to dose reduction. Carefully monitor nonsignificant increases in blood pressure, particularly in clients with preexisting hypertension.

Uncommon but Potentially Serious Effects. Psychostimulants carry the potential for abuse, dependence, and addiction. Generally, individuals abuse these medications in order to achieve a "high." Pemoline has the lowest abuse potential. Prevention of abuse is the best strategy. Therefore, they are not prescribed to individuals with alcohol and substance abuse.

Children have been reported to develop mild growth and weight suppression, but this effect is rarely severe. The best intervention is a "drug holiday." Psychostimulants can be discontinued on weekends, school vacations, and during the summer to help restore adequate weight and growth.

Rarely, psychostimulants lead to tachyarrhythmias and severe liver dysfunction. Baseline and regular monitoring of pulse and ECG are necessary to detect severe cardiac problems. Pemoline appears to pose the greatest risk of hepatic dysfunction; therefore, baseline measurements and regular monitoring of liver function are necessary. As a result, pemoline is not the first agent of choice. Monitor clients for signs of liver toxicity: severe anorexia, weight loss, vomiting, lethargy, jaundice, and edema. Discontinue stimulants if hepatic dysfunction develops.

Clinically Significant Interactions

In combination with MAOIs, psychostimulants may lead to a hypertensive crisis or seizures. Their use with other antidepressants, such as TCAs and SSRIs, should be avoided because of the potential for increased stimulant effects. Conversely, antipsychotic medications diminish stimulant effects. Psychostimulants may also decrease the hypotensive effects of guanethidine. Decreased seizure threshhold is possible with concurrent anticonvulsant therapy.

CASE STUDY

Jeffrey is a 12-year-old fourth-grade student. He presents for evaluation on the recommendation of his teacher who reports that Jeffrey has difficulty paying attention in the classroom. His behavior is generally disruptive, and he appears disorganized and easily distracted. He does not appear to be listening to instructions. He has difficulty sitting still, talks constantly, and is impatient with his friends, and his grades are dropping. His parents report he is often unable to sit still long enough to eat dinner or watch a favorite television show. Jeffrey is diagnosed with ADHD and started on methylphenidate.

The nurse can reassure Jeffrey that he will probably find it much easier to concentrate at school and home once the medication is started. His parents may need support in understanding that Jeffrey's behavior was not volitional or a reflection of their parenting ability. Teaching them that this disorder has biological and genetic components and is responsive to treatment can lessen the emotional impact on both the child and the parents. Methylphenidate is generally well-tolerated in children. Educate the family about possible side effects, including decreased appetite, decreased sleep, headache, or changes in

"NEW GENERATION" MEDICATIONS FOR OBESITY

Several medications have been introduced to treat weight gain. Some, however, have been associated with severe, life-threatening effects. Once known as appetite suppressants, these antiobesity medications are not indicated for people who want to lose 5 or 10 pounds; they are effective treatments for obesity. D(dex)-fenfluramine (Redux), recently removed from the U.S. market, was the first weight-loss medication to be introduced in the U.S. in over 20 years. D-fenfluramine works as a serotonin-agonist, boosting levels of the neurotransmitter serotonin, known to be involved in eating behavior, food cravings, and satiety. Its more common side effects are appetite loss, insomnia, sexual dysfunction, agitation, and sedation. A rare, serious side effect is the risk of heart valve damage and primary pulmonary hypertension (PPH), which is hard to detect and leads to death in most cases. Because of these concerns, the manufacturer of D-fenfluramine voluntarily withdrew it from the U.S. market.

Many clinicians have also raised concerns about the overuse and misuse of medications to treat obesity. Based on clinical studies, most people lose only about 10% of their weight, even with diet and exercise programs. Many gain the weight back after the medication is discontinued. However, other practitioners have pointed out that continued obesity poses serious risks and increases the chances of death; therefore, these benefits of antiobesity medications far outweigh the risks.

Two medications, available for over 20 years but only recently used in combination also successfully reduce weight in obese clients. Fenfluramine (Pondimin), similar to D-fenfluramine, combined with phentermine (Ionamin), increases the release of serotonin and dopamine, respectively. However, fenfluramine also can cause serious heart valve defects and is no longer available for use. Phentermine alone is used to treat obesity and may show some benefits when combined with other medications. Two other medications, sibutramine (Meridia) and orlistat (Xenical) may hold some promise as effective treatments. Leptin, a naturally occurring substance in the body that is associated with obesity, is now being studied. Theoretically, increased leptin levels may send a signal to the brain to stop eating.

Despite their role in treating severe obesity, the role of weight loss medications in other conditions remains unanswered. Their use in eating disorders such as bulimia has not been established; studies are underway to determine their risks and benefits. At this point, they should not be used for clients with eating disorders.

mood. These side effects can be managed symptomatically or by reducing the dose of medication. Jeffrey may come off the medication on weekends and during school vacations. The nurse can be integral in providing education and support to parents and the child.

SYNOPSIS OF CURRENT RESEARCH

The last decade has witnessed a major shift in psychopharmacology. Several new antidepressants were introduced that carry different and more beneficial side effect profiles. Much of the current research is aimed at introducing "better" agents, those with continued efficacy and fewer side effects. The use of mood stabilizers has expanded from traditional treatment with lithium carbonate to the effective use of anticonvulsants. Anxiolytics, sedative-hypnotics, and psychostimulants continue to be used frequently and are developing potential alternative indications.

New antipsychotic medications are now available with increased efficacy for many clients with treatment-resistant conditions. Olanzapine, quetiapine, and sertindole are new atypical agents that show promise in treating the positive and negative symptoms of schizophrenia with fewer side effects, particularly EPS, and without the life-threatening risk of agranulocytosis associated with clozapine. The research evidence suggests that these medications are well tolerated. Olanzapine was more effective than placebos and haloperidol in a study of nearly 3000 clients with psychotic symptoms.[9] Common side effects included somnolence (sedation), dizziness, weight gain, headache, and akathisia, whereas those treated with haloperidol experienced more EPS, nervousness, somnolence, headache, and higher prolactin concentrations. In another study, three different doses of sertindole were compared with placebo and three doses of haloperidol; only sertindole, in doses of 20 mg daily, treated negative symptoms effectively.[10] Common side effects were nasal congestion, dry mouth, decreased ejaculatory volume, and vaginitis. Clients who are prescribed sertindole need gradual dose titration to about 20 mg daily, whereas those who receive olanzapine can be started and remain on 10 mg daily. Both medications appear to have few interactions with other medications.

Indications have been expanded for several medications. Bupropion is in a sustained-release form for the treatment of major depression, with expanding use for smoking cessation. Paroxetine is approved for use in major depression and panic disorder and is being used for OCD. Venlafaxine is being studied for ADHD and generalized anxiety disorder. Fluvoxamine may be approved for treatment of depression, whereas risperidone is being studied for add-on therapy in acute mania and psychotic disturbances in dementia.

Continued growth in pharmacotherapy is expected into the twenty-first century. As seen in Table 6–15, several new medications are under investigation and may receive approval for use before the end of the century. As pharma-

TABLE 6–15. Characteristics of Psychopharmacologic Agents under Development

Medication	Hypothesized Pharmacologic Action
Antipsychotics	
Quetiapine	Dopamine (D_2) blockade
Ziprasidone	Serotonin ($5-HT_{2A}$) and dopamine (D_2) blockade
Pramipexole	Presynaptic dopamine (D_2, D_3) agonist
Mazapertine	Dopamine (D_2, D_3, D_4) and serotonin ($5-HT_{1A}$) blockade
Fananserin	Dopamine (D_4) and serotonin ($5-HT_2$) blockade
Mood Stabilizers	
Lamotrigine	Kindling
Antidepressants	
Citalopram	Serotonin (5-HT) blockade
Flesinoxan	Serotonin (5-HT) agonist
Moclobomide	Reversible MAO-A inhibitor
Anxiolytics	
Adinazolam	Binds to GABA receptors

Note: Medications that are agonists stimulate the receptor, as opposed to antagonists, which block it.

cotherapy evolves, psychiatric nursing will continue to play a key role in helping clients with its positive and negative effects.

AREAS FOR FUTURE RESEARCH

- What are the most effective ways to ensure compliance in clients with various psychiatric disorders?
- Could assessment tools be developed to differentiate treatment-emergent side effects and worsening of illness-related behaviors?
- What are the key aspects of a medication teaching plan that promote medication compliance?
- How could psychiatric nursing activities surrounding medication monitoring be reimbursed differently in the changing health-care arena?
- What is the family's role in medication assessment and monitoring?
- What factors predict therapeutic efficacy in different client populations?
- What effects does gender have on drug absorption and metabolism?
- Do women respond differently to pharmacotherapy than men?
- What are the differences in effects between psychopharmacologic agents and over-the-counter medications?
- How does smoking affect the properties of psychotropic medications?

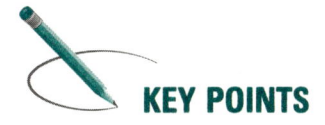

KEY POINTS

- The field of psychopharmacology has focused on developing effective agents with fewer side effects.
- Each medication is associated with common, occasional, and uncommon but potentially life-threatening adverse effects. However, not every client experiences side effects.
- Nurses can help clients and their families distinguish between side effects and worsening symptoms.
- Most antidepressants block the reuptake of serotonin, norepinephrine, or both within hours of their administration. However, these acute alterations in neuronal function do not fully explain how these medications work. Long-term adaptive changes in the synapse relate more to their mechanism of action.
- Several classes of antidepressants are available: tricyclic antidepressants (TCAs), monoamine oxidase inhibitors (MAOIs), selective serotonin reuptake inhibitors (SSRIs), and several novel antidepressants. The SSRIs are now the most common class of antidepressants prescribed.
- Antidepressants are indicated for the treatment of major depression, the depressed phase of bipolar disorder, and dysthymia. Expanding uses include chronic pain syndrome, panic disorder, obsessive-compulsive disorder (OCD), borderline personality disorder, attention-deficit and hyperactivity disorder (ADHD), bulimia, migraine headaches, peptic ulcer, fibromyalgia, and nocturnal enuresis in children.
- Mood stabilizers include lithium carbonate, carbamazepine, and valproic acid. These agents treat mania, prevent recurrent episodes of mania and depression, and maintain and balance the individual's level of functioning.
- Mood stabilizers work by inhibiting kindling. Less frequent and less severe mood states result. Like throwing water on a fire, these medications may extinguish the phases of bipolar disorder.
- Antipsychotic medications are indicated for the treatment of schizophrenia, schizoaffective disorder, acute psychotic states (including drug-induced psychosis), mania (while awaiting the effects of a mood stabilizer), psychotic depression (in combination with an antidepressant), pervasive development disorder, severe nausea and vomiting, Tourette's disorder, and intractable hiccups.
- Antipsychotic medications are classified as either "typical" or "atypical." Clozapine, olanzapine, quetiapine, sertindole, and possibly risperidone represent "atypical" antipsychotic medications that are likely to produce few to no extrapyramidal side effects.

- Typical antipsychotics have primary effects on dopamine. They block a specific dopamine (D_2) receptor located on the postsynaptic neuron that transiently increases levels of dopamine. With ongoing treatment, dopamine levels are reduced.
- Atypical antipsychotics selectively block dopamine (D_2) and serotonin ($5\text{-}HT_2$) receptors. They act on the limbic system, the area of the brain responsible for antipsychotic effects.
- Clozapine, olanzapine, quetiapine, and sertindole treat both the positive and negative symptoms of schizophrenia.
- Antianxiety agents include benzodiazepines and buspirone. Several specific benzodiazepines are also sedative-hypnotics and are used to treat insomnia.
- Benzodiazepines facilitate the transmission of GABA, decrease serotonin turnover, and decrease the activity of serotonergic neurons.
- Methylphenidate, dextroamphetamine, and pemoline are psychostimulants indicated for ADHD in adults and children, narcolepsy, and certain forms of depression.
- Psychostimulants act directly on neuronal synapses to increase the release of norepinephrine, serotonin, and dopamine.
- Psychiatric nurses offer hope that treatment will be successful in stabilizing the client's symptoms and limiting the potentially devastating effects of an untreated psychiatric disorder. The nurse, through education and support that enhances compliance, serves a vital function in positively affecting the outcome.

REFERENCES

1. Hyman, SE, Nestler, EJ: Initiation and adaptation: A paradigm for understanding psychotropic drug action. Am J Psychiatry 153:151, 1996.
2. Pastusek, A, et al: Pregnancy outcome following first-trimester exposure to fluoxetine (Prozac). JAMA 269:2246, 1993.
3. Potter, WZ, et al: Tricyclics and tetracyclics. In Schatzberg, AF, and Nemeroff, CB (eds): Textbook of Psychopharmacology. American Psychiatric Press, Washington, DC, 1995, p. 141.
4. Sternbach, H: The serotonin syndrome. Am J Psychiatry 148:705, 1991.
5. Teicher, MH, Glod, CA, and Cole, JO: Antidepressant drugs and the emergence of suicidal tendencies. Drug Safety 8:186, 1993.
6. Tollefson, GD: Selective Serotonin Reuptake Inhibitors. American Psychiatric Press, Washington, DC, 1995, p. 161.
7. Cohen, LS: A reevaluation of risk of in utero exposure to lithium. JAMA 271:146, 1994.
8. Teicher, MH: Biology of anxiety. Med Clin North Am 72:791, 1988.
9. Beasley, CM, et al: Olanzapine versus placebo and haloperidol: Acute phase results of the North American double-blind olanzapine trial. Neuropsychopharmacology 14:111, 1996.
10. Schultz, SC, et al: Efficacy, safety, and dose response of three doses of sertindole and three doses of Haldol in schizophrenic patients. Schizophr Res 18:133, 1996.

CHAPTER 7

Cognitive-Behavior Therapy

CHAPTER 7

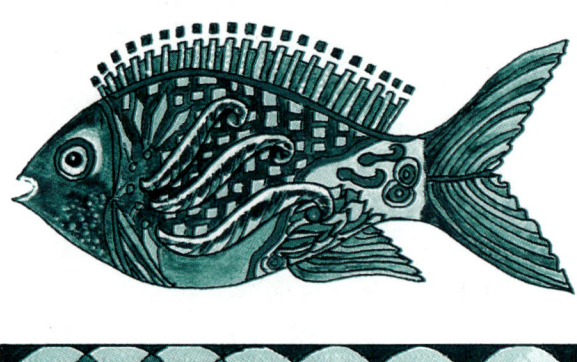

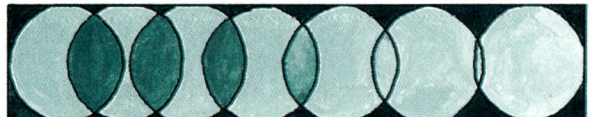

CHAPTER OUTLINE

Purpose of Cognitive-Behavior Therapy
The Nurse's Role
Behavioral Theories
   Conditioning
Behavioral Assessment and Outcome Measurement
Cognitive-Behavior Therapy
Behavior Therapy Procedures
   Relaxation Exercises
   Biofeedback
   Systematic Desensitization
   Token Economies
   Shaping
   Extinction and Punishment
   Modeling
   Exposure-Response Prevention
   Social Skills Training
   Assertiveness Training
Expected Outcomes
Synopsis of Current Research
Areas for Future Research

LEARNING OBJECTIVES

After completing this chapter, the reader should be able to:

- Identify the major techniques used in cognitive-behavior therapy and the differences among them.
- Describe the major components of cognitive-behavior therapy.
- Explain the nurse's role in using cognitive-behavior techniques.
- Understand the steps used in a behavioral analysis.
- Name the conditions for which cognitive-behavior therapy is frequently used.
- Apply cognitive-behavioral techniques to nursing practice.
- Distinguish between cognitive-behavior and other forms of therapy.

Philip G. Levendusky, PhD, FAClinP
Carol A. Glod, RN, CS, PhD
Thröstur Björgvinsson, MA

Cognitive-Behavior Therapy

KEY TERMS
A-B-C model
behavioral analysis
biofeedback
cognitive-behavior therapy
cognitive restructuring
extinction
negative reinforcement
operant conditioning
positive reinforcement
progressive muscle relaxation
punishers
punishment
reinforcers
response prevention
shaping
systematic desensitization

Cognitive-behavior therapy attempts to modify, change, correct, or eliminate maladaptive thoughts and behaviors manifested in depression, anxiety, smoking, shyness, and other problems. Increasingly, the cognitive-behavior therapist is the clinician of choice for individuals whose major symptoms are "in the mind," such as obsessive-compulsive disorder (OCD) and major depressive disorder. Although psychiatric nurse generalists are not cognitive-behavior therapists, they often use these techniques to help clients with a variety of psychiatric disorders deal with feelings and thoughts that overwhelm them.

Cognitive-behavior therapy is a set of wide-ranging procedures that differ in how they are applied to individuals with various emotional, physical, and psychological difficulties. The techniques of cognitive-behavior therapy are derived from scientific research. Objectives based on the client's presenting problem assess progress and outcome. The specific techniques used are based on analysis of the problem behavior, the resources available to the individual to deal with the problem, and the context of the problem behavior. For instance, specific phobias like fear of flying can be treated with cognitive-behavior procedures such as progressive relaxation, systematic desensitization, cognitive restructuring, modeling, contingency management, or assertiveness training, to mention a few. Other clients may need all of these procedures to treat a complex behavioral problem. No single technique is effective for everyone, particularly for those with anxiety disorders. Fortunately, there are a variety of effective techniques for training clients to control anxiety. Psychiatric nurses commonly teach and encourage cognitive-behavior strategies to help clients manage their behavior.

PURPOSE OF COGNITIVE-BEHAVIOR THERAPY

The purpose of cognitive-behavior therapy is to help clients change maladaptive thoughts and behaviors by substituting more adaptive ones. The therapist and client agree on a goal or an end point of treatment and work toward behavior change in the intended direction. For a phobic client, the goal of treatment is to become more able to approach or interact with the feared object, environment, or individual; for example, for fear of flying, the end point is the ability to fly on an airplane. If the client can behave in a nonphobic fashion, then the goal of the therapy has been achieved, regardless of whether the client knows why, how, or when the phobia developed. This orientation stands in contrast to other forms of therapy, particularly those based on Freudian or psychoanalytical models. Instead of exploring the effects of early childhood experiences and resulting conflicts, cognitive-behavior therapy focuses on ways to change thoughts and behavior.

THE NURSE'S ROLE

Nurses frequently confront and manage clients' problematic and maladaptive behaviors. Knowledge of learning theories and cognitive-behavior techniques underlies many nursing interventions. As a member of the interdisciplinary team, part of the nurse's role is to devise behavioral objectives with the client. The nurse may outline those behaviors the client identifies as needing change and break them down into small and manageable segments. The nurse, client, and, at times, the family can develop specific goals for behavior, such as reduced anxiety or increased socialization; in this way, the client and family can be active members of the treatment team. The nurse also advocates for clients, identifying behaviors that are appropriate, constructive, and amenable to change, whatever the treatment setting.

Before beginning to teach and encourage behavioral techniques, the clinician performs a behavioral analysis of the client. The nurse may take an active role in observing, documenting, and outlining behaviors targeted for change.

Nurses teach and reinforce cognitive-behavior techniques, particularly in inpatient or community settings with a behavioral orientation. The nurse may teach progressive relaxation to the client with anxiety; model, shape, and reinforce appropriate behavior (e.g., praise a client as a reward for following through on a task or acting appropriately); or initiate and lead groups that focus on developing social skills and assertive behaviors.

Another major part of the nurse's role is to refer clients for cognitive-behavior therapy. This form of therapy is commonly used to treat adjustment disorders (e.g., those that may follow bereavement) that are characterized by anxiety and depression. It is also used to help people develop more effective coping skills. For instance, individuals who have suffered a recent loss, have been diagnosed with a chronic medical condition, or are experiencing stress from unemployment or relationship difficulties can benefit from cognitive-behavior therapy. Recent research suggests that cognitive-behavior therapy is effective for major depressive disorder, panic disorder, generalized anxiety disorder, posttraumatic stress disorder (PTSD), and OCD. It is the most common treatment for excessive fears and phobias, such as fears of going out of the house alone. Cognitive-behavior techniques are used increasingly to treat long-term conditions such as personality disorders, substance-related disorders, eating disorders, childhood conduct disorders, and attention-deficit/hyperactivity disorder (ADHD). Nurses are in a key position to identify clients who have been diagnosed with these disorders and to suggest a referral for cognitive-behavior therapy. For many, therapy is focused and briefer than other forms of therapy; 6 to 20 sessions may be effective.

BEHAVIORAL THEORIES

Cognitive-behavior techniques are based on learning theories. Behavior therapy developed as a distinct discipline based on Pavlov's principles of conditioning, Watson's theories of behaviorism, and Skinner's theories of learning (Table 7–1).

Watson[1] is credited with being the first to advocate, in the study of the mind, attention to observable behavior and avoidance of introspection. His most famous experiment was his study on conditioning fear in a child. Watson and his wife taught "little Albert," a child with no fear of rats, to fear rats by presenting a rat to the child along with loud, distressing noises. The pairing of the rat and the noises was repeated many times over a series of "conditioning" trials. Following conditioning, not only did little Albert fear the rat without any noise but also he reacted fearfully to white rabbits and similar furry objects.

B. F. Skinner[2] is clearly a seminal and salient proponent of behavioral therapy. In his *Science and Human Behavior*, Skinner simultaneously extended to humans the principles of classical conditioning made famous by the Russian researcher Ivan Pavlov[3] and presented a stinging rebuke of the psychoanalytic approach. Skinner's radical behaviorism and his outline for a psychotherapy based exclusively upon behavioral, experimentally developed and validated concepts paved the way for what is presently the basis of all clinical behavior therapy. Skinner's view of neurotic or problem behavior was quite simple: "the variables to be considered in dealing with a probability of response are simply the response itself and the independent variables."[2]

CONDITIONING

Operant conditioning, based on the work of Skinner, is the cornerstone of most clinical behavior therapy techniques. Essentially, operant conditioning investigates how the events that follow a particular (target) behavior result in that behavior occurring more or less frequently in the future. Events that follow a behavior and result in its occurring more frequently are reinforcers; those that cause it to happen less

TABLE 7–1. Comparison of Behavior Theorists

Theorist	Major Theory	Major Contribution
Pavlov	Classic conditioning	Paired presentation of stimuli (e.g., bell and food) to a learned response (salivation).
Watson	Behaviorism	Advocated studying observable behavior in place of introspection in psychology.
Skinner	Radical behaviorism	Focused on observable stimuli, responses, and effects of reinforcement.

frequently are punishers. **Reinforcers** increase the likelihood that a behavior will recur in the future at an increased frequency. **Punishers** decrease the likelihood that a behavior will be repeated in the future.

Positive reinforcement rewards a behavior to increase its frequency in the future. In behavioral terms, positive reinforcers are "contingent on" a behavior. For example, Skinner demonstrated that pigeons will peck at a light more frequently and at greater rates if bits of grain are presented contingent on pecking. Thus, a bit of grain, desired by a pigeon, serves to reinforce pecking.

Parents are behaviorists. They unconsciously know and try to carry out principles of positive reinforcement. One behaviorally oriented mother found that giving a small toy to her son after he tucked himself into bed without crying increased the frequency of tantrum-free evenings. For this particular boy, any item from a stimulus group of desired objects (toys) served as a reinforcer for not crying when he went to bed at night.

Negative reinforcers also increase the rate of a target behavior in a contingency model. **Negative reinforcement** is not punishment. In fact, as with positive reinforcement, the individual desires the consequences of negative reinforcement, which is why the target behavior increases. For example, many conditioning experiments involve subjecting a laboratory animal to an aversive stimulus until it emits a desired response; rats learn to press a bar in their cage because that response terminates a painful electric current. The target behavior (bar pressing) terminates a noxious experience (electric shock) resulting in a desired outcome (termination of pain). In this example, ending the electric shock is the negative reinforcement contingent on the target behavior of bar pressing.

BEHAVIORAL ASSESSMENT AND OUTCOME MEASUREMENT

Before cognitive-behavior therapy is instituted, a **behavioral analysis** is performed. The behavioral analysis guides the selection of an individualized program of behavior change. Traditionally, the cognitive-behavior therapist completes the analysis; however, psychiatric generalist nurses contribute to it by, for instance, collecting data relevant to the problem behavior and defining problematic behavior.

Behavioral analysis focuses on problems in behavior, in direct contrast to other models of mental illness that assume the cause of disordered behavior is early childhood experiences or biological factors. Through the behavior analysis, the therapist identifies events that maintain problem behaviors and then decides how to alter the behaviors. A behavioral analysis begins by assessing the antecedents (those behaviors and feelings that occur prior to the problematic behavior) and the consequences of the problem behavior to determine the factors that sustain it. The behavioral analysis model is known as the **A-B-C model** because it identifies the antecedents (A) and the events consequent (C) to the target behaviors (B) to promote more adaptive behaviors. Nursing care plans, particularly for clients with psychiatric disorders, often require a behavioral analysis.

A 40-year-old man presents for treatment because of his frequent bouts of binge drinking. He wants to break this drinking pattern because he and his wife will soon be adopting a child, but he has no desire to become totally abstinent. Following several sessions of evaluation, many interesting twists to this particular case begin to emerge. First, the client drinks each weekday evening at a local social club for men. He leaves work, goes directly to the club most evenings, and leaves roughly on time to arrive prior to the dinner hour. Second, on weekends, when socializing with his wife and friends, the client always drinks to excess and is unable to function normally at night's end. Third, the client's drinking has always infuriated his wife and is beginning to get him into trouble at work because he arrives late some mornings and sometimes fails to return to work after "three-martini" lunches. Last, 1 month prior to entering therapy, his employer had received complaints from two female coworkers that he was "behaving in a lecherous manner."

Psychiatric nurses use the following steps to analyze the client's problematic behavior, based on the work of Zifferblatt and Hendricks.[4]

1. *State the problem in behavioral terms.* Describe the presenting problem in terms of observable, quantifiable behaviors, with specified limits, durations, and contents. A behavioral analysis describes the behavior and makes no reference to personality traits or psychodynamic constructs.

The nurse and therapist conduct an extensive behavioral analysis to ensure that this client receives an appropriate treatment program for his problem, which surpasses the chief complaint of alcohol abuse. The problem, stated in behavioral terms, is that the client's drinking occurs in periodic binges, with greatest intensity on weekends, and prior to being alone with his wife. It leads to the understanding that interactions with his wife sustain the client's drinking binges.

2. *Perform a functional analysis of problem-related behaviors.* Another way to phrase this step is to analyze the problem behavior in terms of its antecedents and consequences. It includes a detailed description of what occurs immediately before and after the problematic behavior. Complex problems are broken into smaller component behaviors that are easier to change, thus promoting progress.

The analysis of the binge-drinking client confirms that the events prior to drinking—one-on-one interactions with his wife—are aversive. Essentially, the longer he drinks, the longer he avoids an aversive consequence; that is, he avoids the relationship with his wife. In terms of conditioning theory, this man's binge-drinking behavior is maintained by negative reinforcement: an avoidance of an aversive event (his wife) accomplished by emitting a target behavior (drinking with the boys or other couples).

3. *Designate the target behavior.* The exact behavior targeted for treatment in a behavioral intervention depends upon the first two steps.

For this client, the target behavior was improving the marital interaction.

4. *Formulate behavioral objectives.* Develop clear, precise, and, if possible, written behavioral goals. The client and family are often active partners in the process. At times, the client signs a "behavioral contract," outlining these behaviors. Examples of behavioral objectives include practicing assertiveness skills, learning anxiety-reduction skills, and using these skills to change problem behaviors.

The client, nurse, and therapist develop a written behavioral contract. A series of behavioral goals include developing a normalized marital relationship, practicing assertiveness skills when angry or anxious with his wife or coworkers, and learning alternative anxiety-reduction skills to substitute for avoidant drinking behavior.

5. *Develop an intervention strategy.* Apply principles of behavior theories. Available procedures are selected, based on which will be most effective in achieving the behavioral objectives.

The nurse teaches the client progressive relaxation as a self-control strategy, the therapist helps the client institute the behavioral plan, and the client joins a group to learn and practice assertiveness training. The client and his wife are referred for couples therapy to improve marital communication.

6. *Implement the intervention strategy.* Put the actual strategies into effect.

The nurse meets with the client periodically to teach and encourage relaxation. The client meets weekly with his therapist, participates in his group, and practices the skill exercises outside the treatment setting.

7. *Evaluate the intervention strategy.* Did the strategies accomplish the therapeutic objective for this client?

The client is able to initiate assertiveness skills when angry or anxious with his wife or coworkers and learns progressive relaxation as a substitute for avoidant drinking behavior. The client and his wife continue in couples therapy to improve their marital relationship.

COGNITIVE-BEHAVIOR THERAPY

Cognitive therapists are fond of quoting the Greek philosopher Epictetus (AD 60): "Men are disturbed not by things, but by the views they take of them." Cognitive-behavior therapy combines aspects of **cognitive restructuring**, that is, changing negative thoughts by means of behavioral procedures, based on the idea that thoughts influence feelings and behaviors. Cognitive-behavior therapy has two components: (1) creating situations in which clients alter their thinking about environmental stimuli that previously affected their ongoing behaviors through changes in self-efficacy or coping skills and (2) working with clients to directly confront their "inappropriate views," thereby changing their problematic behavior. If negative and maladaptive thoughts can be changed, so can the behaviors associated with anxiety, depression, and other problematic conditions.

Cognitive-behavior therapy is based on the work of Aaron Beck,[5] who believes that depression is the direct result of *cognitive distortions*. Changing these distorted thoughts is cognitive restructuring. The cognitive distortions with a negative tone initiate "self-talk," literally, negative statements or thoughts about oneself that lead to depressive feelings. Beck and his students (for example, Burns[6]) have identified examples of cognitive distortions that precipitate depression:

RESEARCH NOTE

Kroll, L, Harrington, R, Jayson, D, Fraser, J, and Gowers, S: Pilot study of continuation cognitive-behavioral therapy for major depression in adolescent psychiatric inpatients. J Acad Child Adolesc Psychiatry 35:1156–1161, 1996.

Findings: In this study, adolescents had all received an average of 10 weeks of acute cognitive-behavior therapy, which led to remission of their depressive symptoms. The purpose of the study was to see if they continued to maintain their positive response with ongoing treatment. Fewer of these adolescents relapsed than those in a similar group of remitted, depressed adolescents who did not receive ongoing cognitive-behavior therapy. In particular, continued therapy appeared to be most effective during the first 3 months of long-term treatment.

Application to Practice: Relatively brief courses of cognitive-behavior therapy are effective for both adults and children. This study extends the previous research by exploring the effects of continued therapy, so-called maintenance therapy. Teenagers and adults can be referred for cognitive-behavior therapy for the treatment of depressive disorders and should be encouraged to continue therapy to prevent relapse. They can be shown that discontinuing cognitive-behavior therapy is more likely to lead to re-emergence of depressive symptoms.

- *Overgeneralization:* A single negative event leads to a conclusion concerning the individual's fixed personal disposition; for example, a single mistake leads to the conclusion that the person can never perform the task correctly.
- *Elective abstraction:* An individual dwells on one negative detail from a complex behavioral sequence and ignores confounding, disconfirmatory positive data; for example, a person presumes that a date will find him or her totally unattractive because of 5 extra pounds but refuses to consider that he or she runs a profitable business and was voted person-of-the-year by the local community.
- *Polarized thinking:* A client views events in "all-or-nothing" terms; for example, two best friends argue over the site of a shared vacation and one feels totally rejected by the other.
- *Personalization:* Individuals blame themselves for causing some negative event external to them, despite their having had nothing to do with it; for example, a man's boss walks past him in a huff and fails to reply to a memo he sent 2 days ago. He concludes that his boss is angry with him and that he caused the bad mood, although there are hundreds of other logical explanations to account for the negative behavior.

Cognitive therapy has been used most often to help clients with depressive disorders identify and challenge the assumptions of cognitive distortions. It also is used for many other conditions, including anxiety disorders, substance-related disorders, eating disorders, and personality disorders. The following two examples illustrate applications of cognitive techniques.

> A client with interpersonal anxiety avoids a party because he has failed in similar past situations or he assumes that he will be rejected by others or will make "foolish" mistakes. The cognitive-behavior therapist challenges the thoughts or "labels" and helps the client substitute more adaptive alternatives. For example, the therapist helps the client realize that he can succeed in future situations and teaches him to substitute the following thoughts: "I can meet new people and not be rejected; nobody's perfect; and past events don't have to predict future failure."

> A depressed middle-aged woman, faced with a divorce, career change, and her children needing her less, reports feeling "trapped in a room with four doors, each locked and leading to oblivion." Each door represents a conflict area. She could never get a job and be self-sufficient because she often "felt incompetent" at work. She felt this despite the fact that she had several years of increasingly responsible experience as a teacher. She believes she is a failure as a mother because her children are leaving home. She expresses being "forever" alone. With these negative thoughts about her life, she feels pessimistic and futile in her efforts to problem-solve for the future. Her cognitive distortions include overgeneralization, elective abstraction, polarized thinking, and personalization. The cognitive therapist helps the client identify these cognitive distortions and recognize that assumptions based on these distortions can only result in a depressive outcome.

BEHAVIOR THERAPY PROCEDURES

RELAXATION EXERCISES

Therapists and psychiatric nurses often use relaxation exercises, particularly for clients with anxiety disorders, phobias, insomnia, tension headaches, muscle cramps, and tics. Progressive or deep muscle relaxation is a specific type of relaxation exercise. **Progressive muscle relaxation** training teaches individuals to alternatively tense and relax different major muscle groups in sequence. By systematically contrasting tension and relaxation, the client can learn to better differentiate between tension and relaxation and control the onset of these states. Ultimately, the client learns to substitute more relaxing sensations for unwanted tension.

Progressive relaxation is based on Watson and Raynor's learning theory[1]: anxiety is often learned. If a person learns to respond to conditioned stimuli with anxiety reactions, the ability to control, cope with, or extinguish that anxiety response can also be learned. Thus, anxiety management is presented to the client as a skill that can be developed, much like learning to drive a car or play a sport. Instructions for teaching progressive muscle relaxation are listed in Table 7–2.

BIOFEEDBACK

Biofeedback is literally immediate feedback about a biological function provided to a client by a mechanical device. This feedback is generally presented by changing tones, flashing lights, or graphic presentations of various response patterns. Biofeedback is based on the work of Neal Miller[7] and coworkers, demonstrating that laboratory animals could learn to control physical responses such as heart rate and blood pressure through contingent reinforcement and punishment of these responses. When studies showed that humans could control physiological responses previously thought to be involuntary, biofeedback became widely used. Most significant among these findings was the ability to lower high blood pressure.

Dozens of biofeedback devices are currently available. They range from simple thermometers taped to a finger to elaborate monitoring devices that detect minor variations in muscle tension. The common denominator is that they tell clients how well they are controlling their visceral responses. The critical feature of both biofeedback and progressive relaxation is that, through practice, clients learn to generate sensations of relaxation and reduce sensations that cause or

TABLE 7–2. Instructions for Teaching Progressive Muscle Relaxation

First, present clients with the general principles and rationale for progressive relaxation training, namely, that they can "re-learn" to control their response to anxiety and other conditions. Inform them that their initial attempts may be fraught with clumsiness, an inability to master the technique, and odd sensations to which they are not accustomed. Remind them that, as in any learning experience, one golden rule holds true: practice makes perfect. Teach them to practice the technique in order to ultimately control its outcome.

The next step is to review the major muscle groups that will be the focus of the progressive relaxation training: hands, forearms, upper arms; face, neck, head; shoulders, chest, back; buttocks, legs, feet. At this point, instruct the client in the procedure for tensing and relaxing each of these muscle groups; lead him or her through the tension-relaxation sequence in an orderly and systematic fashion.

Actual training procedures are conducted in a variety of ways, including a three-component technique. The first component consists of carefully and painstakingly taking the client through a tensing and relaxing of each muscle group through explicit instructions, derived from Goldfried and Davison:

"Now, settle back as comfortably as you can, close your eyes, and listen to what I'm going to be telling you. I'm going to make you aware of certain sensations in your body and then show you how you can reduce these sensations. First direct your attention to your left arm, your left hand in particular. Clench your left fist. Clench it tightly and study the tension in the hand and in the forearm. Study those sensations of tension. And now let go. Relax the left hand and let it rest. . . . "

Repeat this procedure for each and every muscle group noted above; it takes about 20 minutes to complete. Following several weeks of practicing the first component, instruct the client in the second component, a version of the above without the client tensing and relaxing the muscles. He or she is instructed to concentrate on the same order of muscle groups but now to just *attempt* to imagine the feeling of "letting go" felt after clenching. This totally cognitive or "thinking" component takes approximately 10 minutes to complete.

Instruct the client to shorten this second component even further with practice. The goal is to develop ultimate relaxation as a coping skill, wherein the client can apply the relaxation procedure to rapidly release tension. The goal of such rapid induction is not to achieve a state of deep relaxation, but rather to increase a client's sense of being able to cope with anxiety-provoking situations and not to let such situations spiral out of control. Relaxation training can be a useful intervention in and of itself. It increases the client's perceived sense of control of physical tension.

Source: Goldfried, MR, and Davidson, GC: Clinical Behavior Therapy. Holt, Rirehart & Winston, New York, 1976.

occur with tension. Biofeedback can be used to reduce muscle tension, which often accompanies anxiety disorders and migraine headaches.

SYSTEMATIC DESENSITIZATION

Creating sensations of relaxation to contrast with incompatible sensations of tension is the defining feature of **systematic desensitization**, a common method used to manage and reduce anxiety. Systematic desensitization is based on the work of Joseph Wolpe.[8] His procedure, *counterconditioning*, is used to help individuals substitute one response—namely, relaxation—for another, usually anxiety.

Systematic desensitization effectively treats a variety of problems that derive from anxiety but is most consistently effective for one-symptom phobias—that is, anxiety or fear reactions conditioned to one specific situation or event. Systematic desensitization is the treatment of choice for fear of objects, such as snakes, of situations, such as claustrophobia, or of tasks, such as public speaking.

If more complex phobias are present, additional behavior therapy techniques are used in conjunction with systematic desensitization. For example, treating other anxiety-based disorders such as sexual dysfunction or agoraphobia calls for the use of systematic desensitization along with behavioral interventions such as modeling and cognitive-restructuring procedures.

Table 7–3 lists the components of desensitization: relaxation, hierarchy, visualization, item presentation, and in vivo homework assignments. The client is initially taught progressive relaxation. Then the client outlines an anxiety or phobia hierarchy, a step-by-step approximation of the feared situation in which the client, with guidance from the therapist, lists the lowest anxiety situation to the highest.

In the case of a woman who is afraid of flying, a low-level anxiety item on a hierarchy might be sitting in the living room on a Sunday afternoon when the boss calls to say that in a month she is going to have to fly to St. Louis. Because a month seems so far away, it provokes little anxiety. A situation higher on a flying-phobia scale takes place a week before the woman is to leave for St. Louis, and she is going to the travel agency to pick up her airline ticket.

During visualization training, clients imagine themselves in a variety of situations. For example, a client may be taught to imagine walking in a supermarket, visualizing and feeling the scene. Next, during item presentation, clients relax and

TABLE 7–3. Desensitization Steps

- Relaxation
- Hierarchy
- Visualization
- Item presentation
- In vivo assignments

then imagine themselves in each of the phobic situations on the hierarchy they have created. This presentation is done in a slow, covert, and systematic fashion: one item at a time. The rate of progression through situations is determined by the client's response and ability to cope with the anxiety. As clients work through the hierarchy, in vivo assignments, in which clients approach the feared stimulus or situation in a gradual fashion, are encouraged. Compliance with these in vivo assignments is a critical part of systematic desensitization.

The typical desensitization takes 15 to 20 sessions. Initial sessions are focused on assessment, relaxation training, and identification of hierarchy items. The bulk of the remaining sessions are implementation of the desensitization protocol. Desensitization works as clients confront the stimuli that create their anxieties or fears without experiencing the catastrophic outcomes they anticipate.[9]

Linehan[21] developed a cognitive-behavior therapy program for patients with borderline personality disorder called *dialectical behavior therapy (DBT)*. It uses techniques such as exposure, problem solving, and cognitive restructuring and emphasizes teaching emotion regulation, interpersonal effectiveness, mindfulness, and distress tolerance. Preliminary empirical support for DBT demonstrates its superiority in effectively reducing borderline personality symptoms, such as parasuicidal behavior, as compared with traditional individual psychotherapy over a 1-year period.

TOKEN ECONOMIES

Although used only in a limited way today, some of the earliest interventions based on behavior therapy reinforced or shaped the behavior of clients institutionalized in psychiatric hospitals.[10] In fact, shaping is a core component of what has long stood as the most salient application of conditioning principles to psychiatric treatment: the *token economy program*. Token economies are treatment programs for severely to moderately ill psychiatric populations. They include specific treatment goals, ongoing observation of the desired behaviors, trained staff who reinforce behavior, and, where successful, adaptive behaviors. They are called token economies because actual tokens are used to promote desired behaviors. Clients save and exchange tokens for incentives or rewards, such as TV-watching time, access to restricted areas of the hospital, or candy.

Token economies strive to promote specific client behaviors such as personal hygiene and obedience to hospital rules. If clients function appropriately in these target areas—for instance, groom themselves, do required jobs, and socialize appropriately—they earn tokens according to prearranged schedules. Certain behaviors earn a set number of tokens, and a certain number of tokens are exchanged for food or other rewards.

Research on token economies has generally demonstrated their effectiveness in changing simple behaviors such as grooming skills[11] in populations of institutionalized patients functioning at severely restricted levels. However, token economies[12] may do little to facilitate any other behaviors beyond the concrete target behaviors of the structured program and do not develop the higher levels of coping skills needed to function outside the psychiatric institution. State-of-the-art behavior therapy now provides clients with a variety of individually tailored programs selected from the rapidly expanding wealth of behavioral procedures.[13]

SHAPING

Shaping is a method of conditioning behavior that incrementally reinforces small behavioral steps until the individual reaches the target behavior. Take the example of teaching an animal to jump through a hoop. The first step in shaping is reinforcing the animal by giving the animal small treats every time it engages in behavior that is a part of the desired "jumping through the hoop" process. For instance, when the animal randomly approaches the hoop, it receives a treat. Then behaviors are reinforced that closely approximate jumping, resulting in its eventually jumping through the hoop. Because all steps in the pattern of successive approximations to jumping through hoops have been reinforced, combining the sequential steps in the routine becomes quite natural for the now-trained subject. For clients with psychiatric disorders, appropriate and desirable behaviors can be shaped by encouraging and reinforcing small steps toward a larger defined goal.

EXTINCTION AND PUNISHMENT

Behavior therapists also try to decrease the frequency of a target behavior or the likelihood that it will occur. Both punishment and extinction can decrease the client's problematic behavior. **Punishment** is accomplished by following a target behavior with an undesired event. Clients may be asked to spend time alone in a quiet, low-stimulus room—time outs—after exhibiting verbally aggressive or destructive behavior. However, punishment is a controversial technique not commonly used on psychiatric inpatient units. Because punishment has the potential to become destructive and abusive to clients, ethical concerns have been raised about its negative effects.

In **extinction**, a desired event is removed when an unwanted behavioral response occurs. In other words, the reinforcer for a behavior is removed and then the frequency of the behavior decreases. Sometimes, the undesirable behavior increases briefly, which does not imply that the program has been ineffective. For example, a client's disruptive behavior may be reinforced by nursing staff attention. The staff decides to use extinction and no longer attend to the client's disruptive behavior, and initially the behavior frequency increases as the client continues to seek attention this way. If the staff is consistently able to avoid paying attention to the disruptive behavior, its frequency will decline after the initial "extinction burst."

MODELING

Before learning more adaptive coping skills, the client must be presented with appropriate or adaptive beliefs, attitudes, or perspectives. *Modeling* refers to two factors: the behavior of the individual whom clients are instructed to imitate and the actual acquisition of new behaviors that occurs as a result of this imitation.[14] Modeling is a component of virtually all cognitive-behavior therapy programs that treat difficulties in interpersonal relationships, including mood and anxiety disorders, psychiatric disorders of childhood, and personality disorders. Therapists and nurses frequently use modeling to present more appropriate behaviors to clients.

A client who is reluctant to confront her spouse about her unhappiness in the marriage can practice the necessary skills through role playing. Modeling procedures are straightforward; clients enact a behavior or set of behaviors immediately after the nurse or therapist demonstrates what the appropriate behavior should be.

Modeling procedures may change maladaptive behaviors or present individuals with a new behavioral repertoire. In most circumstances, modeling provides clients with ways to enhance their social skills. It also facilitates socially appropriate behaviors by inducing clients to act in more appropriate ways, at more appropriate times, or for more appropriate audiences.[14]

EXPOSURE-RESPONSE PREVENTION

Cognitive-behavior techniques also effectively treat conditions such as OCD through exposure, modeling, and response prevention. **Response prevention** prevents the client from engaging in rituals such as hand washing. Before beginning exposure treatment, the client has to understand the rationale for the treatment. It should be clearly explained that the OCD is maintained through both passive and active avoidance. The exposure part is directed at the client's passive avoidance, whereas the response prevention deals with the active avoidance. For example, treatment of compulsive cleaning has two elements. First, the client is exposed to "dirt" or "contaminated" material and not allowed to clean. The exposure to distressing stimuli must last until the client's anxiety and tension are reduced. Modeling is often used in these situations: The clinician shows clients how to put dirt on themselves, and they are then expected to do the same thing. Second, clients are taught how to clean in a nonritualistic way. Several studies indicate that exposure, modeling, and response prevention, coupled with instruction to refrain from carrying out compulsive rituals, can bring about significant improvement in relatively short time periods.[15]

SOCIAL SKILLS TRAINING

In this method, modeling is used to enhance social skills. Social skills training is commonly used to help individuals with schizophrenia or social phobia, two conditions in which social skills are minimal or deficient. The first step is to identify the deficits in behavioral terms: Poor eye contact, a soft voice, and a slumped or indifferent body posture are examples. The client, using modeling procedures, gradually develops and practices new behaviors. Social skills training can take place in individual or group sessions. Videotapes of clients can demonstrate their successful new behaviors. Clients are encouraged to continue practicing the desirable behaviors at home.

ASSERTIVENESS TRAINING

Modeling and role playing are core components of *assertiveness training*,[16] the goal of which is to enable an individual to engage in the assertive behavior. Central components of assertive behavior are ability to express negative feelings such as anger and resentment without being aggressive and ability to express positive feelings without embarrassment, anxiety, or humor.

Increased assertiveness skills are essential to improved social functioning for most clients, regardless of the disorder. Socially phobic, anxious, avoidant, or antagonistic clients often lack the ability to get their feelings heard and understood by others. They may not interact easily because they feel "misunderstood" or believe that their actions are "misinterpreted." Assertiveness training attempts to train clients to present themselves in a fashion that neither evokes anger in the listener nor denies the client's own rights.

The key features of assertiveness training programs are "feeling talk" and "I statements."[16] The goal of feeling talk is, quite simply, to have the client begin to express *any* feeling. Too often clients with assertive skill deficits speak in terms of "shoulds," offending others with their adherence to externalized rules and their insistence that others follow suit. By using feeling talk, clients learn to take personal responsibility for their feelings. For instance, "That man's a fool" avoids responsibility, whereas "I think that man's a fool" demonstrates more appropriate assertiveness skills.

The most common technique is behavior rehearsal,[14] in which the client acts out problematic interpersonal interactions with the nurse or therapist. After this role playing, specific maladaptive behaviors are identified, and the client's behaviors can be adapted.

EXPECTED OUTCOMES

The goal of cognitive-behavior therapy is to change behavior. Its distinguishing feature is defining the problem behaviors in terms of quantifiable behaviors and objective interventions. Outcome data are compared with initial or baseline assessments of the target behavior both during and after treatment. Ideally, cognitive-behavior therapy helps clients change the way they view themselves and the world. For instance, for the individual with depression, the expected outcomes are normalization of mood, sleep and activity patterns, appetite, concentration, and energy; these outcomes

TABLE 7–4. Cognitive-Behavior Techniques Used in the Treatment of Major Psychiatric Disorders

Disorders	Examples of Techniques	Expected Behavioral Outcome
Anxiety Disorders		
Panic disorder with or without agoraphobia	Systematic desensitization Cognitive restructuring Modeling	Decreased panic attacks and fears of going out of the house
Simple phobia	Systematic desensitization	Decreased anxiety of the feared object or situation
Social phobia	Systematic desensitization Social skills training	Decreased fears of speaking, eating, and being with others
Obsessive-compulsive disorder	Exposure Response prevention Modeling	Decreased obsessions and compulsions
Mood Disorders		
Major depressive disorder	Cognitive restructuring Assertiveness training	Decreased depressed mood, improved energy, sleep, appetite; absence of suicidal ideation
Eating Disorders		
Anorexia nervosa	Systematic desensitization Cognitive restructuring	Restoration of normal body weight
Bulimia nervosa	Cognitive restructuring Assertiveness training	Decreased binging and purging behaviors
Psychiatric Disorders of Childhood		
Conduct disorder	Shaping Extinction and punishment	Reduced deviant behaviors
Attention deficit hyperactivity disorder	Token programs	Normal activity patterns and improved academic performance
Personality Disorder		
Borderline personality disorder	Emotional regulation Distress tolerance Mindfulness	Reduced self-destructive behaviors and parasuicidal behaviors

are sought with cognitive-behavior techniques such as cognitive restructuring, to stop negative thoughts, and relaxation exercises. Table 7–4 lists expected behavioral outcomes for specific psychiatric problems.

SYNOPSIS OF CURRENT RESEARCH

Researchers have studied desensitization techniques in individuals with a variety of anxiety disorders. In particular, 80% of individuals with agoraphobia, who have difficulty going out of the house alone, have improved significantly after treatment with systematic desensitization.[17] The treatment appears to be more effective when a family member or friend is also involved. For clients with panic attacks and agoraphobia, combining pharmacotherapy and desensitization is associated with even greater improvement than either technique alone.[18] However, most of the research has used tricyclic antidepressants such as imipramine rather than the newer antidepressants. Antianxiety agents such as alprazolam, used along with cognitive techniques to change distorted thoughts leading to panic attacks, are also more effective than either treatment used alone.

Pharmacotherapy and cognitive-behavior therapy have also been compared in treating individuals with major depressive disorders. Although both are effective, the combination appears to be the most effective.[19] Studies on the effectiveness of cognitive-behavior therapy for bulimia have found that it is more effective than either medications alone or combined with pharmacotherapy.[20] Cognitive-behavior therapy has also shown some effectiveness for borderline personality disorder, substance abuse, obesity, hypertension, migraine and other severe headaches, insomnia, autism, and ADHD.

AREAS FOR FUTURE RESEARCH

- How does cognitive-behavior therapy compare to treatment with the selective serotonin reuptake inhibitors (SSRIs) in the treatment of panic attacks and agoraphobia?
- Are behavioral techniques effective in the treatment of individuals with dementia?
- What is the long-term effectiveness of cognitive-behavior therapy in depression and anxiety disorders?

- How does the nursing process overlap with cognitive-behavior therapy?
- What are the differences between behavior techniques used for children and those used for adults?
- How effective is cognitive-behavior therapy in the treatment of adjustment disorders?
- Do cognitive-behavior techniques decrease the length of hospitalization?

CASE STUDY

Jim R., a 26-year-old single man, is referred for behavior therapy to treat his phobia—fear of snow. In the initial assessment, the client presented with a one-symptom phobia. He indicated that his phobia began about 2 years before he started therapy. Before then, he had not experienced any anxiety in snow. The onset of the phobia was during a snowstorm, when Jim received a message that his father had suffered a massive myocardial infarction. He experienced considerable difficulty in his attempts to get to the hospital because of snow-related conditions. By the time he arrived at the hospital, his father had died. From that time on, he has felt considerable anxiety and upset whenever there is snow or the prospect of snow. What was initially a general feeling of discomfort evolved to the point of major anxiety any time snow is forecast.

Jim sought treatment for this condition and was diagnosed by a psychoanalytically oriented consultant as having a specific phobia. Through an interview, his Beck Depression Inventory score, and other behavioral instruments, it became clear that a number of factors contribute to his snow phobia. In addition to his general anxiety in relation to snow, the client also reported generalized depression. Jim indicated he felt particular conflict at the time of his father's death because of a long-standing negative interaction with his father. He described a troubled adolescence, with his father as his particular "nemesis," but he felt that he was in the process of resolving these conflicts when his father died. Because Jim's father's death was unexpected, however, he was unable to finish resolving the conflicts. The presenting problem of snow phobia, therefore, represents one aspect of what evolved into a complicated clinical situation.

The behavioral analysis reveals several maintaining variables for the condition: (1) the traumatic coincidence of his father's death while Jim was trapped in the snow, (2) Jim's inability to resolve his conflict with his father, leading to a general, low-level depression, (3) the conflict with his father that led to other problems in his life's circumstances, including unhappiness at work and inability to develop meaningful interpersonal relationships, and (4) his need to be in control. Jim's life was out of control at the time of the snowstorm; he remembers how helpless he felt in trying to get to his father, and he never wants to experience that feeling again.

Although the snow phobia represents one condition, a so-called *monosymptomatic phobia*, clearly this treatment problem is multifaceted. The following treatment plan was established for Jim: initially, a desensitization program to facilitate the client's ability to cope with his concern about snow; second, a cognitive restructuring strategy and problem-solving strategy to facilitate his ability to control circumstances related to the snow situations; third, an ongoing cognitive restructuring program to help Jim work toward the resolution of conflicts in his relationships with his father as manifested in his interpersonal and vocational dissatisfaction.

Jim initially responded to systematic desensitization and reported that he experienced some decline in snow phobia. Unfortunately, after approximately 45 days of treatment, the snow season passed and he had to make a decision on whether to continue treatment or to wait until the following fall to resume. Jim decided to pursue continued treatment. Systematic desensitization, therefore, transitioned into an ongoing cognitively oriented psychotherapy, with the goals of self-exploration and resolution of the conflict with his father. This cognitive restructuring identified his tendency to overgeneralize, personalize, and engage in elective abstraction. Ultimately, the client resolved the snow phobia in approximately 15 sessions. Jim remained in therapy for approximately 2 years and was able to make significant gains; he was able to change his job, return to school, graduate with a master's degree, and "weather" a difficult time seeking new employment. In addition, he reported that his understanding of his conflict with his father had greatly improved, and he did not feel that these conflicts were major motivators in his current ability to function. Modeling and social skills training augmented desensitization and cognitive interventions.

CRITICAL THINKING QUESTIONS

1. What factors would lead you to recommend cognitive-behavior therapy for Jim?
2. How does a behavioral analysis explain his symptoms?
3. How do systematic desensitization and cognitive-restructuring techniques differ from traditional "talk" therapy?
4. Identify the short- and long-term goals in Jim's treatment plan.
5. Explain how cognitive-behavior therapy treats Jim's symptoms.
6. Identify behaviors that show Jim is responding to treatment.

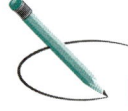

KEY POINTS

- Psychiatric nurse generalists are not cognitive-behavior therapists; however, they often use cognitive-behavior techniques to help clients deal with overwhelming feelings and thoughts.
- The purpose of cognitive-behavior therapy is to help clients change maladaptive thoughts and behaviors by substituting more adaptive ones.
- Cognitive-behavior techniques are based on learning theories.
- Cognitive-behavior therapy attempts to modify, decrease, or eliminate maladaptive behaviors and introduce or increase adaptive and desirable behaviors.
- Before therapy is instituted, a clinician performs behavioral analysis to develop an individualized program of behavior change.
- Progressive or deep muscle relaxation is a behavioral technique that teaches individuals to alternatively tense and relax different major muscle groups in sequence. It is used

to treat anxiety disorders and related problems such as phobias, insomnia, tension headaches, muscle cramps, and tics.

- Biofeedback is, literally, immediate feedback about a biological function, provided to a client by a mechanical device.
- Cognitive-behavior therapy helps individuals directly confront distorted negative thoughts and thereby change their behavior.
- Negative thoughts, also known as *cognitive distortions*, include overgeneralization, elective abstraction, polarized thinking, and personalization. They influence mood and behavior.

REFERENCES

1. Watson, JB, and Raynor, R: Conditioned emotional reactions. J Exp Psychol Gen 3:1, 1920.
2. Skinner, BF: Science and Human Behavior. Macmillan, New York, 1953.
3. Pavlov, IP: Conditioned Reflexes: An Investigation of the Physiological Activity of the Cerebral Cortex. Oxford University Press, New York, 1927.
4. Zifferblatt, SM, and Hendricks, CG: Applied behavioral analysis of societal problems. Am Psychol 29:750, 1974.
5. Beck, AT: Cognitive Therapy and the Emotional Disorders. International Universities Press Inc, New York, 1972.
6. Burns, OD: Feeling Good. William Morrow & Co, New York, 1980.
7. Miller, NE: Biofeedback and visceral learning. Ann Rev Psychology 29:373, 1978.
8. Wolpe, J: The Practice of Behavior Therapy, ed 2. Pergamon, Oxford, 1973.
9. Wilson, GT, and O'Leary, KO: Principles of Behavior Therapy. Prentice-Hall, Englewood Cliffs, NJ, 1980.
10. Lindsley, OR, Skinner, BF, and Solomon, HC: Studies in behavior therapy: Status report I. Metropolitan State Hospital, Waltham, MA, 1953.
11. Kazdin, AE, and Bootzin, R: The token economy: An evaluative review. J Appl Behav Anal 5:343, 1972.
12. Levine, F, and Fasnacht, G: Token rewards may lead to token learning. Am Psychol 29:816, 1974.
13. Levendusky, P, Berglas, S, and Dooley, C: Therapeutic contract program: Preliminary report on a behavioral alternative to the token economy. Behav Res Ther 21:137, 1983.
14. Rimm, DC, and Masters, JC: Behavior Therapy: Techniques and Empirical Findings, ed 2. Academic Press, New York, 1979.
15. Emmelkamp, PM, and Beens, H: Cognitive therapy with obsessive-compulsive disorder: A comparative evaluation. Behav Res Ther 29:293, 1991.
16. Salter, A: Conditioned Reflex Therapy. Farrar, Straus & Giroux, New York, 1949.
17. Taylor, CB, and Arnow, B: The Nature and Treatment of Anxiety Disorders. New York, Free Press, 1988.
18. Telch, MJ, et al: Combined pharmacological and behavioral treatments for agoraphobia. Behav Res Ther 23:325, 1985.
19. Hollon, SD, et al: Cognitive therapy and pharmacotherapy for depression: Singly and in combination. Arch Gen Psychiatry 49:774, 1992.
20. Agras, WS, et al: Pharmacological and cognitive-behavioral treatment for bulimia nervosa: A controlled comparison. Am J Psychiatry 149:82, 1992.
21. Linehan, MM: Cognitive-Behavioral Treatment of Borderline Personality Disorder. New York, Guilford Press, 1993.

CHAPTER 8

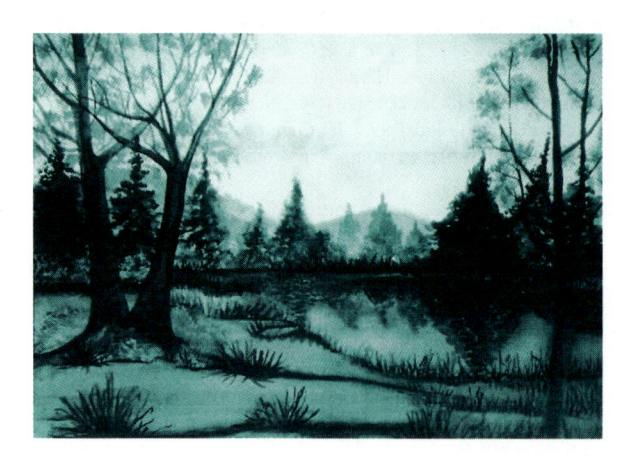

CHAPTER OUTLINE

The Purpose of Crisis Intervention
  The Nurse's Role
  Historical Evolution
Crisis Defined
  Characteristics of a Crisis
  Developmental Phases in a Crisis Situation
  Types of Crises
Crisis Intervention and the Nursing Process
  Assessment
  Diagnosis
  Planning and Implementing Interventions
  Evaluation of the Nursing Process and Expected Outcomes
  Coping with Crisis Work
Implications for Education and Research
Areas for Future Research

LEARNING OBJECTIVES

After completing this chapter, the reader should be able to:

- Define *crisis* and *crisis intervention*; name four types of crises that individuals, families, and communities may encounter.
- Describe the historical evolution of crisis intervention as a treatment modality.
- Analyze the biopsychosocial, cultural, and environmental issues that affect an individual's response to crisis, crisis intervention, and crisis resolution.
- Discuss the role of coping mechanisms related to crisis resolution.
- Apply the nursing process when caring for individuals, families, and communities in crisis.
- Identify and describe the diversity of settings in which crisis intervention may be practiced.

KEY TERMS

anticipatory intervention
changes
coping mechanisms
crisis
crisis intervention
critical incident stress
  debriefing
critical social thinking
fight or flight
general adaptation
  syndrome
precipitating factor
precrisis state
sociocultural crisis

Anne Bateman, RN, EdD
Cindy Peternelj-Taylor, RN, MSc

Crisis Intervention

Whenever one distraught person turns to another person for help or advice, crisis intervention begins. Throughout history, families, friends, and communities have provided assistance to one another in times of crisis. However, **crisis intervention** is a structured therapeutic modality.

THE PURPOSE OF CRISIS INTERVENTION

An individual's ability to cope with and manage crisis is influenced by past and present experiences. Unresolved crises and the associated feelings of helplessness and fear frequently result in regression to previous methods of coping. Adjustment will be maladaptive if the individual has been unsuccessful in resolving past conflicts and developing better methods of coping with change, loss, and trauma. Those who have effectively resolved a crisis and developed adaptive coping mechanisms are more likely to experience future crises as less hazardous and to quickly reestablish homeostasis.[1-3]

THE NURSE'S ROLE

Health professionals working with individuals in crisis must view crisis as a time of opportunity as well as danger and approach those who need assistance as having potential for growth.[2,3] Nurses must understand not only the immediate response and emotional tension created by the crisis but also the biopsychosocial, cultural, and environmental factors that influence how people respond to stressful life events. This chapter outlines the nurse's role as a provider of supportive and therapeutic crisis interventions.

HISTORICAL EVOLUTION

Numerous researchers have contributed to the contemporary understanding of crisis and crisis intervention. Lindemann's[4] model of the grief response and Caplan's[1] model of preventive psychiatry provide the foundation of crisis theory, which is that early intervention at the onset of a **crisis** can reduce the residual negative long-term effects of the crisis experience. Left unresolved, the issues resulting from the stressful event could have repercussions such as emotional distress, mental illness, addictive behavior, suicide, or violence against others.

Stress is an inevitable fact of life; every individual, family, and community experiences anticipated or unanticipated stressors at some point in the life span. The human reaction to stress includes a complex interaction of hormones and neurotransmitters, as well as other physiological changes. Although these processes help people manage the stressful event, they may lead to emotional or psychological pathology. Hans Selye[5] identified a three-stage process of response to stress known as the **general adaptation syndrome**:

1. *The alarm reaction.* Stimulation of the sympathetic nervous system is the immediate response during the alarm reaction as the body attempts to respond and adjust to the stress or stressors. Behaviors associated with this stage are often classified as **fight-or-flight** responses.
2. *Stage of resistance.* Some resistance to the stressor occurs; however, the individual functions at a lower than optimal level and requires more energy than usual for survival.
3. *Stage of exhaustion.* This stage is characterized by total expenditure of the individual's energy, and the ability to adapt fails. Death can result if the demands continue to exceed the person's resources and ability to cope.

Through his pivotal studies on stress, Selye[5] concluded that the residual effects of prolonged stress and unresolved trauma can often be more devastating than the critical event itself.

Anticipated reactions and the potential for maladaptive coping are contingent on how the individual has coped with crisis and stressful events in the past, the significance of the particular event, and the presence of concurrent stressors.[1-4] Baldwin[6] has identified ten corollaries to crisis theory that provide an understanding of the emotional response to the crisis experience (Box 8-1).

CRISIS DEFINED

The scope and nature of the stressors may precipitate a crisis in one or all of the individuals exposed to a particular stressor. Simply stated, *a crisis* is defined as a point that re-

Box 8–1. Baldwin's Ten Corollaries to Crisis Theory

1. Because each individual's tolerance for stress is idiosyncratic and finite, emotional crises have no relationship per se to psychopathology and occur even among the well-adjusted.
2. Emotional crises are self-limiting events in which crisis resolution, either adaptive or maladaptive, takes place within an average period of 4 to 6 weeks.
3. During a crisis state, psychological defenses are weakened or absent, and the individual has cognitive or affective awareness of issues and memories previously well defended against and less accessible.
4. During a crisis state, the individual has enhanced capacity for both cognitive and affective learning because of the vulnerability of this state and the motivation produced by emotional disequilibrium.
5. Adaptive crisis resolution is frequently a vehicle for resolving conflicts that have in part determined the emotional crisis or that interfere with the crisis resolution process.
6. A small external influence during a crisis state can produce disproportionate change in a shorter period than therapeutic change that occurs during noncrisis states.
7. Resolution of emotional crisis is not necessarily determined by previous experience or character structure but rather is shaped by current and perhaps unique sociopsychological influences operating in the present.
8. Inherent in every emotional crisis is an actual or anticipated loss to the individual that must be reconciled as part of the crisis resolution process.
9. Every emotional crisis is an interpersonal event involving at least one significant other person who is represented in the crisis situation directly, indirectly, or symbolically.
10. Effective crisis resolution prevents similar future crises by removing vulnerabilities from the past and by increasing the individual's repertoire of available coping skills that can be used in such situations.

CHARACTERISTICS OF A CRISIS

There is a direct correlation between increased stress related to the crisis response and the degree of biological, cognitive, emotional, and behavioral disorganization experienced. The individual in crisis becomes less and less able to problem solve and accurately interpret the circumstances surrounding the crisis event. Precipitating events of a crisis include actual or perceived losses, threats of losses, or challenges. Maladaptive responses and behavior can occur because of stress or multiple stressors from an unresolved crisis. The nurse working with an individual in crisis needs to consider crisis as a subjective experience and seek an understanding of the circumstances from the perspective of the individual.[2,3] The theoretical perspective of **critical social thinking** is an effective guide to understanding a person's lived experience.[7] Furthermore, the sociocultural, political, and personal forces that affect access to health care services can influence the factors that precipitate a crisis.

Research[1,3,8,9] suggests that crisis, by definition, is self-limiting. People in crisis are unable to function at extreme levels of anxiety for extended lengths of time. On average, the state of disequilibrium known as crisis lasts 4 to 6 weeks. Whether the crisis experience results in growth and enrichment or in increased psychological vulnerability is contingent on the individual's problem-solving abilities, cultural values, and current levels of social and economic support. Although each individual experiences a crisis differently, some level of resolution eventually occurs. The person adapts and returns to the previous level of functioning (the **precrisis state**), develops a new repertoire of coping mechanisms, or decompensates to a lower level of functioning.

Outside Western culture, a crisis is often viewed as a time for movement and growth. The Chinese symbol for crisis quires a change in the usual method of functioning. The change requires adaptation, learning, and growth.[1] Aguilera[3] purports that all individuals exist in a state of emotional equilibrium or balance. When something that has a positive or negative impact, such as a change or a loss, happens, a state of disequilibrium is created, and the individual strives to regain and maintain the previous level of equilibrium. In essence, the individual, family, or community in crisis is at a turning point, and commonly used coping mechanisms fail to solve the problem. Tension and anxiety increase and contribute to the difficulty of finding a tolerable solution. A person in this position experiences great emotional turmoil and is unable to take independent action to solve the problem.

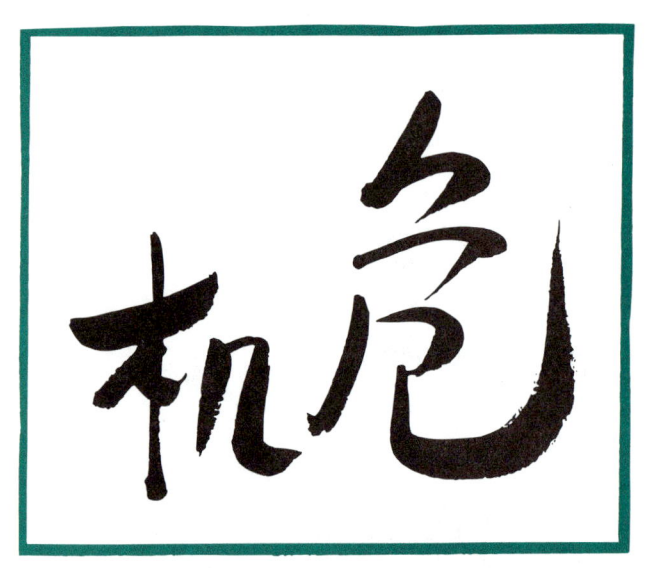

Figure 8–1: Chinese symbol for crisis.

consists of the characters for *danger* and *opportunity* (Figure 8–1). When a crisis is viewed as an opportunity for growth, those involved are much more capable of resolving related issues and more able to move toward positive changes. When the crisis experience is overwhelming because of its scope and nature or when there has not been adequate preparation for the necessary changes, the dangers seem paramount and overshadow any potential growth. The results are maladaptive coping and dysfunctional behavior.

DEVELOPMENTAL PHASES IN A CRISIS SITUATION

Crises, like most human experiences, do not occur in a vacuum. Distinct biopsychosocial phases lead to an active crisis state. The stages of crisis were first described by Tyhurst[10] in a study of individual responses to community disaster. In this milestone study, survivors experienced three overlapping phases:
- a period of *impact*, when the individual realizes the actuality of the event
- a period of *recoil*, when the distress resulting from the event becomes overwhelming and the individual struggles to cope
- a *posttraumatic* period, when the individual experiences disruption in normal functioning

This outline applies most appropriately to crises originating from shocking events such as rape and other violent attacks, the death of a child from sudden infant death syndrome, or sometimes the diagnosis of a terminal illness.[2,6]

Caplan[1] describes a four-phase paradigm that is useful for understanding crises that develop more gradually, such as divorce, and those that result from catastrophic stressors, such as a natural disaster.
- In the *first phase,* the traumatic event causes an initial rise in the individual's level of anxiety. The individual responds with familiar problem-solving mechanisms in an attempt to reduce or eliminate the stress and discomfort. If coping mechanisms are effective, the crisis is averted.
- If the individual's usual problem-solving abilities fail, the individual enters *phase two,* and the stimulus that caused the initial rise in tension continues.
- In the *third phase,* the individual's anxiety continues to rise, and the increased tension moves the individual to reach out for assistance and use every available resource to solve the problem and reduce the increasingly painful state of anxiety.
- *Phase four,* the state of active crisis, results when internal strength and social supports are insufficient, the problem remains unresolved, and tension and anxiety rise to an unbearable level. The individual experiences the continuation of the crisis and severe anxiety or panic that predisposes him or her to psychological disorganization.

The following example illustrates how complex the crisis experience can be.

Liz B. has recently returned to the city to attend graduate school and start a new job. She feels anxious about the changes in geographic location, school, and her employment status. After several months, she starts experiencing extreme fatigue and irritability and misses time from work and school. Because of her short duration of employment, she does not qualify for health insurance. A visit to an urgent care provider produces a diagnosis of anemia. She starts iron-replacement therapy and almost immediately feels better. The crisis is resolved in *phase one*.

Unfortunately, Liz feels better for only a short period. She returns to the urgent care center, where more extensive tests are ordered, and her prescription is changed. Because of the cost of the visit and the tests, she is left without enough money to purchase her prescription. Following a brief discussion of her financial problems with the nurse practitioner, Liz leaves the center with a free sample of her prescribed medications. She begins to feel better, and the crisis is resolved in *phase two*.

The results of the tests reveal that Liz has a form of leukemia, and she will require extensive and costly treatment. Her energy is depleted, and she decides to take a leave of absence from school. She continues her job, and her health benefits are activated, so that the costs of her treatment are now covered. Because she may need assistance with activities of daily living, she consults her parents about the possibility of moving home until her health crisis is resolved. By redefining her goals of going to graduate school and living independently, while at the same time drawing on her existing social supports, she reduces the long-term residual effects of this traumatic event, and the crisis is resolved in *phase three*.

As time progresses, Liz's situation moves into a state of active crisis, *phase four*. Although she was able to draw on social and family supports in phase three, she did not get the professional help she needed to resolve her issues related to the drastic lifestyle changes experienced as a result of her diagnosis. She is at a loss about how to deal with the stress in her life and begins to feel helpless and hopeless. All of the issues that she experienced when she previously lived at home begin to surface again. With professional intervention at this time, Liz may be able to reframe the issues at hand and move on to the business of restoring equilibrium in her life and managing her illness.

Although crisis is not a pathological condition, the disequilibrium that accompanies crisis causes biological, cognitive, affective, and behavioral distortions (see Box 8–2). The inability to problem solve rationally or process information around possible solutions following a crisis event is referred to as *cognitive distortion*. The individual is easily distracted, irritable, and emotionally labile. The stress may be manifested in somatic symptoms such as loss of appetite or inability to sleep. The individual may regress to former, less effective types of behavior such as withdrawal or aggressiveness. These reactions are often difficult for nurses and family members to understand and easy to personalize.

TYPES OF CRISES

In crisis theory, four types of crises are described in the literature: situational, maturational, adventitious, and more recently, sociocultural.[2,3] However, regardless of the type of crisis, the crisis experience produces changes that require new or expanded coping mechanisms. The timing contributes to the potential for a negative outcome. When an individual, family, or community encounters multiple **changes** in a short period, there is an increased risk of maladaptive coping. Multiple losses and stressors reduce one's ability to adapt to the changes that are part of life transitions. The inevitable adjustments to the experiences of birth, death, marriage, geographic relocation, alterations in employment and financial status, and acute or chronic illness predictably contribute to a period of adjustment and the potential for crisis development. Even when the change results from the sudden loss of a loved one or a natural disaster, the ability to adapt and cope with the residual effects is contingent on how the individual, family, or community has managed change in the past.[1-3]

Situational Crisis

The majority of crises that nurses experience on the job can be classified as situational crises, which result from an external event or environmental influence that upsets the individual's or group's biopsychosocial equilibrium. Situational crises are characterized by a sudden, unexpected onset and generally have a singular, rather than a multifaceted, origin. An accident or a diagnosis of a terminal illness, an unexpected pregnancy, a death of a loved one, a sexual assault, witnessing a crime, changes in employment status, and geographic changes are all examples of actual and potential situational crises.[2,3]

Pam B., a 35-year-old high school teacher has recently given birth by cesarean section to a son born 4 weeks premature. Immediately after the delivery, the baby was taken to the neonatal intensive care unit for further assessment and observation. Pam had experienced mild preeclampsia the week prior to delivery and is placed on constant observation following the birth of her son because of an increase in her symptom profile, putting her at risk for convulsions and a hypertensive crisis. Despite his small size, her son, Jacob, is making good progress, and her parents go away on a winter holiday as planned. Twelve days following his delivery, neonatologists determine that Jacob has extensive brain damage. Instead of experiencing the joy and excitement of his birth as she had always imagined it, Pam, a single parent by choice, is devastated. As she attempts to cope with the magnitude of her situation, she is overcome with mixed emotions. She is thankful that her baby is alive, yet is unable to comprehend the significance of his diagnosis. She vacillates between calm and rationality one moment and uncontrollable crying the next.

Any situation may be potentially stressful for one individual but not for another. When intervening in situational crises, it is important to accept and not negate individual responses. Sociocultural and environmental influences further affect the response to changes created by a crisis. The report of a suspicious mammogram likely will be handled better by an individual who is in a supportive relationship, surrounded by family and friends, than by the individual who has recently left a relationship and relocated to a distant geographic location. In essence, the predictable fear and stressors that accompany a specific situational crisis can be further complicated by the other changes in the individual's living situation.

Box 8–2. Dysfunctional Responses to Crisis

Physical	Emotional	Cognitive	Behavioral
Headaches	Anger	Forgetfulness	Crying
Backaches	Disbelief	Confusion	Overeating or
Fatigue	Irritability	Shock	undereating
Insomnia	Lability	Intrusive	Nightmares
Diminished	Apathy	thoughts	School problems
sexual	Numbness	Self-doubt	Work difficulties
drive	Sadness	Helplessness	Substance abuse
GI distress	Survivor	Hopelessness	Social
	guilt	Suicidal thoughts	withdrawal
	Flashbacks	Poor	
		concentration	

Maturational Crisis

Maturational crises are developmental events, or life transitions, requiring significant role changes. Maturational crises occur in predictable successive stages of growth and development: infancy and early childhood, preschool, prepuberty, adolescence, young adulthood, adulthood, late adulthood, and old age.[2,3,8,11,12] Considered part of normal growth and development, crises can happen during each developmental stage and are influenced by the individual's unique biopsychosocial stressors. Erikson's[11] psychosocial theory of development provides a basis for comprehending the magnitude of changes at every life stage. Individuals experiencing maturational crises generally experience increased anxiety and tension as they strive to meet the de-

> **RESEARCH NOTE**
>
> Murray, RB: Needs and Resources: The Lived Experience of Homeless Men. J Psychoso Nurs Ment Health Serv: 34(5): 18–23, 1996.
>
> **Findings:** Interviews were conducted with a stratified convenience sample of 150 homeless men who attended a day treatment program in a Midwestern metropolitan area. This exploratory descriptive study was designed to delineate the needs, resources, and services for homeless men who were either in a situational crisis, severely and persistently mentally ill, or alcohol and drug dependent.
>
> The questionnaire was based on literature review and personal experiences with homeless individuals and specifically designed to obtain information about the participants' experiences of being homeless, their health status and care, the meeting of basic needs, and the available and needed services. Researchers collected all data through face-to-face interviews to ensure consistent use and interpretation of the tool. Contrary to popular methods of data collection in descriptive studies such as this, audiotaping was not used because it was believed that this approach could add to clients' suspicion or delusional thinking. However, participants were told that the investigator would write notes during the interview to ensure accuracy of data collection and because their answers were important. Each interview lasted approximately 1 hour.
>
> Responses to the question, "What is your most pressing or greatest need since you became homeless?" included security, love, respect, privacy, a sense of peace, a job or worthwhile activity, and self-actualization. All groups consistently reported shelter in the form of permanent housing, a job, and income as their most pressing needs. Contrary to the popular myth, none of the homeless people in this study preferred the streets to housing. Furthermore, the men demonstrated much creativity in how they approached and used community resources to meet their needs for food, sleep, elimination, clothing, hygiene and laundry, safety, privacy, and income.
>
> **Application to Practice:** Psychiatric–mental health nursing interventions can be most beneficial when the nurse is knowledgeable of the clients' perceived needs. The results of this study provide the nurse with a greater understanding of the diversity of needs experienced by homeless individuals and stress the importance of effective crisis intervention. The overall findings of this study could be useful to those who provide services, who advocate for the homeless, and who engage in efforts of policy and legislative change. The importance of listening to what the homeless population has to say is perhaps the first step in meeting their health care needs. Then, and only then, can the homeless population be realistically considered in health care reform.

mands and expectations of changes in their roles, sense of self, body image, and attitudes toward others. A person's lifestyle is continuously changed by maturational development. These changes could occur during concomitant biological and social role transitions such as the transition from being a student to an employee, entering marriage, becoming a parent, beginning menopause, and retiring. They usually evolve over an extended period and frequently require the individual to make many changes.[3] The following example illustrates one type of maturational crisis:

> Grant F., a 57-year-old widowed health-care executive seeks help from a private mental health center on the advice of a good friend. Two months earlier, owing to corporate downsizing, he was forced to take an early retirement from his upper management job. Since that time, he has had difficulty sleeping, states that he can't "think clearly," and feels the same way he did when his wife died. After losing his job, he has secluded himself from his former colleagues and says, "What are we going to talk about? They still have their jobs!" He has always been a successful businessman who took pleasure from his work accomplishments. When his wife died 5 years earlier, he immersed himself totally in his career and lost contact with most of his friends outside of work. Although always a confident and self-assured man, he now fears that he is "old" and "useless."

Adventitious Crisis

Adventitious crises are generally described as accidental, uncommon, and unexpected tragedies that disrupt entire communities, often natural disasters such as hurricanes, fires, floods, and earthquakes. The monumental stress from this type of crisis may quickly deplete or overburden existing support systems, including multiple family members, emergency personnel, clergy, friends, neighbors, and disaster relief organizations. Adventitious crises often have deleterious, far-reaching effects upon members of the general population who may fear similar experiences.[12,13] Left untreated, the effects of these crises may lead to acute or posttraumatic stress reactions (Chapter 22).

In addition, war and the unexpected events of mass murders, kidnappings, random shootings, riots, and bombings of public buildings are in this category. Shock and generalized anxiety strike the entire community. The effects of an adventitious crisis do not end with the event itself. Recovery is influenced by a complex interaction of variables related to both the event and the people exposed. Resulting biopsychosocial problems are often severe; without timely intervention, long-term residual effects and psychopathology are likely.[3,10]

> On April 19, 1995, a bomb was detonated at the Alfred P. Murrah Federal Building in Oklahoma City. For weeks people throughout the world were glued to their television sets, looking for answers to this crime. The

> **RESEARCH NOTE**
>
> Coffman, S: Parent's struggles to rebuild family life after Hurricane Andrew. Issues in Mental Health Nursing 17:353–367, 1996.
>
> **Findings:** To gain a deeper understanding of the meaning of everyday experiences following a natural disaster, the author studied 13 parents 2 to 3 months after Hurricane Andrew ravaged their southern Florida homes. Hermeneutic phenomenology provided the method for the study. Through the use of tape-recorded interviews, photographs, newspaper and journal articles, and the researcher's field notes, "struggling to rebuild family life" emerged as the essence of the study.
>
> Coffman concluded that this struggle was an ongoing process, connected to their lives before the hurricane. Participants described how problems created by the hurricane were magnified by the daily ongoing stressors such as divorce, job responsibilities, chronic illness, and unemployment. There were seven descriptive themes: (1) thankful for what we have, (2) overwhelmed by damage and demands, (3) limited by aftereffects, (4) responsible for children's well-being, (5) balancing needs and roles, (6) constantly changing amidst uncertainty, and (7) finding meaning and growing stronger.
>
> For the parents in this study, the time of data collection was a time of coming together and reaffirming the importance of children and family. Parents mentioned different types of support that were helpful at different times in the recovery period. Material support (food and shelter) was seen as particularly important after the storm. Informational support was critical for decision making with regard to relocation and financial assistance. Last, ongoing emotional support from spouses, friends, and family members helped them cope with loss and the cumulative frustrations involved in recovery.
>
> **Application to Practice:** This study provides nurses with an increased understanding of parents' experiences in a natural disaster. Nurses who work with families after a disaster need to determine the exposure of the family to the event itself. Psychiatric–mental health nursing interventions can be most effective when the nurse is knowledgeable of the personal history and meaning each individual attaches to the event. Data from this study indicate that family members bring their own unique background and concerns to the postdisaster situation. The study findings further support the need for nursing interventions that address family needs, support strengths, and involve parents as active decision makers regarding how these needs can best be met.

primary victims of the Oklahoma City bombing were the individuals directly affected, specifically those killed or injured in the bombing and collapse of the building. Numerous others were indirectly affected: those who witnessed the collapse, those who had friends and loved ones killed or injured, those who normally would have been there but were not, those responsible for the security of the building, and those involved as part of the rescue team.

In the aftermath of the Oklahoma City bombing, many individuals likely experienced acute stress disorder (ASD) or posttraumatic stress disorder (PTSD)—someone who narrowly missed being seriously injured or a paramedic who felt responsible for not having saved the life of a child who died. Additionally, many others likely experienced distress manifested in physiological, emotional, cognitive, and behavioral symptoms. Others may have reexperienced the terror of old traumas, even though they were not directly affected by the bombing. Unfortunately, crises of this nature leave their victims both traumatized and grieving.[3,4] In disasters, rescue team members, paramedics, police officers, and firefighters frequently experience fear for their own lives, as well as intense guilt or inadequacy for not having been able to save more lives. Some rescuers experience ASD or PTSD, whereas others may experience less intense symptoms. Last, the community of Oklahoma City and the whole of the American people experienced a crisis regarding government's ability to protect its citizens, and many directed inappropriate blame toward community leaders.

Sociocultural Crises

Hoff[2] describes a **sociocultural crisis** as one arising from the cultural values that are embedded in the social structure. The loss of a job stemming from discriminatory practices based on age, race, sex, sexual preference, or class is a primary example of a sociocultural crisis. This type of job loss varies markedly from job loss due to illness or poor performance. Additionally, crises that relate to deviant acts of others whose behavior violates social norms, such as robbery, rape, and incest, may be classified as a sociocultural crisis. Other examples are the institutionalization of the elderly, which relates to the value of old people and the nuclear family; violence against women and children, which relates to values about discipline and the place of women in society; and residential dislocation, which relates to economic class, ethnic issues, and displacement of the poor during urban upgrading.[2]

Crises from sociocultural sources are generally less amenable to control by individuals, who may be reluctant to confront the system to resolve their crisis. Very often, cultural views and public social policies may be a component of either the identification or the resolution of these crises.

Whenever a crisis originates outside the individual, it is usually beyond the ability of the individual alone to control and manage.

> David T. is a 40-year-old gay employee of a conservative international bank who suspects that he has been dismissed on the basis of sexual orientation discrimination. He is reluctant to publicly confront his employer or go to the human rights commission for fear of unwanted exposure of his homosexuality. Only within the last 2 years has he come to terms with his sexuality, and he is particularly concerned about the response of his aging parents and preteen children, should information surrounding the circumstances of his dismissal become public. He begins to experience overwhelming feelings of inadequacy and low self-esteem but does not consult his nurse therapist until he begins to think that things would be better for everyone if he wasn't around.

CRISIS INTERVENTION AND THE NURSING PROCESS

During times of crisis, people need support and help that is goal directed and purposefully focused. The steps in crisis intervention parallel the steps of the nursing process. Through assessment, diagnosis, planning, and intervention, the nurse supports the process of crisis resolution (Box 8–3). Although individuals' experiences cannot be placed in clearly defined categories, a typical crisis and subsequent intervention would pass through a fairly predictable sequence.[2,3]

Crisis intervention in the early stages focuses on accurately describing the circumstances surrounding the event: the who, what, when, and how. The process of reviewing the details of the event helps clarify the extent of the problem and corrects any misinformation. Often those involved are unable to cognitively understand the connection between the stressful experience and their current emotional state. Aguilera[3] reports that the minimum goal of crisis intervention is to resolve the individual's immediate crisis and restore the level of functioning to the precrisis state. Optimally, the function will improve to above the precrisis level through increased knowledge gained from the process of psychoeducation and enhanced insight.[3,8]

ASSESSMENT

During the initial step of crisis intervention, the nurse collects data regarding the scope and nature of the crisis and its effects on those involved. This information helps the nurse formulate a method of intervention. Immediate intervention is undertaken in situations where the individual's physical or psychological state is life threatening. Acute physical complaints, such as chest pain or breathing difficulties, require immediate medical evaluation. Similarly, threats of suicide or homicide require consideration of the individual's risk of harm to self or others.[2,3]

Assessment of Balancing Factors

Aguilera[3] stresses the importance of assessing whether balancing factors are present or absent. Balancing factors are important to assess because they affect the way an individual perceives and responds to a precipitating stressor. The assessment of balancing factors includes perception of the event, situational supports, and coping mechanisms (see Figure 8–2). Whenever a stressful event occurs, these identified balancing factors can bring about a return to equilibrium, and a crisis is avoided. However, the absence of one or more of these balancing factors may increase disequilibrium and precipitate a crisis. Assessment of these factors is critical for crisis intervention to decide how and when to intervene and whom to call.[3]

Precipitating Events. Insight into how the crisis began, the **precipitating factor**, is necessary to identify accurate methods of intervention. Assessing precipitating events helps clients connect life events with how they are feeling. Because the client's subjective experience of the crisis event is critical, questions should be asked in a matter-of-fact manner that enables a client to discuss the crisis situation[2,3]:

> In what areas of your life have you experienced changes?
> What recent experiences have been upsetting?
> When did you begin to feel anxious? Experience sleep disturbances?
> Describe for me in your own words what caused this situation.
> How long have you been experiencing these problems?

Perception of the Events. Hand in hand with identification of the precipitating events must be exploration of the meaning of the crisis to those involved. Often the symbolic meaning of the crisis far outweighs the reality of the situation. Current issues are sometimes connected to past issues of concern, and together with the client, the nurse looks for a recent event that may be connected to an underlying theme. The subjective meaning of a stressful event plays a major role in determining the nature and degree of coping behaviors. If the

---

Box 8–3. Comparison of the Nursing Process to the Stages of Crisis Intervention

Nursing Process	Crisis Intervention
Assessment	Assessment
Nursing diagnosis	Determination of scope and impact of the crisis experience
Planning	Planning therapeutic intervention
Intervention	Intervention
Evaluation	Resolution of the crisis and anticipatory planning

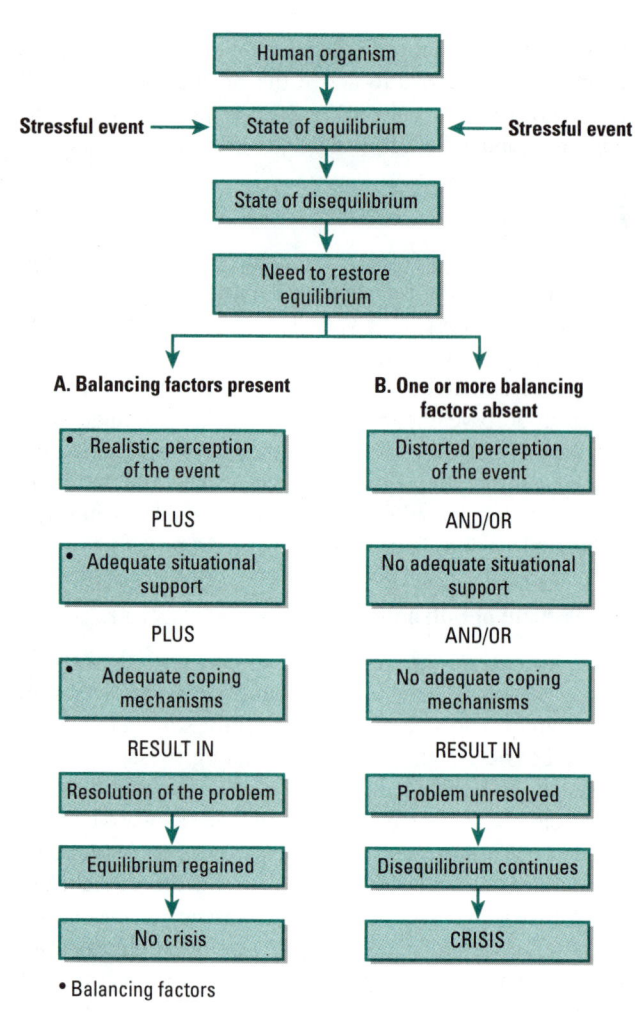

Figure 8–2: Aguilera's paradigm: The effect of balancing factors in a stressful event.

perception of the event is distorted, the relationship between the event and the feelings of stress may not be recognized. Conversely, if the event is perceived realistically, then the relationship between the event and the feelings of stress is recognized, and problem solving can be oriented toward reduction of tension and resolution of the stressful problem.[3] Asking the following questions will help clients discuss their feelings and reactions to the crisis experience:

What does this crisis mean to you?
How do you see what has happened affecting you personally?
How will this situation affect your future?
In what way has this crisis affected your ability to cope?
Tell me what is the most difficult part of the problem now.

Presence of Environmental Supports. In assessing for the presence of environmental supports, the nurse looks for resources that can be depended on to help resolve the crisis at hand. Significant relationships with others not only provide nurturance and support but also are vital resources for coping with stressors. Sudden or unexpected social isolation results in the loss of usual social supports, leaving the individual vulnerable to the stressors of daily living. Confrontation with a stressful situation, combined with lack of support, may lead to a state of disequilibrium and potential crisis.[3,14] The following questions can help the nurse mobilize environmental supports:

Explain in detail for me what help is available to you.
From whom do you seek help or assistance when you are having problems?
Whom can you contact to help you?
Are you employed?
Do you live alone? With family? With a roommate?

Previous Experiences with Problem Solving and Current Coping Ability. Some people are able to problem solve and effectively resolve a crisis, whereas others resort to more dysfunctional methods of coping. In assessing these individuals' normal responses to stress and present **coping mechanisms,** the nurse helps clients identify what problem-solving skills were effective in the past and what they can currently do. The individual in crisis is often overwhelmed and unable to clearly think through what options are available.

The nurse also needs to gain an understanding of those aspects of a person's life that are working well, a process that can be very empowering for clients. Questions that can help the nurse assess past and current coping mechanisms include the following:

Describe for me how you have managed problems in the past.
What do you usually do when you are having problems or experiencing stress?
What has been helpful for you in resolving past problems?
Tell me what it has been like since this problem started.
What aspects of your life are working well?

Caplan[15] describes four methods of coping in response to a crisis or stressful event: (1) behaving in a way that changes the stressful environment or enables the individual to escape from it, (2) acquiring new capabilities to handle the crisis event, (3) intrapsychically defending against dysphoric emotional arousal, and (4) intrapsychically coming to terms with the event and the sequelae by internal readjustment.

Sociocultural Assessment

In addition to assessing the balancing factors, the nurse must consider the sociocultural influences on how individuals communicate their needs in times of crisis. Cultural values affect the process of giving, asking for, and receiving help. Specific sociocultural factors to consider in crisis assessment include:

- Migration and citizenship status
- Gender and family roles
- Religious belief systems
- Child-rearing practices
- Use of extended family and support systems[16]

Eliciting information about the individual's attitudes toward help-seeking behaviors is facilitated with open-ended questions, such as "Tell me about how you manage the household chores and caring for the children" or "Describe for me how you go about getting help when you are having difficulties." Open-ended questions allow people to describe the situation from their lived experience and minimize the influence of the nurse's preconceived ideas about how the problem should be managed.

DIAGNOSIS

After the nursing assessment is complete, the nurse can formulate a nursing diagnosis that will lead to effective nursing interventions. Although many individuals with mental illness experience crisis, crisis is not a psychiatric illness, and even though the disequilibrium that accompanies crisis causes biological, cognitive, affective, and behavioral distortions, the uniqueness of the individual's experiences must not be understated (see Box 8–2). North American Nursing Diagnosis Association (NANDA) nursing diagnoses relevant to those experiencing crisis are listed in Box 8–4.

PLANNING AND IMPLEMENTING INTERVENTIONS

Interventions associated with crisis focus on rapid stabilization and return to the precrisis state. In most cases, the nurse makes a referral for further intervention. The method and site of the intervention are determined by the nature of the crisis and the resources available to the individual, and frequently the nurse refers those affected to the most appropriate setting (e.g., rape crisis center or homeless shelter). Knowledge of intervention resources available to the population served in the nurse's practice area is critical to competent nursing practice.

Although the methods of crisis intervention have generally been classified as generic and individual, these approaches are complementary and not mutually exclusive.

The Generic Approach

The generic approach focuses on the course of the particular kind of crisis that is due to predictable life events. Preventive psychiatry developed this method of intervention to respond to the reactions caused by predictable types of crises: It is designed to reach high-risk individuals and large groups as quickly as possible with specific interventions that are effective for the general population. Generic approaches to crisis intervention include debriefing, trauma response, direct encouragement of adaptive behavior, general support, environmental manipulation, and anticipatory intervention.

Environmental Manipulation. These interventions directly change the client's physical or interpersonal situation, provide situational support, or simply remove the source of the stress.
- Obtaining shelter for a homeless individual
- Offering sick leave to an individual
- Finding shelter for abused women and their children
- Encouraging a client to move in with a friend or sibling while coping with a particular stressor[2,3,6]

Anticipatory Intervention. Anticipatory intervention is a form of primary prevention. Using this approach, the nurse helps the client foresee and predict potential problems or difficulties; this preparation ultimately decreases a client's stress and averts a crisis. This type of intervention is particularly useful for maturational crises that generally are predictable and occur gradually. Types of anticipatory intervention include[1–3]
- Premarital counseling
- Childbirth preparation classes
- Parenting classes
- Preparation for retirement
- Respite care for families with a multiply handicapped child
- Preoperative teaching

The Individual Approach

The individual approach emphasizes a professional's in-depth assessment of the client's own specific biopsychosocial needs. Information from the individual's current lived experience, including all aspects of the social, cultural, and environmental influences, is relevant and provides clues that may result in better understanding of the present crisis situation. It differs from the generic approach in that it is planned to meet the unique needs of the individual, not just the characteristic course of a particular kind of crisis.

The focus of the individual approach is the immediate causes of disturbed equilibrium and the processes necessary for regaining a precrisis or higher level of function-

---

Box 8–4. Common Nursing Diagnoses for Individuals in Crisis

Anxiety
Family Processes, altered
Role Performance, altered
Thought Processes, altered
Self Esteem, chronic low
Self Esteem, situational low
Fatigue
Fear
Hopelessness
Coping, individual, ineffective
Family Coping: ineffective, compromised
Social Interaction, impaired
Knowledge Deficit
Post-Trauma Response
Violence, risk for, directed at self/others
Self Care Deficit
Sleep Pattern Disturbance
Spiritual Distress
Rape-Trauma Syndrome

ing.[3] Crisis resolution includes the supportive resources for the individual and family. The nurse must understand the circumstances that led to the current crisis and adopt an approach that is most likely to help the client respond adaptively. A clear understanding of the dynamics of crisis and the effects unique to the individual, coupled with knowledge of the available resources, gives the nurse the skills necessary for effective intervention.

Planning for effective treatment involves helping the individual and significant others explore what problem-solving techniques were effective in the past and which are available to them now. It focuses on the immediate problem with the goal of reestablishing equilibrium. Unlike extended psychotherapy, the individual approach deals relatively little with the developmental past of the individual in crisis, except to collect relevant data that may result in a better understanding of the client's present circumstances. The plan must be time-limited, concrete, and realistic, as well as consistent with the individual's thinking, feeling, behavior, lifestyle, and sociocultural concerns. The nurse establishes the parameters of the plan with those involved:

What are the agreed-upon immediate solutions?
Where and when will the solutions be implemented?
Who is responsible for what and when?
What is the plan for follow-up?

> **Box 8–5. Attitudes Essential to the Individual Approach to Crisis Intervention**
>
> 1. The therapist must guard against viewing the work as "second best" and view crisis intervention as the treatment of choice for those in crisis.
> 2. Rather than a thorough diagnostic evaluation, accurate assessment of the individual's presenting problem is the foundation of effective crisis intervention.
> 3. Treatment is sharply time-limited in crisis intervention. Both the nurse and the client should direct their energies toward resolution of the presenting problem.
> 4. Dealing with events and issues not directly related to the presenting problem should be avoided because they have no place in this type of treatment modality.
> 5. The nurse frequently needs to take an active and sometimes directive role when working with individuals in crisis. The slower-paced approach common to more traditional therapies is not appropriate when working with people in crisis.
> 6. Maximum flexibility is encouraged. The nurse may serve as a resource person, information giver, and agent of referral to connect with other mental health services and helping resources.
> 7. The goal of this approach to intervention is very explicit. All energy is directed to returning the individual to at least the precrisis level of functioning.
>
> Adapted from: Aguilera, D: Crisis Intervention: Theory and Methodology, ed 7. Mosby, St. Louis, 1994, p. 19–20.

To be most effective, the nurse should adopt a crisis-orientation philosophy when intervening with those in crisis (Box 8–5).

The nurse as a crisis clinician is an active participant in the process who helps the client bring feelings into the open, explore past and present coping mechanisms, find and use situational supports, and make anticipatory plans to reduce the possibility of future crises. Effective early intervention has the financial advantage of providing resolution before more costly treatment may be required.

Therapeutic Techniques. Clients commonly look to the nurse for guidance and direction. Theoretical concepts appropriate to working with individuals in crisis include empathy, authenticity, immediacy, and active listening. The following guidelines will help the nurse respond in a competent and caring manner.[5,14]

- Be specific, use concise statements, and avoid overwhelming the client with irrelevant questions or excessive detail. A calm, controlled presence reassures the client that the nurse can help.
- Listen for facts and feelings: Seeking clarification, paraphrasing, and reflection are effective strategies. Stay with the topic and refocus as necessary.
- Allow sufficient time for the individuals involved to process information and ask questions.
- Help clients legitimize feelings by letting them know that others in similar situations have experienced comparable emotions.
- Clarify distortions by getting clients to look at the situation realistically, focusing on what can be changed versus what cannot.
- Work together with the client. Mutually negotiate and renegotiate plans. Empower clients by allowing them to make informed choices.

Pharmacologic Intervention. For excessive anxiety and somatic complaints, a psychopharmacologic intervention may be indicated. A brief course of treatment with a benzodiazepine, such as lorazepam, is often effective in helping the individual stabilize emotionally and reducing sleep disturbances. Be cautious that the individual is not sedated to the point of being numbed and unable to express emotions necessary to the grieving process. Psychopharmacologic intervention is provided by an MD, preferably a psychiatrist, or a psychiatric–mental health clinical nurse specialist licensed in the expanded role that includes prescribing medications.

Types of Crisis Intervention Programs

Nurses frequently see individuals in crisis. Crisis intervention is provided in a variety of settings and designed to meet the individual needs of a specific population. The setting may be a hospital, an outpatient clinic, a mental health center, or other community setting, ranging from the client's home to a street corner. Often the setting gives specific focus to the intervention, such as in cases of acute psychological disorders; domestic violence, including spousal and partner battering, child or elder abuse; and alcohol and substance abuse. Disaster response and critical incident stress debriefing are provided when the crisis affects large segments of the population. The modality of crisis intervention may involve on-site crisis counseling, mobile outreach, home visits, and telephone counseling.[2,3,16]

Crisis Counseling. This method of brief, problem-focused therapy works on solving the immediate problem. It lasts from one to six sessions and can include individual, group, or family treatment. The concepts of empathy, authenticity, immediacy, and active listening are very important during crisis counseling. Additionally, nurturing, exploring, encouraging, reinforcing new ways of coping, and linking the client to a larger supportive social network are the techniques of this type of intervention.[2]

Mobile Crisis Team. These teams vary from one jurisdiction to another, as do the services they provide. The crisis evaluation is generally provided by a mobile team of interdisciplinary clinicians who go to the location of the critical event. These mobile teams extend services to the community and provide on-site evaluation of the individuals involved in the crisis as well as the circumstances surrounding the event. Crisis management, with community support and education, is the goal of this method of intervention. Home visits for crisis intervention may be provided when the team determines that the individual or significant others would be better served in this environment. Conversely, the individuals involved may be unable to seek assistance elsewhere. Problems commonly encountered by mobile response teams revolve around domestic violence, psychiatric emergencies, and medical emergencies. The goal of mobile response teams is assessment and evaluation, crisis management, and referral.[3,14]

Telephone Counseling or Hotline. Suicide prevention and crisis intervention centers rely heavily on telephone counseling, which is structured to provide intervention to individuals with specific issues. One such hotline is the Battered Women's Hot Line. This service is often community based and staffed by clinicians or volunteers who have been trained to follow specific protocols, with the goal of supporting and stabilizing the immediate crisis and then referring to the most appropriate follow-up assistance. The caller is able to maintain anonymity while exploring what resources are available for the particular problem. Calls generally fall into four categories: (1) crisis calls; (2) ventilation calls to release anger, frustration, fear, and anxiety; (3) combination ventilation and information calls; and (4) information only calls.[2,3,6,15]

Nurses working in environments that provide emergency telephone access must provide supportive intervention and guidance without the help that visual cues give in a face-to-face evaluation. Listening skills are the primary skills of telephone counseling, and after determining the degree of safety risk and suicidal potential, the nurse allows the individual to vent feelings. The following dialogue with a crisis nurse illustrates the adaptation of skills necessary for telephone counseling.

> It was really hard when I first started working for the crisis line. I had a difficult time adapting to telephone counseling. I am such a visually oriented person that I had a hard time feeling confident with the assessments that I was doing over the phone. In my previous job, I relied a lot on visual cues, facial expressions, and body language to assist me with communicating effectively with my clients. With time and experience, I was able to engage the client over the phone and pick up on the subtle nuances in the client's voice. I think the most important piece of advice that I would give to individuals wanting to do crisis counseling is for them to learn the skill of paraphrasing. This is essential to this kind of work; it is critical that you continually paraphrase and check out your understanding with the client, in order to be sure you are certain what the problem is, and how you might be able to assist through to crisis resolution.

Disaster Response and Critical Incident Stress Debriefing. Disaster response and critical incident stress debriefing are methods of helping large groups of individuals affected by an adventitious crisis. *Disaster response* is an organized plan of intervention provided to large segments of the population following such disasters as hurricanes, floods, or accidents. Following disasters of this magnitude, a broad-based "postvention" or trauma response is required and includes the following:

- Crisis intervention and support
- Identification of trauma and grief issues
- Assessment of the severity of those issues
- Short- and long-term support and treatment for grief and trauma issues
- Trauma debriefing for individuals, families, groups, and appropriate follow-up as necessary
- Information and education
- Community "postvention" meetings.[12,13]

Critical incident stress debriefing is a specific method of intervention aimed at specific groups, such as medical first responders, police, hospital personnel, and those affected by a crisis through work, school, or community affiliation. The goal of such debriefings is to reduce the impact of a crisis event on those directly involved in the critical situation or event. Generally, debriefing meetings follow a psychoeducational format in small groups, with a professional facilitator (preferably someone removed from the event) who assists in identifying stressors, venting feelings, and discussing the roles of the individuals involved, with the aim of putting the event into context and allowing the crisis workers to receive peer support.[14,16]

Other Settings. Nurses and other members of the health care team working in acute care settings, birthing centers, schools, outreach centers, clinics, long-term care facilities, hospices, and elsewhere all participate formally and informally in identifying the potential for maladaptive coping and the problem-solving activities that crisis work requires. Through the nursing process, the nurse working with clients experiencing trauma, acute or chronic illness, or death of a loved one is in a position to observe, analyze, evaluate, and identify interventions specific to the situation that will enhance effective adaptation and coping. In essence, the nursing process is the vehicle by which nurses assist the individual in crisis.

EVALUATION OF THE NURSING PROCESS AND EXPECTED OUTCOMES

The last phase of crisis intervention is evaluation. Often it is difficult to evaluate the effectiveness of the intervention because of the nature of the crisis and the number of people involved. The nurse in acute or short-term settings is not always able to evaluate the long-term outcome of the intervention; however, he or she can review how the interventions were implemented and note the effectiveness at the time. Asking "Have positive behavioral changes occurred?" or "Have the individuals involved developed new coping mechanisms?" will guide the nurse in evaluating the effectiveness of the actions taken. The nurse reinforces adaptive coping mechanisms that worked to decrease tension and anxiety. Expected outcomes of crisis intervention include reduced stress and anxiety related to the crisis event and a gradual return to the precrisis level of functioning. Evaluation takes place at many levels, and together with the client, various health care professionals contribute to the resolution of the client's crisis.[3,14]

As the client's coping abilities increase and changes occur, ongoing intervention may include summarizing the progress made to date and allowing the individual to reexperience and reconfirm the positive outcomes. The nurse assists in making realistic plans for the future and in helping the client understand how the present difficulties may help him or her cope with future crisis. Follow-up and evaluation of the intervention assess the need for further intervention and referrals.[2,3]

COPING WITH CRISIS WORK

Ongoing self-reflection and self-awareness on the nurse's part are essential for adaptation to the realities of crisis work. The affective responses of the nurse are frequently intensified because of the nature of the work, which is not always easy or comfortable. The nurse must possess the courage to deal with the tragedies of human suffering. To work successfully with individuals in crisis, the nurse must demonstrate both calmness and empathy in responding to clients' needs. Anger and blame are frequent reactions to stressful events, and the nurse needs to acknowledge these client responses but not personalize them. The role of the nurse is to assist people toward crisis resolution and to stand by them until their problem is resolved.[2,3]

Nurses also need to be sensitive to their own vulnerabilities and be aware of the cumulative impact of listening and witnessing horrific situations. Frustration, apprehension, anger, and fear are common responses, even for the most experienced nurse.[2,3] Develop strategies for coping with crisis work to deal with concerns before, during, and after they arise to maintain optimal mental health. Methods for coping with the stress of crisis work include personal methods, group methods, and employer methods (Box 8–6).

Box 8–6. Coping with Crisis Work

Personal Methods
- Strive for balance between professional and personal life.
- Talk to friends about stressful issues; be careful not to breech confidentiality.
- Consult a colleague whose opinions you respect.
- Formulate your own outlet for stress and anger.
- Seek professional assistance.

Group Methods
- Develop support networks.
- Use self-help groups within the work environment to debrief.
- Ask professionals to lead support groups.
- Employ a supervision group to discuss issues related to the dynamics of caring.

Employer Sanctioned Methods
- Hold clinical case conferences.
- List policies and procedures.
- Educate staff and provide role modeling.
- Educate the community (e.g., trauma response, domestic violence).
- Participate in research.

IMPLICATIONS FOR EDUCATION AND RESEARCH

Bateman[17] observes that a growing number of individuals and families seek mental health services because of the stress and anxiety of a crisis. Often the crisis emerges from a person's inability to access services needed to manage changes that are part of actual or perceived losses, threats of loss, or challenges to security and self-esteem. Understanding the nature, scope, and impact of the crisis for those involved is the key component of crisis intervention.

Access to services during a crisis depends on the response of the service system, the individual's degree of psychopathology, and the presence of an actual or perceived supportive environment. Crisis intervention and social services must be structured to meet the needs of a changing population. Many disciplines are involved with individuals experiencing crisis; a seamless continuum of services must be available to clients to prevent them from falling through the cracks. Education of the general public and enhanced critical social thinking in the curriculum of health care professionals can improve others' understanding of the needs of individuals and families who are experiencing emotional and psychological reactions to a crisis.

AREAS FOR FUTURE RESEARCH

- What are the effects of managed care in mental health services for individuals and families in crisis?
- What is the impact of reduced access to inpatient mental health services for individuals and families?
- What anticipatory interventions can be used to assist families who are in crisis because of the downsizing of corporate America?
- What is the best way to prepare nurses to intervene effectively in crisis situations?

CASE STUDY

Marguerita S., a 19-year-old mother of a 1-year-old daughter, states that her marriage of 2 years is fairly good and that her relationship with her husband is on an "even keel"; outsiders describe her marriage as troubled. She rationalizes that his bouts of anger and threats to "shut her up" are the results of the stress he is feeling with his work. He is an intense and easily frustrated man. However, he constantly reassures her that he loves her (generally following intercourse), and as long as she is good to him and doesn't anger him, she believes everything will be okay.

She grew up in a large city, the eldest of eight children. As the eldest, she had many family responsibilities within her home. Her father was frequently unemployed, and her mother was very busy raising her younger siblings. Although a bright student in school, she quit school following grade nine to work to help support her parents and younger siblings.

At 17, she became pregnant and married her boyfriend, Alberto, against her mother's wishes. His job took them away from her family to a neighboring suburb, approximately 2 hours' commute by bus.

Before her daughter was born, she worked at menial jobs, mostly in the hotel and restaurant industries. Following the birth of her daughter, she found working difficult and was unable to help out with money problems because the cost of day care seemed to take most of her money. Her mother was unable to assist her because she continues to grapple with issues in her own family.

Marguerita and Alberto have struggled along the best they can until she finds that she is pregnant again. Alberto is enraged and demands that she get an abortion, something that is completely unthinkable to Marguerita. The relationship is severely impaired. He stays out late after work and refuses to talk to her unless it is to have sex. She is sickly during the pregnancy and is unable to work at all.

The baby, a son, is born prematurely and requires extensive medical care. Alberto is unsupportive and blames her for everything that has happened. She has no close friends nearby, and her mother is overwhelmed with her own problems. She tries to draw support from Alberto despite his general unavailability and his constant threats to leave her. She is psychologically and economically dependent on Alberto and has no other means of financial support.

The situation escalates to a critical event when he strikes her across the mouth. She sadly begins to realize that she cannot manage the marriage while coping with a sick baby and toddler. She experiences episodes of crying, anxiety, and insomnia. She is physically exhausted and fears that she will not be able to care for her daughter and premature son. The nurse in the neonatal follow-up clinic suggests that the family seek help at the local crisis center.

CRITICAL THINKING QUESTIONS

1. Describe the impact of the multiple stressors in this young mother's life that limit her ability to cope with her current situation.
2. What additional information does the nurse need to collect at this time?
3. How would you describe the type of crisis that this young woman is experiencing? What would be the immediate goal of crisis intervention? What might be the long-term goals?
4. As the nurse working with this family, how might crisis intervention guide your work?
5. What crisis services and community resources exist in your own community?

KEY POINTS

- The experience of crisis is universal to every individual, family, and community.
- The foundation of crisis theory is the concept that early intervention at the onset of a crisis has the potential to reduce the residual negative effects resulting from the crisis experience.
- The experience of crisis is self-limiting and lasts from 4 to 6 weeks. There is a period of transition that includes the danger of psychological vulnerability and the potential opportunity for change.
- A crisis occurs when the individual's internal and external resources are depleted because of the immediate situation or the cumulative effects of multiple stressors. Four types of crises are situational, maturational, adventitious, and sociocultural.
- In part because of the social nature of human beings, during times of crisis, planned biopsychosocial support from others in the immediate environment is needed.
- The steps in the nursing process directly parallel the steps in crisis intervention.
- Data collected during the assessment are the basis for effective crisis intervention. Specifically, the nurse is concerned with the client's perception of the event, situational supports, and coping mechanisms.

- The focus of crisis intervention is to provide support and guidance, with consideration for the lived experience of the individual, family, and group. Two approaches to crisis intervention are the generic approach and the individual approach.
- The minimum goal of crisis intervention is to resolve the individual's immediate crisis and restore the person's level of functioning to the precrisis state.
- Nurses in all areas of practice are in a unique position to respond to those in crisis by offering supportive and therapeutic interventions. A variety of crisis intervention programs are discussed.

REFERENCES

1. Caplan, G: Principles of Preventative Psychiatry. Basic Books, New York, 1964.
2. Hoff, L: People in Crisis, ed. 4 Jossey-Bass, San Francisco, 1995.
3. Aguilera, D: Crisis Intervention: Theory and Methodology, ed 7. Mosby, St. Louis, 1994.
4. Lindemann, E: Symptomatology and management of acute grief. Am J Psychiatry 10:141, 1944.
5. Selye, H: The Stress of Life. McGraw-Hill, Inc New York, 1954.
6. Baldwin, B: Crisis intervention: An overview. In Burgess, AW, and Baldwin, BA (eds): Crisis Intervention Theory and Practice. Prentice Hall, Englewood Cliffs, NJ, 1981, p 29.
7. Stevens, P: A critical social reconceptualization of environment in nursing: Implications for methodology. Advances in Nursing Science 11(4):56, 1989.
8. Janosik, E: Applied crisis theory. In Janosik, E (ed): Crisis Counseling: A Contemporary Approach. Jones and Bartlett, Boston, 1986.
9. Jacobson, G, Strickler, M, and Morley, W: Generic and individual approaches to crisis intervention. Am J Public Health 58:339, 1968.
10. Tyhurst, J: Role of transitional states—including disasters—in mental illness. Paper presented at Symposium on Preventative and Social Psychiatry, sponsored by Walter Reed Institute of Research, Walter Reed Medical Center and National Research Council, Washington, DC, April 15–17, 1957. US Government Printing Office.
11. Erikson, E: Children and Society. WW Norton & Co Inc, New York, 1963.
12. Weaver, J: Disasters: Mental Health Interventions. Professional Resource Press, Sarasota, Fla, 1995.
13. Frederick, C, and Garrison, J: Disaster and mental health: An overview. Behav Today, 12:32, 1981.
14. Arnold, E: Communicating with clients in crisis. In Arnold, E, and Boggs, K (eds): Interpersonal Relationships in Nursing. WB Saunders Company, Philadelphia, 1995, p. 491.
15. Caplan, G: Mastery of stress: Psychosocial aspects. Am J Psychiatry, 138:413, 1981.
16. Cohen, R: Training mental health professionals to work with families in diverse cultural contexts. In Austin, L (ed): Responding to Disaster: A Guide for Mental Health Professionals. American Psychiatric Press, Washington, DC, 1992.
17. Bateman, A: Access Barriers to Outpatient Mental Health Services for Individuals in Crisis. University Press, Amherst, Mass, 1993.

CHAPTER 9

Group Therapy and Therapeutic Groups

CHAPTER 9

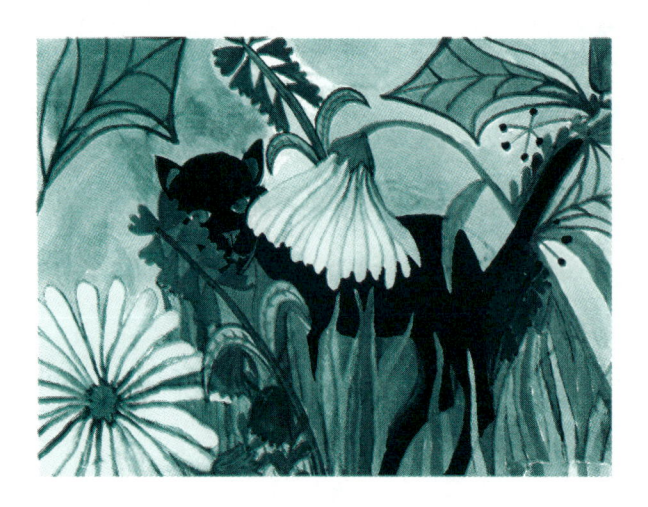

CHAPTER OUTLINE

Defining Group Therapy
Purpose of Group Therapy
   Therapeutic Factors
Creation of the Group
Group Purpose and Goals
   The Nurse's Role
   Membership Selection
   Group Environment
   Client Preparation for Group
Group Intervention Strategies
   Observing for Defensive Maneuvers
   Fostering Connections to Other Members
   Being Empathetic and Supportive
   Being Curious about Group Behavior
   Balancing Group-as-a-Whole Interpretations with Individual
      Interpretations
Stages of Group Development
   Initial Phase
   The Responsive Phase
   The Focused Phase
   The Termination Phase
Expected Outcomes
The Role of the Nurse in Group Therapy
   Educational Preparation
   Supervision
   Type of Group Leadership
   Leadership Styles
Areas for Future Research

Joyce Dagnal Shields, RN, MS, CS, CGP
Cindy Peternelj-Taylor, RN, MSc

Group Therapy and Therapeutic Groups

LEARNING OBJECTIVES

After completing this chapter, the reader should be able to:
- Define group therapy.
- Discuss the role of therapeutic factors as the mechanisms of change in therapeutic groups.
- Review issues related to the selection and preparation of clients for group therapy.
- Identify factors affecting group development.
- Describe the diversity of groups that the psychiatric–mental health nurse may work with in the clinical setting.
- Explain the role of the nurse in working with individuals in groups.
- Apply group concepts in the psychiatric–mental health milieu.
- Identify questions and clinical problems related to group therapy that require further nursing research.

KEY TERMS

consensual validation
group-as-a-whole
group content
group dynamics
group process
group therapy
norms

Group membership is a natural experience in the everyday lives of most human beings. Individuals are born into family groups, are educated in groups, worship in groups, and work, live, and socialize in groups. Individuals over the age of 5 are estimated to belong to an average of five or six groups.[1] Groups are essential to society; they provide a way of relating to other people and are a means through which tasks are accomplished.

Working with groups of clients is an integral component of both inpatient and outpatient psychiatric–mental health nursing. Understanding human behavior in general—and group process in particular—is essential for effective group leadership in the psychiatric–mental health milieu. This chapter provides an overview of group therapy as a treatment modality and highlights the types of groups that nurses usually work with, factors affecting group development, principles of group intervention, and the dynamic role of the nurse in responding to clients' needs in an ever-changing health-care system.

DEFINING GROUP THERAPY

In its simplest form, a group is three or more individuals who are to some degree interdependent. This interdependence—or coming together to achieve a task or a common goal—is what makes these individuals a group.[2] As members of society, nurses participate in groups. They may be members of a neighborhood watch, organized to keep their streets safe; they may be members of the home and school association to provide liaison between parents and the local school board; they may volunteer in an environmental group that reviews waste management in their local community.

As members of a profession, nurses may be actively involved in their professional association, an ad hoc multidisciplinary task force to study health-care reform, and, more commonly, work-related committees, such as the policy and procedure committee, continuous quality control committee, or a staff-development committee.

As mental health professionals, nurses have the privilege of working with clients individually and in groups. In general, **group therapy** can be broadly defined as a treatment modality for two or more individuals who meet on a regular, predetermined basis, with one or more therapists, for the purpose of achieving health-related goals. More specifically, group therapy is a helping process designed to explore psychiatric and emotional difficulties in order to bring about relief of symptoms, an increase in self-esteem and insight, and improvement of behavior and social relationships. Frequently, the focus of group therapy is interpersonal, cognitive, or behavioral changes.

Yalom[3] states that since group therapy was first introduced in the 1940s, it has grown and evolved, along with clinical practice. The number of groups in existence today complicates the search for a single definition of group therapy, and he chooses to speak of "group therapies" rather than group therapy as a singular entity. There are groups to assist individuals with eating disorders and cancer, survivors of sexual assault, adult children of alcoholics, clients with bipolar disorder, the confused elderly, the bereaved, those with chronic fatigue syndrome, and many others.

The settings of group therapy are also diverse: a group for convicted sexual offenders in a correctional facility is group therapy, as is a group for chronically mentally ill clients that meets weekly at the community mental health center. Groups may also be made up of professional women who meet with a therapist in private practice to cope with the stress of trying to be all things, to all people, all of the time.[3]

The theoretical orientations and the technical styles are also very different. Group therapists may practice from a cognitive-behavior model, a psychodynamic model, or a psychoeducational model. These and many others are included in group therapy.[3]

People also receive therapeutic benefits from self-help or mutual-help groups such as Alcoholics Anonymous (AA), the National Alliance for the Mentally Ill (NAMI), or Weight Watchers.[3]

PURPOSE OF GROUP THERAPY

Groups are frequently seen by managed-care companies as a more economical mode of intervention than individual therapy because therapists can see a larger number of clients at one time and thus use their time and energy more efficiently. For example, in a 1-hour period, a nurse could spend the whole hour teaching a variety of relaxation techniques to a small group of six clients, or the same nurse could spend 10 minutes with each client individually and attempt to cover the same material.

However, the primary purpose of group therapy as a treatment modality extends well beyond economics to the strength of the group itself. A group experience can be a meaningful forum for individuals to develop feelings of trust and connectedness to other human beings. Groups can be a refuge from the confusion, anxiety, and discouragement clients feel as they try to make sense of a complicated healthcare system that is focused on managed care. A group therapy experience can offer its members an opportunity to study defenses that are preventing them from achieving personal goals. A group experience is more multidimensional than the dyadic relationship and hence allows for further exploration of multiple perspectives, resulting in both primary (direct) and secondary (indirect) benefits to the client.[2-4]

Crane, Kirby, and Kooperman[5] developed an innovative medication management group to address the diverse needs of an inpatient psychiatric population. The primary purpose of the group was to deal with the problem of compliance with psychotropic medication. Sharing experiences in group resulted in secondary benefits to the group as a whole. Members helped each other by offering suggestions on coping with side effects and, more important, expressed their feelings related to the stigma surrounding mental illness and the need to take medication. Because of these reasons, a group experience is viewed as an extraordinarily powerful event that offers opportunities for change and growth in the lives of its members.

THERAPEUTIC FACTORS

Yalom[3] describes therapeutic change as a complicated process that occurs through the sophisticated interplay of human experiences. Intrinsic to all groups are 11 interdependent therapeutic factors that are the basic mechanisms of change (Box 9–1). Originally identified as "curative factors," they were renamed to reflect the change and growth that individuals can achieve through the interpersonal interaction of a group experience. Because of the uniqueness of the individuals participating in groups, all members may not perceive these factors equally. Likewise, depending on the type of group and its stage of development, some factors may appear more useful than others.

Instillation of Hope

Instillation and maintenance of hope are critical to the success of any therapy. By observing the progress of people who have experienced similar problems, group members gain confidence that their problems, too, can be resolved. Invariably, group members are at various points of wellness along the health continuum, and those who are having difficulties coping can be inspired by those who have benefited from the group experience. Group leaders who draw attention to the progress of group members can further enhance this therapeutic factor. Instillation of hope is critical to therapy and is significantly correlated with positive therapy outcomes. Group leaders need to do whatever they can to increase clients' belief and confidence in the efficacy of the group modality of treatment.[3]

Box 9–1. Yalom's Therapeutic Factors

1. Instillation of hope
2. Universality
3. Imparting information
4. Altruism
5. The corrective recapitulation of the primary family group
6. Development of socializing techniques
7. Imitative behaviors
8. Interpersonal learning
9. Group cohesiveness
10. Catharsis
11. Existential factors

Source: Yalom, ID: The Theory and Practice of Group Psychotherapy (ed 4). Basic Books, New York, 1995.

Universality

Through the support and understanding of others in the group who share similar thoughts, feelings, and experiences, members come to realize that they are not alone and that their problems are not unique. Simply knowing that others are in the same boat relieves clients and reduces their feelings of isolation and anxiety. Although universality is an important concept in individual therapy, group therapy provides more opportunities for **consensual validation** because of the number of people sharing experiences within the group.[3]

Imparting Information

Formal and informal learning occurs in groups. Information may be taught with aids or shared more informally by giving advice. Advice among group members is inevitable and appears to be more helpful as a series of alternative suggestions about how to achieve a goal than as a direct suggestion.[3]

Altruism

Through helping others in group, members experience therapeutic benefits. Human beings need to feel they are needed and useful, and group members receive personal rewards through the genuine act of giving. By learning that they can be useful by offering support, reassurance, suggestions, and insight, members experience self-growth and increased self-esteem.[3]

Corrective Recapitulation of the Family Group

Everyone's behavior is influenced more or less by past family experiences. After members overcome the initial apprehension of being in a therapy group, interactions among group members frequently resemble patterns of communication with significant figures such as parents, siblings, teachers, and peers. Group therapy resembles a family in many respects because of the presence of authority figures (parents), group peers (siblings), and intense emotional responses, including intimacy, hostility, and competitiveness. In therapy, patterns of dysfunctional behavior are identified, evaluated, and changed through feedback and exploration.[3]

Development of Socializing Techniques

Interacting with others in a group setting ultimately produces social learning. Social learning is often explicit, as in the case of a social skills training group for seriously and persistently mentally ill clients. Conversely, social learning may be an indirect result of membership in a group that promotes open feedback, resulting in considerable information about the maladaptive behaviors of group members. Through feedback and role playing, two common techniques used to promote social skill development, members often develop very sophisticated social skills.[3]

Imitative Behavior

In a group setting, the imitative process is much more diffuse than individual therapy because of the number of people who may serve as potential role models. In addition to the group leader, an individual who has mastered a particular skill or developmental task can be an invaluable role model for others. Although this therapeutic factor appears to be more important in the earlier stages of therapy, individuals may imitate selective behaviors that they wish to develop in themselves throughout therapy. Furthermore, clients may gain therapeutic benefit vicariously by witnessing the therapy of another individual with similar problems. This phenomenon is sometimes referred to as *spectator therapy*.[3]

Interpersonal Learning

The group experience offers many opportunities for interacting with others. Interpersonal learning occurs in two ways: feedback from others in the group or insight into oneself. Insight is gained not only by how one perceives but also by how one is perceived by others. Through giving and receiving feedback and gaining insight into themselves, members learn to identify, clarify, and modify maladaptive behaviors. This learning that occurs in groups can easily be modified to other aspects of clients' lives, enabling them to give to others, trust others, and assert themselves.[3]

Group Cohesiveness

Cohesiveness is the sense of belonging that separates the individual (I am) from the group (we are). From it comes the common feeling that both individual members and the total group are of value to each other. Cohesiveness, or the glue that holds groups together, can further be defined as all the forces that influence members to stay in the group. It is enhanced when members feel they are an important part of the group, that their contributions are valued, and that the group work is purposeful.[3]

Catharsis

Simply stated, *catharsis* is the release of intense emotions. In group therapy, members are encouraged to express positive and negative emotions within the safety of the group. This open expression of feelings benefits the individual and the group; individually, members experience the immediate relief that catharsis can bring, and collectively group members learn that they can express their emotions and survive. This therapeutic factor is particularly effective when followed by insight and behavior change.[3]

Existential Factors

Group members learn that loneliness, death, and the meaning of human existence are issues common to all human

> **RESEARCH NOTE**
>
> Hastings-Vertino, K, Getty, C, and Wooldridge, P: Development of a tool to measure therapeutic factors in group process. Arch Psychiatr Nurs 10(4):221–228, 1996.
>
> **Findings:** Group therapy, long considered an efficient and effective means of therapeutic intervention, is based on the premise that the interactional processes within the group are the most important means by which therapeutic changes in group members can be promoted. In response to the need to measure therapeutic aspects of group process in various client groups and across a variety of treatment settings, the Therapeutic Group Interaction Factors Scale (TGIF) was developed to systematically and objectively measure the extent to which Yalom's therapeutic factors are present or absent.
>
> Yalom's conceptualization of therapeutic factors was selected as the framework. Operational criteria including verbal and behavioral indicators were developed to identify therapeutic and nontherapeutic occurrences for each of the 11 factors. A score of +2, +1, 0, −1, or −2 is assigned to each session for each factor based on evaluation of the content expressed (individual and group), taking into account both the amount of content salient to the factor in question and the degree to which therapeutic (positive scores) and nontherapeutic (negative scores) behaviors are dominant.
>
> Two pilot applications of the TGIF are reported. In the first, 10 sessions of a support group for persons with work-related injuries were evaluated; the second was conducted on a nurse-facilitated "psychosocial club."
>
> From these pilot applications, the researchers concluded that the TGIF has high face validity; however, only preliminary tests of its reliability and validity have been conducted.
>
> Although deemed very useful, further refinement and testing are necessary. Recommendations for further use include using two or more raters who (1) are familiar with Yalom's work, (2) receive training in the use of the tool, and (3) concurrently observe and rate the group phenomena.
>
> **Application to Practice:** With continued refinement of this tool, psychiatric–mental health nurses who work as leaders or facilitators of therapeutic groups will be able to study the relationship between Yalom's therapeutic factors and therapeutic outcomes of the group more objectively, rather than relying solely on participants' subjective evaluation of the contribution of each factor. The tool has potential in collaborative interdisciplinary education and research because Yalom's theoretical framework is widely known by mental health professionals. In addition, the researchers conclude that the TGIF is an easy and useful way of keeping track of the prominent aspects of each group session and of making process assessments of the quality of the therapy provided.

beings. Through group membership, individuals learn to take direction for their own lives and to accept responsibility for the quality of their existence.[3]

Nurses must recognize that these therapeutic factors are present to varying degrees in all groups, regardless of the type of group, the setting, the clinical disorder, or the theoretical orientation of the leader. These factors help to explain how people change in groups and offer ways for the group leader to use the **group process** to therapeutic advantage.

CREATION OF THE GROUP

The meaning of therapeutic factors and their significance to clients cannot be underestimated in planning and developing group modalities of treatment. The effectiveness of the group depends a great deal on the conditions surrounding its creation—the practical or structural variables that need to be taken into account.

GROUP PURPOSE AND GOALS

The function of a group depends on the reason the group was formed. The purpose of the group is the foundation or the infrastructure of the group's existence. It facilitates the establishment of group goals, the structure required to attain the goals, and norms that are consistent with the group's purpose. Knowing the focus of the group enables the nurse to make realistic plans; intervention strategies are significantly different for an activity group, for example, than for a psychotherapy group.[6]

After the purpose of the group is clearly established, the goals of the group can be developed to meet the needs of the individual and the group as a whole. Group goals need to be achievable, measurable, and within the capabilities of the group members. Identifying the goals as either long-term or short-term assists with establishing the time frame and type of membership. Furthermore, the goals of the group vary according to the theoretical orientation of the group.

A model for conducting a psychodynamic therapy group for assaultive men was developed by Lanza and associates[7] to help clients (1) identify, understand, and deal with underlying problems resulting in aggressive behavior; (2) improve interpersonal relationships; and (3) find more appropriate ways of expressing feelings.

In contrast, a psychoeducation workshop, designed to help family members living with mental illness, is described by Peternelj-Taylor and Hartley.[8] It was planned (1) to provide families with information about mental illness, including treatment options; (2) to provide liaison with community resources; and (3) to provide a forum to foster mutual support among workshop participants.

A clearly defined purpose facilitates appropriate group goals and provides a sound rationale for the group's existence.

THE NURSE'S ROLE

Psychiatric–mental health nurses can be involved in therapy groups and other types of groups. For the purposes of this chapter, groups are discussed under the following headings:
- Activity groups
- Teaching and behavioral change groups
- Psychotherapy groups
- Peer-support groups
- Self-help groups

Activity Groups

Activity groups facilitate patient communication and interaction and are common in the inpatient milieu and long-term community setting. Clients who are experiencing acute symptoms of their illness or are withdrawn or regressed can benefit a great deal from activity groups. The more emotionally disabled a client is, the more structured the group must be. Clients in activity groups tend to respond best to the structure of a regular time, place, and purpose clearly defined at the outset of the group. Activity groups also require an actively involved group leader; if the leader is neutral or silent, clients may seek shelter in their delusions or hallucinations or withdraw interpersonally from the group. The goals of activity groups include increasing clients' self-esteem, decreasing social isolation, and improving interpersonal communication[2,3] (Box 9–2).

The types of activity groups in which nurses can be involved are limited only by their imaginations. Common activity groups include the following:
- Arts and crafts groups
- Storytelling group therapy
- Current events groups
- Leisure skills groups
- Remotivation therapy groups

CASE STUDY

A psychotherapy group of eight members has been running for 3 years. Six of the members started when the group began, and two members joined 5 months ago. Although originally designed to be a coed group, all group members are female because the therapist has not had male referrals to the group. The group therapist is a clinical nurse specialist in private practice. Group members have consented to be observed through a two-way mirror by undergraduate students in psychiatric–mental health nursing. The stated purpose of the group is to enhance the group members' abilities to build and maintain interpersonal relationships and to increase their capacity for intimacy. One member recently left after being part of the group for 2 years, and a new member is present tonight for her first meeting.

Abigail P, a 38-year-old single woman, is chronically unemployed. The referring therapist described her as an extremely self-centered and self-absorbed individual who has long-term depression unresponsive to medication. Experiments with massage therapy and acupuncture to alleviate her anxiety have been only moderately successful. When she joined the group 5 months ago, she was chronically late and stated that she had struggled with this problem "all of her life." Her mother used to write notes to her teachers stating Abigail could be expected at school "when she decided to arrive." Her lateness to group ended after 3 weeks when the group reminded her that a commitment to be on time was a part of the contract in the group. She was pleased to gain some mastery of this problem, which had alienated her all her life from friends. Her father, a "distant intellectual," owns a very successful printing company. Her mother is an avid reader and a homemaker. Abigail was raised by a nanny and has one brother who is an accountant in Colorado. He avoids visiting his parents as much as possible because it is "too smothering there." She often says it doesn't matter who is present at group because she is willing to talk to "anyone who will listen." She has few friends and says men like her because she can "afford to pay their way."

Karen S, a 33-year-old nursing supervisor, was recently divorced and has sole custody of her 7-year-old son. When she was 10 years old, her brother died of an "accident." He was struck by a car on a major highway after wandering away from a psychiatric hospital where he had been a patient for 3 weeks. No one in her family ever discusses this incident (most likely a suicide). Karen is the only member of her family who does not live in her home state. Her father, a very successful physician who died of a heart attack 6 years ago, was a demanding man who expected a lot of attention from his children. Her mother, who worked at home caring for her six brothers and sisters, is still alive, but she and Karen are not particularly close. A sister with whom she is very close recently confided that she is a lesbian. All her brothers and sisters are successful as lawyers, graphic artists, teachers, and financial consultants. All have some degree of depression, but few have sought treatment. Karen is bright, attractive, and very talented as a nursing supervisor. However, she tends to deal with painful emotions with actions and feels exhausted most of the time. Her son was recently diagnosed as having attention-deficit/hyperactivity disorder (ADHD) and is in therapy with a psychologist. She had been in individual therapy with the group leader for 3 years but currently is participating only in group therapy. She has a new boyfriend she rarely discusses in group.

Aimee W, a 33-year-old single woman, lives alone and is currently employed as a researcher. She has a history of chronic depression dating back to her early 20s. She tends to have chronic problems at work and typically feels "unnoticed and unappreciated by her boss." She grew up in an unsettled environment. When Aimee was 17 years old, her mother was raped in her home by an intruder. Aimee claims that her house was "never the same after that event." Her mother, who never received any form of counseling following the rape, continues to have problems coping with everyday events and is frequently depressed. Her father is an alcoholic who has been physically and emotionally abusive to her. Aimee experienced severe panic attacks and was treated with medication and individual therapy with a social worker, thereby avoiding inpatient hospitalization. She had difficulty participating in individual therapy and remained depressed. She was referred to the group when individual therapy was at an impasse. Over the course of several years in group, she has learned that she is very vague in describing how she feels, and when she does, she rarely feels she is understood. The group has encouraged her to be more specific about what she needs from them. She always sits beside the group therapist and tends to look to her rather than to the group members when she makes comments.

Gerri D, a 36-year-old single woman with a master's degree in business administration, works part-time as a marketing consultant. Her father, to whom she was very close, died 8 years ago, leaving her independently wealthy. She is not close to her mother, who is "impossible" to live with because of her self-centered and self-righteous attitude. Gerri has a long history of depression and has made a great deal of progress in individual therapy with a psychologist she had seen for 8 years. She joined the group several years ago and overall has experienced fewer symptoms of depression. She used to talk a great deal to mask her anxiety. Only once in group did she discuss a man she was dating.

Marilyn L, a 54-year-old married mother of eight, is employed as a legal secretary. She has a long history of migraine headaches, depression, and panic attacks (treated with alprazolam [Xanax], on which she became dependent). She started individual therapy with the group leader, and the panic attacks and the migraines stopped. Unfortunately, she periodically continues to struggle with depression. Her mother was a nurse who worked nights, leaving Marilyn responsible for taking care of her sister and brother and for keeping the house quiet during the day while her mother slept. She was close to her dad, who had depression but never sought treatment. She states that she has a "1950s kind of marriage" where the woman is expected to manage the household and the husband works outside the home. She often passively comments that her husband forgets that she also has a job. Her 27- and 29-year-old sons have both divorced and moved back home; members are constantly chastising her for doing their laundry. While in group, she was able to sign up for her own credit card and drive alone to her summer house in Vermont. For her, these are monumental accomplishments. She feels the group gives her "independence." She has just decided to leave the group to care for her sister who has terminal breast cancer.

Caroline K, a 34-year-old single lesbian, has a long history of depression beginning in adolescence and peaking in young adulthood, when she began to abuse drugs and alcohol. She is employed as an account executive but struggles with chronic job dissatisfaction; she always discovers that her bosses are "totally inadequate." She has had a series of unsatisfying lesbian relationships in which she typically feels alone, isolated, and generally "taken advantage of financially and emotionally." During individual therapy with the group leader, she became suicidal after a breakup with her lover. Hospitalization was averted with intensive individual therapy and a short course of antidepressants. She decided to join the group to decrease her isolation and enhance her ability to build closer interpersonal connections. She has a rather distant mother whom she refers to as the "ice queen" and a father, a wealthy entrepreneur who is frequently verbally abusive to her. She states, "He casts a spell of control over me that I can't ignore." She has never discussed being lesbian with her family, although she thinks it is "a given that everyone ignores." Likewise in group, she has never disclosed that she is lesbian. The group frequently notices that she unconsciously rolls her eyes to defuse the power of any of the interpretations made by the group therapist. She and Marilyn always comment that they started group on the same night and were "there when the group first began." She is always present for all group meetings, except when on vacation. She recently decided to leave the group and terminated over 5 weeks.

Megan J, a 38-year-old recently divorced mother of a 9-year-old son. Her ex-husband suffered from posttraumatic stress disorder following the Vietnam War. His parents were both alcoholics and frequently depressed. Her parents were very strict Irish Catholics who insisted that she shine her "white buck" shoes every day. She experiences some mild depression, which is overshadowed by a very obsessional character style. When Megan was a child, other parents in the neighborhood would send their children to her house for discipline from Megan's mother. They felt that Megan and her sister were "perfect...never out of line." They hoped their children would be the same. She is a very competent office manager in the legal department of a large teaching hospital. Her dad was a police officer who worked long hours. Megan misses him and feels he loved her more than her mother, who was often unhappy and depressed. She has been in individual therapy with the group leader for about 2 years and is managing her divorce reasonably well. She wishes to be less socially anxious and more comfortable with intimacy. She has completed her individual therapy and has joined the group for the first time. She is attractive, articulate, and always well dressed.

Anna S, a 38-year-old, very competent intensive care nurse, is overweight and chronically depressed. She deals with her depression by working long hours and avoids social relationships outside work hours. She is unable to set limits on the numerous requests made of her to increase her professional responsibilities. She is estranged from her mother, who has been both physically and emotional abusive to her throughout her life. Her father died of a heart attack when she was 10 years old. Although she has had a long history of chronic depression with occasional suicidal ideation, she has made a great deal of progress in her individual therapy with a male psychiatrist. Initially she was skeptical about joining group and annoyed at her therapist for suggesting that she join. Since joining, she states that she is less depressed. Group helps her with her feelings of loneliness and isolation, and she sees the group as an antidote for her depression. Most recently, she has rewritten her job description and delegated some of her responsibilities to her staff.

CASE STUDY QUESTIONS

1. What effect does the absence of male members in this group have on each of the members? What effect does it have on the group as a whole? How might the group leader deal with this?
2. Describe the ways in which the group members are well matched as a group. In what ways are they poorly matched?
3. Which members of the group are most likely to pair off unconsciously? What might be the reasons for this?
4. What hypotheses do you have regarding the reasons why Marilyn and Caroline left the group?
5. Which member would be difficult for you to have in group? Discuss.

Teaching and Behavioral Change Groups

The primary concern of teaching and behavioral change groups is to affect the health behavior of clients by helping them deal effectively with their life problems and emotional distress. These groups center around group relations, interactions among group members, and the consideration of a selected issue. Frequently they are time limited or of a fixed duration; for example, an assertiveness group might meet 2 hours per week for 8 weeks. In teaching and behavioral change groups, members learn not only from the group leader but also from one another. The likelihood of clients following through with behavior change is often enhanced when clients commit to a change within the group setting[4] (see Box 9–2).

Clients across the continuum of health-care settings—from traditional inpatient units to independent community living—can benefit immensely from these groups. Information learned in the safety of the group can assist clients to function more comfortably and effectively in their personal lives. Many of the groups psychiatric–mental health nurses run fall into these categories:

- Social skills training groups
- Stress management groups
- Medication management groups
- Illness management groups

Psychotherapy Groups

The goal of psychotherapy groups is treatment of emotional, cognitive, or behavioral dysfunction. In these groups, clients develop an understanding of and insight into their thoughts, feelings, behaviors, and roles in social relationships. How the goals of psychotherapy groups are stated depends on the theoretical orientation and educational preparation of the therapist. Loomis[4] observes that psychiatric–mental health nurses are particularly good psychotherapists because of their ability to integrate biopsychosocial perspectives into the holistic care of clients in groups. Although the objective of group psychotherapy is insight orientation, behavioral change, or both, psychotherapy is most successful in clients who want to develop awareness of their problems and who are motivated and willing to change (see Box 9–2). Psychotherapy groups that nurses may be familiar to include:

- Psychodynamic group therapy
- Cognitive-behavior group therapy
- Insight-oriented therapy

Self-Help Groups

In self-help groups, members share the same problem and help each other by offering support and encouragement. These groups may or may not have a professional leader or consultant; they are frequently run by the members, with rotating leadership responsibilities. Although these are not formal therapy groups per se, they straddle the blurred boundaries between personal growth, support, education,

---

Box 9–2. Goals of Therapeutic Groups

Activity Groups
- Development of socialization techniques
- Imitative behavior
- Imparting of information
- Interpersonal learning

Teaching and Behavioral Change Groups
- Imparting information
- Imitative behavior
- Instillation of hope
- Universality
- Development of socialization techniques
- Group cohesiveness

Psychotherapy Groups
- Instillation of hope
- Universality
- Interpersonal learning
- Group cohesiveness
- Catharsis
- Existential factors
- Corrective recapitulation of the primary family group

Peer Support Groups
- Universality
- Group cohesiveness
- Existential factors
- Imparting of information

Self-help Groups
- Instillation of hope
- Universality
- Altruism
- Imparting of information

---

and therapy and provide many therapeutic benefits for group members.[3]

Nurses may become involved with self-help groups voluntarily or because they have been asked by group members. Three ways that nurses can foster self-help are (1) helping clients identify and share effective coping strategies, (2) consistently giving clients the message that they are the masters of their own destiny, and (3) acting as a liaison between organized self-help and the professional mental health system.[9] The roles of the nurse in self-help groups include referral agent, resource person, member of an advisory board, leader, co-leader, or group facilitator.

When referring clients to self-help groups, the nurse needs to be informed about the purpose of the group, membership criteria, leadership, benefits, and any potential problems the client might experience. Lego[10] reports that many individuals are drawn to support groups because they are tired of dealing with the "system" and prefer to help themselves. The upsurge of managed care may contribute further to the number of people looking for self-help groups. Well-known self-help groups include the following:

- Alcoholics Anonymous (AA)
- Narcotics Anonymous (NA)
- National Alliance for the Mentally Ill
- Overeaters Anonymous (OA)

Peer Support Groups

Peer support groups are becoming increasingly popular. These groups can be very effective ways for professionals to share stresses and work-related problems. Nurses in private practice, who may at times feel professionally isolated, may join a peer support group for the purpose of case consulting, sharing educational opportunities, and providing business information.[10a] Conversely, peer support groups may meet to deal with the emotional turmoil and stress created by the nature of nursing. A group of palliative care nurses may meet formally or informally to discuss their feelings and offer each other support in coping with the grief and multiple losses in their work. Likewise, leaders of groups that work with survivors of childhood sexual assault frequently feel the need for support and encouragement from others who are able to comprehend both the sensitivity and the intensity of the material discussed in groups (Box 9–2).

MEMBERSHIP SELECTION

Membership selection, sometimes referred to as *group composition*, is the first and perhaps most important task of the group leader or therapist. It depends on the type of group, its purpose, and its objectives. In general, group therapists concur that clients with adequate ego integrity and healthy defenses can benefit immensely from the group experience, because of their ability to (1) form a therapeutic alliance with the therapist and (2) process the meaning of their conflicts within the group, with both the therapist and peers.

Homogeneous versus Heterogeneous Groups

Group membership may be described as homogeneous or heterogeneous. In a *homogeneous group*, all members share preselected criteria. For example, all members are men who have problems managing their anger[7] or elderly clients participating in a life experiences group.[11] Group therapy for trauma survivors is most beneficial when the other clients are survivors with similar backgrounds and similar symptoms.[12] Cohesion is often enhanced in homogeneous groups because members quickly identify with each other. Furthermore, members are in a better position to confront each others' dysfunctional behaviors because of their firsthand knowledge of the situation. A potential hazard in homogeneous groups is that members sometimes see themselves only in the context of their disorder and avoid any deeper exploration of their problems.

In *heterogeneous groups*, members share an essential characteristic, such as alcoholism, but age, sex, education, and family background vary significantly. Some authors argue that cohesion, or the groups' ability to "gel," should serve as the primary guide for selection of group members; others focus on a similar level of interpersonal development. Heterogeneous groups more accurately mirror the real world, and members should be specifically chosen to provide demographic variation.[3]

However, a commonsense approach must prevail in the pursuit to select the ideal group. One-of-a-kind characteristics, such as gender, race, or significant differences in age, can serve to isolate an individual within a group. In such cases, select at least two individuals who share the common characteristic, for example, two males in an otherwise all female group.[13]

Cultural Considerations

The cultural background of individual members is an important factor. Members of ethnic and racial minorities make up approximately 22% of the American population. Communication, in general, varies greatly between cultures, and differences may be noted in an individual's use of the spoken language, vocalizations, and body language. Cultural groups vary in their use of space, gestures, facial expression, eye contact, and listening style. Clients who speak English as a second language often require more time to process group communication, particularly when they are anxious or tense. Nurses need to model respect for multiple perspectives in group; however, cultural differences may lead to misunderstandings among group members and impede group functioning.[14]

The Acutely Ill Client

Clients who are experiencing acute symptoms of illness, such as hallucinations, delusions, or confusion related to dementia, are not good candidates for insight-oriented group therapy. A mixture of clients who are acutely agitated or psychotic and those who have progressed to later stages of treatment is often unmanageable for the group leader. However, structured task-oriented groups, such as activity groups, community meetings, and remotivation therapy groups, where the goals are more readily comprehended, can be a bridge to reality for the acutely ill client.[15,16]

Open versus Closed Groups

Deciding whether a group is open or closed should be determined prior to screening potential group members. In a closed group, no new members are added after the group has started. Conversely, in an open group, members can be added at any time. Consistency of leadership, norms, and expectations are among the advantages of a closed group. However, the addition of new members can be like a breath of fresh air as they come with new ideas and new insights.

GROUP ENVIRONMENT

Physical Arrangements

The actual physical environment can have a profound effect on the group's overall functioning. Regardless of the type of group, the right atmosphere requires a location that can meet the overall needs of the group. Although the reality of the practice setting often dictates where groups are held, factors to consider include the furnishings, the room temperature, appropriate lighting, space, sound, privacy, and geographic location. A room that is too cold or too hot is a barrier to learning that limits member participation. A "Please do not disturb" or "Meeting in Session" sign can prevent unwanted intruders from disrupting the group.[6] Seating in most psychotherapy groups allows for maximum exposure of each member within the group, and chairs arranged in a circle is the most common seating arrangement. Classrooms with fixed seating are inappropriate for a psychotherapy group but fine for a teaching and behavioral change group, particularly if participants are required to take notes.

Stigma surrounding mental illness is still so profound that attendance may be enhanced when meetings are held in "neutral" locations such as church halls or community recreation facilities. Likewise, a family support group may choose to meet away from the hospital rather than face the constant reminder of how devastating mental illness can be.

Resources

The available resources influence the group's ability to meet its objectives. Often, teaching and behavioral change groups use teaching materials. Some may need only a blackboard or flip chart; others require an overhead projector, camcorder, television, or videocassette recorder. Social skills training groups often videotape members during sessions to (1) provide immediate feedback to clients and (2) serve as a reference point to evaluate a particular client's progress. Additionally, with client permission, audio or video recordings may be used for the therapist's professional supervision. Regardless of the type of group, it is the group leader's responsibility to ensure that all the required equipment or materials are present and in proper working order.

Group Size

The size of the group is determined by the type of group, the skill of the therapist, the presence of a co-therapist, and the behavior of the members. Most group therapists would agree that the ideal size for interpersonally oriented groups is 8 to 10 members. Groups of this size promote a sense of participation and allow for consensual validation and member-to-member interaction. If the group is too large, there may not be time for all members to take part, and then only the most verbal or aggressive members engage in the group process.

Conversely, if the group is too small, interactions decrease, and the group leader may be conducting individual therapy within the context of the group. Insufficient sharing robs members of the multiple perspectives necessary to analyze or discuss group interactions. In small groups, anxiety can increase because of the perceived pressure to perform. Education groups and many support groups can function effectively with large numbers of people.

Frequency of Meetings

The duration of the group and the length of the sessions vary according to the type of group, its purpose and goals, the setting (inpatient versus outpatient), and the members themselves. Meeting times must be selected to promote regular attendance. Running groups on an inpatient unit is distinctly different from running a group on an outpatient basis with fully motivated, less acutely ill clients. Groups designed for acutely ill or chronically ill clients (sometimes referred to as *lower functioning* groups) may be scheduled to meet daily for 20 to 40 minutes. Some problems specific to inpatient units are identified in Box 9–3.

For higher functioning groups, like psychotherapy groups that meet on an outpatient basis, 60 to 120 minutes once a week may be necessary for members to share and discuss their experiences within the group. Consistently beginning and ending group according to the mutually agreed-on time further contributes to an atmosphere of trust and predictability. Groups may be time limited and meet only for 6 weeks and then disband, or the group may meet for several years, like a classic psychotherapy group.

Suggested guidelines for developing a group proposal are identified in Box 9–4.

Box 9–3. Problems Indigenous to Inpatient Groups

- Client turnover is considerable. Many clients attend the group meetings for only one or two meetings, preventing planned termination; discharge occurs as soon as the client is out of the acute phase of illness, resulting in someone terminating almost every meeting.
- There is little therapist stability. Many of the therapists have rotating schedules and cannot attend all group meetings, thereby limiting continuity of care.
- The group therapist has little time to screen or prepare the clients for group, thereby limiting control over group composition.
- A greater heterogeneity of psychopathology exists. Clients of varying ages manifesting various signs and symptoms of illness are all present in the same group.
- Frequently, groups are made up of many unmotivated clients who are psychologically unsophisticated, who do not want to be in groups, or who do not agree that they even need therapy.
- There is often little sense of cohesion in the group; not enough time exists for members to learn to care for or trust one another.
- Group therapy is only one of the many therapies in which the client participates; some of their activities are with the same clients, and often with the same nurse. They frequently see their therapist in other roles throughout the day.

Source: Adapted from Yalom, ID: Inpatient Group Psychotherapy. Basic Books, New York, 1983, p 50.

> **Box 9–4. Guidelines for a Group Proposal**
>
> 1. Name the proposed group. Identify the need for this group.
> 2. List the purpose of the group.
> 3. Identify the group leader.
> 4. Describe the theoretical orientation that will be used by the group leader.
> 5. Make an assessment.
>   - What are the client needs?
>   - How can a group meet these needs?
>   - State the objectives for the group.
>   - What are the expectations of the system relative to the group?
>   - What resources will be needed for the group?
> 6. Determine group structure.
>   - What is the location of the group?
>   - When will the group meet, and for how long?
>   - What is the duration of the group?
>   - Define the roles and responsibilities for the leader and the members.
> 7. Decide on evaluation methods.
>   - How will the effectiveness of the group be evaluated?
>   - What criteria will be used to measure individual outcomes?

CLIENT PREPARATION FOR GROUP

Preparing clients for the group experience is of utmost importance. Most group therapists meet with prospective clients one to three times in a pregroup interview, with each client individually, or with several new members in a group setting.[17]

During these meetings, the client and therapist explore how the group modality of treatment may benefit the client. The therapist takes a careful history and explores the client's personal goals for joining the group. By meeting with the group therapist, clients have the opportunity to address some of their anxiety and to determine their interest in pursuing a working relationship with the therapist. Discussing the client's previous experiences with groups in general (for example, therapy, work, or school) can unmask some of the tension the client may feel upon beginning group therapy.

> During a pregroup interview, Donald asks the therapist if there will be any beautiful women in the group. When the therapist responds by asking, "What if there are?" Donald discusses his tendency to become easily distracted from his personal goals by becoming overly flirtatious. When the therapist explores this concern further, she learns that Donald's mother, a beautiful woman who abandoned him emotionally, is the center of many issues in Donald's life. At the end of the interview, he feels quite relieved to have discussed his anxiety before entering the group.

Each therapist develops a style of dealing with the pregroup phase of group treatment. As much time as possible should be taken in the pregroup interviews to answer a client's questions, address the client's anxiety, review the group contract, examine the client's readiness to undertake this type of therapy, and briefly explain how the group works. On completion of a pregroup interview, both the client and the nurse should be able to state clearly what they expect from each other and how they will evaluate progress. The nurse will have a beginning relationship with the client that can be transferred to the group setting and a plan for how to work with the client within the group. An individual who is unable to make a commitment to the group at the time of the pregroup interview is unlikely to come to the group.

The Group Contract

When group members and the leader know what to expect from each other, they have the beginning of a group contract. Group therapy contracts facilitate the activities of the group by outlining the formal conditions for the group. The process of developing a contract for a therapy group begins with the selection and preparation of group members, evolves, and is renegotiated throughout the life of the group. Written contracts legitimize the components of the contract and provide clients with concrete information they can keep. As a reference point, the contract can measure the group's progress. In general, the following elements of the contract are introduced at the time of the pregroup interview:

- Goals and purposes of the group
- Location, time, and frequency of the meetings
- Statement regarding the addition of new members
- Attendance expectations
- Roles and responsibilities of group members
- Statement regarding fee schedule
- Statement of confidentiality

Contracts are tailored to address the features unique to a particular group. A limit-setting contract about physical violence or touching within group may be required in a psychodynamic group developed to treat aggressive male inpatients[7] (Box 9–5).

Confidentiality. Confidentiality is a universal norm in all therapy groups and is fundamental to effective group functioning. Members need to feel secure that their identities and the contents of their discussions will be protected and that any violation of this rule requires the permission of the group. In comparison to the health-care professional, clients may not have the same understanding of the ethics of confidentiality. The following statement can assist clients to appreciate how to broach this topic: "What you see in here, what you say in here, stays in here, when you are not in here." The **group content** also needs to be kept in confidence, and clients can sometimes get caught up in the "sensationalism" of the disclosures.

Frequently, the therapist's employer requires documen-

> **Box 9–5. Sample Group Contract**
>
> 1. To be present each week, to be on time, and to remain for the duration of each group meeting.
> 2. To actively work on the problems that brought you to group.
> 3. To put feelings into words, not actions.
> 4. To use the relationships made in the group for therapeutic purposes and not social purposes.
> 5. To remain in the group until the problems that brought you to group have been resolved.
> 6. To be responsible for your bills.
> 7. To protect the names and identities of group members.
>
> **Source:** Rutan, JS, and Stone, WN: Psychodynamic Group Psychotherapy. Guilford Press, New York, 1993.

tation of the individual's progress in group, and any client concerns regarding who will have access to information need to be explored. Clients may also have their own issues and concerns about confidentiality that need to be addressed. Mutually agreed-on rules can be incorporated into the group contract.

GROUP INTERVENTION STRATEGIES

The therapeutic communication skills the group leader uses in group are not necessarily unique to the group setting; rather, they are similar to those of individual therapy. Within the formal therapeutic context of the group, group therapists use basic principles of interpersonal communication. The difference lies in the numbers of interactions that are possible. Bryant, cited by Ormont,[18] observes that:

> Two people in a conversation really amount to four people talking. The four are what one person says, what he wanted to say, what his listener heard, and what he thought he heard. Multiply this by ten or so group members, and there is so much going on that even the great Indian mathematician Ramanujon could spend a lifetime unable to summarize the number of interactions in a group, real and imagined.

For this reason, beginning therapists need to keep interventions simple and allow the process to unfold. One fascinating aspect of group treatment is the variety of ways the same leader is treated by different groups. Discerning their various roles in group helps members understand their past experiences as members in other important groups, such as their families.

Before strategies are chosen, the purpose of the group and the nature of its membership need to be taken into consideration. Some specific intervention strategies common to group therapy are observing for defensive maneuvers, fostering connections with other members, being empathetic and supportive, being curious about group behavior, and balancing **group-as-a-whole** interpretations with individual interpretations.

OBSERVING FOR DEFENSIVE MANEUVERS

In developing a sense of the defense mechanisms that members in the group use and assisting them in being curious, the therapist is guided by the question: "How does this defense mechanism block the individual from achieving his or her goal of building and maintaining relationships?" By adding these data to the history of each individual, the therapist can help each member develop insight into his or her internal life.

Monopolizing

Monopolizing is a common defense mechanism in groups. It can be understood as an attempt to avoid both fear and the wish to be the center of attention. The client who monopolizes the group session may talk incessantly because of underlying anxiety or because of a domineering and controlling personality. Monopolizers are often late, infuriating other members further. Other clients may feel that they do not have the opportunity to participate and may be reluctant to speak up or confront the individual who is monopolizing the group's time. The approach taken depends on the type of group. In an activity group or teaching and behavioral change group, the leader may simply respond by thanking the client for his or her input and asking for other's input. In a psychotherapy group, wondering why the group is allowing itself to be monopolized may be more important. The goal of intervention is not to silence the monopolizer but to hear from more of the group.

FOSTERING CONNECTIONS TO OTHER MEMBERS

Helping members make connections to one another is a useful intervention. Instead of answering a question directly, the therapist may redirect the question to the group for discussion. Frequently, members ask a lot of questions of other members but really haven't joined the group. Their behavior is often an effort to avoid exploring how they feel about being in the group and a way of deflecting the focus from themselves onto other members.

> Abbey says very little about herself in group but tends to interview other group members. She repeatedly asks others if they "feel alienated? . . . feel guilty? . . . feel lonely?"

The leader can ask, "Is this a subject you might know something about?" This question allows the member an opportunity to explain the source of his or her expertise on guilt, anxiety, or shame, elaborate on his or her past experiences, and link them to what may be happening in the group.

BEING EMPATHETIC AND SUPPORTIVE

The task of the group therapist is to help individuals build and maintain meaningful relationships. Empathy is the heart of that process and necessary to create an environment that is safe for all group members.

BEING CURIOUS ABOUT GROUP BEHAVIOR

For many individuals in group therapy, little curiosity existed in their family of origin, frequently because of severe depression or alcoholism of primary caregivers. Shapiro[19] observes:

> In many families where individuals manifest severe personal problems, the members have a striking lack of curiosity about one another. Instead, they are often remarkably certain that they know, understand, and can speak for other family members without further discussions. If individual members attempt to challenge assertions about who they are, they encounter bland denial, unshakable conviction, or platitudinous reassurance. (p. 11)

To wonder, along with a group member, why a certain subject is being discussed or why an individual moved to another chair at a particular time is often a simple and useful intervention.

BALANCING GROUP-AS-A-WHOLE INTERPRETATIONS WITH INDIVIDUAL INTERPRETATIONS

Individuals seek treatment for their personal problems and hence need to feel that they are progressing toward their goals. Therefore, the group therapist has to balance group-as-a-whole interpretations with individual interpretations.

STAGES OF GROUP DEVELOPMENT

Group development is the coming together of individual members interacting with the leader to create an environment that stimulates everyone's learning. Without fail, members demonstrate through their behavior in group what it is like to walk in their shoes. Individual values, beliefs, fears, prejudices, and anxieties emerge as the group develops. Although much has been written about the stages of group development, group development does not necessarily occur in discrete stages. Rather, it is the fine blend of therapist and group members that makes each and every group a unique experience.

This chapter discusses four phases of group development: the initial phase, the responsive phase, the focused phase, and the termination.

INITIAL PHASE

From the moment the individual group members enter the room, group development begins. Most people are concerned about entering new situations, and group members' fears and characteristic ways of dealing with anxiety appear. As a result, communication at this stage tends to be fairly superficial, and the members experience a heightened sensitivity about issues of trust. As they approach the first meeting, they may be asking themselves, "What should I reveal about myself?" "Will there be people here that I like?" "Can I allow myself to be known?" "Will this be a safe place?" "Is it worth the risk of exposure?"

Beginnings are very important, and, to gain insight into how the group might develop, the therapist needs to carefully observe what each member does under stress. The content of the conversations is important, and so is the activity of the group. Who is talking? Who is not talking? Who is late? Where do people sit? What are they discussing? What are they doing? What are the metaphors for anxiety in their conversation? In the initial phase, the therapist needs to encourage participation and convey a sense that in the group feelings, memories, and problems can be examined, appreciated, and understood. All groups are unique in how they develop and thus cannot be defined by any time limit. In some psychotherapy groups, the initial phase may last for weeks or months. In groups of a fixed duration, the initial phase may last only one or two meetings.

Members start out cautiously. As they get acquainted with each other, they may search for similarity between themselves and other group members in an attempt to determine what their role will be in relation to the group process.

> A new group for women is meeting for the first time. One member, Donna, arrives 15 minutes early. As the group leader reviews the group contract, she indicates that the group meeting will begin when the first person talks. Mary is the first to introduce herself and volunteers that she is divorced and lonely. She also mentions briefly that she is tired of being "perfect" all the time. Another member, Kathy, says she is tired of always feeling "guilty" and casually mentions that she is married. Karen, who is lesbian, avoids indicating in her introduction whether she is married; another member sits silently eating a candy bar, while Jean arrives late, sweating and out of breath.

In this example, members respond with familiar defenses in their attempt to "get it right"; some deal with anxiety by arriving early, others by arriving late, while others eat. Some may feel guilty for taking care of themselves by coming to the group. Several define themselves by their marital status. Going slowly in the first group meeting allows the group to experience the anxiety of how to say hello without the pressure of going beyond that task. The therapist's gentle exploration of the tension surrounding the hello may be all that is necessary in the first meeting.

The leader becomes attentive to the needs of the members and is more active in the first meeting than in later stages of group development. The group will feel less anxious and begins to talk. In this early phase, the therapist and members have a window into how the members relate to authority,

going back to their early connections to parents. Insight can come from noticing:
- Do they ask where to sit as if to get permission?
- Do they sit in opposition to the leader or beside the leader?
- Do they make eye contact with the leader or with peers?
- How do they ask questions of the leader?
- Are they demanding, defiant, deferring, or compliant?
- Members also have many questions and will want to know what material is okay to discuss.
- Are past events the focus of the meetings?
- Do they focus only on what is happening in the meeting?
- Do they tell their secrets in group?
- Will it be possible to have their issues kept confidential?

In answering these and other questions, the group members together with the leader are creating the culture and norms of the group.

Group Norms

Group **norms** are the standards for behavior that are expected in group. Norms facilitate effective group functioning and goal achievement by providing some order to govern the group meetings. If everyone talked and no one listened, the group would never achieve its tasks. Every group has rules regarding the behavior that it will and will not tolerate. Sometimes these are explicit (spoken rules) and formalized in the group contract. At other times they are so implicit (unspoken rules) that they are realized only when someone in the group is in violation. Norms may center around risk-taking behaviors, tolerance of humor, decision making, and the like. Initially, the group may look to the leader to develop the group norms, but as the group develops its own identity, members become more actively involved in developing and modifying the group's behavioral standards. Group functioning is disrupted when members deviate from the norms.[6]

Group Cohesion

Group cohesion begins with the "shared survival" of the members in their first meeting, when anxiety is high. The sharing of this anxiety helps group members feel a connection. In surviving this first meeting, they have done something together for the first time. The therapist at this phase attempts to establish norms in the group using the group contract and attends to the goal of establishing a feeling of safety for all members. Leaders play a significant role in the development of cohesiveness because of their influence in clarifying group norms and goals. With guidance from the leaders, members can agree on means of achieving goals as well as expectations for the roles of each person in the group. In this way, group cohesiveness becomes an essential determinant of group effectiveness. This powerful benefit of an effective group is realized when positive and negative feedback can be given in an atmosphere of acceptance without group disintegration.

Manifest and Latent Content

Because there is no right or wrong way to run a group, new group therapists might focus on keeping the early meetings as simple as possible and allowing the process to unfold gradually. Therapists must take the time to listen for developing themes with individuals, as well as with the entire group. Group therapists learn to listen on two levels: the *manifest content*—what is immediately being discussed in the room by way of spoken words—and the *latent content*—or what is not being discussed in the group. Communication in group is most effective when latent content and manifest content are similar.

> Jane talks about the slap in the face she received as a child from her dad, who was an alcoholic. She mentions it over and over again. Finally the therapist wonders about the "slaps in the face" the group might have felt they endured with the therapist's 2-week vacation, as well as her decision to add another member to the group. The group agrees and is then free to discuss each individual's reactions to these events.

Here the manifest content is a literal "slap in the face" endured by the group member as a child. The latent content is the "slap in the face" as a metaphor for the anger the group may be feeling about the therapist's vacation and the addition of the new member.

THE RESPONSIVE PHASE

In this phase of group development, members have established themselves in the community of the group and feel safe enough to begin to share more of their conflicts, disappointments, and reenactments. Members now become responsive to group events such as the addition of a new member, a disagreement with another member, or the therapist's vacation. Often a period of disruption occurs before the group event can be fully discussed.

> A psychotherapy group meets for the first time after the therapist's 2-week vacation. Just prior to group, one member cancels, claiming she would rather "go for a long walk." On the same evening, an additional member calls to say she is unable to get away from work. Neither of these members previously missed group. During group, another member reports that she will be absent next week to have dinner with a friend. Two weeks later, when all group members are present, they are able to explore how their absence symbolized an effort to "vote with their feet" about the therapist's vacation. The member who had dinner with a friend mentions she had scheduled that dinner the week the therapist was away. She had "surprised herself that she had decided to go." She later says she missed hav-

> ing the group and "must have chosen to schedule the dinner to upset the leader." Another member then says she was initially relieved that the group was canceled for 2 weeks because she would "save money." However, she acknowledges the feelings of disconnection from the group and decides the group is an important part of her life. The therapist comments that it sounds as if she has truly joined the group.

During this phase of group development, the therapist continues to become familiar with each member's defenses in the context of the person's history. Members who ask questions of other members while volunteering little of themselves may really be inquiring about themselves.

> Karen, who has shared virtually nothing about herself, asks Margaret if she ever feels guilty. Following Margaret's response, the therapist asks, "Is that a subject about which you might know something?" to which Karen replies, "Yes, of course." The therapist pursues this matter further and asks, "Could you say more about it?" Karen replies that she feels guilty always keeping her mother's alcoholism a secret, and the group is given an opportunity to explore this very important topic with Karen.

The group leader must honor the client's wish not to discuss the matter. Another opportunity will present itself when the member feels more comfortable and ready to address the matter. Asking the member if he or she wishes to work on the subject at this time is a respectful way to proceed. All members have their own time frame regarding intimacy, and the group therapist must become accustomed to a gradual unfolding of progress.

Adding New Members

The addition of new members may occur at any time. Although it is best to begin a group with as many of the total members present as possible, reality often dictates that some will join later or that members will leave and new members will then be added. In a long-term psychotherapy group, several weeks are generally required for the group to process the notion of a new member. In many groups run by nurses, this luxury does not exist, but the principles governing the ideal framework are useful as a reference.

The arrival of a new member should be anticipated as a major event for the group regardless of how long they have been together because the group as they have come to know it will no longer be the same. A new group member rekindles old conflicts about sharing, competition, and the question of sufficient supplies or resources for all concerned. Such a group event allows the therapist to see how each member deals with the stress of change.

THE FOCUSED PHASE

The focused phase of therapy represents the heart and soul of group treatment. In this phase, the group is focused on the twofold task of processing individual and group-as-a-whole events. At this point in development, the group is effective in exploring the needs of members and offering alternative solutions to previously dysfunctional behaviors. Members have shared and survived a variety of experiences together.

Members are more sophisticated about the way they individually deal defensively with life events. For example, they are less likely to tolerate member absences. They begin to remind one another that a particular response is "typical," and an "envelope"—a symbolic membrane that holds the group intact—has developed.[20] Members learn that their sadness, anger, and competition may reenact past experiences; they may more clearly understand themselves. They develop curiosity about each other's behaviors and work to piece together the puzzle of each other's lives. They take on different roles and feel pride in doing so.

> Marie tells Amy that last year at this time she shared the story of her terrible trip to New York with her mother, and it was then that she was able to confront her mother for the first time about her disappointments in their relationship. Amy had forgotten all about it. Marie has become the historian for the group. She has remembered an important event that is now a part of the group's shared experience.

The role of the leader in this phase is now consultant. As the members take bigger risks in the room, the leaders can expect to hear more details about their shortcomings. Because this feedback provides the members with an opportunity to understand how they respond to authority figures, the leader should welcome it. There is a strong sense of meaning in the interconnections. Values and norms emerge in the group. For instance, the importance of honoring the group contract is evident. The group now has a culture that is the foundation of the group.

Group Culture

Group culture is the unique interrelationships among a particular group's purpose, norms, roles, status, and distinct ways of interacting. In how it develops its culture, each group is unique and because of the interdependence of group members, it is easy to observe how each member's behavior influences the other group members. Specific members carry the culture and help new members learn how to function in the group.

> Julie has just joined a group that has been in existence for 4 years. She announces that she is likely to be late each week, states she has had this problem for years, and implies that very little can be done about it. Another member politely states, "This group begins at 5:00 PM and ends at 6:30 PM." Julie replies that she will do the best she can but is late for the second meeting. Other members begin to talk metaphorically about how they hate missing announcements at the begin-

Group Therapy and Therapeutic Groups **173**

> **Box 9–6. Indications of a Mature Group**
>
> 1. Mature working groups emphasize the intragroup responses and interactions as the primary source of learning and cure.
> 2. Despite the primacy of in-group interactions, flexibility develops that allows discussion of relevant events in the members' lives.
> 3. In mature groups, members develop a more collegial relationship with the therapist.
> 4. Members have developed confidence in their ability to tolerate anxiety and to examine problems themselves.
> 5. Through repeated experiences, members gain a deep understanding and appreciation of one another's strengths and weaknesses.
> 6. Members have learned that transactions involve the intrapersonal and the intrapsychic. In other words, behavior is not always what it appears to be and that there are personal meanings that might produce particular behaviors.
>
> **Source:** Rutan, JS, and Stone, WN: Psychodynamic Group Psychotherapy. Guilford Press, New York, 1993, p 44.

ning of meetings at work and how annoying it is when coworkers are late. At the third meeting, Julie arrives just barely on time and is sweating. Members assume she was sweating after rushing in an effort to arrive on time. She devalues this idea and states she was "exercising" but is on time for all subsequent meetings. Later she is able to discuss how being late as a child was a way of being noticed. She is now pleased to find other ways of getting noticed in group.

Bion[21] refers to this stage of group development as a *work group* because the members are clear about their task and seem to be successful in accomplishing it. Rutan and Stone[22] refer to this stage of group development as a *mature group*. The key issue here is that the behavior of individuals in a group is determined by many factors. The work of the therapist is to attend as much as possible to the meanings emerging from these various components. Features of mature groups are described in Box 9–6.

THE TERMINATION PHASE

The termination phase of a group represents important opportunities for individuals to develop insight into their characteristic ways of dealing with loss and separation. An individual who can learn to "work it" will be able to look at old stressors that contribute to fears of intimacy. Sometimes an ending inspires a new interpersonal beginning.

Group members usually decide to leave a group long before they announce it to the membership. If a member has set certain goals at the pregroup interview and now feels the goals have been achieved, it may be a realistic time to leave the group. Generally, the other group members and the leader have a sense of whether this is a reasonable time for the member to leave. Soliciting feedback from other group members is useful for the leader when a member decides to leave a group. This process can help the terminating member make a clearer decision about the timing of the departure.

If the entire group is ending, as in time-limited groups, it is up to the leader to continue to remind the members of the number of sessions remaining. It is often helpful to review with members what they have accomplished as well as how they have changed interpersonally. Questions that assist members to review their progress in groups include the following:

"What new ways have you learned to cope with your issues?"
"What work remains to be done and in what areas?"

Departing members should allow several sessions of the group to review what they have accomplished and to say goodbye to each of the other group members. Most members typically attempt to avoid prolonged goodbyes because it reminds them of previous losses in their lives.

EXPECTED OUTCOMES

Evaluating the group and individual members is an ongoing process that begins during the selection interview. In determining group effectiveness, the nurse is most concerned with the group outcomes. The following questions can serve as guidelines for evaluating group outcomes[4]:

- Has the group accomplished its original objectives?
- What other accomplishments does the group have as a result of the group experience?
- Have the needs of the individual members been met?

Depending on the type of group and its purpose, the expected outcomes may be evaluated informally through subjective participation of the group members. Questions such as "How do you feel as a result of the group?" "What would you like to see stay the same?" and "What would you like to see change?" can assist the nurse in the overall evaluation of the effectiveness of the group. These questions may be answered verbally or evaluated more formally. Frequently, written evaluations use Likert-type scales, wherein the group members answer questions that range from "strongly agree" to "strongly disagree."

In teaching and behavioral change groups, group outcomes may be measured with a pretest and posttest, particularly if increased knowledge is one measure of effectiveness. Similarly, if the goal of a particular group is to change behavior, then maintenance of the new behaviors would be a good test of the group's effectiveness. For example, success in a group designed to treat aggressiveness could be that group participants showed decreased expression of anger, increased effort to control anger, and a decrease in aggressive behavior.

Psychotherapy groups, peer support groups, and self-help

groups are often more difficult to evaluate because the objectives are not necessarily behaviorally oriented. In these cases, the focus of the evaluation tends to be more process oriented. Loomis[4] offers the following questions as a way of evaluating this type of group:
- What did the members like or dislike about the group?
- Did they feel supported?
- Did they enjoy the group experience?

Attendance at meetings can also be a measure of the group's success, as noted in Crane, Kirby, and Kooperman's[5] psychotropic medication group. On evaluation, the leaders concluded that inpatient satisfaction was indicated by excellent group attendance, discussions that easily filled the hour, and feedback that the group was the most useful on the unit. Unfortunately, the nurses did not pursue a research design or formal evaluation of the group and cannot address client compliance to psychotropic medication, which would be the true measure of the group's effectiveness.

Evaluation is an integral component of the nurse's role in the psychiatric–mental health milieu and must be integrated into all phases of group development.

THE ROLE OF THE NURSE IN GROUP THERAPY

Although the nurse is well prepared to participate in group work and uniquely situated within the health-care delivery system, group experiences are often underutilized as a treatment modality. In general, clinicians and clients alike often resist working in groups, perhaps because of the tension that an individual feels when joining a group. Shields and Lanza[23] note that clinicians considering a role as a group leader also experience anxiety and may reject the role for the following reasons:
- Anxiety
- Idealization of the dyadic relationship in individual therapy
- Struggles with autonomy in private practice
- Fears of exposure as a group leader
- Institutional resistance to group treatment

EDUCATIONAL PREPARATION

Psychiatric–mental health nurses conducting group psychotherapy are generally required to be prepared at the master's level, with clinical practice completed under the guidance and supervision of an accomplished professional. Many pursue additional training, certification, or credentials in group psychotherapy and frequently base their approach to a particular clinical problem on a specific theoretical orientation. Several psychiatric–mental health nurses have been certified by the American Group Psychotherapy Association and are actively involved in professional associations such as the Northeastern Society for Group Psychotherapy in Boston.

The American Nurses Association (ANA)[24] *Statement on Psychiatric–Mental Health Clinical Nursing Practice and Standards of Psychiatric–Mental Health Clinical Nursing Practice* identifies group psychotherapy within the domain of the advanced practice nurse. Although not all nurses pursue graduate education and run psychotherapy groups, all nurses participate in groups on a daily basis as members of work groups or as leaders of therapeutic groups. As a result, a solid foundation in groups as a treatment modality is necessary for all nurses. Knowledge of **group dynamics**, group process, group development, and group leadership facilitate the development of nurse therapists who are competently prepared to conduct groups at a level commensurate with their education, knowledge, skills, and abilities.

SUPERVISION

Nurses have access to the intimate lives of the clients in their care. With this privilege comes the responsibility of safe, competent, and ethical practice, which extends beyond the basic theoretical underpinnings necessary to conduct groups. Supervision is recommended for all group leaders, including experts, to provide constructive feedback and facilitate self-awareness and self-evaluation in the leader, particularly around issues of countertransference.

Supervision offers nurses a unique opportunity to gain important information about their clients and, perhaps more important, to learn about themselves. Supervision should be a regular part of all group therapy, conducted under the watchful eye of an experienced group therapist. If supervision is not available in the workplace, private supervision or a peer supervision or consultation group is important for advanced learning. Because supervision entails guiding and mentoring the practice of another in a safe, nonthreatening relationship that fosters examination of thoughts and feelings without fear of repercussions, a supervisor ideally has no direct authority over the therapist being supervised.

TYPE OF GROUP LEADERSHIP

Groups can be led by an individual therapist working alone or by cotherapists who assume joint responsibility for leadership of the group.

Single Therapist

The single therapist mode of operation is common in clinical practice. Groups led by individual therapists are often considered by managed-care companies to be economically sound and a more efficient use of the nurse's time and energy in private practice and in mental health care systems. An obvious disadvantage to this approach is the lack of opportunity for immediate debriefing with a colleague. However, the choice of single therapist–led groups versus coleadership should be determined on the basis of the goals and purposes of the group, not solely on economy. Careful documentation immediately following a group is the best way to track group process. Videotaping group sessions can help a single therapist review both the content and the process of a particular session.

Cotherapist

Groups led by two therapists who are jointly responsible for the leadership of the group are becoming increasingly popular. Cotherapists can monitor and facilitate group development, and may be better able to supervise disruptive members. This approach is particularly useful in illness management groups that simultaneously teach clients and their family members. Male and female coleadership mirrors family situations and may offer a group an opportunity to see a man and woman working together without sexualizing, exploiting, or putting each other down.

Cotherapy can be an effective strategy for training new group leaders, or both therapists may share the role equally. Frequently, groups that employ a cotherapy model are run by a nurse and another member of the mental health team (e.g., psychologist, social worker, psychiatrist). This collaborative arrangement can be very effective in practice.

Disadvantages to the cotherapy model of group leadership relate to difficulties that may arise between the leaders. When members are from different disciplines, there is the additional threat of territoriality. Competition between leaders, philosophical differences, and variance in style or experience can affect how the group will work. An alliance of members with one particular leader may result in splitting, which is common in psychotherapy and not, in itself, the problem. However, how splitting is handled can be problematic. If group leaders do not get along, conflict may not be dealt with openly in the group.

LEADERSHIP STYLES

Leadership styles are influenced by the philosophy of treatment, personality of the leader, nature and purpose of the group, and the degree of mental, emotional, and cognitive impairment of the group members. The style of leadership the psychiatric–mental health nurse adopts is often dictated by the demands of the clinical situation, and nurses must be flexible in modifying their approaches to the situation in which they find themselves. Three general styles of leadership are autocratic, democratic, and laissez-faire.

Autocratic

Leadership in an autocratic type of group is centralized around the leader, who exercises power and control within the group. Group members become dependent on the leader for problem solving and decision making. Although members suggestions may be elicited, they are rarely used. As a result, groups led by autocratic leaders characteristically experience low group morale, scapegoating and hostility among members, and dependence on the leader. In task-oriented groups, productivity may be high under close supervision; however, any potential growth and creativity in the individual group members are thwarted.

Democratic

The focus of the democratic type of leadership is on the group members. The democratic leader welcomes all ideas and actively encourages group participation in problem solving and decision making. As a result, groups led by democratic leaders tend to be characterized by high morale, cohesiveness, and creativity. The group leader provides guidance and expertise as needed but relies on the creative and spontaneous input of all members to achieve the group's goals and objectives. Although running a democratic group takes more time and effort, participants experience a high level of satisfaction and achievement by being an integral part of the group process.

Laissez-faire

In groups led by laissez-faire leaders, members are free to participate as they choose, with neither the leader nor the group taking leadership responsibility. Individuals who are typically highly motivated, task-oriented, and highly knowledgeable may thrive under this type of leadership. More commonly, though, group work remains undone under this type of leadership because members are unclear about the group's purpose and objectives, and there is confusion, frustration, and apathy. Due to the uninvolved approach of the laissez-faire leader, groups can be very time consuming and inefficient in achieving the desired tasks.

AREAS FOR FUTURE RESEARCH

Contemporary issues and trends in psychiatric–mental health nursing have been identified as (1) the rapid expansion of biological science and technology, (2) demographic shifts in the population, and (3) changes in the delivery of mental health services.[24] Because of these significant changes, psychiatric–mental health nurses have been challenged to expand their roles in clinical practice and to work collaboratively and cooperatively with other disciplines in the delivery of mental health services. Issues for further research include:

- The impact of shortened length of stay on the type of group therapy that can be conducted in the inpatient milieu needs to be determined.
- There is a need for nursing research to explore the phenomenon of group commitment with various client groups in different settings.
- Very little research exists on whether the pregroup interview is an adequate predictor of a client's retention in a group and how anxiety can influence an individual's decision about joining the group.

KEY POINTS

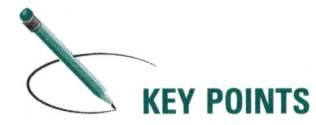

- A group is defined as three or more individuals who are to some degree interdependent.
- Group therapy can be broadly defined as a treatment modality for two or more individuals who meet on a regular predetermined basis with one or more therapists for the purpose of achieving health-related goals. Members accomplish their goals through interactions with other members and with group leaders.
- Group therapy is an effective and economical mode of intervention. Yalom[3] has identified 11 therapeutic factors that are considered the basic mechanisms of change in all types of groups.
- The psychiatric–mental health nurse has the opportunity to work with a great diversity of groups in the psychiatric–mental health milieu: activity groups, teaching and behavioral change groups, psychotherapy groups, self-help groups, and peer support groups.
- When planning groups, the nurse needs to consider the following factors: the type of group, its purpose and goals, membership selection, the size of the group, the frequency of meetings, and the physical environment, including resources.
- Four stages of group development have been identified: the initial phase, the responsive phase, the focused phase, and the termination phase.
- Group therapists use interpersonal communication skills in working with groups of clients. The significant difference between individual therapy and group therapy is the numbers of interactions that are possible in the group.
- Nurses participate as leaders and co-leaders of groups in many health-care settings. The ANA has identified group psychotherapy within the domain of the advanced practice nurse.
- A group contract can facilitate the activities of the group by clearly outlining the formal conditions. Contracts are relevant to all groups and may be written or verbal.

REFERENCES

1. Nakagawa, H: Group theory in nursing practice. In Anderson, CA (ed): Psychiatric Nursing 1974 to 1994: Report on the State of the Art. Mosby, St. Louis, 1995, p 91.
2. Loomis, ME. Group dynamics theory. In McFarland, GK, and Thomas, MD (eds): Psychiatric Mental Health Nursing. JB Lippincott Co, Philadelphia, 1991, p 67.
3. Yalom, ID. The Theory and Practice of Group Psychotherapy, ed 4. Basic Books, New York, 1995.
4. Loomis, ME. Group therapy. In McFarland, GK, and Thomas, MD (eds): Psychiatric Mental Health Nursing. JB Lippincott Co, Philadelphia, 1991, p 767.
5. Crane, K, Kirby, B, and Kooperman, D: Patient compliance for psychotropic medications: A group model for and expanding psychiatric unit. J Psychosoc Nurs Ment Health Serv 34(1):8, 1996.
6. Arnold, E: Communicating in groups. In Arnold, E, and Boggs, K (eds): Interpersonal Relationships in Nursing, ed 2. WB Saunders Company, Philadelphia, 1995, p 259.
7. Lanza, ML, Satz, H, Stone, J, and Kayne, HL: Developing psychodynamic group treatment methods for aggressive male inpatients. Issues in Mental Health Nursing 17:409, 1996.
8. Peternelj-Taylor, CA, and Hartley, VL: Living with mental illness: Professional family collaboration. J Psychosoc Nurs Ment Health Serv 31(3):23, 1993.
9. Quarrington, D: The power of self-help. Canadian Nurse 88(2):26, 1992.
10. Lego, S: Group therapy in nursing practice. In Anderson, C (ed): Psychiatric Nursing 1974 to 1994: Report on the State of the Art. Mosby, St. Louis, 1995, p 40.
10a. Shields, JD, et al: Peer Consultation in a Group Context: A Guide for Nurses. Springer, New York, 1985.
11. Wood, A, and Seymour, LM: Psychodynamic group therapy for older adults: The life experiences group. J Psychosoc Nurs Ment Health Serv 32(7):19, 1994.
12. Applegate, M: Outpatient group therapy for dissociative trauma survivors. J Am Psychiatric Nurses Association 2(2):37, 1996.
13. MacKenzie, KR: Classics in Group Psychotherapy. Guilford Press, New York, 1992.
14. Kavanaugh, KH: Transcultural perspectives in mental health. In Andrews, MM, and Boyle, JS (eds): Transcultural Concepts in Nursing Care. Lippincott, Philadelphia, 1995, p 253.
15. Murphy, MC, Conley, J, and Hernandez, MA: Group remotivation therapy for the 90s. Perspectives in Psychiatric Care 30(3):9, 1994.
16. Yalom, ID: In-Patient Group Psychotherapy. Basic Books, New York, 1983.
17. Gauron, EF, Steinmark, SW, and Gersh, FS: The orientation group in pre-therapy training. Perspectives in Psychiatric Care 15:32, 1977.
18. Ormont, LR: The Group Therapy Experience: From Theory to Practice. St. Martin Press, New York, 1992, p 83.
19. Shapiro, E, and Carr, AW: Lost in Familiar Places. Yale University Press, New Haven, 1991.
20. Day, M: Process in classical psychodynamic groups. Int J Group Psychother 31:153, 1981.
21. Bion, W: Experiences in Groups. Basic Books, New York, 1959.
22. Rutan, JS, and Stone, WN: Psychodynamic Group Psychotherapy. Guilford Press, New York, 1993.
23. Shields, J, and Lanza, M: The parallel process of resistance by clients and therapists to starting groups: A guide for nurses. Arch Psychiatr Nurs 5:300, 1993.
24. American Nurses Association: A Statement on Psychiatric–Mental Health Clinical Nursing Practice and Standards of Psychiatric–Mental Health Clinical Nursing Practice. ANA, Washington, DC, 1994.

CHAPTER 10
Family Therapy

CHAPTER 10

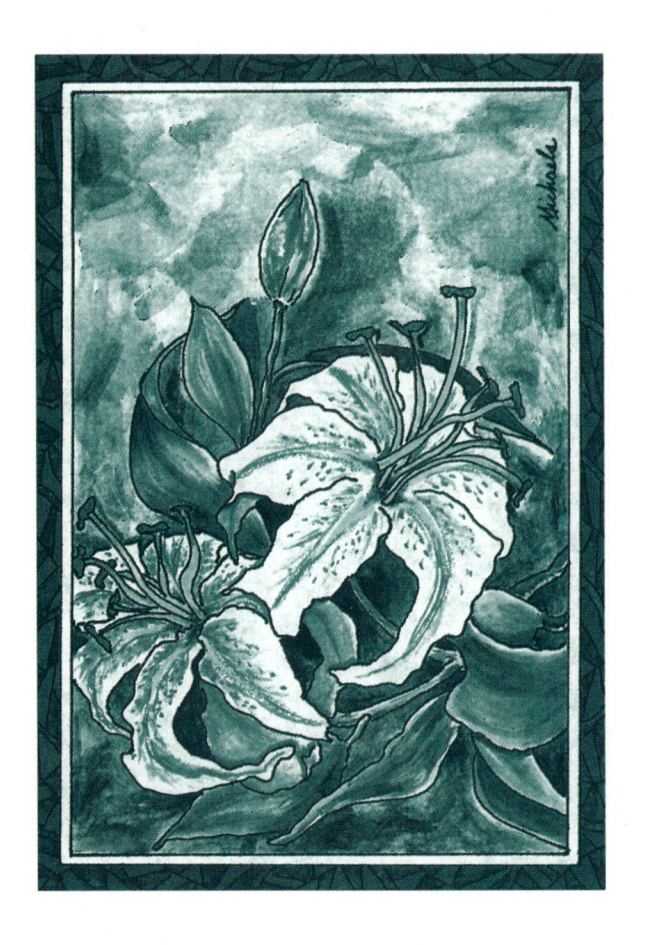

CHAPTER OUTLINE

Purpose of Family Therapy
The Nurse's Role
Assessing the Family System
   Genogram
   Structural Mapping
   Family Assessment Guide
Nursing and Psychiatric Diagnoses
Family Therapy Approaches
   Multigenerational Theories and Therapies
   Structural and Systemic Family Therapy
Expected Outcomes
Synopsis of Current Research
Areas for Future Research

LEARNING OBJECTIVES

After completing this chapter, the reader should be able to:

- Explain the reasons for referring people to family therapy.
- Differentiate family therapy from other forms of intervention.
- Identify the major theoretical frameworks of family therapy.
- Describe classifications of families in relation to nursing and psychiatric diagnoses.
- Apply the nursing process to clients seen in family therapy.

KEY TERMS

family
family boundaries
family of origin
family process

family structure
family system
nuclear family

Margery Chisholm, RN, EdD, CS, ABPP

Family Therapy

Family therapy is the recommended therapy of choice for a variety of family-related problems. The **family** as a whole is the focus of treatment; changing family interaction and functioning is the goal. This therapy is particularly helpful when an individual's symptoms reflect a family's disturbed interactions. Interventions affect each member of the family and the family as a unit. Nurses can help distinguish whether a family has a chronic or serious problem or difficulty in adjusting to a normal developmental stage. Family therapy is conducted by one or two therapists specifically trained in family therapy. Psychiatric nurse generalists are not family therapists; however, some psychiatric clinical nurse specialists specialize in treating families.

Family therapy is *clearly* indicated when
- The family system is significantly involved in some type of psychosocial problem
- The family's ability to perform basic tasks is inadequate
- There are complaints of "behavior problems" and "poor performance"
- There is marital dissatisfaction and conflict
- A child or adolescent is the identified client
- There is a recent clear stressor for the family such as an illness or developmental milestone
- The family defines the problem as a family issue.

Family therapy *may* be indicated when
- A family member is in a hospital or other institutional setting
- Death or desertion causes the loss of a family member
- The family is in the process of a divorce or separation
- A physical illness in one member of the family has created stress and changed family functioning
- A member of the family has an addiction.

As seen in Table 10–1, family therapy is distinguished from individual and group therapy in several important ways: (1) Confidentiality varies because of the relatedness and shared experience of family life; (2) members in families are in extended interaction after a therapy session; and (3) verbal, nonverbal, and behavioral sequences are the focus of concern. The goal of therapy is improved functioning of the family as a whole.

Family-level interventions may be the primary treatment or added to other forms of individual or group therapy in the following situations:
- There is no improvement in individual therapy
- Stress or symptoms develop in other family members as a result of one member's illness or treatment
- An individual is unable or unwilling to use interpretive or individual approaches and could benefit from action approaches
- An individual client spends most of the individual therapy session talking about a family member.

PURPOSE OF FAMILY THERAPY

The purpose of family therapy is to foster more effective communication and ways of relating among family members. The specific goals of most family therapy interventions include
- Improving communication
- Facilitating autonomy and individuation of members
- Increasing empathy
- Fostering flexible leadership
- Improving role agreement and enactment
- Reducing conflict
- Facilitating symptomatic improvement
- Enhancing individual task performance.

THE NURSE'S ROLE

Nurses are often the first health-care professionals to recognize family problems. Nurses may also use family techniques to facilitate a client's recovery from a psychiatric or medical illness. Clients are likely to approach nurses with concerns about a family member and request information, offer important background data, or reveal problems. As a result, assessment and referral for family therapy are key parts of the nurse's role.

Before family therapy is instituted, a family assessment is necessary. The nurse may take an active role in the assessment process, particularly in community and child psychiatric treatment settings. Nurses can determine the appropriateness of a family therapy approach with the questions outlined in Table 10–2. The answers help the nurse decide whether a referral for family therapy is indicated, whether all members should be seen together, the seriousness of the situation, and the availability of members to attend family meetings.

The assessment should address the identified family problem and indicate why the family needs treatment at this particular time. The referral source may be a family doctor, min-

TABLE 10–1. Differences: Individual, Group, and Family Therapy

Form of Therapy	Clients	Confidentiality	Mode of Facilitating Change	Goal of Therapy
Individual	One person; no prior history	Between client and therapist; little contact between meetings	Primarily verbal; sympathetic and supportive environment.	Changes in symptoms, mood, thinking, and behavior of client; relationship intended to end.
Group	Six to eight clients who are unrelated; no prior history	Between therapist and clients and clients with each other; contact between meetings discouraged; power and status equal among members	Primarily verbal and interactional; sympathetic and supportive environment.	Effective interpersonal functioning of members of the group; relationships intended to end.
Family	Two or more related members; prior history affects interaction	Lack of confidential exchanges between members in meetings; extensive contact of clients with each other between meetings. Unequal power and status among members of the family group	Verbal, nonverbal, interactional, and behavioral (tasks and assignments). Environment is stressful and emotional for members in the family.	Effective communication, role taking, interaction, expressions of intimacy, and functioning of members of the family; family has a future together and relationships not intended to end.

ister, school, court system, or self-referral. The referral route often indicates the family's initial view of the problem and its approach to problem solving.

ASSESSING THE FAMILY SYSTEM

During the assessment, the nurse or therapist brings together all members of the family unit who may be affected by the identified problem. For example, a married couple complains of fighting and competition when the family gets together. They have children from previous marriages residing with them as well as children from this marriage. The relevant family members are the couple and each of the children in the new family structure. A key part of the assessment is to form a therapeutic alliance with each member of the family and inquire about their views of the family's problems and strengths.

Family assessment has two components: (1) the interview and (2) factual and observational data. The factual and observational categories are outlined in Table 10–3.

Circular questioning is another assessment method used in family therapy. These questions are intended to demonstrate the relationship pattern and the family's definition of the problem.

1. Verbal and Analogic Information

   Identify cue words such as "guilty," "communication," and "rebellious" that are turned into statements about relationships and differences in relationships. Note eye messages, changes in posture, tone, and redundancies.

   Examples: Who worries most when dad is depressed?
   Who communicates least in the family?
   Who feels guilty when mom stays home?

2. Definition of the Problem
   The family defines the relationships around the problem related to the present.

TABLE 10–2. Preassessment Questions

1. Is the problem stated as a symptom in a family member or is it stated in terms of a relationship?
2. Is the problem seen as a crisis?
3. Has there been a recent important milestone (birth, death, illness) in the family?
4. Is there an outside referral source and what is the reason for the referral?
5. Are there any precipitating events?
6. Is the problem a recent one or has it been a concern for a period of time?
7. What has been the pathway for seeking help? Who has been consulted?
8. Can the problem be managed or is it out of control (e.g., is there a potential for violence)?
9. Who in the family knows about the problem and who would be willing to come to discuss their concerns?
10. Is there a problem with alcohol or drug addiction?
11. Is there a history of sexual or physical abuse?

TABLE 10–3. Family Assessment Guide

I. **Demographic Factors**
   Composition of nuclear family group
   Composition of extended family
   Living arrangements? Individuals in current household
   Health of family members
   Age of family members
   Composition of the parental unit
   Other significant relationships for the family

II. **Sociocultural Factors**
   Ethnicity
   Religion(s)
   Sexual orientation of family members
   Occupation(s)
   Financial status
   Socioeconomic status
   External social constraints (e.g., neighborhood or environmental impact on lifestyle)

III. **History of Family Unit**
   Prior help-seeking for the problem
   Prior psychiatric history of family members
   Prior medical history of all family members
   History of parental relationship, including sexual
   History of difficulties in the couple's relationship
   History of the family as a unit
   History of the family of origin of both parents

IV. **Developmental Factors**
   Adult developmental issues (e.g., parents and adult children)
   Development of children
   Couple's development
   Family's life cycle development

V. **Transactional Factors**
   Communication
   Roles
   Boundaries
   Power (e.g., structure and expression)
   Problem-solving skills

VI. **Affective Factors**
   Level of trust
   Mood or tone
     (Intimacy and affiliation)
     (Conflict resolution)
   Meanings
     (Values)
     (Goals)
   Relational integrity

Examples: What is the problem in the family now? What is the problem that everyone is worried about?

3. Coalition Alignments in the Present
   Use questions to identify family members who are aligned with each other.

   Examples: Who is upset when mother is sad?
   Who feels helpless when dad is angry?
   Who notices first when Johnny is naughty?

4. A Different Sequence
   Track the sequence of behavior of members to show how family actions help enact the problem. This sequence shows the cycle of behavior that the family is unable to change. The sequence is the "solution" to the original problem that has become the new problem. Use questions to alter the family's solution by disrupting the sequence.

   Examples: What do different family members do when Matt says he is running away from home?
   What does dad do?
   What does mom do?
   What would happen if he did run away?
   How does this differ from what used to happen?
   Who agrees with whom?

GENOGRAM

Psychiatric nurses often draw a genogram during the assessment to understand the family. A *genogram* is a diagram of the family constellation that denotes family structure and functioning (Figure 10–1). It gives a "picture" or overview of the family situation, background, and relationships. Important information about members, such as illnesses, occupation, and suicide, is written on the diagram. Families generally are interested in completing the genogram and may be surprised by some of its content.

The genogram represents members in the family tree and their relationship to other family members. The family members are placed horizontally to designate the generations. Vertical lines designate children, with the eldest child on the left, and the remaining children ordered by age. Squares represent males; circles represent females. The symbols contain each individual's name and age. A horizontal line between two symbols designates marriage; a slash on this line marks separation or divorce. The year of a family member's death is placed above the symbol.

STRUCTURAL MAPPING

Although the genogram is derived from historical information about generations, the *structural map* deals with present interactions and patterns. A structural assessment also identifies the relationship patterns and **family process** related to hierarchy, alliances, and coalitions in the family. Structural maps illustrate the current interactions and identify steps to help them change, such as promoting appropriate family structure with clear boundaries and generational hierarchies.

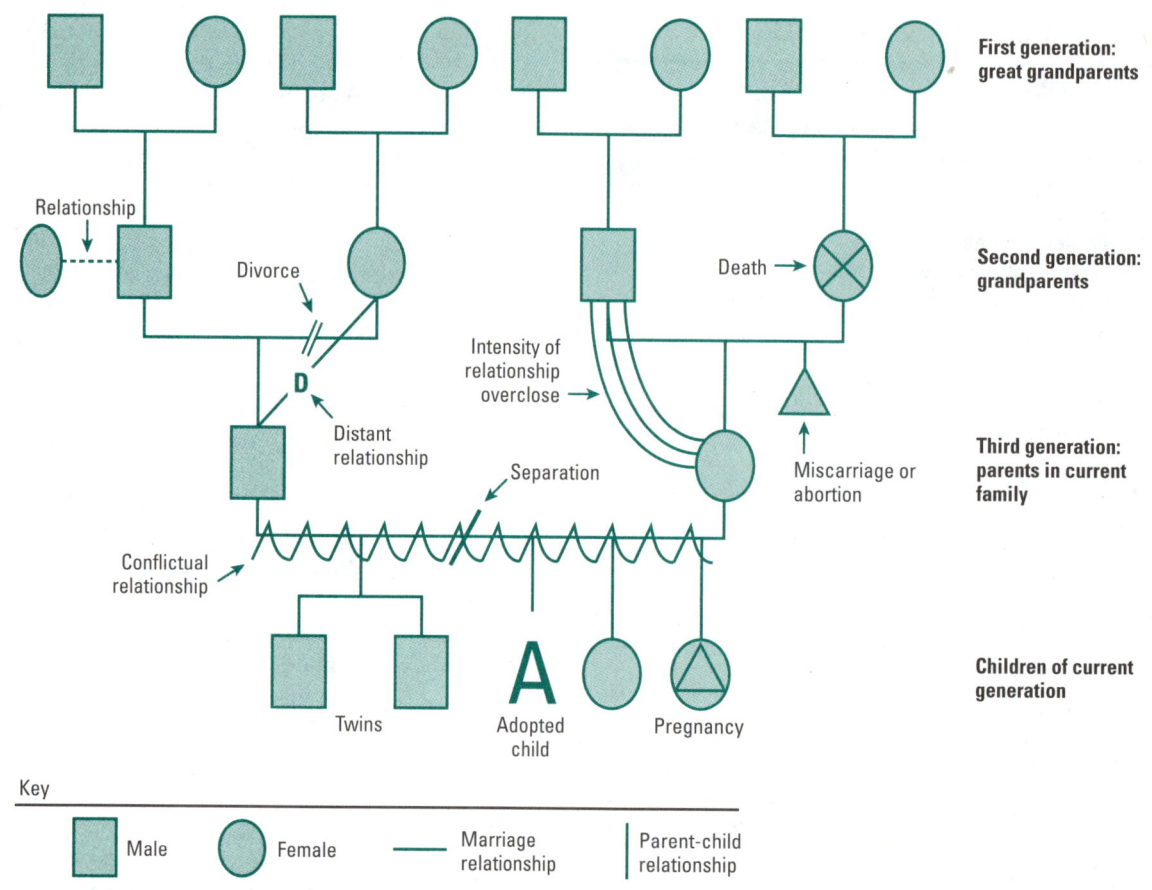

Figure 10–1. Basic genogram with symbols. The diagram depicts the parents of the current generation in a conflictual relationship in which they have separated. The family consist of first-born twins, an adopted child, a third natural daughter, and the mother, who is pregnant. The father comes from a family in which he felt distant with his mother, his parents divorced, and his father had another relationship. The mother comes from a family in which her mother had a miscarriage and had also died. She maintained an overly close relationship with her father. Little is known about the parents' parents. (Adapted from McGoldrich, M, and Gerson, R: Genograms in Family Assessment. Norton, New York, 1985.)

Figure 10–2 shows structural mapping used to assess the interactions and patterns and to facilitate changes within the family and the external environment.

FAMILY ASSESSMENT GUIDE

Demographic Factors

Demographic factors include information about the family composition such as the size of the **nuclear family** or unit, those living contiguously in the home, those living nearby, those living out of the home and the dates of their departures, members of the extended family, health of members in the immediate and extended families, and composition of the family unit. Determine parental composition, such as single parent, biological parents, stepparents, or foster parents. Obtain the number of children and their ages, genders, and biological relationships in the family. Inquire about other significant people living in the home, such as grandparents, baby-sitters, or live-in help.

Sociocultural Factors

Social and cultural parameters define beliefs, traditions, and values of family life that in turn affect behavior. Expectations embedded in cultural assumptions regarding age, ethnicity, sexuality, religion, occupations, and gender influence interactions between family members. For example, a family of mixed religion, race, or ethnicity may struggle to integrate multiple values or deal with cultural stereotypes and prohibitions. Socioeconomic status can also affect family life, manifested in a crowded living space or unsafe neighborhood.[1]

Historical Factors

Three kinds of history are essential in a family assessment: prior physical or mental illness in a family member and help-seeking attempts, history of the family as a unit, and family of origin history. Concerning past physical or mental illness in any family member, ask when it happened, its impact on

BOUNDARY KEY

───── RIGID BOUNDARY

── ── CLEAR BOUNDARY

- - - - DIFFUSE BOUNDARY

EXAMPLES

In a rigid family structure, father is overinvolved with son and in conflict with mother who has a weak boundary with the son.

In a rigid family structure, mother and daughters are in a coalition against the father.

AFFILIATION KEY

{ COALITION

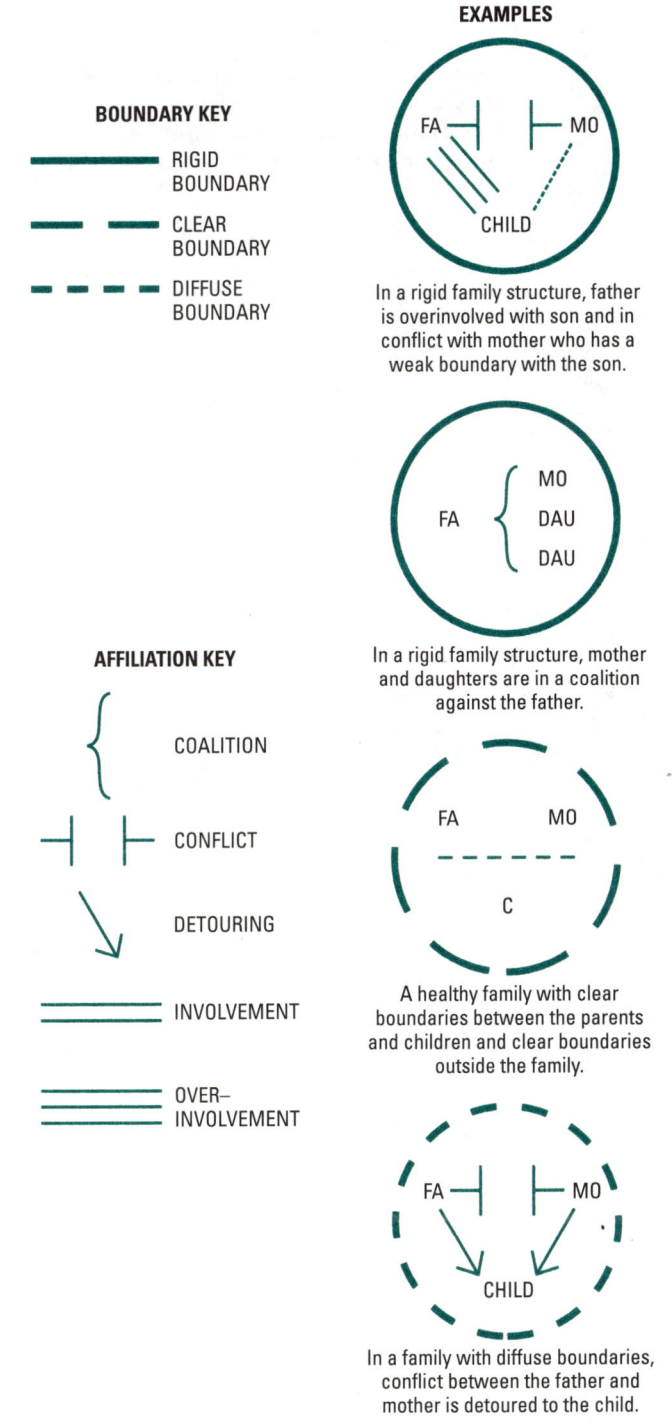

─┤ ├─ CONFLICT

↓ DETOURING

══ INVOLVEMENT

≡ OVER-INVOLVEMENT

A healthy family with clear boundaries between the parents and children and clear boundaries outside the family.

In a family with diffuse boundaries, conflict between the father and mother is detoured to the child.

Figure 10–2. Based on Structural mapping: family assessment. (From Minuchen, S: Families and Family Therapy, Harvard University Press, Cambridge, MA, 1974.)

family members, the duration of the illness, and adjustments the family has made. Evaluate the history of the family as a unit, including when the couple met and how, when they married, and their families' reactions. Ask if the births of all children were planned or unplanned and correlate the births with normal life events and crises; for example, did the birth occur around the time of job loss or promotion, physical or mental illness, death or illness of a family of origin member, or changes of locations?

Ask about the **family of origin**, the family into which each person was born, to understand current problems in the family. Belief systems, emotional cues, and learned behavioral responses are drawn from earlier relational processes; they influence current family interactions and the development of symptoms.

A boy who is slight in build and interested in artistic pursuits is expected to excel in sports because all his male relatives played on the city sport teams. He becomes nauseous and dizzy whenever his school team competes.

Developmental Factors

Development of the family is affected by adult developmental issues of either parent, the developmental shifts and demands of children, development of the couple-parent relationship, and phases of the family life cycle. During a transitional period, such as a "midlife crisis," individuals may reassess their lives, establish new priorities, or seek new skills and interests. At this time, individuals may feel bored and restless and want to change aspects of their lives, relationships, and identity. This transition period may lead to extramarital affairs, separation, or divorce.[2] Transitions of adult children who are leaving home or returning can create stress in family functioning and couple interaction.

Development of Children

Assess children in a family to determine if they are mastering the normative physical, emotional, and intellectual challenges for their ages. In a large family, the infant's and the adolescent's sleep-wake cycles conflict. Assess if each child is meeting age-appropriate developmental expectations and acting in age-appropriate ways in family interactions. Determine whether children assume certain roles, for instance, the "baby," the caretaking child, or the one who misbehaves. Children can put strain on the typical roles of the parents, challenge them in areas where they had difficulty in their own development such as sexuality or separation, and influence the time and energy available for family interests.[3]

Couple Development

The couple's relationship can be viewed in early-, middle-, or late-phase development. Early-phase relationships tend to be unstable and emotionally close, with shared interests and sexual relatedness. Partners are likely to forgo autonomy or separateness. Partners in middle-phase relationships struggle with issues of being their own person and defining aspirations that are different from those of the partner. Emotional distancing, reclaiming of individual interests, sexual boredom, and disillusionment may characterize this phase. As one factor in coming to terms with both individual and partnership needs, late-phase relationships are often stable and satisfying. Alternately, the relationship may stagnate into chronic, unfulfilling, antagonistic, or isolating interactions or dissolution of the relationship.[4]

Family Life Cycle Development

Throughout the life of the family, addition, exit, and aging of members—the family life cycle[5]—are normal and inevitable. Events that require adjustment of the typical emotional and interaction patterns include the following[6]:
- Beginning the couple relationship and leaving the family of origin
- Choosing one's partner as the primary relationship choice among other peer or friendship possibilities
- Marrying and developing of a new family
- Deciding to have children and the pregnancy and postpartum periods
- Parenting infants and preschool children
- Entering children in school with expectations of the broader culture's impact on the family
- Coping with children in adolescence and the related challenges to parental norms
- Downsizing as children leave home
- Being alone again as a couple
- Caring for aging parents of either partner
- Retiring
- Facing death or illness of the partner.

Transactional Factors

Transactions are behavioral exchanges between and among family members that become patterns of interaction over time. Transactions include communication, roles, boundaries in the family, power, and problem solving. Assess both verbal and nonverbal patterns of behavior. Include intuitive hunches and impressions about how the relationship does or does not work.

Communication

Observe if communication is direct, clear, and respectful of differences of opinion. Assess communication style. Is it *congruent* (feelings match the content)? Note the ability to disagree, respond, and listen. Determine the sequence, such as who speaks to whom, and open or closed patterns of interaction.[7] In *open patterns*, the communication is directed to all members. In *closed patterns*, communication takes place only between subsets of the family. For example, children from the original family may have private conversations that exclude adoptive or stepchildren.

Roles

Evaluate how family members describe various roles, such as spousal, parental, occupational, student, and friend, and how much they share similar perceptions of roles. Roles can become polarized and rigid, allowing little spontaneity or change, or they can become exclusive. For example, a young mother may maintain intense and exclusive interaction with a new infant.

RESEARCH NOTE

Waring, EM, Chamberlaine, CH, Carver, CM, Stalker, CA, and Schaefer, B: A pilot study of marital therapy as a treatment for depression. American Journal of Family Therapy 23(1):3–10, 1995.

Findings: Marital discord may increase the risk of a mood disorder in one or both spouses. These authors studied 17 couples, in which the wife was diagnosed with depression, who were given 10 structured, time-limited sessions of Enhancing Marital Intimacy Therapy (EMIT), which was designed to facilitate their self-disclosure. Steps in the intervention included
- Encouraging both spouses to offer an explanation of the depression
- Modeling listening that attends carefully to a spouse's point of view
- Contracting for self-disclosure by both spouses and avoiding interruptions during the process of disclosure
- Focusing on the meaning of experiences and the expression of both affection and anger
- Encouraging spouses to comment on each other's disclosures and provide additional information
- Broadening the perspective of spouses about relationships by encouraging self-disclosure of the following:
  - Each spouse's parents' marriage
  - Reflections on how the couple first met and how the courtship evolved
  - Reflections on the impact of earlier relationships that failed to develop into close confiding relationships.

After treatment, the researchers found that wives were less depressed, healthier, and less symptomatic overall. Wives also thought that their relationship improved, whereas husbands expressed more affection.

Application to Practice: The relationship between depression and marital discord is complicated. Unhappiness in a couple may progress to major depression, or major depression may lead to problems in the relationship. In addressing a couple's complaint of marital problems, nurses should assess the broader aspects of the relationship, for example, psychiatric conditions such as depression that can affect their interactions. This study suggests that addressing relationship issues may help the partner with depression. It implies that specific therapeutic interventions may reduce conflict, promote disclosure of personally stressful experiences, and encourage intimacy.

Boundaries

Family boundaries are the invisible lines of demarcation in a family that separate members or subsets of members. They can be diffuse or rigid, emphasize individual rights and little "togetherness," or reflect extreme togetherness such as "We are totally one and speak for each other." Assess how consistently boundaries operate and how easy it is to break through them.

Power

To assess the power structure, observe a family resolving a conflict or solving a problem, if possible. Relationships are *symmetrical* when partners share power equally, differences are minimized, and roles are similar. Relationships are *asymmetrical* when they are based on a hierarchical structure and are authoritarian, domineering, and nonegalitarian; for example, one partner assumes a parental role toward the other. Observe how children respond to their parents' interactions around power, look at their role in facilitating or thwarting their parents' power positions, and at parental responses. In some families, parents become ineffective and allow children to usurp their power. Children may also become parental, carrying out adult caretaking responsibilities to fill a void. Evaluate *coalitions,* when two people join together against another, and *triangulation,* when a third person is drawn into a conflict in a dyad to diffuse tension.

Problem Solving

The way a family defines a problem influences how they solve it. For example, if parents define their child's wakefulness at night and entering their bed as an indication of illness, then they are less likely to put the child back in his own bed, wait for him to calm himself, or go back to sleep; they are more likely to tolerate the interruption and attend to the child. Conversely, a child's refusal to eat may be defined as stubbornness rather than as a health problem. Before intervening, assess the way families explain problems and problem-solving attempts. Determine whom the family consults, the kind of information they seek, the way they communicate about the problem, and who addresses the problem and carries out the solution.

Affective Factors

Affective factors in the life of the family are values, meanings, and emotions generated by experiential and interactional events that are shared among current family members or are important in the history of the family.

Trust

A climate of respect for different views of members and acknowledgment of individual contributions generates trust in the family. Assess fair distribution of tasks, give and take, so-called reciprocity, and collaboration in role fulfillment. Trust requires a respect for the competence and limitations of each person and implies freedom from coercion, exploitation, or manipulation. Keeping in mind how the needs and goals of individuals mesh with family goals, assess family expectations for individual members.

Mood and Tone

The predominant family mood may be quick paced with anger, hostility, and excitement, or slow paced with depression, withdrawal, and despair. Signs of affection such as hand holding and discussion of emotional events provide clues about the degree of empathy, closeness, or anger. Evaluate intense emotional interactions that can end in abusive exchanges, isolation, or distancing.

Meanings

Determine the meanings that family members attach to events influenced by ethnic, religious, cultural, age, and gender considerations. Meanings may be based on earlier experiences in the family history or reflect similar events in the family of origin. For example, a son's boisterous behavior may be perceived as similar to an alcoholic uncle's.

Relational Integrity

Relational integrity, acting for the interests of oneself and others, involves perceptions of fairness and unfairness in relationships. Assess members' perceptions about what is given and taken, their obligations, and their loyalty to one another.

NURSING AND PSYCHIATRIC DIAGNOSES

After completing the assessment, the family therapist derives a diagnosis and determines a plan of care. Nursing diagnoses clarify the family's particular functional or emotional difficulty; the North American Nursing Diagnosis Association (NANDA)–approved diagnoses that relate to families and family therapy are listed in Box 10–1.

Box 10–2 lists "V code diagnoses," conditions such as relational problems, abuse, or neglect that are the focus of clinical attention and are included in the *Diagnostic and Statistical Manual of Mental Disorders, Fourth Edition (DSM-IV)* but are not mental disorders per se.[8]

FAMILY THERAPY APPROACHES

Family therapy is a common term that implies a systematic set of concepts, therapeutic strategies, and principles of assessment and care. However, the field has spawned competing approaches with different conceptualizations of the family, interventions, and desired outcomes. Two major

> **Box 10–1. NANDA-Approved Nursing Diagnoses Related to Family Therapy**
>
> **Diagnoses of Family Functioning**
> Family Coping: potential for growth
> Family Coping: ineffective, compromised
> Family Coping: ineffective, disabling
> Family Processes, altered
> Parental Role Conflict
> Parenting, altered
> Parenting, altered, risk for
>
> **Individual Diagnoses Relevant to the Family Unit**
> Anxiety
> Communication, impaired verbal
> Grieving, anticipatory
> Grieving, dysfunctional
> Growth and Development, altered
> Home Maintenance Management, impaired
> Protection, altered
> Role Performance, altered
> Social Interaction, impaired

> **Box 10–2. *DSM-IV* Psychiatric Diagnoses**
>
> **Relational Diagnoses**
> Relational problem related to a mental disorder or medical condition
> Parent-child relational problem
> Partner relational problem
> Sibling relational problem
> Relational problem not otherwise specified
>
> **Abuse or Neglect Diagnoses**
> Physical abuse of child
> Sexual abuse of child
> Neglect of child
> Physical abuse of adult
> Sexual abuse of adult
>
> **Additional Conditions**
> Child or adolescent antisocial behavior
> Bereavement
> Academic problem
> Occupational problem
> Acculturation problem
> Phase of life problem
>
> **Individual Response to Psycho Social Stress in the Family**
> Adjustment disorder
>   With depressed mood
>   With anxiety
>   With mixed anxiety and depressed mood
>   With disturbance of conduct
>   With mixed disturbance of emotions and conduct
>   Unspecified

Adapted from the Diagnostic and Statistical Manual of Mental Disorders, Fourth Edition. Copyright 1994 American Psychiatric Association.

family therapy approaches are multigenerational therapies and systems therapies. As seen in Table 10–4, these approaches have different goals, interventions, and roles for the therapist. Table 10–4 identifies the participants, the goals, the role and techniques of the nurse clinician, and the family problem best addressed by the particular approach.

MULTIGENERATIONAL THEORIES AND THERAPIES

Multigenerational approaches obtain a historical account of family life covering three generations. Practitioners emphasize that the past can influence the present and should be taken into account in understanding family dynamics. These multigenerational models include Bowen's theory, contextual family theory, and the object relation theories.

Bowen's Family Emotional System Therapy

In this multigenerational view, individuals deal with anxiety as did past generations, resulting in lack of self-individuation. Anxiety is easily transmitted among family members, and one member often speaks for another. The goal of Bowen's therapy is to help members differentiate from the family's emotional "togetherness" and to help them distinguish feelings from thoughts. The therapist helps adult family members become separate or *differentiate* from their own family of origin. Children are excluded. This form of therapy is helpful for couples, particularly those considering marriage or their first child or those with a symptomatic child.

This family therapy focuses on the family of origin of one or both spouses and is aided by the genogram. In this approach, partners are encouraged to talk to the therapist and not to each other. They are asked to state their thoughts and ideas as the other spouse listens. The therapist attempts to remain neutral by being verbal, taking opposite sides of an issue, and using humor. Partners are encouraged to take "I" positions and state their own ideas, values, and opinions.

> When Mr. C hears from the police that his preadolescent sons have been picked up for shoplifting, he shouts that he will use a belt on them to teach them a lesson. Mrs. C disagrees calmly, "I think that the boys should return the stolen items, apologize for their behavior, and be helped to identify how they can make amends. I think we should find out what they took and why it was important to them."

The therapist acts as a coach, encouraging partners to respond to their spouse's thoughts with a deemphasis on feelings. In this therapeutic process, spouses hear each other for the first time. As one spouse begins to focus on himself or herself and differentiate, the other may struggle to maintain togetherness. Eventually, the remaining spouse starts to differentiate as well.

Contextual Family Therapy

Contextual therapy focuses on what people do in relationships and emphasizes caring, concern, and crediting of pos-

TABLE 10–4. **Comparison of Theoretical Views of the Family**

Theory	Participants	Goals	Role of Clinician	Family Problems
Bowen	An individual or a marital couple	• Differentiate from family origin • Improve cognitive functioning • Decrease emotional reactivity • Modify family relationships, e.g., detriangulation, repair emotional cut-offs	Active, low-keyed, coach, directive Takes cognitive stance emphasizing thinking Techniques: • Genogram • Plan focused approach to change self in relation to family • Reduce anxiety	• Premarital problems • Couples establishing a new family • A symptomatic child is focus of problems in couple's relationship • Couples with high emotionality in interactions • Spouse becoming dysfunctional in role performance
Contextual	Whole family, subsystems of family, and extended family members	• Increase trustworthy relationships • Balance issues of fairness • Confront loyalty obligations • Foster relationship reconstruction and reunion • Foster individual and family growth	Low-keyed exploratory, coach Techniques: • Partial to all family members • Explores legacies and ledgers from family of origin • Facilitates exoneration of parents • Coaches about fairness and loyalty • Fosters trustworthy interactions • Initiates reunions	• Abusive families (sexual and physical, adult and child) • Power imbalances • Estranged families • Unresolved attachment to family of origin • Extramarital affairs • Substance-abusing families • Parentified children in the family • Families caring for aging parents • All life cycle phases
Object Relations	Whole family including children or parents separately	• Increase empathy • Increase esteem of members • Reduce projective communications • Free members of unconscious restrictions • Develop understanding of feelings in relation to oneself • Free children from meeting unmet needs of parents	Active teacher, interpreter, empathic listener Techniques: • Exploration of family histories • Interpretation to increase insight • Empathy training • Decrease of projection processes • Modulation of conflicts and conflictual cycles • Fostering emotional containment of members • Teaching ways to cope with rage and injury	• Child or adolescent symptomatic outside the home • Chronic marital dissatisfaction and fighting • Depression and poor self-esteem in members • Interactions that end in emotional outbreaks • Families unable to solve problems or make decisions • Families where members feel like a victim or victimized in interactions
Structural	Whole families and others impinging on the family; subsystems of the family	• Reorganize family structure: • Create clear flexible subsystems and boundaries • Create effective hierarchy • Foster cohesive executive subsystem • Encourage growth in individual members • Preserve mutual support of members • Promote more adaptive coping	Director, active intervenor, manipulator, coach Techniques: • Use of power and action to shift interaction patterns: Joining family Problem enactment Mapping structures Planned stages of restructuring • Task assignments • Paradoxical interventions • Direct manipulation of interactions	• Families with school-age children; • Families with compliance problems, e.g., asthma, diabetes, anorexia • Life-stage transitions • Divorced and remarried families with children • Families without a workable hierarchy • Families with a chronically ill member • Single-parent families

Continued on following page

TABLE 10–4. Comparison of Theoretical Views of the Family (Continued)

Theory	Participants	Goals	Role of Clinician	Family Problems
Systematic and Strategic	Entire family	Solve the presenting problem: • Specific behaviorally defined objectives • Change behavior to eliminate presenting symptom Social reinforcement: • Acknowledgment • Approval of adaptive behavior Establishing generational boundaries	Director, responsible for creating change, manipulative, action-oriented Techniques: • Joining the family • Giving directives • Substituting new behavior patterns to interrupt feedback cycles • Relabeling, reframing the problem and symptoms • Planning to change symptom-maintaining behavioral sequence • Using paradoxical interventions • Giving homework assignments • Using team approach	• Families with acting-out adolescents • Highly resistant families; symptom-focused families • Families having difficulty establishing a hierarchy • Families struggling with control over relationships • Families with an unhealthy alliance between parent and child with symptoms in the child • Families having trouble coming together (therapy occurs in monthly meeting)

itive interactions. Two key concepts form the basis of concerns and determine the dynamic process in the family: *loyalty* and *justice*. Loyalty includes expectations, commands, and obligations from one's family of origin. Justice involves the balance of fairness in relationships and includes an individual member's merits and obligations. The goal of family therapy is to loosen the invisible loyalties and obligations so each individual can explore new options and give up symptomatic behaviors. It aims to establish trustworthy relationships. This form of therapy helps families who have difficulties such as sexual abuse, extramarital affairs, substance abuse, and other crises. It is useful for all phases of the family life cycle.

> Mrs. A, a 50-year-old woman, cares for an aging mother. Her adult daughter is planning a wedding and wants her to take a weekend to visit. Mrs. A's mother becomes upset and feels that Mrs. A should not be gone so long. Mrs. A feels conflict between her obligations and loyalties to her mother and her daughter.

The family therapist develops a context of trust and fosters trust between family members by emphasizing fairness, siding with one member when the other needs to be accountable, and attending to the needs of all. The therapist acknowledges the contributions members have made to relationships in the family. In a contextual approach, one strategy is *multidirectional partiality*—directing attention to all family members and modeling the right to have each experience heard and understood.[9] Partly by helping family members see that past generations influence loyalty and behavior, the therapist also facilitates acknowledgment that injustices have occurred and that involved parties are coming to terms with the resulting sadness and anger.

Object Relations Theory in the Family

Object relations theory, applied to families, attempts to explain how satisfying relationships with others, so-called objects, are developed and sustained. According to this model, past relationships unconsciously influence current relationships.

Applying these ideas to marriage relationships, Dicks[10] believed that stressed marriages are characterized by mutual projections and attributions. Partners deny feelings that they learned were unacceptable but foster the expression of the feelings in their partner.

> Mrs. L has difficulty allowing herself to be angry. She accuses Mr. L of being angry, and he, in turn, is critical and aggressive and responds irritably to her. Mrs. L corrects his behavior but secretly enjoys the expression of her own "disowned" angry feelings.

The goal of object relations therapy is to free family members of unconscious restrictions so that their relations are based on current realities rather than images from the past. Family therapy helps people understand the vulnerability of parents in relation to unresolved feelings about themselves and helps free children from fulfilling their parents' unmet needs. This form of therapy is helpful for families with children with conduct problems, chronic marital dissatisfaction, depression in one of the parents, or an inability to problem solve.

The family therapist initially establishes an empathic relationship and context. The therapist teaches parents how to contain their emotions and to delay responding to attacks, accusations, and idealizations. The couple is helped to reflect on the meaning of projections. Later, empathy training includes having one member recognize words or actions that aroused hurt feelings in the other. The hurt member is also encouraged to identify desirable alternative responses and behaviors from family members. As therapeutic confrontation occurs, family members are taught to observe aspects of family members they have been ignoring and understand their personalities.[3,4] The therapist interprets individual conflicts to promote change. For example, the therapist may show how a parent's own self-criticism leads to critical behavior toward family members. The ultimate goal is for parents to get in touch with the unconscious roots of misperceptions about other family members and be more empathic to their feelings and experiences.

STRUCTURAL AND SYSTEMIC FAMILY THERAPY

Three theoretical approaches to family therapy conceptualize families as systems; structural family therapy, systemic and strategic family therapy, and the psychoeducational approach. Homeostasis and positive feedback, concepts drawn from general systems theory, underlie these models. Behavior is understood in the context of the family, and an individual's behaviors change as the family context changes. Interventions focus on present interactions within the family and on changing repetitive behavioral sequences. Therapy is brief, symptom-oriented, and directive, using therapeutic contracts and behavioral tasks. Rather than understanding the behavior, relabeling or reframing is emphasized.

Structural Family Therapy

The focus of structural family therapy is to reorganize **family structure**. Structure is the organized pattern in which family members interact; it determines when, how, and to whom family members relate. It includes subsystems, groupings of family members who join together to perform various functions. The overarching goal of structural therapy is to alter family structure so that the family can solve its problems. Structural therapy is favored for families facing life-stage transitions or with school-age children, a chronically ill member, or a member who fails to comply with treatment.

> Billy, the oldest child in the family and a model student, brought home a failing report card since his father's promotion, which requires long absences from home. His mother has relied more on Billy to help her with the younger children; he is the parental child in his father's absence. To help the mother and father reestablish their parental roles and to help Billy return to his status as child, the therapist restructures the family relationship.

The structural family therapist works to change the family structure by changing the way members relate to each other.

> Members of the Z family always agree with each other and are *enmeshed*; they are encouraged to practice stating differing views. Members in the D family have difficulty finding time to be together and are *disengaged*; they are encouraged to draw a picture of the family doing something together.

The therapist actively works in the present, uses direct and indirect interventions, and attempts to highlight and modify interactions. The therapist focuses on the sequences in interactions: when someone speaks, who speaks next, who distracts, and who seeks attention. Important information includes emotions, repetition of behaviors, and duration of interactions; interventions include manipulation of space and moving distant members closer to each other. For example, by having parents sit side by side to discuss an issue and removing the talkative child from between them, the therapist modifies transactional patterns to support the parents. Boundaries are also reinforced when the therapist encourages family members to talk to each other and not about one another. The structural therapist assigns tasks to members—for example, indicating how and to whom family members should communicate—and provides education and guidance such as teaching parents how to take charge or respond differently to children.[11]

Systemic and Strategic Family Therapy

Strategic therapists focus on the present, sequences of interaction, the presenting problem, and symptoms, rather than on understanding, personal growth, past history, or seeing every member of the family. According to this model, interventions focus on changing behavior; a behavior becomes a "problem" depending on how family members respond to it.

> Whenever Amy and her mother disagree, her father protects Amy by scolding her mother and telling her to leave Amy alone. Amy then becomes weepy. Amy also interrupts conversations between the parents and attempts to keep the attention on herself. The family therapist uses directives—tasks with a therapeutic intent—to change inappropriate sequences of behavior. The therapist may ask the parents to discuss the disagreement with Amy by helping her mother to argue with her father.

Used appropriately, these interventions can help change the **family system**; however, they can be harmful if misapplied.[12] The goals of strategic therapy are to reorganize the family, get them "unstuck" from repetitive problem-maintenance cycles, and increase their flexibility. Strategic therapy is helpful for families who have difficulty coming together frequently, symptom-focused families, and those with parent-child conflicts.

Systemic therapists develop hypotheses regarding the rules in the family that maintain interactions and behavior. They emphasize alternative ways of knowing for the family by creating an environment in which new information is introduced into the family system. The pieces of behavior of each family member can be compared to the moves of a player in a conventional game. The therapeutic task is to break the rules and alter the game. Systemic therapists believe in a team approach. The therapist who interviews the family is observed behind a two-way mirror by the team, which focuses on the family interaction and designs the message that will be given to introduce new information to the family. Specific interventions then facilitate change.

Psychoeducational Approach

The psychoeducational model assists families with a seriously and persistently mentally ill member. Both nurse generalists and nurse specialists commonly use the psychoeducational approach to help rather than blame families for their children's psychiatric problems. It focuses on relapse prevention and on maximizing the coping and functioning abilities of clients and families.

By not seeking a cause, the psychoeducational model helps families of clients with schizophrenia more than other therapies. Studying schizophrenia and relapse, Brown, Birley, and Wing[13] coined the term *expressed emotion* (EE) to refer to how a family shows both positive and negative feelings. Clients with schizophrenia are more likely to relapse in families with high EE because they are highly reactive to and easily overwhelmed by stress in their environment, characteristics of high-EE homes. When family members are hypercritical or intrusive, clients become overloaded and decompensate. This form of psychoeducation teaches families how to reduce EE and bypass stress.

The psychoeducational model is applied to families with a wide range of psychiatric disorders and chronic medical illnesses such as multiple sclerosis and diabetes.[14] It challenges beliefs about illness and develops ways families can improve their lives.

The focus of the psychoeducational model generally includes
- Seeking a collaborative partnership with families, including empathy, support, and empowerment
- Identifying and emphasizing family strengths instead of deficits
- Sharing information about the nature and course of the illness
- Emphasizing the role of medication in preventing relapse.

Because family members are the primary caretakers, include them as members of the treatment team. Stress realistic hopes that life can be better for themselves and their ill family member. Help family members lower their expectations and reduce pressure on the client to function normally. In this major shift in family therapy, the search for a cause or cure is replaced with ways to cope with the illness and prevent relapse.

EXPECTED OUTCOMES

Evaluation is an ongoing process in family therapy. Each meeting can be different because of which members attend. Families vary in their participation in and ambivalence about treatment. On one hand, they want to alleviate the pain of the dysfunction, but on the other they may show fear and resistance. Expected outcomes are based on predefined goals. Goals are either immediate or reflect lasting changes in the family over the series of therapeutic meetings. Each family session is evaluated in terms of its impact on long-term goals. For example, an assignment for a parent to teach a sibling of a chronically ill child how to ice skate has the immediate goal of aligning the parent and healthy child in

---

RESEARCH NOTE

Riesch, SK, Tose, CB, Thurston, CA, Forsyth, D, Kuenning, TS, and Kestly, J: Effects of communication training on parents and young adolescents. Nurs Res 42(1):10–15, 1993.

Findings: The purpose of this study was to compare families who attended communication training with those who did not in their perceptions of communication, satisfaction with the family system, and skill in conflict resolution. Three hypotheses were developed: Parents and young adolescents who participate in communication training will have (1) greater satisfaction with the family system, (2) increased open communication, and (3) improved conflict resolution at 2 weeks and 6 months after the training. The results were based on 459 families. Master's prepared nurses facilitated the intervention, 6 weeks of communication training. The results indicated that mothers, fathers, and adolescents receiving the training were more satisfied with the family system than those in the control group. Mothers and adolescents also perceived more open communication. Antisocial behavior decreased significantly among fathers, sons, and daughters in the intervention group, whereas it increased slightly for members of the control group.

Application to Practice: This research illustrates the importance of positive family adjustment to life-cycle changes. These challenging transitions in family life can either offer opportunities for growth and healthy adaptation or present pitfalls that lead to unhealthy coping strategies. Adolescents are challenged to become more adaptable, cohesive, and able to address conflicts. Intervention strategies that address the individual family member, the family context, and education and training in new skills can be important in prevention. The authors cautiously recommend that communication training, aimed at both parents and adolescents, be available for families with children entering middle school. This preventive measure, preparing a child for adulthood, is as relevant as preparation for childbirth.

an enjoyable activity. It may help the family normalize their activities and lessen overinvolvement with the ill child, the long-term goal.

Specific outcomes should be based on predefined goals.

A couple married in their early 40s after a short-term courtship, and the wife became pregnant within 2 months. They disagreed about who should have primary responsibility for caring for the baby and whether the wife should leave her successful career. For this couple, possible goals are

- Facilitating communication
- Addressing decision-making strategies
- Clarifying each spouse's family-of-origin experiences and the impact of parental values and expectations on the couple's choices
- Evaluating spousal roles and expectations drawn from loyalty to family-of-origin values
- Facilitating skills to manage conflict and to improve self-esteem
- Clarifying emerging roles for the couple and for the extended family members.

SYNOPSIS OF CURRENT RESEARCH

Research on the effectiveness of family treatment began in the 1970s. Minuchin and his colleagues[15] were among the first family therapists to investigate the effects of treatment. They studied outcomes of family therapy on children with anorexia nervosa, intractable asthma, and labile diabetes. Based on objective changes such as weight gain, number of asthmatic attacks, and blood sugar levels, 83 to 100% of children responded to treatment. Other studies addressed the effectiveness of family therapy approaches with clients with major mental disorders. Miklowitz and Goldstein[16] studied the effects of psychoeducational family treatment in families with mood disorders. They found that psychoeducation was effective in preventing relapse: only 11% relapsed, whereas 61% relapsed when no psychoeducation was provided. Other research has compared different forms of therapy. One study found that individual therapy may be more effective than family therapy for individuals older than 18 with bulimia and anorexia.[17] Joanning and colleagues[18] found that a family systems approach was more effective in stopping adolescent drug use than adolescent group therapy or a family drug education model. Overall, recent research is rigorously testing the effectiveness of family therapy. No one model has received enough systematic research to clearly state it is the "best" approach; however, these emerging results suggest that many family methods are effective.

AREAS FOR FUTURE RESEARCH

- What are the best ways to measure the effectiveness of family approaches?
- How do the different forms of family therapy vary in clinical outcome?
- What are the effects of nurse-provided psychoeducation to families with a member who has psychiatric or medical illness?
- What standardized tools or self-report instruments best measure the outcome of family therapy?
- What are the most effective interventions for couples with marital problems?
- What are the effects of culture on the outcome of family interventions?
- How do economic and social conditions affect violence in the family?
- How do nurses promote healthy family functioning?
- What are the best ways for divorced and remarried families to function effectively?
- How do family patterns affect teenage parenthood?
- What is the effect of dual-career couples on family functioning?

CASE STUDY

Mrs. C, seen in a community health center for a routine mammogram, told the nurse about tensions in her family, in particular, her children's fighting. The nurse found out that Mrs. C has four children: John, age 23; and three daughters, Sarah, age 21; Amy, age 17; and Beth, age 10. When the nurse asked about any potential violence in the family, Mrs. C revealed that her husband had pushed their 17-year-old daughter on the back. She was concerned that he would "lose it" again. The nurse spoke with Mrs. C about how family therapy might be useful, and Mrs. C agreed to see a family therapist.

Although the therapist invited the whole family to the first session, the father was absent. The son was very vocal, frequently spoke for his mother, and complained bitterly about his father. The daughters were silent except for their discussion of a recent fight between the father and Amy. The two older daughters disagreed about the father's role in the fight. Mrs. C appeared angry at both her husband and Amy. Beth remained silent.

Because so much discussion revolved around the father, the therapist concluded that he must be present in future sessions. Although everyone protested that he would not attend, the therapist assigned them the task of finding a way to have him join them in the sessions. On the second visit he joined the family. The family then related the recent incident that had led to his alienation from the family: He had hit his 17-year-old daughter when she challenged his rules for her dating an older man, age 23. Different members of the family appeared frightened by his loss of control.

Because of the physical abuse, the therapist established rules for safety and assessed the potential for violence. The father expressed regret over losing his temper and indicated that this behavior was unusual. He said he felt stressed because his wife was concerned that Amy was staying out past curfew. Mr. C believed that Amy was acting defiantly. The therapist reviewed methods to curb anger, such as leaving the scene and taking deep breaths. She also discussed the need to have a contract for safety—an agreement that hitting would not be allowed as a way to settle disagreements—and suggested that Mr. C speak to his daughter about the incident so they might reconcile. As Mr. C spoke to his daughter, the therapist encouraged the others to listen quietly to the discussion. The son became angry and loud and said that Amy had a right to make decisions and grow up; he blamed his father for being too strict. Mrs. C said she agreed with her son. The parents were at odds about how to handle Amy's dating and challenge to authority.

With two young adult children, an adolescent, and a younger child, the family appeared to be in a transitional stage of development. Parents need to set different rules for the various children; older children need to separate and move on in their lives. This high-stress period requires adaptation to a new family structure, parents with fewer children, and an eventual return to living alone for the couple. Based on the interactions she saw, the therapist concluded that the family was resisting necessary changes during a transition of the family life cycle.

In the next session, John was asked to sit by the therapist and be an observer-cotherapist while the older sisters developed dating rules that they thought would be fair. At the end of their discussion, John was asked to relay their ideas to Mr. C and to share his thoughts about them with his father. This intervention served two purposes: It aligned the older sisters in a mutually supportive role and encouraged John to address rules with his father in an abstract, less threatening way. He was asked to participate as the oldest child with valuable thoughts to share. During the older sisters' discussion, Mrs. C was encouraged to discuss with Beth plans for an activity they would do together during the coming week, which prevented the mother from undermining the father's authority and also linked her with the youngest child, who appeared to need attention. At the end of this session, the parents were assigned the task of discussing curfew hours and rules during the following week. They were asked to return alone to the next therapy session.

In the individual session with the parents, Mrs. C was sad and depressed and blamed her husband for their daughter's potential promiscuity. She also appeared to be jealous of the attention her husband gave to Amy. The therapist explored the parents' relationship, courtship, and current sexual relationship and discovered that the parents had discontinued any intimate relations two years previously. Amy's dating behavior raised anxieties about their own relationship. Work with the couple continued to address their parenting skills, previous family history, and the difficulty in their sexual relationship. The children were brought in for two more sessions, at which time John indicated that he had found an apartment and Sarah was engaged; Amy was the maid of honor and enjoying her new relationship of sharing with her sister.

CRITICAL THINKING QUESTIONS

1. What concerns led the nurse to refer Mrs. C for family therapy?
2. Who becomes the client in family therapy?
3. What is the immediate goal for family therapy?
4. Identify reasons why family therapy is a more useful approach than either individual or group therapy for the C family.
5. Develop a care plan, including short- and long-term goals for the C family.
6. Identify how family therapy interventions change the family system and pattern of interactions.

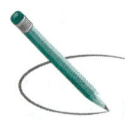

KEY POINTS

- Family therapy has competing approaches with different conceptualizations of the family, foci for intervention, and expected outcomes.
- Family therapy grew out of research focusing on interactions in families with a disturbed member.
- Later research focused on understanding the family as a system in which all members influence each other.
- In a family perspective, conflicts between individuals rather than internal conflicts influence mental health.
- Family therapy is concerned with the whole family and attempts to change family interaction and functioning.
- Family therapy is appropriate for family life-cycle adjustments such as adolescent children and aging parents, normal life crises such as birth of a child, and unexpected crises in the family such as death of a child and divorce.
- Nursing assessment of the family considers demographic, sociocultural, historical, developmental, transactional, and affective factors.
- Assessment data guide the nurse in referral for family therapy, goal setting, and identifying interventions.
- Bowen's theory of family therapy focuses on helping adult family members differentiate from their own family of origin.
- The contextual theory of family therapy views fairness and loyalty as the key issues that influence interactions. It focuses on building trusting relationships among family members.
- Object relation theories focus on establishing empathic understanding between family members by helping them listen, communicate, and control angry, hurtful exchanges.
- The structural theories focus on modifying interactions and establishing appropriate boundaries by assigning tasks, teaching, and guiding.

References

1. Skolnick, AWS, and Skolnick, JH: Family in Transition. HarperCollins Publishers, New York, 1992, p 379.
2. Levinson, D: The Seasons of a Man's Life. Alfred A. Knopf Inc, New York, 1978.
3. Anthony, JE, and Benedek, T (eds): Parenthood: Its Psychology and Psychopathology. Little, Brown & Company, 1970.
4. Anderson, CM, Dimidijian, SA, and Miller, A: Redefining the past, present, and future: Therapy with long-term marriages at midlife. In Jacobson, N, and Gurman, S (eds): Clinical Handbook of Couple Therapy. The Guilford Press, New York, 1995, p 247.

5. Carter, B, and McGoldrick, M: The Changing Family Life Cycle: A Framework for Family Therapy, ed 2. Gardner Press Inc, New York, 1988.
6. Glick, ID, and Kessler, DR: Marital and Family Therapy, ed 2. Grune & Stratton, New York, 1980, p 36.
7. Watzlawick, P, Beavin, JH, and Jackson, DD: Pragmatics of Human Communication. WW Norton, New York, 1967.
8. American Psychiatric Association: Diagnostic and Statistical Manual of Mental Disorders (ed 4). American Psychiatric Association, Washington, DC, 1994.
9. Boszormenyi-Nagy, I, Grunebaum, J, and Ulrich, D: Contextual therapy. In Gurman, AS, and Kniskern, DP (eds): Handbook of Family Therapy, vol II. Brunner/Mazel Inc, New York, 1991.
10. Dicks, HV: Marital Tensions. Basic Books, New York, 1967.
11. Minuchen, S, and Fishman, HC: Family Therapy Techniques. Harvard University Press, Cambridge, MA, 1981.
12. Fisher, L, Anderson, A, and Jones, J: Types of paradoxical intervention and indications/contraindications for use in clinical practice. Fam Process 20:25–35, 1981.
13. Brown, GW, Birley, JLT, and Wing, JK: The influence of family life on the course of schizophrenic disorders: A replication. Br J Psychiatry 121:241, 1992.
14. Rolland, JS: Helping Families with Chronic and Life Threatening Disorders. Basic Books, New York, 1994.
15. Minuchen, S, Rosman, B, and Baker, L: Psychosomatic Families. Harvard University Press, Cambridge, MA, 1978.
16. Miklowitz, DJ, and Goldstein, MJ: Behavioral family treatment for patients with bipolar affective disorder. Beh Mod 14:457, 1990.
17. Dare, C, et al: The clinical and theoretical impact of a controlled trial of family therapy in anorexia nervosa. J Marital Fam Ther 16:3, 1990.
18. Joanning, H, et al: Treating adolescent drug abuse: A comparison of family systems therapy, group therapy, and family drug education. J Marital Fam Ther 18:345, 1992.

CHAPTER 11

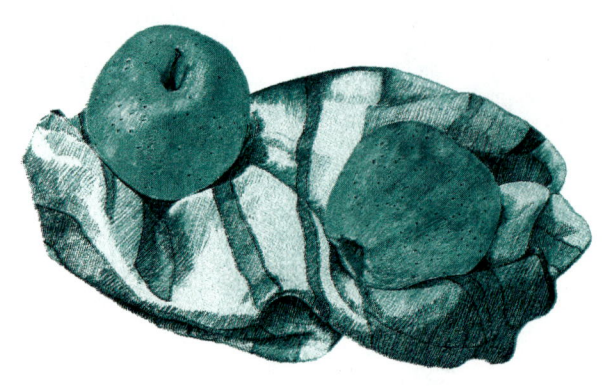

CHAPTER OUTLINE

Purpose of Sexual Therapy
Nurse's Role
  Assessment of Sexual Functioning
  Referral for Sexual Therapy
Sexual Therapy
  Types of Sexual Therapy
Expected Outcomes
Synopsis of Current Research
Areas for Future Research

LEARNING OBJECTIVES

After completing this chapter, the reader should be able to:
- Define the steps and barriers to taking a sexual history.
- Describe the guidelines for a sexual interview.
- Understand the reasons for referral for sexual therapy.
- Identify different types of sexual therapy.

KEY TERMS

healthy sexual functioning
orgasm
sexual arousal
sexual desire
sexual dysfunction

Margery Chisholm, RN, EdD, CS, ABPP

Sexual Therapy

Sexual difficulties recently ranked fourth in a survey of the top problems families face today.[1] Problems with sexual functioning are often underreported, underdiagnosed, and unstudied. Individuals and their partners may be embarrassed to seek help, see the problem as less important than other aspects of their health, or see sexual therapy as a luxury. Nurses and other health-care professionals may be uncomfortable asking questions about intimate behavior and sexual practices. As a result, both professionals and clients may avoid discussing the feelings, thoughts, and activities associated with sexual health. Nonetheless, promoting **healthy sexual functioning** is an important part of the nurse's role.

Sexual difficulties may be temporary, secondary to illness or treatment, or a permanent consequence of a chronic illness or injury. They can be related to medical illness, alcohol or substance abuse, medications, or reflect stressors or marital discord. Nurses are in a key position to assess the presence of an organic cause and, if it is ruled out, refer clients and their partners for sexual therapy.

PURPOSE OF SEXUAL THERAPY

Sexual therapy is a specialized form of therapy, based on cognitive-behavior, systems, and psychodynamic approaches, that assists individuals and couples in their sexual functioning and in understanding their sexual health. Psychiatric nurse generalists do not conduct sexual therapy. Psychiatric clinical nurse specialists, social workers, psychologists, and psychiatrists, often with specialized postgraduate training, are sexual therapists. Nurses can assess the need for further treatment and help resolve sexual difficulties caused by medical illness and the limitations it creates.

NURSE'S ROLE

The nursing role encompasses four main areas.[2]
- Understanding clients' behaviors and reactions to sexuality in health and illness
- Serving as a resource about sexuality, sexual norms, and differences in cultural and individual attitudes about sexuality
- Helping clients develop healthy sexual functioning
- Referring clients with more complex sexual dysfunctions and disorders

ASSESSMENT OF SEXUAL FUNCTIONING

Everyone holds beliefs about acceptable and restricted sexual behaviors and feelings, and societal taboos foster secrecy and privacy. These attitudes may prevent people from revealing sexual behaviors, fantasies, thoughts, and feelings. Therefore, the nurse should strive to create an accepting, nonthreatening atmosphere in which the client and partner can share concerns. Because of their own sexual experiences, lack of appropriate language, or awkwardness in discussing sexual functioning, however, nurses may have difficulty addressing this important part of emotional and physical health. Seek out supervision if personal feelings or difficulties impede the sexual evaluation of clients. Possible nurses' reactions are listed in Table 11–1.

Gather specific sexual information as part of the nursing assessment. Ask about relationships as a way to gradually discuss sexual functioning. Because one or both partners may be experiencing a sexual problem, assessing both members of the couple determines the best treatment plan. Define any areas that the client or family wants kept confidential.

Table 11–2 lists questions nurses can ask to assess sexual health, especially sexual dysfunction.[2] They can help to assess sexual dysfunction in individuals with recent medical illness or who are adapting to a chronic condition.

Several self-report scales—paper-and-pencil questionnaires that the client fills out rather quickly—are also available to assess sexual functioning. Inexpensive and easily scored, they help clients organize their thoughts, disclose sensitive information, and stimulate further exploration of individual sexuality. Some examples of self-report questionnaires are the Marital Satisfaction Inventory,[3] the Sexual Opinion Survey,[4] the Sexual Interaction Inventory,[5] and the Derogatis Sexual Functioning Index.[6] The first scale provides a measure of general marital satisfaction, whereas the others focus on sexual satisfaction and functioning. These scales can be used to gather further information as part of the nursing assessment.

TABLE 11–1. Possible Nurses' Reactions

- May be shy or insecure about the sexual aspects of their professional role even though they are sanctioned to touch others in an intimate and personal manner and to ask personal questions, including questions about sexual matters, related to their patients' health.
- May experience anxiety, even revulsion, when dealing with sexual questions or behaviors while caring for their patients.
- May deny their own or their patients' sexuality by avoiding any verbal or behavioral interaction regarding sexual function, for instance, avoiding the subject of sex, responding to sexually oriented questions in a vague manner, or using euphemistic expressions such as "private parts" or "down below" when referring to genitalia.
- May use hospital rules to sidestep patients' sexual concerns. For example, they may assign male staff to male patients when sexual behaviors or concerns develop.
- May not recognize or may actually encourage patients' becoming emotionally involved with them.
- May experience pity for patients who are unable to perform some sexual acts following injury, such as spinal cord injury. May feel insulted, denigrated, or angered by some patient behaviors, such as flirting, pinching, and exposing body parts.
- May feel uncomfortable dealing with sexual dysfunction in patients.
- May have a mistaken belief that the seriously ill do not have sexual needs or desires, and may show a lack of tolerance and empathy for a patient's sexual concerns during illness.

Source: Gorman, LM, Sultan, DF, and Raines, ML: Davis's Manual of Psychosocial Nursing. FA Davis, Philadelphia, 1996, p 317.

TABLE 11–2. Guidelines for a Sexual Interview

These questions serve as a guideline. Adjustments in the focus and depth of the assessment depend on the nature of the patient's problem and the nurse's level of comfort discussing sexual concerns.

1. Does the patient's current physical condition affect his or her level of sexual function?
2. Does the patient have concerns about body image or self-esteem related to illness, injury, or surgery?
3. What does the patient know about potential or expected changes in sexual function related to the illness, injury, surgery, or medications?
4. What significance does the physical change or limitations have on the patient's perceptions and understanding of sexual function?
5. What are the patient's previous sexual patterns?
6. What does the patient's spouse or significant other understand and believe about the patient's sexual function and the impact of the illness, injury, surgery, or medications?
7. What are the patient's outlook and prognosis regarding sexual function?
8. What is the patient's level of comfort and willingness to discuss sexual function with health professional, spouse, or others?
9. Would the patient or significant other benefit from more education, counseling, or therapy?

Source: Gorman, LM, Sultan, DF, and Raines, ML: Davis's Manual of Psychosocial Nursing. FA Davis, Philadelphia, 1996, p 319.

REFERRAL FOR SEXUAL THERAPY

Before referral for sexual therapy, an assessment of sexual functioning is necessary. Among the factors that influence sexual health are medical problems such as diabetes and hormonal disruption, psychiatric disorders such as major depression, and sociocultural influences such as religious or ethnic teachings. Poor communication between partners or limited physical contact may affect sexuality. Chapter 23 details the medical and pharmacologic contributions that may affect sexual functioning (see Table 11–3).

Sexual therapy is most commonly used to treat the **sexual dysfunctions** (discussed in detail in Chapter 23) disorders that include problems with **sexual desire**, physical components of **sexual arousal** and **orgasm**, and pain. Sexual pain, which may be recurrent or prolonged, features discomfort in the organs and tissues stimulated during sexual activity. Part of the nurse's role is to refer clients, when necessary, for sexual therapy.

Explain to clients that the primary goal of sexual therapy is to create or restore mutual sexual satisfaction, comfort, and pleasure.[7] Inform them about the types of approaches available. Instruct them that a change in their sexual relationship depends on both partners working in the therapy.

SEXUAL THERAPY

Sexual therapy is a deliberate, scientific, and collaborative approach that assists individuals and couples in their sexual functioning and in understanding their sexual health. It combines interventions from cognitive-behavioral, systems, and psychodynamic models. Sexual therapy may involve a single consultation or long-term weekly visits to uncover underlying causes of the problem.

As an extension of marital and family approaches, sexual therapy addresses sexual desire, performance, and satisfaction in sexual encounters between partners. The therapist discusses the relationships among communication patterns, feelings, sexuality, and the couple's interactional patterns. The sexual therapist evaluates four areas of sexual functioning: psychosexual development, psychosocial environment during sexual development, current sexual functioning, and medical history, past and present. Specific dimensions of the sexual functioning assessment are listed in Table 11–4.

TABLE 11–3. Drugs That Alter Sexual Behavior

Drugs (Classification)	Probable Effects
Antihypertensives	Produce vasodilation and decreased cardiac output; depress CNS. Cause impotence in men and decrease vaginal lubrication in women.
Antidepressants	Anticholinergic side effects can cause impotence, premature ejaculation, delayed orgasm. Decrease depression.
Antihistamines	Anticholinergic side effects can cause impotence, premature ejaculation, delayed orgasm.
Antispasmodics	Smooth muscle relaxation can cause impotence.
Sedatives and tranquilizers	Depress CNS. Produce tranquilization and relaxation. Depress libido.
Oral contraceptives	Remove fear of pregnancy.
Alcohol	In small amounts, may increase libido. In large amounts, impairs neural reflexes involved in erection and ejaculation. Chronic use may cause impotence.
Opioid narcotics	Central sedation causes impotence in chronic users.
Cancer chemotherapy agents	Possible temporary or permanent testicular and ovarian failure causing impotence, lack of desire.
Estrogen	Suppresses sexual function in men.
Diuretics	Chronic use may cause impotence.

Source: Gorman, LM, Sultan, DF, and Raines, ML: Davis's Manual of Psychosocial Nursing. FA Davis, Philadelphia, 1996, p 316. Reprinted with permission.

TYPES OF SEXUAL THERAPY

Cognitive-Behavioral Model

The essential components of the cognitive-behavioral model are enhancing communication skills, changing attitudes, decreasing anxiety through exercises, changing the environment, and doing homework assignments to practice new techniques under less stressful conditions. Masters and Johnson, pioneers in the field of sexual therapy, were the first to use this model with clients. They used a dual-sex therapist team with the couple to build the alliance and facilitate behavioral interventions.

The model emphasizes how learning affects healthy and unhealthy sexual functioning. Role models, rules in upbringing, sexual information and misinformation, and peer and family experiences affect sexual performance. Practice exercises and teaching about sexual stimulation can help people "relearn" healthy sexual functioning. As seen in Table 11–5, sensate focus and desensitization are common behavioral interventions. Exercises focus on physical sensations, sexual stimulation, techniques for sexually stimulating the partner, and ways to produce sexual fantasies. These exercises are usually assigned as homework outside the therapy session.

Psychodynamic and Psychosexual Model

Helen Singer Kaplan[8,9] developed a sexual therapy model that integrates psychodynamic theories with behavioral interventions and interpersonal processes. According to the *psychosexual therapy* model, anxiety causes sexual problems. Anxious feelings may be caused by recent or remote, mild or serious, or internal or relationship-related factors. The goal of the psychosexual model is to relieve anxiety related to sexual desire or performance.[9] This therapy begins with an extensive sexual assessment and evaluation. For clients over age 40, the effects of medications or undiagnosed illness are important considerations.

Key components of this approach are changing the immediate causes of the sexual problem and providing symptom relief by using experiential techniques called *sexual tasks*,[9] which are tailored to the specific sexual dysfunction. Each couple proceeds at their own pace based on their decreasing anxiety and increasing comfort with the behavioral tasks.

Once treatment progresses and a trusting alliance is built, the therapist helps the couple look at underlying "deeper causes" for the sexual difficulties.[9] The deeper causes are related to the client's past history and previous sexual experiences. For instance, sexually abused clients usually do not benefit from sexual therapy until their abuse history is uncovered and treated. Clients with hostile or neglectful parents may not progress in therapy until these underlying issues are addressed.

Systems Model

The systems model of sexual therapy is an extension of family therapy theories. Sexuality or sexual difficulties are viewed as symptoms that reflect an underlying family issue. How the sexual problem fits into the relationship is key. The presenting complaint of sexual dysfunction is caused by basic problems with communication, commitment, or intimacy.[10] In therapy, current patterns of interaction are assessed, including how the couple deals with conflict, stress, and anger. For instance, one partner may withhold sex when angry. In the systems model, couples establish set dysfunctional patterns or rules around the relationship issues. To effect change, the sex therapist in this model asks:

- Who initiates sexual activity?
- Who expresses anger?
- Are sexual desires expressed indirectly or directly?

TABLE 11–4. Sexual Functioning Assessment Guide

Psychosocial Dimensions
Family Influences on Sexual Development
- Quality of relationships in family (parents, parents and children, siblings)
- Attitudes toward males, females
- Communication of emotions (methods of expression of affection, anger)
- Teachings about sex (which parent, what aspects, at what age)
- Parents' attitudes and behavior (regarding modesty, privacy, nudity)
- Unusual circumstances (abuse, neglect, substance use)

Sociocultural Influences
Cultural or Ethnic Group Teachings
- Rites of passage
- Attitudes toward gender and role expectations

Religious Teaching and Values (explanations for deviance)

Psychosexual Dimensions
Childhood
- Memory of first sexual feelings
- First sexual experience (pleasant or upsetting)
- When masturbation discovered
- Any sexual experimentation with other children
- Sexual attractions to others? Who? Age?
- Participation in or witnessing of an uncomfortable sexual experience
- Childhood sexual theories or myths

Adolescence
- Age of puberty, menarche, wet dreams
- Reaction to body changes
- Relationships with peers (same sex, opposite sex)
- Self-esteem, body image
- Dating as compared to peers
- Sexual behavior and age at onset
- Importance of sexuality
- Sexual fantasies and pursuits
- Substance use
- Sexual behaviors uncomfortable for self or others

Adulthood
- Significant love relationships after age 20
- Persons with whom sexual
- Marriage and relationship history
- Sexual problems in any of these relationships
- Any unusual sexual experiences
- Sexually transmitted diseases
- Approaches to safe sex and contraception

Current Sexual Functioning
- Sexual and nonsexual activities in current relationship
- Satisfaction in frequency, quality of encounters
- Flexibility in sexual attitudes
- Variability in sexual behavior
- Strengths, weaknesses of partner
- Likes and dislikes of sexual behavior of partner
- Themes of fantasies or daydreams
- Recent changes in sexual functioning? desire? arousal? orgasm?
- Problem always present or reflect a change?
- Frequency of occurrence of problem
- Situations in which problem occurs
- Current engagement in any troubling sexual behavior

Medical History
- Significant childhood and teenage diseases
- Accidents, injuries
- Surgical procedures
- Congenital disorders
- Current diagnosed diseases (acute and chronic)
- Any medical complications
- Births, miscarriages, abortions
- Menstrual difficulties and/or menopause
- Medication
- Psychiatric care
- Any hospitalizations

Source: Adapted from Risen, C: A guide to taking sexual history. Psychiatr Clin North Am 18:39, 1995; Wincze, JP, and Carey, MP: Sexual Dysfunction: A Guide for Assessment and Treatment. The Guilford Press, New York, 1991; and Group for Advancement of Psychiatry, Report # 88, 1977.

- How is affection expressed?
- What does a partner do when feeling stressed?

The goal of treatment is to help clients understand the meaning of the sexual problem and how it affects their relationship in the context of previous and current life experiences.

EXPECTED OUTCOMES

The outcomes of sexual therapy are related to the clinical issues of a particular couple and usually reflect one of the following:

- Increased knowledge about sexual functioning and health
- Transformed attitudes that were destructive, avoidant, and negative, interfering with love making
- Increased acceptance of limitations in sexual functioning due to medical or aging factors
- Increased dialogue and empathy in confronting difficult stressors
- Enhanced communication in all areas of the relationship including sexual areas
- Expanded techniques and strategies in sexual repertoires
- Lessened performance anxiety and body-image anxiety

TABLE 11–5. Cognitive-Behavioral Techniques Used in Sexual Therapy

Sensate Focus

Technique. This method encourages couples to be sensual through body exploration and massage of each other. The first step involves no caressing of genitals or breasts. It is followed by encouraging pleasure to erotic areas.

Goal. To interrupt the couple's anxious interactions and lower expectations and pressure for sexual performance.

Desensitization

Technique. The couple imagines progressively more anxiety-arousing situations or experiences the situation while remaining relaxed.

Goal. To decrease anxiety while simultaneously promoting relaxation.

The Squeeze Technique

Technique. Stimulation of the penis by the partner until sensations of orgasm occur. The partner then squeezes the lower part of the penis with the thumb and first finger of both hands for 3–4 seconds.

Goal. To maintain erection and prevent premature ejaculation.

- Increased feelings of attachment
- Lowered barriers to intimacy and added opportunities for sexual expression.

In addition, the individual's and couple's progress can be evaluated with self-report measures.

SYNOPSIS OF CURRENT RESEARCH

Sexual therapy is a relatively new clinical field that has received little scientific study. Masters and Johnson[11] conducted the first landmark research on sexual dysfunction, described in their 1970 book *Human Sexual Inadequacy*. Because sexual therapy draws on multiple dimensions—namely, the physical, emotional, cognitive, and interactional aspects—it is difficult to describe the treatment and identify what factors cause specific outcomes. Some recent studies have looked at how to conduct research on sexual therapy. The focus has shifted from studying physical aspects of sexual response to include an individual's thinking patterns, sociocultural constraints, and lived experience of therapy. There is little research to support one specific therapeutic approach over another. Most of the research to date has focused on the positive benefits of sexual therapy in several couples, rather than large systematic studies.

AREAS FOR FUTURE RESEARCH

- What is the long-term impact of sexual therapy on sexual functioning?
- What is impact of sexual therapy on quality of life?
- What are the most effective treatments for sexual dysfunctions?
- What client and therapist characteristics correlate with successful treatment?
- How does sexual therapy affect marital happiness and family functioning?
- What is the role of biological and physiological factors in treatment outcome?

CASE STUDY

Mr. and Mrs. C entered therapy for a family problem, the provocative behavior of their adolescent daughter, who broke curfews and displayed other oppositional problems. As the family incident resolved, it became apparent that Mr. and Mrs. C had difficulties in their relationship; they had not had intercourse for several years. The nurse decided to meet with each of them alone and then together to obtain more information.

The nurse assessed their past and current relationship. The couple had been high school sweethearts. Neither had had another serious relationship or sexual encounter. Mrs. C was raised in a strict Catholic family. Mr. C's father was a Protestant minister. Their parents' disapproval of their dating led them to sneak off at nights to meet away from their home town, which added to their excitement. During these dates, they engaged in heavy petting, were rushed in their sexual activity, and always had the anticipation of being found out.

Both were interviewed alone as part of the assessment. Mrs. C had stopped sleeping with Mr. C 2 years previously and moved into the bedroom with their youngest daughter. Mrs. C expressed anger toward him; he didn't seem to care that she had stopped sleeping with him and made no effort to discuss it with her. She thought that he would become more responsive to her if she let him know how upset and unhappy she was. His lack of interest and support left her feeling worse about their problems and their marriage.

Mr. C stated that he felt that his wife was strict and critical with the children. He believed that she was putting too much emphasis on their daughter's dating and turning it into a problem. Although he did not like the age of the boyfriend, he believed that his wife acted hysterically in setting limits and prying into what was happening on their dates. Overall, Mr. C felt that he could not please his wife no matter what he tried. He also described some setbacks in his work in the last few years and said he had to attend to these problems.

When interviewed together, the nurse asked each of them to discuss how their sexual life had been before things seemed to turn for the worse. Mrs. C started to cry and indicated that sex had become frustrating. She was reluctant to indicate why and asked Mr. C to share his view about their sexual life. Mr. C said that he had a problem with premature ejaculation that had made their encounters unsatisfying for his wife. This problem had started when they were dating. He always felt rushed and became tense with sexual excitement. Mrs. C felt confused and thought that he did not love her. She was also uncomfortable with prolonged touching and found it difficult to relax. She said that she had periodic enuresis, was embarrassed by this symptom, and thought that it contributed to their sexual problem.

The nurse then made a referral for sexual therapy. Somewhat reluctantly, Mr. and Mrs. C went to a psychiatric clinical nurse specialist who treated individuals with sexual dysfunctions. After ruling out a medical condition, medication, or substance that affected their sexual functioning, the therapist explored each of their anxious feelings about their sexual relationship, as well as the effect of their daughter's dating relationship on the couple. He suggested *sexual tasks* to decrease anxiety and improve performance. Although they initiated intercourse, Mrs. C remained less satisfied with their relationship. As the treatment progressed, the therapist helped the couple address underlying "deeper causes" for the sexual difficulties, including their parents' disapproval of their relationship and marriage and their religious upbringing. The couple continued to work on these issues weekly for about 1 year. Their marital and sexual relationship improved. Mrs. C continued to have issues related to her parents' behaviors and beliefs. She decided to continue in individual therapy to work on these issues.

CRITICAL THINKING QUESTIONS

1. What sociocultural and familial influences may contribute to this couple's sexual dysfunction?
2. Explain how the daughter's behavior may be linked to the couple's problem.
3. In the assessment of the couple, what further information would you seek? Are there any biological or physiological problems you would want to rule out?
4. Identify reasons for referring the couple for sexual therapy.
5. What behavioral tasks should be assigned as homework? How would you help the couple carry out any homework?
6. What would be your outcome measures at the termination of therapy?

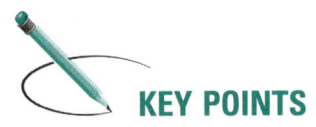

KEY POINTS

- Gathering specific sexual information is best done early in the nursing assessment after establishing rapport and a relaxed climate.
- The sexual assessment interview includes psychosexual development, psychosocial environment during sexual development, current sexual functioning, and current and past medical history.
- Paper-and-pencil tests of sexual attitudes and functioning can facilitate gathering clinical information and also measure outcomes of sexual interventions.
- Medical problems and hormonal levels in men and women can affect sexual functioning.
- Sexual therapy focuses on the individual's physical functioning, relationship issues, and deeper psychological issues.
- Sexual therapy is a deliberate, scientific, and collaborative approach that assists individuals and couples in their sexual functioning and in understanding their sexual health.
- The types of sexual therapy include those based on cognitive-behavior, psychosexual, and systems models of treatment.
- The goals of sexual therapy are based on the areas of difficulty identified in the assessment and determined collaboratively with the couple.

REFERENCES

1. Bazar, J: Family problems alike in U.S., Soviet Union. Am Psychol Assoc Monitor, 34, 1989.
2. Gorman, LM, et al: Davis's Manual of Psychosocial Nursing. FA Davis Co, Philadelphia, 1996.
3. Snyder, D: Marital Satisfaction Inventory: Manual. Western Psychological Services, Los Angeles, 1981.
4. Fisher, WA: The sexual opinion survey. In Davis, CM, Yarber, WL, and Davis, SL (eds): Sexuality-related Measures: A Compendium. Graphic, Lake Mills, IA, 1988, p 34.
5. LoPiccolo, J, and Steger, JC: The sexual interaction inventory: A new instrument for assessment of sexual dysfunction. Arch Sex Behav 3:585, 1974.
6. Derogatis, LR, and Melisaratos, N: The DSFI: A multidimensional measure of sexual functioning. Sex Marital Ther 5:244, 1979.
7. Wincze, JP, and Carey, MP: Sexual dysfunction: A Guide for Assessment and Treatment. The Guilford Press, New York, 1991.
8. Kaplan, HS: The New Sex Therapy. Brunner/Mazel Inc, New York, 1974.
9. Kaplan, HS: Disorders of Sexual Desire. Brunner/Mazel Inc, New York, 1979.
10. Heiman, JR: Treating sexually distressed marital relationships. In Jacobson, NS, and Gurman, AS (eds): Clinical Handbook of Marital Therapy. The Guilford Press, New York, 1986.
11. Masters, WH, and Johnson, JE: Human Sexual Inadequancy. Little, Brown, Boston, 1970.

CHAPTER **12**

Reminiscence Therapy

CHAPTER 12

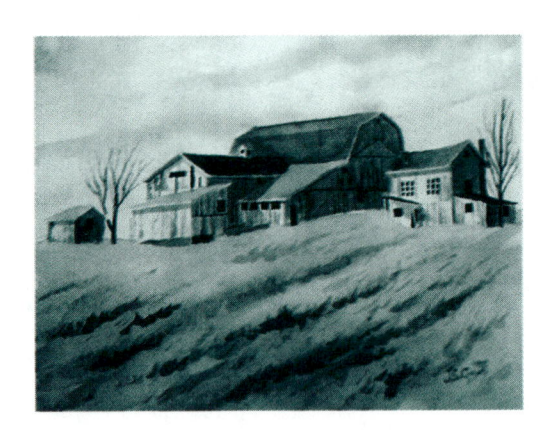

CHAPTER OUTLINE

Types of Reminiscence
   Simple Reminiscence
   Informative Reminiscence
   Life Review
   Oral History and Autobiography
Definition of Reminiscence Therapy
Purposes of Reminiscence Therapy
Nurse's Role in Reminiscence Therapy
Intervention Strategies
Expected Outcomes
Areas for Future Research

LEARNING OBJECTIVES

After completing this chapter, the reader should be able to:

- Differentiate between reminiscence therapy and life review therapy.
- Identify clients for whom reminiscence therapy is an appropriate intervention.
- Discuss the nurse's role in individual and group reminiscence therapy.
- Describe the current state of knowledge about reminiscence therapy based on a review of recent research.

KEY TERMS

informative reminiscence	reminiscence therapy
life review	remotivation therapy
reminiscence	simple reminiscence

Barbara A. Jones, RN, DNSc

Reminiscence Therapy

Reminiscence, the act or process of recalling the past, is a complex phenomenon believed to occur in all people throughout the life span. Havighurst and Glasser[1] noted it in children as young as 10 years old. The amount of time spent reminiscing appears to increase as we age and then to decline in the very old. Reminiscence may be silent or spoken, solitary or interactive, spontaneous or structured.

Prior to publication of Robert Butler's[2] seminal work on reminiscence among the elderly, it was considered a maladaptive behavior. Reminiscence was interpreted as a form of escapism, distracting the elder from unpleasant realities, particularly the multiple losses associated with advanced age, typically, loss of health, spouse, friends, job, residence, and social status. Living in the past seemed understandable because, for the elder, it was preferable to confronting a present characterized by grief, social isolation, and frailty. Reminiscence was devalued yet tolerated because dwelling on the past was a behavior congruent with society's stereotypic view of the elderly.

Butler, using the work of Carl Jung as a framework, interpreted reminiscence as the product of a subtle intrapsychic shift toward increased introspection in aging. Even the most extroverted adults, when confronted by the losses and physical changes that remind them of their own mortality, begin to spend more time reflecting on the meaning of their past and present life experiences. Butler proposed that life review is a major developmental task of the older adult. It enables the elder to resolve the final developmental crisis,[3] achieving a sense of integrity or despair after considering the meaning of one's life. Butler interpreted reminiscence as a purposeful activity through which life review is accomplished. Although more recent interpretations of life review question its universality, purpose, and outcomes, mental health professionals in diverse disciplines concur that reminiscence is a valuable, purposeful behavior among all age groups, especially the elderly.

Reminiscence is an adaptive mechanism that increases the elder's sense of security despite escalating change, enhances self-esteem, preserves self-concept, and reduces stress.[4] Reminiscence therapy may be conducted with individuals or groups wherever elders receive care.

TYPES OF REMINISCENCE

Merriam[5] describes the following types of reminiscence.

SIMPLE REMINISCENCE

The recollection of past experiences without analysis or evaluation is **simple reminiscence.** It can be triggered spontaneously by a sensory stimulus or current event; for example, the scent of lilacs on a warm spring day may trigger memories of lilac bushes in the backyard of one's childhood home, or an approaching holiday might evoke memories of holidays long past. Simple reminiscence may also occur in response to a request for the sharing of memories, for example, someone else saying, "Tell me about your first job." Remembered events are often recounted in rich, colorful detail and positive or negative emotions.

INFORMATIVE REMINISCENCE

Storytelling, through which elders pass on their experience and knowledge to younger generations, and oral history in the form of autobiography, genealogy, or the history of a specific event or region are known as **informative reminiscence.** In preliterate societies that had no written historical records, it was prized, and today oral histories are still priceless legacies for families and rich sources of historical research data for others. Gustafson[6] reminds us that "the personalization of history can provide insight, information, and clarification that otherwise is at risk of being lost forever." Audiotaping or videotaping stories and oral histories adds to their vividness.

LIFE REVIEW

Life review differs from simple and informative reminiscence in its structure, purpose, and intensity. It covers the entire life span in an attempt to integrate all of one's life's experiences into a whole or *gestalt*.[7] It is evaluative in nature, a spontaneous soul-searching. Life review analyzes the meaning of a person's life experiences and attempts to resolve old conflicts. Its impetus is usually impending death. As Butler[2] unequivocally states, "The biological fact of approaching death, independent of—although possibly reinforced by—personal and environmental factors, prompts the life review." This intense, often urgent, process takes an emotional toll on the elder and can generate both negative and positive feelings. Anxiety, regret, guilt, depression, and fear can coexist with enhanced acceptance of self, others, and one's life. A positive self-appraisal is characterized by forgiveness of self and others, acceptance and appreciation of a

> **RESEARCH NOTE**
>
> **Merriam, SB: The structure of simple reminiscence. Gerontologist 29 (6):761–767, 1989.**
>
> **Findings:** This qualitative theory-building study was designed to address the need for a better conceptualization of the phenomenon of reminiscence.
>
> Transcripts of one-to-one reminiscence sessions conducted with 25 older Virginians with a mean age of 71 were examined for recurrent regularities in the data. The patterns identified were refined and consolidated into a set of categories that describe the structure of simple reminiscence.
>
> Merriam identified four phases of elicited reminiscence: selection, immersion, withdrawal, and closure. During the selection phase, the elder mentally sorts through his or her memory files and selects a memory that has special meaning either because of its accompanying feelings or the elder's central role. During immersion, the memory is shared in rich detail. Events and associated emotions are discussed in logical sequence. During the withdrawal phase, the reminiscer reflects on the event often, comparing it to some aspect of his or her present life. Closure is an abrupt summation, often accompanied by a perceived truth or nugget of wisdom.
>
> **Application to Practice:** The four-part structure of simple reminiscence suggests it is an orderly, logically coherent process. The researcher emphasized that similar phases may not be found in spontaneous reminiscence or life review.

person's unique identity and life journey, acceptance of the inevitability of death, and manifestation of such attributes as serenity, wisdom, and candor. As Black and Haight[7] express metaphorically, "The life review is like the weaver, it is the instrument that helps to form the pattern, to find the meaning, and to arrive at a complete sense of one's self." The tapestry woven by all the threads of a life is finally done and the completed picture revealed. Conversely, a negative resolution of life review is characterized by difficulty expiating guilt and relieving intrapsychic conflict, high death anxiety, and chronic depression. Some elders, in profound despair, may attempt suicide.

ORAL HISTORY AND AUTOBIOGRAPHY

Also covering the entire life span but differing from life review in their primary purpose, oral history and autobiography communicate life experiences to an audience to teach, admonish, inspire, or even create myth. The purpose of life review is to find meaning in one's life through self-evaluation and integration of past conflict.[2]

DEFINITION OF REMINISCENCE THERAPY

Reminiscence therapy is the use of simple and informational reminiscence as a nursing intervention for treatment of specific psychosocial nursing diagnoses. Although the client shares memories about himself or herself as well as about remembered persons, events, and places, it is not synonymous with life review therapy, which is a more formal and intense process, covers the entire life span, and is generally conducted one to one. In life review therapy, the client must talk about self, critical choices, and the meaning life events had for him or her. In reminiscence therapy, the client may choose to talk about feelings and life's meaning or choose not to soul-search. Whereas reminiscence therapy may be conducted with clients of any age, it is usually a nursing intervention for older adults.

PURPOSES OF REMINISCENCE THERAPY

Reminiscence therapy is a life-enhancing process. Its goals are to provide opportunities for socialization, diversion, pleasure, and communication; to prevent or alleviate isolation and depression; and to increase life satisfaction and self-esteem by validating the client's worth, uniqueness, and achievements. Romaniuk and Romaniuk[8] identified four functions of reminiscence.

- The client's self-image is enhanced by informing others about the challenges and accomplishments of his life.
- Reminiscence is frequently a pleasurable, comforting activity that passes unoccupied time in an enjoyable manner.
- Reminiscence can increase the client's self-understanding and acceptance of his or her past and present life by stimulating life review, a potentially healing process.
- Reminiscence can be a problem-solving technique, a means for working through a troublesome past or present event.

Reminiscence escalates following a loss and facilitates mourning. It provides an opportunity for *catharsis,* the discharge of intense emotions related to present and past losses, which is especially important for institutionalized elders, who often feel they must keep their emotions in check. Memories of a loss are likely to be bittersweet, involving unresolved conflicts and past wounds both inflicted and received. Reminiscence therapy provides opportunities for resolving such conflicts and completing grief work. Reminiscing reinforces a sense of self in institutionalized older adults who are at risk for depersonalization because of their lack of intimacy and their routinized care.

Sherman[4] emphasizes that reminiscence therapy provides unique opportunities for client assessment. What is remem-

> **RESEARCH NOTE**
>
> Sherman, E: Reminiscence and the Self in Old Age. Springer Publishing Co Inc, New York, 1991.
>
> **Findings:** This descriptive study was designed to validate the four functions of reminiscence previously identified by Romaniuk and Romaniuk.[8] A questionnaire developed by the researcher to measure older adults' perceptions of the functions of reminiscence was distributed to 104 volunteers aged 60 to 91 residing in four senior housing complexes in upstate New York.
>
> Analysis of responses validated the typology of functions of reminiscence developed by Romaniuk and Romaniuk. However, only 54% of participants specified that self-understanding was a function of reminiscence.
>
> Older adults agreed that reminiscence enhances self-image; provides comfort, pleasure, and diversion; and facilitates working through troublesome past or present events. Not all elders agreed that reminiscence increases self-acceptance and self-understanding. Sherman concluded that self-acceptance and self-understanding are functions of life review. Elders themselves appear to recognize a distinction between reminiscence and life review.
>
> **Application to Practice:** Nurses who implement reminiscence therapy should recognize that clients may not expect discussion of the past to be accompanied by self-evaluation or analysis of the meaning of events and experiences. Some elders find self-evaluation uncomfortable, distressing, or highly personal and may withdraw from reminiscence therapy because they do not wish to scrutinize their lives. For this reason, reminiscence therapy should focus on simple and informative reminiscence.

and Snadowsky[10] describe a stepladder approach for deciding on appropriate psychosocial therapeutic modalities with elders (Fig. 12–1). Clients who are severely cognitively impaired or who are apathetic and regressed benefit most from sensory training and validation therapy.[11] For the moderately cognitively impaired client, *reality orientation* and **remotivation therapy** are the recommended modalities. Remotivation therapy is also effective for the profoundly depressed client. Reminiscence therapy is most appropriate for clients who meet one or more of the following criteria:

- Normal cognition or mild cognitive impairment
- Mild to moderate depression
- Withdrawn, socially isolated, understimulated behavior.

Maas, Buckwalter, and Hardy[12] recommend reminiscence therapy for clients with the following nursing diagnoses:

- Self-care deficit due to depression
- Diversional Activity Deficit due to monotonous environment, immobility, decreased activity tolerance, sensory impairment, and social isolation
- Altered Thought Processes due to stage 1 or 2 dementia. These stages are characterized by loss of recent memory, progressive loss of instrumental activities of daily living, depression, and dysfunctional behavior evoked by stress, fatigue, change in routine, or illness.

Rantz[13] agrees that reminiscence therapy may aid memory in the client with mild cognitive impairment. She explains that "the process of sharing may bring latent memories to the surface and connect missing links in memory chains." Reminiscence therapy should be a supportive, nonthreatening experience for the cognitively impaired client. The accuracy of memories cannot be validated readily; therefore, the client's mentation is not under scrutiny.[14] In fact, some of what is shared by any client in reminiscence therapy may be myth or hyperbole[4] for the purpose of maintaining self-esteem or obtaining attention.

Reminiscence therapy can take place with individual clients or in a group. Sherman[4] reported on the benefits of the group approach, noting that "group reminiscing had either captured or triggered a process in a number of participants that seemed to lead to change in the quality and content of their reminiscing as well as in their morale and self-concept."

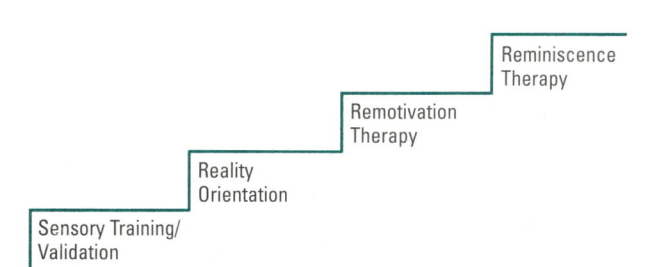

Figure 12–1. Stepladder approach to psychosocial care of the older adult. (Adapted from Weiner, MB, Brok, AJ, and Snadowsky, AM: Working with the Aged: Practical Approaches in the Institution and Community, ed. 2. Appleton-Century-Crofts, Norwalk, CT, 1987.)

bered and shared reveals the client's psychological states and generally reflects his or her present mood or concern. Hamilton[9] suggests that much can be learned about clients by noting both the content of memories and the accompanying affects. Topics repeatedly avoided should also be noted. Those who emphasize memories of family traditions and special events involving family and friends may be reflecting the importance of belonging. Those who stress their achievements and accolades may be reflecting needs related to self-esteem.

NURSE'S ROLE IN REMINISCENCE THERAPY

The nurse's first task is to determine whether reminiscence therapy is appropriate for a particular client. Weiner, Brok,

The group approach is the most appropriate for all clients meeting the inclusion criteria except the homebound, bedbound, and the severely hearing impaired. Clients who have a severe hearing deficit that cannot be corrected are generally poor candidates for a reminiscence group.[15] They experience frustration because of their inability to follow the conversation, and the need to repeat what is being said is disruptive to both the group leader and other members. Clients with severe hearing impairment respond best to one-to-one reminiscence therapy. Their needs for socialization must be addressed through their inclusion in group activities where the emphasis is not on listening.

> **RESEARCH NOTE**
>
> Wallace, JB: Reconsidering the life review: The social reconstruction of talk about the past. The Gerontologist 32(1):120–125, 1992.
>
> **Findings:** Wallace used a qualitative research approach to challenge the widely accepted views of Robert Butler (1963) about the propensity of older adults to talk about the past. Butler[2] proposes that with advanced age, increased talk about the past is expected, universally occurring, and purposeful. It is an outward manifestation of an intrinsic psychodevelopmental process.
>
> One-to-one, unstructured life narrative interviews were conducted with 30 older adult volunteers with a mean age of 91 years. Respondents were asked to tell their life stories, including or omitting whatever they wished. Analysis of transcripts focused on story production rather than on the story itself.
>
> Most respondents had difficulty complying with a general request to tell their life stories and preferred a question-and-answer format. Many respondents indicated they rarely thought about the past.
>
> Rejecting Butler's interpretation of talk about the past, Wallace instead proposes that talking about the past is a social activity prompted by narrative challenges or younger persons' requests for information about the past. The positive effects of reminiscence result from the social reinforcement it provides rather than from conflict integration.
>
> **Application to Practice:** Some elders, given the opportunity to reminisce, may choose not to because they rarely think about past events and feel no need to reconsider them. Wallace's findings contradict those of most researchers who affirm the universality of reminiscence. Instead, he views reminiscence as primarily a social activity. Some clients who perceive that their social needs are met or who have difficulty socializing may decline to participate in reminiscence therapy. The nurse should accept the client's right to refuse yet should also carefully assess that client's social needs and resources.

Box 12–1. Sample Instruments for Baseline Assessment of Potential Group Members

- Global Assessment of Function Scale
- Mini–Mental State
- Brief Cognitive Rating Scale
- Zung Self-Rating Depression Scale
- Beck Depression Inventory

The nurse should complete a baseline assessment of affect, attention span, concentration, and orientation on each potential group member. Many valid and reliable instruments are available for use as assessment tools.[16] The nurse may also assess clients less formally on the basis of observation and interaction and on the perceptions of other staff. Clients assessed to be appropriate for the reminiscence group should be approached and asked to participate. Because the word *group* can be intimidating to some elders who associate that term with psychotherapy, the nurse can refer to a *meeting*. Clarify the group's purpose: to share memories with other group members in response to a selected topic or theme. Those who seem reluctant to participate should be encouraged to attend the initial session as listeners until they feel more comfortable.

The nurse planning a reminiscence group should consider working with a co-leader who can assist with physical arrangements, transportation issues, and monitoring group processes and outcomes.[14] Members should be given a list of the dates and times of the group sessions; however, they should also be given additional reminders on the day before and at the end of the session. Clients who use hearing aids or corrective lenses should be reminded to bring them to the group.

Group size is an important issue. Having fewer than four clients in the group puts too great a demand for participation on the members. Eight members are ideal.[15]

Leaders should give careful consideration to the space where the group will be held. A quiet, well-lit room with a table and comfortable chairs is ideal. Sessions typically are held for 1 hour once or twice weekly. The importance of beginning and ending on time cannot be overemphasized. Failure to start on time diminishes the importance of the group in the eyes of its members and creates anxiety. When the group runs beyond its stated time, it conflicts with other activities and inconveniences both group members and staff.

Based on assessment of the prospective group members, the nurse should select for the initial group session a topic or theme likely to be nonthreatening and appealing (Table 12–1). An alternative is planning groups focusing on each decade of life or on early childhood memories, school days, jobs and careers, marriage and parenting, and retirement years. Music and memorabilia trigger reminiscence and pro-

TABLE 12–1. Sample Topics For Reminiscence Therapy Group

Favorites (vacation, dress or outfit, song)	Fashions
Firsts (date, car, job)	Pets
Hobbies	Sports
Holidays	Tools
Family traditions	

vide sensory stimulation. While almost any stimulus can induce reminiscence, photographs and music are among the most powerful stimuli. For example, a book on "Olde Philadelphia" delighted elders participating in a reminiscence group in a Philadelphia suburb. All had grown up in the city and migrated to the suburbs to raise their children. They pored over photographs of stores, churches, restaurants, theaters, and baseball parks, sharing vivid memories of their experiences in these places, many of which were since demolished. A group held in a long-term care facility sponsored by the Catholic church responded enthusiastically to hymns of their youth that are now no longer popular.

The leaders often serve refreshments appropriate to the chosen theme. For example, at a reminiscence group session for elderly Jewish clients, which was devoted to the Jewish holiday of Purim, *hamentashen* were served. These traditional triangular fruit pastries are served on Purim to symbolize the tricornered hat worn by the king's viceroy, Hamen, whose plan to slay the Jewish people was turned upon himself by Queen Esther's clever strategy. As children, these elderly clients probably dressed up in costumes and reenacted the story of Purim. A well-chosen refreshment can function as a trigger for reminiscence.

To decrease members' anxiety, the initial group sessions should be highly structured, and the leaders directive. As the group members begin to know one another and what to expect in the group, they feel more comfortable sharing memories and typically assume more of the leaders' functions. They may suggest a theme or a refreshment or volunteer to bring a cherished object. In a long-term care setting, the nurse may be astonished to discover that residents have shared a common space for years yet know little about one another. The first few sessions may seem stilted as elders politely take turns speaking to the leaders with little member-to-member interchange. As cohesion develops, members talk more to one another rather than to the leaders. The nurse's goal during these early sessions is to make each member feel welcome, comfortable, and appreciated.

INTERVENTION STRATEGIES

Throughout the life of the reminiscence therapy group, the nurse uses principles of group dynamics and group process.[15] All members require acknowledgment and attention from the leader to prevent attrition from the group. The nurse can facilitate interaction by encouraging each member to speak, while adding that members who prefer not to talk are most welcome to continue attending. The nurse may be able to establish member-to-member connections by emphasizing common bonds among members.

For example, Carolyn M, a reminiscence group member, stated that she never did much traveling because she worked 12 hours a day in a family-owned bakery. However, she had read extensively and included James Michener's stories of faraway places among her favorites. The leader knew that Eunice L, one of the group's quietest members, was born in Doylestown, Pennsylvania, where James Michener grew up. She asked Eunice about him. The group and its leader were surprised to learn that timid Eunice had been Michener's high school classmate. She had many interesting stories to share but would never have done so without prompting. The positive feedback Eunice received from the other members led to future self-initiated group participation.

Pace is a critical issue in reminiscence therapy. The nurse should refrain from hurrying the group. Time is needed for memories to surface and be articulated; silence must be accepted and expected. Often leaders feel uncomfortable with silence and fill it with their own reminiscence or a change of topic. Rushing can cause anxiety and irritation. The leaders must take their cue from the members' responses. If members indicate discomfort with silence by fidgeting, laughing, or complaining, the nurse can respond with an example or restate her question. Otherwise, silence is purposeful and must be permitted.

Because monopolizers can disrupt the group process by frustrating and alienating other members, the nurse should intervene by validating the monopolizer's contribution to the group and then directing attention to another group member.[15] If, after several trials, this intervention is not effective in modifying the monopolizer's behavior, the nurse should meet with the member outside the group to restate the group's purpose and perhaps allow additional time for the member's oral history. Clients who ramble should be gently refocused.

Cognitively impaired clients should be assessed for signs of anxiety. The inability to remember or excessive stimulation by the group can cause the cognitively impaired member to lose self-esteem or trigger a catastrophic reaction. The leader who notes anxiety may diffuse it by offering the client additional information or one of the objects brought to group to prompt reminiscence. A gentle touch or prompting can communicate reassurance and acceptance.

Not all remembrances are pleasurable. Some may evoke sadness, regret, disappointment, grief, or anger. The nurse should comment on the affective quality accompanying the shared memory in order to validate the feelings of the older adult.[9] The nurse should be present for the distressed client to convey empathy and provide support. When a client is struggling with a painful memory, words may come haltingly. If the leaders or members urge the client to move on or provide negative feedback, the client feels alone and unaccepted; catharsis and healing are blocked. The nurse must help the group acknowledge the member's pain and provide support. All present have had times of sadness and should be able to empathize. For many group members, holiday memories seem to be particularly poignant.

The nurse must be patient when a client continually reworks certain themes or brings up the same issue. Such repetition is essential in order to resolve and integrate some life experiences. If it seems to impede the group process, the nurse should meet individually with this member to explore the possibility of one-to-one reminiscence therapy or life review therapy.

Both the nurse and the group can assist the client to reframe life events when memories lead to a self-appraisal that is harsh and unforgiving.

> William R shared his perception that he had been a terrible father who spent little time with his children. He described his present relationship with his daughter as superficial and said he was estranged from his two sons. The nurse asked a question about William's relationship with his father. He shared that his father died when he was 9 years old. His mother remarried when he was 14. The marriage was a troubled one, and William's stepfather took little interest in him. The connection between his own lack of a father and his difficulties in parenting was clarified. Another male group member discussed the demands of supporting a wife and several children; he complimented William for fulfilling his role as provider. A female member urged William to talk with his sons about his feelings or, if easier, write to them.

The nurse should evaluate the quality of the reminiscences shared by group members. Sherman[4] suggests a rating scale for this purpose (Table 12–2).

Sherman[4] writes that the "lack of first-person pronouns in reminiscing cannot be overemphasized in terms of its importance or significance. It can be indicative of an attempt to block, forget, or disown an experience from the past." When a client's communication within the reminiscence group remains at levels 1 and 2, the likelihood of experiencing the life-enhancing benefits of reminiscence therapy is reduced. The nurse should attempt to elicit emotional expression from the client by asking about feelings associated with the memory being shared. If the client remains unable to discuss feelings, the nurse should respect this apparent need for distance and control.

Three additional levels of reminiscence, reflecting progressively higher ownership of affective responses, may be experienced by clients but are more likely in one-to-one reminiscence and particularly in life review therapy than in reminiscence groups. Most discourse in reminiscence therapy groups is at levels 1 through 4.

TABLE 12–2. Evaluating the Quality of Reminiscence

- Level 1 discourse. Reminiscence is superficial and impersonal. The client talks about the past with detachment as though the events recounted happened to someone else.
- Level 2 discourse. Personal pronouns (I, me, my) are used by the client; however, communication focuses on sharing ideas, events, and actions. Feelings are not addressed.
- Level 3 discourse. The client briefly refers to feelings without elaboration.
- Level 4 discourse. Reminiscence primarily focuses on feelings about and perceptions of events, actions, and relationships.

EXPECTED OUTCOMES

The positive outcomes of reminiscence therapy include a decrease in depression and self-absorption, increased stimulation and diversion, and "the sheer pleasure of discovery or rediscovery of some forgotten aspect of the self or history of the self that can now be recalled."[4] Clients with early dementia can experience enhanced self-esteem, enabling them to better cope with their illness.[17] Other indirect benefits of reminiscence therapy, such as improved self-care, appetite, and sleep, can be attributed to the energizing effects of higher morale and enhanced quality of life.

When reminiscence occurs in a group, additional benefits are realized. The client can experience the curative or therapeutic factors[18] that can occur in all groups (Table 12–3). Increased socialization within the reminiscence group has the potential to carry over into participation in social activities outside the group. Some clients, through participation in the reminiscence group, may find a confidant. The relationship between client and confidant compensates for former close friends the client has lost due to their death or relocation.

The nursing staff also benefits from reminiscence therapy, which enables them to see their clients as individuals with unique histories and life experiences.[19]

Information about clients' health beliefs, coping skills, and cultural perspectives can be acquired readily. Appropriate self-disclosures made by staff leading the group can eliminate the imprisonment model[20] that is frequently operative in institutional settings. Clients sometimes see themselves as incarcerated, dependent upon staff with whom they have an adversarial relationship. By knowing their clients better and becoming better known by them, staff can prevent or reverse such negative effects of institutionalization as infantilization and depersonalization (see Table 12–3).

Although extremely rare, two negative outcomes of reminiscence are possible. In retentive reminiscence, the past is

TABLE 12–3. Positive Feelings Reported by Some Reminiscence Group Members

Altruism	• Putting others' needs ahead of mine
	• Helping others and being important in their lives
Cohesiveness	• Feeling alone no longer
	• Revealing things about myself and still being accepted by the group
Universality	• Learning I'm not the only one with my type of problem
Interpersonal Learning—Input	• Learning how I come across to others
Interpersonal Learning—Output	• Feeling more trustful of the group and other people
	• Learning to work out difficulties with members within the group
Guidance	• Group members giving definite suggestions about a problem
	• Group leader offering suggestions
Catharsis	• Getting things off my chest
	• Learning how to express positive and negative feelings
Identification	• Seeing that others could reveal thoughts and feelings and benefit from this experience
Family Reenactment	• Being in the group was like being in an accepting, understanding family
	• Through the group experience, better understanding past relationships with parents and relatives
Self-understanding	• Discovering and accepting previously unknown or unacceptable parts of myself
Instillation of Hope	• Seeing positive changes in the other group members inspires me
Existential Factors	• Recognizing that life is at times unfair and unjust
	• Recognizing that ultimately there is no escape from some of life's pain

Source: Modified from Yalom, I: The Theory and Practice of Group Psychotherapy (ed 3). Basic Books, New York, 1985.

RESEARCH NOTE

Lappe, JM. Reminiscing: The life review therapy. J Gerontological Nursing 13(4): 12–16, 1987.

Findings: Lappe compared the psychological benefits of participating in a reminiscence group to participating in another type of group to determine whether group process alone or reminiscence as an intervention produced the positive effects observed. Eighty-three elders, with a mean age of 82.6 years, who had resided in four nursing homes for an average of 33 months, were randomly assigned to either reminiscence therapy or a current events group and then pretested with the Rosenberg Self-Esteem Scale (RSE). Four groups met weekly, and four groups met twice each week to compare the effects of meeting frequency. All groups met for 10 weeks. The RSE was again administered to the group members within 24 hours of their final group session.

Posttest results indicated that the reminiscence group members exhibited a significantly greater increase in self-esteem scores than current events group members. Groups that met twice a week did not show a significantly greater increase in self-esteem than groups that met weekly.

Lappe concluded that the intervention of reminiscence therapy, rather than the group process alone, produced the increase in self-esteem scores.

Application to Practice: Lappe verified the unique benefits of group reminiscence therapy as an intervention to increase the self-esteem of institutionalized elders. Time spent by elders talking with one another and with the nurse about the past is purposeful activity. Conducting reminiscence therapy is a major professional nursing function in long-term care settings.

---

viewed as so superior to the present that the client wishes to remain there. The client withdraws further and further from present reality, choosing instead to reenter and relive an idealized and glorified past.

In reparative reminiscence, the client, through recollection of the past, experiences a severe sense of guilt accompanied by anxiety and a need for forgiveness and restitution.[2,4] Working through reparative issues within the group is hard; other members begin to feel uncomfortable or try to talk the client out of the negative self-appraisal. The nurse may need to intervene outside the group or refer the client for psychological or spiritual counseling, perhaps with life review therapy. The client's perceived need to atone should never be minimized.

AREAS FOR FUTURE RESEARCH

Much of the research to date concerning reminiscence therapy is conceptually flawed, ambiguous, and of limited usefulness. According to Black and Haight,[7] in more than 85 articles published since 1964, researchers have used the terms *reminiscence therapy* and *life review therapy* interchangeably. Nurse researchers are urged to clearly define their terms in future studies.

Burnside and Schmidt[15] discuss the lack of quasi-experimental research, with random assignment and control groups, to measure outcomes of reminiscence therapy. Such studies can be difficult to implement because of institutional constraints and the ethical dilemma of denying an intervention associated with enhanced quality of life. Burnside and Schmidt[15] recommend a single-subject, or case-study, design in which information about a client is collected preintervention and postintervention.

Nurse researchers should also consider qualitative approaches to study the phenomenon of reminiscence. Older adults' perceptions of its meaning need to be described and explored. Researchers emphasize the pleasure, socialization, and diversion reminiscence therapy provides. Do older adults themselves perceive these benefits and others?

CASE STUDY

Evelyn H, 89 years old, recently sold her lifelong home and moved to the personal care unit of a nearby continuing-care retirement community. She could no longer live independently because of limitations imposed by Parkinson's disease. A quiet, serious woman, Evelyn had difficulty forming relationships with residents. Her visitors were few because she had never married or had children, all but one of her siblings were deceased, and her surviving friends were either distant or had impaired mobility.

The unit's nurse became increasingly concerned over Evelyn's isolation and depressive symptoms. She invited Evelyn to participate in a reminiscence group held each Wednesday morning. Evelyn was silent during her first two sessions but appeared to enjoy herself. The third group meeting focused on hobbies. The nurse had brought in needlework, a fishing rod, a stamp collection, and some ceramics to stimulate reminiscence. Evelyn admired the handiwork, adding that she had not done much sewing at home because she was employed for 42 years as a tailor of custom-made ladies' suits. She shared the name of her former employer.

Ralph H, an 84-year-old man with mild cognitive impairment, responded excitedly that his brother had worked for the same business. Their ensuing conversation revealed many shared acquaintances, experiences, and memories. At the conclusion of the group session, Ralph approached Evelyn and invited her to join him and his friends at lunch in the dining room.

Over the next few months, Evelyn developed supportive relationships with both group members and Ralph's friends. Ralph also benefited because reminiscing with Evelyn stimulated the unwounded areas of his mind and provided much affirmation and pleasure.

CRITICAL THINKING QUESTIONS

1. Should reminiscence groups be organized homogeneously according to clients' nursing diagnoses or would a heterogeneous group be more productive?
2. Evelyn has been attending reminiscence therapy group for 2 months. At this morning's session, devoted to the theme of school memories, she very haltingly reveals a memory of an early romance and the severe emotional pain of rejection. She begins to weep. How would you handle this within the group? Would you intervene outside the group?
3. Ralph monopolizes the reminiscence group. He is very entertaining, and the other members enjoy listening to him. When you attempt to refocus the group, the other members urge Ralph to continue. How would you intervene in this situation?
4. Critics of Erikson and Butler[2,3] suggest that at least half of older adults fail to resolve the last developmental crisis of integrity versus despair. They also believe that many elders never question the meaning of their lives. How important do you believe it is to address with clients the developmental task of achieving integrity?
5. The nurse manager asks you to relinquish leadership of the reminiscence therapy group so that you can allocate more time to quality assurance activities. She suggests that a certified nurses' aide take over the group. Develop an effective argument supporting the nurse's role as leader of the reminiscence therapy group.

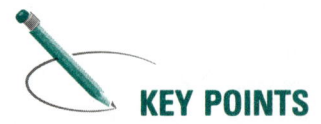

KEY POINTS

- Reminiscence therapy is a nursing intervention that enhances the older adult's sense of identity, security, and self-esteem while reducing stress.
- Reminiscence therapy may be conducted with individual clients or in groups in any setting where elders receive care.
- Life review and reminiscence are not synonyms. Life review involves consideration of the client's entire life for the purposes of self-appraisal, conflict resolution, and self-acceptance. It is generally conducted individually with clients who desire to undertake this evaluative process. In contrast, reminiscence therapy uses simple and informative reminiscence to provide socialization, diversion, and pleasure to increase the client's life satisfaction and sense of self-worth. It is a supportive, nonthreatening, therapeutic process.
- Reminiscence therapy is recommended for most elders, especially those who are withdrawn or mildly to moderately depressed.
- Reminiscence therapy can be enhanced with music, photographs, other memorabilia, and refreshments.
- Sometimes memories shared during reminiscence therapy are accompanied by intense emotion. The nurse should be prepared to validate the elder's feelings while offering empathy and support.

REFERENCES

1. Havighurst, RJ, and Glasser, R: An exploratory study of reminiscence. 17: 245–253, 1972.
2. Butler, R: The life review: An interpretation of reminiscence in the aged. Am J Psychiatry 26:65–76, 1963.
3. Erikson, E: Childhood and Society. New York, 1950.
4. Sherman, E: Reminiscence and the Self in Old Age. Springer Publishing Co Inc, New York, 1991.
5. Merriam, SB: The structure of simple reminiscence. Gerontologist 29 (6):761–767, 1989.
6. Gustafson, M: Reminiscence, her way. Am J Nurs 94 (6):64–65, 1994.
7. Black, G, and Haight, B: Integrality as a holistic framework for the life review process. Holistic Nursing 7(1):7–15, 1992.
8. Romaniuk, M, and Romaniuk, JG: Looking back: An analysis of reminiscence functions and triggers. Exp Aging Res 7:477–481, 1981.
9. Hamilton, DB: Reminiscence therapy. In Bulechek, G, and McCloskey, J (eds): Nursing Interventions: Treatments for Nursing Diagnoses. WB Saunders Company, Philadelphia, 1985.
10. Weiner, MB, Brok, AJ, and Snadowsky, AM: Working with the Aged: Practical Approaches in the Institution and Community. Prentice-Hall, Englewood Cliffs, NJ, 1987.
11. Feil, N: The Validation Breakthrough: Simple Techniques for Communicating with People with Alzheimer's Type Dementia. Paul H Brookes Publishing Co, Baltimore, 1993.

12. Maas, M, Buckwalter, K, and Hardy, M: Nursing Diagnoses and Interventions for the Elderly. Addison-Wesley Publishing Co Inc, Redwood City, CA, 1991.
13. Rantz, M: Diversional activity deficit. In Maas, M, Buckwalter, K, and Hardy, M (eds): Nursing Diagnoses and Interventions for the Elderly. Addison-Wesley Publishing Co Inc, Redwood City, CA, 1991.
14. Huber, K, and Miller, P: Reminiscence with the elderly—do it! Geriatric Nursing 5(2):84–87, 1984.
15. Burnside, I, and Schmidt, MG: Reminiscence group therapy. In Working with Older Adults: Group Processes and Techniques (ed 3). Jones & Bartlett Publishers Inc, Boston, 1994.
16. Kane, RA, and Kane, RL: Assessing the Elderly: A Practical Guide to Measurement. Lexington Books, Lexington, MA, 1981.
17. Soltys, FG, and Coats, L: The SolCos model: Facilitating reminiscence therapy. Gerontological Nursing 20(11):11–16, 1994.
18. Yalom, ID: The Theory and Practice of Group Psychotherapy, ed. 3. Basic Books, New York, 1985.
19. Lappe, JM: Reminiscing: The life review therapy. Gerontological Nursing 13(4):12–16, 1987.
20. Wolanin, MO, and Phillips, LR: Confusion: Prevention and Care. Mosby, St. Louis, 1981.

CHAPTER 13

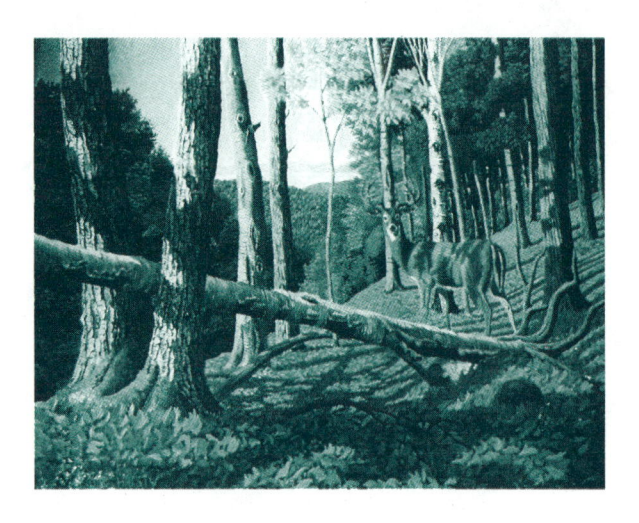

CHAPTER OUTLINE

Purpose of Milieu Therapy
Functions of the Milieu
  Containment
  Support
  Structure
  Involvement
  Validation
Nurse's Role as Milieu Manager
Expected Outcomes
Areas for Future Research

LEARNING OBJECTIVES

After completing this chapter, the reader should be able to:

- Differentiate between therapeutic community and milieu therapy.
- Describe the history of milieu therapy from the 1700s to the present.
- Define the nurse's role as milieu manager.
- Identify areas for nursing assessments, nursing interventions, and expected client outcomes within the context of a short-term inpatient milieu.

KEY TERMS

containment	support
involvement	therapeutic community
milieu therapy	validation
structure	

Karen Hogan King, RN, MS, CS, PC

Milieu Therapy

Through the course of this century, the concept of **milieu therapy** has ranged from the foundation of inpatient treatment to an afterthought in planning acute care. As somatic therapies, length of stay, severity of illness, and cost containment have become prominent factors in the inpatient psychiatric setting, the notion of milieu therapy as an essential modality has come into question.[1] This therapy is important to nursing because the "milieu" traditionally has been the domain of the nurse.[2]

Milieu therapy traces its origins to late–eighteenth century France, when Philippe Pinel struck the chains from insane clients under his care.[3] Pinel attempted to use scientific methods to demonstrate that clients treated with kindness and compassion improved. His theory found social interest in early–nineteenth century England, which was concerned with humanitarian reform. In 1806, William Tuke's "moral treatment" created a milieu that combined kindness and structured activities for psychiatric clients.[4] Quakers transported this philosophy to the United States.

During the Freudian era, as society became more focused on the individual, the moral approach receded. Intrapsychic issues were of more interest than the effect of the milieu on the individual.[5]

After World War II, Maxwell Jones's concept of the therapeutic community gained prominence.[6] The emphasis on the effect of the environment on behavior was reminiscent of the nineteenth-century moral treatment era.

PURPOSE OF MILIEU THERAPY

The **therapeutic community** specifically emphasized health and rehabilitation instead of mental illness. The community members included all staff as well as clients (when the term *client* instead of *patient* was first used). Democracy and egalitarianism were deliberately employed to erode the barriers between staff and clients. A focus on group processes rather than on individual therapy was maintained, and the concept of a multidisciplinary team was introduced.[4]

The concept of the community meeting was also introduced in the therapeutic community model. Unlike most "community meetings" in the structure of today's milieu, this meeting expected free expression of affect from both staff and clients.[7] Because permissiveness, egalitarianism, emphasis on group rather than individual, and community self-regulation were the prime characteristics of the community, any differences in roles or power structures between staff and clients were de-emphasized.

In Maxwell Jones's therapeutic community at the "Industrial Unit" of Belmont Hospital in Sutton, Surrey, England, the clients were carefully screened. They were primarily war veterans with substance-abuse problems or character disorders, and there was very little psychosis. The length of stay was very long as well.

Although the therapeutic community was designed as a specific social setting, it is considered to be the foundation for milieu therapy, or the therapeutic milieu, as it is defined today. Certain elements of the therapeutic community are still valid:

- Viability of the multidisciplinary team concept
- The assumption that clients and staff have a meaningful impact on each other
- The belief that support and structure are helpful to client recovery
- The belief that the unit milieu is dynamic and evolving and that unit culture needs to be monitored.

These elements do not depend on length of stay or severity of illness. However, elements of the therapeutic community are no longer valid in a cost-contained, psychopharmacologic-based treatment setting (Table 13–1). The concept of milieu therapy grew from the therapeutic community—with an important conceptual difference. The therapeutic milieu was consciously sculpted to promote structured interactions and communication, and ultimately staff retained authority and responsibility for the milieu.[8]

FUNCTIONS OF THE MILIEU

In 1978, Gunderson[9] defined five essential functions of the therapeutic milieu: **containment, support, structure, involvement,** and **validation** (Table 13–2). Even in today's inpatient milieu, which "serves as a brief, intensive waystation for client, family, and ambulatory providers,"[10] these functions are valid.

TABLE 13–1. Invalid Beliefs of the Therapeutic Community Still Present in Current Settings

- The belief that staff has ultimate authority in the milieu. (The belief that clients have power to self-regulate is critical.)
- The belief in permissiveness as promoting cure. (Behavior that was once considered healthy is now considered unhealthy acting out. Containment, safety, and limit-setting are now important.)
- The belief that all pathological behavior is due to faulty social interactions and that corrective social interactions are required to cure all clients.
- The belief that cure is based on examination of processes going on in the group rather than individual therapy.
- The belief that all clients should receive "the same treatment" regardless of diagnosis.

CONTAINMENT

Containment maintains the safety of the milieu. Physical integrity is paramount, both in terms of preventing injury through assault or suicidal acts and in terms of providing medical care and proper nutrition for clients. The environment is contained literally through locked doors and windows. Staff know the whereabouts of each client and keep track of visitors and other people who enter the unit. Certain items universally considered dangerous (for instance, razors or sharp knives) are housed in a staff area and are accounted for at each shift.

Clients are expected to maintain appropriate boundaries regarding personal space, personal belongings, social behavior, and attire. The staff must be nonjudgmental in determining what is appropriate, keeping in mind the goal of containment.

TABLE 13–2. Functions of the Milieu

- *Containment*: maintaining the safety of the milieu
- *Support*: maintaining a sense of connection, worth, and hope in the milieu
- *Structure*: defining the milieu in terms of time and orientation
- *Involvement*: addressing clients' active participation in treatment and in other interactions within the milieu
- *Validation*: Affirming a person's individuality within the milieu

Source: Sederer, LI: Brief hospitalization. In American Psychiatric Press: Review of Psychiatry 2:518, 1992.

SUPPORT

A sense of connection, worth, and hope in the milieu is provided by support. Clients feel supported in an environment in which they believe they are understood and cared for without being infantilized or feeling dependent.

Even in a fast-paced inpatient setting, groups can provide an opportunity for clients to be empathic to each other, to give advice, and to provide reality testing for each other in a nonthreatening way. Supportive groups incorporate Yalom's[11] curative factors, in particular, instillation of hope, universality, imparting of information, altruism, development of socialization techniques, imitative behavior, interpersonal learning, and group cohesiveness.

STRUCTURE

The milieu is defined in terms of time and orientation through structure. Structure provides a sense of organization and concreteness in the milieu and gives clients a comfortable way to feel attached to the unit.

Traditionally, the unit expectations and norms could be passed along to new clients by incumbents' directions and role modeling. The "history" of the unit could be held within the client group. In many units, hall policies regarding structure (for example, visiting hours and medication times) could be discussed or even amended at community meetings.

INVOLVEMENT

Involvement addresses clients' active participation in treatment and in other interactions within the milieu. In the short-term setting, the milieu is an essential foundation for goal setting, discharge planning, medication treatment, and client education.

The nurse involves the client in treatment from the outset, forming an alliance by helping him or her to identify the crisis that resulted in hospitalization.[12] Then the nurse involves the client in setting some very specific goals for the hospitalization, which may differ from the treatment team's goals in scope and specificity. Clients who are actively involved in setting goals are more likely to be involved in the milieu and in the treatment process.[13]

VALIDATION

Validation affirms a person's individuality within the milieu. The individual relationship between the nurse and the client is, in itself, validating. The nurse can enhance this affirmation by developing specific interventions for the client's care. In interviews with the client, the nurse can encourage the expression of affect, reaffirm the client's sense of self, and focus on the client's relationship to the outside world. In the short-term setting, clients may not experience such a loss of connection to the outside world by virtue of being separated from their usual milieu only briefly.

> **RESEARCH NOTE**
>
> LeCuyer, E: Milieu therapy for short stay units: A transformed practice theory. Arch Psychiatr Nurs 6(2):108–116, 1992.
>
> **Findings:** Principles of milieu therapy have been applied to inpatient psychiatric settings for many years. The author demonstrates that nursing practice related to milieu therapy can be adapted to meet the needs of clients in short-stay inpatient units. The author defines traditional components of milieu therapy, identifies current client needs, and develops nursing actions to meet short-term treatment goals.
>
> Concepts basic to the milieu—containment, support, validation, structured interaction, open communication, arrangement of client environment, and ties with family and community—are still valid in today's inpatient settings to meet client needs. Traditional inpatient goals of resocialization and ego development are seen as long-term outpatient goals. Current outcomes include symptom resolution, increased or restored coping, hope and sense of direction for treatment, willingness to engage in treatment after discharge, sense of confidence in treaters, and knowledge of resources. The nursing role becomes clearer in the more concrete, clearly defined short-term setting. Nursing actions include providing or coordinating structured activities, limits, and controls as needed; setting up appropriate treatment experiences; maintaining therapeutic activity levels; facilitating open communication; and coordinating or participating in policy development and implementation.
>
> **Application to Practice:** Concepts developed as the foundation of the therapeutic milieu can be applied to today's short-stay units. Nurses can continue to manage the milieu effectively and provide specific interventions for clients in a brief hospitalization.

NURSE'S ROLE AS MILIEU MANAGER

Although milieu therapy is no longer the primary treatment philosophy of inpatient units, recognize that inpatient work cannot be carried out effectively without a well-functioning milieu. The nurse as a milieu manager is mindful of keeping a safe and respectful environment of open communication; flexibility in programming to meet different developmental, educational, and diagnostic needs; predictability in structure; and active involvement of clients and families. In maintaining this environment, the nurse provides a trusting atmosphere of care, competence, and safety for clients. By providing a milieu with these attributes, the nurse makes it possible for clients to ally with their treatment team and successfully plan for the next level of care.

In a brief hospitalization, the treatment team's goals include crisis intervention, diagnosis, initiation of a treatment plan, acute symptom stabilization, discharge planning, and consultation with clients, families, and others in the client's outpatient network.[10] Client and family education are an essential part of the consultation as well. The nurse can facilitate the client's relationship with the milieu and the treatment team as a whole by representing the clients to the team and helping them to negotiate the course of hospitalization.

For the milieu to feel safe—in other words, contained but not oppressed or coerced—there needs to be agreement among the nursing staff regarding what constitutes containment. To be kept physically safe, a particular client may need to be closely observed by staff and have potentially dangerous objects (for example, a glass vase) removed from the milieu. If the nurse responds to this individual's needs by increasing observation and keeping the client away from such objects, that individual feels safe in the milieu. If the staff members decide that vases (or belts or pencils, and so forth) are potentially dangerous and ban such objects from the unit, however, then the atmosphere in the milieu may become one of oppression and danger rather than safety and containment.

To reinforce support, the nurse creates an atmosphere of respect, nurturance, and reassurance among clients and between staff and clients. Nursing staff can lead supportive groups.

The nurse can provide structure by orienting new clients to the unit routine and guiding them concretely through each day's agenda and expectations. A written client handbook with group schedules, unit expectations, visiting hours, medication times, staff schedules, and a description of privileges is useful. The nurse needs to provide a predictable and consistent environment, achieved through keeping to a defined schedule, starting and ending meetings on time, and having clear expectations with specific consequences. Communication must be clear among staff and between clients and staff. A setting that is uncluttered and well organized, without being inflexible, also contributes to a sense of an adaptive structure. As with containment, the nurse needs to assess each client to determine his or her ability to negotiate the unit structure independently and to provide assistance if it is needed.

To create involvement, the nurse works actively to draw clients into treatment by encouraging attendance at groups, prescribed medications, and interaction with other clients. Groups for goal setting, discharge planning, and education can be developed. In a short-term setting, the milieu should be responsive to individuals' differences in education needs, treatment goals, and ability to tolerate stimulation. As with structure in the short-term unit, written materials can be helpful.

In creating a validating milieu, the nurse supports negotiation and flexibility within the context of the unit structure. The nurse encourages clients to help each other in identifying strengths, both present and future. As with other functions of the milieu, validation can be done effectively in milieu groups, particularly those groups related to setting treatment goals.

EXPECTED OUTCOMES

All clients, regardless of psychiatric diagnosis, are expected at discharge to be able to:
- Manage self-destructive and homicidal feelings
- Have fewer acute symptoms (such as psychosis, dissociation, or drug or alcohol toxicity)
- Manage in a less restrictive setting.

Regarding a client's presenting problem, the nurse plans for client statements and behaviors that reflect:
- No intention or desire to harm self or others
- A more realistic self-perception
- Participation in a daily schedule
- More appropriate interactions.[14]

Outcomes for physical and self-care activities include:
- Six or more hours of sleep, or client report of feeling rested
- Adequate nutritional intake and regular elimination
- Hygiene and grooming with minimal assistance.[14]

Expected educational outcomes for client and significant other include their ability to identify:
- Precipitants
- One sign or symptom of illness
- Medication
  - Name, dose, time
  - Purpose
  - Common side effects
  - Reasons to call a physician
  - Diet modifications
  - Drug-drug interactions
  - Drug-food interactions
- Crisis plan
- Aftercare plan.[14]

AREAS FOR FUTURE RESEARCH

- As care moves to outpatient and partial hospital settings, it will be important to track the evolution of Gunderson's five functions of the milieu[6] in their adaptation to these less formal settings.
- No current research supports the assumption that length of stay is affected by a well-functioning milieu. A study comparing length of stay in clients actively participating in a goal-focused milieu versus clients being treated by medications and containment could clarify the validity of this assumption.
- Similarly, a study of clients treated with the previously named approaches could give information about the milieu's effect on recidivism.

CASE STUDY

Mary M is a 32-year-old single female student in an MBA program who presents for her first psychiatric admission. Her chief complaint is "People around me are afraid I will kill myself."

History of Present Illness. Mary has been experiencing lack of motivation, decreased concentration, and performance anxiety for about 6 months. Since that time she has been in therapy with a psychologist at her college clinic. About 2 months ago, her depression became more severe following the breakup of her relationship with a boyfriend and a job rejection. She began to experience suicidal ideation with no plan, psychomotor retardation, decreased sleep, decreased appetite, and hopelessness.

About 1 month prior to admission, Mary cut her left wrist in a suicide attempt. She was referred to a psychopharmacologist who prescribed fluoxetine (Prozac) 20 mg per day. She began to feel increased energy and for a time was free of suicidal ideation. Two weeks later, Mary again lacerated her left wrist. Two days prior to admission, she attempted to asphyxiate herself by placing a plastic bag over her head and securing it with a rubber band around her neck. She removed the plastic bag prior to losing consciousness. Although she did not report this episode to her therapist, she did tell a friend, who encouraged her to seek admission.

Past Psychiatric History. One previous episode of depression at age 19, without suicidality, psychopharmacology, or hospitalization.

Past Medical History. Tonsillectomy at age 6.

Drug and Alcohol History. Mary stated that she smoked marijuana once a week for a year at age 19. She does not use alcohol or other drugs.

Family History. Mary is the youngest of three daughters. Her sisters are ages 34 and 37. Her parents are both alive and well, mother age 62 and father age 63. Her sisters are high school graduates, both married with no children. Her parents are retired. Her father was a foreman at an electric company in the Midwest. Mary reports depression in her maternal grandmother, now deceased, who was treated with a course of electroconvulsive therapy in the 1980s.

Social and Developmental History. Mary reports a "happy" childhood, appropriately achieving developmental milestones, and doing well in school. She was raised in a suburban neighborhood in the Midwest. She reached menarche at age 12.

Mental Status Examination at Admission. Mary M was a casually dressed woman who appeared her stated age. She had psychomotor retardation, poor eye contact, and slow, soft, and unslurred speech. She was cooperative in the interview. She had logical, goal-directed thought processes. Her thought content included suicidal ideation with a plan to overdose on over-the-counter medication. She denied thought insertion, thought blocking, ideas of reference, delusions, and hallucinations. She was alert and oriented to person, place, and time. She recalled three of three objects at 5 minutes. She correctly spelled *world* backward and could name presidents from Clinton to Franklin Roosevelt. She could perform serial 7s. She was able to abstract an interpretation of proverbs.

Her admission diagnosis was Major Depression, Recurrent Episode, Severe, Without Psychotic Features (*DSM-IV* 296.33).

Hospital Course

Mary was admitted to the inpatient unit by her primary nurse, Eric. Because she was assessed to be acutely suicidal, she was placed on 5-minute checks and supervised sharps. She appeared to Eric to be able to verbalize her suicidal thoughts rather than impulsively act on them. Eric encouraged Mary to agree to a structured schedule of brief meetings with the nursing staff. He assisted her in developing a plan to inform staff of intrusive thoughts of suicide. He recommended several groups including goals group, medication group, and here-and-now group. He planned to assess Mary each shift and record documentation in areas of physical concerns, activity pattern, cognitive-perceptual patterns (especially important in assessing suicidal potential), role-relationship pattern, and coping-stress tolerance pattern. Mary was prescribed an increase in her Prozac to 40 mg a day at the time of admission, so Eric reviewed the common side effects of selective serotonin reuptake inhibitors with Mary (nausea, diarrhea, agitation, insomnia, headache, sexual dysfunction, and akathisia).[15]

Over the next 24 hours, Mary attended the medication education group, in which she evidenced knowledge of her medication's name, dose, purpose, and side effects. After attending the goals group, she set as a goal an increase in her outpatient support by contacting the local Manic Depressive and Depressive Association and by accepting a referral to an outpatient group therapy. In talks with her nurse, she identified an issue for her outpatient therapy—that is, her need to overachieve, her use of increased work hours as an alleged means of support, and her sense of failure when she could not live up to her own unrealistic expectations. She began to see a pattern of isolation and disappointment that would lead to suicidal ideation. She discussed these concerns in the here-and-now group and received support for her insight from the other clients.

By the second 24 hours of hospitalization, Mary was no longer feeling she would be unsafe if she left the hospital. She was able to articulate ways she could ask for help. Eric's nursing assessment found Mary to be alert and oriented; having no side effects from her medication, improved sleep, and adequate intake and output; and able to manage all self-care activities. She continued to have normal thought processes and content. Her mood was "positive" and her affect was calm. She had actively participated in the milieu groups on the unit and set up an aftercare plan that included weekly psychotherapy with her previous therapist, Prozac 40 mg a day, weekly attendance at MDDA meetings, a group psychotherapy meeting weekly, and a return to her school program and apartment.

Because all expected outcomes were met, Mary was able to be discharged 2 days after admission.

CRITICAL THINKING QUESTIONS

1. How were Gunderson's five functions of the milieu demonstrated in this inpatient setting?
2. What symptoms led to the diagnosis of depression in Mary?
3. How did Mary meet the psychiatric, physical, and client education outcomes?
4. What elements of milieu therapy can remain viable in ever-decreasing lengths of stay of inpatients?
5. What does a milieu have that can be transferred to a community-based setting?
6. In what ways does the role of the nurse as milieu manager remain essential even in times of cost-cutting and downsizing?
7. What can be anticipated as the future philosophy of mental health care?

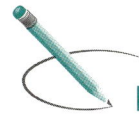

KEY POINTS

- The therapeutic community is the foundation for milieu therapy.
- Clients and staff in the milieu have a meaningful impact on each other.
- The five essential functions of the milieu remain helpful to client recovery in today's inpatient treatment settings.
- The nurse as milieu manager keeps a safe and respectful environment of open communication, flexibility in programming, predictability in structure, and active involvement of clients and families.
- Goals for brief hospitalization include crisis intervention, diagnosis, initiation of a treatment plan, acute symptom stabilization, discharge planning, and consultation to the client's outpatient network.

REFERENCES

1. LeCuyer, E: Milieu therapy for short stay units: A transformed practice theory. Arch Psychiatr Nurs 6:108, 1992.
2. Cumming, J, and Cumming, E: Ego and Milieu. Aldine de Gruyter, New York, 1962.
3. Macalpine, I, and Hunter, R: Three Hundred Years of Psychiatry, 1535–1860. Oxford University Press Inc, London, 1963, p 603.
4. Devine, B: Therapeutic milieu/milieu therapy: An overview. JPN and Mental Health Service 19:20, 1981.
5. Gutheil, T: The therapeutic milieu: Changing themes and theories. Hospital Community Psychiatry 36:1279, 1985.
6. Sederer, LI: Inpatient psychiatry: What place the milieu? (edit). Am J Psych 141:673, 1984.
7. Jones, M: The Therapeutic Community. Basic Books, New York, 1953.
8. Tuck, I, and Keels, M: Milieu therapy: A review of development in this concept and its implications for psychiatric nursing. Issues in Mental Health Nursing 12:51, 1992.
9. Gunderson, JG: Defining the therapeutic processes in psychiatric milieus. Psychiatry 41:327, 1978.
10. Sederer, LI: Brief hospitalization. In American Psychiatric Press: Review of Psychiatry 2:518, 1992.
11. Yalom, I: Inpatient Group Psychotherapy. Basic Books, New York, 1985.
12. Aguilera, D: Crisis Intervention: Theory and Methodology. Mosby, St. Louis, MO, 1986.

13. Carr, V, Varran, C, and Maxson, E: Development of a model for short-term psychiatric hospitalization. Arch Psychiatr Nurs 2:153, 1988.
14. McLean Hospital Department of Nursing Standard of Care for the Patient with Bipolar Disorder, Department of Nursing Process Standards Manual, December 1991, Revised July 1995.
15. McLean Hospital Department of Nursing Protocol for the Management of Patient Who Is Taking Selective Serotonin Reuptake Inhibitor (SSRI) Medication. Department of Nursing Process Standards Manual, July 1995.

CHAPTER 14

Electroconvulsive Therapy and Other Biological Therapies

CHAPTER 14

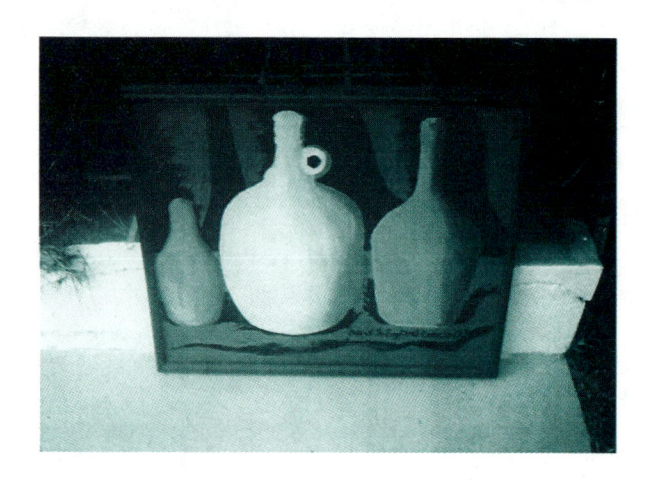

CHAPTER OUTLINE

Types of Biological Therapies
 Electroconvulsive Therapy (ECT)
 Psychosurgery
 Phototherapy
 Sleep Deprivation Therapy
Synopsis of Current Research
Areas for Future Research

LEARNING OBJECTIVES

After completing this chapter, the reader should be able to:

- Identify the major indications for electroconvulsive therapy (ECT) and the rationale for instituting treatment.
- Explain the mechanism of action of ECT and other biological therapies.
- Discuss the contraindications and risks for the individual receiving ECT.
- List the possible predictors of response and the outcome criteria for biological therapies.
- Implement the nursing process in planning care for the individual receiving ECT or another biological therapy.
- Devise a teaching plan for the client receiving a biological treatment.
- Analyze the controversies about these biological therapies.

KEY TERMS

anterograde amnesia
capsulotomy
cingulotomy
lux
phototherapy
psychosurgery

retrograde amnesia
seasonal affective disorder (SAD)
sleep deprivation
sleep restriction
subcaudate tractotomy

Carol A. Glod, RN, CS, PhD

Electroconvulsive Therapy and Other Biological Therapies

Biological therapies such as electroconvulsive therapy (ECT), psychosurgery, phototherapy, and sleep deprivation have been surrounded by controversy. Sensationalized accounts of ECT and psychosurgery have at times portrayed these treatments as cruel and inhumane, and the effectiveness of phototherapy and sleep deprivation has been questioned.

With any intervention, careful assessment and selection of clients who may derive benefit is necessary. These treatments are no exception. While they are not indicated for every individual with a psychiatric disorder, severe, debilitating, and intractable problems may require extraordinary measures such as ECT or psychosurgery to improve dysfunctional behaviors and enhance functioning. Phototherapy and sleep deprivation are two new biological interventions that are effective for certain psychiatric disorders, such as seasonal affective disorder (SAD) and major depression, respectively.

TYPES OF BIOLOGICAL THERAPIES

ELECTROCONVULSIVE THERAPY (ECT)

ECT is indicated for those very few individuals who are extremely ill. For those with intense, severe, and intractable behaviors at imminent risk for suicide, unable to tolerate the side effects of medications, or nonresponsive to medications, ECT can be a lifesaver. This relatively safe treatment involves low-energy electrical stimulation of the brain to cause a seizure that lasts about 1 minute. During the procedure, the client is anesthetized with a short-acting general anesthetic agent, such as methohexital or sodium thiopental and receives succinylcholine for neuromuscular blockade. One hundred percent oxygen is delivered under continuous pressure until spontaneous breathing resumes. The individual is monitored continuously during the treatment, including pulse, blood pressure, ECG, and EEG. There are two basic forms of ECT: it may be administered to the right temple and top of the head (unilateral ECT) or to both temples (bilateral ECT).

Treatments are usually administered 2 to 3 times weekly, for a course of 6 treatments. There is substantial individual variation in the number received, but usually 6 to 10 treatments are required for the full therapeutic effect. If no significant therapeutic response occurs by the sixth treatment, most patients are switched to bilateral ECT, which is continued to the twelfth treatment and beyond if noticeable improvement is noted. Twelve to 15 procedures are usually considered an adequate trial. Figure 14–1 shows a client about to receive ECT.

Theory of Action

The exact mechanism of action of ECT is not fully understood; however, effects may be related to the seizure. During the seizure, virtually all levels of neurotransmitters are altered: norepinephrine, serotonin, acetylcholine, dopamine, and γ-aminobutyric acid (GABA). ECT also affects the neuroendocrine system, and thus hormones such as corticotropin-releasing factor (CRF), adrenocorticotropic hormone (ACTH), thyrotropin-releasing hormone (TRH), and prolactin levels are affected. Neurophysiologically, the blood-brain barrier becomes more permeable, and regional cerebral blood flow and neurometabolism are reduced. The specific effects of these neurobiological changes on the way ECT works and on how it affects the client are still not fully understood.

Selection Criteria

Although ECT is an effective form of treatment for major depression and some other major Axis I psychiatric disorders, it is usually reserved for clients who do not respond to medication trials. It may be used as the initial treatment for clients with severe or psychotic depression, those who have failed to respond to other treatment such as several antidepressant trials, depressed individuals with medical con-

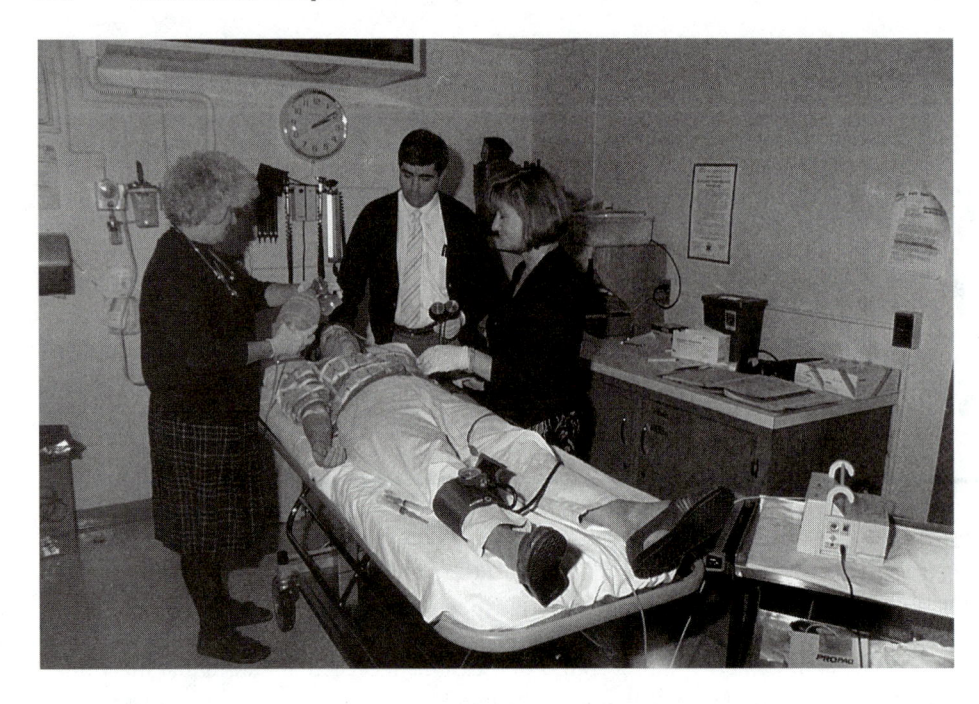

Figure 14–1. A client about to receive ECT.

ditions precluding the use of medication, and those who require a rapid response.[1] In younger, nonpsychotic clients with major depression, it is not the first line of treatment. ECT is more often used for the elderly because they meet so many of the criteria. Other severe and intractable major psychiatric disorders that may benefit from ECT are listed in Table 14–1.

Certain factors such as melancholic or psychotic features during depression or a past positive response to ECT may predict a good response to ECT. Studies have shown that individuals with major depression with psychotic features have a better response to ECT or to a combination antidepressant-antipsychotic medication than to antidepressant treatment alone. Individuals with severe catatonia, as part of an acute exacerbation of schizophrenia, may stop eating and drinking. Catatonia may rapidly abate with ECT, minimizing the risk of dehydration. Some clients with schizophrenia may benefit from ECT, reducing positive and negative symptoms and the need for rehospitalization.[2]

Contraindications

There are no absolute contraindications to ECT. Individuals with preexisting cardiac disease, gastroesophageal reflux, or compromised airways require a complete medical workup before ECT. Recent myocardial infarction or intracranial lesions such as tumors may be a contraindication because of the risk of cardiac arrest or prolonged seizures. ECT has been used and appears safe in all trimesters of pregnancy, although further study is necessary. Preexisting neurological problems such as aneurysm may prolong seizure duration, and cardiac conditions such as unstable hypertension may lead to cardiac arrest. These and other possible contraindications to the use of ECT are listed in Table 14–2.

Medications should not be administered concurrently with ECT. Tricyclic antidepressants, bupropion, and some

TABLE 14–1. Conditions for Which ECT May Be Beneficial

1. Severe major depression
2. Severe major depression with psychotic features
3. Bipolar disorder (manic, depressed, or mixed phase), unresponsive to pharmacologic treatment
4. Severe mood disorder during pregnancy
5. Major depression in older adults
6. Schizophrenia, particularly with catatonic or affective symptoms
7. Postpartum psychoses

TABLE 14–2. Possible Contraindications to the Use of ECT

Contraindication	Rationale
Intracranial pressure	May prolong seizure duration
Intracranial lesions	May prolong seizure duration
Uncontrollable hypertension	May increase risk of cardiac arrest
Recent myocardial infarction	May increase risk of cardiac arrest
Recent intracerebral hemorrhage/unstable aneurysm	May increase risk of cerebral hemorrhage
Disorders with increased anesthetic risk	May increase risk of respiratory arrest

other antidepressants lower the seizure threshold, and anticonvulsants and benzodiazepines raise it, making treatment more difficult. Medications that successfully treat an underlying physical illness such as hypoglycemics, antihypertensives, and motility suppressants may minimize complications associated with anesthesia. Concomitant treatment with monoamine oxidase inhibitors (MAOIs) is usually contraindicated; MAOIs cannot be given along with epinephrine, which is needed if complications arise during anesthesia. Lithium should be avoided because it may lead to a neurotoxic syndrome characterized by confusion and decreased responsiveness.[3] ECT is not commonly administered to children or adolescents. Clozapine should be used cautiously during ECT because it may increase the risk of seizures.

Adverse Reactions

Immediately after ECT, disorientation, attention difficulty, and transient neurological abnormalities may occur. Usually they resolve within a few hours or days. The most notable adverse effect is short-term anterograde and retrograde memory loss. **Anterograde amnesia** is loss of the ability to retain newly learned information, and this type usually resolves within the first few weeks after treatment.[4] **Retrograde amnesia** is difficulty in recalling information learned prior to ECT. This type may last longer, particularly loss of personal information. Permanent gaps in memory for the months around the treatment have been reported.[5] Bilateral administration of ECT, high-intensity current, shorter duration of time between treatments, and possibly advanced age increase the risk of memory loss. The risk of long-term, retrograde memory loss increases with a second course of treatment. Poor cognitive status prior to ECT and greater disorientation immediately afterward seem to predict more impairment in retrograde memory loss.[6]

Headache and muscle pain commonly occur after ECT. For severe muscle pain, some centers pretreat clients with curare in addition to succinylcholine to diminish this reaction. Myocardial infarction, arrhythmias, congestive heart failure, tachycardia, and hypertension may occur during ECT, and bradycardia and hypotension may occur after the seizure. Other side effects include risks of anesthesia, such as aspiration and CNS depression. Prolonged seizures, status epilepticus, and death rarely occur.

Nursing Considerations

The nurse should ensure that the client understands the procedures fully and then signs a statement of informed consent. Questions or misunderstandings should be clarified before ECT is administered. Most individuals are anxious, particularly because of frightening accounts of ECT in the past or in popular movies such as *One Flew over the Cuckoo's Nest*. Using therapeutic listening, the nurse can allow clients to discuss their fears and provide accurate information.

Before treatment, a complete physical examination, blood count (CBC), urinalysis, and ECG may be ordered. Individuals with concurrent medical disorders may require additional consultation and medical workup. For instance, those with diabetes may require blood glucose monitoring on the day of each treatment, and individuals with respiratory difficulties will need a chest x-ray.

In preparation for the first treatment, clients must refrain from taking food or fluid (NPO) for 8 hours prior to treatment to prevent aspiration. Nurses should carefully observe clients and instruct them to avoid accidental ingestion and potential complications. In the morning, atropine is administered intramuscularly to prevent bradycardia or asystole and to reduce oral secretions. Immediately following the procedure, monitor the client for recovery from anesthesia, including vital signs and orientation to time, place, and person. It is important to take vital signs every 5 minutes until the individual awakens, then every 15 minutes until alert, and then when necessary, every 2 to 4 hours until stable. Recovery may take only a few minutes, yet substantial sedation may continue for hours afterward. Allow the client to rest peacefully for several hours after a treatment.

Clients commonly show slight and brief improvement in mood and behavior after their first few treatments. These transitory benefits are a good prognostic sign for sustained response. Reassure clients that the temporary improvement will probably continue after more treatments, and encourage individuals to continue treatment, even if they have not yet benefited.

Often ECT is administered during hospitalization, but increasingly it is performed on an outpatient basis. In either case, the individual requires several hours to recover from the treatment. Instruct clients and families to expect fatigue and drowsiness after the treatment. Allow individuals who appear sedated to sleep. There are rarely complications. Outpatients will need a ride home.

Tell the client and family to expect some memory loss, particularly for events prior to ECT, which usually resolves within a few hours, days, or weeks. Teach clients and their families to report any memory problems that persist after a few weeks.

Families and friends need reassurance and psychoeducation about the procedures, benefits, and potential risks of ECT. Client and family education should focus on what happens during the treatment. Tell them that ECT is an extremely effective, safe, painless procedure, performed under anesthesia, with constant monitoring of the body's reaction. Instruct clients and families that ECT differs from shocks delivered to animals or humans as part of behavior modification. Stress the realities and safety of the procedure. Educate clients and families about the number of treatments necessary (usually about 10 to 12); they may notice benefit after a few treatments. Emphasize the need for continued long-term follow-up and antidepressant therapy. Medication is necessary to prevent relapse and recurrence of symptoms after ECT is discontinued.

Expected Outcome

The expected outcome of treatment with ECT is resolution of the behaviors associated with the major psychiatric disorder, restoration of functioning, and improved quality of life. At times, only partial benefit may be derived. In addition, the lasting effects may be short term, and continued treatment may be necessary. For some, this will involve monthly maintenance ECT treatments on an outpatient basis. More commonly, medication treatment with an antidepressant is necessary to sustain an ongoing response.

PSYCHOSURGERY

Psychosurgery (prefrontal leukotomy) for treating psychiatric disorders was first described decades ago. These early surgical procedures, largely frontal lobotomy, were associated with severe reactions and led to mixed results. With the advent of psychopharmacology, neurosurgical procedures waned, but recently several studies have demonstrated the effectiveness of psychosurgery in *select* individuals. Basically, these procedures are surgical manipulation of normal brain tissue, similar to neurosurgery for intractable pain or uncontrollable seizures, to treat severe psychiatric disorders unresponsive to conventional methods. Only a few institutions offer psychosurgery, and some countries have banned it altogether because of extreme human rights violations.

During surgery, an exact neuroanatomical structure is lesioned, guided by magnetic resonance imaging (MRI) to visualize the specific region. **Cingulotomy** is the most common psychosurgical procedure for anxiety disorders, intractable pain, and major depression. It involves inserting heated electrodes into two adjacent bilateral holes into the cingulate bundle, creating lesions. **Subcaudate tractotomy**, used for treatment-resistant affective disorders, targets an area beneath the caudate nucleus, the substantia innominata. Limbic leukotomy is aimed at several brain regions and produces 10 lesions via heated electrodes. **Capsulotomy**, developed in Sweden, consists of one of two methods. One involves lesioning the brain by gamma irradiation; the other, performed under local anesthesia, targets the anterior limb of the internal capsule. Psychosurgery is carried out by specialized neurosurgeons, located in only a few centers internationally.

Theory of Action

All forms of psychosurgery share a neurosurgical basis: that a confined manipulation or dissection of connections between brain regions produces demonstrable changes in mood and behavior. The purpose of the surgery is to sever connections in the frontal lobes or between the limbic area and brain stem. However, the mechanism of action of these procedures is not well understood.

Selection Criteria

The following selection criteria were adapted from Mindus and Jenike,[7] who outlined specific guidelines for the use of psychosurgery in obsessive-compulsive disorder (OCD) (Table 14–3). Eligible candidates for psychosurgery must have severe or intractable depression (often psychotic depression), bipolar disorder, schizophrenia, schizoaffective disorder, or OCD. These individuals have often tried every psychopharmacologic intervention available, as well as ECT, and not responded. Severe suicidal behavior and severe impairment in functional status are further criteria. A review of nearly 1300 psychosurgeries reported that the suicide rate dropped from 15% preoperatively to 1% postoperatively.[8]

Contraindications

Individuals younger than 20 years or older than 65 years are generally not candidates for psychosurgery; however, children with intractable seizures have been successfully treated with temporal lobectomy. Clients who have brain pathology such as atrophy or tumor, a major personality disorder (borderline, paranoid, antisocial, histrionic), or substance abuse are not candidates because of the potential for noncompliance, serious adverse reactions, or worsening behaviors.

Adverse Reactions

Early surgical procedures, largely frontal lobotomy, were associated with hemorrhage, seizures, infection, and profound personality changes. The majority of personality changes were dulling and poor judgment. More recently, reviews of

TABLE 14–3. General Guidelines for the Use of Psychosurgery

1. The client fulfills criteria for a major psychiatric disorder (bipolar disorder, major depression, schizophrenia, schizoaffective disorder, OCD).
2. The duration of illness is greater than 5 years.
3. The disorder causes marked suffering.
4. The disorder leads to substantial impairment in psychosocial functioning.
5. Current treatment options have been tried systematically for at least 5 years without significant effect on behavior, or were discontinued because of intolerable side effects.
6. The prognosis, without neurosurgical intervention, is considered poor.
7. The client gives informed consent.
8. The client willingly agrees to participate in the preoperative evaluation and to the postoperative rehabilitation program.
9. The treatment team will be responsible for the long-term management of the client.

Source: Adapted from Mindus, P., and Jenike, M.A.: Neurosurgical treatments of malignant obsessive compulsive disorder. Psychiatr Clin North Am 15:922, 1992.

the effects of psychosurgery have found that negative personality changes are unlikely to occur.[7] Alterations in personality are a risk and typically include behaviors associated with frontal lobe dysfunction, such as impulsivity, hostility, aggression, or general psychopathology. Reduced intellectual ability is not considered a substantial risk because many clients have shown either improvement or no change in IQ following psychosurgery.

Other adverse reactions include those associated with major neurosurgery—infection, hemorrhage, hemiplegia, seizures, suicide, and weight gain—but are generally uncommon. One review found no deaths resulted from nearly 700 cingulotomies performed over a 25-year period.[9]

Nursing Considerations

Prior to considering psychosurgery, clients must be capable and willing to give informed consent to the procedure by documenting their full knowledge of the risks and benefits. During and after surgery, typical nursing interventions follow guidelines for other neurosurgical procedures. Infection, intracerebral hemorrhage, and edema are potential consequences. Clients should also be closely monitored for hemiplegia, seizures, cognitive and personality changes, and weight gain. Assessing the potential benefits in the weeks and months postsurgery is essential.

The nurse has to remember that psychosurgery is often the last resort for individuals with intractable psychiatric disorders. As such, profound hopelessness and suicidal ideation may be present. Carefully assess the presence of suicidal thoughts or plans.

Families and friends need reassurance and psychoeducation about the specific type of psychosurgery and its potential benefits and risks. Clients and families should be told that psychosurgery is different from the lobotomies performed several decades ago and that psychosurgery is reserved only for those clients who have failed virtually all other interventions. Sophisticated neuroimaging techniques and discoveries about the relationship between brain abnormalities and severe psychiatric disorders have refined the procedures. Educate clients and families about the uncommon personality changes that may occur, such as impulsive, hostile, or aggressive behaviors. Emphasize the need for continued long-term follow-up. Assure them that immediate benefits are uncommon and that positive effects may take weeks or months to emerge.

Expected Outcome

Reduction in severe, intractable behaviors, enhanced functioning, and improved quality of life are the outcomes. Because of the controversy associated with its use, studies on psychosurgery have carefully evaluated outcomes based on reliable rating scales. One, the Pippard postoperative scale, rates improvement on five levels: "A" indicates total remission, "B" notes much improvement, "C" is for those with slight improvement (relief of symptoms that continue and necessitate medication), "D" designates persons without improvement, and "E" denotes worsening.[7] These ratings are commonly used to assess the outcome of psychosurgery.

PHOTOTHERAPY

Phototherapy, or light therapy, involves the direct administration of a high-intensity light treatment. Initially, light therapy was 6 hours of daily exposure to a light unit that delivered 2500 **lux** (a measure of light intensity); however, since then, phototherapy has evolved to more intense and convenient units. Three different forms of phototherapy units have been developed and are commercially available: traditional "light box" therapy (displayed in Figure 14–2); the phototherapy visor, a head-mounted light unit; and the dawn simulator. For the treatment of **seasonal affective disorder (SAD)**, a subtype of major depression, the light box is generally most effective and convenient at an intensity of 10,000 lux for at least 30 to 60 minutes daily. Ten thousand lux, when measured by a light meter, is equivalent to being outside at dawn looking at the sky on a sunny spring day. In contrast, more than 100,000 lux could be expected on a sunny beach day in the summer, versus only 100 to 400 lux for indoor light. Indoor light is well below the threshold necessary for light therapy to be effective. Opposite to antidepressant therapy, phototherapy produces a rapid onset of action, with a response developing after just a few days of treatment.

The second alternative, the phototherapy light visor, contains halogen light bulbs, is convenient and portable, and allows more freedom of movement. Although many different intensities have been investigated in the treatment of SAD (from 60 to over 6000 lux), surprisingly, a positive response has been reported using *all* of these intensities. Recent studies have called into question the effectiveness of the light visor.[10] Compared to the phototherapy light box, light-visor treatment appears less effective.

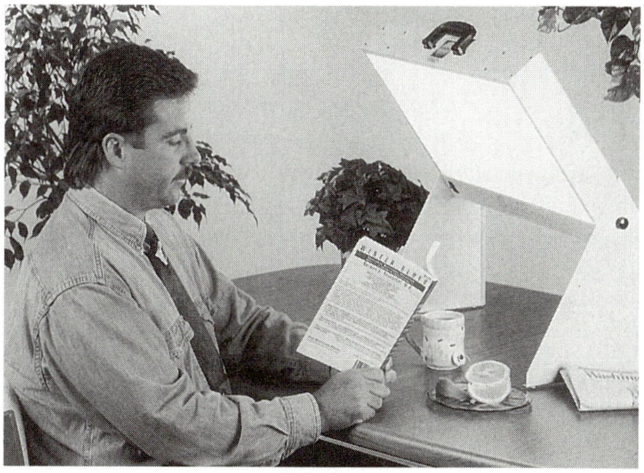

Figure 14–2. A person receiving phototherapy.

Third, the dawn simulator is a timing device that is connected to a bedside lamp, containing a halogen light bulb (about 75 watts). Generally, the device "turns on" the light bulb at a very low intensity, and gradually over the course of 2 hours, the light bulb reaches its full intensity. The individual is sleeping while the light is very slowing illuminating the room, during the early morning hours from about 5:00 to 7:00 am. In the few studies conducted to date, the dawn simulator has successfully reversed the symptoms of SAD in most clients. Whereas its intent is to mimic the dawn light signal usually received in the sunny months, this device has led to further evidence for "resetting" the body's internal clock as the mechanism of action of phototherapy.

Theory of Action

Several theories attempt to explain the effectiveness of phototherapy, particularly in treating SAD. The shortening of the winter day, with fewer hours of sunlight, was thought to lead to "hibernating" behaviors, similar to that of many animals. According to the *photoperiod effect*, light therapy was proposed to work by lengthening the winter day to mimic a summer day. In the initial studies of light therapy, 6 hours of daily exposure to 2500 lux of light—3 hours in the morning and again in the evening—were effective in treating SAD. Shortly thereafter, the total time was reduced to 2 hours with sustained efficacy, resulting in little support for this theory.

Then disruption in melatonin was investigated. Melatonin, a hormone normally secreted at night, induces sleep. Early studies on the effect of bright light found that melatonin secretion could be suppressed with bright light exposure. Although several studies revealed mixed results about the relationship between melatonin and the action of light therapy, one study proved pivotal. If phototherapy worked by suppressing melatonin secretion, light would have beneficial effects only at certain times of the day (early morning or late evening). Instead, there was no difference in the timing of light therapy, suggesting that melatonin was not critical in the mechanism of action of phototherapy.

Several researchers hypothesized that the eyes are the crucial link to the actions of light therapy, but no clear results have emerged. Dysregulation in key neurotransmitters, such as serotonin, is another theory about the effectiveness of phototherapy.

The most prominent theory in recent years involves the action of bright light on biological rhythms. Light therapy with a dawn simulator is effective, despite being delivered when the individual is sleeping, with eyes closed. In addition, phototherapy is effective for a variety of conditions associated with a disruption in body rhythms (see the following). Alfred Lewy first proposed the phase-shift hypothesis, which suggested that administering phototherapy in the morning would shift the 24-hour rhythm of melatonin earlier in persons with SAD. In contrast, phototherapy delivered in the evening should not be effective; however, this is not the case. Two other complicated theories have been proposed. Charles Czeisler, a researcher who has investigated

---

RESEARCH NOTE

Teicher, MH, Glod, CA, Oren, DA, Schwartz, PJ, Luetke, C, Brown, C, and Rosenthal, NE. The phototherapy light visor: There is more to it than meets the eye. Am J Psychiatry 1995, 152:1197–1202.

Findings: Phototherapy is the most common treatment for SAD. Over 20 double-blind studies have found that bright artificial light therapy, delivered by a light box, is effective in this condition. Recently, light treatment was redesigned to provide a more comfortable and portable head-mounted device, the phototherapy light visor. In this study, the researchers tested the effectiveness of the light visor in 57 individuals with SAD. Specifically, they compared a visor delivering 600 lux of white light to one that delivered dim red light. Dim red light has been shown to be a placebo (inactive) treatment.

Both the red and white visors were effective. Thirty-nine percent of clients who received red light benefited from treatment. Forty-one percent of clients who received white light also benefited from treatment. Overall, there were no differences between individuals treated with red or white light visors. These results were similar to other studies that studied the effectiveness of phototherapy light visors. No differences have been found between visors of different light intensities and light colors. Based on the results of this and other studies, the researchers concluded that the light visor was "nothing more than an elaborate placebo." They suggested that the novelty of trying a unique light treatment was enough to produce a response in about 40% of the clients, regardless of the intensity or color of the light. They concluded that the visor appears to be less effective than traditional light box treatment.

Application to Practice: This study points to the need for careful study of new phototherapy devices as they are released. The conclusions suggest that light visors are not as effective as light boxes for the treatment of SAD. Why the visor is less effective is poorly understood. However, phototherapy is gaining increasing popularity as an effective and "holistic" treatment, especially for SAD. Nurses should educate clients and the public about the latest research so that the most effective treatment is selected. Several light units are available from many different manufacturers, and currently no prescription is necessary. Before investing in a phototherapy device, clients should have a complete evaluation to determine if light therapy is indicated. They should also be warned about the risks and adverse effects. Once light therapy is recommended, the light box is probably the best option. If clients are going to invest several hundred dollars in treatment, nurses can guide them in their selection to avoid potential pitfalls. Further research is needed on the light visor and on another device that appears effective, the dawn simulator. More research is also needed on the efficacy of different phototherapy units in the treatment of other conditions such as phase-delay sleep disorder, jet lag, and changes secondary to shift work schedules.

biological rhythms, suggested that light therapy reduces the amplitude of our 24-hour rhythms, but no studies have found evidence to support this theory. Another theory is that light therapy works like a metronome to keep the body's biological rhythms in sync with a 24-hour day.[11] Further research is needed.

Selection Criteria

Originally designed to treat SAD, phototherapy remains the treatment of choice for individuals with this disorder. It has also been useful for some nonseasonal depression, particularly in combination with other therapies, such as antidepressants, and for sleep disorders and disturbances in circadian rhythms. For instance, in clients with phase-delayed sleep disorder, in which sleep patterns shift later into the night and day, phototherapy seems to be able to shift the sleep cycle to an earlier time. Problems associated with jet lag and frequent changes in working hours can also be treated with phototherapy. Interestingly, it may have a positive effect for some women with premenstrual syndrome.

Adults seem to benefit the most from phototherapy. It has been used successfully in older adults with depression, sleep disorders, and dementia. There are reports of clients over 80 years old who have had a paradoxical reaction, however, experiencing intense nightmares, bad memories, and plaguing thoughts of past losses.

A recent study on children and adolescents suggested that a combination of light box and dawn simulator effectively treated SAD[12] and phase-delayed sleep disorder.

Contraindications

Individuals with cataracts and glaucoma are usually advised to avoid phototherapy. They may be at greater risk during the use of light box or light visor study (rather than dawn simulation); however, no systematic study has been done. Phototherapy should also be used cautiously in individuals with migraine headaches because of the potential to induce or worsen the headaches.

Adverse Reactions

Generally, light therapy is well tolerated and associated with few adverse effects, among them headache, insomnia, slight agitation or irritability (similar to excess caffeine stimulation), hypomania, or eyestrain. Lessening the duration of exposure to the light source diminishes these problems. Early morning awakening has been associated with use of the dawn simulator.

One potential concern is whether light therapy will cause cataracts or other eye problems with repeated chronic exposure. Light therapy has been available for over 13 years, and to date no ophthalmologic conditions have been reported; however, the potential problems are still being investigated. Medications that have photosensitizing effects, making the eyes more sensitive to the sun and to eye damage, may pose a greater risk for individuals who use phototherapy. Animal studies have found that lithium-treated rats developed retinal damage secondary to ongoing prolonged light exposure.

Nursing Considerations

One of the most important roles for nursing is to promote a balanced view of the treatment of various disorders and to educate clients and the public in the uses, benefits, and risks of phototherapy. When used correctly for appropriate conditions, light therapy is a beneficial treatment that may avoid the use of pharmacologic or more costly therapeutic interventions. The cost of a light box or dawn simulator varies, but they can be obtained for about $300 to $400. Because light units require no prescription, anyone can purchase and use them incorrectly without knowing the full risks. Timing, duration, distance from the light source, angle of exposure, and viewing of the light source are crucial components of proper treatment. Encourage clients to be carefully assessed and instructed in the use of this treatment, like any major intervention. A resource for clients is the book *Winter Blues* by Norman Rosenthal[13] or, for those who travel frequently, *How to Beat Jet Lag*, by Dan Oren and his colleagues.[14]

Individuals who perform light therapy regularly should be carefully monitored by an expert trained in the use of this procedure. In particular, depressed clients should be assessed for the response to phototherapy and their side effects monitored. Educate clients and families that phototherapy, like any treatment, is associated with certain risks. Instruct them to report regular headaches, agitation, insomnia, or eyestrain. Warn older adults that they may experience a rare side effect of severe agitation and reliving of past bad memories, which they should report immediately.

Although no severe ophthalmological difficulties have been reported, individuals require baseline eye examinations to rule out cataracts or glaucoma, conditions that might be worsened by phototherapy. After clients have been cleared to receive light therapy, instruct them to obtain yearly eye examinations.

For the treatment of SAD, light therapy is the most common intervention. Educate clients and families that whichever form of artificial light treatment they perform, treatment begins in the fall, continues throughout the winter, and is discontinued in the spring. Light therapy is not needed during the summer because the typical SAD sufferer is without symptoms. Light treatment is administered daily, and usually individuals respond within a few days. Stress the need to continue light therapy each day to receive ongoing benefit. Evaluate compliance and educate clients and families that symptoms generally return after several days of missed treatment.

Educate clients and families that 2 weeks of light therapy are necessary to determine antidepressant response. Changing the timing, duration of exposure, or light device may promote response. For those who fail to respond to phototherapy, other options exist, such as antidepressant therapy, alone or in combination with light therapy.

Expected Outcome

The benefits of phototherapy for SAD include restoring appetite and improving eating, sleep, mood, and social and occupational functioning. For the treatment of depression, at least 2 weeks of daily light therapy are considered an adequate trial. The positive outcome for the treatment of sleep and circadian rhythm disorders would be normalizing sleep-wake cycles, mood, and energy levels.

SLEEP DEPRIVATION THERAPY

Restricting sleep to various times during the night (**sleep restriction**) or eliminating sleep (**sleep deprivation**) is another effective treatment for major depression. Many individuals find this surprising because insomnia and feeling tired are key behaviors associated with depression. However, emerging evidence suggests that both total and some forms of partial sleep deprivation for several nights can reverse symptoms. Sleeping from about 9:00 pm to 1:00 am and being *deprived* of sleep for the remainder of the night appears to have antidepressant effects. Sleep deprivation in the first half of the night has little benefit. One of the unfortunate drawbacks is that continued deprivation of sleep is necessary to sustain the response, making it difficult for many clients to continue. One study found that depriving depressed individuals of rapid-eye movement (REM) sleep alone was effective yet cumbersome.

Theory of Action

Sleep deprivation is proposed to affect biological rhythms. The sleep-wake cycle follows a 24-hour rhythm, and within the sleep cycle are discrete periods of light, deep, and REM sleep. The amount of REM sleep normally increases later in the sleep cycle; however, in depression, the onset of REM occurs earlier in the night. Sleep deprivation may affect the timing and frequency of REM sleep and hence be responsible for its therapeutic effect. Because other circadian processes, such as temperature and neuroendocrine levels, coincide with the sleep cycle, a disruption in these measures may account for some of the action of sleep deprivation.

Selection Criteria

Sleep deprivation therapy is indicated for individuals with major depression who are willing to consent to this procedure. Those who demonstrate substantial diurnal variation in mood or energy may be more likely to respond. They feel better as the day progresses, and sleep deprivation may help this process by continuing it uninterrupted during the night. Some preliminary evidence suggests that sleep deprivation may be effective for clients whose depression is in partial remission, to augment or hasten antidepressant response, and in some women with premenstrual syndrome.

Contraindications

Individuals with bipolar disorder may be at high risk for mania if treated with sleep deprivation therapy.

Adverse Reactions

The major adverse reaction is mania, a state of increased mood, energy, speech, and activity. Overall, sleep deprivation therapy is well tolerated.

Nursing Considerations

Although sleep restriction or deprivation is effective for treating depression, initiating and maintaining the precise protocol for sleep and waking is essential for beneficial effects. One of the main nursing considerations is to encourage and monitor this schedule. For sleep restriction, instruct clients to sleep only in the early part of the night, from about 9:00 pm to 1:00 am. Changing the timing of sleep or wake times interferes with obtaining positive effects. Clients must strictly comply with these procedures each night in order to receive benefit. Emphasize that while sleep restriction or deprivation is effective, the schedule may be impractical and difficult to follow consistently. Because depressed clients often have difficulty with fatigue, lack of energy, and sleep disturbance, maintaining any regular sleep schedule, especially one that leads to decreased sleep, is demanding. Suggest that the client or family consider alternative treatments such as antidepressant therapy in the case of noncompliance.

As for other treatments for major depression, assess the response to sleep deprivation or sleep restriction. The individual should have normal appetite, energy, and activity patterns, good concentration ability, and absence of depressed mood and suicidal ideation.

Expected Outcome

Sleep deprivation therapy can be expected to restore mood, energy, appetite, functioning, and other depressed behaviors.

SYNOPSIS OF CURRENT RESEARCH

Much of the research is focused on investigating the precise mechanism of action of somatic treatments. For example, although ECT has been associated with dysregulation of neurotransmitters, several substances are implicated and no one clear explanation has emerged. Recent studies on the effects of ECT have focused on clearly determining who is at highest risk for developing severe side effects such as amnesia.

Recently, a long-term study investigated whether individuals with OCD had lasting effects of cingulotomy.[15] Of 33 individuals, four had committed suicide; however, at least 25% demonstrated benefit from this procedure.

Although a review of sleep deprivation studies found substantial methodological problems with the majority, they did appear to demonstrate its effectiveness in depression, particularly when combined with medication.[16]

In the investigation of SAD, much of the current research focuses on determining the effectiveness of phototherapy on children and older adults. Some investigations have found that children and adolescents are affected by SAD and that the combination of phototherapy and dawn simulation is effective in reversing the symptoms.[12] Other investigations have explored whether light therapy may treat "sundowning," depression, or behaviors associated with Alzheimer's disease in older adults, with mixed results.

AREAS FOR FUTURE RESEARCH

- What are the most effective ways to explain ECT to clients?
- What is the client's experience of receiving a somatic treatment?
- What other disorders are responsive to treatment with phototherapy?
- What measures help ensure compliance with sleep-deprivation treatment?
- What is the relationship between controversy and use of ECT?
- What is the stigma associated with receiving psychosurgery?
- What are the most important ethical issues for clients receiving psychosurgery?
- What is the nurse's role in long-term treatment with clients who have received psychosurgery?
- What are the long-term risks of daily exposure to phototherapy?
- What are the most useful forms of light treatment for children and adolescents with SAD?

CASE STUDY

Eleanor A is a 60-year-old woman with long-term chronic major depression. At age 19, she was first hospitalized in a state facility for depression, suicidal ideation, and her concerns that others were poisoning her. She had stopped caring for herself. She spent several years in the state hospital, recovered, and eventually married and had two children. After the birth of her first child, she became severely depressed with severe sleep disruption, lost 25 lb, and lacked the energy to care for her child or herself. She became paranoid and suicidal, was hospitalized again, and was treated with a variety of antidepressant and antipsychotic medications.

Eleanor never worked and played a secondary role to her husband in raising the family. Although her behavior improved somewhat, she remained depressed for many years. Recently, her husband passed away. Her daughter, now a physician, brought her mother for further evaluation and assessment of treatment options.

At the time of evaluation, she weighed 110 lb, said very little, and had poor hygiene. She stated that "life had long ended" for her and she had always wished that her husband would outlive her. Eleanor reported depressed mood, lack of energy, sleeping only 5 hours each night, and suicidal thoughts. She appeared profoundly depressed and displayed psychomotor retardation. No precise suicide plan was evident, but she admitted that she wanted to "join her husband." She also revealed that she had been hearing her late husband's voice and seeing images of him. Eleanor's daughter thought that her mother was paranoid; her mother had made comments that others were stealing from her.

After a complete assessment, the treatment team recommended hospitalization and ECT. Eleanor was initially resistant. She remembered seeing "a line of people waiting to have ECT" in the state hospital who emerged as "zombies." The nurse reassured her that ECT was safe, painless, and administered differently today. The nurse also told Eleanor and her family that the procedure was very effective for severe forms of depression like hers. Eleanor later met other clients who were receiving ECT. When she noticed that they did not seem like "zombies" and told her that ECT was helpful, she agreed to start treatment.

After a few ECT treatments, Eleanor's mood was brighter and her energy and sleep improved. After the treatment she couldn't remember receiving the atropine or going to the center to receive ECT. No other memory impairments were evident. She continued to miss her husband, but she felt more hopeful about the future. Slowly, the suicidal thoughts abated. She appeared more interested in things and began to make plans for the future. Eleanor completed 10 ECT treatments and was discharged on antidepressant medication.

CRITICAL THINKING QUESTIONS

1. Design a teaching plan to enhance the client's and family's understanding of benefits and risks of ECT.
2. Explain the mechanism by which ECT treats severe psychiatric disorders.
3. Develop a care plan, including short-term and long-term goals for Eleanor's hospital stay.
4. Identify behaviors that Eleanor is responding to treatment.
5. Select the most appropriate therapeutic approaches for treating Eleanor as an outpatient.
6. What community resources could the nurse suggest to support Eleanor's functioning after discharge?

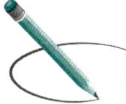

KEY POINTS

- As with any procedure or pharmacologic intervention, the benefits should outweigh the risks in the decision to institute biological therapy for a particular client.
- Once associated with cruel and inhumane circumstances, biological therapies such as ECT and psychosurgery have been refined to provide safe and effective treatment to individuals with severe psychiatric illness.
- ECT is a relatively safe procedure indicated for individuals with severe psychiatric disorders such as major depression with psychotic features, major depression or bipolar

disorder nonresponsive to several medication trials, or other conditions with intense, severe, and intractable behaviors in clients at imminent risk for suicide.

- The mechanism of action of ECT is not completely understood. It may affect the neurobiology of the brain by altering levels of neurotransmitters, changing the neuroendocrine system, or reducing cerebral blood flow.
- The most common side effects of ECT are headache and disorientation immediately following treatment and short-term anterograde and retrograde memory loss, which usually resolves within a few days or weeks.
- Psychosurgery involves surgical manipulation of normal brain tissue, similar to neurosurgery for intractable pain or uncontrollable seizures. It is used to treat severe or intractable depression (often psychotic depression), bipolar disorder, schizophrenia or schizoaffective disorder, and OCD, when virtually every psychopharmacologic intervention and ECT have failed.
- Phototherapy involves the administration of artificial light treatment. It is commonly used to treat SAD, jet lag, and sleep disorders such as phase-delayed sleep disorder.
- Phototherapy appears to work by "resetting" the body's clock to keep the body's rhythms in sync with a 24-hour day.
- Phototherapy devices include the light box, light visor, and dawn simulator. The most effective and well-studied are phototherapy light boxes that deliver 10,000 lux of bright light.
- Adverse effects of phototherapy are minimal; they include headache, agitation, eyestrain, insomnia, and hypomania.
- Total sleep deprivation and partial sleep deprivation (sleep restriction) are biological therapies used to treat depression; however, continued compliance is needed to maintain the positive effects.

REFERENCES

1. Depression in Primary Care: vol 2. Treatment of Major Depression. Agency for Health Care Policy and Research. Publication No. 93-0551. Rockville, MD, 1993.
2. Sajatovic, M, and Meltzer, HY: The effect of short-term electroconvulsive treatment plus neuroleptics in treatment-resistant schizophrenia and schizoaffective disorders. Convuls Ther 9:167, 1993.
3. Coppen, A, et al: Lithium continuation therapy following electroconvulsive therapy. Br J Psychiatry 139:284, 1981.
4. Sackeim, HA: The cognitive effects of electroconvulsive therapy. In Moos, WH, Gamzu, ER, Thal, LJ (eds): Cognitive Disorder: Pathophysiology and Treatment. Marcel Dekker, New York, 1992.
5. The Practice of Electroconvulsive Therapy: Recommendations for Treatment, Training, and Privileging: A Task Force Report of the American Psychiatric Association. APA, Washington, DC, 1990.
6. Sobin, C, et al: Predictors of retrograde amnesia following ECT. Am J Psychiatry 152:995, 1995.
7. Mindus, P, and Jenike, MA: Neurosurgical treatment of malignant obsessive compulsive disorder. Psychiatr Clin North Am 15:921, 1992.
8. Bridges, PK, et al: Psychosurgery: stereotactic subcaudate tractomy. An indispensable treatment. Br J Psychiatry 165:599, 1994.
9. Ballantine, HT, et al: Treatment of psychiatric illness by stereotactic cingulotomy. Biol Psychiatry 22:807, 1987.
10. Teicher, MH, et al: The phototherapy light visor: There is more to it than meets the eye. Am J Psychiatry 152:1197, 1995.
11. Teicher, MH, et al: Circadian rest-activity disturbances in seasonal affective disorder. Arch Gen Psychiatry, in press.
12. Swedo, SJ, et al: A controlled trial of light therapy for the treatment of pediatric seasonal affective disorder (SAD). J Am Acad Child Adolesc Psychiatry, in press.
13. Rosenthal, NE: Winter Blues. The Guilford Press, New York, 1993.
14. Oren, DA, et al: How to Beat Jet Lag: A Practical Guide for Air Travelers. Holt Rinehart & Winston, Inc, New York, 1993.
15. Jenike, MA, et al: Cingulotomy for refractory obsessive-compulsive disorder. A long-term follow-up of 33 patients. Arch Gen Psychiatry 48:548, 1991.
16. Leibenluft, E, and Wehr, TA: Is sleep deprivation useful in the treatment of depression? Am J Psychiatry 149:159, 1992.

UNIT FOUR
Psychiatric Disorders

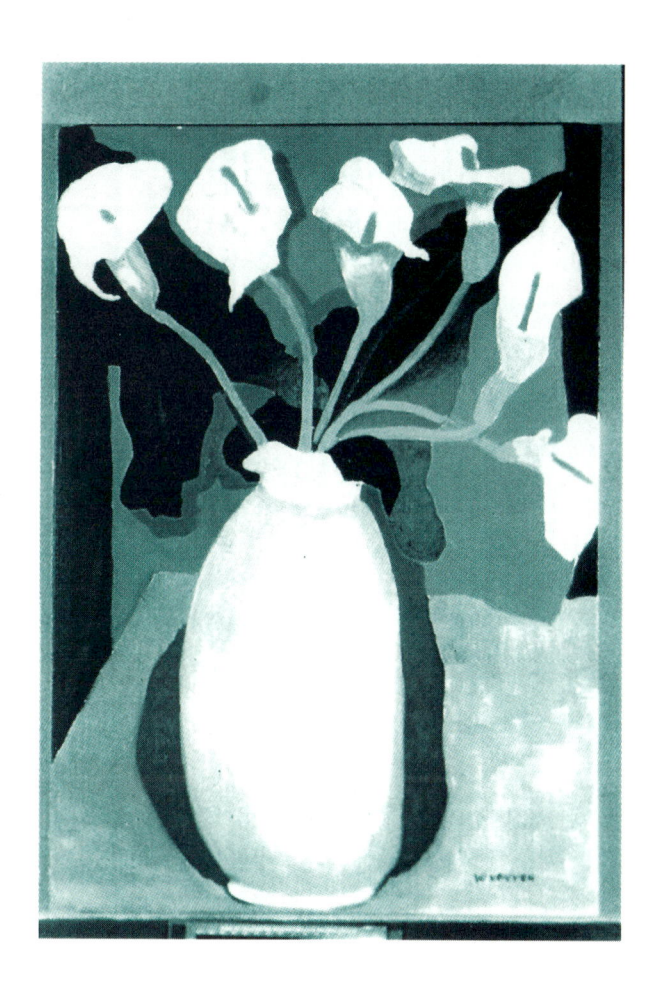

CHAPTER 15
Delirium, Dementia, Amnestic, and Other Cognitive Disorders

CHAPTER 16
Mental Illness due to a General Medical Condition

CHAPTER 17
Substance-related Disorders

CHAPTER 18
Schizophrenia and Other Psychotic Disorders

CHAPTER 19
Mood Disorders

CHAPTER 20
Anxiety Disorders

CHAPTER 21
Somatoform Disorders

CHAPTER 22
Posttraumatic and Dissociative Disorders

CHAPTER 23
Sexual and Gender Identity Disorders

CHAPTER 24
Eating Disorders

CHAPTER 25
Sleep Disorders

CHAPTER 26
Adjustment Disorders

CHAPTER 27
Personality Disorders

CHAPTER 28
Attention-Deficit/Hyperactivity Disorder

CHAPTER 15

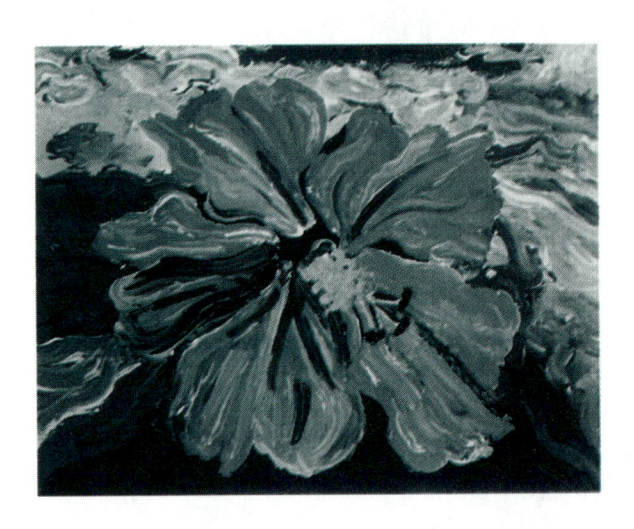

CHAPTER OUTLINE

Normative Aging and Cognition
Delirium
   Definition
   Characteristic Behaviors
   Culture, Age, and Gender Features
   Etiology
   Prognosis
   Assessment
   Interventions for Hospitalized Clients
   Expected Outcomes
Dementia
   Definition
   Characteristic Behaviors
   Diagnostic Aids
   Culture, Age, and Gender Features
   Etiology
   Prognosis
   Assessment
   Planning Care
   Interventions for Clients in the Community
   Client and Family Education
   Expected Outcomes
   Differential Diagnosis
Amnestic Disorders
   Definition
   Characteristic Behaviors
   Diagnostic Aids
   Culture, Age, and Gender Features
   Etiology
   Prognosis
   Planning Care
   Interventions for Clients in the Community
   Expected Outcomes
Synopsis of Current Research
Areas for Future Research

Gail Montague Schober RN, CS, MS
Carol A. Glod, RN, CS, PhD
Barbara A. Jones RN, DNSc

Delirium, Dementia, Amnestic, and Other Cognitive Disorders

LEARNING OBJECTIVES

After completing this chapter, the reader should be able to:
- Identify the characteristic behaviors of dementia, delirium, and amnestic disorders.
- Recognize the diagnostic criteria for dementia and delirium.
- Apply the nursing process when caring for clients with cognitive disorders.
- Describe the prevalence of cognitive disorders by age, gender, and ethnicity.
- Discuss appropriate nursing interventions for clients with cognitive disorders.
- Specify strategies to decrease caregiver burden in family members of clients with cognitive disorders.
- Identify outcome criteria to evaluate nursing interventions for clients with both acute and chronic cognitive disorders.

KEY TERMS

Alzheimer's disease
amnesia
amnestic disorders
anterograde amnesia
apraxia
catastrophic reaction
CCU-psychosis
confabulation
Creutzfeldt-Jakob disease
delirium
dementia
Huntington's disease
reality orientation
remotivation therapy
validation therapy
vascular dementia

Although clients of any age can experience alteration in cognition, age is the primary risk factor for the development of acute and chronic changes in intellectual functioning. As the twenty-first century approaches, the United States' burgeoning population of older adults will be the major consumers of nursing services. Today, one in eight Americans is over age 65, and life expectancy beyond age 65 has increased significantly. Centenarians are the most rapidly growing age cohort.[1] One in 12 Americans over the age of 65 will experience chronic, irreversible intellectual decline; by age 85, this rate rises to 1 in 2 people. Currently, 2.4 million Americans suffer from dementing illnesses; by the year 2040, this number is projected to escalate to 7.3 million as the last of the baby boomers reach their 80s.

Changes in cognition or memory signal a change from usual functioning. Delirium, dementia, amnestic disorders, and other cognitive disorders are commonly caused by medical conditions, medications, substances, or a combination of these factors.

Cognitive impairment may be acute or chronic. Acute alteration in mental status, **delirium**, is often the earliest sign of illness in older adults. With appropriate management, the client experiencing delirium can regain normal mental status. Nurses caring for clients experiencing acute or chronic alteration in cognitive function must be prepared to assess, intervene, and assist them to achieve and maintain their maximum level of independence, while ensuring client safety. Nurses commonly assume the roles of advocate, researcher, coordinator, and teacher while working with this population. Because most elders reside in the community, attention to family dynamics and concerns is also paramount if institutionalization of the cognitively impaired elder is to be delayed or avoided.

NORMATIVE AGING AND COGNITION

Part of normal aging includes anatomical and physiological changes in the nervous system, such as loss of neurons, decrease in brain weight, decrease in dendritic growth, pigment changes, and reduction in neurotransmitters. Despite these changes, most elders do not experience cognitive deterioration as they age. Longitudinal studies of elders using the

BOX 15–1. Psychiatric Effects of Medications on Older Adults

Drug Class	Drug	Possible Effects
Analgesics/Anti-inflammatories	Aspirin	Confusion, paranoia
	Indomethacin	Delusions, emotional dissociation, hallucinations, hostile behavior, hypomania, paranoia
	Sulindac	Bizarre behavior, depression, illusions, paranoia
Anticonvulsants	Carbamazepine	Loose associations, psychosis
	Phenytoin	
	Primidone	
Antidepressants	Amitriptyline	Delusions, forgetfulness, illogical thoughts, paranoid delusions, sleep disturbances
	Amoxapine	Delusions, mania
	Imipramine	Forgetfulness, illogical thoughts, paranoid delusions, sleep disturbances
	Nortriptyline	Paranoid delusions
	Trazodone	Increased activity, paranoia, pressured speech
Antiparkinson agents	Amantadine	Agitation, illusions
	Bromocriptine	Delusions, paranoia
	Levodopa	Hallucinations, illusions, insomnia, psychotic symptoms
Benzodiazepines	Diazepam	Delusions
	Flurazepam	Depression
	Triazolam	Paranoia
Cardiac/cardiovascular drugs	Digitoxin	Agitation, delusions, paranoia
	Digoxin	Delusions, depression, fatigue, incoherency, paranoia, social withdrawal
	Disopyramide	Agitation, depression, insomnia
	Methyldopa	Depression, inability to concentrate
	Nadolol	Guilt, insomnia, sadness
	Procainamide	Delusions, hallucinations
	Propranolol	Depression, decreased energy and sleep, paranoia, paranoid delusions, visual and perceptual disorders
	Thiazides	Depression
H_2 Blockers	Cimetidine	Agitation, confusion, depression, insomnia, lethargy, manic symptoms
	Ranitidine	Depression
Steroids	Prednisolone	Hallucinations, paranoid delusions
	Prednisone	Depression, euphoria, hypomania, illusions

Source: Adapted from Wood, K, Harris, M, Morreale, A, and Rizos, A: Drug-induced psychosis and depression in the elderly. Psychiatr Clin North Am 11:167–193, 1988.

Weschler Adult Intelligence Scale (WAIS) indicate that intellectual decline is minimal, of late onset, and mainly confined to timed performance measures. However, the aging brain is increasingly vulnerable to changes in its internal and external environment. Infection, dehydration, drugs, and other stressors can dramatically affect the cognitive function of older persons. Box 15–1 lists some of the major psychiatric effects of medications on older adults.

DELIRIUM

Definition

Delirium is an acute disorder of cognition characterized by disturbances in attention, perception, thinking, memory, psychomotor behavior, and the sleep-wake cycle.[2] It is a time-limited syndrome of acute onset that is highly treatable when recognized in time. This acute confusional state that impairs all mental processes can result from any condition that disrupts the metabolic or structural integrity of the brain. Risk factors for delirium are summarized in Table 15–1.

Characteristic Behaviors

One symptom alone does not constitute delirium. Instead, a constellation of symptoms, the risk factors, and the sudden onset of symptoms suggest its presence.[3]

Delirium fluctuates over the course of the day and is the direct result of an underlying medical condition, exposure

TABLE 15–1. Risk Factors for Delirium

- Chronic end-stage illness dehydration
- Electrolyte and acid-base disorders
- Neurological disorders including head trauma, subdural hematoma, temporal lobe epilepsy, and dementia
- Cultural or language barriers
- Personality type—active, dominant personality is associated with increased risk
- Advanced age
- Decreased sensory ability
- Cerebrovascular events including hemorrhage, thrombus, embolus, myocardial infarction, arrhythmia, and cardiac failure
- Metabolic disorders including diabetes and thyroid disease
- Pain
- Sleep deprivation
- Urinary retention and fecal impaction
- Medications

Source: Coyle, MK: Organic illness mimicking psychiatric episodes. Journal of Gerontological Nursing 13:31–35, 1987.

to a toxin, drug withdrawal, or a combination of these problems. Electroencephalogram (EEG) findings are also abnormal and show either slow or rapid activity.[4]

Factors such as sensory deprivation or sensory overload can increase agitated behavior in the susceptible client. An environment where there is isolation, unfamiliar staff, uncomfortable procedures, lack of sleep, and the potential use of medications or restraints that can cause confusion can lead to delirium. Misperceiving objects or actions as something to fear, clients may attempt to protect themselves by attacking caregivers who approach them, call out, or moan throughout the night.

Delirium develops in clients in critical care environments so commonly that the term **CCU-psychosis** has been coined to describe it; its incidence is estimated at 30%. CCU-psychosis includes agitation, delusions, and hallucinations. Possible causes include sensory deprivation, overstimulation, and drug reactions.[5] Drake and Romano[6] reported that adverse drug reactions result in 163,000 cases of drug-induced mental alteration annually.

Atypically, clients may present with "quiet" delirium, a marked deviation from baseline cognitive function not accompanied by symptoms of psychosis. Because delirium that presents in this manner is frequently a missed diagnosis or caregivers erroneously conclude that the client is demented,[1] the nurse must be aware of clients' baseline level of functioning.

Culture, Age, and Gender Features

Delirium may occur at any time in life but is most prevalent in children and in those over age 60. According to the *Diagnostic and Statistical Manual of Mental Disorders (DSM-IV)*,[4] children may be more prone to delirium than adults, particularly delirium due to medications or a febrile response. With increasing age, the risk is greater for women than men.

Etiology

The most common causes include medical disorders, medications, illicit substances, and drug withdrawal. Table 15–2 lists medications that can contribute to delirium.

Prognosis

Delirium is a medical emergency[1] that is reversible if diagnosed and treated in time. Some cases remit spontaneously; others progress into dementia and more chronic problems. Even when the underlying cause is treated, delirium may last from 1 to several weeks. As a general rule, the older the clients and the longer they have been exhibiting signs of delirium, the longer the delirium takes to abate. Delirium in medical-surgical clients is associated with longer hospital stays and higher mortality rates.[7] About 10% of clients with delirium progress to coma and death.[8]

Assessment

To accurately identify delirium, the nurse should incorporate a mental status examination into client assessment. Many brief, reliable, and valid questionnaires are available for this purpose. Examples include the Mini–Mental Status Examination (see Chapter 2), Digit Span Test, Vigilance "A" Test, Clinical Assessment of Confusion, and the Confusion Assessment Method.[9] Alternatively, the nurse may assess clients through observation and by engaging them in conversation. When interviewed, the delirious client has difficulty in recounting events in a logical sequence and shifts from one subject to another in rapid succession. During the course of the interview, assess memory, thought processes, attention, and concentration.[3] Family members and significant others can be very helpful in providing information about the client's baseline mental status, health history, medications, and other risk factors.

Interventions for Hospitalized Clients

Delirium usually requires immediate intervention and therefore is treated in urgent care settings, emergency rooms, and the hospital. Treatment is based on the cause of the client's delirium. For example, if delirium is the result of sensory deprivation due to the inconsistent use of glasses or hearing aid during hospitalization, staff should ensure that these are worn. If sensory overload is the problem, the environment should be modified to reduce stimulation. Softening lighting, decreasing the number of staff who interact with the client, providing for rest, and decreasing noise are examples of interventions to reduce sensory overload.

Attention to client safety to prevent falls and other traumatic injuries is a nursing priority. The delirious client re-

Diagnostic Criteria for Delirium

Diagnostic Criteria for 293.0 Delirium Due to . . . [Indicate the General Medical Condition]

A. Disturbance of consciousness (i.e., reduced clarity of awareness of the environment) with reduced ability to focus, sustain, or shift attention.

B. A change in cognition (such as memory deficit, disorientation, language disturbance) or the development of a perceptual disturbance that is not better accounted for by a preexisting, established, or evolving dementia.

C. The disturbance develops over a short period (usually hours to days) and tends to fluctuate during the course of the day.

D. There is evidence from the history, physical examination, or laboratory findings that the disturbance is caused by the direct physiological consequences of a general medical condition.

CODING NOTE: If delirium is superimposed on a preexisting Dementia of the Alzheimer's Type or Vascular Dementia, indicate the delirium by coding the appropriate subtype of the dementia, e.g., 190.3 Dementia of the Alzheimer's Type, With Late Onset, With Delirium.

CODING NOTE: Include the name of the general medical condition on Axis I, e.g., 293.0 Delirium Due to Hepatic Encephalopathy; also code the general medical condition on Axis III (see Appendix G for codes).

Diagnostic Criteria for Delirium Due to Multiple Etiologies

A. Disturbance of consciousness (i.e., reduced clarity of awareness of the environment) with reduced ability to focus, sustain, or shift attention.

B. A change in cognition (such as memory deficit, disorientation, language disturbance) or the development of a perceptual disturbance that is not better accounted for by a preexisting, established, or evolving dementia.

C. The disturbance develops over a short period (usually hours to days) and tends to fluctuate during the course of the day.

D. There is evidence from the history, physical examination, or laboratory findings that the delirium has more than one etiology (e.g., more than one etiological general medical condition, a general medical condition plus Substance Intoxication or medication side effect).

CODING NOTE: Use multiple codes reflecting specific delirium and specific etiologies, e.g., 293.0 Delirium Due to Viral Encephalitis; 291.0 Alcohol Withdrawal Delirium.

Diagnostic Criteria for Substance Withdrawal Delirium

A. Disturbance of consciousness (i.e., reduced clarity of awareness of the environment) with reduced ability to focus, sustain, or shift attention.

B. A change in the cognition (such as memory deficit, disorientation, language disturbance) or the development of a perceptual disturbance that is not better accounted for by a preexisting, established, or evolving dementia.

C. The disturbance develops over a short period (usually hours to days) and tends to fluctuate during the course of the day.

D. There is evidence from the history, physical examination, or laboratory findings that the symptoms in Criteria A and B developed during, or shortly after, a withdrawal syndrome.

NOTE: This diagnosis should be made instead of a diagnosis of Substance Withdrawal only when the cognitive symptoms are in excess of those usually associated with the withdrawal syndrome and when the symptoms are sufficiently severe to warrant independent clinical attention.

Code [Specific Substance] Withdrawal Delirium: (291.0 Alcohol; 292.81 Sedative, Hypnotic, or Anxiolytic; 292.81 Other [or Unknown] Substance)

Diagnostic Criteria for Substance Intoxication Delirium

A. Disturbance of consciousness (i.e., reduced clarity of awareness of the environment) with reduced ability to focus, sustain, or shift attention.

B. A change in cognition (i.e., memory deficit, disorientation, language disturbance) or the development of a perceptual disturbance that is not better accounted for by a preexisting, established, or evolving dementia.

C. The disturbance develops over a short period (usually hours to days) and tends to fluctuate during the course of the day.

D. There is evidence from the history, physical examination, or laboratory findings of either (1) or (2):
 (1) the symptoms in Criteria A and B developed during Substance Intoxication
 (2) medication use is etiologically related to the disturbance.*

NOTE: This diagnosis should be made instead of a diagnosis of Substance Intoxication only when the cognitive symptoms are in excess of those usually associated with the intoxication syndrome and when the symptoms are sufficiently severe to warrant independent clinical attention.

Continued on following page

> *The diagnosis should be recorded as Substance-Induced Delirium if related to medication use. Refer to Appendix G for E-codes indicating specific medications.
>
> Code [Specific Substance] Intoxication Delirium: (291.0 Alcohol; 292.81 Amphetamine [or Amphetamine-Like Substance]; 292.81 Cannabis; 292.81 Cocaine; 292.81 Hallucinogen; 292.81 Inhalant; 292.81 Opioid; 292.81 Phencyclidine [or Phencyclidine-Like Substance]; 292.81 Sedative, Hypnotic, or Anxiolytic; 292.81 Other [or Unknown] Substance [e.g., cimetidine, digitalis, benztropine])
>
> **Source:** Reprinted with permission from the Diagnostic and Statistical Manual of Mental Disorders, Fourth Edition. Copyright 1994 American Psychiatric Association.

quires continuous nursing supervision. Because physical restraints are likely to increase confusion and the risk of accident, alternatives should be employed. Miles[10] describes how improper management of a restless, elderly woman with cognitive and physical disabilities resulted in asphyxiation by her physical restraint. She was unable to free herself or call for help.

Reorient the client to time, place, and person. To avoid escalating anxiety, approach clients unhurriedly. Remind them repeatedly that their symptoms will subside with time. To reduce social isolation and assist with reorientation, encourage family members to remain with the client if possible and to bring in familiar objects to reinforce the client's sense of identity.

A client with ongoing problems may need referral to a home care agency or rehabilitation center to restore compromised function.

TABLE 15–2. Medications That Can Cause or Contribute to Dementia or Delirium

Analgesics	*Cardiovascular*
Narcotics	Atropine
Codeine	Digitalis
Meperidine	Diuretics
Morphine	Lidocaine
Pentazocine	
Propoxyphene	*Hypoglycemics*
Nonnarcotic	Insulin
Indomethacin	Sulfonylureas
Antihistamines	*Psychotropic Drugs*
Diphenhydramine	**Antianxiety drugs**
Hydroxyzine	Benzodiazepines
Antihypertensives	**Antidepressant drugs**
Clonidine	Lithium
Hydralazine	Tricyclics
Methyldopa	**Antipsychotics**
Propranolol	Haloperidol
Reserpine	Thiothixene
	Thioridazine
Antimicrobials	Chlorpromazine
Gentamicin	
Isoniazid	**Hypnotics**
	Barbiturates
Antiparkinsonism drugs	Benzodiazepines
Amantadine	Chloral hydrate
Bromocriptine	
Carbidopa	**Others**
L-Dopa	Cimetidine
	Steroids
	Trihexyphenidyl and other anticholinergics

Source: Kane, RL, Ouslander, JG, and Abrass, IB: Essentials of Clinical Geriatrics, ed 2. McGraw-Hill, New York, 1989, p. 90.

PHARMACOLOGIC INTERVENTIONS

Low doses of antianxiety agents such as benzodiazepines can help the client who is agitated and in distress. Typically, the effective dose for an elderly client may be only one-third to one-fourth the dose prescribed for a younger adult. It is most effective when given 1 to 2 hours before the client tends to become agitated. Because longer-acting agents can cause excessive drowsiness in some clients, shorter-acting benzodiazepines such as lorazepam (Ativan) and oxazepam (Serax) are recommended.

Buspirone (BuSpar) is an alternative to treatment with benzodiazepines. It is an anxiolytic that has few known sedating effects and a short half-life. Neuroleptics also may be prescribed to decrease delusions and hallucinations, if present. Monitor elderly clients' responses carefully because they are prone to paradoxical reactions to neuroleptics; agitation may intensify rather than diminish, and oversedation may occur.[2]

Expected Outcomes

For the individual with delirium, improvement will be demonstrated by:
- Return to baseline level of cognitive functioning
- Appropriate reality testing
- Ability to communicate thoughts and needs appropriately
- Ability to understand others
- No injuries.

Diagnostic Criteria for Dementia

Diagnostic Criteria for Dementia Due to Other General Medical Conditions

A. The development of multiple cognitive deficits manifested by both
  (1) memory impairment (impaired ability to learn new information or to recall previously learned information)
  (2) one (or more) of the following cognitive disturbances:
    (a) aphasia (language disturbance)
    (b) apraxia (impaired ability to carry out motor activities despite intact motor function)
    (c) agnosia (failure to recognize or identify objects despite intact sensory function)
    (d) disturbance in executive functioning (i.e., planning, organizing, sequencing, abstracting).

B. The cognitive deficits in Criteria A1 and A2 each cause significant impairment in social or occupational functioning and represent a significant decline from a previous level of functioning.

C. There is evidence from the history, physical examination, or laboratory findings that the disturbance is the direct physiological consequence of one of the general medical conditions listed below.

D. The deficits do not occur exclusively during the course of a delirium.

294.9 Dementia Due to HIV Disease
  CODING NOTE: Also code 043.1 HIV infection central nervous system on Axis III.

294.1 Dementia Due to Head Trauma
  CODING NOTE: Also code 854.00 head injury on Axis III.

294.1 Dementia Due to Parkinson's Disease
  CODING NOTE: Also code 332.0 Parkinson's disease on Axis III.

294.1 Dementia Due to Huntington's Disease
  CODING NOTE: Also code 333.4 Huntington's disease on Axis III.

290.10 Dementia Due to Pick's Disease
  CODING NOTE: Also code 331.1 Pick's disease on Axis III.

290.10 Dementia Due to Creutzfeldt-Jakob Disease
  CODING NOTE: Also code 046.1 Creutzfeldt-Jakob disease on Axis III.

294.1 Dementia Due to . . . [Indicate the General Medical Condition not listed above]

For example, normal-pressure hydrocephalus, hypothyroidism, brain tumor, vitamin B_{12} deficiency, intracranial radiation.
  CODING NOTE: Also code the general medical condition on Axis III.

Diagnostic Criteria for 290.4x Vascular Dementia

A. The development of multiple cognitive deficits manifested by both
  (1) memory impairment (impaired ability to learn new information or to recall previously learned information)
  (2) one (or more) of the following cognitive disturbances:
    (a) aphasia (language disturbance)
    (b) apraxia (impaired ability to carry out motor activities despite intact motor function)
    (c) agnosia (failure to recognize or identify objects despite intact sensory function)
    (d) disturbance in executive functioning (i.e., planning, organizing, sequencing, abstracting).

B. The cognitive deficits in Criteria A1 and A2 each cause significant impairment in social or occupational functioning and represent a significant decline from a previous level of functioning.

C. Focal neurological signs and symptoms (e.g., exaggeration of deep tendon reflexes, extensor plantar response, pseudobulbar palsy, gait abnormalities, weakness of an extremity) or laboratory evidence indicative of cerebrovascular disease (e.g., multiple infarctions involving cortex and underlying white matter) that are judged to be etiologically related to the disturbance.

D. The deficits do not occur exclusively during the course of the delirium.

Code based on predominant features:
  290.41 With Delirium: if delirium is superimposed on the dementia.
  290.42 With Delusions: if delusions are the predominant feature.
  290.43 With Depressed Mood: if depressed mood (including presentations that meet full symptom criteria for a Major Depression Episode) is the predominant feature. A separate diagnosis of Mood Disorder Due to a General Medical Condition is not given.
  290.40 Uncomplicated: if none of the above predominates in the current clinical presentation.

Continued on following page

Specify if:
   With Behavioral Disturbance
   CODING NOTE: Also code cerebrovascular condition on Axis III.

Diagnostic Criteria for Dementia Due to Multiple Etiologies

A. The development of multiple cognitive deficits manifested by both
   (1) memory impairment (impaired ability to learn new information or to recall previously learned information).
   (2) one (or more) of the following cognitive disturbances:
      (a) aphasia (language disturbance)
      (b) apraxia (impaired ability to carry out motor activities despite intact motor function)
      (c) agnosia (failure to recognize or identify objects despite intact sensory function)
      (d) disturbance in executive functioning (i.e., planning, organizing, sequencing, abstracting).
B. The cognitive deficits in Criteria A1 and A2 each cause significant impairment in social or occupational functioning and represent a significant decline from a previous level of functioning.
C. There is evidence from the history, physical examination, or laboratory findings that the disturbance has more than one etiology (e.g., head trauma plus chronic alcohol use, Dementia of the Alzheimer's Type with the subsequent development of Vascular Dementia).
D. The deficits do not occur exclusively during the course of a delirium.

   CODING NOTE: Use multiple codes based on specific dementias and specific etiologies, e.g., 290.0 Dementia of the Alzheimer's Type, With Late Onset, Uncomplicated; 290.40 Vascular Dementia, Uncomplicated.

Diagnostic Criteria for Substance-Induced Persisting Dementia

A. The development of multiple cognitive deficits manifested by both
   (1) memory impairment (impaired ability to learn new information or to recall previously learned information)
   (2) one (or more) of the following cognitive disturbances:
      (a) aphasia (language disturbance)
      (b) apraxia (impaired ability to carry out motor activities despite intact motor function)
      (c) agnosia (failure to recognize or identify objects despite intact sensory function)
      (d) disturbance in executive functioning (i.e., planning, organizing, sequencing, abstracting).
B. The cognitive deficits in Criteria A1 and A2 each cause significant impairment in social or occupational functioning and represent a significant decline from a previous level of functioning.
C. The deficits do not occur exclusively during the course of a delirium and persist beyond the usual duration of Substance Intoxication or Withdrawal.
D. There is evidence from the history, physical examination, or laboratory findings that the deficits are etiologically related to the persisting effects of substance use (e.g., a drug of abuse, a medication).

Code [Specific Substance]-Induced Persisting Dementia: (291.2 Alcohol; 292.82 Inhalant; 292.82 Sedative, Hypnotic, or Anxiolytic; 292.82 Other [or Unknown] Substance)

Source: Reprinted with permission from the Diagnostic and Statistical Manual of Mental Disorders, Fourth Edition. Copyright 1994 American Psychiatric Association.

DEMENTIA

Definition

Dementia refers to a constellation of symptoms resulting in impairment of short- and long-term memory. Its onset is slow or insidious, yet progressive, and it ends in death. Often individuals can mask their beginning symptoms for long periods. Because this syndrome is associated with deterioration in judgment and abstract reasoning, social and occupational functioning are significantly affected. The most common cause of dementia is **Alzheimer's disease**. Other types of dementia include vascular dementia and dementia due to head trauma, substances, and medical conditions such as human immunodeficiency virus (HIV), Parkinson's disease, **Huntington's disease**, and Pick's disease.

Mrs. W, 79 years old, lives with her daughter and son-in-law. Recently, her daughter noticed that her mother is more demanding and seems to be afraid of being alone. She often insists that she is hungry and when her daughter patiently explains that she has just eaten, her mother flies into a rage. Mrs. W enjoys taking frequent walks around her immediate neighborhood; however, on two recent occasions she has been unable to find her way home. When asked about these inci-

Critical Pathway: Dementia

Care Needs	1st 24 hours	Days 2-5

Assessment/Evaluations	Past psych hx
	Medication hx
	    Medical hx
	    Suicide risk
	    Self-care ability
	    Mental competence
	    Mental status
	    Psychiatric eval
	    Nursing assessment
		Family interview
		Social work eval
		    Evals by physical/occupational, activity, group therapies

Diagnostic Tests/Workup	Physical exam by NP, internist/gerontologist
	    Lab tests inc CBC, chem panel, drug screen, other as indic by medical hx
	    CAT scans, MRIs, other tests as indicated
		Review results of evaluations, lab work
		    Implement appropriate interventions
		    Implement further workup as needed
		    Psychological testing as indicated

Treatment	Orient to unit Initial activity orders	Participate in PT, OT, activities, group therapies 1:1 psychotherapy if able Participate in family sessions as approp
Medications	Order initial drug doses for psych and medical symptoms prn meds for agitation ordered	Monitor responses & side effects Adjust as approp
Safety/Self-care	Establish unit rules Monitor for wandering, self-injury, agitation Monitor eating, elimination, hygiene and sleep needs	Continue to monitor, per column 1 Institute interventions as approp Implement reality orientation measures throughout environment, fall precautions Assist with self-care needs
Education	Unit orientation Patient rights	Begin education on dementia and meds within abilities Reorientation
Discharge Plan	Identify initial concerns of pat/family	Identify pat/family issues Identify caregiver needs Identify possible resources/living
Outcomes	____ Patient assessed by MD and nurse ____ Initial activities/orders in place ____ Patient does not harm self Progressing per pathway? Yes ____ No ____ If no, referred to _____	____ Assessments by all disciplines complete ____ Workups completed ____ Multidiscipline tx plan developed and implemented ____ Meds adjusted as needed ____ Pat begins to participate in tx plan ____ Patient does not harm self Progressing per pathway? Yes ____ No ____ If no, referred to _____

Care Needs	Days 6–10+	Discharge
Assessment/Evaluations	Ongoing reassessment	—
Diagnostic Tests/Workshop	All results available and implemented in tx plan	Need for follow-up medical care established and appointments made.

Treatment	Continues in tx plan
	    Outpatient plan established.
	    Caregiving needs after discharge being evaluated.
		Outpatient tx appointments in place
		    Issues r/t insurance, transportation complete
		    Caregiving arrangements in place

Medications	Continue to monitor doses, side effects	Establish doses at discharge

Continued on following page

Critical Pathway: Dementia (Continued)

Care Needs	Days 6–10+	Discharge
	Establish outpatient medication regimen	Ensure medications, instructions available Ensure caregivers aware of medication needs
Safety/Self-care	Continue to monitor for self-injury, wandering, agitation Ensure nutrition, hygiene, sleep needs met Monitor continence Establish care needs at discharge	Ensure caregivers able to maintain pt safety Ensure pat has resources for food, hygiene
Education	Continue to educate pat/caregivers on dementia Educate on patient safety Educate on meds, side effects Food/drug interactions Nutritional counseling Community resources Educate caregivers on pat care needs and safety	Instructions and pat education materials in writing
Discharge Plan	Outpat tx plan complete Readmission criteria in place Identify caregiver support program Determine need for placement	Social worker completes outpatient care inc living arrangements, caregivers, insurance, activities, placement Medical equipment, home health care, transportation arranged
Outcomes	____ Pat demonstrating improvement and stabilization of symptoms ____ Stabilization of medication doses ____ Appropriate discharge plan developed ____ Patient does not harm self	____ Leaves hospital demonstrating plan to comply with outpat plan ____ Caregivers verbalize awareness of patient needs ____ Pat and/or caregivers able to verbalize resources for help ____ Pat and/or caregivers demonstrate knowledge of meds and side effects
	Progressing per pathway? Yes ____ No ____ If no, referred to _____	Progressing per pathway? Yes ____ No ____ If no, referred to _____

dents, Mrs. W denies being lost and accuses her daughter of treating her like a child.

Characteristic Behaviors

Symptoms of dementia range from mild cognitive deficits that interfere slightly with daily life to severe, life-threatening alterations in neurological functioning. Because the onset is insidious, diagnosis typically does not occur for years following the initial symptoms. The client may use **confabulation**, fabrication of events or experiences, in an effort to compensate for memory loss. Frequently, uninhibited behavior is the family's first clue that something is wrong. One elderly man shocked his wife by masturbating in the hallway of their apartment house. When other residents brought this behavior to his attention, he seemed perplexed that others viewed it as a problem.

The client may also engage in risk-taking behavior, perhaps while driving. Family members may seek help because the client's personal hygiene has declined or because of sleep disturbances. Prinz and Vitello[11] note that dementia is accompanied by sleep fragmentation, less efficient sleep, and decreased total sleep time. As dementia progresses, night-wandering episodes or sundowning may occur. Table 15–3 lists the common symptoms of sundowning.

Dementia of the Alzheimer's Type

Characteristically, Alzheimer's disease progresses in three broad stages (see Table 15–4) and seven discrete stages, as seen in Table 15–5. The Global Deterioration Scale (GDS) helps nurses and other clinicians determine the client's stage of cognitive decline.[12] Stage 1 represents normal cognition. During stage 2, cognitive decline is more subjective than

TABLE 15–3. Sundowners

```
Sick
   Urinary retention/fecal impaction
      New environment
         Demented
            Old
               Writhing in pain
                  Not adequately evaluated
                     Eyes and ears
                        Rx—therapeutic drug intoxication
                           Sleep deprived
```

Source: From Leskoff, SE, Besdine, RW, and Wetle, T: Acute confusional states (delirium) in the hospitalized elderly. Annual Review of Gerontology and Geriatrics 6:1–26, 1986.

TABLE 15–4. The Early-, Middle-, and Late-Stage Symptoms of Alzheimer's Disease

Early-Stage Symptoms
- Difficulty performing well-known duties
- Confusion
- Gradual forgetfulness
- Moodiness
- Trouble expressing thoughts
- Problems with sleeping
- Impaired judgment
- Difficulty adapting to new situations
- Anxiety
- Fear

Middle-Stage Symptoms
- Overwhelming confusion
- Decreased attention span
- Short-term memory impairments
- Motor restlessness
- Decreased comprehension
- Aphasia
- Problems with recognizing others
- Depression
- Anger
- Repetition
- Gait disorders
- Decision-making difficulties
- Difficulties with two or more step procedures

Late-Stage Symptoms
- Regression
- Significantly impaired ability to perform ADLs
- Incontinence
- Swallowing difficulties
- Weight loss
- Seizures
- Aggression
- Hallucinations
- Inability to recognize family or self
- Long-term memory loss
- Personality changes

objective. Elders may complain that they have difficulty remembering names or locating objects. They may have problems finding the right words to express their thoughts and have difficulty concentrating.[13]

At stage 3, the client becomes increasingly unable to perform in complex social and work situations. Signs may still be subtle at this stage. For example, a caterer may be unable to plan the menu for a client's wedding even though he or she has completed this task successfully many times before. During this stage, family, friends, and coworkers may express concern about the client's level of functioning. Short-term memory, concentration, and the ability to calculate are affected. The client may become lost while driving in familiar areas. When given a blank piece of paper and asked to write a sentence, a literate client may be unable to comply because of thought impoverishment or may write a sentence that does not contain a noun and a verb or does not make sense. The client may be reluctant to undergo health assessment because the interviewer is likely to expose memory deficits that the client has been denying. The client also may appear anxious and inattentive.

I tried to tell my family that something was wrong with Mom. At first, she just didn't seem as sharp as before. But when she'd call me, she'd ask the same questions over and over again—it was like it was the first time for her. I was very frustrated. Dad said it was just a sign of getting old. Then she started forgetting really important things; She didn't pay the bills, and she would get lost when she went out. When we finally got her evaluated, she was in a moderate stage of Alzheimer's disease. It was too late to try some of the medications that can be effective if started early on. Now she needs help with all sorts of things—cooking, bathing, dressing—and she doesn't sleep well at night. She's starting to forget who I am. It's like she's just a shell of the person she once was; and I now have a mother who doesn't know I exist.

Obvious memory impairment and an inability to travel or handle finances independently characterize stage 4. Clients who retain sufficient cognitive function to be aware of their decline may be depressed, with flat affect. To preserve self-esteem, the client is likely to withdraw from social situations and avoid complex tasks that might expose his or her impairment.

By stage 5, clients are frequently disoriented to time and place but still know their own names and the names of significant others. Typically, they are unable to recall major, relevant aspects of their current lives. They can no longer survive without assistance because of impairments in judgment and in instrumental activities of daily living.

Severe cognitive decline is evident in stage 6. Clients are largely unaware of recent life events and experiences. They forget the names of spouses or caregivers on whom they depend. Assistance with activities of daily living is required.

TABLE 15–5. Global Deterioration Scale (GDS) for Age-Associated Cognitive Decline and Alzheimer's Disease

GDS	Clinical Characteristics	Diagnosis
1 No cognitive decline	• No subjective complaints of memory deficit. • No memory deficit evident on clinical interview.	Normal

2
Very mild cognitive
	• Subjective complaints of memory deficit, most frequently in the following areas:
	  (a) forgetting where one has placed familiar objects.
	  (b) forgetting names one formerly knew well. No objective evidence of memory deficit on clinical interview.
	• No objective deficit in employment or social situations.
	• Appropriate concern with respect to symptoms.
		Age-Associated Memory Impairment (AAMI)

3
Neurocognitive
Mild cognitive decline
	• Earliest clear-cut deficits; manifestations in more than one of the following areas:
	  (a) patient may get lost while traveling to an unfamiliar location.
	  (b) coworkers become aware of patient's relatively poor performance.
	  (c) word and name-finding deficits become evident to intimates.
	  (d) patient may read a passage or book and retain relatively little material.
	  (e) patient may demonstrate decreased facility remembering names upon introduction to new people.
	  (f) patient may lose or misplace objects of value.
	  (g) concentration deficit may be evident on clinical testing.
	• Objective evidence of memory deficit may be obtained only with an intensive interview.
	• Decreased performance in demanding employment and social settings.
	• Denial begins to be manifest in patient.
	• Mild to moderate anxiety frequently accompanies symptoms.
		Mild Disorder

4
Moderate cognitive decline
	• Clear-cut deficit on careful clinical interview.
	• Deficit manifest in following areas:
	  (a) decreased knowledge of current and recent events.
	  (b) some deficit in memory of one's personal history.
	  (c) concentration deficit evident on serial subtractions.
	  (d) decreased ability to travel, handle finances, etc.
	• Frequently no deficit in these areas:
	  (a) orientation to time and place.
	  (b) recognition of familiar persons and faces.
	  (c) ability to travel to familiar locations.
	• Inability to perform complex tasks.
	• Denial is dominant defense mechanism.
	• Flattened affect and withdrawal from challenging situations occur.
		Mild Alzheimer's Disease

5
Moderately severe
	• Patient can no longer survive without some assistance.
	• Patient is unable to recall a major, relevant aspect of his or her current life during interview, for example:
	  (a) address or telephone number of many years.
	  (b) names of close family members (e.g., grandchildren).
	  (c) name of high school or college from which graduated.
	• Frequently some disorientation to time (e.g., date, day of the week, season) or to place.
	• An educated person may have difficulty counting backward by 4s or from 20 by 2s.
	• Persons at this stage retain knowledge of many major facts regarding themselves and others.
	• They invariably know their own names and generally know their spouse's and children's names.
	• They require no assistance with toileting or eating but may have difficulty choosing the proper clothing to wear.
		Moderate Alzheimer's Disease

Continued on following page

TABLE 15–5. Global Deterioration Scale (GDS) for Age-Associated Cognitive Decline and Alzheimer's Disease (Continued)

GDS	Clinical Characteristics	Diagnosis

6
Severe cognitive decline
	• May occasionally forget the name of the spouse upon whom he/she is entirely dependent.
	• Is largely unaware of all recent life events and experiences.
	• Retains some knowledge of surroundings, e.g., the year, the season, etc.
	• May have difficulty counting by 1s from 10, both backward and sometimes forward.
	• Requires some assistance with ADLs:
	  (a) may become incontinent.
	  (b) will require travel assistance but occasionally will be able to travel to familiar locations.
	• Diurnal rhythm frequently disturbed.
	• Almost always recalls his or her name.
	• Frequently continues to be able to distinguish familiar persons in their environment.
	• Personality and emotional changes occur; these are quite variable and include:
	  (a) delusional behavior, e.g., patients may accuse spouse of being an impostor; may talk to imaginary figures in the environment.
	  (b) obsessive symptoms, e.g., person may continually repeat simple cleaning activities.
	  (c) anxiety symptoms, agitation, and even previously nonexistent violent behavior may occur.
	  (d) cognitive abulia, e.g., loss of willpower because an individual cannot carry a thought long enough to determine a purposeful course of action.
		Moderately Severe Alzheimer's Disease

7 Very severe cognitive decline	• All verbal abilities are lost over the course of this stage. • Early in this stage words and phrases are spoken but is circumscribed. • Later, no speech remains; only grunting occurs. • Incontinent of urine; requires assistance toileting and feeding. • Basic psychomotor skills (e.g., ability to walk) are lost as this stage progresses. • Ultimately, the brain can no longer tell the body what to do. • Generalized and cortical neurological signs and symptoms are frequently present.	Severe Alzheimer's Disease

Source: Reisberg, B, et al: The global deterioration scale for assessment of primary degenerative dementia. Am J Psychiatry 139:1136–1139, 1982.

Incontinence may develop. Personality and emotional changes may include delusions, obsessions, anxiety, agitation, and belligerence.

During stage 7, all verbal abilities are gradually lost; however, clients retain the ability to vocalize. They are incontinent of urine and feces and basic psychomotor skills such as walking and swallowing deteriorate. Ultimately, because the brain can no longer tell the body what to do, total care is required. Generalized and cortical neurological signs are present.[12]

Vascular Dementia

Approximately 20% of all dementias are caused by multiple cerebral infarctions.[13] In this type of dementia, clients display behaviors similar to those with Alzheimer's; however, the onset is typically more sudden than in Alzheimer's disease. The diagnosis of **vascular dementia** can be made by observing multiple lesions of the cerebral cortex and the subcortical structures in the brain by computed tomography (CT) scan and magnetic resonance imaging (MRI). Laboratory findings may demonstrate cardiac and vascular changes.

Recent research suggests that vascular dementia is more common than thought and may be preventable.[14] These researchers propose that cognitive decline and cognitive impairment are associated with the risk of stroke as people age. They conclude that declining scores on mental status tests are early risk factors for subsequent strokes in the elderly with a history of cerebrovascular disease. Beginning aggressive treatment at that point may reduce the incidence and severity of vascular dementia.

> **RESEARCH NOTE**
>
> McCarty, E: Caring for a patient with Alzheimer's disease: Process of daughter caregiver stress. J Adv Nurs 23:792–803, 1996.
>
> **Findings:** This research explored the process of how women care for their aging parents with dementia. Seventeen women, caring for their parents with Alzheimer's disease, were studied. Daughters were faced with making decisions for parents and reviewing medication and medical interventions. The researcher found that certain factors increase or decrease the stress associated with caregiving. Those with mixed feelings or conflictual relationships with their parents may have more stressful experiences. Daughters who care for both parents, one with the disease and the other parent who is coping with its effects, are also at higher risk for caregiver stress. Those with siblings or spouses may use them as a source of social support, thereby decreasing the stress in their lives.
>
> The participants struggled with a sense of powerlessness and vulnerability about their parents' fate. They also expressed concern about their own future and the risk of developing Alzheimer's disease.
>
> **Application to Practice:** This study supports the idea that nursing interventions should be aimed at both clients and their families. The consequences of debilitating disorders such as dementia have profound effects, especially on those who care for clients. Daughters may assume the major role of caretaker; more support from others may decrease the stress associated with their caretaking experience. Nurses can help families monitor the elder's care and provide resources to promote effective coping strategies. Psychoeducation can be aimed at helping them understand the stages of Alzheimer's disease, its effects, and its causes. They also need time to discuss their own feelings and reactions to the caregiving experience.

Dementia due to Medical Conditions

Dementia is common in Parkinson's disease, Huntington's disease, and **Creutzfeldt-Jakob disease,** a transmissible, progressive, neurological disease caused by the same slow-acting virus that produces mad cow disease. The viral cause of this disease led to the hypothesis that a virus may play a part in the etiology of Alzheimer's disease.

In one condition, a rare but potentially curable cause of dementia occurs when obstruction to the flow of ventricular fluid produces a classic triad of **apraxia,** urinary incontinence, and dementia. This syndrome may follow head trauma or result from an infection.

Symptoms of dementia may also accompany infectious processes such as syphilis, tuberculosis, subacute bacterial endocarditis, and acquired immunodeficiency syndrome (AIDS).

Multiple Dementias

Several formal diagnoses of dementia often coexist. Clients may have both Alzheimer's disease and vascular dementia, or the symptoms of Alzheimer's may be exacerbated by an acute infection, sensory deprivation, or a change in their medication regimen.

Diagnostic Aids

Mental status examinations, laboratory tests, CT scans, and MRI assist in the diagnosis of dementia. These procedures may reveal reversible causes of confusion such as hypothyroidism and brain tumors. The diagnostic workup also includes checking serum electrolyte, B_{12}, and folate levels; a complete blood count (CBC); and thyroid function tests to rule out nutritional deficits.

Neuroimaging studies may reveal changes due to Alzheimer's disease. Cerebral atrophy and white matter changes in the ventricles may extend into the white matter of the frontal, parietal, and occipital lobes. Although several promising diagnostic tests exist, there are no consistent identifiable brain changes that can definitely confirm the diagnosis of dementia of the Alzheimer's type.

The mental status examination reveals memory deficits and the inability to think abstractly. Clients are typically unable to explain the meaning of proverbs except in concrete terms. For example, "a rolling stone gathers no moss" may be discussed via a detailed explanation of why moss will not adhere to a stone.

Clients may have changes in mood and psychotic thoughts. Assess clients for depression, which may mimic or enhance symptoms of cognitive decline. Personality changes are not often seen in the early stages of dementia but become more common as the disease progresses. Delusions of persecution may be manifest as clients accuse others of taking things they themselves have misplaced. If delusions produce fear, clients may become agitated and violent toward others who are misperceived as wanting to do harm.

Culture, Age, and Gender Features

Culture

Different types of dementia may present differently based on the individual's culture. Because some people may not be familiar with information used in memory assessment, consider each client's cultural background.

Age

Box 15–2 lists the prevalence of dementia and other cognitive disorders. Early-onset Alzheimer's disease occurs before age 65 and is relatively uncommon. The percentage of clients over age 65 residing in the community who exhibit symptoms of Alzheimer's disease increases with age. In the group 65 to 74 years of age, 3.9% are estimated to have probable Alzheimer's. Those 74 to 85 years of age have a 16.4% prevalence rate. Among those over age 85 years, the probability

Diagnostic Criteria for Alzheimer's Disease

Diagnostic Criteria for Dementia of the Alzheimer's Type

A. The development of multiple cognitive deficits manifested by both
   (1) memory impairment (impaired ability to learn new information or to recall previously learned information)
   (2) one (or more) of the following cognitive disturbances:
      (a) aphasia (language disturbance)
      (b) apraxia (impaired ability to carry out motor activities despite intact motor function)
      (c) agnosia (failure to recognize or identify objects despite intact sensory function)
      (d) disturbance in executive functioning (i.e., planning, organizing, sequencing, abstracting).

B. The cognitive deficits in Criteria A1 and A2 each cause significant impairment in social or occupational functioning and represent a significant decline from a previous level of functioning.

C. The course is characterized by gradual onset and continuing cognitive decline.

D. The cognitive deficits in Criteria A1 and A2 are not due to any of the following:
   (1) other central nervous system conditions that cause progressive deficits in memory and cognition (e.g., cerebrovascular disease, Parkinson's disease, Huntington's disease, subdural hematoma, normal-pressure hydrocephalus, brain tumor)
   (2) systemic conditions that are known to cause dementia (e.g., hypothyroidism, vitamin B$_{12}$ or folic acid deficiency, niacin deficiency, hypercalcemia, neurosyphilis, HIV infection),
   (3) substance-induced conditions.

E. The deficits do not occur exclusively during the course of a delirium.

F. The disturbance is not better accounted for by another Axis I disorder (e.g., Major Depressive Disorder, Schizophrenia).

Code based on type of onset and predominant features:
With Early Onset: if onset is at age 65 years or below:
290.11 With Delirium: if delirium is superimposed on the dementia.
290.12 With Delusions: if delusions are the predominant feature.
290.13 With Depressed Mood: if depressed mood (including presentations that meet full symptom criteria for a Major Depressive Episode) to a General Medical Condition is not given.
290.10 Uncomplicated: if none of the above predominates in the current clinical presentation.
With Late Onset: if onset is after age 65 years:
290.3 With Delirium: if delirium is superimposed on the dementia.
290.20 With Delusions: if delusions are the predominant feature.
290.21 With Depressed Mood: if depressed mood (including presentations that meet full symptom criteria for a Major Depressive Episode) to a General Medical Condition is not given
290.0 Uncomplicated: if none of the above predominates in the current clinical presentation.

Specify if:
With Behavioral Disturbance.

CODING NOTE: Also code 331.0 Alzheimer's disease on Axis III.

Source: Reprinted with permission from the Diagnostic and Statistical Manual of Mental Disorders, Fourth Edition. Copyright 1994 American Psychiatric Association.

---

of being diagnosed with dementia of the Alzheimer's type is 47.55%.[15] It is estimated that as many as half of nursing home residents have some form of dementia.

Dementia is uncommon in childhood or adolescence.

Gender

Dementia of the Alzheimer's type is more common in women than in men.

Etiology

Neuroanatomical Changes

Alois Alzheimer first described the symptoms of the dementia that was named after him. Along with cognitive changes, he also identified characteristic plaques and tangles, specific types of proteins that accumulate in the brains of people with Alzheimer's disease. *Plaques* are sphere-shaped structures that have amyloid protein cores. *Tangles* are abnormal bundles of protein also found in the brain. Whereas tangles attack the inside of the neuron, plaques attack from the outside, engulfing the axons and dendrites. Plaques and tangles represent deterioration of the brain, leading to the symptoms of the disease.

Biological Theories

Amyloid Cascade Hypothesis. Alzheimer's disease may be due to too much of the protein β-amyloid. β-amyloid protein is present in the brain and other parts of the body

Nursing Care Plan: DEMENTIA

Nursing Diagnosis #1: Altered thought processes evidenced by disorientation, memory deficits, inability to perform activities of daily living, poor judgment related to cerebral degeneration, Alzheimer's disease

Client Outcome Criteria
- Demonstrates improved reality orientation.
- Responds coherently to simple requests.
- Follows simple directions.

Interventions
- Establish a baseline assessment of the client's mental status and functioning. Be aware of the client's attempts to disguise memory loss by confabulation, avoidance, or rambling.
- Avoid making demands of the client that he or she is unable to handle. This will only add to confusion and anxiety.
- Break down tasks in small steps. Give verbal, visual, and written cues to keep the client on track.
- Ask only one question or make only one request at a time.
- Provide a structured routine.
- Provide familiar objects of the client's in the environment.
- Avoid agreeing with the client's confused thinking, but also do not get into arguments challenging a fixed belief. Rather try to distract the client or consider acknowledging the feelings associated with the confusion.
- Incorporate orientation cues throughout the environment, e.g., large clocks, calendars, signs on doors, large daily schedule posted in client's room.
- Reduce distractions when talking to client. Keep environment simple and uncluttered.

Nursing Diagnosis #2: Risk for injury evidenced by falls, wandering related to confusion, lack of understanding of environmental hazards, poor coordination

Client Outcome Criteria
- Remains injury free.
- Demonstrates appropriate actions to avoid injury.
- Demonstrates reduced wandering behavior.

Interventions
- Maintain safe environment, e.g., arrange furniture to accommodate any disabilities, keep bed in low position, assign room near nurses' station, maintain adequate lighting, supervise client in bathroom, at meals, and when ambulating.
- Monitor closely for responses to medication such as confusion or sedation that may increase risk of injury.
- Make sure the client uses needed assistive devices like hearing aids or glasses as appropriate.
- Take the client to the bathroom before going to sleep to reduce the risk of getting up during the night. If the client is on diuretics or laxatives, administer them early in the day and provide additional supervision as needed. Keep bathroom lights on.
- Monitor facility or home exits to ensure the client cannot leave unsupervised. Use alarms. Make sure the client is always wearing identification that cannot be removed. Teach family and home caregivers about safety.
- Consider use of restraints as a last resort if the client remains at risk for injury and wandering.
- Provide an area where the client can walk safely, such as a dayroom or physical therapy gym.

Nursing Diagnosis #3: Impaired social interactions evidenced by inappropriate social behavior, emotional lability related to altered thought processes, confusion, Alzheimer's disease

Client Outcome Criteria
- Demonstrates appropriate behavior in social situations.
- Demonstrates reduced emotional liability in social situations.
- Increases participation in social interactions.

Interventions
- Determine the client's response to social situations.
- Make sure the client uses a hearing aid, dentures, or glasses, as needed, as well as good hygiene and appropriate dress.
- Recognize that the client may revert to inappropriate behavior such as crude remarks or hostility when anxious. Ignore these responses and distract the client to other topics. Avoid arguing or criticizing the client. Identify situations that are threatening and make efforts to reduce the client's exposure to these.
- Use medications, e.g., antipsychotics or anxiolytics, appropriately to reduce anxiety and agitation.
- Keep social situations brief. Engage client routinely in brief social situations with others. Use concrete language and simple topics to keep anxiety low.

Nursing Diagnosis #4: Self-care deficit evidenced by poor hygiene, poor nutrition, dehydration, noncompliance with taking medications related to confusion, Alzheimer's disease

Client Outcome Criteria
- Receives adequate nutrition and hydration.
- Demonstrates ability to feed self.
- Demonstrates appropriate personal hygiene.

Interventions
- Assess the client's ability to care for self including personal hygiene, elimination, eating, and drinking.
- Provide the needed assistance to ensure basic needs are met. Allow plenty of time to work with the client with a minimum of distractions.
- Observe the client's eating and drinking patterns and assist as needed with opening containers and cutting up food. Make sure food is allowed to cool. Reduce distractions at mealtime. Ensure that the client is able to chew and swallow food. Make adjustments in diet if there are chewing or swallowing problems, and evaluate if there is a need for dental work or dentures. Offer fluids on a regular schedule.
- If the client is at home, determine if prescribed medications are being taken appropriately. Work with family and home caregivers to set up an improved system to monitor medications. Determine if the client is using over-the-counter medications, and be aware of the impact of these on cognitive functioning.
- Create a schedule for elimination by taking the client to the bathroom regularly. Determine the need for laxatives.
- Gently correct inappropriate behavior. Reinforce what is appropriate. If the client persists in inappropriate behavior, focus on distracting him or her from the situation.
- Ensure the client dresses appropriately for the situation. Provide assistance with bathing and mouthcare.

Box 15-2. Prevalence of Cognitive Disorders

Disorder	Prevalence
Delirium	10%*
Dementia of the Alzheimer's type	2–4%**
Vascular dementia	Uncommon
Amnesia	Uncommon

*Of hospitalized clients over age 65
**Of people over age 65

Source: Based on data from the Diagnostic and Statistical Manual of Mental Disorders, Fourth Edition. Copyright 1994 American Psychiatric Association.

in all individuals. It helps in the development and maintenance of the central nervous system. Overproduction of β-amyloid destroys neurons, leading to the symptoms of cognitive decline.

What causes excess β-amyloid? Some clients with Alzheimer's disease may have an abnormal gene that forms a substance called amyloid precursor protein, APP. APP then forms amyloid deposits, which in turn form the characteristic plaques and tangles found in the brains of people with Alzheimer's disease. The plaques and tangles eventually cause the neuron to die.

Another potential cause of excess β-amyloid is that clients with Alzheimer's disease have a gene that makes a defective protein, apo E.[16] There appear to be two types of apo E: "good" and "bad." "Good" apo E binds to β-amyloid and then removes it so that β-amyloid doesn't build up. Because "bad" apo E cannot remove β-amyloid from the neuron, excess amyloid accumulates, forms plaques and tangles, and causes neuronal death.

Cholinergic Theories. The cholinergic-deficiency hypothesis suggests that decreased levels of acetylcholine cause Alzheimer's disease. Figure 15–1 shows how acetylcholine is affected. Acetylcholine, a neurotransmitter, is usually formed in cholinergic neurons. The enzyme that makes acetylcholine is choline acetyltransferase; normal levels of this enzyme are decreased by 90% in clients with Alzheimer's disease. When levels of this enzyme are decreased, the result is reduced levels of acetylcholine, which is especially apparent in a group of neurons found in the basal forebrain. More than 75% of cholinergic neurons in the basal forebrain are lost during the last stages of Alzheimer's disease. The degree of cognitive impairment in Alzheimer's disease is related to the decreased amount of acetylcholine in cholinergic neurons in the cortex.[17] Medications that build up acetylcholine such as tacrine slow down the process of cognitive decline, especially for clients in the early stages of the disease.

Norepinephrine and Serotonin Theories. Other neurotransmitters are also altered in Alzheimer's disease. For example, norepinephrine levels are reduced in the cortex of

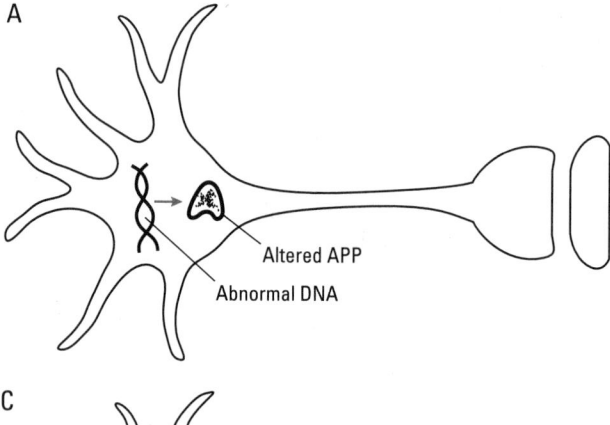

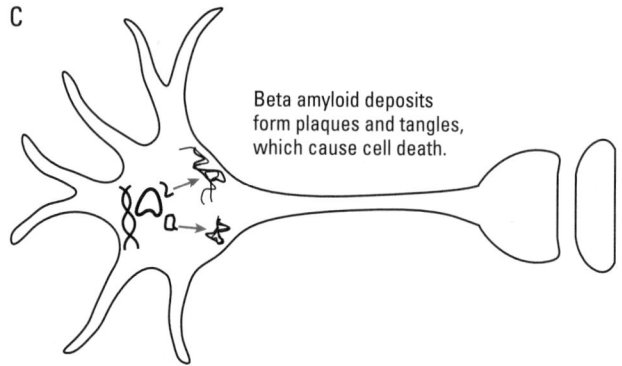

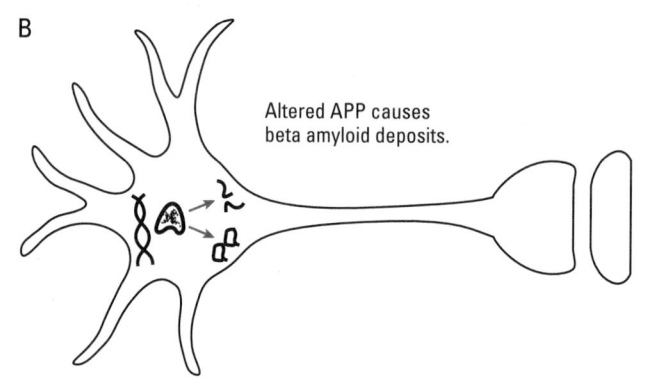

Figure 15-1. The amyloid cascade hypothesis of Alzheimer's disease. *(A) Part 1:* A leading contemporary theory for the biological basis of Alzheimer's disease centers around the formulation of beta amyloid. Perhaps Alzheimer's disease is essentially a disease in which the abnormal deposition of beta amyloid gets to the point that it destroys neutrons. Thus, Alzheimer's disease may be essentially a problem of too much formation of beta amyloid or too little removal of it. One idea is that neurons in some patients destined to have Alzheimer's disease have an abnormality in the DNA that codes for a protein called amyloid precursor protein (APP). The abnormal DNA starts a lethal chemical cascade in neurons, beginning with the formation of an altered APP. *(B) Part 2:* Once APP is formed (see Figure 15–1A), it leads to the formation of beta amyloid deposits. *(C) Part 3:* Once beta amyloid deposits are formed from abnormal APP, beta amyloid deposits form plaques and tangles in the neuron. From Stahl, SM: Essential Psychopharmacology. Cambridge University Press, New York, 1996, pp. 294–295.

nearly 50% of clients. Loss of serotonin seems to produce alteration in sleep patterns early in the course of the disease. When the brains of individuals with Alzheimer's are compared to the brains of normal subjects, three amino acids with neurotransmitter functions believed to play a role in memory are also reduced: asparate, γ-aminobutyric acid (GABA), and glutamate.[17] The "excitotoxic hypothesis" proposes that too much glutamate may cause neurons to degenerate. *Excitotoxicity* refers to overexcited neurons; the neurons are literally excited to death. This hypothesis may help explain the loss of neurons in Alzheimer's disease, Parkinson's disease, Huntington's disease, and other neuropsychiatric disorders.

Genetic Theories

Alzheimer's disease can be genetically transmitted. Mutations in three genes have been linked to one genetic transmittable form of the disorder: presenilin-1 (PS1), PS2, and amyloid precursor protein genes. Research demonstrates that family members who inherit two of the less common variants of the apo E protein (apolipoprotein E), apo E-IV, are eight times more likely to develop Alzheimer's disease than are family members who inherit adenosine triphosphate (ATP) E-III genes, the more common variant. Affected clients who have the mutant PS1 genes have double the number of plaques that lead to degeneration.

Dementia of the Alzheimer's type is inherited as a dominant trait with linkage to chromosomes 21, 14, and 19.[4] Researchers have discovered that gene coding for the brain protein found in tangles and plaques can be traced to chromosome 21. In some families with positive histories for Alzheimer's disease, a specific gene sequence on chromosome 21 is inherited. Down's syndrome is also more common in these families.[18] When the exact sequence of inheritance is discovered, it may become possible to intervene to prevent expression of Alzheimer's disease.

Prognosis

Although the prognosis of some dementias such as the Alzheimer's type is progressive and deteriorating, some dementias can be treated and others are reversible. Table 15–6 lists treatable dementias and disorders that can be reversed.

The course of dementia differs from that of depression and delirium. Table 15–7 lists the difference in progression between these disorders.

Assessment

Medications or medical illness may be responsible for cognitive changes. Nurses are in a prime position to help clients and their families receive a complete evaluation. Use a mnemonic, based on the word *dementia*, to help with assessment.

D–drugs
E–emotional illness, pseudodementia
M–metabolic, endocrine disorders
E–eye, ear, environment
N–nutritional, neurological
T–tumors, trauma
I–infection
A–alcoholism, anemia, atherosclerosis

Dementia can be distinguished from delirium and depression, even though clients' behaviors may appear similar. Box 15–3 lists some differences.

Planning Care

Nurses planning care for clients with dementia should emphasize two priorities: maintaining the client's maximum level of functional independence and ensuring safety. Formal and informal caregivers frequently conclude that doing things for the client is more efficient and less frustrating than encouraging self-care. However, to maintain functional abilities and promote self-esteem, clients should be encouraged to bathe and dress themselves, exercise, and assist with meal preparation or other household chores within the limits of their abilities. Cueing and task segmentation may be necessary to enable clients to perform activities of daily living. For example, they may retain the ability to feed themselves but may not eat without cueing and encouragement.

RESEARCH NOTE

Damasio, A, Damasio, H, Grabowski, T, Tranel, D, and Hichwas, R: A neural basis for lexical retrieval. Nature 380:499–505, 1996.

Findings: These researchers present intriguing findings into Alzheimer's disease. They examined writing samples from a group of nuns, from their early 20s to their 80s. The researchers hypothesized that the most educated nuns would be least likely to develop Alzheimer's disease; however, the data did not support their prediction. They discovered that they could predict with 90% accuracy which nuns would manifest the disease. Nuns whose early writing demonstrated grammatically complex sentences and were rich in ideas were still cognitively sharp in their 80s. Like atherosclerosis, Alzheimer's disease may be a lifelong illness to which one is genetically predisposed, yet symptoms are not manifest until late adulthood.

Application to Practice: This research suggests that individuals who are predisposed to dementia may show writing deficits early in adulthood. Cognitive assessment can be incorporated into physical examinations throughout the life span to provide baseline information for detecting beginning declines associated with aging. Families may wait for the emergence of dramatic unmanageable symptoms of dementia before seeking assistance. Nurses can take an active role in early intervention.

TABLE 15–6. Diseases Presenting as Dementia

Alzheimer's Disease
With or without vascular disease
With or without Parkinson's disease
With or without dementing illness
Other Progressive Dementias
Degenerative Diseases
Pick's disease
Huntington's disease
Progressive supranuclear palsy
Parkinson's disease
Diffuse Lewy body disease
Cerebellar degenerations
Amyotrophic lateral sclerosis (ALS)
Parkinson–ALS–dementia complex of Guam and New Guinea
Rare genetic and metabolic diseases
Vascular Dementias
Multi-infarct dementia
Cortical microinfarcts
Lacunar dementia
Binswanger's disease
Cerebral embolism by fat or air
Anoxic Dementia
Cardiac arrest
Cardiac failure (severe)
Carbon monoxide
Traumatic
Dementia pugilistica (boxer's dementia)
Head injuries (open or closed)
Infections
Acquired immunodeficiency syndrome (AIDS)
Creutzfeldt-Jakob disease
Progressive multifocal leukoencephalopathy
Postencephalitic dementia
Behçet syndrome
Treatable Dementias
Infections
Herpes encephalitis
Fungal meningitis or encephalitis
Bacterial meningitis or encephalitis
Parasitic encephalitis
Brain abscess
Neurosyphillis
Normal-pressure Hydrocephalus
Space-occupying Lesions
Chronic or acute subdural hematoma
Primary brain tumor
Metastatic tumors

Multiple Sclerosis (some cases)
Autoimmune Disorders
Disseminated lupus erythematosus
Vasculitis
Toxic Dementia
Alcoholic dementia
Metallic poisons
Organic poisons
Other Disorders
Concentration camp syndrome
Whipple's disease
Heat stroke
Reversible Causes of Dementia
Psychiatric Disorders
Depression
Sensory deprivation
Other psychoses
Drugs
Sedatives
Hypnotics
Antianxiety agents
Antidepressants
Antiarrhythmics
Antihypertensives
Anticonvulsants
Digitalis and derivatives
Drugs with anticholinergic side effects
Nutritional Disorders
Pellagra (vitamin B_6 deficiency)
Thiamine deficiency (Wernicke syndrome, acute phase)
Cobalamin deficiency (Vitamin B_{12}) or pernicious anemia
Folate deficiency
Marchiafava-Bignami disease
Metabolic Disorders
Hyperthyroidism and hypothyroidism
Hypercalcemia
Hypernatremia and hyponatremia
Hypoglycemia
Hyperlipidemia
Hypercapnia
Kidney failure
Cushing's syndrome
Addison's disease
Hypopituitarism

Source: Adapted from Katzman, R, and Rowe, JW (eds): Principles of Geriatric Neurology. FA Davis, Philadelphia, 1992, p. 170.

Interventions for Clients in the Community

The majority of nursing care occurs in the community, whether the client is living at home, in assisted living, or in a long-term care facility. Use the clinical management tips listed in Table 15–8.

Maintaining Independence

Regardless of setting, an important goal is to maintain the client's maximum independence and to keep experiences failure-free. Staff or family must be ready to step in to assist when the client shows mounting frustration. If such frustration is unchecked, a **catastrophic reaction** may result, an

TABLE 15–7. A Comparison of the Course of Depression, Delirium, and Dementia

Depression	Delirium	Dementia
Cause may be identified	Cause may be identified	Cause may be unknown
Time limited	Time limited	Can become chronic
Insidious	Acute onset	Insidious
Usually treatable	Always treatable	Not often treatable or reversible

outburst of rage with possible violence directed toward self or others that is often followed by a period of withdrawal and depression.

Maintaining Safety

Because of lack of insight and poor judgment, individuals are at risk for harming themselves or others. Caregivers must be aware of the potential dangers of leaving clients alone or permitting them to engage in activities that they can no longer handle safely. If they wander, they should be permitted to wander within the limits of a safe, supervised area and wear an identification bracelet at all times. The home or nursing unit must be altered to compensate for the cognitive and physical losses of the client.

Structure

Clients respond positively to structure and a predictable daily routine. Clients in the early stages of dementia can benefit from **reality orientation**, frequent reminders of date, time, and whereabouts.

Box 15–3. Ways to Distinguish Depression from Dementia

Symptom	Depression	Dementia
Depressed mood	++++	+
Severe guilt	+++	−
Worsening over time	−	++++
Consistently poor performance	−	+++
Object naming difficulties	−	+++
Impaired drawing ability	−	+++
Client concerned	++++	−
Sundowns	−	+++
Abnormal CT scan	−	+++

Key: − absent, + possible, ++ likely, +++ common, ++++ very common.

Source: Adapted from Yesavage, J: Differential diagnosis between depression and dementia. Am J Med 94 (suppl 5A), 23S–28S, 1993.

TABLE 15–8. Clinical Management Tips for Working with Clients with Dementia

Communication Strategies
- Look directly at clients when speaking to them.
- Identify yourself prior to each interaction.
- Use simple, short phrases.
- Ask specific rather than general questions: "Does your stomach hurt?" rather than "How are you?"
- Distract clients who ask the same question repeatedly.
- Assist clients in word-finding difficulties; suggest words or try to determine their underlying feelings.
- Strive to take a calm and consistent approach.
- Reassure clients that you are there to help.
- Avoid arguing and confrontative statements.
- Convey a patient and understanding attitude.

Ways to Decrease Confusion
- Establish a regular and predictable routine.
- Break down complex tasks into small, simple steps.
- Strive for consistent care by regular staff.
- Use a large clock and calendar, crossing off each day.
- Decrease distraction and stimulation; avoid clutter or unnecessary objects.
- Post lists of daily activities.
- Have the client wear glasses or a hearing aid, if needed.
- Avoid medications, if possible.
- Check client frequently.

Ways to Promote Safety
- Have client wear an identification bracelet.
- Install special locks and safety devices on doors, stove, and other potentially dangerous objects.
- Provide night lights and reflective tape in the shape of arrows to direct clients to the bathroom.
- Check the client frequently for burns, bruises, or abrasions.
- Assess the client for any signs of abuse.
- Use restraints only after other methods are ineffective.

Ways to Promote Physical and Emotional Well-Being
- Encourage regular exercise.
- Ensure that clients receive adequate nutrition and hydration.
- Allow client as much independence as possible.
- Provide assistance with feeding, dressing, and personal hygiene as needed.
- Assess frequently for physical pain, constipation, and discomfort.
- Evaluate agitation and worsening behavior carefully; worsening behavior may reflect physical decline.
- Suggest day treatment for clients living at home.

Family Education
- Teach ways to control uncooperative behavior.
- Teach about the causes and course of dementia.
- Encourage families to read resources on caring for clients with dementia.
- Monitor and assess the level of stress on the family.
- Encourage their use of social support to decrease caregiver stress.
- Help families mourn the loss of their loved one.

Source: Adapted from Gorman, LM, Sultan, DF, and Raines, ML: Davis's Manual of Psychosocial Nursing for General Patient Care. FA Davis, Philadelphia, 1996, pp. 193–203.

Catastrophic reactions can occur when clients are experiencing sensory overload. Staff and family should closely monitor clients' level of stimulation and their response to it. For example, clients who can feed themselves and enjoy conversation during a routine weekday dinner may be unable to adapt to the hectic pace, noise, and presence of extended family and guests at a holiday meal.

Frequent Assessment

Assess changes in both physical and mental health status frequently. All staff caring for clients with dementia should know what is normative or baseline behavior for that individual. Clients can experience a sudden exacerbation of symptoms that requires immediate intervention but is mistakenly attributed to resistance or a catastrophic reaction. Many clients with depression respond well to pharmacologic intervention. Some may be unable to inform the nurse that they are in pain or have other symptoms of acute or chronic physical illness. One nursing home resident died as a result of peritonitis missed by staff who reported an increase in agitation but did not explore potential causes for the client's distress.

> **RESEARCH NOTE**
> Rovner, BW, Steele, C, Shmuely, Y, and Folstein, M: A randomized trial of dementia care in nursing homes. J Am Geriatr Soc 44:7–13, 1996.
>
> **Findings:** The researchers conducted a study to determine the efficacy of an experimental program for managing dementia clients in nursing homes. The intervention involved "Activities, Guidelines for Psychotropic Medications, Education Program," A.G.E. Clients participated in an activity program weekdays from 10:00 am to 3:00 pm and had their medications managed by a psychiatrist rather than a primary care physician. The psychiatrist also made education rounds with the staff to discuss each client's behavioral problems, use of antipsychotics, physical restraint use, activity level, and functional and cognitive status. Results suggested that the A.G.E. program decreased behavioral disorders and reduced the use of psychiatric medications.
>
> **Application to Practice:** Because dementia clients have a progressive, irreversible illness, they are at risk for receiving minimal treatment. This study demonstrates that clients benefit from a well-designed program of activities and judicious management with psychiatric medications administered under the supervision of psychiatric specialists. Despite their decline, these interventions can help treat problem behaviors and perhaps avoid medications in some clients. Nurses can advocate for this vulnerable group to ensure that they receive effective treatment.

Developing behavior plans requires ingenuity. Nursing care should change to take into account the client's functional stage and behavioral responses. The actions or behaviors that clients adopt as the disease progresses, though at times cryptic, are their way of communicating with the world.[19] So-called problem behaviors should be interpreted as attempts to communicate needs.

Care plans that emphasize interdisciplinary collaboration are critical to address the needs of dementia clients and their caregivers.[20] These clients' complex needs cannot be met by one professional group alone. For example, strategies to facilitate independence in eating could be developed jointly by nursing, dietary, and occupational therapy. When planning care, recognize that cultural differences influence caretaking behavior.[21]

Validation Therapy

As dementia progresses, reorientation strategies become ineffective and may increase the client's agitation. **Validation therapy** is one approach that is often used.[22] In validation therapy, nursing staff attempt to enter the client's world rather than force him or her to relate to an external world he or she can no longer comprehend.

> An 86-year-old female client with dementia refused to participate in a reminiscence therapy group because she feared that the baby doll she always carried with her would require feeding, changing, or other care. She also felt that her "baby" might catch a cold from group members. Attempts to force this client to abandon the doll and attend the group or to accept that the doll was not real provoked a catastrophic reaction. Instead, staff praised the client for her excellent caregiving and assured her that they would care for her "baby" while she took a much needed break to visit with friends. She happily complied.

Feil[22] emphasizes that nurses initially may be uncomfortable with validation therapy because they fear they are fostering delusional behavior. She stresses that when a client has an irreversible, degenerative cognitive impairment, quality of life issues are paramount. Validation strategies increase the client's sense of being understood by others and reduce the incidence of agitation and catastrophic reaction, thereby enhancing quality of life.

Remotivation Therapy

Remotivation therapy is also widely used with cognitively impaired elders. In stage 1, emphasis is placed on experiencing the world and deriving pleasure and sensory stimulation from a structured group welcoming each member and assisting him or her to feel safe and comfortable. In stage 2, the group's theme is introduced and perhaps illustrated by a brief, appropriate poem or musical selection. Examples of popular remotivation themes are favorite flowers and baseball. During stage 3, group members become involved in a simple task or sensory experience related to the chosen theme. They might touch and smell various flowers or handle baseballs and gloves. During stage 4, clients are encouraged to reminisce in relation to the group's theme. Ham and Sloane[1] emphasize that demented clients retain much long-term memory; accessing and using it can improve quality of life. Stage 5 focuses on establishing a climate of appreciation; the nurse thanks the client for attending and for his or her unique contribution. The purpose of remotivation therapy is to interrupt self-absorption and isolation, to create a bridge to external reality, and to provide pleasure and sensory stimulation.[23]

PHARMACOLOGIC INTERVENTIONS

All medications should be considered individual therapeutic experiments, and the client's response should be carefully monitored. The goal is to enhance quality of life rather than to produce a malleable client more readily cared for by staff.

Memory Enhancers

When initiated early in the course of the illness, tacrine, a centrally acting anticholinesterase agent, is effective in slowing the progression of Alzheimer's disease. Figure 15–2 shows how tacrine and other medications under development increase levels of acetylcholine by inhibiting the enzyme acetylcholinesterase.

Low doses of tacrine, 25 mg tid, are given initially and then increased as indicated to a maximum daily dose of 200 mg to achieve the drug's maximum beneficial effects. Because hepatotoxic effects have been observed, liver function is monitored every 1 to 2 weeks, and the dosage is decreased or discontinued if liver enzymes are elevated. Tacrine may lead to improved memory and functioning especially for individuals in the early stages of the disease.

Another cholinesterase inhibitor, donepezil (Aricept), was recently introduced for the treatment of mild to moderate Alzheimer's disease. Initial doses of 5 mg may be increased after 4 to 6 weeks to a total daily dose of 10 mg. Common side effects may include nausea, diarrhea, and insomnia; uncommon side effects may include fatigue, vomiting, muscle cramps, and anorexia. Rare but potentially serious side effects may include syncope or gastrointestinal bleeding, particularly in those at risk for developing ulcers. Donepezil can enhance mental abilities by improving memory, reasoning, orientation, and language, especially for clients in the early stages of dementia.

Medications Used to Treat Agitation and Aggression

Antipsychotic medications are used judiciously in the management of dementia. Ham and Sloane[1] report that many clinicians are reluctant to prescribe these drugs because of accusations that they chemically restrain the client. However, their use is sometimes essential to humane management of the frightened, agitated, or hallucinating client who fails to respond to behavioral management strategies. Dosage is carefully titrated to produce calmness without oversedation. The most commonly used agents are high-potency antipsychotics such as haloperidol and risperidone. Very low doses, for example, 0.5 mg of haloperidol, are indicated; high doses may cause worsening of behavior, particularly increased restlessness or stupor. Olanzapine, a new atypical antipsychotic, is currently being investigated for the treatment of agitation and aggression associated with dementia.

Antipsychotics may be given in conjunction with low doses of short-acting benzodiazepines such as lorazepam

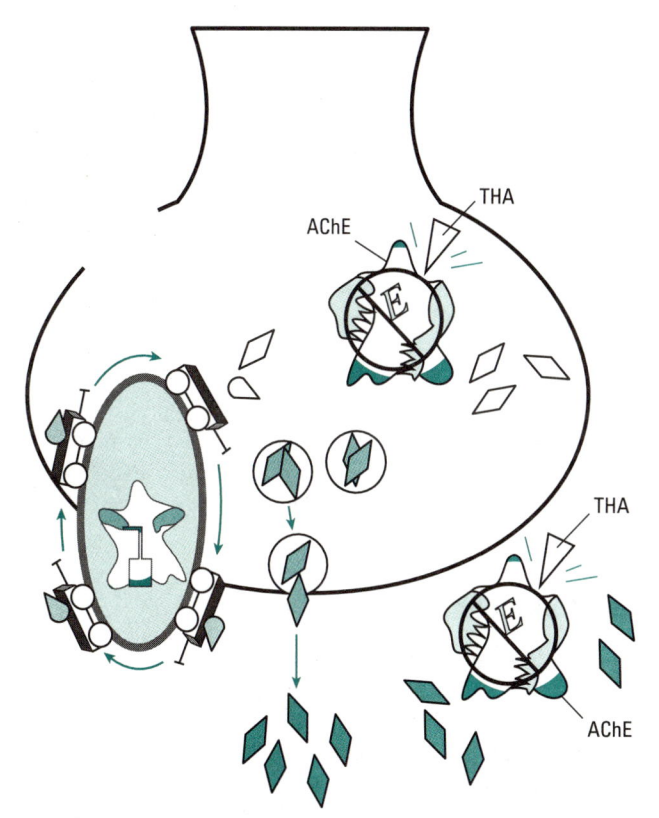

Figure 15–2. Cholinesterase inhibitor treatment for Alzheimer's disease. Numerous investigations suggest that deficiency of cholinergic functioning may be linked to memory disturbances. Some investigators believe that this underlies the memory disturbance of Alzheimer's disease, while others believe that it may be more related to the memory changes of age-associated memory impairment. At any rate, levels of acetylcholine (ACh) synthesis and levels of its synthetic enzyme CAT are reduced in brains of Alzheimer's disease patients. A powerful and successful mechanism of boosting ACh in the brain is to inhibit ACh destruction by inhibiting the enzyme acetylcholinesterase (AChE). This causes the buildup of ACh, which is no longer destroyed by acetylcholinesterase. This approach has led to the only therapy approved specifically for the treatment of Alzheimer's disease in the United States, namely tetrahydroaminoacridine (THA) or tacrine. Other similar agents are in late clinical testing. Since these agents appear to depend on the presence of intact cholinergic neurons, they may be most effective in the early stages of Alzheimer's disease, while cholinergic neurons are still present, since there is no evidence that these agents alter the course of the underlying demoting process. From Stahl, SM: Essential Psychopharmacology. Cambridge University Press, New York, 1996, p. 304.

(Ativan). This combination is used for severe agitation and insomnia. For clients whose disrupted sleeping patterns prevent them from achieving the restorative benefits of sleep, the short-acting hypnotic zolpidem (Ambien) is occasionally prescribed.

Antidepressants

Sedating antidepressants such as trazadone (Desyrel) and nefazodone may be prescribed for clients with concurrent depression and possibly for those with agitation. Sedation may help calm the client, whereas the antidepressant effects are necessary to treat depressed mood and other symptoms. The selective serotonin reuptake inhibitors (SSRIs), particularly those with short half-lives, are indicated for depression. Recent research suggests that sertraline (Zoloft) may help treat both depression and agitation in clients with dementia.

Client and Family Education

> The wife of a client with dementia cried as she disclosed that she felt she was living with a stranger. Her previously placid, affable husband now exhibited aggression and hostility. She reported that if she altered his breakfast menu in any way, he would pick up his plate and throw it at the wall. If she left the house to run errands, he would accuse her of infidelity when she returned. Most distressing of all was the response of her two adult sons, one a minister and the other a corporate executive. They were so upset by the changes in their father that they coped by distancing themselves. Their mother perceived herself as abandoned as she struggled to meet the changing needs of her husband. As he lost function, she stated that caring for him was like "going to a funeral every day."

Despite the sense of burden experienced by caregivers, they are often reluctant to ask for help from either informal sources or community agencies. Drew[21] reported that African-American families felt comfortable asking neighbors to help with small tasks such as going to the supermarket or pharmacy. They felt, however, that basic daily care was the responsibility of the primary family caregiver who felt a strong sense of duty and the need to sacrifice self for the benefit of another. Hispanic caregivers indicated that asking for help was seldom acceptable; they stated, "In our culture, you don't ask for help. You take care of your own."[21] These caregivers emphasized values about caregiving that centered on their respect for others, a sense of obligation to preserve the client's dignity and pride, patience, and tolerance.

Many support services are available for families caring for clients with dementia. Official agencies such as the local Agency on Aging provide case management services, homemakers and home health aides, respite care, referral for adult day care, and caregiver support groups. Additional resources are available from the Alzheimer's Disease and Related Disorders Association (ADRDA) and Children of Aging Parents (CAPS). Frequently, families coping with the care of a client with dementia are either unaware of these and other resources or reluctant to use them. They fear invasion of privacy, a negative response from the client, or a quality of care inferior to that which they are delivering.

Encourage families to consider available services on a trial basis. It is critical that caregivers attend to their own physical and emotional well-being. Zarit and colleagues[24] report that often caregivers have more physical health problems than the client, take more medications, and experience symptoms of chronic stress that erode both their health and coping abilities. Families may also benefit from a number of excellent, comprehensive books, such as *The 36 Hour Day*[25] and *Another Name for Madness*.[26]

Expected Outcomes

For the individual with dementia, improvement will be demonstrated by:
- Being able to communicate basic needs
- Receiving adequate nutrition and hydration
- Functioning at the highest level possible
- Not showing assaultive behavior
- Remaining safe
- Displaying less agitation.

Differential Diagnosis

Medications
- Medications may cause a decline in cognitive functioning.
- Psychiatric effects of medication are ruled out prior to diagnosis of dementia.

Pseudodementia
- Pseudodementia describes clients who have the capacity to perform a task but are prevented from performing at their actual level by lack of desire, negativity, and apathy.[27]
- Clients may refuse to bathe or dress yet still be able to choose clothing. In Alzheimer's disease, the individual always loses the ability to select clothing prior to losing the capacity to bathe or dress.

Sensory Impairments
- Vision or hearing impairments contribute to social isolation, suspiciousness, and functional decline of elders.
- These impairments often go undetected.
- Sensory problems are readily remediated.
- Behaviors may be misinterpreted by others as symptoms of dementia.

Substance Abuse
- Alcoholism is also associated with progressive irreversible cognitive decline.
- Establish if the client has had a prolonged history of alcohol abuse.

- Alcohol may be used to manage anxiety related to early symptoms of Alzheimer's disease.
- Recent patterns of excessive alcohol consumption may represent a response to memory loss rather than its cause.

Nutritional Deficits

- Undernutrition resulting in inadequate intake of B vitamins can produce a neurotoxicity that results in cognitive loss.
- Deficits often occur in elders whose daily food intake falls markedly below the Recommended Dietary Allowances.
- Deficits may occur in those with pernicious anemia or other absorption problems.
- Nutritional deficits are common in alcohol abuse.

Delirium

- Dementia and delirium may overlap in symptoms.
- Symptoms are distinguishable.
- The courses of dementia and delirium differ.

AMNESTIC DISORDERS

Definition

Individuals with **amnestic disorders** present with a memory disturbance that causes impairment in social or occupational functioning.[4] They have difficulty learning and recalling new material. The cause for the memory impairment is a general medical condition such as head trauma or ingestion of a substance such as medication, alcohol, or toxins. Problems with remembering previously stored information vary according to the location and amount of brain damage. Only after excluding memory impairment that occurs during an episode of delirium or dementia is the diagnosis made.

Characteristic Behaviors

Changes in personality such as apathetic behavior, emotional blunting, and lack of initiative may be evident. Other clients, especially those with global amnesia, may appear agreeable but are bewildered by the world around them. During the early stages of **amnesia**, it is common to find individuals using confabulation to fill in gaps in their memory. This coping mechanism tends to go away in time. The ability to remember information across a delay of time is also profoundly affected.

Depending on the area of the brain that has been affected, clients may have difficulty recalling the names of political personalities or historical figures. They may display a lack of insight about their memory loss and may deny its presence altogether. Some may agree that they have a problem but appear unconcerned by it.

Normal age-related changes in memory differ from memory changes related to amnesia. As one ages, it is normal to

---

Diagnostic Criteria for Amnesia

Diagnostic Criteria for 294.0 Amnestic Disorder Due to . . . [Indicate the General Medical Condition]

A. The development of memory impairment as manifested by impairment in the ability to learn new information or the inability to recall previously learned information.

B. The memory disturbance causes significant impairment in social or occupational functioning and represents a significant decline from a previous level of functioning.

C. The memory disturbance does not occur exclusively during the course of a delirium or a dementia.

D. There is evidence from the history, physical examination, or laboratory findings that the disturbance is the direct physiological consequence of a general medical condition (including physical trauma).

Specify if:
  Transient: if memory impairment lasts for 1 month or less.
  Chronic: if memory impairment lasts for more than 1 month.
  CODING NOTE: Include the name of the general medical condition on Axis I, e.g., 294.0 Amnestic Disorder Due to Head Trauma; also code the general medical condition on Axis III.

Diagnostic Criteria for Substance-induced Persisting Amnestic Disorder

A. The development of memory impairment as manifested by impairment in the ability to learn new information or the inability to recall previously learned information.

B. The memory disturbance causes significant impairment in social or occupational functioning and represents a significant decline from a previous level of functioning.

C. The memory disturbance does not occur exclusively during the course of a delirium or a dementia and persists beyond the usual duration of Substance Intoxication or Withdrawal.

D. There is evidence from the history, physical examination, or laboratory findings that the memory disturbance is etiologically related to the persisting effects of substance use (e.g., a drug of abuse, a medication).

Code [Specific Substance]-Induced Persisting Amnestic Disorder:
  (291.1 Alcohol; 292.83 Sedative, Hypnotic, or Anxiolytic; 292.83 Other [or Unknown] Substance)

Source: Reprinted with permission from the Diagnostic and Statistical Manual of Mental Disorders, Fourth Edition. Copyright 1994 American Psychiatric Association.

forget names on occasion or to misplace keys. It is not normal for people to forget what the keys represent or who are the members of their own family.

Diagnostic Aids

History, mental status examinations, and imaging studies may be used to identify amnesia. Magnetic resonance imaging (MRI) findings include structural atrophy in the medial temporal lobes of the brain. There may also be an enlargement of the third ventricle or temporal horns.

Amnestic clients have severe difficulties remembering everyday events even though they may perform in the normal range on standardized tests of language, perception, and intelligence.[28,29] Because some profoundly affected amnestic individuals can remember immediate memories and reproduce a span of digits or letters, they can be distinguished from clients with delirium who do not have the attention span necessary to remember the order or even the numbers themselves.

Culture, Age, and Gender Features

Age of onset depends on the primary pathological process causing the disorder. For example, when the cause is a medication, symptoms are rarely seen before the age of 20. Most clients are over 40 years old and have long histories of alcohol abuse.

Etiology

Biological Theories

Hypoxia, herpes-simplex encephalitis, thiamine deficiency, and chronic use of ethanol are possible causes of amnesia.

Amnesia is usually associated with bilateral damage to the temporal lobe or other parts of the limbic system. Damage to specific areas of the brain can produce different symptoms in amnestic clients. Those with difficulty recognizing fear and emotions may have problems in the amygdala. Clients with damage to the basal ganglia may have trouble with learning skills. Injury to Broca's area and Wernicke's area may affect how language is understood and spoken.

Neuropharmacologic Theories

Benzodiazepines such as triazolam (Halcion) have been implicated in **anterograde amnesia,** which involves profound forgetfulness for new material. In a study that compared triazolam to other benzodiazepines, researchers found that there were no differences between medications; triazolam did not cause more negative reactions or memory problems.[30] Further research is needed to determine if benzodiazepines cause memory loss.

Prognosis

The prognosis depends on the cause of the amnesia. If the memory loss is due to a head trauma, it may be temporary. Memory loss is usually greatest directly after the injury has occurred and then gradually improves over the next 2 years. Memory for events that occurred during the amnestic period is not totally restored. Amnestic disorders from cerebral infarction, surgery, or malnutrition can result in the destruction of middle temporal lobe structures, and the amnesia can persist indefinitely.

Planning Care

Planning care involves supporting the client's remaining abilities while maintaining emotional support and safety. Neuropsychological testing should be done to assess deficits and intact abilities. If individuals deny impairment or show signs of lack of insight, modify the environment to meet their safety needs. Educate the family about the client's requirements and abilities so that they can help create a supportive environment.

Interventions for Clients in the Community

Similar to that for dementia or delirium, the care plan addresses the client's need for assistance with daily living issues, including making a living and functioning in a family and society. Some do very well with slight modifications to their routine, whereas others require institutionalization.

Nursing care includes teaching activities that emphasize habit and repetition. The treatment goal is to prevent further deterioration of brain structures while providing the individual with a secure environment. Thus, interventions that use the declarative memory system are needed. Task groups that are small and structured groups that break down tasks into sequential steps are helpful.

Long-term care is tailored toward safety, supporting remaining abilities, retraining within the scope of clients' abilities, and enlisting family and community support. The goal may be to assist living in a group home or a day-care facility in the community.

Expected Outcomes

For the individual with an amnestic disorder, improvement will be demonstrated by:
- Remaining safe
- Performing activities of daily living at the optimal level
- Demonstrating positive coping skills.

SYNOPSIS OF CURRENT RESEARCH

Overview

Current research regarding cognitive disorders includes:
- Uncovering the secrets of the brain's memory systems
- Studying the effects of neurotransmitters in the brain and the effect of drugs on them
- Analyzing the effects of aging on the brain and memory

- Finding genetic links in Alzheimer's clients
- Using estrogen therapy to decrease behaviors in demented clients
- Improving diagnostic tests for suspected Alzheimer's disease
- Measuring intervention outcomes with cognitively impaired clients.

Socialization

One research study looked at the effects of socialization and music-therapy intervention on self-esteem and loneliness in spouse caregivers of Alzheimer's clients.[31] The majority of caregivers had increased self-esteem at the end of the program. Using music, some couples had reestablished some of the emotional intimacy that was lost from their relationship. The music made it feasible for individuals with dementia to improve verbal and nonverbal interactions.

Outcomes

Documenting positive outcomes for demented elders in nursing homes is the focus of other research. Rovner and associates[32] developed a randomized trial of negative behavior in nursing home clients with dementia. They used an activity program weekdays from 10:00 am to 3:00 pm, psychotropic drug management by a psychiatrist rather than the primary care physician, and educational rounds to discuss each client's behavioral, functional, and medical status. Measurement tools for the study were documentation of behavior disorders, antipsychotic drug and physical restraint use, patient activity levels, and functional and cognitive status. These interventions decreased the negative behavior disorders and the use of antipsychotic drugs in this population.

Genetics

Advances in genetic testing have led to the identification of two genes involved in the early stages of Alzheimer's disease. Apo E, the gene associated with increased risk for late onset of Alzheimer's disease, is the basis for a genetic test to distinguish this disorder from other types of dementia. Researchers have also found that injecting certain Alzheimer's genes, PS1 and PS2, doubles the amount of β-amyloid protein. This suggests that overproduction of amyloid is the cause of the disease. In other studies, tests to detect a certain protein, tau, in spinal fluid, hold promise as a diagnostic aid.

Medications

Several new medications are being tested for their effectiveness in dementia. *Nootropics,* sometimes called "smart drugs," target the neurotransmitter glutamate and may enhance memory. Ampalex is the name of one medication currently being studied. In addition to selegiline (Deprenyl), the one approved effective treatment for Parkinson's disease, several new medications are being tested.

AREAS FOR FUTURE RESEARCH

- What is the impact of chronic illness on the spouse of the cognitively impaired client?
- What are measurable outcomes for nursing interventions for the cognitively impaired client?
- What are the most effective care plans for the cognitively impaired client living in the community?
- What is the effectiveness of advanced directives for cognitively impaired clients?
- What are the most cost-effective ways to care for the cognitively impaired client?
- What are the most effective components of end-stage care?

CASE STUDY

A visiting nurse was sent to a home in the community for an initial visit to 76-year-old Jane, who required post–hip fracture assistance. Jane's husband greeted the nurse at the door with a smile, said he was happy to see her, and ushered her into the living room. The client was seated on the family sofa with her right leg positioned perilously close to the edge of the hassock placed in front of her. She began to rise, and both the husband and the nurse immediately cautioned her to remain where she was sitting. Jane didn't question why the nurse was in her living room; she didn't appear disturbed by her presence. Her face was blank, and her affect was subdued. When the nurse introduced herself and explained the reason she had come, the woman appeared uninterested. She looked underweight and unkempt. Upon questioning Jane, the nurse soon discovered that she was unable to follow along with the interview.

Jane's husband was able to describe the events leading up to the fall that caused the hip fracture. Jane had been alone in the late afternoon and had tried to reach a high shelf by fashioning a makeshift stool out of a cardboard box. She had been trying to reach a liquor bottle that the husband had placed there. There had been no head trauma involved in the incident. Jane's husband told the nurse that his wife's memory had been steadily worsening and that she had been having difficulty remembering events that recently occurred. Upon further questioning, the husband confided that his wife had a long history of being alone in the house while he was on the road as a salesman. He also stated that he had noticed that she was less personable and quieter than she used to be in the past. The husband confided that he was thinking of leaving his wife after she recovered from the fracture because she didn't seem to notice that he was there and that he was repulsed by her slovenly appearance. After the nurse asked the husband for a more complete history, he confided that his wife had been a "social drinker" for years.

CRITICAL THINKING QUESTIONS

1. What behaviors suggest that Jane has serious errors in judgment and memory problems?
2. What are the clues in the client's appearance that make the nurse suspect that there is more to Jane's story than the husband is telling her?

3. What community resources are available for Jane's family?
4. Specify two interventions that Jane's husband could implement to increase Jane's safety without seriously compromising her independence.
5. Design a teaching plan to help Jane remain safely at home.
6. What are the short- and long-term goals for Jane?

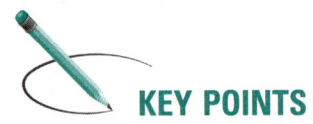

KEY POINTS

- Changes in cognition or memory signal a change from usual functioning; individuals with delirium, dementia, amnestic disorders, and other cognitive disorders show these changes.
- Most elders do not experience cognitive deterioration as they age.
- Delirium is a time-limited and acute disorder of cognition characterized by disturbances in attention, perception, thinking, memory, psychomotor behavior, and the sleep-wake cycle. When recognized in time, it is highly treatable.
- Delirium fluctuates over the course of the day and is the direct result of an underlying medical condition, exposure to a toxin, drug withdrawal, or a combination of these problems. The delirious client requires continuous nursing supervision.
- Delirium develops in about 30% of clients in critical care environments and is called "CCU-psychosis." Causes of CCU-psychosis include sensory deprivation, overstimulation, and drug reactions.
- Dementia includes a constellation of symptoms resulting in impairment of short- and long-term memory. Its onset is slow or insidious, yet progressive, and ends in death. The most common type is Alzheimer's disease. Other types of dementia include vascular dementia and dementia due to head trauma, substances, and medical conditions such as AIDS, Parkinson's disease, Huntington's disease, and Pick's disease.
- Alzheimer's disease progresses in seven discrete stages; the GDS helps nurses determine the client's stage of cognitive decline.
- Recent research suggests that vascular dementia is more common than has been thought and may be preventable.
- Mental status examinations, laboratory tests, computed tomography (CT) scans, and MRIs assist in the diagnosis of dementia.
- Specific types of proteins, plaques and tangles, accumulate in the brains of people with Alzheimer's disease and lead to the symptoms of the disease.
- Alzheimer's disease may be due to too much of a protein, β-amyloid, or due to too little removal of it. Another hypothesis, the cholinergic-deficiency hypothesis, suggests that decreased levels of acetylcholine cause this disease.
- Alzheimer's disease is genetically transmitted. Mutations in three genes have been linked to one genetically transmittable form of the disorder: PS1, PS2, and amyloid precursor protein genes.
- Although the prognosis of some dementias such as the Alzheimer's type is progressive and deteriorating, some dementias can be treated, and others are reversible.
- Nursing care for clients with dementia should emphasize two priorities: maintaining the client's maximum level of functional independence and ensuring safety.
- Treatment of dementia may include validation therapy, remotivation therapy, and pharmacotherapy, particularly with memory enhancers, antidepressants, and antipsychotics.
- Dementia and cognitive disorders have profound effects on families and their caregiving abilities. Nursing care is targeted at supporting and intervening with families.
- Amnestic clients have severe difficulties remembering everyday events, usually because of bilateral damage to the temporal lobe or other parts of the limbic system. Head trauma, hypoxia, herpes-simplex encephalitis, thiamine deficiency, and chronic use of alcohol are possible causes.

REFERENCES

1. Ham, RJ, and Sloane, PD: Primary Care Geriatrics: A Case Based Approach, ed 3. Mosby, St. Louis, 1997.
2. Morency, C, Levkoff, S, and Lipsitz, L: Delirium or Dementia? A Nursing Challenge. A program sponsored by the National Institute on Aging as part of the MA Alzheimer Research Center and the Harvard Geriatric Education Center, 1992.
3. Inaba-Roland, KE, and Maricle, RA: Assessing delirium in the acute care setting. Heart Lung 27:48, 1992.
4. American Psychiatric Association: Diagnostic and statistical manual of mental disorders, ed 4. American Psychiatric Association, Washington, DC, 1994.
5. Wood, KA, et al: Drug induced psychoses and depression in the elderly. Psychiat Clin North Am 11:167, 1988.
6. Drake, AC, and Romano, E: How to protect your patient from the hazards of polypharmacy. Nursing '95 25(6):34, 1995.
7. Fulop, G, et al: Impact of psychiatric comorbidity on length of hospital stay for medical surgical patients: A preliminary report. Am J Psychiatry 144:878, 1987.
8. Kaplan, HI, and Sadock, B: Synopsis of Psychiatry, ed 6. Williams & Wilkins, Baltimore, 1991, p 243.
9. Pompei, P, et al: Detecting delirium among hospitalized older patients. Arch Intern Med 155(3): 301, 1995.
10. Miles, S: A case of death by physical restraints: New lessons from a photograph. Am Geriatr Soc 44:291, 1995.
11. Prinz, PN, and Vitello, MV: Sleep in demented and in healthy, non complaining seniors. Proceedings from the National Institute of Health Consensus Development Conference on The Treatment of Sleep Disorders in Older People, 1990, pp 41–46.
12. Reisberg, B: The global deterioration scale for assessment of primary degenerative dementia. Am J Psychiatry 139:1136, 1982.
13. Crook, T, et al: Age-associated memory impairment: Proposed diagnostic criteria and measures of clinical change: A report of a National Institute of Mental Health Work Group. Dev Neuropsychology 2:261, 1986.

14. Feruccia, L, et al: Cognitive impairment and risk of stroke in the older population. J Am Assoc Geriatr 44:237, 1996.
15. Evans, D, et al: Estimated prevalence of Alzheimer disease in the United States. Milbank Q 68:267, 1990.
16. Marieb, E: The central nervous system. In Human Anatomy and Physiology, ed 3. The Benjamin-Cummings Publishing Co, Redwood City, CA, 1995.
17. Tariot, P: Neurobiology and treatment of dementia. In Salzman, C (ed): Clinical Geriatric Psychopharmacology, ed 2. Williams & Wilkins, Baltimore, 1992, p 278.
18. Luo, YQ, et al: Physiological levels of beta-amyloid increase tryosine phosphorylation and cytosolic calcium. Brain Res (1995 May 29) 681(1–2):65–74.
19. Kitwood, T: Dementia care psychology: Analyzing your caregiving commitment. Proceedings of the Fourth National Alzheimer Disease Education Conference Section (A11): July 1–15, 1995.
20. Carty, A, and Day, S: Interdisciplinary care: Effect in acute hospital settings. J Gerontol Nurs 19:22, 1993.
21. Drew, JC: Cultural variations in the dementia experience. Proceedings of the Fourth Annual Alzheimer Disease National Education Conference Section (A11), July 1–9, 1995.
22. Feil, N: Validation: The Feil Method. Feil Productions, Cleveland, OH, 1992.
23. Burnside, I, and Schmidt, M: Working with Older Adults, ed 3. Jones & Bartlett Publishers Inc, Boston, 1994.
24. Zarit, S, et al: Comparative effectiveness of individual and group interventions to support caregivers. Soc Work 35:207, 1990.
25. Mace, N, and Robins, P: The 36 Hour Day. The Johns Hopkins University Press, Baltimore, 1981.
26. Roach, M: Another Name for Madness. Houghton Mifflin, Boston, 1985.
27. Reding, MJ, et al: Follow-up of patients referred to a dementia service. J Am Geriatr Soc 32:265, 1984.
28. Schater, DL: Memory Systems of the Brain: Animal and Human Cognitive Processes. Weinberger, N, Lynch, G, and McGaugh, J (eds). The Guilford Press, New York, 1985, p 351.
29. Squire, L, and Zola-Morgan, S: Memory: Brain systems and behavior. Neuroscience 11:2, 1987.
30. Rothschild, AJ: Disinhibition, amnestic reactions, and other adverse reactions secondary to triazolam: A review of the literature. J Clin Psychiat (supp): 69, 1992.
31. Clair, A, Tebb, S, and Berstein, B: The effects of socialization and music therapy interventions on self-esteem and loneliness in spouse caregivers of those diagnosed with dementia of the Alzheimer type: A pilot study. Am J Alzheimer Care and Related Disorders and Research 8:24, 1993.
32. Rovner, BW, et al: A randomized trial of dementia care in nursing homes. J Am Geriatr Soc 44:7, 1996.

CHAPTER 16

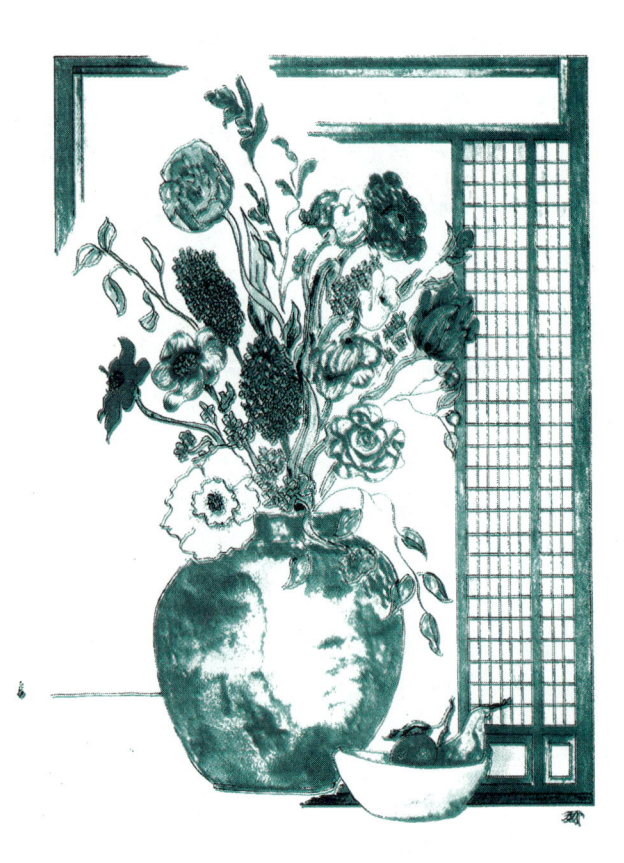

CHAPTER OUTLINE

Common Mental Illnesses due to General Medical Conditions
  Characteristic Behaviors
  Culture, Age, and Gender Features
  Etiology
  Prognosis
  Planning Care
  Interventions for Hospitalized Clients
  Intervention for Clients in the Community
  Expected Outcomes
  Differential Diagnosis
Critical Care Unit Psychosis
  Characteristic Behaviors
  Culture, Age, and Gender Features
  Etiology
  Prognosis
  Interventions for Hospitalized Clients
  Expected Outcomes
  Differential Diagnosis
Synopsis of Current Research
Areas for Future Research

LEARNING OBJECTIVES

After completing this chapter, the reader should be able to:

- Discuss the incidence of mental illness in general medical conditions.
- List the common causes of these symptoms.
- Describe the appropriate assessment of a psychiatric client who presents with new symptoms that may be related to a general medical condition.
- Differentiate between clients with delirium, depression, and personality disorders due to general medical conditions.
- Formulate nursing diagnoses and interventions for the depressed, agitated, and hallucinating client.
- Describe three environmental factors that contribute to CCU-psychosis.
- Describe nursing interventions to prevent CCU-psychosis.

Linda M. Gorman, RN, MN, CS, OCN, CRNH

Mental Illness due to a General Medical Condition

KEY TERMS

critical care unit (CCU) psychosis
delirium
disinhibitions

COMMON MENTAL ILLNESSES DUE TO GENERAL MEDICAL CONDITIONS

Mental illnesses due to a general medical condition are frequently overlooked in the psychiatric and medical-surgical setting because the onset of these disorders is often subtle with complex etiologies. The nurse is in a key role to identify such behaviors as subtle personality changes like irritability or use of foul language, intermittent confusion, or a paranoid response to a routine question. These changes can progress to severe depression, delirium, or psychosis. All of these can occur in an individual with a known medical condition or prior to physical symptoms that would indicate a medical condition.

These changes can be seen in someone who is in an acute care hospital for treatment of a known medical condition, in an emergency room when the client presents with atypical psychiatric symptoms, or in a client in a psychiatric clinic or hospital for whom a medical condition has not been suspected.

The *Diagnostic and Statistical Manual of Mental Disorders, Fourth Edition (DSM-IV)*[1] now recognizes the importance of this diagnosis. The 1994 edition eliminated the term "organic" because it implies that nonorganic or functional mental illnesses are unrelated to ones with physical causes. *DSM-IV* recognizes that these disorders may, in fact, be related and cannot be looked at as opposites.

Because these symptoms are often unrecognized, statistics on the frequency are limited. Hall and colleagues[2] found that 9% of psychiatric clients in outpatient settings had medical disorders producing depression, confusion, anxiety, and speech or memory impairment. In 1981 his group found that of 100 state hospital psychiatric clients, 46% had unrecognized medical disorders that either caused or exacerbated their psychiatric illness.[3] Hall's studies reinforce the need for routine laboratory testing and physical examination as part of any psychiatric workup.

DSM-IV identifies 11 forms of psychiatric conditions due to general medical conditions (Table 16–1). By far the most frequently seen is **delirium** due to a general medical condition, which can contribute to mental changes in consciousness, confusion, perceptual disturbances, and agitation. Foreman[4] found that up to 70% of clients who become delirious are never recognized by physicians or nurses as being in a delirious state.

Any mental disorder due to a general medical condition can lead to delayed diagnosis of medical conditions, especially if the symptoms are assumed to be caused by a psychiatric disorder or general emotional stress. At times, the only initial symptoms are psychiatric. Time may be lost as symptoms are tolerated, then treated with tranquilizers or antipsychotics, and finally referred for a psychiatric consult. When possible physical causes are not investigated, the result can be increased mortality rates due to a delayed diagnosis as well as longer stays in the hospital. Less obvious sequelae might include self-injury due to falls when the confused client tries to ambulate, injuries and complications from restraints including thrombi and strangulation, and side effects from the medications given to control the psychiatric symptoms.

In the mental health setting, psychiatric symptoms are generally assumed to be part of a psychiatric disorder, and further workup is not considered until the symptoms become much worse or new physical symptoms occur. Another marker may be atypical psychiatric symptoms that do not respond to treatment. Because these symptoms can be so easily overlooked, consider a medical workup with the onset of any new psychiatric symptoms. These symptoms can develop over hours or days and may also be intermittent. Once the cause is identified and treated, the symptoms will usually resolve quickly as well.

Characteristic Behaviors

Mental illness due to a general medical condition can be one of the most difficult and frustrating diagnoses to make. Early signs may include sudden onset of confusion in a previously oriented client, intermittent personality changes such as angry outbursts, anxiety, mood changes such as euphoria or

TABLE 16–1. DSM-IV Mental Disorders That May Be the Result of a General Medical Condition

- Delirium
- Dementia
- Amnestic disorder
- Psychotic disorder
- Mood disorder
- Anxiety disorder
- Sexual dysfunction
- Sleep disorder
- Personality change
- Catatonia
- Mental disorder not otherwise specified

Source: Reprinted with permission from the Diagnostic and Statistical Manual of Mental Disorders, Fourth Edition. Copyright 1994 American Psychiatric Association.

Diagnostic Criteria for 293.0 Delirium due to a General Medical Condition

A. Disturbance of consciousness (i.e., reduced clarity of awareness of the environment) with reduced ability to focus, sustain, or shift attention.

B. A change in cognition (such as memory deficit, disorientation, language disturbance) or the development of a perceptual disturbance that is not better accounted for by the preexisting, established or evolving dementia.

C. The disturbance develops over a short period (usually hours to days) and tends to fluctuate during the course of the day.

D. There is evidence from the history, physical examination, or laboratory findings that the disturbance is caused by the direct physiological consequences of a general medical condition.

Source: Reprinted with permission from the Diagnostic and Statistical Manual of Mental Disorders, Fourth Edition. Copyright 1994 American Psychiatric Association.

RESEARCH NOTE

Inouye, SK, and Charpentier, PA: Precipitating factors for delirium in hospitalized elderly persons. JAMA 275(11):852–857, 1996.

This study sought to develop and validate a predictive model for delirium based on precipitating factors during hospitalization and then to examine the interrelationships of precipitating factors and baseline vulnerabilities. To identify the predictive factors, 196 clients over 70 years old admitted to a general medical floor with no delirium at baseline were followed. Trained researchers conducted structured interviews with the clients and their primary nurses from admission to the unit until discharge. A variety of factors were evaluated and risk factors for delirium were determined.

Findings: The greatest potential for developing delirium occurred by day 9 of hospitalization. In this group, 18% met the diagnostic criteria for delirium. Those who developed it were more likely to have the following variables from most to least frequent: use of physical restraints; malnutrition; more than three medications added during the 24 to 48 hours before the onset of delirium; use of a bladder catheter; and any iatrogenic event such as hospital-acquired infection, unintentional injury like a fall, or complications of diagnostic or therapeutic procedure.

Application to Practice: The authors present this information in hopes of developing a predictive model in which delirium can be addressed and treated when risk factors are present. This model would encourage earlier identification of delirium and provide a validated instrument to accurately diagnose clients.

---

depression, and **disinhibitions** (for example, swearing, taking off clothes in public, and sexual behavior). Later signs may include evidence of psychotic behavior such as hallucinations, paranoid delusions, and manic or suicidal behavior. Nightmares, sleep disruption, panic attacks, or catatonia may also occur. Very often the psychiatric symptoms are not those normally seen in primary psychiatric disorders.[1]

Diagnostic Criteria for 293.xx Psychotic Disorder due to a General Medical Condition

A. Prominent hallucinations or delusions.

B. There is evidence from the history, physical examination, or laboratory findings, that the disturbance is the direct physiological consequence of a general medical condition.

C. The disturbance is not better accounted for by another mental disorder.

D. The disturbance does not occur exclusively during the course of a delirium.

Source: Reprinted with permission from the Diagnostic and Statistical Manual of Mental Disorders, Fourth Edition. Copyright 1994 American Psychiatric Association.

> **Diagnostic Criteria for 293.83 Mood Disorder due to a General Medical Condition**
>
> A. A prominent and persistent disturbance in mood predominates in the clinical picture and is characterized by either or both of the following:
>   (1) depressed mood or markedly diminished interest or pleasure in all or almost all activities
>   (2) elevated, expansive, or irritable mood.
> B. There is evidence from the history, physical examination, or laboratory findings that the disturbance is the direct physiological consequence of a general medical condition.
> C. The disturbance is not better accounted for by another mental disorder.
> D. The disturbance does not occur exclusively during the course of a delirium.
> E. The symptoms cause clinically significant distress or impairment in social, occupational, or other important areas of functioning.
>
> **Source:** Reprinted with permission from the Diagnostic and Statistical Manual of Mental Disorders, Fourth Edition. Copyright 1994 American Psychiatric Association.

> **Diagnostic Criteria for 310.1 Personality Change due to a General Medical Condition**
>
> A. A persistent personality disturbance that represents a change from the individual's previous characteristic personality pattern.
> B. There is evidence from the history, physical examination, or laboratory findings that the disturbance is the direct physiological consequence of a general medical condition.
> C. The disturbance is not better accounted for by another mental disorder.
> D. The disturbance does not occur exclusively during the course of a delirium and does not meet criteria for a dementia.
> E. The disturbance causes clinically significant distress or impairment in social, occupational, or other important areas of functioning.
>
> **Source:** Reprinted with permission from the Diagnostic and Statistical Manual of Mental Disorders, Fourth Edition. Copyright 1994 American Psychiatric Association.

> **Diagnostic Criteria for 293.89 Anxiety Disorder due to a General Medical Condition**
>
> A. Prominent anxiety, panic attacks, or obsessions or compulsions predominate in the clinical picture.
> B. There is evidence from the history, physical examination, or laboratory findings that the disturbance is the direct physiological consequence of a general medical condition.
> C. The disturbance is not better accounted for by another mental disorder.
> D. The disturbance does not occur exclusively during the course of a delirium.
> E. The disturbance causes clinically significant distress or impairment in social, occupational, or other important areas of functioning.
>
> **Source:** Reprinted with permission from the Diagnostic and Statistical Manual of Mental Disorders, Fourth Edition. Copyright 1994 American Psychiatric Association.

For example, a client presenting with new onset of schizophrenic symptoms would be unlikely to be diagnosed with schizophrenia at age 75. This client may or may not have signs of a medical condition at the time the psychiatric symptoms occur. *DSM-IV* recommends considering a general medical condition as the cause if the symptoms cannot be better accounted for by a mental disorder. The key to linking these symptoms to a general medical condition is often the sudden behavior changes in someone with no history of psychiatric disorder, or at least of that type, and the ability to diagnose the medical condition rather than assume it is psychiatric. See Diagnostic Boxes 16–1 through 16–5 for the *DSM-IV* diagnostic criteria for the most common mental conditions due to general medical conditions.

A thorough medical and psychiatric history and examination with mental status examination, including current prescribed medications and over-the-counter (OTC) drugs, are essential. Nurses need to be familiar with how to perform mental status examinations to assess the broad range of cognitive functions.

Investigate a history of recent head injuries and exposure to toxins. The presence of visual hallucinations may be an indicator of exposure to some toxic substance. Interview family members and caregivers about stresses the client may be experiencing. Ask about the client's behavior or falls. Listen to family and caregivers when they report subtle personality changes that the health-care team might not note as

TABLE 16–2. Mental Status Changes due to Endocrine Disorders

Name of Condition	Cause of Disorder	Changes in Mental Status
Addison's disease (hypoadrenalism)	Deficiency in adrenocortical hormones of the adrenal cortex due to disturbed hypothalamic, pituitary, or adrenal functioning	Depression Negativism Suspiciousness Apathy
Cushing's syndrome (hyperadrenalism)	Excessive amounts of adrenocortical hormones (ACTH) of the adrenal cortex due to diseases of the hypothalamus or pituitary that produce excessive amounts of ACTH or to hyperplasia of the adrenal cortex; can also be caused by steroid drugs	Excitement Acute anxiety Emotional instability Depression (when disorder is result of internally caused elevated levels) Euphoria (when disorder is result of steroid drugs)
Hyperthyroidism	Excessive secretion of thyroid glands; basal metabolic rate is elevated	Nervousness Excitability Emotional instability Insomnia Psychosis (in acute stages)
Hypothyroidism (myxedema)	Deficiency of thyroid secretion; basal metabolic rate is decreased	Apathy Sluggishness Irritability Delusions and paranoid thinking (in acute stage); can sometimes persist for months
Hyperparathyroidism	Excessive secretion of parathyroid glands results in increased levels of calcium and phosphorus	Mixed levels of anxiety and depression Weakness Irritability Psychosis
Hypoparathyroidism	Deficient parathyroid secretions	Apathy (if onset is rapid) Depression (if onset is slow) Psychosis
Hyperinsulinism	Adenoma of Langerhans' islets; excessive insulin in bloodstream due to overdosage or undereating	Anxiety attacks Confusion Emotional lability
Pituitary problems of any kind, depending on etiology and course; can also cause psychiatric symptoms		Mixed, depending on etiology, course of the disease

Source: Adapted from Barry, PD: Psychosocial Nursing, ed 3. JB Lippincott Co, Philadelphia, 1996.

significant. For example, a formerly quiet, soft-spoken elderly man may become more animated. This behavior may appear "normal" to others, but his family are aware they have never seen the client like this. In addition, awareness of alcohol or illicit drug use is important. Rule out electrolyte imbalances and other metabolic disorders with appropriate laboratory testing. More involved testing including computed tomography (CT) scans, electroencephalograms (EEGs), and spinal taps can be done, depending on the client's symptoms, to rule out possible medical conditions. In the acute hospital setting, a psychiatric consultation is often requested to conduct a thorough mental status examination as well as to assess for psychiatric diagnoses.

Culture, Age, and Gender Features

DSM-IV[1] notes that 10 to 15% of people over 65 years old admitted for a medical condition exhibit delirium on admission, and another 10 to 15% develop it over their hospital course. This statistic indicates that one-third of elderly patients in the acute care hospital are potentially at risk for these symptoms! Risk factors include being physically restrained, bed bound, and socially isolated, and having a poor relationship with caregivers.[5,6] In addition to delirium, the elderly are at high risk for psychiatric symptoms from multiple medical problems.[7] Labeling elderly clients who present with confusion as having dementia rather than assuming an acute problem can delay diagnosis. It probably occurs less often with younger clients.

No research indicates that culture or gender plays a role in the development of these symptoms.

Etiology

These psychiatric symptoms have hundreds of possible causes. Very often combinations of causes, concurrent psychiatric problems, or current stress levels can be additional factors. Psychiatric symptoms in general medical conditions demonstrate the very close connection between behavior and physiological functioning. They occur because some noxious agent or physiological process is influencing brain functioning.

Metabolic

Endocrine. Metabolic causes include changes in functioning of the endocrine glands including the thyroid, parathyroid, adrenals, and insulin-producing cells of the pancreas. Fluctuation in hormone levels generally has a major influence on normal brain functioning. Because the affective state is particularly sensitive to hormone levels, endocrine disorders are especially prone to precipitate mood disorders (see Table 16–2).

Hyperthyroidism is particularly well known for causing psychiatric symptoms such as phobias and manic behavior. It may first present as a psychiatric disorder such as paranoid schizophrenia, major depression, or bipolar disorder.[8] Initial symptoms often include sleeplessness, anxiety, emotional lability, and difficulty concentrating.

Nutritional. B-complex vitamins are associated with psychological well-being because they are needed for normal brain metabolism. Vitamin B_{12}, folic acid, thiamine, and nicotinic acid deficiencies, which all present with changes in psychological functioning, may be due to long-term alcohol use, malnutrition, or specific disorders such as pernicious anemia (lack of vitamin B_{12} absorption).

Electrolyte Imbalance. Sudden increases or decreases in many electrolytes can cause mental symptoms. Brain tissue is sensitive to abnormal levels of the electrolytes shown in Table 16–3.

Clients with metastatic breast, lung, and prostate cancers often have hypercalcemia. Depression, fatigue, and irritability are very common early signs of abnormally high levels that can become life threatening. Because cancer is often associated with depression, hypercalcemia can be easily overlooked.

Cancer

The diagnosis of a malignancy with its many possible complications can contribute to a variety of psychiatric symptoms. Pasacreta and Massie[9] note that depression, anxiety, and delirium are the most prevalent disorders. Causes can include pain and metabolic complications such as malnutrition, electrolytic imbalances, and paraneoplastic syndromes, in which the tumor itself secretes a substance that influences brain function. Because the diagnosis of cancer is often associated with an intense emotional response, the onset of a mental disorder caused by the physical effects of the cancer is easily confused with the emotional response of depression or anxiety.

Vascular

Any condition that leads to reduced blood supply to the brain brings on sudden changes in mental status as well as other mental symptoms. The specific symptoms depend on the extent and location of the insult. For example, in a cerebrovascular accident (CVA), the area of the brain that is damaged determines the type of mental symptoms. Emotional lability, irritability, depression, and personality changes are the most common changes with a CVA, especially when the damage is in the left frontal area. More gradual mental changes, such as loss of memory, impaired intellectual functioning, and impaired social interactions, can occur in arteriosclerosis because of generalized reduced circulation to the entire brain.

Neurological

Head Trauma. Depending on the area of injury, amount of edema, and intracranial pressure (ICP), head injury can bring on a variety of mental changes. Initial symptoms may include confusion and amnesia. Hallucinations, delusions, personality changes, and labile emotions as sequelae to the brain insult may be of longer duration. The head trauma client may also experience anxiety and phobic responses related to confusion and amnesia. Acute onset of schizophrenia has occurred immediately after a traumatic head injury. Elderly clients who sustain a head injury in a fall and do not report it can develop a chronic, subdural hematoma with a slow-onset deteriorating mental status and other mental symptoms that can be confused with dementia.

Chronic Neurological Conditions. Neurological conditions such as multiple sclerosis and Parkinson's disease are associated with psychiatric symptoms. Though 20 to 30% of clients with Parkinson's disease also have dementia, less obvious and often underdiagnosed mental changes include depression and anxiety that are believed to be due to brain deterioration rather than a reactive psychological response to a chronic illness.[10] Antiparkinson drugs such as levodopa can also cause depression.

Multiple sclerosis is associated with persistent euphoria, labile emotions, and depression, which are believed to be caused at least in part by the demyelinating process in the specific central nervous system (CNS) region involved.

Seizure disorders can also be a chronic problem leading to personality changes and other mental symptoms. Because

TABLE 16-3. Mental Status Changes due to Electrolyte Imbalance

Electrolyte	Normal Level	Abnormal Level	Cause	Changes in Mental Status
Calcium	8.5–10.5 mg/dL	+Hypercalcemia	Hyperparathyroidism	Loss of energy Depression Irritability
		−Hypocalcemia	Hypoparathyroidism; deficiency of calcium or vitamin D in the diet	Psychosis in acute CMD caused by surgical removal of gland; nutritional deficiency results in less acute symptoms: b concentration, b intellectual functions, emotional lability, depression
Sodium	135–145 mEq/L	+Hypernatremia	Dehydration due to excessive water loss from body (vomiting, diarrhea) Diabetes insipidus Restricted fluid intake Excessive diuresis	Irritability Hyperactivity in intellectual ability Stupor
		−Hyponatremia	Severe dietary restriction of sodium Addison's disease Excessive water consumption (polydipsia)	Depression Lethargy Withdrawal Anorexia
Phosphorus	2.6–4.5 mg/dL	−Hypophospatemia	Gram-negative septicemia Alcohol withdrawal Hyperalimentation Poor nutritional status	Apprehension Irritability Numbness Stupor
Potassium	3.5–5 mEq/L	+Hyperkalemia	Renal disease Potassium-sparing diuretics Level of potassium in intravenous fluids	Weakness Dysphasia
		−Hypokalemia	Renal disease Cushing's syndrome Loss of potassium due to diuretics Self-induced vomiting Gastroenteritis	Changes in mood and personality Tearfulness Hopelessness Helplessness
Base bicarbonate	Blood pH 7.38–7.42, bicarbonate level 24 mEq/L	+Alkalosis	Prolonged vomiting Taking large amounts of bicarbonate Hyperventilation	b Intellectual functioning Apathy Delirium Stupor
		−Acidosis	Severe respiratory illness: emphysema, status asthmaticus Renal failure Diabetes mellitus with ketosis	b Intellectual ability Drowsiness Confusion Delirium

Source: Adapted from Barry, PD: *Psychosocial Nursing*, ed 3. JB Lippincott Co, Philadelphia, 1996.

an epileptic disorder is so complex, a thorough neurological and psychiatric evaluation is necessary when mental changes occur. Symptoms may include confusion, hallucinations, irritability, and aggressive behavior. These changes may occur just before a seizure or may be longer lasting.

Brain Tumors. Any brain tumor, whether it is a primary brain tumor or metastatic, can produce psychiatric symptoms. With any brain tumor, edema is the major cause of symptoms, which can include personality changes such as disinhibitions, anger, emotional lability, confusion, anxiety, and depression.

Other Causes

Other conditions that can contribute to these symptoms include infections such as sepsis (confusion and restlessness

Drug Side Effects and Drug Interactions

Both prescription and OTC drugs, even when used according to prescribed instructions and dosages, can cause psychiatric symptoms (see Tables 16–4 and 16–5). The more drugs a client is taking, the greater the risk of mental symptoms. The incidence of these symptoms emphasizes the need for a thorough assessment of all the medications the client is taking.

The elderly are at especially high risk because of their use of more prescribed and OTC medications, reduced renal and liver function that increases the chance of drug accumulation, increased adipose tissue that promotes retention of fat-soluble drugs, and multiple chronic illnesses. Psychiatric symptoms may be overlooked because they are assumed to be due to dementia. Children, too, are vulnerable to side effects because they are more sensitive to inappropriate dosing.

One of the best-known drug categories to cause psychiatric symptoms is corticosteroids. Steroids are frequently prescribed for inflammations, cancer, asthma, and brain tumors. Travlos and Hirsch[12] note that 6% of clients taking steroids are at risk for psychotic reactions. Initial symptoms often include hyperactivity, euphoria, insomnia, and rest-

> **RESEARCH NOTE**
>
> Pasacreta, JV, and Massie, MJ: Nurses' reports of psychiatric complications in patients with cancer. Oncol Nurs Forum 17(3):347–353, 1990.
>
> This study surveyed 100 nurses working in inpatient units in a large cancer research hospital on one day for psychiatric problems present in their clients. The increasing acuity of hospitalized clients with cancer has created a greater demand on nurses, and the presence of psychiatric symptoms makes that demand even greater. Being aware of the number of clients with psychiatric symptoms may give information to administrators on staffing needs, needs for psychiatric consultation services, and areas for inservice education.
>
> The authors developed a questionnaire asking nurses about specific psychiatric complications of clients under their care. Twenty-five psychiatric symptoms or problems listed on the survey were generated from a log of problems identified when psychiatric nurse consultations were requested in the previous year. Categories included depression, anxiety, mixed depression and anxiety, delirium, eating problems complicated by emotional factors, behavioral problems, and family problems.
>
> **Findings:** Eleven percent of the clients were reported to have a history of psychiatric problems prior to the current hospital admission. Hospitalwide, the surveyed nurses perceived 264 (55%) clients as having symptoms requiring psychiatric consultation. The most frequent symptoms were anxiety, depression, and delirium. Only 13% of the clients were currently being followed by a psychiatric consultant.
>
> **Application to Practice:** Results reinforce the frequency of psychiatric problems, the need for psychiatric consultation services, and the need for oncology nurses to receive education on the psychiatric problems of cancer clients.

can be one of the earliest signs), complications from acquired immunodeficiency syndrome (AIDS), and even urinary tract infections, particularly in the elderly. Hypoxia, lung conditions, and liver and renal failure are other major causes of these problems. Liver failure causing hepatic encephalopathy can contribute to depression and confusion.

The postoperative elderly client is particularly at risk because of exposure to anesthetics, not eating, pain, lack of oxygen, and the other causes listed previously.[11] Depression and cognitive changes such as loss of memory and linguistic ability following coronary artery bypass surgery in all age groups were originally thought to be due to the length of time on the bypass pump.[11] Microemboli released into the circulation during surgery when the aorta or carotid artery is clamped are now believed to be the cause.

TABLE 16–4. Drugs That Cause Depression

General Drug Categories	
Anticonvulsants	
Barbiturates	
Benzodiazepines	
Beta-blockers	
Contraceptives, oral	
Corticosteroids	
Digitalis	
Opioids	
Procaine derivatives	
Sedative-hypnotics	
Sulfonamides	
Thiazides	
Thyroid hormones	
Specific Drugs	**Trade Name**
Acyclovir	Zovirax
Clonidine	Catapres
Disulfiram	Antabuse
Isoniazid	INH
Isosorbide dinitrate	Isordil
Levodopa	L-Dopa
Methyldopa	Aldomet
Metoclopramide	Reglan
Nifedipine	Procardia
Reserpine	Serpasil
Tamoxifen	Nolvadex
Trimethoprim/sulfamethoxazole	Bactrim

Source: The Medical Letter. Drugs that cause psychiatric symptoms. Med Lett 35(65), 1993, with permission.

TABLE 16–5. Commonly Used Drugs That Cause Psychotic Symptoms

Generic name or drug category	Reaction
Amphetamines	Hallucinations, paranoia
Albuterol	Hallucinations, paranoia
Anticholinergics (atropine, scopolamine)	Confusion, delirium, hallucinations
Anticonvulsants	Confusion, delirium
Antidepressants	Hallucinations
Antihistamines	Hallucinations
Benzodiazepines	Rage, paranoia, hallucinations
Beta-blockers (Inderal, Timoptic)	Confusion, hallucinations
Ciprofloxacin (Cipro)	Delirium, psychosis
Corticosteroids (prednisone, dexamethasone)	Confusion, paranoia
Cyclosporine	Hallucinations
Digitalis	Nightmares, confusion
Disulfiram (Antabuse)	Delirium, psychosis
Histamine H$_2$-receptor antagonists (Tagamet, Pepcid, Zantac)	Hallucinations, paranoia
Interferon	Delirium, paranoia
Meperidine (Demerol)	Agitation, nightmares, hallucinations
Opioids	Hallucinations, nightmares
Procaine derivatives (Pronestyl)	Confusion, psychosis
Promethazine (Phenergan)	Hallucinations
Pseudoephedrine (in cold remedies)	Hallucinations
Ritalin	Hallucinations, paranoia
Sedatives-hypnotics	Confusion, hallucinations
Sulfonamides	Confusion, hallucinations
Tamoxifen	Delusions
Thyroid hormones	Hallucinations
Trimethoprim-sulfamethoxazole (Bactrim)	Hallucinations, delusions
Zidovudine (AZT)	Paranoia, hallucinations

Source: The Medical Letter: Drugs that cause psychiatric symptoms. Med Let 35(65) 1993, with permission.

lessness. These symptoms can progress to hallucinations, delusions, and suicidal behavior. At increased risk are clients with preexisting affective disorders and those who need high doses of steroids because of trauma such as head and spinal cord injury or spinal cord compression caused by metastatic cancer. The mental changes can put these clients at risk for other complications if they are unable to comply with instructions and take inappropriate doses or stop steroids abruptly, precipitating acute withdrawal reaction.

Prognosis

Because psychiatric symptoms caused by a medical disorder can delay diagnosis, complications and death are probably more likely if psychiatric symptoms are present. In addition, because these conditions are often complex with multiple complications, the prognosis is certainly affected. Delirium has been documented to increase mortality by 10 to 15%[13] because its presence indicates the severity of the illness and a poorer prognosis.[12]

Planning Care

Nursing care of the client with mental illness due to a general medical condition must focus on astute observation, maintenance of client safety and reality testing, emotional support, and education for the client and family on what is causing the client's often disturbing symptoms. Nursing diagnoses may include Sensory/Perceptual Alterations, Altered Thought Processes, Anxiety, Knowledge Deficit, and Risk for Injury, as well as diagnoses that would relate to the client's medical condition.

Psychiatric complications seen in the acute hospital setting are a challenge because the staff may feel unprepared to deal with these symptoms.[14] Unprepared staff sometimes overlook symptoms or avoid dealing with them until they become extreme.

Interventions for Hospitalized Clients

After an accurate diagnosis of the medical condition is made and treatment is started, the psychiatric symptoms often abate quickly. It is during the diagnosis period that the nurse is usually faced with a confusing picture of new symptoms and behavior changes. Nursing interventions need to be focused on physical assessment, monitoring of vital signs, and maintenance of fluid and nutrition intake, sleep-wake cycle, and skin care. Client and family education is most important because the new onset of these psychiatric symptoms is es-

> **RESEARCH NOTE**
>
> Morency, CR, Levkoff, SE, and Dick, KL: Delirium in hospitalized elders. J Gerontological Nursing 20(8):24–30, 1994.
>
> In an acute care teaching hospital 325 clients were interviewed within 48 hours of admission. The interview included a Delirium Symptom Interview tool. The results of this interview were then compared with an interview with the client's nurse and a review of the medical record.
>
> **Findings:** Of the 325 subjects, 125 were found to have delirium on admission or during their stay. When compared with the nurse and chart sensitivity to the assessment of delirium, the interview tool was found to be significantly different from what the nurses assessed. Nurses were particularly deficient in identifying perceptual disturbances, speech disturbances, and fluctuating behavior as delirium.
>
> **Application to Practice:** In addition to finding a high frequency of delirium (38% of subjects), this study also found that nurses seemed deficient in their assessment of delirium symptoms. The authors suggest that nurses need more education about the components of the mental status examination and the variety of symptoms associated with delirium in the elderly population in an acute care setting. Nurses were proficient in assessing for disorientation and sleep-wake cycle disturbance but frequently did not recognize the more subtle symptoms.

pecially distressing. Reinforce that these symptoms will dissipate after appropriate treatment is found. Remind the family not to take personally behavior that the client cannot control. Another focus of nursing interventions is to promote the completion of diagnostic tests such as x-rays and laboratory tests. This intervention can be difficult when the client is agitated or uncooperative.

For the client who is agitated, combative, or hostile, gear interventions to providing a calm, safe environment and setting limits. Reassure the client that you are there to help, but also remember that he or she is probably frightened and will have difficulty trusting. Intervene early to prevent aggressive behavior from getting out of control. If the nurse observes the client closely and uses reality orientation, and the medication is effective, physical restraints can sometimes be avoided. When they are needed, keep reinforcing the reason for the restraints and promote the respect and dignity of the client. Maintain a trusting, calm, nonthreatening relationship. Remind all staff not to take the client's behavior personally.

To respond to the hallucinating client, listen to his or her descriptions of experiences, and then reinforce how frightening these are, but explain the possible causes. Maintain frequent contacts with the client to develop a trusting relationship. Reinforce that you are not experiencing the hallucinations, but do not challenge or argue with the client about them. Focus conversations on what is happening in the immediate environment. Provide a calming environment with some structure by maintaining a daily routine.

For the confused client, a major intervention is frequent reorienting to time, place, and situation. Make sure the client has his or her own hearing aid (with working batteries) or glasses available. Because of the client's shortened attention span, repeat information frequently. All staff must make efforts to communicate clearly and simply. Present instructions unambiguously, and present multiple topics one at a time. Cut down distractions by closing the door and turning down the volume on the television while talking to the client. If the client has a hearing deficit, speak slowly while making eye contact and write out information. Avoid yelling at the client, who may feel threatened. Make the environment as easy to maneuver as possible by posting large signs on doors as a reminder of locale, and make sure the path to the bathroom is free of obstacles. Sometimes familiar objects from home can assist with orientation.

The depressed client needs a supportive, reassuring environment, reinforcement of strengths and skills, physical activity, and realistic goals. Avoid false reassurance or criticism for not accomplishing goals. Encourage venting of feelings and social interaction. Assess for suicide potential.

Clients with personality changes such as inappropriate behavior need to be reminded of what is appropriate (for example, to speak more softly and keep a gown on). Set limits on inappropriate behavior. Educate the client and family about the cause of these changes and reassure them that they are temporary. Family may need assistance on controlling the client's behavior. Role model acceptable behavior. Avoid yelling or arguing, which the client will interpret as threatening behavior.

For the delusional client, listen to the concerns but avoid arguing about the content of the delusions. Focus conversations more on reality, here-and-now issues. Be aware that this client may be very sensitive to your behavior and will read into your facial expressions. For example, if you are abrupt with the client, he or she will take that personally and react negatively to it. Delusional clients may also be sensitive to other conversations overheard outside their rooms and think the conversations relate to them. The delusional client who overhears a nurse talking about needing keys for the narcotic drawer may think he or she is going to be locked up. Because the client's environment cannot be completely controlled in a hospital, the nurse can best intervene by being sensitive to these conversations and try to anticipate client concerns.

The very anxious client needs reassurance and a calming environment. Limiting intrusions to a client's room, keeping noise levels down outside the room, explaining all interventions and procedures, and encouraging calming techniques like deep breathing and relaxation can help.

Pharmacologic interventions for the specific behaviors

Nursing Care Plan: MENTAL ILLNESS DUE TO A GENERAL MEDICAL CONDITION

Nursing Diagnosis #1: Altered thought processes evidenced by disorientation, exaggerated responses, poor judgment, hallucinations, delusions related to a mental illness due to a general medical condition.

Client Outcome Criteria
- Demonstrates reduced evidence of hallucinations or delusions.
- Demonstrates improved reality orientation.
- Demonstrates more appropriate behavior.

Interventions
- Provide a quiet, calm environment, and approach client in a calm, reassuring manner.
- Explain all procedures in a clear, concrete manner, avoiding jargon. If the client becomes distressed, clarify any concerns.
- Plan a schedule for the client's day and provide as much structure as possible.
- Routinely incorporate orienting cues in all contacts with the client, e.g., time, place, and date. Provide clocks and calendars.
- Reassure the client and family that psychiatric symptoms will most likely abate when the medical condition improves.
- Make brief, frequent contacts with the client without threatening or challenging his or her beliefs.
- If delusional or hallucinating, let him or her know you realize these are frightening, but do not react to them as if they are real. Never talk to the client's voices or get involved in the delusion.
- Focus on real events. Avoid listening to long confusing stories that are not based on reality. Direct conversation to here-and-now events.
- Provide consistent staff who are familiar with the client's responses.
- Educate staff that they should not take the client's behavior personally and ensure that they understand the cause of the behavior.

Nursing Diagnosis #2: Risk for injury evidenced by confusion, falls, poor judgment related to confusion, and agitation from mental illness due to a general medical condition.

Client Outcome Criteria
- Remains safe from injury.
- Demonstrates appropriate action and judgment to avoid injury.

Interventions
- Identify safety hazards in the client's environment and implement measures to reduce the risk of injury, e.g., keep walker at bedside, clear path to bathroom, and keep call light in reach.
- Make frequent rounds to observe the client's behavior. Ensure that all staff and family are aware of the client's needs.
- Ensure the client has glassess, hearing aids, canes, etc., as needed.
- Reinforce compliance with medical treatment to resolve these symptoms.
- Set limits on destructive behavior.
- Structure activities during the day.
- Be aware of sudden changes in the client's mental status that could lead to pulling out IVs, catheters, etc. Anticipate this by reducing the number of tubes the client needs where possible, covering IV side with large dressing, administering antipsychotic medications, and using wrist restraints as a last resort.
- Check the client routinely for cuts, bruises, and burns.
- Supervise any situation where there is higher risk for injury such as meals.

Nursing Diagnosis #3: Sleep pattern disturbance evidenced by day-night reversal and inadequate sleep periods; confusion related to critical illness, CCU setting, and care routines that disrupt sleep.

Client Outcome Criteria
- Is able to sleep adequate amount of time.
- Wakes up feeling refreshed.
- Is able to rest between care needs.

Interventions
- Establish a schedule for sleeping and ensure that all staff are aware of it. Prioritize procedures that must be done and delay others until later. Try to promote sleep at night as much as possible.
- Ensure visitors are instructed on the need for the client to sleep.
- Provide environment more conducive to sleep, e.g., darken room, play soft music, put a sign on door not to disturb the client, try to reduce noise from equipment in room if possible, and offer herbal tea or another soothing drink if possible.
- Ensure the client is not taking in any caffeine or other stimulants.
- Encourage the family to bring in the client's pillow, blanket, and favorite items.
- Ensure pain and other uncomfortable symptoms are treated.
- Reassure the client and family that symptoms will abate after the client's condition is stable.
- Reorient the client to time, place, and person as needed.
- Provide clocks and calendars in the room to enhance orientation.
- Use sedatives and hypnotics as needed.
- Talk to the client about his or her fears and concerns. Provide reassurance.

may be needed until appropriate treatment is started. Medication use usually should be minimized because of the fear of masking symptoms or causing a worsening of the physical condition, such as in a head injury. Short-acting antianxiety drugs like Porazepam and antipsychotic medications such as haloperidol may be used to control symptoms that are particularly distressing or disruptive. Antidepressants may be tried for the depressed client, but because they take several weeks to completely lift symptoms, they usually are avoided. If a medical condition is suspected, the fewer new medications the client takes, the clearer the clinical picture. In addition, the lowest dosages to achieve the response may reduce the possibility of side effects.

Another important factor in pharmacologic intervention is to treat the symptom correctly, especially for pain. In a confused or agitated client who is unable to verbalize pain, treatment with antianxiety drugs may be inadvertently used rather than the appropriate analgesic. Such use could lead to the client being overtreated with tranquilizers and still being in pain. Be aware that long-acting drugs such as slow-release analgesics or tranquilizers or even antihypertensive medications are more prone to side effects than immediate-release drugs. For those clients who are at risk for psychiatric symptoms, long-acting drugs should probably be avoided.

Interventions for Clients in the Community

Diagnosing and treating a client in the community can be more difficult because of the limited opportunity health-care professionals have to observe the behaviors. Seeing a client intermittently in the office or clinic requires skilled observations as well as precise documentation of behavior observations by the client, family, and staff. The family must be closely involved in keeping track of behavior changes and medication compliance. Home health supervision can also be helpful.

For a client who is agitated or confused, the family or other home caregivers must be involved in providing reality orientation and maintaining a safe environment. Evaluation by a home health agency social worker can determine if this client can be maintained safely at home or if hospitalization or placement in a more supervised setting is needed. The nurse must educate the family and caregivers on what to look for, how to provide interventions in the home, and when to call for more help.

Expected Outcomes

Improvement will be demonstrated by:
- Maintenance of client safety and dignity
- Resolution of all psychiatric symptoms
- Verbalization by the client and family that they understand the causes of these symptoms

Differential Diagnosis

An accurate diagnosis of mental illness due to a general medical condition can be difficult to make because once a psychiatric diagnosis is made, the medical workup may stop. Excellent diagnostic skills are essential.

Symptoms can be confused with dementia, especially of the Alzheimer's type, in the elderly client; substance abuse; or a primary psychiatric disorder such as schizophrenia, bipolar disorder, or depression. In the client with a known medical condition, the stress of coping could produce psychiatric symptoms such as panic attacks or depression.

CASE STUDY

Cynthia T, a 56-year-old woman, had recently become increasingly fatigued and depressed. Normally an energetic, upbeat person, she was now sad, tearful, and had trouble getting herself up in the morning to go to work. Her husband and son became concerned and encouraged her to see a psychotherapist. She agreed but after three sessions found the symptoms to be intensifying. She was barely able to get out of bed, and the therapist recommended a psychiatric evaluation for medication.

The psychiatrist found out that in addition to her current depressive symptoms, Cynthia had been diagnosed with breast cancer 3 years ago. After a lumpectomy, radiation therapy, and 6 months of prophylactic chemotherapy, she was given a "clean bill of health." Cynthia initially followed up with her internist and oncologist for regular checkups and mammograms, but in the past year she found excuses to avoid seeing her doctors. In fact, her husband didn't realize that she had not been pursuing medical follow-up. After taking her psychiatric history, the psychiatrist contacted her internist, who saw Cynthia immediately. He found her calcium level to be 11.5, which is moderate hypercalcemia.

She was admitted to the hospital where aggressive intravenous hydration was started as well as appropriate medications including pamidronate (Aredia) to combat hypercalcemia. The presence of hypercalcemia is a common condition in metastatic breast cancer. Her calcium level had been rising over the past few months, and the symptoms of fatigue and depression were typical of this rising level. A bone scan revealed cancer in the hips and vertebrae.

When her therapist visited her in the hospital, she found Cynthia in much better spirits. She admitted that over the past months she had suspected that the breast cancer had advanced. She was aware of a constant backache and fatigue. She realized she was avoiding facing that the cancer had metastasized but never suspected that symptoms of depression could be caused by the hypercalcemia. In some ways, Cynthia was relieved that her symptoms were now improved and she was beginning treatment for the metastasis. Her emotional and cognitive functioning continued to improve.

CRITICAL THINKING QUESTIONS

1. What factors contributed to Cynthia's new onset of depressive symptoms?

2. What could the therapist have done to further evaluate contributing factors to Cynthia's depression?
3. What emotional issues may Cynthia have been struggling with in regard to her breast cancer?

CRITICAL CARE UNIT PSYCHOSIS

Critical care unit (CCU) psychosis is often unrecognized and poorly understood. It is the sudden onset of severe delirium that is multifocal. It may also be known as intensive care unit (ICU) syndrome or ICU delirium. It was initially identified in the 1960s when CCUs were new entities in hospitals. Clients who entered the CCUs with their intact mental status and no evidence of psychiatric symptoms were becoming confused and agitated, hallucinating, and demonstrating personality changes. Although the stress of the environment was initially blamed, it is now believed that multiple causes contribute to the altered cerebral metabolism and imbalance of neurotransmitters and some enzymes that characterize it. Symptoms usually occur within 2 to 5 days after admission to the unit.[15] Approximately 30 to 40% of CCU clients experience CCU-psychosis, but the percentage increases to up to 50% in the elderly.[15,16]

Some experts believe the term CCU-psychosis should be avoided because it implies a cause-and-effect relationship to the CCU, when, in fact, a life-threatening condition such as hypoxia or bleeding may be the cause and be overlooked.[17]

Characteristic Behaviors

Early symptoms often include either hyperactivity, restlessness, and combativeness or slow responses, withdrawal, and apathy. Other symptoms include memory impairment, hallucinations, delusions, personality changes such as disinhibitions, hostility, confusion, and fluctuating mental status. Careful assessment, as noted previously in this chapter, needs to include a thorough medical and psychiatric history, noting medication use, and assessment of coping styles. After discharge from the CCU, many clients have limited memory of what happened to them or their behavior in the CCU, but memories can occasionally return in the form of dreams.

Culture, Age, and Gender Features

Clients over 60 years old with multiple illnesses, including chronic brain disorders like Alzheimer's disease, are at highest risk for CCU-psychosis. These clients are more susceptible to mental status and behavioral changes from the stress of the CCU environment, as well as the impact of multiple illnesses and complications. However, all age groups are vulnerable. Culture and gender do not seem to play a role.

Etiology

Sleep Deprivation

Because of the client's critical condition, procedures are performed around the clock, making it difficult for CCU clients to sleep.

Sensory Overload and Deprivation

The CCU client is continually bombarded with beeping monitors, alarms, and other stimuli. For example, the client might have a ventilator with an alarm, bubbling sounds from water in the ventilator tubing, three or more IV pumps each with its own alarm, bubbling chest tubes, and constant sound from the suction machine. Combined, they are well above the recommended noise levels for hospitals. Staff conversations near the client as well as outside of the room also help to create a tremendously stressful environment. The client does not know if it is night or day because units rarely have windows, clocks, or calendars. In addition, lack of privacy, limited visiting from family, and close proximity to other critically ill clients contribute to the sensory overload. Despite the stimuli, the client's reality testing is limited and thought processes impaired to the extent that the stimuli have no meaning, and sensory deprivation results. The high-technology environment with multiple pieces of equipment around the client also creates a frightening, dehumanizing atmosphere.

Prolonged Immobilization

Being bound to bed for days with numerous tubes, lines, and restraints creates tremendous feelings of powerlessness. Clients on ventilators given paralytic drugs to reduce movement are still aware of their immobilization.

Because CCU clients have multiple diagnoses and metabolic conditions, they are susceptible to all the causes listed previously for general medical conditions that cause psychiatric symptoms and CCU-psychosis.

Prognosis

CCU-psychosis is associated with prolonged CCU and hospital stays as well as more complications from client injuries, self-extubations, and the need for more sedation among other factors. However, once the client leaves the CCU and stablizes medically from any sequelae, the prognosis remains consistent with the medical condition, and CCU-psychosis is not a factor.

Interventions for Hospitalized Clients

Nurses play an important role in reducing the impact of CCU-psychosis by astute observation for early signs of mental changes. CCU nurses can prevent or reduce the extent of this syndrome by promoting sleep even in the most critically ill by coordinating care so that several procedures are done at one time (allowing at least 2 to 3 hours of uninterrupted sleep); educating other health-team members and visitors about the client's need for sleep; reducing noise where possible by turning down the volume of alarms; reducing talking by staff outside the client's room; frequent orienting to time, place, and situation; and humanizing the high-tech environment by using touch, promoting privacy, using eye contact, and encouraging family to bring in personal items like photos or a watch. Promote orientation by having the client wear his or her own glasses and hearing aids as needed. Provide structure by following a schedule for client care where possible, and teach the client and family about the environment to provide some meaning.

When the client is transferred to a lower level of care, inform nurses in these areas about the client's need for sleep and about his or her psychiatric symptoms. Communicate the sleep schedule to night staff.

Avoid using medical jargon and abbreviations around the client because this can cause misunderstandings. Try to give information to the client in very small amounts because of the shortened attention span. Remember to repeat information because the client's short-term memory is poor. When the client is found trying to get out of bed, do not yell angrily, which will frighten and feed into possible delusions.

Pharmacologic treatment includes use of haloperidol, lorazepam, analgesics (for physical distress), and other drugs for treatment of the physical causes.

Expected Outcomes

For the individual with CCU-psychosis, improvement will be demonstrated by:
- Fewer hallucinations
- Less anxiety
- Less aggressive behavior
- Increased sleep
- No injuries.

Differential Diagnosis

The symptoms of CCU-psychosis are most often confused with delirium, dementia, and psychiatric diagnoses. When a client suddenly develops unusual or bizarre behaviors in the CCU, knowledge of the client's baseline personality and history of psychiatric disorders is essential. In addition, recent intake or abuse of drugs or alcohol may also be a factor. All of the causes of psychiatric symptoms in general medical conditions that were discussed previously in this chapter must also be ruled out.

CASE STUDY

Norman, an 85-year-old man, was admitted to the CCU after emergency surgery for a ruptured diverticulum. The client had been healthy and active before admission for sudden onset of severe abdominal pain. In the CCU, he continued on a ventilator for several days because it was difficult to wean him off it. On the third postoperative day, the nurses noted that Norman seemed restless, pulling at his endotracheal tube and requiring wrist restraints. He was awake and alert; however, his eyes darted around the room and he appeared anxious. On the fourth day, he pulled out his endotracheal tube; fortunately he didn't require reintubation.

When his wife visited him, she found her husband talking about the CCU staff trying to kill him. He demanded to leave and tried to get out of bed while his wife was there. He refused to listen to her reassurances and required administration of lorezepam and a vest restraint. Blood gases tests indicated Norman was hypoxic.

After he rested, his blood gases improved and he seemed calmer but continued to state that the staff was holding him against his will. Staff instituted more efforts to establish trust as well as a sleep schedule. The staff reinforced information about his environment in short segments. During visiting hours, his wife talked about future plans once he improved. She was allowed to spend more time with him. She and the staff reinforced what had happened to him with the surgery.

Within 2 days Norman was still questioning what staff were doing but seemed much more amenable to following instructions. He was transferred to a step-down unit and was discharged to home 5 days later. When seen in his surgeon's office for follow-up care, he had little memory of his time in the CCU. He exhibited normal mental functioning.

CRITICAL THINKING QUESTIONS

1. What factors contributed to Norman's apparent CCU-psychosis?
2. What nursing interventions were instituted to reduce Norman's response?
3. What client and family education was needed with Norman and his wife?

SYNOPSIS OF CURRENT RESEARCH

Current research seems to be focused on identifying factors that contribute to delirium in the elderly population with general medical conditions. Evaluating the effectiveness of mental status rating tools and documenting the psychiatric symptoms in specific medical conditions such as cancer are other current areas of interest.

AREAS FOR FUTURE RESEARCH

A review of current literature indicates a lack of nursing research on this entire subject. Because nurses are at the forefront of identifying clients with these mental changes, nurses need to consider the following areas of research:

- Developing nursing assessment or rating tools that can better identify and follow symptom changes in these clients in the psychiatric and acute care setting.
- Identifying specific environment factors in the CCU that increase or decrease CCU-psychosis, and determining what nursing staff interventions influence development of CCU-psychosis.
- Determining the frequency of mental disorders in specific populations such as cancer, dialysis, or open-heart surgery clients. This could better predict staffing needs and education needs of staff working in these areas.
- Examining specific interventions as alternatives to physical restraints.
- Studying client response to psychotropic medications used to treat these symptoms.
- Examining the clinical preparation of psychiatric nurses and other mental health professionals to assess these symptoms accurately.
- Looking at nurses' preparation for conducting mental status examinations.

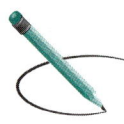

KEY POINTS

- Depression, delirium, and psychosis can occur in individuals with a known medical condition or prior to the onset of physical symptoms.
- *DSM-IV* identifies 11 forms of psychiatric conditions that result from medical conditions; delirium is the most common.
- Sudden onset of psychiatric symptoms such as confusion, mood changes, and disinhibitions are common clues.
- Hundreds of possible causes of psychiatric symptoms exist, including endocrine, nutritional, and electrolyte imbalances; cancer; vascular changes; medication effects; and neurological condiitions such as head trauma, multiple sclerosis, and brain tumors.
- Nursing interventions are tailored to the individual client, and based on presenting symptoms. For instance, for agitated and aggressive clients, provide a calm and safe environment and set limits. For confused clients, reorient frequently to time, place, and situation.
- Medications are used cautiously in the treatment of mental illness due to a general medical condition; they may mask symptoms or worsen behaviors.
- Critical care unit (CCU) psychosis, often unrecognized, is the sudden onset of severe delirium that occurs 2 to 5 days after admission to the unit.
- Early symptoms of CCU-psychosis include hyperactivity, restlessness, and combativeness, or conversely, withdrawal and apathy. Psychotic symptoms, personality changes, confusion, and mental status changes are also common.
- The most common causes of CCU-psychosis include sleep deprivation, sensory overload and deprivation, prolonged immobilization.
- Key nursing interventions for CCU-psychosis include early observation and detection of symptoms, promoting sleep, reducing noise, personalizing treatment, orienting frequently, and providing structure.

REFERENCES

1. American Psychiatric Association: Diagnostic and Statistical Manual of Mental Disorders, ed 4. APA, Washington, DC, 1994.
2. Hall, RCW, et al: Physical illness presenting as psychiatric disease. Arch Gen Psychiatry 35:1315–1320, 1978.
3. Hall, RCW, et al: Unrecognized physical illness prompting psychiatric admission: A prospective study. Am J Psychiatry 138(5):629–635, 1981.
4. Foreman, MD: The cognitive and behavioral nature of acute confusional states. Sch Inq Nurs Pract 5(1):3–16, 1991.
5. Inouye, SK, and Charpentier, PA: Precipitating factors for delirium in hospitalized elderly persons. JAMA 275(11):852–858, 1996.
6. Morency, CR: Mental status change in the elderly: Recognizing and treating delirium. J Prof Nurs 6(6):356–363, 1990.
7. Barry, PD: Psychosocial Nursing: Care of Physically Ill Patients and Their Families, ed 3. JB Lippincott Co, Philadelphia, 1996.
8. Steinberg, PI: A case of paranoid disorder associated with hyperthyroidism. Can J Psychiatry 39(3):153–155, 1994.
9. Pasacreta, JV, and Massie, MJ: Nurses' reports of psychiatric complications in patients with cancer. Oncol Nurs Forum 17(3):347–353, 1990.
10. Caine, ED, Grossman, H, and Lyness, JM: Delirium, dementia and amnestic and other cognitive disorders and mental disorders due to a general medical condition. In Kaplan, HI, and Sadock, BJ: Comprehensive Textbook of Psychiatry, ed 6. Williams & Wilkins, Baltimore, 1996.
11. Neelon, VJ: Postoperative delirium. Nurs Clin North Amer 2: 579–587, 1990.
12. Travlos, A, and Hirsch, G: Steroid psychosis: A cause of confusion on the acute spinal cord injury unit. Arch Phys Med Rehabil 74:312–315, 1993.
13. van Hemert, AM, van der Mast, RC, Hengeveld, MW, and Vorstenbosch, M: Excess mortality in general hospital patients with delirium: A 5-year follow-up of 519 patients seen in psychiatric consultations. J Psychosom Res 38:339–346, 1994.
14. Francis, J, and Kapoor, W: Delirium in hospitalized elderly. J Gen Intern Med 5:65–79, 1990.
15. Gorman, LM, Sultan, D, and Raines, L: Davis's Manual of Psychosocial Nursing for General Patient Care. FA Davis Co, Philadelphia, 1996.
16. Geary, SM: Intensive care unit psychosis revisited: Understanding and managing delirium in the critical care setting. Crit Care Nurs Quar 17(1):51–63, 1994.
17. Lipowski, ZJ: Delirium: Acute Confusional States. Oxford University Press Inc, New York, 1990.

CHAPTER 17
Substance-related Disorders

CHAPTER 17

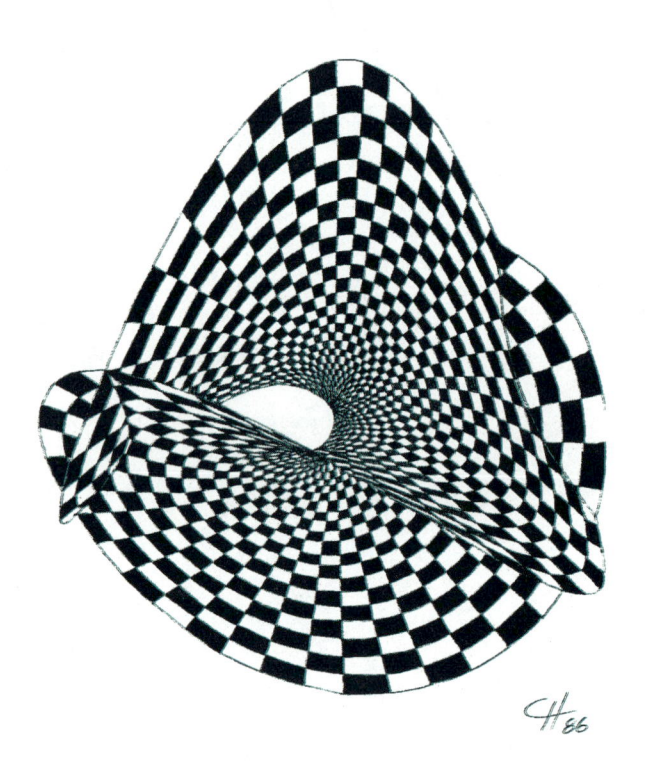

CHAPTER OUTLINE

Definition
Characteristic Behaviors
  Substance Abuse
  Alcohol Abuse
  Substance Dependence
  Enabling
  Intoxication and Withdrawal
Culture, Age, and Gender Features
  Culture
  Age
  Gender
Etiology
  Biological Theories
  Imaging Studies
  Genetic Theories
  Behavioral Theories
Prognosis
Assessment
  Short Alcohol and Drug History
  Screening Tools
  Family and Significant Others
  Physical Findings and Mental Status Examination
  Laboratory Findings
Planning Care
Interventions for Hospitalized Clients
  Acute Intoxication
  Acute Withdrawal
Interventions for Clients in the Community
  Brief Interventions
  Cognitive-Behavior Therapy
  Long-Term Substance Dependence
  Family Interventions
  Pharmacologic Treatments
  Alcohol Dependence
  Benzodiazepines and Sedative-Hypnotic Withdrawal
  Opioids
  Stimulant Withdrawal
  Nicotine Withdrawal
Expected Outcomes
Differential Diagnosis
  Medical Disorders
  Mood Disorders
  Psychotic Disorders
  Anxiety Disorders

Patricia K. Dahme, MSN, ARNP, CS

Substance-related Disorders

CHAPTER OUTLINE (Continued)

Personality Disorders
Attention-Deficit/Hyperactivity Disorder (ADHD)
Common Nursing Diagnoses
Areas for Future Research

LEARNING OBJECTIVES

After completing this chapter, the reader should be able to:

- Define common terms used in diagnosing and treating substance-related disorders.
- Discuss the factors that contribute to substance abuse and dependence.
- Identify the behavioral and physical signs that indicate early substance abuse and dependence.
- List three signs of withdrawal from each drug class.
- List three signs of intoxication from depressants, stimulants, hallucinogens, and opioids.
- Explain effective behavioral and pharmacologic interventions in withdrawal and sobriety maintenance.

KEY TERMS

addiction	psychoactive substances
agonist	psychological dependence
antagonist	substance abuse
intoxication	substance dependence
misuse	tolerance
physiological dependence	withdrawal

No other area in health care affects so many individuals and creates so many social, physical, and psychological problems as **substance abuse** and dependency. In the United States, about 18% of the population experiences a substance-use disorder at some point in their lives. The cost of addictive illness is estimated at $144 billion per year in health care and job loss.[1] Alcohol is the most commonly used drug; marijuana is the most commonly used illegal substance. Fifty percent of all auto accidents and homicides probably involve alcohol (Figure 17–1), and alcohol and other drugs are implicated in social problems such as increased crime and violence. However, these substances, primarily alcohol, have been used widely by many individuals in a recreational manner without related problems or disorders.

Societal views of drug use have vacillated between condemnation of the substance, resulting in prohibition, and condemnation of the individual abusing or dependent on the substance. Unfortunately, society's ambivalent views about drug use may be reflected in the attitudes of many health-care providers, including nurses, who either fail to accurately identify substance-abuse problems or harshly judge others for their abuse and dependence.

Although illegal drugs gain the most media and law enforcement attention, legal drugs have the highest mortality rates. Tobacco-related disorders account for approximately 500,000 deaths a year. One in 10 deaths are related to alcohol. More people die annually from **misuse** of legally obtained prescriptions drugs than from all illegal substances combined.[2]

Definition

Psychoactive substances are drugs or chemicals that, when taken, alter one or several of the following:

- Perception
- Awareness
- Consciousness
- Thinking
- Judgment
- Decision making
- Insight
- Mood
- Behavior

These substances include alcohol, prescription drugs, over-the-counter (OTC) medications, solvents, and illicit drugs. Drug abuse and dependence are characterized by negative effects on physical wellness, finances, sociability, interpersonal relationships, legal problems, driving, occupation, and family.[1] Substance abuse can directly affect health or lead to neglect of nutrition, hygiene, and other aspects of self-care.

The World Health Organization (WHO) changed the terminology from "addiction" to "chemical dependence," to emphasize that the disorder is an illness and to counteract the negative stereotype of the drug addict.

I didn't know it at the time, but I had entered the drinking life. Drinking was part of being a man. Drinking was an integral part of sexuality, easing entrance to its dark and mysterious treasure chambers. Drinking was the sacramental binder of friendships. Drinking was the reward for work, the fuel of

Average Monetary Costs Per Crash (1990 Dollars)

	Blood Alcohol Level		
	Equal to 0%	**Between 0% and 0.1%**	**Greater Than or Equal to 0.1%**
Fatal	$609,000	$755,000	$807,000
Non-Fatal	11,000	20,000	19,000
Any Injury	14,000	33,000	33,000
Uninjured	1,200	1,200	1,200
Property-Damage-Only	1,500	1,500	1,500

Average Comprehensive Costs Per Crash (1990 Dollars)

	Blood Alcohol Level		
	Equal to 0%	**Between 0% and 0.1%**	**Greater Than or Equal to 0.1%**
Fatal	$2,401,000	$2,732,000	$2,785,000
Non-Fatal	33,000	70,000	67,000
Any Injury	46,000	246,000	117,000
Uninjured	1,200	1,200	1,200
Property-Damage-Only	1,500	1,500	1,500

Figure 17–1. Statistics from 1990 show that alcohol-related crashes resulted in over 22,000 fatalities, 1.9 million nonfatal injuries, and about 4.6 million damaged vehicles. When there is no alcohol involved, the average costs for a fatal crash in $609,000; when the blood alcohol level is at least 0.1%, the usual level for the charge of driving under the influence, the average fatal crash costs $807,000. The greater the alcohol involvement, the greater the cost per crash. When other factors are costed out such as lost quality of life, so-called comprehensive costs, fatal crashes cost from $2.4 to $2.7 million.

---

celebration, the consolation for death or defeat. Drinking gave me the strength, confidence, ease, laughter; it made me believe that dreams really could come true.

PETE HAMILL[3]

Characteristic Behaviors

The Diagnostic and Statistical Manual of Mental Disorders (DSM-IV) separates substance-related disorders into two categories: substance-use disorders such as abuse and dependence (Table 17–1), and substance-induced disorders such as **intoxication** and **withdrawal** (Table 17–2). Box 17-1 lists 11 classes of substances with the potential for abuse; Box 17-2 lists 5 general categories of substances.

SUBSTANCE ABUSE

As seen in the Diagnostic Box Criteria for Substance Abuse and Dependence, substance abuse is characterized by several behaviors including difficulty meeting school or work obligations and neglecting responsibilities and relationships.

> People are shocked when I tell them I'm an addict. I can almost read their minds: but you look so pretty and so together. Well that's now. Getting hooked was easy. I was working at a nurs-

TABLE 17–1. DSM-IV Substance-Use Disorders

Alcohol dependence
Alcohol abuse
Amphetemine dependence
Amphetemine abuse
Cannabis dependence
Cannabis abuse
Cocaine dependence
Cocaine abuse
Hallucinogen dependence
Hallucinogen abuse
Inhalant dependence
Inhalant abuse
Nicotine dependence
Opioid dependence
Opioid abuse
Phencyclidine dependence
Phencyclidine abuse
Sedative-hypnotic or anxiolytic dependence
Sedative-hypnotic or anxiolytic abuse
Polysubstance dependence
Other (or unknown) substance dependence
Other (or unknown) substance abuse

Source: Reprinted with permission from the Diagnostic and Statistical Manual of Mental Disorders, Fourth Edition. Copyright 1994 American Psychiatric Association.

TABLE 17–2. *DSM-IV* Substance-induced Organic Mental Disorders

Alcohol intoxication	Hallucinogen-induced psychotic disorder
Alcohol withdrawal	Hallucinogen-induced mood disorder
Alcohol intoxication delirium	Hallucinogen-induced anxiety disorder
Alcohol withdrawal delirium	Inhalant intoxication
Alcohol-induced persisting dementia	Inhalant intoxication delirium
Alcohol-induced persisting amnesic disorder	Inhalant-induced persisting dementia
Alcohol-induced psychotic disorder	Inhalant-induced psychotic disorder
Alcohol-induced disorders (mood, anxiety, sexual dysfunction, sleep, other)	Inhalant-induced mood disorder
	Inhalant-induced anxiety disorder
Amphetamine intoxication	Nicotine withdrawal
Amphetamine withdrawal	Opioid intoxication
Amphetamine intoxication delirium	Opioid withdrawal
Amphetamine-induced psychotic disorder	Opioid intoxication delirium
Amphetamine-induced disorders (mood, anxiety, sexual dysfunction, sleep, other)	Opioid-induced psychotic disorder
	Opioid-induced mood disorder
Caffeine intoxication	Opioid-induced sexual dysfunction
Caffeine-induced anxiety disorder	Opioid-induced sleep disorder
Caffeine-induced sleep disorder	Phencyclidine intoxication
Cannabis intoxication	Phencyclidine intoxication delirium
Cannabis intoxication delirium	Phencyclidine-induced psychotic disorder
Cannabis-induced psychotic disorder	Phencyclidine-induced mood disorder
Cannabis-induced anxiety disorder	Phencyclidine-induced anxiety disorder
Cocaine intoxication	Sedative, hypnotic, or anxiolytic intoxication
Cocaine withdrawal	Sedative, hypnotic, or anxiolytic withdrawal
Cocaine intoxication delirium	Sedative, hypnotic, or anxiolytic intoxication delirium
Cocaine-induced psychotic disorder	Sedative, hypnotic, or anxiolytic withdrawal delirium
Cocaine-induced disorders of mood, sleep, anxiety, sexual dysfunction	Sedative, hypnotic, or anxiolytic-induced persisting dementia
	Sedative, hypnotic, or anxiolytic-induced persisting amnestic disorder
Hallucinogen intoxication	Sedative, hypnotic, or anxiolytic-induced psychotic disorder
Hallucinogen persisting perception disorder	Sedative, hypnotic, or anxiolytic-induced disorders of mood, anxiety, sexual dysfunction, or sleep
Hallucinogen intoxication delirium	

Source: Reprinted with permission from the Diagnostic and Statistical Manual of Mental Disorders, Fourth Edition. Copyright 1994 American Psychiatric Association.

Box 17–1. Eleven Classes of Substances with the Potential for Abuse and Dependence

1. Alcohol
2. Amphetamine or similarly acting sympathomimetics
3. Caffeine
4. Cannabis
5. Cocaine
6. Hallucinogens
7. Inhalants
8. Nicotine
9. Opioids
10. Phencyclidines (PCP) or similarly acting arylcyclohexylamines
11. Sedative, hypnotic, or antianxiety agents

Box 17–2. Five General Categories of Substances

Based on their shared physiological and psychological effects, many of these substances can be classified into five general categories:

1. Central nervous system (CNS) depressants, including alcohol, sedative-hypnotics, antianxiety agents, and volatile inhalants
2. Stimulants, including cocaine and amphetamine, caffeine,* nicotine,† and related substances
3. Opioids including analgesics
4. Hallucinogens including PCP
5. Cannabis.

*Caffeine is not considered to cause either dependence or abuse.
†Nicotine is currently classified as causing dependence but not abuse.

DSM–IV Criteria for Substance Abuse and Dependency

Criteria for Substance Abuse

A. A maladaptive pattern of substance use leading to clinically significant impairment or distress, as manifested by one (or more) of the following, occurring within a 12-month period:
   (1) recurrent substance use resulting in a failure to fulfill major role obligations at work, school, or home (e.g., repeated absences or poor work performance related to substance use; substance-related absences, suspensions, or expulsions from school; neglect of children or household)
   (2) recurrent substance use in situations in which it is physically hazardous (e.g., driving an automobile or operating a machine when impaired by substance use)
   (3) recurrent substance-related legal problems (e.g., arrests for substance-related disorderly conduct)
   (4) continued substance use despite having persistent or recurrent social or interpersonal problems caused or exacerbated by the effects of the substance (e.g., arguments with spouse about consequences of intoxication, physical fights)

B. The symptoms have never met the criteria for Substance Dependence for this class of substance.

Criteria for Substance Dependence

A. A maladaptive pattern of substance use, leading to clinically significant impairment or distress, as manifested by three (or more) of the following, occurring at any time in the same 12-month period:
   (1) tolerance, as defined by either of the following:
       (a) a need for markedly increased amounts of the substance to achieve intoxication or desired effect
       (b) markedly diminished effect with continued use of the same amount of the substance
   (2) withdrawal, as manifested by either of the following:
       (a) the characteristic withdrawal syndrome for the substance (refer to Criteria A and B of the criteria sets for Withdrawal from the specific substances)
       (b) the same (or a closely related) substance is taken to relieve or avoid withdrawal symptoms
   (3) the substance is often taken in larger amounts or over a longer period than was intended
   (4) there is a persistent desire or unsuccessful efforts to cut down or control substance use
   (5) a great deal of time is spent in activities necessary to obtain the substance (e.g., visiting multiple doctors or driving long distances), use the substance (e.g., chain-smoking), or recover from its effects
   (6) important social, occupational, or recreational activities are given up or reduced because of substance use
   (7) the substance use is continued despite knowledge of having a persistent or recurrent physical or psychological problem that is likely to have been caused or exacerbated by the substance (e.g., current cocaine use despite recognition of cocaine-induced depression, or continued drinking despite recognition that an ulcer was made worse by alcohol consumption)

Specify if:
   With Physiological Dependence: evidence of tolerance or withdrawal (i.e., either Item 1 or 2 is present)
   Without Physiological Dependence: no evidence of tolerance or withdrawal (i.e., neither Item 1 nor 2 is present)

Course specifiers:
   Early Full Remission
   Early Partial Remission
   Sustained Full Remission
   Sustained Partial Remission
   On Agonist Therapy
   In a Controlled Environment

Source: Reprinted with permission from the Diagnostic and Statistical Manual of Mental Disorders, Fourth Edition. Copyright 1994 American Psychiatric Association.

---

ing home and had terrible back pain. The harder I worked, the more my back just ached. I'd be out for weeks at a time because I needed total bed rest. That's when I got hooked on pain killers. But they didn't just relieve the pain. It was the "high" that really appealed to me. Then to calm down or just to wash the pills down, I began to drink. At first I could function somewhat at work. The truth is that I was going in to steal pills; drug diversion, as it's called. What was I thinking? I feel really bad about taking the meds from the patients. But nothing mattered except getting high. When I finally got caught, I knew I had to do something. I was facing losing my nursing license and being out on the street. Luckily the state had a program to help addicts like me. Now I'm on the advisory board to help other nurses.

The following signs and symptoms suggest substance-use disorders:

- Problems in areas of life functioning including frequent job changes, marital conflict, separation, divorce, work-related accidents, lateness, absenteeism, legal problems including arrest, decline in academic performance, social isolation, and estrangement from friends and family.

Box 17–3. Prevalence of Substance-related Disorders

Prevalence	Disorder
Alcohol abuse	16%
Males	29%
Females	6%
Substance abuse	18%
Other drug dependency	9%

Source: Data from Miller, NS, and Fine, J: Current epidemiology of comorbidity of psychiatric and addictive disorders. Psychiatr Clin North Am 16:1, 1993, and Regier, DA, et al: Comorbidity of mental disorders with alcohol and other drug abuse. Results from the Epidemiological Catchment Area (ECA) Study. JAMA 264:2511, 1990.

- Driving while intoxicated (more than one incident suggests dependence), leisure activities that involve alcohol or other drugs, and financial problems including those related to spending for drugs.
- Physical findings including trauma secondary to falls, auto accidents, fights, fatigue, insomnia, headaches, vague physical complaints, sexual dysfunction, loss of libido, erectile dysfunction, anorexia or weight loss, seizure disorder and seizures, and looking older than stated age.

Schuckit[4] suggests asking all clients about alcohol-related life problems: marital separation or divorce, multiple arrests related to alcohol, physical evidence that alcohol has harmed health, or a job loss related to drugs. Any of these implies a dangerous drinking pattern that require further assessment.

ALCOHOL ABUSE

Two types of alcoholism have been identified, each with distinct characteristics.[4,5] Type I alcoholism, which affects both men and women,
- is relatively mild
- is influenced by environmental factors such as low economic status
- begins later in life

Type II alcoholism affects only men who have
- a more severe family history of alcoholism
- antisocial personality features
- a strong genetic component
- earlier onset of alcohol problems (before age 25)
- reduced serotonin functioning
- inability to abstain from alcohol
- loss of control while drinking

Much of my memory of those years is blurred because drinking was now slicing holes in my consciousness. I never thought of myself as a drunk; I was, I thought, like many others—a drinker. I certainly didn't think I was an alcoholic. But I was already having trouble remembering the details of the night before. It didn't seem to matter; everybody else was doing the same thing. We made little jokes about having a great time last night—I think. And we'd begun to reach for the hair of the dog.

PETE HAMILL[3]

A study of men found three distinct stages of alcoholism.[6]

Stage I: heavy social drinking of four drinks daily. Drinking in this stage remained stable or decreased for some and essentially caused no symptoms. Some evolved into Stage II.

Stage II: recurrent intake exceeded six to seven drinks daily and included social, medical, or legal complications. Drinking in this pattern lasted approximately 10 years between the ages of 25 and 35. One-third of the men reverted back to Stage I, one-third stayed at Stage II, one-third progressed to Stage III.

RESEARCH NOTE

Wechsler, H, et al: Health and behavioral consequences of binge drinking in college. JAMA 272:1672–1677, 1994.

Findings: Binge drinking, a common occurrence on college campuses, is consuming 5 or more drinks in a row for men and 4 or more on one occasion for women during a 2-week period. The authors studied over 17,000 students from 140 colleges. Binge drinking often results in dangerous behaviors and serious health consequences for the drinkers and others in their environment. Almost one-half of the students (44%) were binge drinkers; 50% of the men and 39% of the women drank excessively. About 1 in 5 students were frequent binge drinkers; they binged 3 or more times in the previous 2 weeks. One in five also engaged in frequent and deliberate intoxication. Students between ages 17 and 24 years had higher binging rates than older students.

Binge drinking was associated with serious problems. Almost half of the frequent binge drinkers had at least five health and behavior problems, including engaging in unplanned and unprotected sex, getting in trouble with campus police, damaging property, driving after drinking, and getting injured or hurt. In addition to these risky behaviors, they created problems for non-binge-drinking students who reported being pushed, hit, or assaulted and receiving unwanted sexual advances.

Application to Practice: Binge drinking is a common occurrence on college campuses. Along with the direct unhealthy effects of alcohol abuse, students who binge have more behavior problems. The nurse can use this information to help assess alcohol abuse in young adults and educate individuals and the community about the risks of binge drinking. Nurses can use this information to assess alcohol-related behaviors and advocate for the treatment of individuals who binge drink.

Stage III: classified as late-stage alcoholism and meets the *DSM-IV* criteria for dependence with consistent loss of control, withdrawal, morning drinking, and detoxification. Dependence led to premature death in more than one-third of the men. Less than one-sixth of men returned to social drinking and one-third of the alcohol-dependent men evolved into abstinence.

SUBSTANCE DEPENDENCE

The hallmarks of **substance dependence** are lack of control over drug use and its increasing importance. Substance dependence is characterized by at least three symptoms within a 12-month period:
- Tolerance
- Withdrawal
- Taking larger amounts
- Inability to reduce use
- Excess time spent on obtaining drugs
- Impairment in functioning
- Continued use despite negative consequences

Individuals may tolerate certain drug effects but not some physical effects. For example, an opioid user who develops **tolerance** may not experience the drug's euphoric effects but still exhibits constricted pupils. Withdrawal symptoms or needing to use the drug to treat withdrawal indicates **physiological dependence**. Dependence indicates impaired control of substance use. People take the drug in larger amounts and over longer periods. The drug becomes the most important thing in their lives.

ENABLING

This term is commonly used to describe the behaviors of individuals in the family or social system who inadvertently promote continued alcohol or drug use. By protecting them from the consequences of their actions, families, friends, and coworkers often "enable" clients to drink or use drugs. Examples of enabling behaviors include ignoring or making excuses for a spouse's behavior or finishing the work of a colleague who is unable to function. Effective treatment requires that significant others recognize and change their behavior.

INTOXICATION AND WITHDRAWAL

The diagnostic boxes describe the *DSM-IV* criteria for withdrawal and intoxication. Acute intoxication usually involves an increase or exacerbation of responses associated with the type of drug used.

In early 1993, in an effort to break this increasingly sad and dangerous pattern [of alcoholism], Eleanor and I persuaded Terry [our daughter] to enter a special treatment program at the National Institutes of Health (NIH) in Bethesda, Maryland. She cooperated, as did Eleanor and I, with the 6-week treatment agenda, which included counseling and group-discussion sessions with family members of other patients. We

---

Criteria for Substance Intoxication and Withdrawal

Criteria for Substance Intoxication

A. The development of a reversible substance-specific syndrome due to recent ingestion of (or exposure to) a substance. **Note:** Different substances may produce similar or identical syndromes.

B. Clinically significant maladaptive behavioral or psychological changes that are due to the effect of the substance on the central nervous system (e.g., belligerence, mood lability, cognitive impairment, impaired judgment, impaired social or occupational functioning) and develop during or shortly after use of the substance.

C. The symptoms are not due to a general medical condition and are not better accounted for by another mental disorder.

Criteria for Substance Withdrawal

A. The development of a substance-specific syndrome due to the cessation of (or reduction in) substance use that has been heavy and prolonged.

B. The substance-specific syndrome causes clinically significant distress or impairment in social, occupational, or other important areas of functioning.

C. The symptoms are not due to a general medical condition and are not better accounted for by another mental disorder.

Source: Reprinted with permission from the Diagnostic and Statistical Manual of Mental Disorders, Fourth Edition. Copyright 1994 American Psychiatric Association.

---

were encouraged by Terry's serious effort, hopeful attitude, and apparent progress into recovery. On the morning of her completion of the program, I drove to the NIH center and brought her to our Washington home. She asked if she could use my car for a few minutes to pick up a prescription at a nearby drugstore. Three hours later I was called by a concerned bartender who informed me that Terry had collapsed from heavy drinking. It pains me even now to recall the sad and bitter disappointment, the personal regret and doubt about my own judgment that followed. And let me be frank about this. I was furious.

GEORGE McGOVERN[7]

During withdrawal, depressant drugs stimulate the CNS, whereas stimulant drugs produce CNS depression. Intoxication and withdrawal follow the adage that what goes up must come down, or what goes down must come up. Table 17–3 lists the common effects of drugs of abuse, signs of intoxication, and their possible effects on the CNS.

TABLE 17–3. Common Drugs of Abuse, Effects, Signs of Intoxication and Theorized CNS Activity

Drug Class	Drug Examples	Drug Effects	Signs of Intoxication	Theorized CNS Activity
CNS Depressants				
Alcohol	Liquor, Beer, Wine	Relaxation, euphoria, release of inhibitions, memory loss (blackouts)	Slurred speech, nausea, vomiting, incoordination, coma	Enhances the action of GABA; stimulates the release of dopamine in the norepinephrine; increases dopamine metabolism
Sedative-Hypnotics	Barbiturates including secobarbital, pentobarbital, Quaaludes; Benzodiazepines, including diazepam, chlordiazepoxide	Euphoria, loss of inhibitions, poor judgment	Drowsiness, sedation, emotional instability	Binds to specific receptors on nerve cell membranes, increases GABA transmission by enhancing the effect of GABA receptor
Inhalants	Amyl nitrate; benzene; hydrocarbons; ketones; glycols; esters found in paint thinner, cleaning fluid, glue, gasoline	Euphoria, drowsiness, headache, fatigue, dizziness; kidney, liver, and brain damage	Giddiness, increased heart rate, ataxia, arrhythmias	
Stimulants				
Amphetamines	Dexedrine, methamphetamine, benzedrine, methylphenidate	Euphoria, relief of fatigue, wakefulness, decreased inhibition, hypersexuality, impaired judgment, appetite suppression, irritability, anxiety, panic attacks, paranoia	Psychomotor activation, sweating, increased blood pressure, increased heart and respiratory rates, tremors, dilated pupils	Cocaine and amphetamines block the reuptake of DA at the nerve endings; amphetamines cause increased DA release
Cocaine	Crack, powder			
Nicotine	Cigarettes, snuff, cigars, chewing and pipe tobacco	Enhanced performance	Increased heart rate and blood pressure, increased oxygen consumption	
Caffeine	Coffee, tea, cola	Stimulation, increased alertness	Increased heart rate and blood pressure	
Opioids	Morphine, codeine, heroin, methadone, oxycodone, propoxyphene, meperidine	Analgesia, euphoria, constipation, drowsiness, reduction in sexual and aggressive drives	Pupillary constriction, sedation, respiratory depression	Opioids bind to specific μ-opioid receptors on nerve cell membranes, inhibit the release of GABA, freeing DA to fire more actively
Cannabis	Marijuana, hashish	Euphoria, mild intoxication, relaxation, sexual arousal	Reddened eyes, increased heart rate, dry mouth, incoordination	
Hallucinogens	LSD, psilocybin, mescaline, MDMA (Ecstasy), phencyclidine (PCP, angel dust)	Euphoria, sharpened perceptions, altered body image, altered perceptions, distortions in judgment and memory, detachment from surroundings, decreased sensory awareness, confusion, brief psychotic reactions, hallucinations	Dilated pupils, flushing, emotional swings, increased blood pressure, increased temperature, sweating, fever, agitation, paranoia	

Culture, Age, and Gender Features

CULTURE

Substance abuse spans all geographic regions, ethnic groups, and social classes. Cultural norms play an important role in substance use, in the designation of abuse, and in the choice of substances used. Cultures with a high rate of alcohol abuse and dependence may condone drunkenness; those with low rates designate the appropriate use of small quantities in celebrations (Jewish and Mediterranean) or condemn it altogether (Muslim, Jehovah's Witness, and Mormons). In cultures where drinking with meals is allowed and generations and genders drink together, lower rates of alcohol abuse are evident. China and Japan have a lower prevalence of alcohol abuse partly because of a negative physiological response.[4] In the *Asian flush syndrome*, the skin becomes warm and flushed, the pulse increases, and blood pressure decreases. Native Americans and Eskimos may have high rates of alcohol abuse because it was introduced into their culture without clear rules about its appropriate use.

Patterns of alcohol use in the United States, similar to northern European countries, reflect a high tolerance for heavy drinking and drunkenness and, as a result, a high rate of alcoholism.

Percent of Population Age 12 and Older Reporting Heavy Alcohol Use in the Past Month, 1993

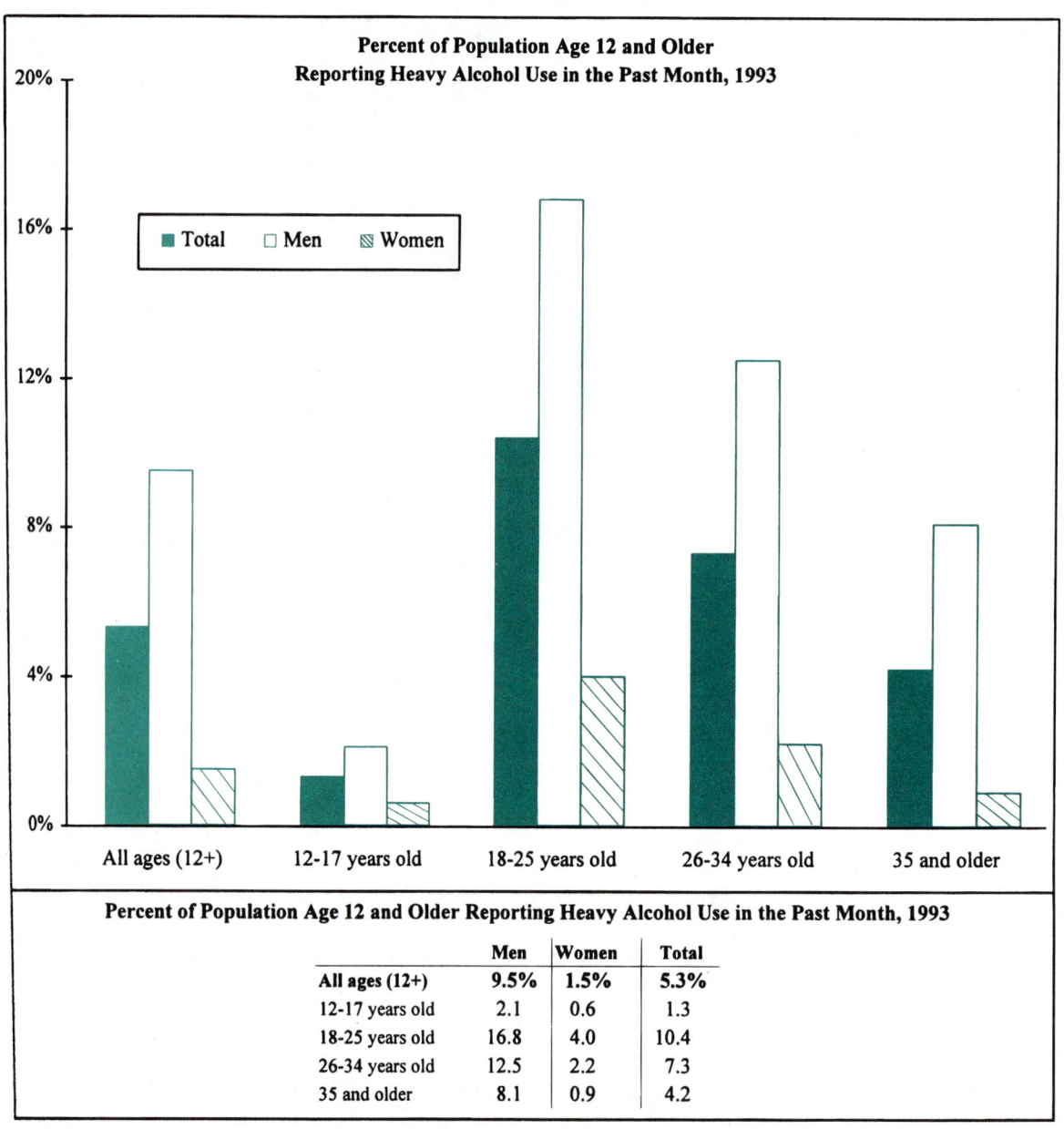

	Men	Women	Total
All ages (12+)	9.5%	1.5%	5.3%
12-17 years old	2.1	0.6	1.3
18-25 years old	16.8	4.0	10.4
26-34 years old	12.5	2.2	7.3
35 and older	8.1	0.9	4.2

Figure 17–2. Young adults ages 18 to 25 are the most likely to report heavy alcohol use in the past month. Men at all ages are more likely to be heavy drinkers. In the total population, men are six times more likely than women to report current heavy alcohol use. Past month heavy alcohol use is defined as drinking five or more drinks per day on each of five or more days in the last 30 days.

AGE

Box 17–3 lists the prevalence of alcohol and substance abuse. As seen in Figure 17–2, the highest prevalence of substance use and abuse is in the 18- to 24-year-old age group, particularly in white men. An abusive drinking pattern, known as *binge drinking*, is common in young adults and a major cause of serious health problems, accidents, and death.

Children of alcoholic parents have a fourfold higher rate of alcoholism than the general population, even if they are adopted and raised by nonalcoholic parents.[4]

GENDER

White males are two to three times more likely than females to become dependent on alcohol.[8] Women are more likely to start drinking later in life than men, but alcohol-related problems usually occur sooner and at lower levels of consumption, perhaps because of physiological differences.[8] After drinking an equal amount of alcohol, women have higher blood alcohol levels than men. In addition, a recent discovery suggests that women have about half the amount of a gastric enzyme, alcohol dehydrogenase, in their systems as men.[9] This enzyme helps to metabolize alcohol; a lower amount may allow more alcohol to circulate in their blood.

The natural history of alcoholism suggests a predictable pattern of alcohol use, particularly in men, over a period of time. Of those who develop alcohol dependence, many start drinking in their teens and experience their first major drinking-related life problems in their late 20s to early 30s.[4] Dependence evolves over an average of 10 years for men, with many periods of abstinence or marked decreases in drinking alternating with periods of drinking problems before they present for treatment in their 40s.[6] Women tend to begin abusing alcohol during periods of transition such as divorce or when they are in relationships with heavy drinkers.

Gender and culture influence alcohol abuse and its consequences. Rates of alcohol abstention are higher among both African-American men (30%) and women (49%) than among non-Hispanic whites. However, alcohol-related morbidity and mortality are significantly increased in African-American men because of alcohol-related liver diseases and esophageal cancer. Heavy alcohol consumption among African-American men is less common than in non-Hispanic whites but increases sharply in men in their 30s.[10]

Because 75% of all prescriptions are written for women, abuse and misuse of prescription drugs are slightly higher in women.[8]

Etiology

BIOLOGICAL THEORIES

Although the exact mechanisms that cause drug dependence are still unknown, recent research has centered on the effects of addictive substances on brain biology and physiology. Because this research is difficult to do in humans, many of the studies are conducted on animals. Animals self-administer the same drugs that have high abuse potential in humans. These drugs act as powerful reinforcers for behavior, similar to food and sex, presumably by providing a pleasurable sensation or mood state and leading to **psychological dependence.**

Alcoholics may lack an internal alarm to stop drinking. People who do not develop alcoholism have a built-in alarm that signals when to quit drinking. One or two drinks often

---

> **RESEARCH NOTE**
>
> Murphy, SA: Coping strategies of abstainers from alcohol up to three years post-treatment. Image J Nurs Sch 25:29–35, 1993.
>
> **Findings:** Little is known about the process involved in maintaining abstinence from alcohol use. The author followed 23 alcohol-dependent individuals for 3 years after treatment to better understand the experiences and coping strategies involved in maintaining abstinence. Using journals, interviews, and mailed questionnaires, the researcher collected data at 12, 18, and 36 months following treatment.
>
> The three aims of the study were to
> - Document the experiences over time of individuals with alcohol dependence who were abstaining from drinking.
> - Identify differences between men and women in managing the transition from drinker to nondrinker.
> - Examine the relevance of the transtheoretical model of change developed by Prochaska and DiClemente.
>
> The results of this study found support for the phases of change described in the transtheoretical model. Phase 1, *precontemplation*, found men reporting secret drinking, behavior usually attributed to women. Women reported that tragic life events contributed to drinking. Women were more likely than men to have spouses or partners who drank and encouraged them to resume drinking. The transition from treatment to home was described as an anxiety-provoking experience. Men were more likely than women to recall and use specific skills learned in treatment in highly stressful situations. Both men and women used other coping strategies including accepting responsibility, information seeking, problem solving, seeking and accepting social support, reframing issues, and positive reappraisal.
>
> **Application to Practice:** The experience of successful alcohol abstainers provides valuable information for nurses to assist clients in initiating and maintaining abstinence. Nurses need to be aware of the differences between men and women in maintaining sobriety, particularly the increased relapse risk caused by drinking spouses. This study suggests that nurses can encourage the early and continuous involvement of family during the ongoing phases of abstinence. Support use of the identified coping strategies employed in this study.

lead to a "high" or pleasant feelings, whereas several drinks depress the CNS and can lead to intoxication. Before intoxication, most individuals' alarms go off.

Addictive substances activate neurotransmitters in the mesolimbic *dopaminergic reward pathway*.[11] Stimulating this nerve pathway leads to the powerful reinforcing properties or "highs." When an addictive substance is absorbed and distributed to the brain, it alters the balance of neurotransmitters that modulate pleasure, pain, and reward.

Depending on the type of chemical taken, other neurotransmitter systems that perform a variety of functions are activated. These neurotransmitters include endogenous opioids, serotonin, norepinephrine, γ-aminobutyric acid (GABA), and glutamate. Once stimulated, they set off a cascade of other effects, such as changes in second messengers that may then affect gene expression.

Cocaine potently stimulates the dopamine reward pathway, as does methylphenidate. Other drugs of abuse affect particular neurotransmitters: nicotine stimulates nicotine receptors, marijuana stimulates cannabinoid receptors, hallucinogens stimulate serotonin receptors, and phencyclidine (PCP) and alcohol stimulate NMDA glutamate receptors.

IMAGING STUDIES

Chronic use of alcohol, sedative-hypnotics, antianxiety medications, marijuana, and inhalants decreases blood flow to the brain.[12] The reverse occurs during withdrawal, when blood flow "rebounds," or increases. Individuals with intense alcohol cravings have increased blood flow to the right side of the brain, particularly in the caudate nucleus.[13] These brain changes also occur when people have other compulsive behaviors such as in obsessive-compulsive disorder (OCD).

GENETIC THEORIES

Researchers have primarily studied people with alcoholism and family patterns of this dependence. Monozygotic (identical) twins have twice the concordance rate for alcoholism of nonidentical dizygotic twins. Adoption studies show that sons of alcoholics raised by adoptive parents became alcoholic more often than sons of nonalcoholics raised by adoptive parents.[14]

Current research suggests that genetic factors, interacting with environmental risks, contribute to alcoholism. There is evidence that young sons and daughters of alcoholics are more sensitive to the effects of alcohol; mood, motor performance, changes in hormones, and disturbances in brain wave patterns are evident (Figure 17–3).[15]

Genes that control certain liver enzymes also appear to play a role in how alcoholism is inherited. Two liver enzymes, aldehyde dehydrogenase (ALDH-2) and antidiuretic hormone (ADH), are more common in alcoholism. When these genes are inactive, people are less likely to develop alcoholism, and their presence predicts a greater risk for alcoholism.[16]

BEHAVIORAL THEORIES

Two behavioral models, *conditioning* and *homeostasis*, may explain abuse, relapse, and dependence. Environments or

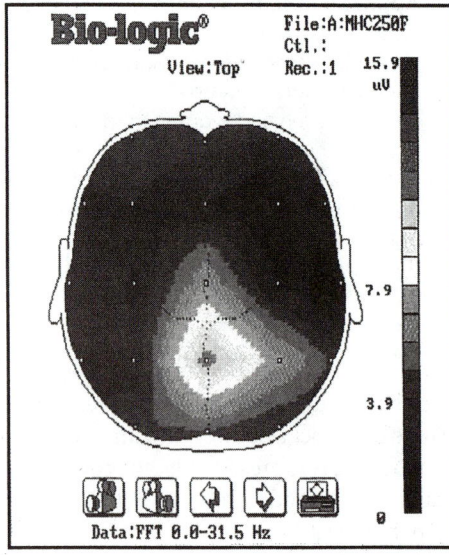

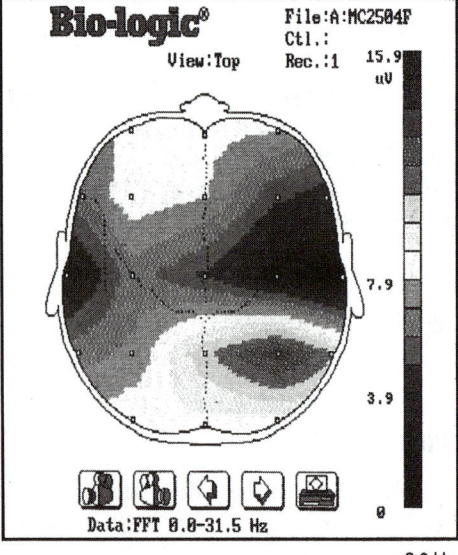

Figure 17–3. EEG topographic map of cocaine-induced alterations in EEG alpha activity. Data are from a representative subject while he was pushing the joystick indicating that he was feeling euphoric.

circumstances that are associated with past substance use may "condition" or reinforce continued drinking and drug abuse. To maintain a homeostatic balance, individuals may also continue to abuse substances; stopping the drug leads to withdrawal symptoms that lead to restarting the drug to reverse the symptoms. In both models, drug cravings "trigger" drug-seeking behavior similar to the way hunger stimulates eating.

Khatzian[17] proposed a self-medicating theory of substance dependence. He studied heroin and other opiate users and found that individuals took drugs to self-medicate emotional states rather than to get high. The choice of drug was not random but corresponded to seeking relief from unpleasant feelings. For example, some people use stimulant drugs to relieve and escape depressed mood.

Although there are probably several causes of drug dependence, genetic, twin, and outcome findings suggest that this syndrome is not just the result of a "general lack of control" or "moral weakness." Past experiences, family history, personality, and social context may interact to promote substance abuse.

Prognosis

Most of the research on substance-use disorders has focused on the effects of alcohol. Because it is legal and more widely used, more is known about the prognosis for alcohol-use disorder than other drug-use disorders. The prognosis for substance abuse is not as well understood because most individuals studied are in treatment for substance dependence. Substance abuse, most prevalent in adolescence and young adulthood, does not always progress to dependence. Some are able to cut back or curtail abusive patterns with minimal intervention or adverse consequences. Others will die because of its irresistible effects.

> ... never once did Terry give up the struggle to move from relapses back to sobriety. With her body crying out in pain for alcohol, her spirit longed for sobriety. Physically she got high temporarily on alcohol and then crashed into despair again. But the high her head and mind craved was simply to feel stable and secure. All the evidence and the testimony of her closest friends leave no doubt that Terry tried until the end to resist the powerful claims of her body against her spiritual longing for a sober, satisfying life. Her sister Susan had noted that Terry's journals tell of a valiant and perceptive nurturing of her soul even while her body was falling victim to alcoholism.
>
> GEORGE McGOVERN[7]

Substance dependence is a chronic illness characterized by frequent remissions and relapses to previous levels of substance abuse.[18] The highest success rates are for those who abstain from all psychoactive substances, have a strong desire to quit, and have previously functioned well. With consistent help, most alcoholics improve; 60 to 70% of the most stable will still be abstinent after 1 year.[4]

The longer the substance dependence, the poorer the prognosis; tolerance develops with continued use, requiring higher doses of the drug. Physical or mental deterioration occurs, along with possible overdose and death. Of those with heroin dependence, 25% die within 10 to 20 years of beginning use.[19] Death may also result from suicide, homicide, and infectious disease such as tuberculosis, hepatitis, and acquired immunodeficiency syndrome (AIDS). Individuals addicted to drugs and alcohol commit suicide at rates 15 to 20% higher than the general population.

RESEARCH NOTE

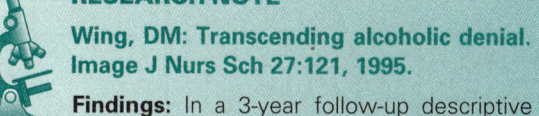

Wing, DM: Transcending alcoholic denial. Image J Nurs Sch 27:121, 1995.

Findings: In a 3-year follow-up descriptive study of 30 alcoholics, this researcher identified a theory of overcoming alcoholic denial in five progressive stages.

In stage I, clients reacting to a critical event began to transcend denial when they
- Ascribed meaning to the critical event that brought them into treatment
- Were able to alter their self-perception
- Related the event to their alcohol use.

When the relationship between the critical event and drinking was perceived, alcoholics moved into stage II, role disaffiliation. In this stage, altered self-perception resulted in feelings of fear and confusion. Strategies for coping with this ambiguity were initiating change and resigning. Individuals who resigned did not have faith in their ability to change and returned to active drinking.

Individuals who initiated change remained abstinent and moved into stage III, ambiguous anticipation. Properties of this stage included hope that life could be better without alcohol and a passive role in recovery.

In stage IV, peer affiliation, individuals allowed themselves to be vulnerable and listened to peer role models in recovery who confronted denial and reinforced that alcohol was a problem. Individuals who did not affiliate were characterized by isolating, distancing, and avoiding.

Stage V was marked by accepting the alcoholic identity, assuming personal responsibility for drinking problems, making a decision to stay sober, and identifying recovery goals that were more internally focused.

Application to Practice: This information provides nurses with a framework for understanding the process that overcoming denial entails. Those who successfully complete each stage progress to abstinence, whereas others may display behaviors suggestive of ongoing denial and relapse. Nurses can identify the stage clients are in and help them set realistic goals. Nurses can also set realistic expectations for themselves and their clients that allow a change in denial over time.

Percent of Population With a Substance Abuse Disorder, Mental Disorder, or Both Disorders in Lifetime, Age 15 to 54, 1991

Only Substance Abuse/Dependence 12.9%

Both Disorders 13.7%

Only Mental Disorder 21.4%

Percent of Population With Substance Abuse, Mental Disorder, or Both Disorders, Age 15 to 54, 1991

	Lifetime	Past Year
Any Substance Abuse or Mental Disorder	48.0%	29.5%
Only Substance Abuse/Dependence	12.9	6.6
Only Mental Disorder	21.4	18.2
Both Substance Abuse and Mental Disorder	13.7	4.7

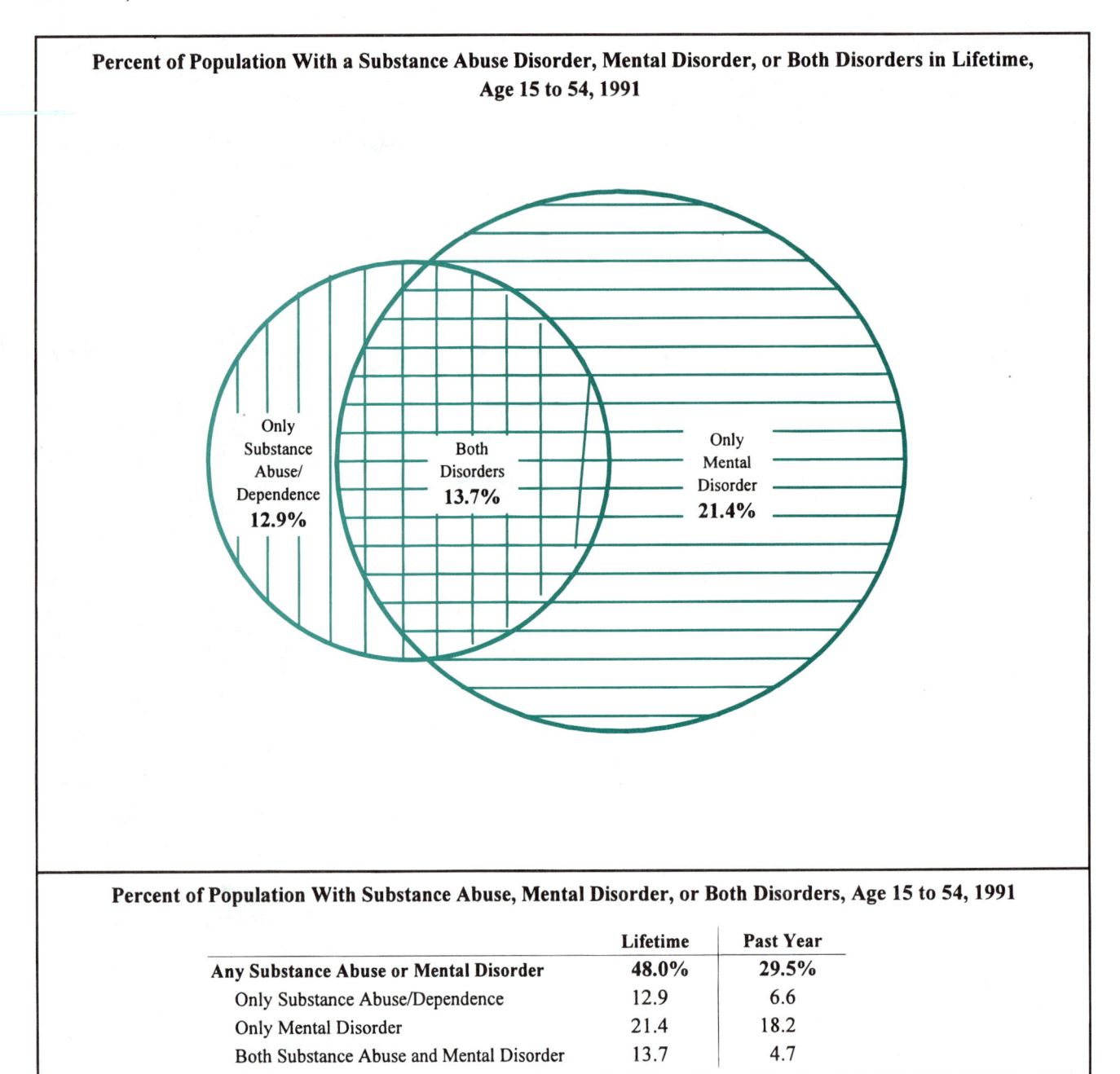

Figure 17–4. About 14% of the population, ages 15 to 54, has had both substance abuse/dependence and a mental disorder in their lifetime. About 5% had both disorders in the past year, according to the National Comorbidity Survey conducted in 1991.

Individuals with substance abuse and dependence commonly have other psychiatric conditions. As seen in Figure 17–4, about 29.5% of the population has a lifetime prevalence of both substance-related and mental disorders.

Assessment

Nurses, because they work in a variety of community and hospital settings, are often the ones to recognize and intervene with clients who exhibit early signs of substance abuse. They are also more sensitive to the health implications of nicotine use. Assessment should include screening for other substances, including prescription, OTC, legal, and illegal drugs. Early detection and intervention may prevent the harmful physical and psychosocial problems associated with dependence.

As the first step, take a thorough history to detect patterns of social, emotional, physical, and behavioral changes or difficulties associated with substance use. Comprehensive assessment includes recognizing early behavioral and physical signs, understanding laboratory test values, and learning community resources for treatment referrals.

The client's report of substance use may affect the accuracy of the history. Clients often minimize or deny the extent of their use and the resulting problems. Many blame others for their current or past vocational, relational, or legal problems rather than recognizing that these problems arise from drug addiction. Be aware of what the client is trying to avoid. When possible, use objective tools and information from family, friends, and coworkers. Focus on substance use, not the client, as the source of the problem.

Discuss what measures you will take to safeguard confidentiality; clients and family members are often reluctant to disclose sensitive information, particularly if the substances are illegal or disclosure might compromise relationships or their work. Know the specific state and institutional reporting requirements and confidentiality laws.

SHORT ALCOHOL AND DRUG HISTORY

As with all nursing assessments, take a straightforward, nonjudgmental approach to elicit accurate information. Begin with "how" rather than "why" questions; start with "How did that affect you?" rather than "Why did you drink?" Clients may see "why" questions as judgmental and become defensive. Tactfully pursue possible substance use even if the client becomes defensive or avoids questions.

Incorporate the following questions about alcohol and drug use into a routine, nonthreatening inquiry about health habits, smoking, or caffeine beverage consumption:

- How often do you use alcohol and other drugs? Include the names of groups, OTCs, prescription drugs, and street drugs.
- How much do you usually use? Give amounts such as the number of joints, ounces per glass, or number of pills at what dosage.
- Have you ever used alcohol or drugs more that you use them now? When? Under what circumstances did you use drugs more heavily?

If you suspect that the client is dependent on drugs or alcohol, ask the following:

- How much do you use, and what are the effects?
- Do you have any withdrawal symptoms?
- Have you ever lost control when you drink or use drugs?
- Have you ever tried to stop using this drug on your own?
- How have you done it? What happened?
- Do you spend much time thinking about drugs or trying not to get caught?

SCREENING TOOLS

A number of brief screening tools can help detect alcohol abuse or dependence. The easiest to remember and administer is the CAGE[20,21] (Table 17–4). Administer the CAGE, particularly in primary care and medical settings.[22] This tool measures lifetime consumption and is easy to remember. A positive response to two or more questions suggests a high possibility of alcohol dependence and requires further assessment.

The Short Michigan Alcoholism Screening Test (SMAST), listed in Table 17–5, is a well-validated screening instrument for detecting alcohol dependence. Its 13 items examine drinking patterns as well as the consequences of drinking.[23]

TABLE 17–4. CAGE Screening Test for Alcoholism

1. Have you ever felt you ought to **C**ut down on your drinking?
2. Have people **A**nnoyed you by criticizing your drinking?
3. Have you ever felt bad or **G**uilty about your drinking?
4. Have you ever had a drink first thing in the morning to steady your nerves or get rid of a hangover? (**E**yeopener)

Scoring: One positive response warrants further evaluation. Two positive responses suggest a high possibility of alcohol dependence and require further assessment.

Source: Ewing, J: Detecting alcoholism: The CAGE questionnaire. JAMA 252:1905–1907, 1984 with permission. Copyright 1984, The American Medical Association.

TABLE 17–5. Short Michigan Alcoholism Screening Test (SMAST)

1. Do you feel you are a normal drinker? (Do you drink less than or as much as most other people?) (No)
2. Does your wife, husband, a parent, or other near relative ever worry or complain about your drinking? (Yes)
3. Do you ever feel guilty about your drinking? (Yes)
4. Are you able to stop drinking when you want to? (No)
5. Do friends or relatives think you are a normal drinker? (No)
6. Have you ever attended a meeting of Alcoholics Anonymous? (Yes)
7. Has drinking ever created problems between you and your wife, husband, parent, or other near relatives? (Yes)
8. Have you ever gotten into trouble at work because of drinking? (Yes)
9. Have you ever neglected your obligations, your family, or your work for 2 or more days in a row because you were drinking? (Yes)
10. Have you ever gone to anyone for help about your drinking? (Yes)
11. Have you ever been arrested for drunken driving, driving while intoxicated, or driving under the influence of alcoholic beverages? (Yes)
12. Have you ever been arrested, even for a few hours, because of other drunken behavior? (Yes)

Scoring: Alcoholism-indicating responses are in parentheses; 3+ points place individuals in an "alcoholic" category; 2 points suggest a problem for further evaluation; <1 is nonalcoholic.

Source: Journal of Studies on Alcohol, vol. 36, pp. 117–126, 1975. Copyright by Journal of Studies on Alcohol, Inc., Rutgers Center of Alcohol Studies, New Brunswick, NJ 08093.

TABLE 17–6. Drug Abuse Screening Test (DAST-10)

The following questions concern information about your possible involvement with drugs *not including alcoholic beverages* during the past 12 months.

In the statements, "drug abuse" refers (1) to the use of prescribed or OTC drugs in excess of the directions and (2) to any nonmedical use of drugs. The various classes of drugs may include cannabis, solvents, antianxiety drugs, sedative-hypnotics, cocaine, stimulants, hallucinogens, and narcotics. Remember that the questions *do not include alcoholic beverages.*

These questions refer to the past 12 months.

1. Have you used drugs other than those required for medical purposes? Yes _____ No _____
2. Do you abuse more than one drug at a time? Yes _____ No _____
3. Are you always able to stop using drugs when you want to? Yes _____ No _____
4. Have you had "blackouts" or "flashbacks" as a result of drug use? Yes _____ No _____
5. Do you ever feel bad or guilty about your drug use? Yes _____ No _____
6. Does your spouse (or parents) ever complain about your involvement with drugs? Yes _____ No _____
7. Have you neglected your family because of your use of drugs? Yes _____ No _____
8. Have you engaged in illegal activities in order to obtain drugs? Yes _____ No _____
9. Have you ever experienced withdrawal symptoms (felt sick) when you stopped taking drugs? Yes _____ No _____
10. Have you ever had medical problems as a result of your drug use (e.g., memory loss, hepatitis, convulsions, bleeding, etc.)? Yes _____ No _____

Scoring: 1 positive response warrants further evaluation.
Source: Skinner, HA: Drug Abuse Screening Test (DAST), copyright 1982, p. 363, with kind permission from Elsevier Science Ltd, The Boulevard, Langford Lance, Kidlington OX5, United Kingdom.

Table 17–6, the Drug Abuse Screening Test (DAST-10), screens for other drug abuse. It is designed to quantify the extent of involvement with drugs.[24] A positive score to one or more questions warrants further assessment.

FAMILY AND SIGNIFICANT OTHERS

Whenever possible, interview family members and significant others to increase the validity of the assessment. Family, friends, or coworkers can be an excellent source of corroborating or getting additional information. However, family members may also minimize or deny problems, partly because of their own problems with drugs or out of fear. Sometimes clients are more open if they are aware that others are participating in the assessment.

PHYSICAL FINDINGS AND MENTAL STATUS EXAMINATION

Suspect possible substance abuse in a client who presents with bruises, burns, or other injuries. Inspect skin on the arms for evidence of scarring, sores, or abrasions for intravenous drug use. Check nasal passages for ulceration from snorting drugs. Note signs of sepsis, nutritional deficiency, or poor hygiene.

Focus the mental status examination on detecting signs of acute intoxication, withdrawal, and delirium. Depressed respirations, tachycardia, hypertension, and sleepiness may signal acute overdose.

LABORATORY FINDINGS

Toxicology testing for drugs of abuse can be an important component of the assessment. Suggest drug screens for suspected or possible drug overdose, during routine examinations of clients with acute mental status changes, and in suspected drug or alcohol problems. Toxicology screening may reveal important information; for example, the client who abuses cocaine may also abuse "downers." However, not all drugs of abuse are detected. To accurately understand the results, one must know when the client's last use probably occurred, the drug's rate of metabolism, and the type of screening used. Toxic screens do not detect inhalant use, and alcohol is detected only within a few hours of ingestion. Blood alcohol levels detect recent alcohol use, but not dependence.

Depending on factors such as number of drinks ingested, blood alcohol levels help establish the degree of intoxication. Table 17–7 lists different blood alcohol levels, the number of drinks commonly associated with each level, and associated behavior signs and symptoms.

> Newspapers reported that a famous 19-year-old woman was arrested following a motor vehicle accident. Her car went off the road and struck a tree. Her blood alcohol level (BAL) was 0.15, well above the legal and physical level of intoxication for a young adult. She later told the press that she had had 3 to 4 drinks, each of which had 3 different types of liquor, the equivalent of 9 to 12 drinks. However, she insisted she was not drunk.

TABLE 17–7. Blood Alcohol Level (BAL) and Common Signs and Symptoms*

BAL	Number of Drinks	Signs and Symptoms
0.02–0.05%	1–3	Impaired mentation and sensory function, decreased coordination, euphoria, changes in mood and behavior
0.100–0.199%	4–6	Ataxia, decreased mentation, slurred speech, impaired judgment, labile mood, impaired driving
0.200–0.299%	7–10	Extreme ataxia, poor judgment, nausea and vomiting, double vision
0.300–0.399%	11–17	Cold clammy skin, heavy breathing, amnesia, anesthesia
0.400–0.499%	18–25	Respiratory failure, coma
0.5%	25–30	Death

*Varies with levels of tolerance, gender, amount of time between drinks, ingestion of food, etc. BAL measures only current alcohol use.

Because other biochemical tests used as screening markers of heavy, regular alcohol use are limited by problems with sensitivity and specificity, a combination of laboratory tests may be most useful. Table 17–8 lists laboratory tests that may indicate heavy alcohol use.

TABLE 17–8. Laboratory Tests That May Indicate Heavy Alcohol Use*

GGT (γ-glutamyltransferase)	Plasma enzyme up to 6 times higher than normal in individuals who consume more than 3 g/kg of body weight Normal limits: Men, 8–38U/L Women, 5–29 U/L (under 45 years of age)
MCV (mean corpuscular volume)	Increases in response to prolonged heavy drinking Normal limits: 86–98 μm³
AST (aspartate aminotransferase; formerly called SGOT)	Liver enzymes that increase in response to excessive alcohol intake
ALT (alanine aminotransferase; formerly called SGPT)	Normal limits: AST, 0.35 U/L ALT, 0.35 U/L

*All laboratory tests are subject to false negatives and false positives.

Planning Care

Substance disorders adversely affect social, emotional, physical, and spiritual functioning. Plan care based on the client's current level of functioning, nursing and medical diagnoses, the holistic assessment, past and current substance use, past history, social support, housing, and employment.

In planning care for clients who are intoxicated or withdrawing from substances, physiological and safety needs are the first priority to avoid injury or medical complications.

Confront and question ineffective coping related to denial of a substance-use problem. Encourage the family and healthy peers, if possible, to confront the client's inability or unwillingness to acknowledge problems. Suggest that clients participate in treatment programs and self-help or peer recovery groups. Both techniques, confrontation and support groups, may help break through denial.

Assist clients who are able to admit they have a problem to set realistic and attainable goals such as staying sober "one day at a time." Help them identify existing community resources, including individual or group psychotherapy. Give positive feedback for initial and continued efforts toward abstinence. Focus on identified strengths, and help the client build self-esteem. Maintain a supportive attitude toward recovery.

Whether treatment is effective depends on the severity of the client's substance-use disorder, the readiness of the client to seek help, and the type of services and setting needed. Assessment and referral are minimum nursing interventions. Use the levels of care for substance dependence, approved by the American Society on Addiction Medicine:[25]

- Level 6: a medically managed chemical dependency unit in a general hospital for clients with a medical or psychiatric diagnosis sufficient for hospitalization. These clients have dual diagnoses of drug dependence plus another serious illness.
- Level 5: a medically supervised residential treatment facility that is located in either a hospital step-down unit or in a residential alcohol and drug treatment facility. Though there is on-call health provider availability, medically or psychologically unstable clients are not treated.
- Level 4: an intensive partial hospitalization setting where the client attends structured programming for 20 hours a week but lives elsewhere.
- Level 3: less intensive contact several times per week, usually 6 to 12 hours for 1 to 3 months, often at night after work.
- Level 2: traditional outpatient contact that might be 1 to 4 hours per month for several months.
- Level 1: peer assistance in Alcoholics Anonymous (AA) or Narcotics Anonymous (NA) without any professional help. Appropriate referral is based on the presence or absence of medical problems, psychiatric problems, detoxification problems, a supportive environment, insight, and the likelihood of relapse.

Clients who are willing to attempt abstinence as a treatment goal require attention to their need for detoxification based on the presence or absence of impending withdrawal symptoms and past history of withdrawal. Referral is based on the level of care needed, and most clients can accomplish withdrawal without any special medical intervention. However, between 4% and 8% of alcohol-dependent clients are at risk for life-threatening withdrawal.[4] These clients would benefit from referral to a level 5 placement.

Further referrals are based on whether the client has a job, residence, and financial or insurance resources to pay for treatment. A client who is employed and married and has low risk for withdrawal might be managed as an outpatient with individual or marital counseling and AA. A client who has no job or family and a long history of drug use or relapses, however, would benefit from placement in a drug-free environment, such as a therapeutic community setting that provides skill training in the areas of work and social relations. A client who has a problem with a drug like heroin and is unwilling to abstain may be referred to a methadone-maintenance treatment program is warranted. At the same time, the nurse can educate the client about the risk factors for AIDS and hepatitis and give information about blood-borne diseases.

Interventions for Hospitalized Clients

ACUTE INTOXICATION

Prioritize interventions based on current health problems. Monitor cardiovascular, respiratory, and neurological functioning, including levels of consciousness, vital signs, toxicology reports, and intake and output. Assess self-harm potential, particularly if the client's drug use was aimed at suicide. Implement suicide precautions if necessary.

> Michael G, a 52-year-old divorced man, was admitted for his sixth detoxification from alcohol and was well known to the staff. The nurses checked his vital signs every 15 minutes. They found that he was confused and disoriented for time and place but otherwise cooperative with care. However, between checks, he managed to put a "belt around his neck and attach it to his bed." The nurse found him hanging from the side of his bed, moaning, cyanotic, and semicomatose.

Create an accepting and supportive environment. Strive to be nonjudgmental in all interactions to minimize anxiety or agitation. Stay with the client if possible, and assess for any potential for violence. Avoid restraints; clients may see them as threatening and react with negative behavior. Communicate with a soothing tone of voice and a nonthreatening posture. Orient the client to place, time, and person. Continuously monitor for signs of impending withdrawal. After the client is physiologically stable, assess the severity of the substance-abuse problems and levels of acceptance for referral.

It can be uncomfortable to work with clients with substance abuse and dependence. Nevertheless, outcomes are generally more favorable in an empathic environment. Conversely, client outcomes suffer when nurses and therapists confront clients in an aggressive manner. Effective communication includes being confrontational, directive, and empathic at the same time.[26] Examine your own awareness, biases, past experiences, and attitudes regarding substance use. If ignored, these feelings may lead to more aggressive responses and get in the way of providing effective nursing care.

> Mary, a second-year nursing student, was assigned to care for Robert K during his hospitalization after overdosing on alcohol and opioids. Mary found it difficult to make eye contact with him and busied herself with tasks outside his room rather than attend to his current care needs. Her nursing instructor noticed Mary's unusual avoidance. She helped Mary identify her reactions and stereotypes; Mary had a grandfather with alcoholism who would get angry and violent while drinking. Her family never dealt with the problem and instead always "walked on eggshells." Her reaction was to avoid and distrust her grandfather; she was also now avoiding Robert K. The instructor helped Mary talk about her attitudes and beliefs about substance abuse. She clarified Mary's misperceptions, identified areas for additional education, and suggested she observe an AA meeting. Mary was then able to interact in a therapeutic way with the client and established an empathic, nonjudgmental relationship with him.

ACUTE WITHDRAWAL

Nursing interventions are similar to those used in acute intoxication. However, specific interventions are based on the type of drug withdrawal. Table 17–9 lists the withdrawal symptoms of depressants, opioids, and stimulants and the corresponding nursing interventions.

After the client is medically stable, share the results of the assessment. Gather sufficient data and confront the client about the identified problem. Language is important; avoid such terms such as "addict" or "alcoholic." Emphasize the problem behavior, such as "heavy drinking" or "problem drug use." Express concern about substance use, regardless of the certainty of the data to support it. Highlight the client's presenting problems such as insomnia, anxiety, marital discord, or fatigue, as well as the health risks associated with continued substance use.

If the client denies a problem, attempt to continue to establish rapport in a nonjudgmental manner. Avoid colluding with the client to deny, avoid, or minimize the actual or potential problems. Avoid arguments. Role play an empathic confrontation with peers to develop confrontational skills. Remember that one interaction may not change drug use but may provide a positive experience for the client to build on.

TABLE 17–9. Withdrawal Symptoms and Nursing Actions

Substance	Withdrawal Symptoms	Nursing Actions
Depressants *Alcohol* Mild. Begins within hours, lasts up to 48 hours after last drink	Mild. Insomnia, irritability, anxiety, headache, mild gastrointestinal distress, mild hypertension, and tremulousness Moderate. Tachycardia, mild fever, sweating, nausea, vomiting, photophobia, and marked tremor	Monitor vital signs and behaviors using alcohol withdrawal scale (e.g., CIWA-Ar: seek and order for medication if score >10), promote rest and sleep, keep environment quiet, assess mental status, orient client as needed, medicate client as ordered, remain with client, offer fluids and light foods during periods of lucidity
Severe. Occurs within the 1st week after stopping or reducing heavy alcohol intake	Severe. Tachycardia, elevated blood pressure, excessive sweating, difficulty sustaining attention, clouding of consciousness, disorientation, hallucinations, seizures, delirium	Maintain quiet, nonstimulating environment, institute seizure precautions, administer anticonvulsant or other medication as ordered
Sedative-Hypnotics, Antianxiety Drugs Withdrawal begins 12–24 h with the shorter-acting drugs; withdrawal from longer-acting drugs peaks at days 5–8	Anxiety, tremors, insomnia, nightmares, irritability, anorexia, nausea, vomiting, hypotension, seizures, delirium, hyperexia, generalized malaise, tachycardia, coarse tremors, excessive sweating, confusion, and hallucinations	Monitor vital signs and behaviors, remain with client, promote rest and sleep, offer fluids and light foods, administer cross-tolerant medication as needed, institute seizure precautions
Opioids Early withdrawal begins 8–10 h after last dose; short-acting opioid withdrawal reaches peak 36–72 h after last dose, acute symptoms subside by the 5th day; longer-acting opioid withdrawal symptoms start 2–3 days after last dose, peak 4–6 days with symptoms up to 10–12 days	Yawning, insomnia, restlessness, abdominal cramps, diarrhea, anorexia, anxiety, craving, dysphoria, fatigue, headache, goose bumps, hot and cold flashes, irritability, rhinorrhea, lacrimation, muscle spasms, diaphoresis, increased blood pressure, increased pulse, low-grade fever, mydriasis, muscle spasms, nausea and vomiting	Monitor vital signs and behaviors, remain with client, offer fluids and light foods, keep environment quiet and nondistracting, medicate client as ordered
Stimulants *Amphetamines* *Cocaine* "Crash" phase usually occurs between 9 and 96 h after last use	Depressive feelings, high drug craving, fatigue with desire for sleep, agitation, paranoia, insomnia or hypersomnia	Promote sleep and rest, monitor vital signs, assess mental status, provide calming support if client is agitated, remain with client if frightened or disoriented, orient client to reality as needed
Nicotine Symptoms begin 30–40 minutes after last use and diminish by 1 mo except for craving, and increased appetite, which can last for 6 mo or more	Withdrawal characterized by craving, irritability, anxiety, restlessness, insomnia, increased appetite, difficulty concentrating	Support and encourage behavioral approaches to avoiding triggers to smoking

TABLE 17–10. Addiction Research Foundation Clinical Institute Withdrawal Assessment for Alcohol (CIWA-Ar)

Patient _____ Date /___/___/___/ y m d	Time _____;_____ (24 hour clock, midnight = 00:00)

NAUSEA AND VOMITING—As "Do you feel sick to your stomach? Have you vomited?" Observation
0 no nausea and no vomiting
1 mild nausea with no vomiting
2
3
4 intermittent nausea with dry heaves
5
6
7 constant nausea, frequent dry heaves and vomiting

TREMOR—Arms extended and fingers spread apart. Observation
0 no tremor
1 not visible, but can be felt fingertip to fingertip
2
3
4 moderate, with patient's arms extended
5
6
7 severe, even with arms not extended

PAROXYSMAL SEATS—Observation
0 no sweat visible
1 barely perceptible sweating, palms moist
2
3
4 beads of sweat obvious on forehead
5
6
7 drenching sweats

ANXIETY—Ask "Do you feel nervous?" Observation
0 no anxiety, at ease
1 mild anxiety
2
3
4 moderately anxious, or guarded, so anxiety is inferred
5
6
7 equivalent to acute anxiety states as seen in severe delirium or acute schizophrenic reaction

AGITATION—Observation
0 normal activity
1 somewhat more than normal activity
2
3
4 moderately fidgety and restless
5
6
7 paces back and forth during most of the interview, or constantly thrashes about

TACTILE DISTURBANCES—Ask "Have you any itching, pins-and-needles sensation, any burning, any numbness, or do you feel bugs crawling on or under your skin?" Observation
0 none
1 very mild itching, pins and needles, burning or numbness
2 mild itching, pins and needles, burning or numbness
3 moderate itching, pins and needles, burning or numbness
4 moderately severe hallucinations
5 severe hallucinations
6 extremely severe hallucinations
7 continuous hallucinations

AUDITORY DISTURBANCES—Ask "Are you more aware of sounds around you? Are they harsh? Do they frighten you? Are you hearing anything that is disturbing to you? Are you hearing things you know are not there?" Observation
0 not present
1 very mild harshness or ability to frighten
2 mild harshness or ability to frighten
3 moderate mild harshness or ability to frighten
4 moderately severe hallucinations
5 severe hallucinations
6 extremely severe hallucinations
7 continuous hallucinations

VISUAL DISTURBANCES—Ask "Does the light appear to be too bright? Is its color different? Does it hurt your eyes? Are you seeing anything that is disturbing to you? Are you seeing things you know are not there?" Observation
0 not present
1 very mild sensitivity
2 mild sensitivity
3 moderate sensitivity
4 moderately severe hallucinations
5 severe hallucinations
6 extremely severe hallucinations
7 continuous hallucinations

HEADACHE, FULLNESS IN HEAD—Ask "Does your head feel different? Does it feel like there is a band around your head?" Do not rate for dizziness or lightheadedness. Otherwise, rate severity.
0 not present
1 very mild
2 mild
3 moderate
4 moderately severe
5 severe
6 very severe
7 extremely severe

ORIENTATION AND CLOUDING OF THE SENSORIUM—Ask "What day is this? Where are you? Who am I?"
0 oriented and can do serial additions
1 cannot do serial additions or is uncertain about date
2 disoriented by date by no more than 2 calendar days
3 disoriented by date by more than 2 calendar days
4 disoriented for place or person

Total CIWA-A Score _____
Rater's Initials _____
Maximum Possible Score 67

Source: Sullivan, JT, et al: Assessment of alcohol withdrawal: The revised clinical institute withdrawal assessment for alcohol scale (CIWA-Ar). Brit J of Addiction 84:1353, 1989.

Depressants

Alcohol. When alcoholic drinking is stopped or reduced, a characteristic withdrawal syndrome often occurs. Insomnia, irritability, anxiety, headache, mild gastrointestinal distress, mild hypertension, and tremulousness occur in mild withdrawal, beginning within hours. Symptoms may be delayed for several days if the individual has taken longer-acting depressant drugs. Severe withdrawal may lead to a medical emergency, delirium tremors or *DTs*; 15% will die if untreated.

Paul V, a 50-year-old self-employed, married lawyer, was hospitalized for surgical repair of his hip that was fractured in a fall. The surgical repair was uncomplicated until 3 days after surgery when he became agitated, diaphoretic, disoriented to time and place, and was seen talking to himself as he tried to climb out of bed and walk. His pulse was 120, and his blood pressure was elevated. After the nurse gathered more information about suspected alcohol abuse from his family and friends, he was diagnosed with severe alcohol withdrawal delirium.

As shown in Table 17-10, alcohol withdrawal symptoms can be measured with the Revised Clinical Institute Withdrawal Scale (CIWA-Ar).[27] This 10-item scale contains criteria that rate the severity of the client's withdrawal at regular intervals.

Benzodiazepine and Sedative-Hypnotic Withdrawal. This type of withdrawal is unpleasant and potentially life-threatening. Symptoms are similar to alcohol withdrawal.

Opioids. Naturally occurring opioids such as opium, morphine, and codeine, semisynthetic opioid derivatives such as heroin, dihydromorphine and dihydrocodeine, and synthetic opioids such as methadone and meperidine are all capable of creating physical dependency and may require detoxification if they were taken in sufficient quantities over a period of time. Less than 3 weeks of daily administration can produce dependence.[28] Clients with chronic pain may become dependent on narcotics after a few weeks of regular use. The more rapidly metabolized the drug, such as heroin, the more severe the withdrawal syndrome.

Stimulants

Cessation of stimulant abuse does not produce a physiological withdrawal syndrome similar to that of depressants or opioids. A "crash" phase usually occurs between 9 and 96 hours after the last use of a high-dose stimulant. Self-medication with depressant drugs such as alcohol and benzodiazepines is common during this phase.

Interventions for Clients in the Community

I didn't join Alcoholics Anonymous. I didn't seek out other help. I just stopped. My goal was provisional and modest; 1 month without drinking. For the first few weeks, this wasn't easy. I had to break the habits of a lifetime. But I did some mechanical things. I created a mantra for myself, saying over and over again, I will live my life from now on, I will not perform it. I began to type pages of private notes, reminding myself that writers were rememberers, and I had already forgotten material for twenty novels. I urged myself to live in a state of complete consciousness, even when that meant pain or boredom.

PETE HAMILL[3]

There is no one treatment that is most effective to quit alcohol or drugs. Brief interventions aimed at reducing substance intake, social skills training, self-control training, stress management, and self-help groups can be useful.[26]

BRIEF INTERVENTIONS

Brief interventions are often helpful for changing the drinking behaviors of individuals who have symptoms of alcohol abuse without dependence. Discuss specific findings from the nursing assessment. Educate clients about the relationship between clinical findings, health problems, and abuse.

The typical elements of a brief intervention for alcohol abuse are represented by the acronym FRAMES:[29]

Feedback regarding a client's drinking that is individualized and objective
Responsibility placed on the client for deciding what to do regarding drinking
Advice to change given
Menu of interventions and options for change presented, including a willingness to negotiate the goals of change
Empathetic style of counseling
Self-efficacy emphasized.

COGNITIVE-BEHAVIOR THERAPY

Self-control Training

Self-control training interventions educate clients with mild to moderate alcohol abuse about the risks of heavy alcohol consumption and how to establish safe moderate levels of drinking.[30–32] Cognitive-behavior theories are the basis for these interventions; alcohol problems are learned behaviors that can be changed. The goal is drinking in moderation. This approach requires continued care in case clients cannot cut back their drinking. The goal is to maintain contact, while emphasizing their responsibility for their actions. The safe drinking guidelines in Box 17-4 are key.

Social Skills Training

Social skills training focuses on teaching clients how to form and maintain interpersonal relationships. It includes the communication skills of listening, problem solving, and assertiveness. Social skills training is usually conducted in groups and accompanies other treatment interventions.

> **Box 17-4. Safe Drinking Guidelines.**[31,32]
>
> **Men:** No more than 2 to 3 drinks* a day (any 24-hour period), 3 days a week; or no more than 2 drinks daily, no more than 12 drinks per week.
>
> **Women:** No more than 1 to 2 drinks a day, no more than 3 days a week; or 1 drink per day, no more than 9 drinks per week.
>
> **Note:** These guidelines must be adapted downward with pregnant women, individuals debilitated by other illnesses, or for those who take other psychoactive drugs.
>
> *One drink = 4 oz of wine, 12 oz of beer, or 1.5 oz of 80-proof beverage.

Stress Management and Other Techniques

Nurses can teach stress management techniques to help individuals reduce tension and manage stress. This approach usually includes relaxation strategies, systematic desensitization to stressors, and cognitive strategies. The client learns how to manage personal responses to stress situations and how to make changes in the external environment.

Other cognitive-behavior interventions include contracting for sobriety, external monitoring of abstinence through urine or blood toxicology screenings, and monitoring laboratory tests in alcohol-abusing clients. Job or legal sanctions may require some clients to receive this type of monitoring. Abstinence is the goal; a comprehensive treatment plan is necessary.

Self-Help Groups

Twelve-Step Programs: AA and NA. Although they are not treatment programs per se, AA and NA are self-help groups that often hold meetings in treatment centers. Many treatment centers follow a Minnesota Model of treatment—that is, a model of care stressing abstinence and the 12 steps. Both AA and NA are successful for many people, and meetings are held daily in most cities and weekly in small towns. Anyone with a desire to stop drinking or taking drugs is welcome. Their philosophy is based on recovery through the support of the fellowship and the 12-step program. Table 17–11 outlines these steps; they stress "powerlessness" over chemicals and turning individuals' "will over to a power greater than ourselves." The belief "Once an alcoholic, always an alcoholic" is central. Key slogans reflect aspects of stress management and psychological support: living "one day at a time," "easy does it," and "let go and let God." After members become sober, they begin sponsoring other new members. This offer of support from someone who is also recovering is vital to the program. Regular attendance at meetings is also essential. Evidence suggests that AA and NA are helpful to many; however, more research is needed.

TABLE 17–11. The Twelve Steps and Twelve Traditions of Alcoholics Anonymous

Twelve Steps of Alcoholics Anonymous

1. We admitted we were powerless over alcohol, that our lives had become unmanagable.
2. Came to believe that a Power greater than ourselves could restore us to sanity.
3. Made a decision to turn our wills and lives over to the care of God as we understood Him.
4. Made a searching and fearless moral inventory of ourselves.
5. Admitted to God, to ourselves, and to another human being the exact nature of our wrongs.
6. Were entirely ready to have God remove all these defects of character.
7. Humbly asked Him to remove our shortcomings.
8. Made a list of all persons we had harmed, and became willing to make amends to them all.
9. Made direct amends to such people whenever possible, except when to do so would injure them or others.
10. Continued to take personal inventory and when we were wrong promptly admitted it.
11. Sought through prayer and meditation to improve our conscious contact with God as we understood Him, praying only for knowledge of His will for us and the power to carry that out.
12. Having had a spiritual awakening as a result of these steps, we tried to carry this message to alcoholics and to practice these principles in all our affairs.

The Twelve Traditions of Alcoholics Anonymous

1. Our common welfare should come first; personal recovery depends upon AA unity.
2. For our group purpose, there is but one ultimate authority—a loving God as He may express himself in our group conscience. Our leaders are but trusted servants; they do not govern.
3. The only requirement for AA membership is a desire to stop drinking.
4. Each group should be autonomous except in matters affecting other groups or AA as a whole.
5. Each group has but one primary purpose—to carry its message to the alcoholic who still suffers.
6. An AA group ought never endorse, finance, or lend the AA name to any related facility or outside enterprise, lest problems of money, property, and prestige divert us from our primary purpose.
7. Every AA group ought to be fully self-supporting, declining outside contributions.
8. Alcoholics Anonymous should remain forever nonprofessional, but our service centers may employ special workers.
9. AA, as such, ought never be organized; but we may create service boards or committees directly responsible to those they serve.
10. Alcoholics Anonymous has no opinion on outside issues; hence the AA name ought never be drawn into public controversy.

Continued on following page

TABLE 17–11. The Twelve Steps and Twelve Traditions of Alcoholics Anonymous (Continued)

11. Our public relations policy is based on attraction rather than promotion; we need always maintain personal anonymity at the level of press, radio, and films.
12. Anonymity is the spiritual foundation of all our traditions, ever reminding us to place principles before personalities.

Source: The Twelve Steps and Twelve Traditions are reprinted with permission of Alcoholics Anonymous World Services, Inc. Permission to reprint the Twelve Steps and Twelve Traditions does not mean that AA has reviewed or approved the contents of this publications, nor that AA is a program of recovery from alcoholism only—use of the Twelve repatterned after AA, but which address other problems, or in any other non-AA context, does not imply otherwise. Steps and Twelve Traditions in connection with programs and activities which are patterned after AA, but which address other problems, does not imply otherwise.

LONG-TERM SUBSTANCE DEPENDENCE

Because substance-use disorders are chronic, clients may have several episodes of relapse alternating with abstinence. Assess where each client is in the course of his or her illness and continue to work empathically toward mutual goal setting to change behavior. Use the clinical management tips listed in Table 17–12.

> *I've now been sober for a year. Again. Coke, pills, vodka, those were my drugs. Coke to get high, downers to sleep at night, and vodka to "party." I started in high school. I guess you could say I was a bad kid. I didn't realize it until later, but my family life stunk. My dad would beat me when he got drunk, my mom would go off and not deal with anything, and us kids were left on our own. I ran away when I was sixteen. I lived on the streets and found myself a pimp. I was stoned all the time. I got tossed in and out of detox centers for years. Then the virus started to get passed around. I hadn't shot up, but I'd been with plenty of guys that had. I think that's what finally helped me quit, at least the first time. My sponsor and my therapist are trying to help me get through this. The longest sobriety I've had is 6 years. I still miss the drugs and know that when life gets real stressful, I'm likely to use. AA and NA help, but a lot of it is just my own willpower. Like they say, "one day at a time."*

People move through predictable stages in changing their unhealthy behaviors such as smoking, drinking, and overeating.[33] Identify where clients are in the process of change (Table 17–13). During the first stage, *precontemplation*, individuals do not think that they have a problem. They have no intention of changing. In the second stage, *contemplation*, they think about changing their behavior but are ambivalent. In the *preparation* stage, individuals intend to quit their habit or **addiction** and start making plans such as tapering down their use or setting a quit date. During the *action* stage, they

TABLE 17–12. Clinical Management Tips

Communication Strategies
- Convey empathy, understanding, and acceptance.
- Strive to maintain a positive attitude, particularly with clients who relapse often.
- Avoid criticism, and criticize blame.
- Recognize "countertransference" feelings or negative reactions to caring for the individual with a substance-related disorder.

Ways to Promote Sobriety
- Encourage moderate exercise and healthy activity patterns.
- Encourage the client to convey feelings and concerns.
- Encourage participation in individual or group therapy.
- Help the client and family structure and plan each day.
- Help clients identify their strengths.
- Suggest social support through psychotherapy groups or self-help groups.
- Jointly establish with the client daily structure and short- and long-term goals.
- Suggest relaxation strategies and other behavioral interventions to cope with anxiety and insomnia, if present.
- For clients in denial, confront the consequences of their substance abuse.
- Involve family and other important people in clients' treatment plans.
- Help clients establish social supports with individuals that will promote their sobriety.
- Reinforce the AA and NA philosophy "one day at a time."
- Set limits on manipulative behaviors.
- Continually evaluate the presence of comorbid conditions such as mood and anxiety disorders.

Client and Family Education
- Teach clients and families that alcoholism and substance abuse are diseases, not moral weaknesses.
- Recognize that substance-related disorders affect all family members.
- Identify "enabling" behaviors, and teach families how to substitute healthier patterns.
- Tell families that they are not responsible for their member's substance abuse.
- Tell the client and family to report any worsening signs of depression or suicidal thoughts.
- Educate about the detrimental effects of alcohol and substance use, including depression and sleep disruption.
- Help the client and family identify community resources such as Adult Children of Alcoholics (ACOA), AL-Anon and other self-help groups.
- Encourage clients to reveal their urges to use substances before they act on them.
- Educate clients about the risks of human immunodeficiency virus (HIV), hepatitis, and other diseases associated with substance abuse.

Source: Adapted from Gorman, LM, et al: Davis's Manual of Psychosocial Nursing for General Patient Care, FA Davis, Philadelphia, 1996, pp 283–289.

TABLE 17-13. **Stages of Behavior Change and Interventions**

Stage	Client Stage	Interventions
Precontemplation	No intention to change; unaware there is a problem with substance use	Raise concern about client's substance usage; educate client about how substance is affecting health
Contemplation Can last 1–3 y	Aware of substance use problems; ambivalent about making change	Explore the pros and cons of continued use versus abstinence or reduced use
Preparation	Intend to quit; making small changes	Affirm and encourage client's decision to change; encourage short-term goals and set time line for behavior change
Action Lasts 1 day–6 mo	Overt changes	Identify obstacles to behavior change and work with client to develop and employ effective coping strategies
Maintenance Begins after 6 mo of change	Stabilizing changes and preventing relapse	Identify at-risk situations that could trigger relapse to substance use
Relapse	Return to an earlier stage	Praise client for past progress, normalize relapse as part of change process, and encourage a plan to change behavior

Source: Adapted from Prochaska, JO, DiClemente, CC, and Norcross, JC: In search of how people change: Applications to addictive behaviors. Am Psychol 47:1102–1109, 1992.

make overt changes and attempt sobriety or try to reduce their behaviors. The *maintenance* phase begins about 6 months after sobriety. The focus is on stabilizing change and preventing relapse. Relapse often occurs several times before change is maintained. Clients with recent sobriety are in the action stage and need continued support, particularly during the first year.

During the maintenance stage of recovery, help the client to identify triggers to substance use and to recognize and manage psychosocial stressors associated with potential relapse. Support the development of new behavioral strategies such as relaxation training, social support, and self-help programs. Educate clients about the relapsing nature of dependence. Help them understand that a brief return to alcohol or drugs can be a temporary "lapse," rather than relapse to regular substance use. Never give permission for occasional drug use. The ultimate goal of relapse prevention for clients with substance dependence is abstinence, not controlled use.[34]

Teach clients skills for anticipating, avoiding, and coping with their personal high-risk situations. Help them to develop constructive responses to cope with lapses when they occur. Remind them about the long-term negative consequences of substance abuse. Suggest the tips from the 12-step programs: "HALT," an acronym meaning to try not to get too Hungry, Angry, Lonely, or Tired, feelings that put clients at high risk for relapse.

In those cases where clients consistently return to their drug-taking behaviors, several detoxification interventions may be required before sustained abstinence is attempted.

Provide care through ongoing management and support for attempts to stay drug-free. Identify support for clients and their families. Maintain a hopeful stance while encouraging abstinence and ongoing recovery. Attend AA or NA meetings with other nursing students to better understand the self-help movement by hearing the stories of those who are attempting to maintain their sobriety.

Assess for the client's readiness to change and the coexistence of other mental health problems. A client case management approach may be useful. In client case management, the nurse develops an ongoing relationship with the client.[35]

FAMILY INTERVENTIONS

Substance-abuse treatment has traditionally focused on the individual.[36] However, family support is necessary to help clients maintain sobriety. Involve the family at every stage. In the past, families were treated as the cause of the problem, but it is more useful to think of the family system as both affecting and being affected by the substance user. Help families identify the problem and sources of support. Teach them about substance dependence and present possible treatment solutions. Al-Anon, a 12-step program for family and friends of alcoholics, is a helpful resource. A referral to family therapy may be necesary to address problems such as adolescents with substance abuse, couples with marital problems, and those who tend to "scapegoat" one member. Ineffective family coping related to the chemical abuse requires intervention by the nurse who can help the family develop realistic expectations of the substance-abusing family member.

We also need to love and share, more than we do, the impact of alcoholism on the family and associates of the alcoholic. Our family probably made every mistake possible in reacting to Terry's disease—including not recognizing it as a disease for a long time. We also did some things right, and we learned a few things from our mistakes.

Alcoholism is indeed a family disease. It is a family disease in that it tends to run in some family trees more than others. It is a family disease also in that the alcoholic's disease will over time affect mental, emotional, financial, and lifestyle factors relating to the rest of the family. In a sense, the alcoholic's disease erupts in ways that threaten the entire family's health and well-being.

GEORGE McGOVERN[7]

PHARMACOLOGIC TREATMENTS

Pharmacologic treatments of substance-use disorders are concentrated in two areas:

- Initial attainment of abstinence by withdrawing the client from the substance(s) used
- Chronic maintenance or the prevention of relapse.

The goal of withdrawal or detoxification is to reduce the duration and severity of the withdrawal syndrome or to reverse the potentially life-threatening effects of alcohol or other drug overdose. Current pharmacology focuses on treating abuse of opioids and depressants because they present potential serious medical complications.

Stimulant withdrawal has few physiological complications; however, depressive symptoms and drug craving often continue as problems. Treatment is primarily psychosocial interventions.

Long-term care often involves maintenance pharmacologic interventions with either blocking agents (**antagonists**) that prevent the abused drug from producing behavioral or physiologic effects, or substitution agents (**agonists**) that maintain the drug-dependent state. Substitution agents are used to prevent illicit drug use. Table 17–14 lists the com-

TABLE 17–14. Pharmacologic Treatment of Substance-related Disorders

Substance Disorder	Medication Generic	Trade	Dosing
Alcohol Dependence			
Acute Withdrawal	Diazepam	Valium	5–20 mg q 4 hr prn
	Chlordiazepoxide	Librium	25–100 mg q 4 hr prn
	Atenolol	Tenormin	50–100 mg/day*
	Clonidine	Catapres	0.05–0.3 mg/day
	Carbamazepine	Tegretol	800 mg/day for 1–2 days; then reduced over the next week
Maintenance	Disulfiram	Antabuse	125–250 mg/day
	Naltrexone	ReVia	25–50 mg/day
Opioid Dependence			
Acute Withdrawal	Clonidine	Catapres	0.05–0.3 mg, increased prn, after 3–4 days is tapered
	Naltrexone	ReVia	12.5 mg/day
	Buprenorphine	Buprenex	2–8 mg/day for 1 mo; then abruptly discontinue and begin IV naltrexone
Acute Overdose	Naloxone	Narcan	0.4–0.8 mg IV q 5–15 min prn
Maintenance	Naltrexone	ReVia	50 mg/day
	Methadone		60–120 mg/day
	Buprenorphine	Buprenex	12–16 mg/day
Cocaine Dependence			
Nicotine Withdrawal	Desipramine	Norpramine	50–200 mg/day
	Clonidine	Catapres	0.05–0.3 mg/day
	Nicotine gum	Nicorette	1 piece prn
	Transdermal nicotine	Nicotrol	15–25 mg patch for 4–12 wk; then lower-dose patch for 8 more wk

*Not given if pulse <50.

mon pharmacologic interventions and doses to treat withdrawal and prevent relapse.

ALCOHOL DEPENDENCE

Acute Withdrawal

Treatment for alcohol withdrawal is aimed at providing rapid substitution of a drug that suppresses signs and symptoms of autonomic hyperactivity such as tremor, tachycardia, and hypertension, as well as preventing seizures, the most serious complication.

Because of their safety, benzodiazepines, antihypertensives such as clonidine and atenolol, and carbamazepine are most commonly used.[27,37–39] The barbiturate phenobarbital is used with clients with mixed alcohol and barbiturate detoxification. Benzodiazepines relieve autonomic arousal symptoms of tremulousness, agitation, insomnia, tachycardia, and hypertension and may help prevent seizures and DTs.

Maintenance

Maintenance pharmacologic treatments prevent relapse; they are effective when combined with psychosocial treatments, particularly relapse-prevention therapies that use cognitive and behavioral techniques and self-help groups such as AA and NA.

Disulfiram (Antabuse) is used to deter drinking. A physiological reaction occurs if alcohol is used with this drug. Disulfiram inhibits an enzyme, aldehyde oxireductase, that breaks down alcohol. If alcohol is ingested when the client is taking disulfiram, a toxic reaction occurs that may include nausea, hypotension, flushing, dizziness, dyspnea, blurred vision, and possibly shock and death. Instruct clients that this reaction may occur up to 2 weeks after stopping the medication.

Naltrexone (ReVia) is used to maintain abstinence in opioid-dependent clients and is now approved for use with alcoholics.[40] Naltrexone, an opioid antagonist, reduces abuse by blocking opioid receptors. Selective serotonin reuptake inhibitors (SSRIs) such as fluoxetine may reduce cravings; however, more research is necessary.[41]

BENZODIAZEPINES AND SEDATIVE-HYPNOTIC WITHDRAWAL

Pharmacologic interventions are similar to those used for alcohol dependence and involve three options.

- The first is to use decreasing doses of the drug of dependence under medical supervision. This requires cooperation with the dosing regimen and abstinence from alcohol or other drugs.
- The second option is to substitute a long-acting barbiturate, such as phenobarbital, and gradually withdraw the substitute medication.
- The third option, for clients with both alcohol and benzodiazepine dependence, involves substituting a long-acting benzodiazepine, such as chlordiazepoxide, with a gradual reduction of this drug over 1 to 2 weeks.

OPIOIDS

Acute Withdrawal

The current method of opioid withdrawal is substitution and subsequent withdrawal of the cross-tolerant medication methadone. Because methadone is a long-acting, orally effective synthetic narcotic, it is used as a substitute for highly addictive narcotics such as heroin, morphine, hydromorphine, or meperidine. Clonidine may facilitate opioid withdrawal because it reduces many of the sympathetic autonomic arousal symptoms such as tachycardia, piloerection, diarrhea, and intestinal hypermotility. Clients may be switched from methadone to clonidine.

A more rapid detoxification from opioids involves the use of naltrexone and clonidine. Starting doses of 12.5 mg of naltrexone are given with clonidine over 4 days.[42]

Buprenorphine is a recently approved alternative to methadone for detoxification.[43] The drug suppresses acute opioid withdrawal and seems to produce less physical dependence than methadone. Clients may taper off buprenorphine more easily than off methadone.

Acute Overdose

Naloxone (Narcan) is an opioid-antagonist medication used to reverse acute overdoses of opioids. Naloxone blocks the uptake of and displaces opioids at their receptor sites in the nerve synapse. Because naloxone is short acting and poorly absorbed orally, it is given intravenously. It reverses the effects of opioid overdose. It may also be used to bring on withdrawal before beginning the long-term therapies described previously.

Maintenance

Current maintenance treatment for narcotic abstinence or preventing relapse involves naltrexone, methadone, or buprenorphine. Naltrexone allows clients to return to their usual environments secure in the knowledge that they cannot get high while on this drug. It is primarily used in combination with a structured treatment program and motivated clients.[44] Methadone decreases criminal and drug-seeking behaviors because opiate craving is satisfied. Clients must show evidence of dependence for a minimum of 1 year and current physical dependence. Those who are more successful also receive rehabilitation services such as job training and vocational counseling.

Buprenorphine is an alternative drug for maintenance because its shorter, less intense withdrawal syndrome allows an easier transition to a drugfree state than methadone. A new long-acting opioid substitution medication under investigation is levo-α-acetylmethadol (LAAM).

STIMULANT WITHDRAWAL

The withdrawal phase from stimulants lasts approximately 8 to 10 weeks after stimulant abstinence. Symptoms include anhedonia, anxiety, lack of energy, and stimulant craving. If relapse is not experienced during the withdrawal phase, the client enters the so-called extinction phase, a return to normal moods with episodic craving.

Pharmacologic treatment for stimulant-related disorders is in the experimental stage. Desipramine and other tricyclic antidepressants have shown some effectiveness; however, more studies are needed.

NICOTINE WITHDRAWAL

The primary pharmacologic approach to nicotine dependence is substitution therapy with nicotine agonist taken in the form of either a chewing gum or a transdermal patch. Both forms are FDA-approved treatment methods for decreasing symptoms of nicotine withdrawal. They are commonly used along with behavioral interventions.

After using these substitution methods for 2 to 3 months, fewer than 25% of individuals are able to remain abstinent for 6 to 12 months.

Because nicotine withdrawal may be associated with increased norepinephrine activity, medications that affect norepinephrine transmission may be effective. Clonidine may suppress hyperactive norepinephrine neurons to successfully treat nicotine withdrawal and promote smoking cessation.[45]

Expected Outcomes

For the client with intoxication or withdrawal, improvement is demonstrated by:
- Adequate sleep duration and continuity
- Adequate nutrition
- Normalization of vital signs
- Orientation to time, place, and person
- Absence of physical injuries
- Clear sensorium; expresses no excessive fears or delirium
- Absence of physical symptoms
- Appropriate behavior and normalization of physical activity.

For the client with substance abuse and dependence, improvement is demonstrated by:
- Participation in immediate detoxification, if necessary
- Acknowledgment of a substance problem
- Initiation of a trial period of abstinence or willingness to decrease use
- Knowledge of a connection between substance and health problems
- Regular attendance at AA or NA meetings
- Recognition of the need for ongoing treatment.

Differential Diagnosis

MEDICAL DISORDERS

- Medications or physical conditions such as chronic pain may precipitate substance-related disorders.
- Neurological conditions such as head trauma may be mistakenly attributed to intoxication or withdrawal.
- Those with infectious diseases such as viral gastroenteritis may appear to suffer from withdrawal symptoms.

MOOD DISORDERS

- Depressed mood may present along with or during substance-related disorders.
- Clients may self-medicate with drugs, particularly stimulants and alcohol, to get "high."
- Alcohol, used to cope with stress, insomnia, mania, and depression, is a depressant that can lead to depression.
- Marijuana, cocaine, and other substance abuse may precipitate or accompany the presentation of depression or mania.
- Stimulant abuse may be confused with symptoms of mania; once discontinued, euphoric mood, high energy, and pressured speech quickly abate.

PSYCHOTIC DISORDERS

- Schizophrenia and other psychotic disorders may be misdiagnosed.
- Psychotic symptoms, such as hallucinations, delusions, and paranoia, occur with both schizophrenia and substance-related disorders, particularly intoxication, and do not differentiate the two illnesses.
- Schizophrenia, schizoaffective disorder, and delusional disorder are all characterized by distinct periods of psychotic symptoms that are not substance induced.
- Psychosis usually remits quickly and spontaneously when related to substance abuse.

ANXIETY DISORDERS

- Common comorbid anxiety conditions include generalized anxiety, panic disorder, social phobia, posttraumatic stress disorder, and OCD.
- Clients may "self-medicate" to treat symptoms of anxiety.
- Anxiety may appear during withdrawal and be misdiagnosed.

PERSONALITY DISORDERS

- Personality disorders, especially borderline personality disorder and antisocial personality disorder, complicate diagnosis or coexist with substance-related disorders.

- Borderline personality disorder is characterized by frequent mood shifts without the other symptoms of depression or mania. Anger is the predominant mood.
- Antisocial personality disorder is often associated with substance-related disorders; drug-seeking behavior can lead to criminal and antisocial behaviors.

ATTENTION-DEFICIT/HYPERACTIVITY DISORDER (ADHD)

- Teenagers and adults with undiagnosed ADHD may abuse alcohol and substances.
- Early identification of persistent hyperactivity, impulsivity, and inattention is necessary.

Common Nursing Diagnoses

Cognitive responses
    Knowledge Deficit
    Thought Processes, altered
    Noncompliance
Biological responses
    Sensory/Perceptual Alterations
    Injury, risk for
    Self Care Deficit
    Infection, risk for
    Sleep Pattern Disturbance
    Sexual Dysfunction
    Nutrition, altered
    Pain
    Growth and Development, altered
Psychosocial responses
    Communication, impaired verbal
    Coping, individual, ineffective
    Anxiety
    Fear
    Social Isolation
    Family Processes, altered
    Social Interaction, impaired
    Parenting, altered
    Growth and Development, altered
    Violence, risk for
Spiritual responses
    Spiritual Distress
    Powerlessness
    Hopelessness
    Grieving

Areas for Future Research

- What are the effective nursing interventions in assessment, detoxification, and prevention of relapse?
- What nursing interventions are effective in reducing clients' distress during withdrawal?
- What are the differences between substance-abusing individuals who progress to dependence and those individuals who do not become dependent?
- How do substances affect women, adolescents, the elderly, and individuals from a variety of ethnic backgrounds?
- What factors place children of alcoholics and other drug addicts at risk for substance dependence?
- What are the effective nursing interventions with dually diagnosed clients?
- How do serotonin-enhancing agents promote abstinence from alcohol and nicotine?
- How do nurses "enable" patients and colleagues to abuse drugs?
- What behaviors constitute positive outcomes of nursing interventions when relapse is quite common?

CASE STUDY

Matt L, a 15-year-old high school sophomore, was taken to the community mental health center's urgent care department by his family. He came home agitated and threatened to kill his parents. His family had never seen that type of behavior from their son, whom they described as quiet and easygoing. Matt's parents noted that his grades had been slipping and that he seemed less motivated than usual for about 2 weeks. The nurse performed a mental status examination; however, Matt was uncooperative. His speech was incoherent and dysarthric; he also had a short attention span. He was not oriented to person, place, or time, and appeared paranoid. Matt was pacing and agitated, and threatened to assault the nursing staff. He was put in physical restraints, and blood was drawn for a toxicology screen. The nurse continually monitored his vital signs; his pulse remained over 120 beats/minute and his blood pressure was 160/100. The nurse also noticed muscle rigidity and that his eyes showed nystagmus.

After several hours in restraints, Matt talked about what happened. He had been smoking marijuana daily for weeks. That day, he was smoking marijuana with friends after school, and one of his friends mentioned that he put some "dust" in the joint. His toxicology screen came back positive for both marijuana and phencyclidine (PCP), also known as "angel dust." These results, in combination with his abrupt behavior and mental status changes, led to the diagnosis of PCP intoxication. Substance abuse, related to marijuana, was a provisional diagnosis.

The nurse supported Matt's openness and helped him tell his family about his drug use. "I can get it under control," he kept repeating to them. The nurse suggested that they see a counselor in the health center and that Matt join a psychotherapy group for teens with substance-abuse problems. He refused. His father began shouting and "ordered" him to go into treatment or face being "kicked out." The nurse helped Matt's parents realize that Matt's denial was common, and that he had taken the first steps toward acknowledging his drug use. She stressed that drug abuse was a disease and that treatment could help him get control over it. She also suggested that "strong arm" tactics were detrimental to helping teens overcome substance-related disorders. The nurse arranged for a drug counselor to meet with the family and Matt before discharge.

CRITICAL THINKING QUESTIONS

1. What behavior and physical clues did Matt exhibit during the health center visit suggesting drug intoxication?
2. What other measures could the nurse have taken to decrease his agitated behavior?
3. Explain the process of denial in substance abuse and its effects on the course of the disorder.
4. Develop a care plan, including short- and long-term goals, for Matt and his family for community-based treatment.
5. Identify behaviors that would indicate that Matt is responding to treatment.
6. Design a teaching plan to assist Matt and his family to deal with substance abuse.

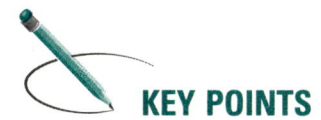

KEY POINTS

- Substance-related disorders, including abuse, misuse, and dependence, occur in a large percentage of medical and mental health problems.
- Substances include depressant agents such as alcohol and sedative-hypnotics, opioids such as meperidine, oxycodone, and heroin, stimulants such as cocaine and amphetamine, nicotine, cannabis, and hallucinogens (such as LSD and PCP).
- Substances of abuse are highly reinforcing and are thought to produce their effects by stimulating a "reward pathway" in the brain. This pathway is rich in endogenous opioids and certain neurotransmitters such as dopamine, GABA, and serotonin.
- Substance abuse is dangerous use of a substance, whereas substance dependence is compulsive use or loss of control over use. Dependence may include physiological symptoms of tolerance and dependence. Once substance dependence develops, frequent relapses to previous uncontrolled use are common despite episodes of abstinence.
- Patterns of behavior that suggest substance-related disorders include problems in relationships and employment, injuries, accidents, legal problems, and physical and mental health disturbances.
- A thorough assessment of substance use is crucial in clients who present with symptoms of psychiatric disturbances such as depression, anxiety, psychosis, and behavior problems.
- Several interview tools (CAGE, SMAST, and DAST-10) are used to detect substance dependence. Laboratory tests (GGT, MCV, AST, ALT) may be useful in detecting heavy drinking; specific drug screening tests can be used to detect alcohol and drug use.
- There is a high comorbidity of substance-related disorders with other psychiatric disorders, including antisocial personality, bipolar, anxiety, and depressive disorders.
- Withdrawal syndromes from addictive substances can be very painful, and withdrawal from regular depressant use can be life-threatening.
- Planning and implementing nursing care for a client with substance-induced disorders necessitate attention to acute physical and safety needs as well as education and support. Interventions for substance-use disorders include feedback, education about the effects of substance use, support, stress management, family interventions, and self-help groups such as AA and NA.
- Substitution medication with gradual detoxification is the primary method used in the treatment of moderate to severe depressant, nicotine, and opioid withdrawal syndromes. Maintenance medications are used in combination with psychosocial treatments for the ongoing treatment of alcohol and opioid dependence and include the antagonist agents disulfiram and naltrexone, and substitution agents such as methadone, LAAM, and buprenorphine.

REFERENCES

1. Galanter, M, and Kleber, HD (eds): Textbook of Substance Abuse Treatment. American Psychiatric Association Press, Washington, DC, 1994.
2. Gold, MS: The Facts About Drugs and Alcohol, ed 3. Psychiatric Institute of America Press, Washington, DC, 1988.
3. Hamill, P: A Drinking Life: A Memoir. Little, Brown & Company Inc, Boston, 1994.
4. Schuckit, MA: Treatment of alcoholism in office and outpatient settings. In Mendelson, JH, and Mello, NK (eds): Medical Diagnosis and Treatment of Alcoholism. McGraw-Hill Inc, New York, 1992.
5. Goodwin, DW: Genetic determinants of alcoholism. In Mendelson, JH, and Mello, NK (eds): Medical Diagnosis and Treatment of Alcoholism. McGraw-Hill Inc, New York, 1992.
6. Vaillant, GE: The Natural History of Alcoholism: Causes, Patterns and Paths to Recovery. Harvard University Press, Cambridge, 1983.
7. McGovern, G: Terry: My Daughter's Life-and-Death Struggle with Alcoholism. Villard, New York, 1996.
8. Warner, LA, et al: Relevance and correlates of drug use and dependence in the United States: Results from the national comorbidity survey. Arch Gen Psychiatry 52:219, 1995.
9. Frezza, M, et al: High blood alcohol levels in women. N Engl J Med 322:95, 1990.
10. Seale, JP, and Muramoto, ML: Substance abuse among minority populations. Prim Care 20:167, 1993.
11. Koob, GF: Drugs of abuse: Anatomy, pharmacology and function of reward pathways. Trends Pharmacol Sci 13:177, 1992.
12. Mathew, RJ, and Wilson, WH: Substance abuse and cerebral blood flow. Am J Psychiatry 148:292, 1991.
13. Modell, JG, and Mountz, JM: Focal cerebral blood flow during craving for alcohol as measured by SPECT. J Neuropsychiatry Clin Neurosc 7:15, 1995.
14. Goodwin, DW: Alcoholism and genetics: The sons of our fathers. Arch Gen Psychiatry 42:171, 1985.
15. Lukas, SE: Brain electrical activity as a tool for studying drugs of abuse. In Mello, NK (ed): Advances in Substance Abuse, vol 4. Jessica Kingsley Publishers, London, 1991.

16. Higuchi, et al: Alcohol and aldehyde dehydrogenase polymorphisms and the risk for alcoholism. Am J Psychiatry 152:1219, 1995.
17. Khatzian, EJ: The self-medication hypothesis of addictive disorders; Focus on heroin and cocaine dependence. Am J Psychiatry 142:1259, 1985.
18. American Psychiatric Association: Diagnostic and Statistical Manual of Mental Disorders, ed 4. American Psychiatric Association, Washington, DC, 1994.
19. Kamerow, DB, Pincus, HA, and McDonald, DI: Alcohol abuse, other drug abuse and mental disorders in medical practice: Prevalence, costs, recognition and treatment. JAMA 225:2054, 1988.
20. Mayfield, DG, et al: The CAGE questionnaire: Validation of a new alcoholism screening instrument. Am J Psychiatry 131:1121, 1974.
21. Ewing, J: Detecting alcoholism: The CAGE questionnaire. JAMA 252:1905, 1984.
22. Kitchens, JM: Does this patient have an alcohol problem? JAMA 272:1782, 1994.
23. Selzer, ML, Vinokor, A, and van Rooijen, LA: A self-administered Short Michigan Alcoholism Screening Test (SMAST). J Stud Alcohol 36:117, 1975.
24. Skinner, HA: Drug abuse screening test. Addic Behav 7:363, 1982.
25. Halikas, JA: Treatment of drug abuse syndromes. Psychiatr Clin North Am 16:693, 1993.
26. Hester, RK: Outcome research: Alcoholism. In Galanter, M, and Kleber, HD (eds): Textbook of Substance Abuse Treatment. American Psychiatric Association Press, Washington, DC, 1994.
27. Sullivan, JT, et al: Assessment of alcohol withdrawal: The revised clinical institute withdrawal assessment for alcohol scale (CIWA-Ar). Br J Addiction 84:1353, 1989.
28. Kleber, HD: Opioid detoxification. In Galanter, M, and Kleber, HD (eds): Textbook of Substance Abuse Treatment. American Psychiatric Association Press, Washington, DC 1994.
29. Miller, WR, and Rollnick, S: Motivational Interviewing. The Guilford Press, New York, 1991.
30. Minicucci, DS: The challenge of change: Rethinking alcohol abuse. Arch Psychiatr Nurs 8:373, 1994.
31. Bradley, KA, Donovan, DM, and Larson, EB: How much is too much? Arch Intern Med 152:2734, 1993.
32. Sanchez-Craig, M, and Israel, Y: Patterns of alcohol use associated with self-identified problem drinking. Am J Public Health 75:178, 1985.
33. Prochaska, JO, DiClemente, CC, and Norcross, JC: In search of how people change: Applications to addictive behaviors. Am Psychol 47:1102, 1992.
34. Marlatt, GA, and Gordon, JR: Relapse Prevention: Maintenance Strategies in the Treatment of Addictive Behaviors. The Guilford Press, New York, 1985.
35. Drake, RE, McHugo, GJ, and Noordsy, DL: Treatment of alcoholism among schizophrenic outpatients: 4-year outcomes. Am J Psychiatry 150:328, 1993.
36. Steinglass, P: Family therapy: Alcohol. In Galanter, M, and Kleber, HD (eds): Textbook of Substance Abuse Treatment. American Psychiatric Association Press, Washington, DC, 1994.
37. Kraus, ML, et al: Randomized clinical trial of atenolol in patients with alcohol withdrawal. N Engl J Med 313:905, 1985.
38. Baumgartner, GR, and Rown, RC: Clonidine versus chlordiazepoxide in the management of acute alcohol withdrawal syndrome. Arch Intern Med 107:880, 1987.
39. Ries, RK, et al: Carbamazepine treatment for benzodiazepine withdrawal. Am J Psychiatry 146:536, 1989.
40. Volpicelli, J, et al: Naltrexone in the treatment of alcohol dependence. Arch Gen Psychiatry 49:867, 1992.
41. Naranjo, CA, et al: Fluoxetine differentially alters alcohol intake and other consummatory behaviors in problem drinkers. Clin Pharmacol Ther 47:490, 1990.
42. Vining, E, Kosten, TR, and Kleber, HD: Clinical utility of rapid clonidine naltrexone detoxification for opioid abusers. Br J Addiction 83:567, 1988.
43. Shi, JM, et al: Three methods of ambulatory opiate detoxification: Preliminary results of a randomized clinical trial. National Institute on Drug Abuse Research Monograph # 132. U.S. Government Printing Office, Washington, DC, 1993.
44. Ling, W, and Wesson, DR: Naltrexone treatment for addicted health care professionals: A collaborative private practice experience. J Clin Psychiatry 45:46, 1984.
45. Covey, LS, and Glassman, AH: A meta-analysis of double-blind placebo-controlled trials of clonidine for smoking cessation. Br J Addiction 86:991, 1991.

CHAPTER 18

Schizophrenia and Other Psychotic Disorders

CHAPTER 18

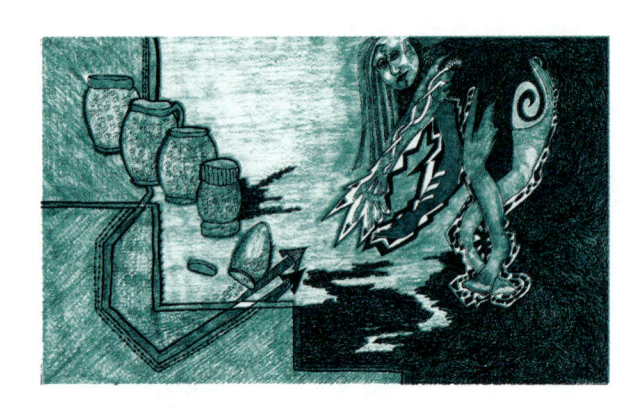

CHAPTER OUTLINE

Schizophrenia
Characteristic Behaviors
Culture, Age, and Gender Features
Etiology
Prognosis
Other Psychotic Disorders
Schizophreniform Disorder
Schizoaffective Disorder
Delusional Disorder
Brief Psychotic Disorder
Assessing Acute Episodes of Illness
Assessing the Prodromal Phase of Schizophrenia in the Community
Planning Care
Interventions for Hospitalized Clients
Interventions for Clients in the Community
Client and Family Education
Differential Diagnosis
Expected Outcomes
Common Nursing Diagnoses
Synopsis of Current Research
Areas for Future Research

Carol A. Glod, RN, CS, PhD
Martin H. Teicher, MD, PhD
Stephanie Stockard Spelic, RN, MSN, CS, CPC, LMHP

Schizophrenia and Other Psychotic Disorders

LEARNING OBJECTIVES

After completing this chapter, the reader should be able to:

- State the criteria that describe schizophrenia, and distinguish it from other major psychiatric disorders.
- Differentiate negative and positive symptoms in psychotic disorders.
- Name the major etiological theories of schizophrenia.
- Distinguish between the different types of schizophrenia.
- Implement the nursing process in planning care for clients with psychotic disorders.
- List communication strategies that are effective with individuals with psychosis.
- Distinguish between symptoms of psychosis and medication-related side effects.
- Educate families about the diagnosis, treatment, and course of psychotic illness.

KEY TERMS

delusions
flat affect
formal thought disorder
hallucinations
negative symptoms
paranoia
positive symptoms
psychosis

Psychotic disorders are some of the most severe, chronic, and intractable psychiatric disorders. Schizophrenia is the most common and widely studied of the psychotic disorders, but also included in this group are schizoaffective disorder, delusional disorder, schizophreniform disorder, brief psychotic disorder, and other psychotic disorders not otherwise specified (NOS). Characteristic features of the psychotic disorders are misperceptions of reality and altered thought processes.

Psychotic disorders may occur at any age and vary in their time of onset and duration of symptoms. Schizophrenia, the most severe and chronic of the disorders, usually begins during adolescence or young adulthood and has a deteriorating course. In schizophrenia, the person is overwhelmed by an onslaught of bizarre thoughts and hallucinations, resulting in inappropriate or bizarre ways of relating and a general disorganization in daily functioning and behavior. At this critical time, when young adults are beginning new stages of life by going off to college, starting employment, or separating from family, their dreams of career, marriage, and family may be shattered by severe deficits in interpersonal relationships, self-care, and occupational functioning.

In the following vignette, a mother describes her 18-year-old daughter's first psychotic episode at the beginning of the overwhelming and debilitating illness that is schizophrenia.

I remember coming home one day from work and seeing my daughter in the backyard. She had become so isolated in recent months. She rarely went out, never spoke to her friends, and had little contact with us. She wouldn't even eat meals with her family. The only thing she seemed to enjoy was smoking cigarettes. When I saw her in the backyard, I could tell that something was really wrong. My heart sank. My daughter had gathered all the knives from the kitchen and was carefully arranging them. She would spontaneously start shouting, although no one was around, and then she darted up a big tree in the backyard. Her behavior had become more bizarre over the last few months. Although she used to whisper to herself sometimes, she was talking and shouting to herself a lot of the time.

I didn't know what to do when I saw all the knives. When I confronted her in the past, she would get angry and whisper something to herself. Sometimes she would take off and I wouldn't see her for hours. But when I saw the knives, I knew there was trouble. All of a sudden she came running in the house and told me they had finally found her and we would all be killed. "We need to get them," she just kept screaming that phrase over and over. As she shouted, she looked all around for the intruders. I finally had to call the police. It broke my heart. The look she gave me was one that said it all; I had betrayed her. I looked out the window again and remembered all the times when she was young and when she climbed that tree. She seemed so happy and carefree. I knew then that those days were gone.

Along with the profound effects of schizophrenia on the individual, families suffer emotionally, financially, and even physically as they attempt to acquire treatment and care for their loved one. With such a chronic and debilitating disease, parents surrender their dreams of their child's education, marriage, family, and career. Brothers and sisters may suffer from the financial and emotional strains placed upon the family and need to assume care for their sibling as their parents age, while also struggling to maintain their own families and careers. Schizophrenia, like many of the psychotic disorders, has devastating consequences for the individual, family, and society.

SCHIZOPHRENIA

In biblical times, individuals with schizophrenia or other mental disorders were thought to be possessed by demons. Exorcising of the demons, shunning, or killing the individual was a common response. In some cultures, however, the person was held in high regard; hallucinations, delusions, and unusual forms of speech were considered to be unusual and special powers.

Emil Kraepelin, an eminent psychiatrist of the early 1900s, proposed that *dementia praecox*, now referred to as schizophrenia, was due to premature deterioration of the brain. He also differentiated schizophrenia from manic-depressive psychosis (bipolar disorder) by noting that schizophrenia had a deteriorating course, whereas manic-depressive illness was characterized by exacerbation and remissions in behavior. This is still a key distinguishing feature.

Later, psychiatrist Eugen Bleuler conceptualized schizophrenia as having four fundamental symptoms: disturbances of association and affect accompanied by ambivalence and autism.

Even as recently as a few decades ago, the prevailing etiologic theory was a disturbance in the mother-child relationship. Popular views were that the individual had a "split personality." Even today, people carelessly refer to contradictory behavior as "schizophrenic."

Recent advances suggest a neurobiological basis. Although the exact etiology of schizophrenia is unknown, evidence from genetic, biochemical, neurological, and brain-imaging studies suggests that this severe and debilitating illness results from multiple factors, including environmental effects.

Characteristic Behaviors

In schizophrenia, characteristic symptoms are readily observed. According to the *Diagnostic and Statistical Manual of Mental Disorders, Fourth Edition (DSM-IV)*,[1] at least two or more of these symptoms must be present for a significant portion of time during a 1-month period. (See Diagnostic Criteria for Schizophrenia.) Table 18–1 lists the characteristics of hallucinations, delusions, and thought disorders.

1. **Delusions** (false beliefs)
2. **Hallucinations** (distorted misperceptions of reality)
3. Disorganized speech (incoherence or verbalizations difficult to follow or understand)
4. Grossly disorganized or catatonic behavior
5. Negative symptoms such as **flat affect,** alogia, or avolition.

As shown in Table 18–2, these symptoms are delineated into two groups, **positive symptoms,** which include hallucinations, delusions, **formal thought disorder,** and odd or

TABLE 18–1. Characteristics of Hallucinations, Delusions, and Thought Disorder

Hallucinations
- Usually experienced as beginning outside the client's head or in the external world.
- Can be simple or complex.
- Auditory most common, experienced usually as "voices," can be one or more voices conversing, commanding (issuing orders), familiar or unfamiliar, heard clearly or mumbled.
- Auditory hallucinations can also be noises or music.
- Visual hallucinations may be images, individuals, animals, or flashes of light.
- Olfactory (smell) and gustatory (taste) hallucinations often occur together leading to unpleasant tastes and odors.
- Tactile hallucinations are physical sensations such as being touched or pulled, or experiencing "electrical," "crawling," or sexual sensations.

Delusions
- Persecutory delusions: beliefs that one is being tormented, attacked, or wronged by others; being followed or spied on by government agencies such as the CIA.
- Grandiose delusions: beliefs that one possesses special abilities, powers, or wealth or is an important person.
- Nihilistic delusions: beliefs that the world is ending, or that one is dead, dying, or doesn't exist.
- Religious delusions: beliefs that one has special religious powers, a special relationship to God, or a religious mission.
- Somatic delusions: beliefs that the body is rotting or disfigured or has a fatal disease; body organs have "stopped" working.
- Sexual delusions: beliefs that masturbation accounts for illness; sexual activity is known to others.

Thought Disorder
- Ideas of reference: beliefs that one is being talked about or "referred" to repeatedly; beliefs that certain events are related or have special meaning to the individual.
- Loose associations: shifting from one topic to another unrelated topic; also called "derailment."
- Thought broadcasting: beliefs that one's private thoughts can be perceived or are "broadcast" to others.
- Thought insertion: beliefs that others are controlling or "injecting" thoughts.
- Thought withdrawal: beliefs that others are controlling thoughts by removing them.
- Concrete thinking: loss of ability to engage in abstraction or to think conceptually.

TABLE 18-2. Key Features of Schizophrenia and Psychotic Disorders

	Definition	Types/Symptoms
Positive symptoms		
Hallucinations	Problems with sensory perception that seem to reflect reality. The individual is convinced that he or she can hear, see, smell, etc., something that is imperceptible to others.	Auditory, voices commenting, voices conversing, visual, olfactory (smell), somatic (physical), tactile (touch), gustatory (taste).
Delusions	False beliefs and disturbances in thinking; firm convictions and thoughts about the world that are not based in reality. When challenged about the unlikelihood of the beliefs, the individual perseveres relentlessly.	Persecutory; jealous, guilty, grandiose, religious, somatic. Delusions of reference, delusions of being controlled, delusions of mind reading. Can involve thought insertion, thought withdrawal, or thought broadcasting.
Formal thought disorder	Disordered thinking or use of language.	Tangentiality, illogical thinking, derailment, nonsensical or incoherent speech, circumstantiality.
Odd or bizarre behavior	Behaviors that are inappropriate to usual social convention; odd mannerisms or gestures.	Agitated, repetitive, immobile, rocking, sexual; odd clothing combinations.
Negative symptoms		
Flat affect	Absence of a range of facial expressions that would occur naturally.	Poor eye contact, facial expression remains unchanged; inappropriate affect; lacks spontaneous movements, vocal inflections, emotional reactions, or expressive gestures.
Alogia	Insufficient thinking, observed through shortage of speech and language.	Concrete replies to questions, poverty of speech, speech lacks content, blocked thinking, protracted silence before response.
Asociality (anhedonia)	Lack of a range of meaningful or social relationships.	Few relationships with friends, impaired intimacy, relationships lack closeness, lacks hobbies or activities.
Avolition	Lack of motivation; apathy; impaired ability to initiate activity.	Poor hygiene and self-care; inert; lacks persistence in daily and occupational activities.
Inattention	Observable impairment in attention.	Misses social cues; inattentiveness during conversations.

bizarre behavior, and **negative symptoms**, which include flat affect, alogia, asociality (or anhedonia), avolition, and inattention.

Positive symptoms clearly interfere with self-care and the ability to relate to others. These symptoms may also threaten the life or safety of clients or others depending upon the nature of the hallucinations, delusions, or other alterations of thought. Negative symptoms such as the shortage of speech and language found in *alogia*, the lack of motivation seen in *avolition*, and inattention and isolation impede clients' ability to work, socialize, and develop intimate relationships.

However, the diagnosis of schizophrenia or other psychotic disorders does not depend solely on the presence of psychotic symptoms, which may also be seen in other disorders such as dementia or mood disorders. In addition to the psychotic symptoms, the diagnosis must include an assessment of the social or occupational dysfunction and self-care deficits that may follow or accompany the "active" phase in which psychotic symptoms are prominent.

Prodromal Phase

The first phase, known as the *prodromal phase*, may be insidious and slow with subtle behaviors, or it may be acute in its onset.[1] Families or teachers may observe the first behavior changes in mid to late adolescence; individuals may become very isolated and either overfocus on schoolwork or completely stop doing their usual activities. Bizarre preoccupations may center on such people as musicians or movie stars or on a particular topic in science or math.

> June K, a 17-year-old, began to listen to the music of a rock group nearly 24 hours a day. She stopped going to school and began following the band around the country. She stopped seeing friends, and her entire life began to revolve around the rock group.

Social withdrawal, work or school impairment, lack of motivation, poor attention to hygiene, and strange ideas may develop slowly over months or years. Eventually these behaviors culminate in an acute episode, as seen in the active phase.

DSM-IV Diagnostic Criteria for Schizophrenia

A. Characteristic symptoms: Two (or more) of the following, each present for a significant portion of time during a 1-month period (or less if successfully treated):
   (1) delusions
   (2) hallucinations
   (3) disorganized speech (e.g., frequent derailment or incoherence)
   (4) grossly disorganized or catatonic behavior
   (5) negative symptoms (i.e., affective flattening, alogia, or avolition)

   NOTE: Only one Criterion A symptom is required if delusions are bizarre or hallucinations consist of a voice keeping up a running commentary on the person's behavior or thoughts, or two or more voices conversing with each other.

B. Social/occupational dysfunction: For a significant portion of the time since the onset of the disturbance, one or more major areas of functioning such as work, interpersonal relations, or self-care are markedly below the level achieved prior to the onset (or when the onset is in childhood or adolescence, failure to achieve expected level of interpersonal, academic, or occupational achievement).

C. Duration: Continuous signs of the disturbance persist for at least 6 months. This 6-month period must include at least 1 month of symptoms (or less if successfully treated) that meet Criterion A (i.e., active-phase symptoms) and may include periods of prodromal or residual symptoms. During these prodromal or residual periods, the signs of the disturbance may be manifested by only negative symptoms or two or more symptoms listed in Criterion A present in an attenuated form (e.g., odd beliefs, unusual perceptual experiences).

D. Schizoaffective and Mood Disorder exclusion: Schizoaffective Disorder and Mood Disorder With Psychotic Features have been ruled out because either (1) no Major Depressive, Manic, or Mixed Episodes have occurred concurrently with the active-phase symptoms; or (2) if mood episodes have occurred during active-phase symptoms, their total duration has been brief relative to the duration of the active and residual periods.

E. Substance/general medical condition exclusion: The disturbance is not due to the direct physiological effects of a substance (e.g., a drug of abuse, a medication) or a general medical condition.

F. Relationship to a Pervasive Developmental Disorder: If there is a history of Autistic Disorder or another Pervasive Developmental Disorder, the additional diagnosis of Schizophrenia is made only if prominent delusions or hallucinations are also present for at least 1 month (or less if successfully treated).

NOTE: *Classification of longitudinal course* (can be applied only after at least 1 year has elapsed since the initial onset of active-phase symptoms):

Episodic With Interepisode Residual Symptoms (episodes are defined by the reemergence of prominent psychotic symptoms); *also specify if:* With Prominent Negative Symptoms
Episodic With No Interepisode Residual Symptoms
Continuous (prominent psychotic symptoms are present throughout the period of observation); *also specify if:* With Prominent Negative Symptoms
Single Episode In Partial Remission; *also specify if:* With Prominent Negative Symptoms
Single Episode In Full Remission
Other or Unspecified Pattern

Diagnostic Criteria for 295.30 Paranoid Type
A type of Schizophrenia in which the following criteria are met:

A. Preoccupation with one or more delusions or frequent auditory hallucinations.

B. None of the following is prominent: disorganized speech, disorganized or catatonic behavior, or flat or inappropriate affect.

Diagnostic Criteria for 295.10 Disorganized Type
A type of Schizophrenia in which the following criteria are met:

A. All of the following are prominent:
   (1) disorganized speech
   (2) disorganized behavior
   (3) flat or inappropriate affect

B. The criteria are not met for Catatonic Type.

Diagnostic Criteria for 295.20 Catatonic Type
A type of Schizophrenia in which the clinical picture is dominated by at least two of the following:
   (1) motoric immobility as evidenced by catalepsy (including waxy flexibility) or stupor
   (2) excessive motor activity (that is apparently purposeless and not influenced by external stimuli)
   (3) extreme negativism (an apparently motiveless resistance to all instructions or maintenance of a rigid posture against attempts to be moved) or mutism
   (4) peculiarities of voluntary movement as evidenced by posturing (voluntary assumption of inappropriate or bizarre postures), stereotyped movements, prominent mannerisms, or prominent grimacing
   (5) echolalia or echopraxia

Diagnostic Criteria for 295.90 Undifferentiated Type
A type of Schizophrenia in which symptoms that meet Criterion A are present, but the criteria are not met for the Paranoid, Disorganized, or Catatonic Type.

Continued on following page

> **Diagnostic Criteria for 295.60 Residual Type**
>
> A type of Schizophrenia in which the following criteria are met:
>
> **A.** Absence of prominent delusions, hallucinations, disorganized speech, and grossly disorganized or catatonic behavior.
>
> **B.** There is continuing evidence of the disturbance, as indicated by the presence of negative symptoms or two or more symptoms listed in Criterion A for Schizophrenia, present in an attenuated form (e.g., odd beliefs, unusual perceptual experiences).
>
> **Source:** Reprinted with permission from the Diagnostic and Statistical Manual of Mental Disorders, Fourth Edition. Copyright 1994 American Psychiatric Association.

Active Phase

The active phase is characterized by delusions, hallucinations, disorganized speech, grossly disorganized or catatonic behavior, and negative symptoms. When onset is acute, this phase is often the first sign that others observe. Certain stressors, such as leaving for college, taking exams, or breaking up a relationship, may precede the active phase. Older adolescents frequently precipitate the episode by experimenting with drugs or alcohol. The active symptoms would occur inevitably, but drugs and alcohol affect neurochemical functioning even more negatively.

> As June K followed the rock group around the country, she became more and more involved in drug use. Although appearing to be a "groupie," she began to display the delusion that the main singer (whom she had never met) was in love with her and wanted to father her child. She claimed that he constantly sent her telepathic messages of his adoration of her and would not stay out of her mind. Many times she expressed frustration and irritation about his constant interference with her mind, but she was pleased that he thought so highly of her and felt she was perfect in every way. She ate very little, smoked constantly, and looked disheveled. Because of her poor judgment about drug use and the people with whom she associated, her safety was constantly in danger. She lived for a time on her parents' credit cards until they were finally able to locate her and bring her home for treatment, which she resisted angrily.

Individuals with schizophrenia may act silly or laugh inappropriately. They may display an emotional response that is not congruent with the present situation (*inappropriate affect*), for instance, laughing at a tragic situation.

They also show lack of motivation or loss of interest, some of the so-called negative symptoms, which are evident in poor personal hygiene and self-care deficits. Clients may fail to eat regularly, obtain adequate nutrition, or seek care when health problems arise and may engage in behaviors such as drug use, wandering the streets, and using poor judgment about safe company and surroundings.

Bizarre movements unrelated to medication, such as rocking, posturing, odd mannerisms, and lack of movement, may occur. Clients with psychotic disorders in general, and particularly in schizophrenia, may appear to be listening to internal "voices" (*auditory hallucinations*), such as the "telepathic" messages that June K believed she received. Often, they may sit very still and appear engrossed in thought, as if they were listening carefully; this is known as the "listening attitude." Auditory hallucinations may contain commands that the client perform some behavior, commonly a dangerous or unsafe act. These "command" hallucinations are important to identify because they may place the client or others in danger.

At other times, clients may respond to imagined individuals or objects. These *visual hallucinations* often frighten clients. They may claim to have seen God, Jesus, the devil, or other powerful or frightening figures. Visual hallucinations may also include snakes, bugs, vermin, and other creatures.

Paranoid hallucinations may be present—voices telling the individual to "trust no one." Paranoid delusions often include being "monitored" by the FBI or IRS. Clients with **paranoia** misinterpret the intentions of others. They may believe that socializing will make it easier for others to "spy" on them. They may look around suspiciously as if they are being followed and question why certain ordinary procedures are being done. Paranoid clients refuse to answer certain questions or discuss certain topics for fear they will reveal "secret" information that may be used to harm them. They may refuse to eat, fearing food has been poisoned or that "ground glass" or other harmful objects have been added.

Clients speech may contain bizarre concepts, digress from usual content, show a paucity of words, or be overly concrete. Asked to explain the expression "a rolling stone gathers no moss" during a mental status examination, a client with schizophrenia might respond, "Stones get messy with moss on them," demonstrating concrete thinking and a lack of abstraction.

Blocking of speech, in which clients lose their train of thought in mid-sentence and cannot continue, may also be present. Some clients exhibit loose associations or tangentiality of speech, such as "My brother is coming to pick me up in the car. I like cars. The automakers in Detroit are cheating us. So is the IRS. It's like the IRA. There should be a rebellion soon."

Clients may use *neologisms*, which are made-up words that

have meaning only to the client: "You are tixicating me." "My medicine rotigets me." *Word salad* may also be evident in schizophrenia: "Over hill over there what's the word behind the trail." Clients may demonstrate stereotyped speech by reverting to or perseverating with the same idea over and over. *Clanging* rhymes words: "Look up at the star. I went to the bar. She drove the car, and it went far. I'm out in the tar."

One of the most difficult aspects of schizophrenia is clients' lack of awareness of symptoms or outright denial that anything is unusual or amiss. Termed "poor insight," this characteristic seriously limits the nurse's opportunity to obtain an accurate history and assessment of current and previous functioning.

Subtypes

Different subtypes further describe schizophrenia: paranoid, disorganized, catatonic, undifferentiated, and residual types.[1] Table 18–3 illustrates the most prominent symptoms that define the subtypes, although certain behaviors may overlap. Paranoid schizophrenia features delusions or auditory hallucinations that have a persecutory (being watched, spied upon, or harmed) or grandiose theme (being a famous person or having special powers or skills).

Disorganized type is characterized by a flat or inappropriate affect with disorganized behavior and speech. In catatonic schizophrenia, individuals exhibit two of the following: motor immobility with *cataplexy* (loss of muscle tone or collapsing), purposeless and excessive motor activity, extreme negativism or mutism, bizarre postures or stereotyped movements, *echolalia* (echoing the words of another), or *echopraxia* (imitating movements).[1]

If none of these features is prominent, or the client has features of more than one subtype, then undifferentiated type is present. A final type is residual, in which there are hallucinations, disorganization of behavior, and speech, but to a lesser extent than found in schizophrenia. Residual type may also be diagnosed when negative symptoms predominate.

TABLE 18–3. Major Features of the Subtypes of Schizophrenia

Subtype	Definition	Examples
Paranoid	• Preoccupation with delusions or auditory hallucinations. • None of the following is present: disorganized speech or behavior, flat or inappropriate affect.	Believing that the FBI or CIA is watching; hearing "messages" from the government that there is a plot to overthrow the president.
Disorganized	• Disorganized speech • Disorganized behavior • Flat or inappropriate affect • No evidence of catatonia	Silliness, laughter; childlike behavior; poor hygiene; grimacing and odd mannerisms and behaviors.
Catatonic	Two of the following: • Severe physical immobility, stupor • Excessive and purposeless motor activity • Mute or extreme resistance to all instructions • Inappropriate and bizarre postures or stereotyped movements • Echolalia (parrot-like repetition of words), echopraxia (imitation of another person's movement).	Odd and peculiar movements such as: • Maintaining rigid posture • Bizarre postures or grimacing • Repeating the phrases or movements of others • Catalepsy (sudden loss of muscle tone and collapsing usually during extreme emotion) • Mutism • Extreme increases or decreases in motor activity • Usually requires constant supervision.
Undifferentiated	Two or more of the following • Delusions • Hallucinations • Disorganized speech • Disorganized or catatonic behavior • Negative symptoms • Does not meet criteria for paranoid, disorganized, or catatonic type.	Hears "God's voice"; makes nonsensical statements; doesn't complete ADLs; stays in apartment and smokes all day; has no friends or social relationships.
Residual	No *prominent* delusions, hallucinations, disorganized speech, or disorganized or catatonic behavior. Negative symptoms predominate, or *mild* positive symptoms remain.	Odd beliefs or unusual perceptions; unmotivated, absence of social contacts or significant relationships, unchanged facial expression, says little.

Source: Adapted from the Diagnostic and Statistical Manual of Mental Disorders, Fourth Edition. Copyright 1994 American Psychiatric Association.

Diagnostic Aids

The Brief Psychiatric Rating Scale (BPRS; Table 18–4)[2] assesses overall psychiatric functioning with particular relevance to psychotic symptoms. Nurses use this scale to evaluate **psychosis** and the impact of symptoms on the individual's daily life.

No specific laboratory tests or identifiable disruptions in dopaminergic (see Etiology section) functioning are currently available to determine the presence of any psychotic disorders, including schizophrenia. However, certain neurological signs, also referred to as "soft signs," may be present in schizophrenia, including poor coordination and confusing left and right orientation.[1]

There may be facial abnormalities in the palate or eye position, such as a highly arched palate and narrow- or wide-set eyes.[1] Clients may drink excessive amounts of water, leading to water intoxication through depletion of electrolytes. Structural or functional brain abnormalities such as enlarged ventricles, decreased temporal and hippocampal size, and abnormal blood flow to the prefrontal cortex have also been reported in schizophrenia. Unfortunately, none of these abnormalities conclusively diagnoses schizophrenia.

Culture, Age, and Gender Features

Culture

Cultural differences are evident in presentation, course, and outcome. For instance, catatonia, immobility, and bizarre posturing is more common in non-Western countries.[1] Although the reason for this unexpected finding remains unclear, people in less-developed countries may better accept and tolerate the symptoms. Schizophrenia is more likely to be diagnosed in certain cultures, such as African-Americans, and in those who are socioeconomically deprived and less educated.[1]

Cultural background is important in assessment. Healthcare professionals may misinterpret beliefs in sorcery and witchcraft, accepted in some cultures, as delusions. Although visual hallucinations are common in schizophrenia, "hearing God's voice" may be a common experience for people who are strongly religious. A good example of cultural differences occurred with a student in the acute care psychiatric setting.

> An African-American woman diagnosed with bipolar disorder had demonstrated no hallucinations or delusions until recently. The staff became concerned when the woman began talking about the "voice of the Lord" speaking directly to her. The student caring for the client talked with the woman and assessed the situation. He reported that her speech reflected her strong religious background. He himself had been brought up in a religious culture in which the minister was perceived as the "Voice of God." This is precisely what the woman meant, and she was relieved that the student understood and communicated this understanding to the staff.

Gender and Age

Schizophrenia occurs equally in males and females, although males tend to be hospitalized at a younger age. Females tend to develop schizophrenia later in life, have more mood symptoms, and yet are able to function better in relationships and occupation.[1]

Schizophrenia is uncommon in children and usually diagnosed between the ages of 15 and 35.

Etiology

Neurophysiological and Neuropharmacologic Theories

Several neurotransmitters have been implicated in the pathogenesis of schizophrenia, including dopamine, serotonin, glutamate, norepinephrine, and γ-aminobutyric acid (GABA). For many years, the dopamine theory of schizophrenia, which suggested that there was an overactivation of the dopamine system, either too much dopamine or too many dopamine receptors, prevailed. The evidence for dopamine overactivity came from pharmacologic research. All of the original classic antipsychotic drugs were found to block (antagonize) dopamine receptors, and the potency with which they blocked dopamine D_2 receptors correlated strongly with their clinical potency (daily dose in milligrams). Furthermore, it was known that chronic high-dose amphetamine abuse could produce a schizophrenic-like state with paranoia and hallucinations. Neuropharmacologists discovered that amphetamines worked by activating the dopamine system, causing dopamine neurons to release too much dopamine. Because antipsychotic drugs worked by attenuating dopamine neurotransmission at the receptor level, and amphetamines produced psychosis by activating dopamine neurons, it was logical to postulate that schizophrenia resulted from excessive dopamine transmission. Autopsy studies of brains from deceased schizophrenics provided partial support for the dopamine overactivity theory.[3]

Although the dopamine system appears to play a significant role in the mechanism of antipsychotic drug effects, more contemporary studies strongly suggest that schizophrenia is not caused by dopamine overactivity.

Despite many efforts, no signs of excess dopamine production (through chemical analysis of cerebrospinal fluid), or an excess number of dopamine D_2 receptors (using positron-emission tomography; PET) have been found in living schizophrenics who had never been exposed to antipsychotic drugs.[4] Some researchers, however, postulate that schizophrenia may be related to an excess number of a dopamine D_2 receptor subtype called D_4.

Another major problem with the dopamine overactivity theory is that antipsychotic drugs block dopamine receptors within minutes of administration but take weeks to exert

TABLE 18–4.

BRIEF PSYCHIATRIC RATING SCALE
Overall and Gorham

DIRECTIONS: Place an X in the appropriate box to represent Level of severity of each symptom.

Patient Name _____ Physician _____

Patient SS # _____ UT # _____ HH # _____ Date _____

Symptom	Not Present	Very Mild	Mild	Moderate	Mod. Severe	Severe	Extremely Severe
SOMATIC CONCERN - preoccupation with physical health, fear of physical illness, hypochondriasis.	☐	☐	☐	☐	☐	☐	☐
ANXIETY - worry, fear, over-concern for present or future, uneasiness.	☐	☐	☐	☐	☐	☐	☐
EMOTIONAL WITHDRAWAL - lack of spontaneous interaction, isolation deficiency in relating to others.	☐	☐	☐	☐	☐	☐	☐
CONCEPTUAL DISORGANIZATION - thought processes confused, disconnected, disorganized, disrupted.	☐	☐	☐	☐	☐	☐	☐
GUILT FEELINGS - self-blame, shame, remorse for past behavior.	☐	☐	☐	☐	☐	☐	☐
TENSION - physical and motor manifestations of nervousness, over-activation.	☐	☐	☐	☐	☐	☐	☐
MANNERISMS AND POSTURING - peculiar, bizarre unnatural motor behavior (not including tic).	☐	☐	☐	☐	☐	☐	☐
GRANDIOSITY - exggerated self-opinion, arrogance, conviction of unusual power or abilities.	☐	☐	☐	☐	☐	☐	☐
DEPRESSIVE MOOD - sorrow, sadness, despondency, pessimism.	☐	☐	☐	☐	☐	☐	☐
HOSTILITY - animosity, contempt, belligerence, disdain for others.	☐	☐	☐	☐	☐	☐	☐
SUSPICIOUSNESS - mistrust, belief others harbour malicious or discriminatory intent.	☐	☐	☐	☐	☐	☐	☐
HALLUCINATORY BEHAVIOR - perceptions without normal external stimulus correspondence.	☐	☐	☐	☐	☐	☐	☐
MOTOR RETARDATION - slowed weakened movements or speech, reduced body tone.	☐	☐	☐	☐	☐	☐	☐
UNCOOPERATIVENESS - resistance, guardedness, rejection of authority.	☐	☐	☐	☐	☐	☐	☐
UNUSUAL THOUGHT CONTENT - unusual, odd, strange, bizarre thought content.	☐	☐	☐	☐	☐	☐	☐
BLUNTED AFFECT - reduced emotional tone, reduction in formal intensity of feelings, flatness.	☐	☐	☐	☐	☐	☐	☐
EXCITEMENT - heightened emotional tone, agitation, increased reactivity.	☐	☐	☐	☐	☐	☐	☐
DISORIENTATION - confusion or lack of proper association for person, place, or time.	☐	☐	☐	☐	☐	☐	☐

Global Assessment Scale (Range 1-100) _____

Source: Reproduced with permission of authors and publishers from Overall, JR and Gorham, DR: The Brief Psychiatric Rating Scale. Psychological Reports, 1962, 10, 799–812. Copyright Southern Universities Press 1962.

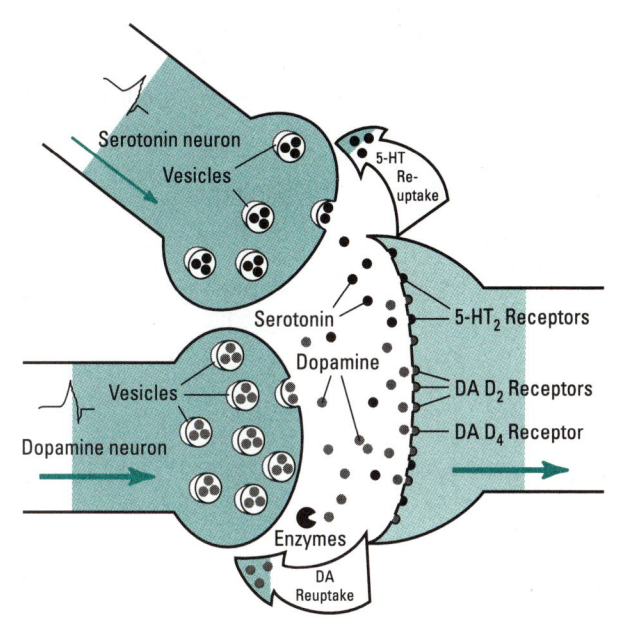

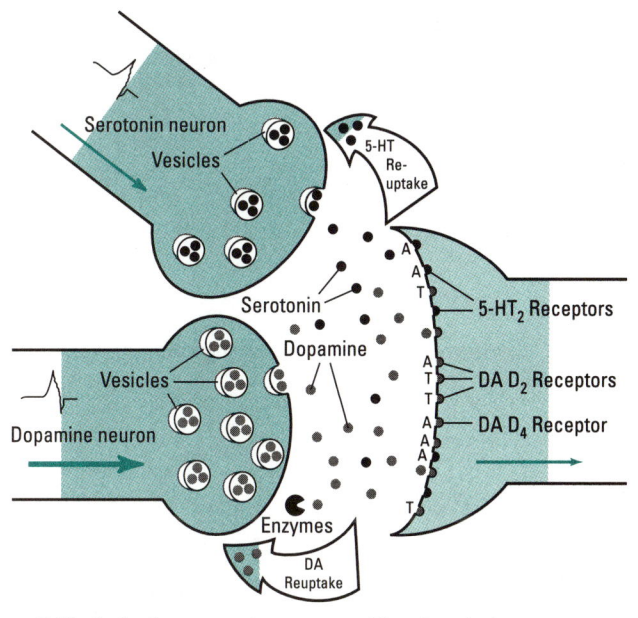

Schizophrenia and Other Psychotic Disorders **315**

tory patients with schizophrenia, even though clozapine is a much weaker dopamine D₂ antagonist than the classic antipsychotic drugs. As a consequence, a great deal of research conducted to find out how clozapine differs from other antipsychotic drugs has led to new theories, which remain to be tested, that focus on dopamine-serotonin balance, dopamine D_4 receptors, or specific serotonin receptors such as 5-HT_7.

Taken together, current research suggests that dopamine and serotonin may be involved in the pathophysiology of schizophrenia, but that a host of other transmitter systems may also be involved (Figure 18–1). Most recently, research interest has focused on the excitatory neurotransmitter glutamine, as phencyclidine (PCP or angel dust) affects this transmitter and can produce an even more convincing schizophrenic-like psychosis than amphetamines. In a syndrome as complicated and varied as schizophrenia, it is unlikely that a disturbance in a single neurotransmitter system can be the cause.

Genetic Theories

Early family, twin, and adoption studies describe genetic vulnerability and clustering of schizophrenia in families. First-degree relatives of persons with schizophrenia have 10 to 15 times the risk[5] of developing schizophrenia. However, most clients with schizophrenia have no close family relatives with the disorder, indicating that the environment is also a crucial factor.

The best evidence on heredity and genetic predisposition comes from studies of twins. If schizophrenia is diagnosed in one twin, there is a 40 to 55% chance that an identical (monozygotic) twin will develop schizophrenia. However, if the twin is not identical (dizygotic), there is only a 10 to 14% chance that they will develop schizophrenia.[5] The high concordance in identical twins is not a consequence of parents treating them more identically. High concordance persists even in twins separated at birth and raised by different families. This type of data provides very strong evidence that schizophrenia has an inheritable genetic component. Nevertheless, a risk factor of 40 to 55% indicates that genetics is not the entire story and that other factors are equally important. Genes apparently provide a predisposition or vulnerability to develop schizophrenia, but something else must occur for the disorder to actually develop.

In this "two-hit" model of schizophrenia, the combination of heredity and environmental factors leads to the disorder. A genetic defect doesn't fully explain schizophrenia but provides an underlying vulnerability, the so-called first hit. Then a life event such as prenatal viral exposure or complications during delivery cause a "second hit." Only those who experience both "hits" develop schizophrenia.

Genetic linkage studies have attempted to find a "schizophrenic gene" in regions of the chromosome that contain the genetic information for creating dopamine and serotonin receptors and the enzymes that produce these transmitters. Although some promising results were initially reported, there are no consistent positive findings.[5]

Figure 18–1. Increased activity in dopamine neurons is hypothesized to underlie schizophrenia. The arrows indicate the strength of activity in each of the neurons. (*A*) Schematic showing how dopamine and serotonin neurons interact. (*B*) The effects of typical (T) and atypical (A) neuroleptics on the postsynaptic site. These agents block dopamine receptors; the typical neuroleptics, such as haloperidol, block D₂ receptors, while the atypical neuroleptics, such as clozapine, olanzipine, and risperidone, block D₄ and D₂ dopamine receptors and serotoninergic 5-HT₂ receptors. (Courtesy of Dr. Susan Andersen.)

their full therapeutic benefits. Their antipsychotic effects may result from more gradual compensatory changes that occur in the brain after their administration.

Finally, the atypical antipsychotic agent clozapine is more effective than classic antipsychotic drugs in treating refrac-

The search for genetic factors in schizophrenia will remain complicated. First, this disorder has "low penetrance," which means that many individuals with high genetic risk will never develop the disorder. Second, there are "phenocopies" of the disorder, which indicates that some clients develop schizophrenia even though they do not carry the genes. Finally, psychiatric diagnosis is difficult, and major theoretical questions arise whether family members with schizoaffective disorder, schizotypal personality, borderline personality, or other similar conditions should be counted as cases.

Environmental and Neurodevelopmental Factors

If genes convey only a vulnerability to developing schizophrenia, what are the other risk factors? The fetal period seems to be a time of risk.[6] There is a modest but significant association between risk of developing schizophrenia and season of birth that can be traced back to the rates with which mothers contracted certain viral infections during their second trimesters of pregnancy. This hypothesis is bolstered by animal studies that suggest that prenatal viral infections can produce alterations in the arrangement of brain neurons that resemble microscopic abnormalities found in schizophrenic brains. Moreover, epidemiological data suggest an association between incidence of obstetrical complications at delivery and risk of developing schizophrenia. Other interesting information comes from studies of identical twins in which one twin has schizophrenia and the other clearly does not. Investigators found that the twin who went on to develop schizophrenia was invariably lighter at birth and had a much greater incidence of perinatal neurological abnormalities. In short, the second major factor in the etiology of schizophrenia may be any one of a number of conditions that injure or impair the developing brain.

Neuroanatomical researchers are becoming convinced that schizophrenic clients have subtle microscopic abnormalities in their brains that must have arisen very early in life. However, clinicians know that schizophrenia is a developmental disorder with peak onset in late adolescence or early adulthood. True cases of childhood schizophrenia are extraordinarily rare. If these abnormalities were present at the time of birth, how could they remain relatively quiescent for 20 years or more, and then become such a terrible problem?

Weinberger[7] has proposed that a fixed brain abnormality (lesion), acquired before birth, is ultimately responsible for schizophrenia. Initially, the consequences of this lesion are "silent." During the adolescent period, the brain goes through very dramatic change, primarily, the elimination of a large number of synapses and neurotransmitter receptors and the increased myelination of nerve fibers. In childhood, the brain produces a very high density of synaptic connections and receptors. Approximately 40% of these connections are eliminated by early adulthood, probably in a process in which the brain sacrifices plasticity and adaptability for increased speed and efficiency. During this phase, it may be that redundant backup circuits are eliminated that normally are no longer important but were providing crucial alternative pathways in schizophrenics. Another theory holds that nerve fiber pathways are becoming increasingly myelinated during adolescence, which increases communication between brain regions. In particular, a pathway connecting the prefrontal cortex with the limbic system does not myelinate until late in adolescence, when certain brain regions may be brought into much closer communication. A defect in one of these regions (producing faulty data or

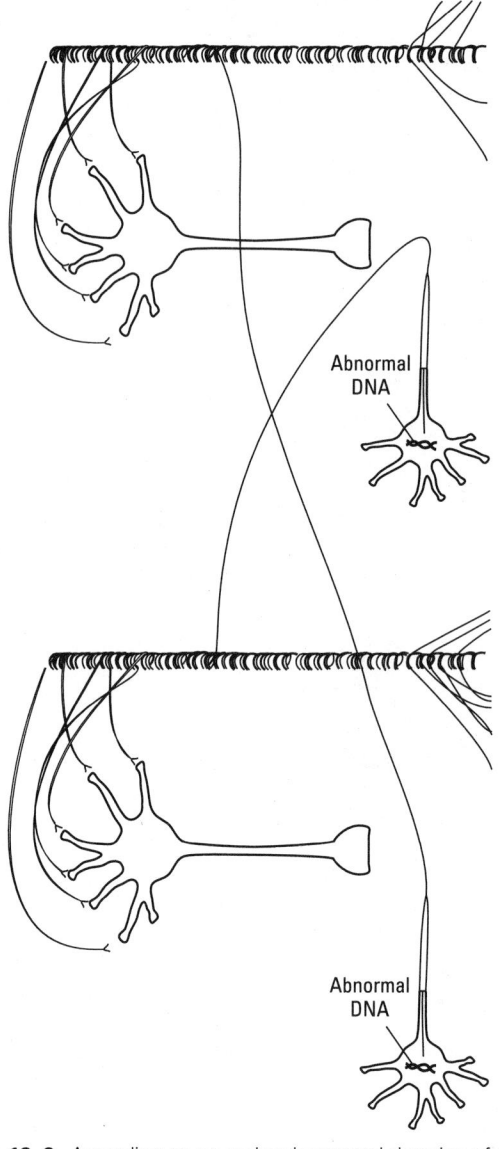

Figure 18–2. According to neurodevelopmental theories of schizophrenia, an abnormality in the DNA of a schizophrenic patient may cause the wrong synaptic connections to be made during the prenatal and early childhood formation of the brain and its connections. Schizophrenia may be the result of abnormal development of the brain from the beginning of life because neurons fail to migrate to the correct parts of the brain, fail to form appropriate connections, and then are subject to breakdown when used by the individual in late adolescence and early adulthood. (From Stahl, 1996, p 286.)

noise) can then produce more interference with other brain regions, leading to an increasing array of difficulties.

Abnormalities in Brain Structure and Function

Researchers have been searching for specific anatomical abnormalities in the schizophrenic brain for more than a century. Until recently, these efforts have been disappointing. Now some consistent and compelling findings have emerged from different laboratories.

Microscopic studies have found abnormal neural migration and abnormal neural orientation in several regions of the schizophrenic brain (Figure 18–2). Neurons migrate to their final destination during fetal development, which limits the problem to this period. Several different brain regions are affected, indicating that the problem is relatively widespread. Neural migration problems are not specific to schizophrenia and have also been observed in autopsied brains from clients with mental retardation and learning disorders.

Functional imaging studies that measure brain metabolism, blood flow, and blood perfusion have suggested that the prefrontal cortex, which serves a primary role in executive functions such as planning and higher-level abstraction, may be cognitively impaired in some people with schizophrenia. Cognitive tasks that use the prefrontal cortex have been found, in some studies, to enhance metabolism and blood flow in this region in healthy volunteers but not in schizophrenics.

Overall, researchers studying the etiology and pathophysiology of schizophrenia are developing complex models that tie together cortical regions (prefrontal cortex and anterior cingulate cortex), limbic regions (hippocampus), and the striatum. These models also integrate neurochemistry because the striatal and cortical regions are highly innervated by dopamine and serotonin (Figure 18–3). Further, these cortical and limbic regions communicate with the striatum through glutaminergic pathways. Damage to different parts of this circuit may produce similar effects. Overactivation of any one of these transmitters through illicit drug use can produce hallucinations or psychosis by disturbing their balance, and it may prove possible to treat these disorders through a variety of different pharmacologic strategies.

Prognosis

Certain factors have been associated with poorer prognosis (Table 18–5). For example, the presence of positive or negative symptoms may predict the ability to function in daily activities. Those individuals with positive symptoms are about nine times more likely to be employed when in the residual phase of their illness.[8] Those with negative symptoms tend to have fewer years of education, a poorer premorbid adjustment, and less likelihood of responding to treatment than those without negative symptoms.[8]

Only about 5 to 15% of clients fully recover, although new treatments such as atypical antipsychotic medications may provide hope in the future. About 40 to 55% of schizophrenic individuals show partial recovery, whereas 20% have a deteriorating, chronic course. The disorganized subtype is associated with the most severe impairment.

Because of altered thought processes, clients are likely to neglect their physical health or develop other concurrent problems such as nicotine, alcohol, or substance abuse (see *Dual Diagnosis*). Studies show that about 10% commit suicide.

OTHER PSYCHOTIC DISORDERS

Other psychotic disorders include schizophreniform disorder, schizoaffective disorder, delusional disorder, brief psy-

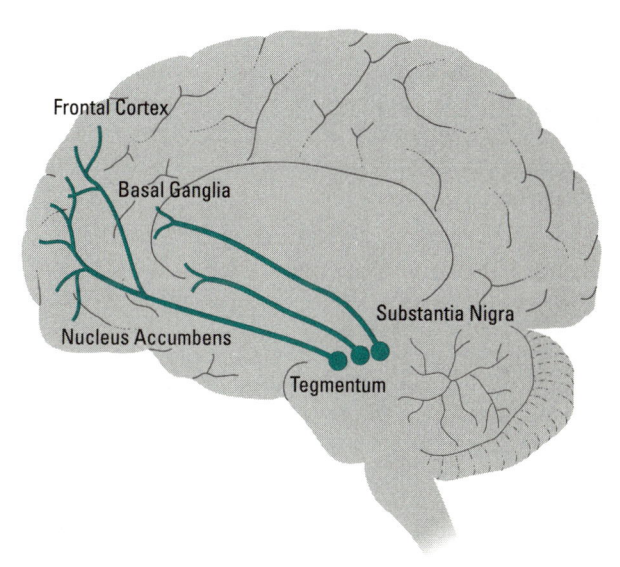

Figure 18–3. Antipsychotic agents target the dopamine system in the brain where they exert therapeutic and unwanted side effects by decreasing dopamine neurotransmission. The mesocortical pathway, which projects from the tegmentum to the front cortex, plays a role in the positive and negative symptoms as well as the cognitive deficits associated with schizophrenia. The nigostriatal dopamine pathway projects from the substantia nigra to the basal ganglia and is responsible for the motor side effects of neuroleptics. The third system, the mesolimbic system, projects from the tegmentum to the nucleus acumbens. Activation of this system is believed to account for the delusions and hallucinations of psychosis.

TABLE 18–5. Factors That Relate to Poor Outcome in Schizophrenia

Early age of onset
Insidious onset
Poor premorbid adjustment
Sustained emotional withdrawal
Inappropriate affective response
Enlarged cerebral ventricles
Reduced blinking rates
Perinatal brain injury
Poor response to medications

DUAL DIAGNOSIS

Dual diagnosis refers to the presence of substance or alcohol abuse and another mental illness. Substance and alcohol abuse can occur with any other major psychiatric condition; however, one of the most debilitating problems is comorbid schizophrenia. The co-occurrence of these disorders is estimated to be from 10 to 70%. In one recent survey, the lifetime prevalence of schizophrenia and alcohol abuse was 47%, whereas the prevalence of schizophrenia and cocaine abuse was 17%.[1] Combined with a psychotic disorder, substance abuse leads to more health and social problems. Individuals with a psychotic disorder who abuse drugs or alcohol are more likely to engage in criminal behaviors, attempt suicide, and become homeless.

Individuals with schizophrenia or psychotic disorders often deny using or abusing substances. Family members are good sources of information for determining whether a potential problem exists. Several risks factors suggest the presence of alcohol or substance abuse: a history of substance abuse, a history of violence, clouding of consciousness, several psychiatric hospitalizations, and having friends who abuse drugs. Other clues to dual diagnosis include poor attention, difficulty responding to questions, disorientation, and misperception of time.

Clients with a dual diagnosis of schizophrenia and substance abuse need an integrated treatment approach, preferably within the same setting. Sequential treatment, for instance, treatment for schizophrenic behaviors and then for substance abuse, is much less effective than combined treatment.[2] The positive and negative symptoms of schizophrenia and substance abuse need to be addressed concurrently, usually through pharmacotherapy, behavioral therapy, supportive therapy, psychoeducation, and case management. Clients with a dual diagnosis also need to have a continuum of care available to them; hospitalization, day treatment, and an outpatient program may be needed, depending on the duration and severity of their symptoms. Treatment goals include recognizing that they need help, establishing a relationship with a case manager or therapist, and understanding the need to maintain sobriety.

Clients with a dual diagnosis need a low-intensity treatment setting because psychotic symptoms worsen in environments with confrontation and high levels of emotion.[2] A highly structured approach is also effective; structure provides the external controls that these clients often lack. Pharmacotherapy generally consists of antipsychotic medications. Psychoeducation can promote medication management: understanding the purpose of medication, need for regular administration, side effects, and what to do about missed or skipped doses. Case management includes helping clients receive benefits such as social security or health insurance, medical care, food, housing, and clothing. Via psychoeducation and supportive therapy, clients are taught about their illness, symptom management, and ways to detect early signs of relapse. Behavioral treatment often includes social-skills training, including methods to deal with other people in a variety of settings. Social-skills training teaches clients how to establish eye contact, make appointments, use public transportation, and get help with everyday tasks, such as banking and food shopping. In order to promote sobriety, some behavioral techniques focus on helping clients refuse drugs from friends or dealers. Other behavioral techniques include issuing a "credit card," used to buy clothes and food, which is earned by taking medications regularly, attending the treatment program and self-help groups, and maintaining daily hygiene.

Clients with a dual diagnosis need to participate regularly in specially designed self-help programs for substance and alcohol abuse. Based on the principles of "12-step" programs such as Alcoholics Anonymous (AA) and Narcotics Anonymous (NA), these groups are designed for individuals who may be paranoid and require long-term medication treatment. Many traditional AA and NA groups strongly discourage the use of any "substances," including prescribed medication; the adapted AA and NA groups assume that pharmacotherapy is an essential part of the treatment plan. Clients choose a sponsor and progress through the 12-step program to achieve and maintain sobriety.

1. Regier, DA, et al: Comorbidity of mental disorders with alcohol and other drug abuse: Results from the Epidemiologic Catchment Area Study. JAMA 264:2511–2518, 1990.
2. Dixon, L, and Rebori, TA: Psychosocial treatment of substance abuse in schizophrenic patients. In Kerr, TA (ed): Contemporary Issues in the Treatment of Schizophrenia. American Psychiatric Press, Washington, DC, 1995.

chotic disorder, and psychotic disorder not otherwise specified (NOS).[1] As seen in *Diagnostic Criteria for Other Psychotic Disorders*, these disorders are all characterized by having some psychotic symptoms similar to schizophrenia. Distinguishing between the psychotic disorders can be difficult, but the key features of all of them are misperceptions about reality or distorted thought processes. They differ in type of symptoms, duration, and extent of functional decline. Carefully assess duration of symptoms, presence or absence of mood symptoms, and overall level of functioning.

SCHIZOPHRENIFORM DISORDER

The diagnosis of schizophreniform disorder is often made when individuals show some symptoms of schizophrenia but for only 1 to 6 months. Functioning may not be significantly impaired, although there may be self-care deficits, social withdrawal, and occupational dysfunction. Although some recover from schizophreniform disorder, the majority go on to develop schizophrenia. Behaviors that predict remission include confusion, absence of flat affect, and a sudden onset of symptoms within 4 weeks of a major change in behavior.

SCHIZOAFFECTIVE DISORDER

Schizoaffective disorder is characterized by an uninterrupted period of illness in which two major criteria are present: criteria A symptoms of schizophrenia and symptoms of mood disorders. Two key symptoms of schizophrenia, such as delusions, hallucinations, disorganized speech, disorganized or catatonic behavior, and negative symptoms, such as affective flattening, avolition, and alogia, are exhibited. In addition, the client has symptoms associated with major depressive disorder, mania, or mixed episodes of bipolar disorder. The major feature that differentiates schizoaffective disorder from schizophrenia is that the mood symptoms co-occur for a prolonged time period with the psychotic symptoms. In schizophrenia, mood symptoms are brief, and psychotic symptoms predominate.[1] Unfortunately, schizoaffective disorder is associated with severe dysfunction, a deteriorating course, social withdrawal, poor occupational functioning, and self-care deficits.

DELUSIONAL DISORDER

The key feature of this disorder is delusions without the hallucinations, disorganized behavior and speech, or negative symptoms characteristic of schizophrenia.[1] In severe forms, delusional disorder may occur with body dysmorphic disorder, where the delusion is extreme but focused specifically on one body part. Delusional disorder is generally characterized by nonbizarre delusions that may have erotic, grandiose, jealous, persecutory, or somatic themes. Clients with delusional disorder are often able to function fairly well, hold down a job, marry, and have a family. They tend to be more extroverted and less socially withdrawn than individuals with schizophrenia.

For many years, my wife has been having an affair. Sometimes I think she's having an affair with my brother, but in the past I knew it was my father. I could just tell by the way they looked at one another. I used to think my mother was cheating on my father, but my family says that was false. Recently, I confronted my neighbor about having an affair with my wife. He said what they all do, "That's ridiculous." My wife is getting more upset with me. She says that these beliefs of mine are not true and are wrecking our marriage. I really love my wife, but I think we're headed for a divorce. I decided to go for some help because I don't want to lose her. She said she'd like to meet with my counselor to help us with this.

This man describes a specific delusion that is, his wife is having an affair. He has had this false belief for several years, with only the partner in the affair changing. No other symptoms were present—no hallucinations, odd behaviors, or mood symptoms to suggest depression or bipolar disorder. He is employed and is an avid gardener. His main difficulty is a circumscribed delusion that his wife is unfaithful.

BRIEF PSYCHOTIC DISORDER

If an individual experiences delusions, hallucinations, disorganization, or catatonic behavior for less than 1 month, a brief psychotic disorder is diagnosed.[1] The onset of the psychotic behavior is abrupt and often in response to a severe and recent stressor, such as loss of a significant other, a natural disaster, or the birth of a child. Although brief psychotic episodes remit within 1 month, during that time, individuals suffer severe symptoms leading to impairment of daily function, self-care, nutrition, and hydration. Poor judgment during this time may result in dangerous and suicidal behaviors. Following the episode, the individual will return to the previous level of function.

Prognosis

Individuals with psychotic disorders have a widely variable course of illness, displaying exacerbations and remissions of symptoms[1] (Table 18–6). In schizoaffective disorder, the prognosis is more hopeful and recovery is more likely. Although one-third of individuals with schizophreniform disorder recover within 6 months, two-thirds develop schizophrenia.[1] The course of delusional disorder varies; some individuals experience a remission of symptoms alternating with delusional periods.[1] Brief and other psychotic disorders usually resolve quickly, within days or weeks, and there is a return to previous levels of functioning.

Assessing Acute Episodes of Illness

An individualized plan of care should anticipate the severe symptoms and deteriorating nature of clients' behavior. First, determine if they are suffering from their first psychotic episode or an acute exacerbation of a chronic disorder. In either case, severe impairment in daily functioning and self-care and particular symptoms or behaviors frequently threaten the safety of the clients or others.

Assess the existence and influence of delusions, hallucinations, and paranoid or disorganized thinking upon safety. Dangerous or assaultive behavior may be a consequence of altered thought processes and disturbed behavior. If the client is assaultive, actively planning suicide, or ignoring basic

DSM-IV Diagnostic Criteria for Other Psychotic Disorders

Diagnostic Criteria for 295.40 Schizophreniform Disorder

A. Criteria A, D, and E of Schizophrenia are met.

B. An episode of the disorder (including prodromal, active, and residual phases) lasts at least 1 month but less than 6 months. (When the diagnosis must be made without waiting for recovery, it should be qualified as "Provisional.")

Specify if:
 Without Good Prognostic Features
 With Good Prognostic Features: as evidenced by two (or more) of the following:
  (1) onset of prominent psychotic symptoms within 4 weeks of the first noticeable change in usual behavior or functioning
  (2) confusion or perplexity at the height of the psychotic episode
  (3) good premorbid social and occupational functioning
  (4) absence of blunted or flat affect

Diagnostic Criteria for 295.70 Schizoaffective Disorder

A. An uninterrupted period of illness during which, at some time, there is either a Major Depressive Episode, a Manic Episode, or a Mixed Episode concurrent with symptoms that meet Criterion A for Schizophrenia.
 NOTE: The Major Depressive Episode must include Criterion A1: depressed mood.

B. During the same period of illness, there have been delusions or hallucinations for at least 2 weeks in the absence of prominent mood symptoms.

C. Symptoms that meet criteria for a mood episode are present for a substantial portion of the total duration of the active and residual periods of the illness.

D. The disturbance is not due to the direct physiological effects of a substance (e.g., a drug of abuse, a medication) or a general medical condition.

Specify type:
 Bipolar Type: if the disturbance includes a Manic or a Mixed Episode (or a Manic or a Mixed Episode and Major Depressive Episodes)
 Depressive Type: if the disturbance only includes Major Depressive Episodes

Diagnostic Criteria for 297.1 Delusional Disorder

A. Nonbizarre delusions (i.e., involving situations that occur in real life, such as being followed, poisoned, infected, loved at a distance, or deceived by spouse or lover, or having a disease) of at least 1 month's duration.

B. Criterion A for Schizophrenia has never been met.
 Note: Tactile and olfactory hallucinations may be present in Delusional Disorder if they are related to the delusional theme.

C. Apart from the impact of the delusion(s) or its ramifications, functioning is not markedly impaired and behavior is not obviously odd or bizarre.

D. If mood episodes have occurred concurrently with delusions, their total duration has been brief relative to the duration of the delusional periods.

E. The disturbance is not due to the direct physiological effects of a substance (e.g., a drug of abuse, a medication) or a general medical condition.

Specify type (the following types are assigned based on the predominant delusional theme):
 Erotomanic Type: delusions that another person, usually of higher status, is in love with the individual
 Grandiose Type: delusions of inflated worth, power, knowledge, identity, or special relationship to a deity or famous person
 Jealous Type: delusions that the individual's sexual partner is unfaithful
 Persecutory Type: delusions that the person (or someone to whom the person is close) is being malevolently treated in some way
 Somatic Type: delusions that the person has some physical defect or general medical condition
 Mixed Type: delusions characteristic of more than one of the above types but no one theme predominates
 Unspecified Type

Diagnostic Criteria for 298.8 Brief Psychotic Disorder

A. Presence of one (or more) of the following symptoms:
 (1) delusions
 (2) hallucinations
 (3) disorganized speech (e.g., frequent derailment or incoherence)
 (4) grossly disorganized or catatonic behavior
 NOTE: Do not include a symptom if it is a culturally sanctioned response pattern.

B. Duration of an episode of the disturbance is at least 1 day but less than 1 month, with eventual full return to premorbid level of functioning.

C. The disturbance is not better accounted for by a Mood Disorder With Psychotic Features, Schizoaffective Disorder, or Schizophrenia and is not due to the direct physiological effects of a substance (e.g., a drug of abuse, a medication) or a general medical condition.

Specify if:
 With Marked Stressor(s) (brief reactive psychosis): if symptoms occur shortly after and apparently in response to events that, singly or together, would be markedly stressful to almost anyone in similar circumstances in the person's culture
 Without Marked Stressor(s): if psychotic symptoms do *not* occur shortly after, or are not apparently in response to events that, singly or together, would be markedly stressful to almost anyone in similar circumstances in the person's culture

Continued on following page

With Postpartum Onset: if onset within 4 weeks postpartum

Diagnostic Criteria for 297.3 Shared Psychotic Disorder

A. A delusion develops in an individual in the context of a close relationship with another person(s), who has an already-established delusion.

B. The delusion is similar in content to that of the person who already has the established delusion.

C. The disturbance is not better accounted for by another Psychotic Disorder (e.g., Schizophrenia) or a Mood Disorder With Psychotic Features and is not due to the direct physiological effects of a substance (e.g., a drug of abuse, a medication) or a general medical condition.

Diagnostic Criteria for 293.xx Psychotic Disorder Due to . . . [Indicate the General Medical Condition]

A. Prominent hallucinations or delusions.

B. There is evidence from the history, physical examination, or laboratory findings that the disturbance is the direct physiological consequence of a general medical condition.

C. The disturbance is not better accounted for by another mental disorder.

D. The disturbance does not occur exclusively during the course of a delirium.

Code based on predominant symptom:

.81 With Delusions: if delusions are the predominant symptom

.82 With Hallucinations: if hallucinations are the predominant symptom

CODING NOTE: Include the name of the general medical condition on Axis I, e.g., 293.81 Psychotic Disorder Due to Malignant Lung Neoplasm, With Delusions; also code the general medical condition on Axis III (see Appendix G for codes).

CODING NOTE: If delusions are part of a preexisting dementia, indicate the delusions by coding the appropriate subtype of the dementia if one is available, e.g., 290.20 Dementia of the Alzheimer's Type, With Late Onset, With Delusions.

Diagnostic Criteria for Substance-Induced Psychotic Disorder

A. Prominent hallucinations or delusions.

NOTE: Do not include hallucinations if the person has insight that they are substance induced.

B. There is evidence from the history, physical examination, or laboratory findings of either (1) or (2):

(1) the symptoms in Criterion A developed during, or within a month of, Substance Intoxication or Withdrawal

(2) medication use is etiologically related to the disturbance

C. The disturbance is not better accounted for by a Psychotic Disorder that is not substance induced. Evidence that the symptoms are better accounted for by a Psychotic Disorder that is not substance induced might include the following: the symptoms precede the onset of the substance use (or medication use); the symptoms persist for a substantial period of time (e.g., about a month) after the cessation of acute withdrawal or severe intoxication, or are substantially in excess of what would be expected given the type or amount of the substance used or the duration of use: or there is other evidence that suggests that existence of an independent non-substance-induced Psychotic Disorder (e.g., a history of recurrent non-substance-related episodes).

D. The disturbance does not occur exclusively during the course of a delirium.

NOTE: This diagnosis should be made instead of a diagnosis of Substance Intoxication or Substance Withdrawal only when the symptoms are in excess of those usually associated with the intoxication or withdrawal syndrome and when the symptoms are sufficiently severe to warrant independent clinical attention.

Code [Specific Substance]-Induced Psychotic Disorder: (291.5 Alcohol, with Delusions; 291.3 Alcohol, with Hallucinations; 292.11 Amphetamine [or Amphetamine-like Substance], with Delusions; 292.12 Amphetamine [or Amphetamine-like Substance], with Hallucinations; 292.11 Cannabis, with Delusions; 292.12 Cannabis, with Hallucinations; 292.11 Cocaine, with Delusions; 292.12 Cocaine, with Hallucinations; 292.11 Hallucinogen, with Delusions; 292.12 Hallucinogen, with Hallucinations; 292.11 Inhalant, with Delusions; 292.12 Inhalant, with Hallucinations; 292.11 Opioid, with Delusions; 292.12 Opioid, with Hallucinations; 292.11 Phencyclidine [or Phencyclidine-like Substance], with Delusions; 292.12 Phencyclidine [or Phencyclidine-like Substance], with Hallucinations; 292.11 Sedative, Hypnotic, or Anxiolytic, with Delusions; 292.12 Sedative, Hypnotic, or Anxiolytic, with Hallucinations; 292.11 Other [or Unknown] Substance, with Delusions; 292.12 Other [or Unknown] Substance, with Hallucinations)

Specify if

With Onset During Intoxication: if criteria are met for Intoxication with the substance and the symptoms develop during the intoxication syndrome

With Onset During Withdrawal: if criteria are met for Withdrawal from the substance and the symptoms develop during, or shortly after, a withdrawal syndrome

Source: Reprinted with permission from the Diagnostic and Statistical Manual of Mental Disorders, Fourth Edition. Copyright 1994 American Psychiatric Association.

Critical Pathway: Schizophrenia

Care Needs	1st 24 Hours	Days 2–5
Assessments/ Evaluations	Past psych history Medication history Medical history Suicide risk Self-care ability Appropriate legal status Psychiatric evaluation Nursing evaluation	Family interview Social work eval Evals by activities, OT, group, other therapies Continue psych and nursing evals

Diagnostic Tests/ Workup	Physical exam by internist, NP
	    Lab tests inc CBC, chem panel, drug screen, others
	    CAT scan, EEG, etc. as approp
		Review results of evals and lab work
		    Implement appropriate interventions
		    Implement further workup as needed
		    Complete psychological testing

Treatment	Orient to unit
	
	Initial activity orders
		Multidisciplinary tx plan developed
		    1:1 psychotherapy
		    Begin OT, activity, group rx as tolerated
		    Participate in family session if approp

Medications	Order inital doses of meds for psych & medical symptoms
	    Prn meds available for agitation, hallucinations
	    Monitor responses, side effects
		Establish appropriate medication doses
		    Adjust doses prn.
		    Ascertain appropriate routes
		    Monitor side effects & responses

Safety/Self-Care	Establish unit rules r/t risk for suicide, elopement, socialization, violence, substance abuse Evaluate need for isolation, restraints Monitor eating, elimination, sleep needs, and ability to care for self	Continue to monitor, as in column 1 Implement interventions for a safe environment Promote appropriate behavior at meals, toileting, hygiene Establish sleep schedule
Education	Unit orientation Client rights	Begin discussion on understanding dx Review connection between behavior, anxiety, stress Overview of meds Impact of Tx and test results. Begin family education re: dx.
Discharge Plan	Identify initial concerns	Identify patient/family concerns. Identify possible resources/living arrangements.
Outcomes	_____ Client assessed by MD and nurse _____ Initial tx plan started _____ Client does not harm self or others Progressing per pathway? Yes _____ No _____ If no, referred to _____	_____ Assessments by all disciplines complete _____ Workups complete _____ Multidiscipline tx plan developed & implemented _____ Meds adjusted as approp _____ Patient begins participating in tx _____ Patient does not harm self or others Progressing per pathway? Yes _____ No _____ If no, referred to _____

Care Needs	Days 6–10+	Discharge
Assessment/ Evaluations	Reassessment ongoing	
Diagnostic Tests/ Workup	All results available and implemented in tx plan	Need for follow-up medical care established and appointments made

Continued on following page

Critical Pathway: Schizophrenia   (Continued)

Care Needs	Days 6–10+	Discharge
Treatment	Tx plan inc 1:1 psychotherapy, groups, OT, activities Outpatient plan established	Outpatient tx appointments in place 　Issues r/t insurance, transportation complete
Medications	Cont monitoring response and adjust doses prn Monitor side effects Establish outpatient medication regimen	Identify discharge meds Ensure access to prescriptions
Safety/Self-Care	Cont to monitor & intervene for high-risk behaviors per days 1–5 Cont to monitor eating and self-care Establish self-care needs at discharge	Establish resources inc home care and caregivers for additional help Ensure patient has resources for food Involve family and caregivers as approp Ensure patient and caregivers know resources for help
Education	Cont to educate on dx, factors that exacerbate symptoms Teach coping skills to manage psychotic symptoms Education on meds and side effects Explain food and drug interactions Provide nutritional counseling List available community resources	Send patient home with written instructions and handouts. Reinforce teaching in outpatient tx
Discharge Plan	Establish outpatient tx plan Establish criteria for readmission Determine need for placement	Social work reviews plan for outpatient tx, living arrangements, insurance, work, leisure, finances Arrange transportation home Put in place access to resources for help
Outcomes	_____ Patient participates in tx plan _____ Patient demonstrates improvement and stabilization of symptoms _____ Stabilization of med doses _____ Requires less supervision _____ Patient does not harm self/others Progressing per pathway? Yes _____ No _____ If no, referred to _____	_____ Leaves hospital demonstrating understanding of D/C plan, prescriptions, knowledge of living arrangements _____ Family verbalizes plan to participate in tx plan _____ Patient verbalizes when to call for help _____ Patient acknowledges plan to comply with tx _____ Patient demonstrates readiness to function more independently Progressing per pathway? Yes _____ No _____ If no, referred to _____

health needs such as nutrition, acute care hospitalization or intensive outpatient treatment is necessary. In extreme states of psychosis, clinicians or police may initiate commitment procedures to protect the client or others from harm. Because of altered thought processes from hallucinations and delusions, clients are often in denial or unaware of their behavior; provide and maintain a safe environment. Table 18–7 describes assessment of self-care deficits related to safety and physical needs. In acute episodes, priority is given to safety and fluid and nutritional intake, followed by less urgent needs.

Mental Status Examination

The mental status examination provides a framework for evaluating the acutely psychotic client. Assessment of ap-

Box 18–1. Prevalence of Psychotic Disorders

Disorder	Prevalence
Schizophrenia	1%
Schizophreniform disorder	0.2%
Schizoaffective disorder	Unknown, less prevalent than schizophrenia
Delusional disorder	0.03%
Brief psychotic disorder	Unknown, but thought to be uncommon

Source: Data from the Diagnostic and Statistical Manual of Mental Disorders, Fourth Edition. Copyright 1994 American Psychiatric Association.

---

pearance may reveal inappropriate dress, neglected hygiene, poor eye contact, or inappropriate affect, such as laughing while relating a serious or upsetting event. Affect may lack spontaneity or appear flat. Bizarre, aggressive, or self-destructive behavior, often caused by hallucinations or delusions, may be readily apparent, or the thought disorder may cause withdrawal, isolation, or fear.

Altered Thought Processes

It is important to assess hallucinations, delusions, or other thought disorders in some detail to understand clients better and provide safe, effective care. Assessment must be based upon clients' willingness to discuss these phenomena, which may be the last thing fearful, paranoid clients wish to do. For example, voices may tell clients that all health-care personnel are "demons" in clever disguise and anything they reveal will be used against them, or clients may believe that staff members are reading their minds or taping everything they do or say. Williams[9] suggests assessment of nine factors regarding hallucinations:

- Identify all sensory aspects of the hallucination, including auditory, visual, tactile, and others.
- Assess how long the client has experienced hallucinations and, if possible, ask the client to describe what happened and when the hallucinations were first experienced.
- Assess how real the hallucinations are to the client, as well as the ability to distinguish reality from the experience of the hallucination.
- Identify the major theme and underlying feelings of the hallucination. For example, if the client has the belief that people wish to harm him or her, the theme is distrust and fear.
- Assess whether command hallucinations are being experienced, whether the client follows the commands, and the potential for harm.
- Note the time of day or situations in which the client is most likely to experience hallucinations.
- Assess the client's response to the hallucinations, for example, fear, despair, suicidal thoughts, or guilt.
- Determine the ways in which the individual has tried to cope with hallucinations, both ineffectively and effectively.
- If the client denies hallucinations, but gives nonverbal indications suggesting them, ask gently if the voices are telling him not to discuss them, or to indicate by a nod if there are voices.

The importance of assessing hallucinations is illustrated in the following example in which staff failed to assess the client's behavior.

Beginning at 2:00 pm, Jerry, a client diagnosed with paranoid schizophrenia, approached the nursing station and asked the time. The staff member responded without following up on this seemingly ordinary re-

---

TABLE 18–6. Differences in the Symptoms and Course of Psychotic Illnesses

Disorder	Positive Symptoms	Negative Symptoms	Duration of Symptoms	Decline in Functioning	Mood Symptoms
Schizophrenia	Present	Present	≥ 6 months	Significant	Few
Schizophreniform Disorder	Present	Present	1–6 months	None	None
Schizoaffective Disorder	Present	Present	Unspecified*	Probable	Common
Delusional Disorder	Present[†]	Absent	≥ 1 month	None	Common
Brief Psychotic Disorder	Present	Absent	1–30 days	None	None

*An "uninterrupted period of illness," probably lasting months to years.
[†]Delusions only.

TABLE 18-7. **Potential Safety and Physical Self-Care Deficits in Psychotic Disorders**

Safety	• Assess for orientation to reality and existence of hallucinations or delusions. • Assess for history of violent behavior. • Assess for side effects or adverse effects of medications.
Oxygenation	• Monitor vital signs for possible untoward side effects of medication: postural hypotension, tachycardia, arrhythmias.
Fluid and nutrition	• Assess ability of client to feed self. • Assess effects of social dining with less stimulating environment • Monitor food and fluid intake. Paranoia may decrease intake; medication may increase appetite leading to weight gain. • Weigh client weekly.
Elimination	• Assess for urinary retention or constipation related to side effects of medication. • Observe extremely psychotic clients for ability to manage elimination hygienically (incontinence, hoarding feces, smearing, etc.)
Sensory and cognitive perception	• Assess ability to interpret and respond to environment. • Assess orientation to reality and altered thought processes. • Assess ability to problem solve, recall, and memory.
Rest and activity	• Monitor sleep patterns. Assess for medication side effects that result in too much drowsiness or restlessness, which prevents sleep. • Assess motor activity; slower motor activity may increase response time resulting in clumsiness or injury. Overactivity can result in exhaustion.
Hygiene	• Assess ability to perform basic hygiene and grooming. • Monitor rituals or beliefs that may interfere with hygiene.
Sexuality	• Assess thought processes related to sexuality or sexual identity that may result in unrealistic fears or bizarre action. • Monitor for medication side effects that may affect sexuality (altered libido, ejaculation problems, male gynecomastia, and menstrual irregularities.)

quest. At 3:00, 4:00, and every hour on the hour, Jerry asked the same question, often of a different staff member. This behavior was not noted or explored or passed along to nurses on the following shifts. At 2:00 am when the night nurse made rounds, she found that Jerry, who had appeared asleep on earlier rounds, had barricaded his door shut with furniture and was in terror that the voices were coming to torture and kill him. The "voices" had told Jerry that at 2:00 am something terrible was going to happen to him, and he had spent the day preparing a plan to defend himself. Had even one of the staff inquired, "Is something special happening that you're interested in the time?" his fears might have been revealed. Also, spending time with Jerry throughout the day would have provided the opportunity to assess and explore the fearful nature of the auditory hallucinations. Fortunately, Jerry was not physically hurt in this episode, but the potential for harm was very serious.

Other aspects of the assessment include observations of the client's participation in or withdrawal from social interactions. For example, in catatonia, the client virtually withdraws, having no contact with others. In paranoid schizophrenia, the client may accuse others of attempting harm, respond aggressively and defensively, or withdraw and become isolated and secretive. The client who is delusional and grandiose may treat others with disdain or disrespect. The altered thought processes of hallucinations and delusions often impair social judgment, and the client may make racial slurs or inappropriate sexual advances or become aggressive toward others. Other people, the psychotic client, and other clients may need protection. In the community, this type of behavior often results in the client being seriously injured because others see only annoying or challenging behavior instead of an illness.

Distinguish behaviors from the side effects of treatment. Often agitation is present; however, this can be confused with motor restlessness (*akathisia*) resulting from antipsychotic drugs. If this uncomfortable side effect of treatment is missed, agitation may be treated with more prn neuroleptics, leading to increased akathisia. When severe, this adverse reaction may lead to aggressive or assaultive behavior.

Assessing the Prodromal Phase of Schizophrenia in the Community

Recently, greater attention has been focused on ways to detect schizophrenia prior to the onset of psychotic symptoms, the so-called preonset phase. In this phase, there are active but nonpsychotic symptoms.[10] Most clients experience functional or symptomatic problems beginning in childhood. Nurses can join other psychiatric professionals to detect and treat individuals before the onset of the full spectrum of schizophrenic symptoms. Beginning clues may include social withdrawal, work impairment, inappropriate affect, lack of motivation, and bizarre ideas. These behaviors may be brought to the nurse's attention by concerned parents or through observation of children or adolescents in the school health setting or in community programs. In these cases, the

Nursing Care Plan: SCHIZOPHRENIA

Nursing Diagnosis #1: Altered thought processes evidenced by hallucinations, delusions, exaggerated responses related to inability to process and synthesize information, inability to evaluate reality.

Client Outcome Criteria
- Demonstrates improved reality orientation.
- Demonstrates improved reality-based thinking.
- Demonstrates reduced evidence of hallucinations or delusions.

Interventions
- Approach the client in a calm manner without showing shock or judgmental responses to the behavior. Promote trust.
- Focus on client's current behavior rather than past behavior or issues.
- Maintain communication with client by making short, frequent contacts without threatening or challenging his or her beliefs. Avoid physical contact and any behavior that could be interpreted as threatening.
- Incorporate reality orientation in all communication.
- Provide structured routine.
- Encourage client to talk about real events. Avoid listening to long, confusing stories that are not based on reality. Rather, direct conversation to here and now events.
- If the client is hallucinating or is delusional, let him or her know you realize these can be frightening but do not react to them as if they are real. Avoid talking back to the client's voices or getting involved in the delusion. For example, let the client know you do not see anyone else in the room or you have no evidence that someone is stalking the client.
- Focus on the feelings generated by the hallucinations or delusion rather than the content such as fear or comfort created by them.
- Distract the client by focusing on less-threatening content.
- Teach client techniques to challenge disturbed thoughts such as thought stopping, use of physical activity, and seeking out support system.
- Encourage client to seek out staff or others when experiencing frightening thoughts.

Nursing Diagnosis #2: Social isolation evidenced by withdrawal, anxiety in social situations, inappropriate behavior, poor attention span related to inability to concentrate, anxiety, preoccupation with own thoughts, delusion, hallucinations.

Client Outcome Criteria
- Demonstrates improvement in appropriate communication with others.
- Demonstrates less anxiety and inappropriate behavior in social situations.
- Expresses pleasure in participating in social activities.

Interventions
- Spend brief periods with client engaging in nonthreatening conversation reinforcing trust.
- Reinforce any attempts at communication and participation in social activities.
- Identify client's interests and focus discussion on that.
- Gradually encourage participation in social activities for brief periods. Offer to be with client during these activities.
- Ensure that client can leave social situation if it becomes too threatening. Teach client specific techniques for coping with increasing tension and anxiety.
- Role model appropriate behavior in social situations. Give client gentle feedback on inappropriate behavior.

Nursing Diagnosis #3: Self-care deficit evidenced by difficulty with grooming, nutrition, hygiene related to regression, withdrawal, and impaired thought processes.

Client Outcome Criteria
- Demonstrates increased ability to care for self.
- Demonstrates increased interest in self-care.
- Reports any need for assistance with personal care.

Interventions
- Assess client's ability to meet basic self-care needs such as nutrition, hydration, and elimination.
- Provide assistance with self-care needs.
- Encourage wearing appropriate clothes for the setting.
- Role model appropriate behavior and give concrete directions on what is expected.
- Develop a structured schedule for client's routine for hygiene, toileting, and meals. Ensure that all staff are aware of the schedule and follow it for consistency.
- If client is not eating, offer food and fluids on a regular schedule.
- Encourage client to ask for assistance.
- Gently correct or assist client when demonstrating inappropriate behavior. Consider limiting social situations until able to do some things for himself or herself such as eating.

Nursing Diagnosis #4: Impaired verbal communication evidenced by flight of ideas, neologisms, word salad, echolalia related to disordered thinking, withdrawal, regression, impaired judgment.

Client Outcome Criteria
- Demonstrates improved ability to express self.
- Identifies factors that influence inappropriate responses.
- Demonstrates reduced incidence of inappropriate communication.

Interventions
- Let client know when you do not understand what he or she is saying. Ask client to clarify or restate communications. Specifically point out words that do not make sense.
- Facilitate trust by communicating your concern about client. Listen and demonstrate interest in his or her concerns.
- Arrange for consistent staff to work with client to facilitate understanding of client and enhance trust.
- Point out incongruous communication that can make the client's message confusing. Role model appropriate and congruous behaviors and messages.
- Assist client in communicating his or her needs to others.
- Demonstrate a calm, patient demeanor especially if the client is unable to communicate his or her needs. Anticipate needs when possible.
- Praise client's attempts at verbalizing.
- Maintain brief but frequent contacts with client to encourage verbal communication.

nurse should advocate and refer for a thorough diagnostic assessment. Accurate diagnosis is essential because schizophrenia is associated with tremendous social stigma, leaving the client with an enduring "label" that can adversely affect his or her entire life.

Planning Care

Planning nursing care must include understanding the client's developmental stage and level of acceptance of the disorder. The client experiencing a first psychotic episode is likely to be an adolescent or young adult. The impairment in thinking processes and judgment causes many clients to fail to acknowledge symptoms. Lack of participation or resistance to treatment is common. It is also difficult, particularly for a young person, to believe that the illness is often lifelong, chronic, and requires ongoing attention and management.

A major part of treatment is convincing the individual that treatment is required. This may be a slow process, especially for clients with a psychotic disorder, because the implications are overwhelming; they are living with an often debilitating illness that impairs cognition, emotion, and behavior.

Supportive therapy with a psychoeducational approach or goal-oriented psychotherapy as part of a behavioral or rehabilitation program is recommended. For clients who meet the full criteria for a psychotic disorder, assist in planning education for a trial of antipsychotic medication. As much as possible, educate and support family and significant others.

In acute states, the nurse may take the lead in planning for basic needs. Care plans should target relevant health needs, such as adequate nutrition, sleep and activity patterns, basic hygiene, and regular medical, dental, and, for female clients, gynecological exams.

Interventions for Hospitalized Clients

Therapeutic Communication

Communication with actively psychotic clients requires patience and understanding because they may seem as though they are "in their own world" and making connections can be frustratingly difficult. With persistence and skill, however, even clients who seem unreachable can learn to communicate effectively. A major challenge, particularly with the paranoid client, is to build trust. This is a difficult task given the severity of an acute episode of psychosis and the current limitations of inpatient hospitalization.

One way to build rapport is to allow clients to express concerns openly at their own pace. Excessive questioning may seem like prying and increase their feelings of suspiciousness. At times, the nurse may become part of the client's delusional system, further impeding effective communication.

It is not helpful to confront false beliefs directly by saying, "That isn't true." Challenging statements may lead to in-

> **RESEARCH NOTE**
>
> **Jensen, LH, and Kane, CF: Cognitive theory applied to the treatment of delusions of schizophrenia. Arch Psychiatr Nurs 10:335–341, 1996.**
>
> **Findings:** Recent research has focused on using cognitive-behavior therapy to treat symptoms of schizophrenia. These authors review the state of the art of this type of therapy in treating psychotic symptoms, particularly delusions. The goal of cognitive interventions in schizophrenia is to replace delusions with more adaptive thoughts. First, the nurse develops rapport and assesses the delusions, including the extent and degree of belief in them. One way to evaluate the certainty of belief in delusions is to write down the client's delusions on pieces of paper, and ask the client to place them on a "thermometer" with ratings of zero (least conviction) to 100 (absolute conviction). Using alternative explanations and reality testing, the therapist can work on the least certain delusion. Reality testing asks the client to actually "disprove" the delusion.
>
> **Application to Practice:** Extending cognitive therapy to delusions is another potentially effective intervention to treat those with psychotic disorders. Therapy is short term and can augment psychopharmacology. The effectiveness of these techniques is currently under investigation but holds promise for helping clients with severe and disturbing beliefs and thoughts. Nurses can encourage individuals and families to consider this treatment to support their efforts to overcome psychotic symptoms.

creased agitation and possibly aggression. Sometimes sidestepping the reality of the situation, for instance, saying that no one is really following them, is more effective. Try gentle and subtle interventions. If the individual is experiencing auditory hallucinations, one strategy is to state, "Sometimes people hear things or voices others can't hear," or, taking it a step further, "Your mind is playing tricks on you." Supportive statements, such as "This must be frightening for you" or "It's hard to understand all that's happening," might be useful.

Overall, take a calm, reassuring, nonjudgmental stance. Simple, short sentences work best. Frequent but brief interactions are less threatening, particularly if the client is paranoid.

The following clinical example involves a nursing student who is talking with a 22-year-old female client diagnosed with acute undifferentiated schizophrenia. The client demonstrated loose associations, ideas of reference, paranoia (two people, her ex-boyfriend and his new girlfriend, want to kill her), and auditory hallucinations. Very little of her conversation is reality based, yet the student picks up on her fear, confusion, and the fact that she hears voices in a very short conversational exchange.

CLINICAL EXAMPLE: PROCESS RECORDING

Preinteraction Phase

Setting. I am sitting at the end of the hallway by the window on the CCU unit. I am talking with my client about her mother coming to visit tonight. It is very quiet and she asked to talk to me.

Unit Milieu. The clients are all very anxious because of a code last night and all the disruption. There were also three new admissions to the unit in the early morning hours. It is now about 8:00 am and most clients are eating breakfast. No clients are around us.

Significant Data Prior to Interaction. This client has had many problems with behavior the last 2 days. She has been laughing inappropriately and yelling at staff and other clients for no reason. She also dumped her breakfast all over the floor and table, and when staff intervened, she became upset and agitated. When a staff member raised his voice to her, she began to cry and went to her room, and this is when she asked me to come and talk to her. We headed for a quiet area at the end of the hall.

Goals.

Student—Have a quiet, nonstimulating setting. Really try and follow her train of thought and be alert for the hallucinations. Listen for themes of T and M wanting to hurt her (ex-boyfriend and new girlfriend). If she does have a hallucination, be able to refocus her on reality.

Client—Be able to focus for short periods of time without distraction.

Interaction	Analysis
1. ST. I am glad you wanted to talk to me. I noticed you were telling P that your Mom visited last night. Can you tell me about the visit?	1. Giving positive reinforcement, indicating interest in her.

Process Recording

2. ST. Did your Mom come and visit last night?	2. Focused question to be concrete.
3. CL. Ya, Ya, she came and came to visit. She did my hair, my mommy did my hair, Mommy, Mommy, are you my Mommy?	3. Responds to question, but becomes confused that I am her Mommy.
4. ST. No, I am not your Mommy. I am J.	4. Reoriented pt. to reality She calls many people Mommy.
5. CL. Oooooh, ya ya ya. You are J, JD. Where is your Mommy?	5. She remembered my name. She understood what I said.
6. ST. My mommy lives in California. Where does your Mommy live?	6. Giving her information and a direct question to get back to reality and back on the topic of visit.
7. CL. (laughing uncontrollably) She lives somewhere out there. Step by step. Hey Michael, you know Michael, remember I told you the story. NO, NO, YOU WERE THERE; YOU DID IT! (Eyes are darting around the room, blank look on face, very anxious.)	7. CL. started to actively hallucinate, very confused; hard to follow and understand.
8. ST. Are you hearing voices? Yes, I think this must be very scary to hear these voices telling you what to do.	8. Direct question to find out if she is hallucinating. Also redirect to reality and express empathy for her feelings.
9. ST. Are you still hearing the voices? If you are, I want you to tell them to go away right now.	9. Trying to help her gain control.
10. CL. GO AWAY! YOU ARE MAKING ME MAD!	10. She is responding to my suggestion to tell them to go.
11. ST. Can you tell me what they were telling you?	11. Trying to get info on voices. Are they commands, noises?
12. CL. THEY WANT TO KILL ME! M IS GOING TO GET YOU. YOU WERE THERE. TELL THEM TO GO AWAY (laughing suddenly and uncontrollably) Can I go to the bathroom? You need to come with me because you won't hurt me like the others.	12. CL. tells what she's thinking. Seems to trust me.
13. ST. Yes I will come but no one wants to hurt you.	13. Empathy and reassurance.
14. CL. (laughing and rolling on the floor) OK, let's go to my room.	

Themes. Fear, afraid others will hurt her. There obviously was something they did that must have been violent. It seems that they had a verbal or physical fight of some kind because every time she has talked about this she always says, "They are going to hurt me; you were there; you saw it happen." This has been consistent in the last 2 days, and she has said this several times.

Goals. Partially met. I was able to have a quiet setting; I was able to refocus the client when she was hallucinating. I do not know if I did a great job of identifying the theme of the hallucination. I was able to keep the client focused for a short period of time.

Maintaining Safety

Because clients with psychotic disorders cannot clearly discern what is real from what is not, there is always the potential for dangerous behaviors stemming from responses to hallucinations or delusions. Reassure them that they are safe and provide a nonstimulating, safe environment. One-to-one interactions may help minimize paranoia and excess stimulation. Avoid challenging or confrontational statements. When possible, let clients know the behavior is dangerous, while expressing your concern for their safety: "Jim, I'm very concerned you might get hurt if you listen to those voices. Please let me know what they are telling you."

It is important to anticipate aggressive behavior and to ask clients whether they are having any thoughts of hurting themselves or others. Maintain a safe distance when clients appear potentially dangerous while continually assessing client safety. If behavior escalates to hurting self or others, consider seclusion and physical and chemical restraint.

Providing Structure

Consistency and structure assist the client in meeting basic needs such as hygiene, nutrition, sleep, activity, and social interaction. Even simple decisions such as what to eat, what to wear, and when to shower can become impaired. Sometimes individuals will drink excessive fluid, smoke excessively, or abuse alcohol or other substances. State clear simple goals and their rationales firmly and repeatedly; avoid ultimatums or threats. Stress the need for regular sleeping patterns and discourage naps. Break down tasks into small, simple steps to help achieve success.

Attempting Milieu Therapy

Milieu therapy provides the external structure and intensive care that clients require. It may be in the form of an acute care hospitalization, intensive outpatient program such as day hospitalization, or residential care. In any situation, safety is the main goal. Until the psychotic processes are under control or lessened, daily functioning and self-care are impaired. Milieu therapy keeps clients safe until their thinking and judgment become clearer and more based in reality.

Continuously monitor clients' potential for dangerous behavior. Extreme paranoia and command hallucinations should be constantly monitored in a nonintrusive fashion. Gently remind clients of the need to shower, eat, and interact with others. A nurse who is consistent and known to the individual is generally more accepted.

Avoid touching clients because physical contact can be extremely threatening. In one case, a male nursing student attempted to provide reassurance by placing his hand on the client's back. The client perceived this contact as sexual, became enraged, and began shouting that the student had tried to rape him because he was homosexual. Touch may be misperceived or seen as beginning "evidence" of an "attack" because of paranoid thinking. Use the clinical management tips listed in Table 18–8.

TABLE 18–8. Clinical Management Tips for Dealing with the Hallucinating or Delusional Client

Effective Communication Techniques
- Use brief, short-word sentences and a nonthreatening tone.
- Avoid ultimatums, arguments, and challenging statements.
- If trust is established, gently point out that clients' beliefs or hallucinations are not real. For instance, "I don't see anyone following you," or "I don't hear any voices."
- Maintain an honest and consistent approach.
- Use supportive statements such as "The world is a scary place," or "It's hard to understand all that's going on."
- Approach the client in a calm manner, and use frequent, short interactions to build trust.
- Explain procedures and the need for medication simply.

Ways to Reduce or Minimize Psychosis
- Engage the client in reality-based activities and short-term plans.
- Provide structure and a daily schedule for meal times, hygiene, sleep, and activity.
- Assist the client in meeting activities of daily living, encouraging as much independence as possible.
- Encourage the client to take antipsychotic medication as directed, and perform "mouth checks" to ensure that they have actually swallowed the medication.
- Monitor the client's judgment and decision making.
- Suggest that the client "not listen to the voices right now," or "not focus on those ideas right now."
- Look for events that lead to an increase in symptoms. Once identified, try to minimize these precipitating factors.
- Ensure that the client receives adequate sleep and rest.
- Assess improvement by determining whether thinking and judgment are clearer and more reality based.
- Give praise and positive reinforcement to the client when reality-based perceptions and thoughts are expressed.
- Use distraction, such as exercise, activities, and listening to music, to help the client cope.

Ways to Prevent Self-Harm or Dangerous Behavior
- Keep clients safe, particularly if "command" hallucinations are present that tell them to hurt themselves.
- Ensure that the client's environment is safe and nonstimulating.
- Continually assess the nature and severity of hallucinations and delusions by asking the client to describe them.
- Reassure clients that they are safe and that you are there to help.

Source: Adapted from Gorman, LM, et al: Davis's Manual of Psychosocial Nursing for General Patient Care. FA Davis, Philadelphia, 1996, pp. 217–220.

Interventions for Clients in the Community

Many of the acute interventions used for clients in the hospital are also helpful for those in the community. In the case of schizophrenia and schizoaffective disorder, nursing interventions are key in managing clients with long-term symptoms or those that are unresponsive to treatment. Despite adequate treatment and several medication trials, some clients will continue to suffer from positive and negative symptoms. Coping with ongoing symptoms is debilitating. The major role of the nurse in the community is to encourage clients to obtain and continue treatment while simultaneously assisting them to maintain structure and functional ability in their lives. Weekly home visits are sometimes necessary. Many clients require supervised living arrangements such as halfway houses; however, these residences are expensive and are not usually covered by insurance. Often clients have been ill so long that they are uninsured, unable to keep a job, and dependent on government assistance. Financial assistance can help them obtain housing and rehabilitation.

The client's frequent denial of illness or need for medication is the major challenge to nursing interventions. These clients are not active consumers; they fail to seek treatment during periods of acute crisis. Many clients are at high risk for homelessness and concurrent safety and health risks.

Jim discontinued his medication, and in less than 1 week his auditory hallucinations returned. These "voices" told him that his apartment was "bugged" and his food was "poisoned." He stopped eating, virtually stopped drinking, and began wandering the streets, afraid to remain in his apartment. He did not seek help and was unaware of the severity of his condition, until he was picked up by the police.

TABLE 18–9. Factors That May Contribute to Discontinuation of Neuroleptic Medication

Medication-related
- Adverse effects
- Route of administration (intramuscular vs. oral)
- Complexity of medication regimen (e.g., timing, number of doses)

Client-related
- Denial of illness
- Distress from adverse effect
- Stigma
- Alcohol or substance abuse

Family Refusal

Difficulty Obtaining or Receiving Care

Source: Weiden, P: Neuroleptics and quality of life: The patient's perspective. Neuropsychopharmacology 10:241, 1994.

A major problem arising from clients' denial of their illness and need for medication is noncompliance. Some studies suggest that 75% of clients stop their medication for at least 1 week.[11] This poses a high risk for relapse. Reasons for discontinuing medication range from adverse effects to difficulty obtaining psychiatric care (Table 18–9).

Nurses are often the first clinicians to identify the problem and intervene. The client or family often know which medications cause adverse effects and which ones can be tolerated.

Steve stopped taking his medication, haloperidol, because it kept him awake. When she assessed him, the nurse discovered that he suffered from terrible akathisia (restlessness with the need to pace) and couldn't stay in bed. Steve told her that chlorpromazine, another antipsychotic, helped him sleep. With this change, the client was able to sleep better and became more willing to take the drug consistently, achieving therapeutic benefit.

Key Nursing Interventions

Assist with the Activities of Daily Living. Assist clients with activities such as paying bills, buying groceries, and making meals. Ensure that the client gets regular physical, dental, and, in the case of women, gynecological examinations and meets other health needs. Jointly devise a regular daily schedule and encourage compliance with it by using frequent reminders and a posted checklist.

Watch for Signs of Relapse. Continually monitor and assess the client for signs of relapse. Prodromal symptoms may indicate a pending relapse. Stress the need for ongoing psychiatric care, including supportive psychotherapy and pharmacotherapy. Ensure opportunities for early intervention to prevent or lessen the severity of relapse. Daily structure and medication monitoring can help prevent acute exacerbations of the illness and prevent hospitalization.

Encourage Socialization. Positive symptoms may be seen more often in early stages of the illness, whereas negative symptoms predominate in the long term. Motivating these clients is extremely challenging and requires a solid basis of trust and persistence. Help them develop social roles and a social support network. Encourage participation in client-based drop-in centers or self-help groups to promote social stimulation. Help clients whose illness is stabilized to receive vocational training or return to a work environment adapted to their current level of functioning if possible. Volunteer jobs, for several hours a week, promote social contact, structure, and purpose in life.

Promote Communication. Refer to group therapy. Groups may promote interpersonal connection, improve social skills, and diminish social withdrawal. They may also be an important educational tool in long-term management of symptoms. One study[12] found that participants in a structured group experienced several positive outcomes. When taught strategies to manage auditory hallucinations, participants felt less distress about hallucinations and tended to use the techniques they learned. The mutual teaching and learning among nurses and clients enhanced their self-esteem and ability to communicate openly about auditory hallucinations. Participants achieved high levels of engagement and tried new ways to manage symptoms and communicate with others.

Understand the Impact of Their Loss. Remain aware of the grieving that occurs because these clients and their families frequently face significant losses, including loss of future dreams of college, career, intimate relationships, and parenting. Financial loss is common, and the individual may need to receive long-term disability.

> Sally, an intelligent woman with a college degree, had her first psychotic episode as a junior in college. She managed to finish college and obtain a banking job, but because of the nature of her illness, she saw her career plans decline to the point that she was able to manage only a part-time filing position. Because the severity of her illness led to severe disability, her grief at the loss of her future intensified over the years. Her therapy included grief work as well as helping her separate and support her self-worth from the ravages of a chronic illness.

Some clients are able to maintain structured part-time work or school. It is essential that the illness be explained to a supervisor, who may be supportive in assisting the client to adapt to a work schedule. Families may need to take on the role of guardian or caretaker to help the client manage everyday life. One of the most profound effects of long-term psychotic illness is decreased self-esteem. The lack of confidence and reduced self-efficacy may be more noticeable when the positive symptoms have abated. Individual or group psychotherapy can help the client maximize capabilities affected by the illness and recognize limitations.

Pharmacologic Treatment: Schizophrenia

Antipsychotics. Antipsychotic medications, also called neuroleptics, are the mainstay of pharmacologic treatment. Although these drugs have the potential to treat some of the most disturbing psychotic symptoms, they may lead to adverse effects and potentially life-threatening reactions.

Antipsychotics are classified as either typical or atypical, based on their pharmacologic effects. Typical antipsychotics are those that lead to extrapyramidal symptoms (EPS), whereas atypical antipsychotics, such as clozapine, cause little to no EPS. All of these medications have been shown to be better than a placebo (inactive treatment); however, some clients may respond better to atypical agents. Table 18–10 lists a comparison of haloperidol and commonly used atypical antipsychotic medications. Figure 18–4 shows how these agents cause beneficial effects or adverse reactions by affecting different regions.

There is no way to predict how a client might respond to an antipsychotic, unless the client has been on the medication before. If possible, ask the client about medications tried previously and his or her response to them. In an emergency state when sedation is needed, antipsychotics may calm ag-

TABLE 18–10. Comparison of Atypical Antipsychotic Medications and Haloperidol

Generic Name Trade Name	Clozapine Clozaril	Risperidone Risperdal	Olanzapine Zyprexa	Sertindole[†] Serlect	Haloperidol Haldol
Dose*					
Initial dose	25–50	1–2	5–10	4	2–5
Common dose	300–600	6–8	10–15	12–20	6–8
Maximum dose	900	12	20	24	20
Common Side Effects					
EPS	+	++	+	+	++++
Anticholinergic	++++	+	++	+	++
Sedation	++++	++	+++	+	++
Hypotension	++++	++	+	+	+
Seizure	++++	+	+	+	+
Weight gain	++++	++	++	++	++
Treatment Effect					
Positive symptoms	Marked	Marked	Marked	Marked	Marked
Negative symptoms	Marked	Moderate	Marked	Marked	Mild

*In mg
[†]Scheduled to be released onto the market in 1997.
NOTE: Risperidone is associated with little to no EPS in daily doses less than 6 mg in adults.
Key: + = very low, ++ = low, +++ = moderate, ++++ = high
Source: Adapted from the Physician's Desk Reference, 1997; and Teicher, MH, and Glod, CA: Neuroleptic drugs: Indications and guidelines for their rational use in children and adolescents. Journal of Child and Adolescent Psychopharmacology, 1:33–56, 1990.

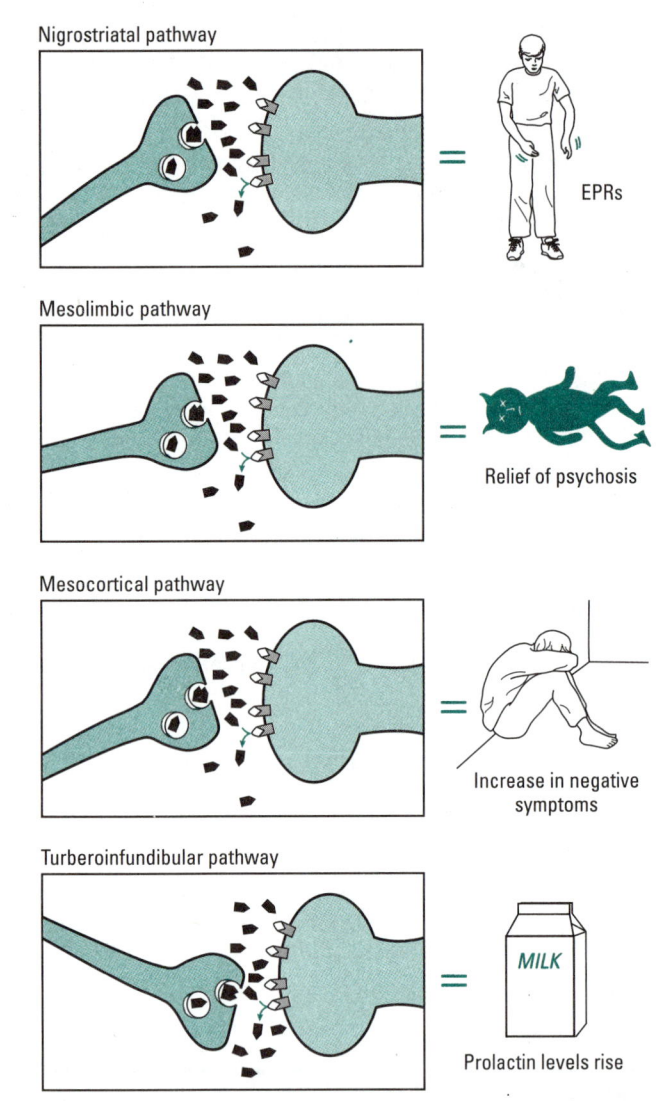

Figure 18–4. Effects of dopamine receptor-blocking neuroleptics in each of the four dopamine pathways. Blocked dopamine receptors in the postsynaptic projects of the nigrostriatal pathway produce disorders of movement that appear similar to those in Parkinson's disease, which is why these movements are sometimes called *drug-induced parkinsonism*. Since the nigrostriatal pathway projects to basal ganglia, part of the extrapyramidal neuronal system of the central nervous system, side effects associated with blockage of dopamine receptors there are sometimes also called *extrapyramidal reactions*. Shutting down the mesolimbic dopamine pathway by blocking the postsynaptic dopamine receptors causes reduction of delusions and hallucinations. Blocked dopamine receptors in the mesocortical dopamine pathway may produce blunting of emotions and various cognitive side effects that actually mimic negative symptoms. Sometimes these cognitive side effects of neuroleptics are called the *neuroleptic-induced deficit syndrome*. Finally, when the dopamine receptors in the tuberoinfundibular dopamine pathway are blocked, prolactin levels rise, sometimes so much that women can begin lactating inappropriately, a condition known as *galactorrhea*. (From Stahl, 1996, p 258.)

itation if given by injection within 30 to 60 minutes; however, there are no antipsychotic effects with this type of dosage.

The nurse must remember the goal of pharmacotherapy: to achieve an adequate dosage with minimal side effects. Most clients require a moderate dose; for instance, a daily dose of 300 to 600 mg of clozapine, 8 to 10 mg of haloperidol, or 10 to 20 mg of olanzapine. Too low of a dose will be ineffective, whereas too high of a dose may lead to severe

RESEARCH NOTE

Weiden, P. Neuroleptics and quality of life: The patient's perspective. Neuropsychopharmacology 10:241, 1994.

Findings: Uncomfortable side effects are a major reason for stopping medication because adverse reactions are more likely to lead to noncompliance. In this study, the author interviewed 72 individuals with schizophrenia after discharge from the hospital. Instead of asking clients to respond to a checklist of adverse reactions, the author asked individuals and families about their experience of side effects and their degree of distress. Clients identified persistent akinesia (stiffness, lack of movement) as the most severely distressing event, as did families. Following akinesia, anticholinergic effects and akathisia were reported commonly, but were less distressing to clients. Other parkinsonian symptoms were infrequent and emerged as less disturbing. One of the major consequences of bothersome side effects is noncompliance. For families bothered by distressing adverse effects, support for continued treatment may be withdrawn. The authors of this study emphasized a careful, nonjudgmental manner in eliciting information about side effects, phrasing questions as if noncompliance was common.

Application to Practice: The approach in this study emphasizes the importance of questioning clients in an open-ended manner about adverse effects and the degree of distress medications produce. It also indicates that family members, important members of the treatment team, have strong beliefs about the effects of antipsychotic medications. Questioning clients and families can enhance compliance. Psychiatric nurses can help individuals anticipate adverse reactions and suggest ways to manage uncomfortable effects. Both pharmacologic and nonpharmacologic interventions can be used. Higher doses are associated with more uncomfortable effects. Thus, lowering medication doses can help reduce the severity of effects. Nurses can also suggest that alternate antipsychotic medications may be considered if adverse effects are severely distressing. The study stresses the importance of approaching individuals about pharmacotherapy; assume that clients will skip doses and experience disturbing effects during antipsychotic treatment.

side effects and worsening of behavior.[13] Clients will require long-term, integrated treatment with both pharmacologic and other interventions.

Because it takes several weeks for the antipsychotics to effectively treat positive symptoms, the client may not feel better initially and want to discontinue the medication. Teach clients and families to wait, often for several weeks, to determine whether the drug will be effective. Assess for noncompliance.

Monitor the potentially dangerous, uncomfortable, or embarrassing side effects that may occur in initial stages of treatment (Table 18–11). For example, higher potency agents, such as haloperidol or risperidone, in doses over 6 mg, are more likely to cause EPS. Lower potency agents are associated with sedation, orthostatic hypotension, and anticholinergic effects, whereas moderate-potency antipsychotics have mixed effects. These drugs can also lead to tardive dyskinesia or the life-threatening effects of neuroleptic malignant syndrome. (See Chapter 6).

Side effects of antipsychotics can be advantageous occasionally. For instance, neuroleptics that have sedation as a primary side effect may help manage aggression or agitation before achieving antipsychotic effects.

A key role for nurses is assessing the client's therapeutic and adverse response to medications. Nurses are also instrumental in differentiating whether the client's behavior is due to worsening symptoms of psychosis or to a negative response to antipsychotic treatment. For example, an EPS symptom such as akinesia (lack of movement, stiffness) may be so disturbing to a client that it leads to noncompliance. Akinesia is also associated with the appearance of a masklike face, which needs to be carefully distinguished from flat affect.

Nurses evaluate both the acute and long-term effects of antipsychotic agents. Clients must be adequately informed, but not so frightened by the effects that they refuse medication. Each individual client's concerns and fears should be addressed when assessing the best approach to take for teaching.

Assist the client in becoming responsible for personal medication management. Continually assess noncompliance by encouraging clients to be honest about how and whether they take their medication. For clients who have difficulty taking their medication consistently, long-acting depot formulations are available for haloperidol and fluphenazine. These medications may be administered intramuscularly, about every 2 weeks, and ensure that the client receives the necessary medication over that time period.

Atypical Antipsychotics. Atypical antipsychotics treat both positive and negative symptoms. They are used for three reasons: (1) lack of response to a typical antipsychotic agent, (2) unmanageable side effects from the other antipsychotics, or (3) presence of negative symptoms.

Clozapine represents a breakthrough for individuals with intractable psychosis and severe negative symptoms. Compared to typical antipsychotics such as chlorpromazine and haloperidol, clozapine is more effective; one major study showed that 30% of clients who failed to respond to typical antipsychotics improved significantly.[14] Clozapine causes little to no EPS or tardive dyskinesia. With the introduction of other atypical agents such as risperidone, olanzapine, and sertindole, clients have several promising options to reduce and possibly eliminate their symptoms.

Recent studies also show that the effects of clozapine have enabled clients to improve their quality of life. One study found that clients made significant gains in working or returning to school after receiving clozapine.[15]

Although clozapine has potential for greater therapeutic efficacy, it carries substantial risks that require careful client monitoring (see Chapter 6). Agranulocytosis, a life-threatening adverse effect associated with clozapine, requires

TABLE 18–11. Extrapyramidal Symptoms: Side Effects of Typical Antipsychotics

Dystonia. Severe and involuntary contractions of muscles caused by antipsychotic drug therapy that may include tics, problems with swallowing, and spasms in major muscle groups; for example, flexion of the trunk muscles or oculogyric crisis, prolonged fixation of the eyeballs in one place.

Dyskinesia. Difficulty and stiffness of voluntary movement, resulting in partial or incomplete movements.

Akathisia. Extreme restlessness and inability to sit still; often confused with anxiety. The client may pace, constantly move the feet, have difficulty concentrating, reading or performing simple tasks. Clients often describe this feeling as if their bodies feel heavy, yet they feel like they could "jump out of their skin."

Parkinsonism syndrome. Symptoms resembling Parkinson's disease that occur after the first week of treatment, but usually before entering the second month of treatment. The client's symptoms will resemble those of a Parkinson's patient, with fatigue, slowness, a feeling of heaviness, amotivation, muscular rigidity, a flat, masklike facial expression, shuffling gait, drooling, pill-rolling movements of the fingers, tremors, and altered movement.

Akinesia. Apathy, fatigue, slowness, lack of motivation. This can also be confused with the amotivation (negative symptom) of schizophrenia.

Choreathetoid movements. Writhing, wormlike movements of the limbs.

Tardive dyskinesia. A syndrome that is seen after long-term use of antipsychotic medication. Symptoms include slow movements of the lips, tongue, and mouth, with chewing, smacking, sucking, tongue protrusion, or lip licking. Other symptoms may include puffing of the cheeks, blinking, and facial grimacing. Choreoform movements of the body and limbs may also be present. The symptoms may intensify with stress and are absent during sleep.

weekly blood monitoring. The medication and monitoring is expensive, costing up to $10,000 per year. It is also difficult for psychotic clients with little motivation, poor judgment, and limited insight into their illness and need for treatment to follow the steps necessary to receive clozapine. They must follow through with laboratory work, make clinic visits to review results on a regular basis, and also obtain medication at the pharmacy. The other atypical agents, without the risk of agranulocytosis, may be a better option for some.

Assist clients and families in obtaining treatment with atypical antipsychotics. For example, the nurse may advocate for a clozapine trial when treatment with typical antipsychotics has not been effective. Families should also be encouraged to take an active role at the initiation of treatment to ensure that clients receive adequate help. The nurse may need to accompany clients to the lab, clinic, or pharmacy. If possible, a one-stop clozapine clinic that offers laboratory testing and medication strengthens the likelihood of compliance, although it may add to the cost.

Nurses also take an active role in monitoring side effects. For instance, weight gain of over 20 lb is not uncommon, and preventive intervention such as an activity and exercise program and nutritional counseling should be initiated at the start of treatment. Carefully assess any signs of infection that signal a drop in white blood cell count (WBC), because clients may fail to observe or report these symptoms. Give patient and supportive encouragement to clients and families, because the initial benefits may be minimal and not evident for more than 6 months.

Before I started taking clozapine, it was like I was in a daze. I just hung around my apartment. I never called anyone because I thought the telephone was bugged. Sometimes I'd forget to eat, and my parents told me I didn't shower for days. My roommate would get on my nerves a lot, and I'd yell at him to shut up. My mother also got on my nerves; once I nearly punched her. I guess she knew I was about to hit her so she called the police. I forget which hospital they took me to—I've been in so many that I lost count. The doctors tried me on all different medications. I remember I used to get shots every 2 weeks or so, but they didn't make me feel good. It seemed like they were just trying stuff out on me. I finally told them I wasn't going to be a guinea pig anymore and stopped going to the clinic.

I was really scared to try the clozapine, and wasn't wild about getting my blood drawn every week. I remember thinking at first that I had acquired immunodeficiency syndrome (AIDS) and had to get my blood checked because I was going to die. That was pretty crazy. My parents took me to the lab and then to the clinic to see the psychiatric nurse. She was the one who suggested the clozapine. She told me that I might not notice any difference, but that some people, like, had gotten better. At first I wet the bed. Boy, that was embarrassing. The clozapine didn't make a big difference right away; it was kinda gradual. I think that I'm still very slowly getting better each day. It's been 2 years now. I started working out again, and I go to a day program 3 days a week. I may even get a volunteer job, working with blind kids. I always wanted to work with them. I also started to play the trumpet again. Now my roommate yells at me! But we worked that out. He still gets on my nerves, so does my mother, but it doesn't get to me like before. I think the best thing about the medication is that I'm alive again. It's like that film "Awakenings" where people come out of their shell. That's how I am, and I think I'm getting a little better every day.

Electroconvulsive Therapy. Occasionally, electroconvulsive therapy (ECT) may be necessary for individuals with psychotic disorders, although this treatment is reserved for treatment-resistant or extreme cases of schizoaffective disorder or schizophrenia. ECT is used along with antipsychotic medication for clients with persistent positive symptoms and can be therapeutic for clients who show mood symptoms or catatonia. A rapid response may be obtained in severely ill psychotic clients who are at risk for dehydration or starvation. Six to 12 ECT treatments are generally administered in the hospital (see Chapter 14). More than 12 treatments are not beneficial and will not prevent worsening or relapse of symptoms.

Pharmacological Treatment: Schizoaffective Disorder and Schizophreniform Disorder

The usual treatment is to administer neuroleptic drugs, at times combined with a mood stabilizer such as lithium, or valproic acid. Individuals who experience an acute onset of symptoms and have a family history of mood disorders may be more likely to respond to a mood stabilizer. These agents may treat disturbances in mood, appetite, sleep, and energy.

Pharmacologic Treatment: Brief Psychotic Disorder and Delusional Disorder

These individuals usually receive short-term treatment with antipsychotics.

Psychosocial Rehabilitation

Several types of community-based rehabilitation programs treat individuals with chronic mental illness (see Chapter 29). Many of these programs use some type of behavior therapy as the basis of their treatment. The goal of psychosocial rehabilitation is to help individuals adjust to community living. Innovative approaches generally include a group of services that encourage clients to practice and take responsibility for their behavior and to ultimately change it. The following are the words of a client, Howie the Harp, who strongly advocates community-integrated care.[16]

When we talk about independent living, we're not talking about leaving people alone to suffer with no help. We're talking about having freedom to make choices; to choose whom and what to be interdependent with; to choose when we need help, how it is to be provided, and by whom ... in short, we're talking about empowerment. We're talking about independent living, with supports and services that enable us crazy folks to make a success of independent living.

HOWIE THE HARP

Resource management, as part of psychosocial rehabilitation, teaches people how to perform certain basic tasks, such as how to manage money, negotiate transportation, deal with getting incorrect change, study for an examination, or interview for a job. Social-skills training or social problem solving can also assist individuals in managing everyday situations. Skills training may include steps necessary to adequately care for personal hygiene, leisure, and recreation. These basic approaches lead clients through a series of steps, including obstacles and problems, in order to reach a new skill or the desired outcome. Actually taking the individual through the situation (for instance, using public transportation) is often necessary for successful implementation. Homework assignments, paced at the individual's level, can also assist in meeting clearly defined goals.

Some community-based programs also stress that many non–health-care providers, such as newspaper carriers, restaurant owners, and postal carriers, could be engaged in a total community effort to intervene successfully with clients with psychotic disorders. The goal is to improve personal, social, and occupational functioning despite the severe neuropsychological deficits associated with psychotic disorders.

Client and Family Education

Educate both clients and families about the diagnosis of a major psychotic disorder. Medication teaching is always necessary because families may not understand the need for neuroleptics and be unaware of possible side effects. Review positive and negative symptoms, resulting behaviors, theories and possible causes, effective treatment, course, and prognosis.

Client Education

Client-centered education occurs when acute symptoms are controlled or moderated, making it easier for the client to learn about the disorder, medications, and symptom management. A consistent and trusting relationship with the nurse facilitates compliance with treatment.

Frederick and Cotanch[17] found that clients could effectively use self-help techniques to deal with auditory hallucinations. Cognitive techniques included talking back to the voices or ignoring them. If the voices were neutral and nonthreatening, some clients found it easier to go along with what the voices wanted and then they would go away. Others found reasoning with the voices worked. Behavioral techniques such as reading, listening to music, drawing, cleaning, or doing yardwork also were helpful. Most clients found that the radio or television was intrusive and made the voices seem louder.

Learning about and managing their illness can give clients a sense of control often absent during the acute stages of illness. A trusting relationship with the nurse and ongoing maintenance of medication and therapy can reassure clients that they will be safe if symptoms reappear and relapse occurs.

Family Education

Often the family is the key to ensuring that the client receives and maintains treatment. Researchers in schizophrenia offer helpful guidelines for assisting families to cope with the ill family member[18]:

- **Clarify roles.** Discuss clearly who in the family will do what for the client, and what the role of the nurse, physician, or other health professional will be in caring for the client. Recognize that families will change and their abilities and willingness to help will change as well.
- **Work together.** Teamwork is essential. Most families want to be part of the team and should be recognized and valued for their contributions.
- **Educate.** Most families are anxious to learn all they can and can then go on to educate relatives, peers, and other professionals.
- **Encourage input.** Involve family members in providing input into program evaluations, planning of programs, ethical issues, and monitoring. States often have consumer boards made up of clients and family members who advocate for various programs and needs of the chronically mentally ill individual.
- **Expect intense feeling.** The nurse must be aware that families have often had long, frustrating, and even abusive experiences with the mental health system and mental health professionals. The intense feelings may come up unexpectedly or be displaced onto current situations. Understanding and compassion, rather than defensiveness, are the most helpful response. The nurse must remember that the family, as well as the client, is dealing with significant loss. Loss of dreams for their child, fears about caring for the adult child in the future, and feelings of failure and humiliation are ongoing concerns.
- **Use local support groups.** Area meetings for support and education exist in larger cities or nearby towns. Mental health agencies and professionals often keep a list of liaison groups for families. Even isolated rural families can receive information and support from the National Alliance for the Mentally Ill, and support through the internet.
- **Recognize different beliefs.** Families have a wide variety of beliefs about mental illness. Mental health professionals vary in their approach to care. Learn to accept the differences and incorporate them into providing care for the client.

- **Acknowledge family strengths.** Consistently point out and support family strengths. Encourage them to share their expertise with other clients and families.
- **Develop professional support.** Working with the chronically mentally ill client can be very draining emotionally. It is essential that the nurse develop a support network to share ideas, successes, and failures and to learn new knowledge and skills.
- **Recognize limitations.** Be honest with families about the limitations of current knowledge and resources, as well as the difficulties engendered by the disorder, to help families to come to terms with their own expectations and limitations.

Differential Diagnosis[1]

Medical Disorders

- Sudden onset of brief psychotic symptoms suggests a physical cause or substance abuse.
- Medications or physical conditions may precipitate psychotic disorders.
- Symptoms are similar to psychotic disorders but are excluded from the diagnosis.

TABLE 18–12. **Medical and Pharmacologic Differential for the Diagnosis of Psychotic Disorders**

Medical
Stroke
Head trauma
Viral encephalitis
CNS tumor
AIDS
Vitamin deficiency
Temporal lobe epilepsy
Porphyria
Syphilis
Systemic lupus erythematosus
Toxic poisoning
Degenerative diseases of the CNS
Cushing's disease
Hypoglycemia
Pharmacologic
Amphetamine
Cocaine
Phencyclidine (PCP)
Steroids
Nonsteroidal anti-inflammatory drugs (NSAIDs)
Alcohol withdrawal
Anticholinergic agents
L-Dopa
Sedative-hypnotic withdrawal

- Medical and pharmacologic conditions are considered before making the diagnosis of a mood disorder, listed in Table 18–12.

Mood Disorders

- Schizophrenia is generally characterized by a chronic deteriorating course, whereas mood disorders are acute episodes followed by remissions.
- Psychotic symptoms occur in mood and psychotic disorders.
- Clients display depressive-like delusions or hallucinations during major depression and grandiose psychotic symptoms during mania.
- Schizoaffective disorder is difficult to distinguish from mood disorders; psychotic symptoms must be present for 2 weeks without mood symptoms.

Alcohol and Substance Abuse and Dependence

- Alcohol or illicit drugs may lead to symptoms of a psychotic disorder or coexist with one.
- Alcohol may lead to abuse and dependence, which complicate treatment.
- Denial of a coexisting abuse or dependence disorder is likely.
- Delusions or hallucinations that occur as a direct physiological consequence of a substance of abuse lead to the diagnosis of substance-induced psychotic disorder.

Obsessive-Compulsive Disorder (OCD)

- Obsessions are repetitive, intrusive, and unwanted thoughts rather than false beliefs (delusions).
- Obsessions may be accompanied by compulsions.
- Compulsions are distinguished from bizarre and inappropriate behavior by their repetition and performance in response to counteract obsessions.
- In OCD, clients generally recognize their exaggerated thoughts and behaviors.

Personality Disorders

- Schizotypal, schizoid, or paranoid personality disorders may predispose an individual to developing schizophrenia.
- Personality disorders are characterized by a pervasive pattern of relating to others.
- Individuals with personality disorders lack distinct delusions, hallucinations, and a formal thought disorder.
- Clients with borderline personality disorder may show transient psychotic symptoms.

Pervasive Developmental Disorders (PDD)

- Disorders such as autism are characterized by disturbances in speech, mood, and the ability to relate to oth-

ers.[1] They differ in the onset and nature of psychotic symptoms.
- Clients with PDD develop symptoms in early childhood but fail to display prominent delusions and hallucinations.
- Minimal speech and significant difficulty relating to others are present in PDD.

Expected Outcomes

The client with a psychotic disorder will:
- Remain safe and not harm self or others.
- Show normalization of thought patterns and hallucinations or other psychotic symptoms, or show evidence for control of these processes.
- Meet basic self-care needs and adequate hygiene.
- Begin to resume interpersonal interactions in an appropriate manner.
- Have adequate nutrition.
- Demonstrate adequate sleep and activity patterns.
- Become more motivated and establish short-term goals.
- Have a beginning understanding of the illness and of ways to manage it.
- Recognize the impact of behavior on relationships.
- Identify impending symptoms of psychosis and stressors that precipitate their onset.
- Continue to follow medication regimen as prescribed.

Common Nursing Diagnoses

Thought Processes, altered
Sensory/Perceptual Alterations (specify): visual, auditory, kinesthetic, gustatory, tactile, olfactory
Self Care Deficit, feeding, bathing/hygiene, dressing/grooming, toileting
Violence, risk for, directed at self/others
Denial, ineffective
Noncompliance (specify)
Communication, impaired verbal
Hopelessness
Sleep Pattern Disturbance
Social Interaction, impaired
Social Isolation
Nutrition: altered, less than body requirements
Nutrition: altered, more than body requirements
Nutrition: altered, risk for more than body requirements

Synopsis of Current Research

Brain Structure. Most of the research currently underway is focused on understanding the neurobiology of psychotic disorders such as schizophrenia, and the effectiveness of serotonin-dopamine antagonists. Recent MRI studies have found reduced cranial capacity, whereas other studies have found enlarged ventricles, dilatation of sulci in the cortex, reduced temporal lobes, and reduced metabolism in the prefrontal cortex during cognitive tasks. Taken together, these investigations suggest that abnormalities in brain structure or function in individuals with schizophrenia. In addition, pioneering studies using PET and single photon emission computed tomography (SPECT) scans have shown that negative symptoms are associated with decreased blood flow and glucose metabolism in the prefrontal cortex of individuals with schizophrenia.

Genetic Causes. Other recent research on schizophrenia suggests a genetic defect on chromosome 15, possibly on a nicotinic receptor. Having too few nicotinic receptors or some dysfunction in these receptors may be a risk factor for the disorder. Defective nicotinic receptors have been linked to positive symptoms such as delusions and hallucinations and the client's inability to filter out problems such as "voices" or noises. The involvement of nicotinic receptors may also help explain why clients with schizophrenia tend to smoke cigarettes; smoking heavily may be a way to "self-medicate" symptoms.

Antipsychotics. The pharmacologic treatment of psychotic illness, particularly schizophrenia, is a major focus of current research. The atypical antipsychotic clozapine has been shown to be superior to other typical antipsychotics in the treatment of schizophrenia. The reason for its increased effectiveness is another area of investigation. Clozapine affects serotonergic functioning, suggesting that imbalances in serotonin may be important in the pathophysiology of schizophrenia. Risperidone, olanzapine, and sertindole, atypical antipsychotics that block serotonin receptors, further implicate the role of serotonin. These agents appear to be less likely to cause side effects, particularly EPS effects, in part because of their effects on serotonin. Effects on the serotonin system may interact with the dopamine system to explain how negative symptoms are treated. In addition, several investigational antipsychotics are being tested to provide other alternatives for the treatment of schizophrenia.

Other Causes. Several other areas of key research have focused on other important issues. The diagnosis and management of the first acute episode of psychosis, or a "first break," is the target of several studies. Gender differences in schizophrenia have suggested important differences in age of onset, premorbid characteristics, course of the illness, treatment response, and side effects. Denial, lack of insight, and prominent behaviors associated with schizophrenia are also under investigation. In relationship to medication noncompliance, denial and poor insight have been identified as major impediments to continued successful treatment and instead are associated with poorer outcomes and recidivism (see Research Note).

Areas for Future Research

- How do antipsychotic medications enhance the quality of life of clients with severe psychotic disorders?

> **RESEARCH NOTE**
>
> Szymanski, SR, Cannon, W, Gallacher, F, Erwin, RJ, and Gur, RE. Course of treatment response in first-episode and chronic schizophrenia. Am J Psychiatry 153:519–525, 1996.
>
> **Findings:** This study compared the course of schizophrenia in clients with their first acute episode to those with chronic schizophrenia. The focus of the research was to examine the effects of antipsychotic medications on outcome after 2 years of treatment. Thirty-six clients with acute schizophrenia were compared to 34 clients with chronic schizophrenia. Each subject in the study received a moderate dose of antipsychotic medication based on clinical decisions by their prescriber. After 6 months of medication treatment, both groups showed significant improvement in positive symptoms. Only those clients with chronic schizophrenia showed improvement in negative symptoms. Clients in this study were also assessed every 6 months for the entire 2 years of study. After 6 months, no substantial improvement was noted.
>
> The researchers also examined what factors predicted who would respond better to medication. Individuals with more severe symptoms prior to treatment, those with shorter duration of illness, and those who complied more consistently with medications improved more. Individuals with prolonged illness were less likely to respond to antipsychotic agents and had a poorer outcome. The study also found that chronic schizophrenic clients do not take longer to recover than acutely psychotic clients. However, the individuals included in the study had no other psychiatric or medical diagnoses or history of substance abuse. These factors are more likely to lead to poorer outcome in clients with schizophrenia.
>
> **Application to Practice:** These findings confirm some of the previous research on the effects of pharmacotherapy in schizophrenia. Positive symptoms generally improve more than negative symptoms, and the benefits are usually evident in the first 1 to 6 months of medication treatment. The more severe the initial symptoms, the better the response. This suggests that improvement of schizophrenic symptoms, particularly positive symptoms, may take weeks to months, but that further response is unlikely after 6 months of treatment. It also suggests that if a client has not responded within 6 months of treatment, switching to a different medication may be necessary.
>
> Compliance with medication appears to be predictive of a better outcome than with intermittent dosing or noncompliance. Part of the nurse's role is to stress the need for continuing antipsychotic medication consistently for 6 months. An adequate duration of consistent medication is necessary to fully determine whether the client has responded.

- What are the most important nursing interventions that diminish negative symptoms?
- What factors help encourage psychotic individuals to take necessary medication consistently?
- What are the most important factors that correlate with positive outcome in the treatment of psychotic disorders?
- How do social and community resources help the individual with schizophrenia?
- What are the most common stressors that lead to relapse, and how can they be measured?
- How do clients with severe psychotic disorders make decisions about their health care?
- Are clients with schizophrenia at higher risk for developing AIDS?
- What basic health-care needs go unrecognized in individuals with psychotic disorders?

CASE STUDY

Stan is a 21-year-old college student. He had attended a small private high school and was committed to doing well. He had a small circle of friends but, because he lived a distance from most of them, he spent much of his time studying and listening to music. He applied to and was accepted by a prestigious university to study engineering.

At college, Stan did little in the way of socializing. Studying was taking more and more of his time just to keep up. Phone calls home were frequent, and he often complained that the professors were trying to keep him from doing well. He had one incident at school where he spent most of the night studying for a test, and when he went in to take the test, he went into a rage, ripped up the test, and ran out of the room screaming. His roommate had recently requested a change of room because Stan was often talking to himself or pacing within the room or hall. He did not do much each day and stopped bathing or washing his clothes. He began missing several of his classes because he did not want to be in the same room with the "friends of the devil" who were trying to trip him up.

While home for Thanksgiving weekend, his parents noticed that he spent much of the day in his room. When they suggested that he call a high school friend and go out for the evening, he began to attack his father, shouting angry words about how they were trying to get rid of him.

When his mother tried to intervene, he threatened her also. The police were called, and Stan was taken to the local emergency department. When he arrived there about 1 hour later, he was still mumbling and pacing, occasionally shouting out at personnel walking by.

When the nurse entered the room, Stan became increasingly agitated and accused her of trying to kill him. At one point, when she asked him how he liked going to college, he threatened her and shouted obscenities. The physician came in just in time to prevent him from physically hurting her. Stan then received haloperidol IM and was admitted to the inpatient psychiatric unit.

CRITICAL THINKING QUESTIONS

1. What behavioral clues did Stan exhibit during the few months preceding the onset of the violent behavior?
2. What measures could the nurse or family have employed to decrease his hostile behavior?
3. Explain the mechanism by which haloperidol reduces psychotic behavior.
4. Develop a care plan, including short- and long-term goals for Stan's inpatient hospitalization.
5. Identify behaviors that indicate Stan is responding to treatment.
6. Select the most appropriate therapeutic approaches for treating Stan as an outpatient.
7. Design a teaching plan to assist the family in caring for Stan when he is discharged.

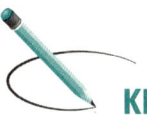

KEY POINTS

- Psychotic disorders are characterized by misperceptions of reality and altered thought processes. They include schizophrenia, schizoaffective disorder, delusional disorder, schizophreniform disorder, brief psychotic disorder, and psychotic disorder not otherwise specified (NOS). They differ in the type of symptoms experienced, their duration, and whether a functional decline is present.

- *Psychosis* is a broad term that refers to misperceptions of reality, false beliefs, disordered thoughts, and lack of insight or awareness into the discrepancy between reality and something that is actually false or unreal.

- Delusions (false beliefs), hallucinations (distorted misperceptions of reality), formal thought disorder (bizarre thoughts), and odd or bizarre behaviors comprise positive symptoms. Negative or deficit symptoms include flat affect, alogia (shortage of speech and language), avolition (lack of motivation), problems with attention, and social isolation.

- Schizophrenia is the most common psychotic disorder and five subtypes are currently recognized: paranoid, disorganized, catatonic, undifferentiated, and residual.

- Schizophrenia and other psychotic disorders were once thought to result from poor parenting and communication during early childhood. Recent theories have shifted to neurobiological underpinnings. One prominent theory proposed that schizophrenia resulted from an excess of dopamine activity (dopamine hyperactivity). Recent research suggests that other neurotransmitter systems such as serotonin, glutamate, norepinephrine, and GABA may play complex roles in the neurophysiology of schizophrenia.

- No specific laboratory or diagnostic tests can identify any of the psychotic disorders. However, structural or functional brain abnormalities such as enlarged ventricles, decreased temporal and hippocampal size, and abnormal blood flow to the prefrontal cortex have been reported in schizophrenia.

- The Brief Psychiatric Rating Scale (BPRS) is used to evaluate psychosis and the impact of symptoms on the individual's daily life.

- Schizophrenia is characterized by three identifiable stages: a prodromal phase with subtle deteriorating behaviors, an active phase of symptoms, and a residual phase.

- Antipsychotic medications remain the mainstay of treatment for psychotic disorders. Atypical antipsychotics, such as clozapine and possibly risperidone, may lead to greater improvement in positive and negative symptoms.

- Individuals with psychotic disorders commonly deny or fail to recognize the severity of their symptoms. Families play a significant role in helping them to obtain and maintain treatment.

- Because of psychotic symptoms, individuals with psychotic disorders may display dangerous, suicidal, or assaultive behaviors. Maintaining the safety of the client and others is paramount.

- Individuals with schizophrenia require long-term integrated treatment with pharmacologic and other interventions.

- Long-term care of individuals with psychotic disorders focuses on developing adequate coping skills, complying with medication, managing daily hygiene and tasks, preventing relapse, and encouraging participation in structured treatment programs.

- Families generally require support and education about psychotic illnesses. The focus is on coping with the diagnosis, understanding the illness and its course, teaching about medication, and learning ways to manage symptoms.

REFERENCES

1. American Psychiatric Association: Diagnostic and Statistical Manual of Mental Disorders, ed 4. American Psychiatric Association, Washington, DC, 1994.
2. Overall, JE: The Brief Psychiatric Rating Scale (BPRS). Recent developments in ascertainment and scaling. Psychopharmacol Bull 24:97, 1988.
3. Clardy, JA, Hyde, TM, and Kleinman, JE: Post-mortem neurochemical and neuropathological studies in schizophrenia. In Andreasen, NC (ed): From Mind to Molecule. American Psychiatric Press, Washington, DC, 1993.
4. Farde, L, et al: D_2 dopamine receptors in neuroleptic-naive schizophrenic patients' positron emission tomography study with [11C] raclopride. Arch Gen Psychiatry 44:634, 1990.
5. Tsuang, MT, Gilbertson, MW, and Faraone, SV: The genetics of schizophrenia current knowledge and future directions. Schizophr Res 4:157, 1991.
6. Knable, MB, Kleinman, JE, and Weinberger, DR: Neurobiology of schizophrenia. In Schatzberg, AF, and Nemeroff, CB (eds): Textbook

of Psychopharmacology. American Psychiatric Association, Washington, DC, 1995.
7. Weinberger, DR: Implications of normal brain development for the pathogenesis of schizophrenia. Arch Gen Psychiatry 44:660, 1987.
8. Pogue-Geile, MF, and Zubin, J: Negative symptoms and schizophrenia: A conceptual and empirical review. Int J Ment Health 16:3, 1988.
9. Williams, CA: Perspectives on the hallucinatory process. Issues in Mental Health Nursing 10: 99, 1989.
10. McGlashan, TH: Early detection and intervention in schizophrenia research. Schizophr Bull 22:327, 1996.
11. Weiden, PJ, et al: Neuroleptic noncompliance in schizophrenia. In Tamminga, CA, and Schultz, SC (eds): Advances in Neuropsychiatry and Psychopharmacology, vol 1, Schizophrenia Research. Raven Press, New York, 1991.
12. Buccheri, R, et al: Auditory hallucinations in schizophrenia. J Psychosoc Nurs Ment Health Serv 34:12, 1996.
13. Baldessarini, RJ, Cohen, BM, and Teicher, MH: Significance of neuroleptic dose and plasma level in the pharmacologic treatment of psychoses. Arch Gen Psychiatry 45:79, 1988.
14. Kane, J, et al: The Clozaril Collaborative Study Group: Clozapine for the treatment-resistant schizophrenic. A double-blind comparison vs. chlorpromazine/benztropine. Arch Gen Psychiatry 45:769, 1988.
15. Meltzer, TY, et al: Effects of 6 months of clozapine treatment on the quality of life of chronic schizophrenic patients. Hosp Comm Psychiatry 41:892, 1990.
16. Carling, PJ: Return to Community: Building Support Systems for People with Psychiatric Disabilities. The Guilford Press, New York, 1995.
17. Frederick, J, and Cotanch, P: Self help techniques for auditory hallucinations. Issues in Mental Health Nursing 16:213, 1995.
18. Spaniol, L, Zipple, A, and Lockwood, D: The role of the family in psychiatric rehabilitation. Schizophr Bull 18:341, 1992.

CHAPTER 19
Mood Disorders

CHAPTER 19

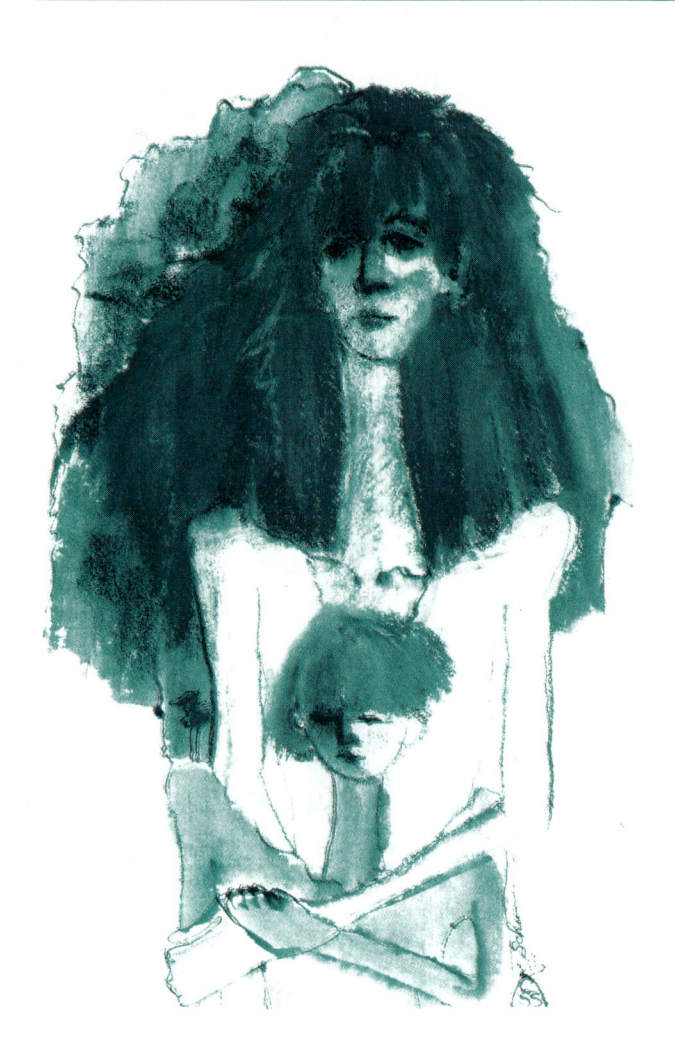

CHAPTER OUTLINE

Major Depression
  Definition
  Characteristic Behaviors
  Culture, Age, and Gender Features
  Etiology
  Prognosis
  Assessment
  Planning Care
  Interventions for Hospitalized Clients
  Interventions for Clients in the Community
  Expected Outcomes
Bipolar Disorder
  Characteristic Behaviors
  Culture, Age, and Gender Features
  Etiology
  Prognosis
  Planning Care
  Interventions for Hospitalized Clients
  Interventions for Clients in the Community
  Client and Family Education
  Expected Outcomes
Differential Diagnosis
Common Nursing Diagnoses
Synopsis of Current Research
Areas for Future Research

Carol A. Glod, RN, CS, PhD

Mood Disorders

LEARNING OBJECTIVES

After completing this chapter, the reader should be able to:

- Describe the symptoms and behaviors of major depression and mania.
- Explain and contrast theories of depression.
- Implement the nursing process in planning care for the individual with depression.
- Analyze the impact of major depression on the individual's daily functioning.
- Compare and contrast depressive and manic behaviors.
- Distinguish between the different subtypes of bipolar disorder.
- Implement the nursing process in planning care for the individual with acute mania.
- Explain theories about the development of bipolar disorder.
- Teach clients and their families about the consequences and management of mood disorders.

KEY TERMS

anhedonia	kindling
bipolar	mania
dysphoria	psychomotor retardation
dysthymia	racing thoughts
euphoria	rapid cycling
euthymia	seasonal affective disorder (SAD)
hypersomnia	
hypomania	unipolar depression

Mood disorders are conditions that have disturbances in mood as the characteristic feature: major depression, bipolar disorder, and dysthymia (Table 19–1).

The term *depression* has several different meanings in popular usage and suggests a range of possibilities. Everyone feels depressed from time to time. In the field of psychiatric nursing, however, depression refers to a specific condition, with a cluster of definable symptoms, that causes significant impairment in someone's life. For nurses and other healthcare professionals, distinguishing between a transient sad feeling, clinical depression, and normal mood can present a significant diagnostic challenge.

Although substantial advances have been made in understanding the neuropharmacology and brain chemistry associated with major depression, no known blood tests or clinical procedures can confirm or refute the diagnosis. Make no mistake, though—clinical depression with its concomitant symptomatology exerts a profound influence on daily life and has potentially devastating consequences if left untreated. William Styron, an accomplished novelist, writes eloquently about his experience of depression.[1] In his book *Darkness Visible,* he chronicles the effects of depression on his career, daily activities, and thinking and describes his experiences with various treatments. His perspective gives a voice to the personal costs of this disorder.

My brain had begun to endure its familiar siege: panic and dislocation, and a sense that my thought processes were being engulfed by a toxic and unnameable tide that obliterated any enjoyable response to the living world. This is to say more specifically that instead of pleasure—certainly instead of the pleasure I should be having in this sumptuous showcase of bright genius—I was feeling in my mind a sensation close to, but indescribably different from, actual pain . . . a form of torment so alien to everyday experience.[1]

WILLIAM STYRON

In contrast to major depression, individuals with **mania** show extremes of mood and behavior that are often opposite to those seen with depression. Both disorders are classified as mood disorders and have affected the lives of many famous and successful people. Abraham Lincoln and Winston Churchill are thought to have suffered from the mood swings and episodic nature of these manic and depressive symptoms. In fact, recent studies have suggested that individuals with mania may be highly creative and ingenious, responsible for many great works of art, literature, and music. Unfortunately,

TABLE 19–1. Prevalence of Mood Disorders

Disorder	Prevalence
Depression	10% of general population 17% of adults
Dysthmia	0.4%–1.6%
Bipolar Disorder	6%

Source: Adapted from the Diagnostic and Statistical Manual of Mental Disorders, Fourth Edition. Copyright 1994 American Psychiatric Association.

Clinical Management Tips for Clients with Mood Disorders

Effective Communication Strategies
- Strive to convey an empathic, respectful, concerned approach.
- Use simple repeated statements, with few words.
- Avoid statements that are inflammatory.
- Do not allow the manic client to talk endlessly; interrupt and redirect as needed.
- Convey an understanding attitude toward repeated complaints, such as somatic complaints, without any physical cause.
- Be accepting even though the client may have little interest in things or appear negative.
- Provide reassurance and avoid minimizing the client's concerns.

Ways to Reduce or Prevent Violence to Self or Others
- Ask about any suicidal thoughts or plans.
- Set firm, unambiguous limits on inappropriate or excessively energetic behaviors.
- Let the individual know when his or her behavior is dangerous.
- Try not to challenge the client directly.
- Provide and monitor a safe environment for the client in the hospital or in the community.

Ways to Promote Physical and Psychological Health
- Encourage moderate exercise and healthy activity patterns.
- Encourage and monitor adequate and balanced food intake.
- Reduce stimulation in the environment to promote concentration and focus.
- Assess social and family support.
- Encourage the client to be as independent as possible.
- Avoid simplistic reassurances such as "things will get better soon."
- Point out any small improvement in symptoms.
- Encourage the client to convey his or her feelings and concerns.
- Encourage participation in individual or group therapy.
- Help the client and family structure and plan each day.
- Help identify their strengths.
- Suggest social support through psychotherapy groups or self-help groups.
- Break down tasks into small steps.
- Jointly establish with the client daily structure and short-and long-term goals.

Client and Family Education
- Educate the family about the impact of untreated mood disorders on the individual's life and functional ability.
- Tell the client and family to report any worsening signs of depression or suicidal thoughts.
- Educate the client and family about mood disorders as illnesses that are not their "fault."
- Teach clients and families about the "lag time" between starting antidepressants and onset of therapeutic effect.
- Explain that self-esteem is influenced by mood disorders and suggest steps to develop enduring self-esteem.
- Review common, uncommon, and potentially dangerous side effects of medication; explain when the client should call the prescriber about side effects.
- Inform the client that several strategies exist to manage uncomfortable side effects including reduced dosages, additional medications, or switching to another medication.
- Tell clients about the need to continue medication and discuss with their prescriber any desire to stop it.
- Teach the client and family about the effects of major depression and mania on functioning; encourage that major decisions be delayed until symptoms abate.
- Educate about the detrimental effects of alcohol and substance use, including depression and sleep disruption.
- Help the client and family identify community resources such as suicide hotlines.

Source: Gorman, LM, Sultan, DF, and Raines, ML: Davis's Manual of Psychosocial Nursing for General Patient Care. FA Davis, Philadelphia, 1996.

---

it is impossible to tap into only the positive and creative aspects of the illness. The negative, self-destructive, and impulsive behaviors that are characteristic of this condition can lead to disastrous consequences, including suicide.

I feel really good, but I don't think I'm manic. I got up at 3:30 this morning and started working around the house, went to work, and got a lot accomplished. What's wrong working so much—I need the money. My wife tells me to slow down, and when she does she says I just blow up. Doesn't she understand?

Kay Redfield Jamison, a prominent researcher who has bipolar disorder, has described its advantages and disadvantages in her book, *An Unquiet Mind*.

My mind was beginning to have to scramble a bit to keep up with itself, as ideas were coming so fast that they intersected one another at every conceivable angle. There was a neuronal pileup on the highways of my brain, and the more I tried to slow down my thinking, the more I became aware that I couldn't. My enthusiasms were going into overdrive as well, although there was some underlying thread of logic in what I was doing. One day, for example, I got into a frenzy of photocopying: I made thirty to forty copies of a poem by Edna St. Vincent Millay, an article about religion and psychosis from the American Journal of Psychiatry, *and another article, "Why I Do Not Attend Case Conferences," written by a prominent psychologist who had elucidated all of the reasons why teaching rounds, when poorly conducted, are such a horrendous waste of time. All three of these articles seemed to me, quite suddenly, to have profound meaning and relevance for the clinical staff on the ward. So I passed them out to everyone I could.*[2]

KAY REDFIELD JAMISON

Dysthymia is a milder chronic form of depression, different from major depression. It is characterized by 2 or more years of depressed mood that occurs most days. The individual with dysthymia has fewer of the related depressive behaviors: poor appetite or overeating, changes in sleep, loss of energy, poor concentration, or feelings of hopelessness.[3] Because the depressive behaviors have been present for years, the client may have difficulty recognizing them.

I get up every morning and drag myself out of bed. I never quite look forward to the day, but I don't feel suicidal or anything like that. Life really isn't so bad, but I wish I could do more. I go to work, come home, and just don't do very much. This is how things have been for years. Maybe other people think that I'm depressed. I think I'm just kinda getting by.

MAJOR DEPRESSION

Definition

Classified as a mood disorder, major depression is sometimes called *clinical,* or *endogenous* depression, meaning that symptoms arise from within and are not influenced by the environment. *Depression* is a period of intense sad mood and other physical symptoms that exist nearly every day for at least 2 weeks. Individuals with major depression experience disturbances in sleep, appetite and weight, energy, concentration, and physical activity and may entertain thoughts of death or suicide. Guilt and anxiety may accompany the depressed mood. This constellation of symptoms interferes with client's ability to complete daily tasks, relate to others, and function professionally. Figure 19–1 shows that depression exerts a greater influence than major medical disorders on physical and social functioning. Seasonal, postpartum, treatment-resistant, and psychotic depression are examples of subtypes of major depression.

Characteristic Behaviors

Early identification of symptoms is important. Children may present with different behaviors or moods, whereas adults may have difficulty concentrating or **anhedonia,** a loss of interest or pleasure in those activities that the individual previously enjoyed. For students, skipping classes, an unwillingness to engage in their usual social activities, or lower grades may be early signs of depression. Some living in the community may become isolated and withdrawn and, as a result, "fall between the cracks."

Left untreated, early warning signs worsen and progress to depressive behaviors. Major depressive disorder is identified by a group of symptoms that usually lead to some difficulty in social, occupational, sexual, or daily functioning. *The Diagnostic and Statistical Manual of Mental Disorders, Fourth Edition (DSM-IV)*[3] requires the presence of depressed mood or markedly diminished interest or pleasure in life activities. In

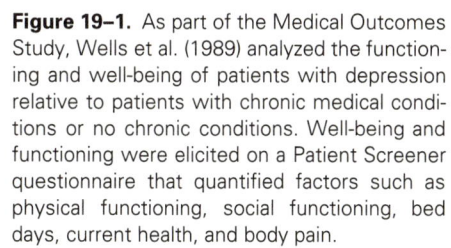

Figure 19–1. As part of the Medical Outcomes Study, Wells et al. (1989) analyzed the functioning and well-being of patients with depression relative to patients with chronic medical conditions or no chronic conditions. Well-being and functioning were elicited on a Patient Screener questionnaire that quantified factors such as physical functioning, social functioning, bed days, current health, and body pain.

Results from this study demonstrated that patients with depressive disorders had significantly greater impairment of physical and social functioning than patients with other chronic general medical illnesses, including hypertension, diabetes, arthritis, and gastrointestinal problems (Wells, et al., 1989). The significant morbidity associated with depressive disorders reinforces the importance of making the proper diagnosis and initiating appropriate treatment (Adapted from Wells, KB, Stewart, A, Hays, RD, et al. JAMA 262:914–919, 1989).

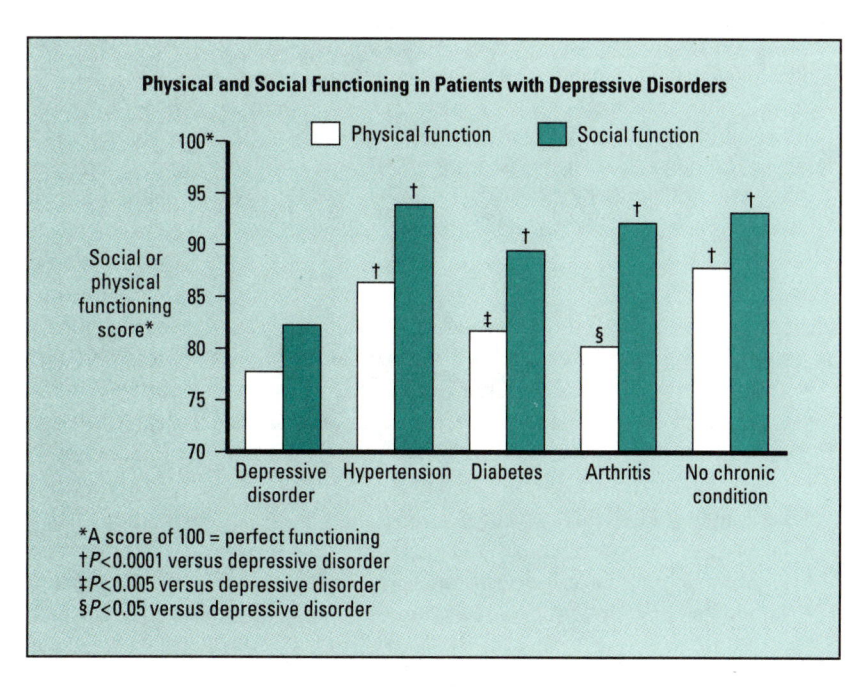

*A score of 100 = perfect functioning
†$P<0.0001$ versus depressive disorder
‡$P<0.005$ versus depressive disorder
§$P<0.05$ versus depressive disorder

> **RESEARCH NOTE**
>
> Beeber, LS, and Caldwell, CL: Pattern integration in young depressed women: Part II. Arch Psychiatr Nurs 10:157–164, 1996.
>
> **Findings:** This report describes preliminary research on six young women with depression. Their depression was theorized to result from problems with self-esteem, with protective and stressful elements in the women's close relationships leading to more severe depression. Using an intervention based on the interpersonal theory of Hildegard Peplau, the women participated in a collaborative program between primary care providers and psychiatric clinical nurse specialists. Based on detailed interviews with the clients, these authors reported four main findings. First, women described themselves as being in the "helpless person" role, whereas the nurse was the "helper person." Second, mutual concerns arose in the nurse-client relationship. For instance, one client kept a journal that was helpful to her treatment and also to the nurse. Third, a pattern called "pursuer-distancer" emerged. The young women would pursue relationships intensely, then would pull away, and eventually would become depressed. Last, clients continued in the relationship with the nurse despite feeling dissatisfied and believing that the interactions were a "poor fit."
>
> **Application to Practice:** Although this data is based on a small number of women, it suggests that Peplau's theoretical notions about the nature of interpersonal relationships are key in depression. Events that occur in the therapeutic relationship between the nurse and client are important in treating major depression. In young women, decreased self-esteem is a major issue affected by the ups and downs of relationships. Nursing interventions should target ways to enhance self-esteem as well as the relationship with the nurse. This study also supports other research on the effectiveness of psychotherapy for depression. Dealing with the problems in relationships, particularly for this age group, is essential for promoting mental health. Furthermore, because depressed women are more likely to present to their primary care providers, links with psychiatric health-care professionals such as psychiatric clinical nurse specialists can promote early assessment and intervention.

See the Diagnostic Box for the full criteria for major depressive episode.

There are several common subtypes and classifications of major depression based on symptom presentation (Table 19–2). The severity of the depression is rated as mild, moderate, or severe. One major subtype, **seasonal affective disorder (SAD)**, generally occurs in the fall in response to shortening days and lack of bright light exposure.

An individual with a past history of major depression or a family history of depression may be more prone to develop depression, particularly given a period of extreme stress or specific life stressor, such as divorce, unemployment, or trauma. Typically, depressive symptoms are very similar to the previous episode, for example, **psychomotor retardation** and hypersomnia. Dysthymia may also be a precursor to the development of depression. The birth of a child may be a factor in the development of depressive symptoms. The "baby blues," a 3- to 7-day period of sadness postpartum, is common, but the onset of the characteristic symptoms of depression for 2 weeks heralds the beginning of postpartum depression. For older adults, placement into a nursing home or severe chronic illness may precipitate major depression.

DIAGNOSTIC AIDS

Dexamethasone Suppression Test

Although there is currently no single diagnostic laboratory or objective test that detects major depression or other mood disorders, the dexamethasone suppression test (DST) has shown the most promise. It is not commonly used, however, because it identifies only about 50% of depressed individuals. As seen in Table 19–3, recent research has shown that the DST may be a biological marker to distinguish individuals with depression and posttraumatic stress disorder (PTSD).[4] Circulating amounts of cortisol, a stress hormone, are increased in some depressed individuals. In PTSD, cortisol levels are decreased. The DST test measures cortisol levels before and after the system is "challenged" with a synthetic steroid, dexamethasone (Decadron). When most healthy adults are given a small dose (1 mg) at bedtime, their systems send a signal to "shut off" production of cortisol so that their cortisol levels are lower. For 40 to 50% of depressed individuals, however, an abnormality in their usual feedback mechanism fails to send the signal to decrease production, and cortisol levels are elevated after the administration of dexamethasone (greater than 5 mcg/dL). Such people are classified as "nonsuppressors"; that is, they fail to suppress cortisol production. Individuals with PTSD suppress cortisol production in response to the DST, but to a greater degree than others. They are classified as "enhanced suppressors."

No specific blood tests exist to accurately detect decreased amounts of neurotransmitters (for example, low serotonin levels); however, efforts are underway to continue to develop other reliable objective tests for the diagnosis of depression and other mood disorders.

addition, at least four of the following symptoms must also be present nearly every day during a 2-week period:
- Changes in weight (increased or decreased)
- Changes in sleep (increased sleep [**hypersomnia**] or insomnia)
- Psychomotor retardation or agitation
- Fatigue or loss of energy
- Feelings of worthlessness or guilt
- Poor concentration or indecisiveness
- Thoughts of death or suicidal ideation or attempt.

DSM-IV Criteria for Major Depressive Episode

A. Five (or more) of the following symptoms have been present during the same 2-week period and represent a change from previous functioning; at least one of the symptoms is either (1) depressed mood or (2) loss of interest or pleasure.

NOTE: Do not include symptoms that are clearly due to a general medical condition, or mood-incongruent delusions or hallucinations.

(1) Depressed mood most of the day, nearly every day, as indicated by either subjective report (e.g., feels sad or empty) or observation made by others (e.g., appears tearful). NOTE: In children and adolescents, can be irritable mood.
(2) Markedly diminished interest or pleasure in all, or almost all, activities most of the day, nearly every day (as indicated by either subjective account or observation made by others)
(3) Significant weight loss when not dieting or weight gain (e.g., a change of more than 5% of body weight in a month), or decrease or increase in appetite nearly every day. NOTE: In children, consider failure to make expected weight gains.
(4) Insomnia or hypersomnia nearly every day
(5) Psychomotor agitation or retardation nearly every day (observable by others, not merely subjective feelings of restlessness or being slowed down)
(6) Fatigue or loss of energy nearly every day
(7) Feelings of worthlessness or excessive or inappropriate guilt (which may be delusional) nearly every day (not merely self-reproach or guilt about being sick)
(8) Diminished ability to think or concentrate, or indecisiveness, nearly every day (either by subjective account or as observed by others)
(9) Recurrent thoughts of death (not just fear of dying), recurrent suicidal ideation without a specific plan, or a suicide attempt or a specific plan for committing suicide

B. The symptoms do not meet criteria for a Mixed Episode.

C. The symptoms cause clinically significant distress or impairment in social, occupational, or other important areas of functioning.

D. The symptoms are not due to the direct physiological effects of a substance (e.g., a drug of abuse, a medication) or a general medical condition (e.g., hypothyroidism).

E. The symptoms are not better accounted for by Bereavement (i.e., after the loss of a loved one), the symptoms persist for longer than 2 months or are characterized by marked functional impairment, morbid preoccupation with worthlessness, suicidal ideation, psychotic symptoms, or psychomotor retardation.

Source: Reprinted with permission from the Diagnostic and Statistical Manual of Mental Disorders, Fourth Edition. Copyright 1994 American Psychiatric Association.

TABLE 19-2. Subtypes of Major Depression and Associated Features

Subtype	Feature
Major Depression, recurrent	Currently meet *DSM-IV* criteria with a previous episode.
Major Depression, single episode	Currently meet *DSM-IV* criteria with no previous episodes.
Major Depression, with psychotic features	Currently meet *DSM-IV* criteria with hallucinations, delusions, or paranoia.
Major Depression, with atypical features	Currently meet *DSM-IV* criteria with hypersomnia (excess sleep), loss of energy, hyperphagia (increased appetite), and increased weight, along with brightening of mood in response to positive events.
Major Depression, with seasonal pattern	Currently meets *DSM-IV* criteria, with regular onset and remission of symptoms; also known as SAD.
Major Depression, with postpartum onset	Currently meets *DSM-IV* criteria, with onset of symptoms 4 weeks postpartum.

Source: Reprinted with permission from the Diagnostic and Statistical Manual of Mental Disorders, Fourth Edition. Copyright 1994 American Psychiatric Association.

SEASONAL AFFECTIVE DISORDER (SAD)

Seasonal depression has been recognized for centuries; however, the cluster of symptoms in Seasonal Affective Disorder (SAD) has only recently been established. SAD is a common disorder, affecting about 6% of the population, including children and adults. This syndrome is characterized by some typical depressive symptoms such as depressed mood, lack of energy, and loss of interest in pleasurable activities.* Most SAD sufferers display atypical depressive symptoms, including increased appetite, weight gain, carbohydrate cravings, increased sleep, severe fatigue, social withdrawal, and diurnal variation type B (afternoon slump in mood or energy). The essential feature of this seasonal depression is the regular occurrence of symptoms, usually with a fall-winter onset and spring-summer remission. This seasonal relationship must have occurred for at least 2 consecutive years. Seasonal summer depressions may also occur (spring-summer onset with fall-winter remission), although the symptoms differ.

There are several theories about the etiology of fall-winter SAD. The initial theory, the *photoperiod effect*, suggested that SAD was due to shortened winter days and the associated lack of sunlight. Many animals hibernate during the winter, triggered by the decreased light. SAD clients were exposed to light therapy to lengthen the winter day, mimicking summer days. Another leading theory of SAD is the *melatonin hypothesis*. The peak release of melatonin, which leads to sleep induction, occurs later in the night in SAD sufferers. Disruption in neurotransmitters may also account for SAD symptoms. Some studies have found that individuals with SAD have reduced levels of serotonin. Biological rhythm theories, which center on disrupted 24-hour (circadian) rhythms, may explain the development of SAD.

As our lives have become more oriented toward indoor activities, it may be that we have regressed to being "cave dwellers." Individuals who have been secluded for days under special research conditions without light or time cues have rhythms that fail to sync with a 24-hour day. Instead, their internal body clock drifts more toward a lunar or 25-hour day. While these theories provide some beginning understanding for the development of SAD and the mechanism of action of light therapy, more studies are necessary to determine the basis for this disorder.

*Source: Rosenthal, NE, Sack, DA, and Gillin, C: Seasonal affective disorder: A description of the syndrome and preliminary findings with light therapy. Arch Gen Psychiatry 41: 72–80, 1984.

TABLE 19–3. Differences in the Hypothalamic-Pituitary-Adrenal Axis (HPA) in Major Depression and Posttraumatic Stress Disorder (PTSD)

	Major Depression	PTSD
Cortisol level	Increased	Decreased
Cortisol level during DST*	Decreased	Increased

*Dexamethasone Suppression Test.

Rating Scales

The Beck Depression Inventory (BDI)[5] and the Zung Rating Scale (Table 19–4) are self-report measures used to assess the presence and evaluate the severity of depression. The Hamilton Depression Rating Scale (HDRS)[6] is an observer-rated instrument that also covers the major symptoms of depression. Although these rating scales are not diagnostic assessments—a complete diagnostic interview is necessary to determine the presence of the disorder—the BDI and HDRS are useful in evaluating the outcome of treatment or assessing whether the client is improving.

Culture, Age, and Gender Features

CULTURE

Depression may be expressed differently in different cultures, and symptoms may also have very different meanings or levels of severity, depending on the individual's culture. For example, some cultures view depressed mood as less debilitating than irritability. Instead of a predominantly depressed or sad mood, clients may present with primarily physical complaints. In Hispanic and Mediterranean cultures, headaches and problems with "nerves" may predominate; in Asian cultures, weakness, tiredness, or "imbalance" may present; in Middle Eastern culture, "problems of the heart" are likely.[3]

AGE

Children and Adolescents. Clinicians once believed that depression did not occur in young children because they were not able to think abstractly. However, depression can strike at any age and is diagnosed with the same criteria as for adults. Prepubertal children, unlikely to suffer from depression, tend to show symptoms of irritability, social withdrawal, and somatic complaints such as headaches and stomach aches. Depression in young children often coexists with anxiety disorders, attention-deficit/hyperactivity disorder (ADHD), and behavioral disorders of childhood such as conduct disorder. More commonly, depression begins in adolescence. Adolescents may show irritable rather than down

TABLE 19–4. Zung SDS*

INSTRUCTIONS

Listed below are 20 statements. Please read each one carefully and decide how much of the statement describes how you have been feeling during the past week. Decide whether the statement applies to you for NONE OR A LITTLE OF THE TIME, SOME OF THE TIME, A GOOD PART OF THE TIME, OR MOST OR ALL OF THE TIME. Mark the appropriate column for each statement.

EXAMPLE

Statement I feel nervous	None or a little of the time	Some of the time	A good part of the time	Most or all of the time
If the statement "I feel nervous" describes the way you have felt "A GOOD PART OF THE TIME", you would mark column 3 "A GOOD PART OF THE TIME" as shown.	[1]	[2]	[3]	[4]

Statement	None or a little of the time	Some of the time	A good part of the time	Most or all of the time
1. I feel downhearted and blue	[1]	[2]	[3]	[4]
2. Morning is when I feel the best	[1]	[2]	[3]	[4]
3. I have crying spells or feel like it	[1]	[2]	[3]	[4]
4. I have trouble sleeping at night	[1]	[2]	[3]	[4]
5. I eat as much as I used to	[1]	[2]	[3]	[4]
6. I still enjoy sex	[1]	[2]	[3]	[4]
7. I notice that I am losing weight	[1]	[2]	[3]	[4]
8. I have trouble with constipation	[1]	[2]	[3]	[4]
9. My heart beats faster than usual	[1]	[2]	[3]	[4]
10. I get tired for no reason	[1]	[2]	[3]	[4]
11. My mind is as clear as it used to be	[1]	[2]	[3]	[4]
12. I find it easy to do things I used to do	[1]	[2]	[3]	[4]
13. I am restless and can't keep still	[1]	[2]	[3]	[4]
14. I feel hopeful about the future	[1]	[2]	[3]	[4]
15. I am more irritable than usual	[1]	[2]	[3]	[4]
16. I find it easy to make decisions	[1]	[2]	[3]	[4]
17. I feel that I am useful and needed	[1]	[2]	[3]	[4]
18. My life is pretty full	[1]	[2]	[3]	[4]
19. I feel that others would be better off if I were dead	[1]	[2]	[3]	[4]
20. I still enjoy the things I used to do	[1]	[2]	[3]	[4]

SCORING

Each question is rated on a 1–4 scale; questions worded positively are reverse scored. A total score is obtained by summing ratings for each question: The more depressed the respondent, the higher the score. Depressed clients usually have scores greater than 60.

Source: Zung, W: A self-rating depression scale. *Arch Gen Psychiatry* 12:334, 1965.

moods, and excess sleep and increased appetite instead of insomnia and loss of appetite. Suicide, particularly impulsive acts, and drug or alcohol abuse are major risks.

Elderly. Older adults are more likely to display insomnia and cognitive complaints such as poor concentration, memory loss, and distractibility. Physical complaints may predominate; clients may experience somatic distress rather than sadness or mood changes. The aches and pains do not have any physiological basis; in extreme cases, older clients may become delusional and believe (falsely) that they have a life-threatening illness.

Although the rate is increasing among adolescents, suicide is more common among older adults, particularly men. In general, those who attempt suicide are younger and usually women, whereas those who succeed are more likely to be older men, who use more lethal methods (Box 19–1).

Box 19-1. Risk Factors for Suicide

- Presence of a psychiatric disorder, particularly major depression
- Major depression with psychotic features
- Previous suicide attempts
- A family history of successful suicide
- Concomitant substance or alcohol abuse
- Lack of social supports
- Stressful life events
- Chronic medical illness

Source: Blumenthal, SJ, and Kupfer, DJ: Suicide over the Life Cycle: Risk Factors, Assessment, and Treatment of Suicidal Patients. American Psychiatric Press, Washington, DC, 1990.

Etiology

BIOLOGICAL THEORIES

Classic theories of depression proposed that it resulted from a deficiency in norepinephrine and serotonin. Recent theories center on the neuropharmacologic effects that occur long term.[7] The dysregulation hypothesis suggests that, instead of a simple decrease in norepinephrine or serotonin transmission in depressed individuals, there is an overall disruption or imbalance in the release of these neurotransmitters.[8] In response to the short-term increases in norepinephrine and serotonin from antidepressant therapy, the brain "adapts" to the outpouring of these neurotransmitters like a thermostat (Figure 19-2). When high levels of norepinephrine and serotonin are released, the postsynaptic neuron "sees" an excess and sends a signal to lower production. Specifically, the receptors to which the neurotransmitters bind decrease in number (down-regulate) or become less sensitive. A signal to produce less norepinephrine or serotonin goes to the presynaptic neuron, which attempts to balance the initial high amounts of neurotransmitters. These effects take weeks to occur. Antidepressants work by balancing (regulating) levels of norepinephrine and serotonin. Depression is then hypothesized to result from poor regulation (dysregulation) of these neurotransmitters.

Genetic Theories

Family and genetic studies provide the leading evidence for the genetic transmission of **unipolar depression**. First-degree relatives of individuals with major depression have about twice the risk for developing this disorder than the rest of the population.[9]

Twins, presumed to have similar genetic makeups, who are reared apart provide an opportunity to determine the contribution of heredity versus parenting and childhood experiences (so-called nurture). Identical twins (monozygotic) have a 54% risk of one twin developing depression if the other has had a diagnosed episode.[9] The risk of developing

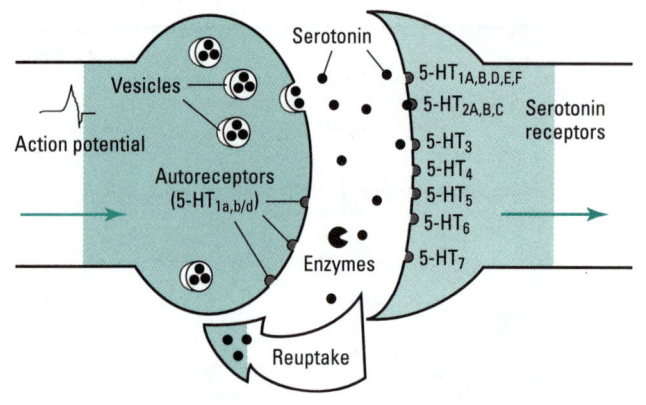

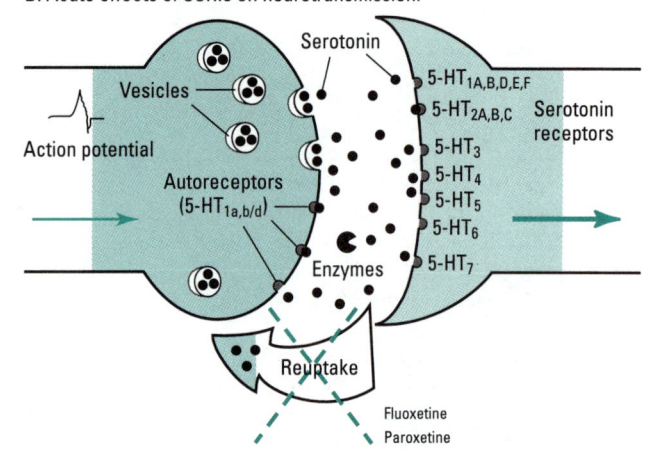

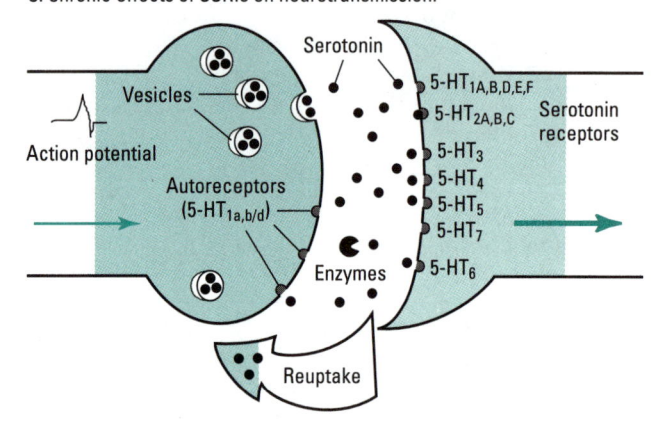

Figure 19-2. The effects of selective serotonin reuptake inhibitors (SSRIs) on neurotransmission. The arrows indicate the strength of the response, both presynaptically and postsynaptically. (*A*) Shows normal neuronal activity of a serotonin neuron. (*B*) The acute effects of SSRIs (like fluoxetine and paroxetine) cause an increase in extracellular (synaptic) levels of serotonin and an enhanced response from the postsynaptic neuron as serotonin exerts its effects. (*C*) The chronic effect of SSRIs is not as strong as the initial response, as presynaptic autoreceptors desensitize and moderate the response. (Courtesy of Susan Andersen.)

depression in nonidentical (dizygotic) twins is about 24% higher than that of the general population but less than that for monozygotic twins. These studies have their limitations. Although they reveal that depression is a complex disorder with a genetic component, they fail to explain the transmission of the disorder.

More recent studies have attempted to explore the complicated nature of contributing factors. They suggest that although family history of depression is a factor, stressful life events, previous depressive episodes, and neuroticism predict the development of depression. Early childhood experiences, such as physical or sexual abuse or loss of a parent, may also help explain the pathogenesis of depression. Despite proof for a genetic vulnerability for unipolar depression, the development of the disorder is complex, affected by many factors.

Circadian and Other Rhythm Theories

The phases of major depression may follow a seasonal pattern or recur every several years. Definable rhythms that occur more than every 24 hours are called *infradian rhythms*. SAD follows an infradian rhythm and is a subtype of major depression. In SAD, the depression recurs each winter and remits in the summer.[10]

Depression may result from a disruption in circadian rhythms, which follow a 24-hour pattern. Simply stated, depressed individuals may be "less circadian," and antidepressants may work by restoring circadian rhythmicity. Examples include a reduction in the circadian rhythm of serotonin, norepinephrine, thyroid-stimulating hormone (TSH), and melatonin. Another important component of this theory is that rhythms of less than 24 hours appear to increase in depression. For instance, depressed children have greater (12-hour) activity rhythms than do normal children.[11] The increased 12-hour rhythm may explain why depressed clients often feel worse in the morning and somewhat better in the evening, about 12 hours later.

Other biological rhythm theories suggest that the timing of rhythms may be altered in major depression. These include the *phase-advance* and *phase-delay* theories. The phase-advance theory suggests that the timing of certain circadian processes, such as core body temperature, rapid eye movement (REM) sleep, and cortisol, occurs earlier (is phase-advanced) relative to the timing of other circadian processes, such as activity patterns, slow-wave sleep, and some psychological functions. The opposite theory is the phase-delay theory. This theory suggests that the timing of certain daily rhythms occurs later (is phase-delayed) than in other circadian processes. The best example is the melatonin theory, which has been examined in SAD. Melatonin, a hormone normally secreted at night, facilitates sleep onset. In some individuals with depression, the timing of melatonin release is phase-delayed; the secretion of melatonin occurs later. Delayed melatonin secretion is related to later onset of sleep and may account for the difficulty depressed clients have in falling asleep.

Psychoanalytic Theories

For many years, the predominant theories about the development of major depression and other psychiatric disorders involved a psychodynamic or psychoanalytic framework. Psychoanalytic theories of depression focus on three major areas: hostility, loss, and conflict. One hypothesis is that hostility turned inward, or anger against the self, is central to the pathogenesis of depressive states. Other psychoanalytic interpretations have focused on the relationship between suffering a major loss and the subsequent development of

> **RESEARCH NOTE**
>
> **Beck, CT: Teetering on the edge: A substantive theory of postpartum depression.**
>
> **Findings:** The study developed a theoretical model based on 12 women who suffered from postpartum depression. Each subject received an in-depth interview after participating in a postpartum depression support group. The author sought to determine the nature of the psychosocial problem in postpartum depression, and how women managed the depression successfully using the grounded theory method. The participants identified loss of control as the major problem during their postpartum depression.
>
> "Teetering on the edge" was the process that subjects confronted during their depression. This concept reflected their feeling of being between sane and insane. They coped with this process through a series of four stages. When they were "encountering terror," women experienced the postpartum depression unpredictably and suddenly. During this stage, anxiety attacks, obsessions, and loss of concentration were overwhelming. In the next stage, "dying of self," women suffered from alarming unrealness, isolation, withdrawal, and suicidal ideation. Women dealt with these powerful feelings during the following stage, "struggling to survive." Women sought professional help, attended postpartum depression support groups, and used their faith and prayer to manage the depression. Finally, women with postpartum depression recovered gradually and inconsistently.
>
> **Application to Practice:** Depression during the postpartum period is a common condition filled with terror. Women are at highest risk for developing this type of depression from days to 6 months following childbirth. After postpartum depression develops, women pass through a series of stages, lasting several months or years. Nurses are in a key position to assess and intervene early with women with postpartum depression. Early intervention is essential to mitigate dangerous consequences such as suicidal behavior and child neglect. Nurses can also initiate postpartum depression support groups to improve outcomes. Spiritual interventions with postpartum depressed women may enhance recovery.

TABLE 19–5. Some Thought Patterns Seen in Depression

Rigidity of Thoughts. Maintaining inflexible fixed rules for behavior, when options are available.

Dichotomous Thinking. Polarizing options without a range of possibilities.

Magnification. Exaggerating events or situations.

Personalization. Assuming too little or too much responsibility for a situation.

Arbitrary Inference. Jumping to conclusions despite evidence to the contrary.

Externalization. Believing one's problems are due to external events.

---

depression. The third viewpoint is that ongoing dynamic conflicts within the self have a major role in the development of depression. It emphasizes early childhood experiences, relationships to primary caregivers, and the caretaker's capacity to form empathic and healthy connections. Finally, psychodynamic theories suggest that certain personality styles, such as borderline personality, may predispose the individual to depression.

Cognitive-Behavior Theories

Cognitive and behavior theories center more on the here and now than on the past. One of the most recent theories about the etiology and treatment of individuals with major depression centers on the relationship of thoughts (cognitions) and behavior to mood states. Cognitive theorists hold that self-deprecating thoughts—feeling stupid, ugly, incapable,

---

What are the trends in death rates due to suicide among adolescents and young adults?

Suicide deaths continue to increase among both men and women age 15–19. Suicide deaths among adults age 20–24 increased from 1950 to 1980 and decreased slightly in 1990. Overall, the suicide death rates continue to be higher among men than women age 15–24.

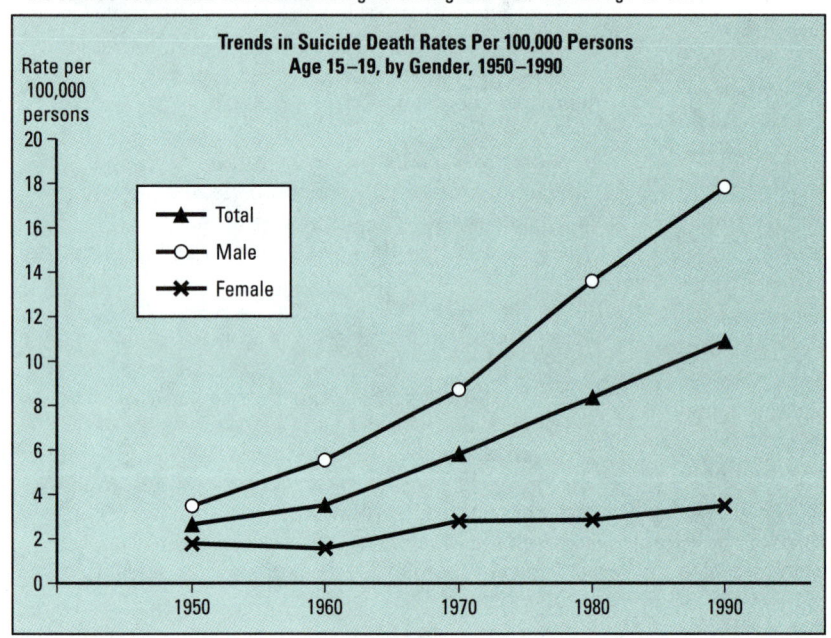

Trends in Suicide Death Rates Per 100,000 Persons Age 15–19, by Gender, 1950–1990

Trends in Suicide Death Rates Per 100,000 Persons Age 15–24 by Gender, 1950–1990

	1950	1960	1970	1980	1990
Total 15 to 24 years	4.5	5.2	8.8	12.3	13.2
Male	6.5	8.2	13.5	20.2	22.0
Female	2.6	2.2	4.2	4.3	3.9
20 to 24 years	6.2	7.1	12.2	16.1	15.1
Male	9.3	11.5	19.2	26.8	25.7
Female	3.3	2.9	5.6	5.5	4.1
15 to 19 years	2.7	3.6	5.9	8.5	11.1
Male	3.5	5.6	8.8	13.8	18.1
Female	1.8	1.6	2.9	3.0	3.7

Figure 19–3. Source notes: CDC National Center for Injury Prevention and Control (1994): Programs for the Prevention of Suicide Among Adolescents and Young Adults. *Mobidity and Mortality Weekly Report* 43(RR-6) 3–7, April 22. Data compiled by the National Center for Health Statistics, Division of Vital Statistics. Cause-of-death statistics are based on information reported on the death certificate. The International Classification of Diseases is used for selecting the underlying cause of death from the reported conditions.

hopeless, incompetent, lazy, undeserving, and so forth—are associated with the development of depressive feelings. Table 19–5 lists examples of depressive thought patterns. The main focus of cognitive therapy is to identify distorted thoughts rather than explore past experiences or inner conflicts.

Behavioral theories are rooted in the initial Pavlovian findings that behavior can be conditioned through manipulation of circumstances. These theories suggest that people also become conditioned to respond because of learned behaviors, although these responses may worsen depression, leading to further isolation and hopelessness.

Prognosis

One of the most significant consequences of major depression is the toll it can exact on day-to-day functioning. Depression affects people's ability to perform their usual activities, is associated with substantial comorbidity, and increases the risk of mortality. In fact, recent studies suggest that the morbidity and limitations caused by depressive disorders are more severe than for most chronic medical conditions, with the exception of cardiac disease.[12] The combination of depression and a major medical disorder multiplies the limitations, resulting in loss of productivity, increased or inappropriate use of health-care resources, and alcohol and substance abuse. If left untreated, individuals with depressive disorder have a 25 to 30% risk of suicide during their lifetime. Death rates from suicide have been rising, particularly among 15- to 19-year-olds (Figure 19–3). Despite these consequences, the social stigma associated with a psychiatric disorder prevents many people from seeking adequate treatment.

Assessment

A common dangerous and often false belief is that individuals who threaten suicide are manipulative and looking for attention. Even if manipulation is the goal, suicide is sometimes the result. An important evaluative and intervention strategy for managing depressed clients, regardless of setting, is to assess their suicidal thoughts and potential for self-destructive actions. Use the suicide assessment listed in Box 19–2. Asking depressed individuals about suicide does not "plant the idea" in their heads. Studies have shown that a suicide assessment does not increase the risk for suicide; rather, avoiding questions about suicide may increase the risk.[13]

A direct, caring approach is the most successful for eliciting whether suicidal ideation is present. Some clients may be relieved that someone has finally cared enough to ask. A whole range of suicidal feelings may be present, from passive thoughts ("I sometimes wake up and wish I hadn't") to more active ones ("I see my pills and think that taking them would solve all my problems"). When precise thoughts are present, ask detailed questions about frequency, intent, plans—

Box 19–2. Suicide Assessment

Initial Questions

- Have you had any thoughts that life isn't worth living, either recently or in the past?
- Do things ever seem so hopeless that you wish you were dead?
- Do you ever think or feel that others would be better off if you died?
- How often do you think these thoughts [or have these feelings]?
- Do [did] you ever feel that you wanted to kill yourself?
- Have you ever tried to kill yourself? How?

If Current Suicidal Ideation Is Present

- Have you thought about ways you might kill yourself? How?
- Who else have you told these thoughts to?
- When did you last have these thoughts?
- Did you feel like acting upon them?
- What stopped you from acting on them?

If Individual Has Potential Plan, Establish Seriousness

- When might you act on these urges?
- Is there someone you can call before acting on them?

specifically, the nature of those plans. Begin with more open-ended questions to elicit mild or passive thoughts and then progress to more pointed questions to determine the individual's safety. Although this assessment is generic, it can be adapted to different developmental levels, like teenagers or adults, or to different cognitive levels.

If a client has an established suicide plan and timetable but refuses to agree to call a professional before acting, hospitalization is definitely indicated. Students may find themselves in situations in which a client expresses suicidal thoughts or feelings spontaneously. Because it can be difficult to assess the seriousness of the intent and to determine whether to refer the individual for professional help or to intervene immediately, the beginning student ought to consult with the staff and get supervision from the instructor before making the treatment plan.

Planning Care

Most clients with depression are overwhelmed by even simple tasks. For them to return to baseline functioning, their symptoms must be resolved. Therefore, the nurse who is planning care has to assess the client's quality of life and the role depression plays before recommending treatment. If the individual does fulfill the full criteria for major depression, an antidepressant trial is generally indicated. If the symptoms are present to a severe degree or the client is actively planning suicide, hospitalization or intensive outpatient treatment is necessary. In addition, individual psychother-

Critical Pathway: Depression

Care Needs	First 24 hours	Days 2–5
Assessments/Evaluations	Past psych hx Medication hx Medical hx Suicide risk Self-care ability Approp legal status Psychiatric eval Nursing assessment	Family interview Social work eval Evals by activities, occupational, group, other therapies Continue psych/nursing evals
Diagnostic Tests/Workup	Physical exam by internist, NP Lab tests inc. CBC, chem panel, drug screen, thyroid panel, others as needed	Review results of evals and lab work Implement approp interventions from problems identified from workup Implement further workup as needed Begin psychological testing
Treatment	Orient to unit Order initial activity.	Develop multidisciplinary tx plan Begin 1:1 psychotherapy Begin group therapy Begin OT and activity therapy Participate in family sessions as approp
Medications	Order initial doses of drugs for psych & medical symptoms Monitor response, side effects	Monitor responses, side effects Adjust doses as approp
Safety/Self-care	Establish unit rules r/t risk for suicide, elopement, substance abuse Monitor eating, elimination, sleep, hygiene	Continue to monitor and implement interventions for safe environment as per column 2 Implement changes in diet as approp Begin interventions to enhance sleep, and promote elimination and hygiene
Education	Unit orientation Patient rights	Begin education on depression Provide overview of meds Explain impact of workup/test results
Discharge Plan	Identify initial concerns	Identify family and patient concerns Identify possible resources/living arrangements
Outcomes	___ Patient assessed by MD and nurse ___ Initial activity orders in place ___ Patient does not harm self Progressing per pathway? Yes ___ No ___ If no, referred to _____	___ Assessments by all disciplines complete ___ Medical workup completed and tx plan implemented ___ Multidisciplinary tx plan implemented ___ Meds adjusted as needed ___ Patient begins participating in tx ___ Patient does not harm self Progressing per pathway? Yes ___ No ___ If no, referred to _____

Care Needs	Days 6–10+	Discharge
Assessment/Evaluations	Reassessment ongoing	
Diagnostic Tests/Workup	Check that all results are available and implemented in tx plan Determine need for further tests	Establish need for follow-up medical care and make appointments

Continued on following page

Critical Pathway: Depression (Continued)

Care Needs	Days 6–10+	Discharge
Treatment	Continue treatment plan Develop outpatient plan	Ensure that outpatient tx appointments are in place Check issues r/t insurance, transportation, work to enhance compliance with outpatient plan
Meds	Continue to monitor response and adjust doses as needed Consider raising doses as approp Monitor side effects Establish outpatient meds	Ensure drug regimen is in place Ensure access to prescriptions
Safety/Self-care	Continue to monitor risks per days 1–5 Establish no-suicide contract Continue monitoring eating, elimination, sleep patterns and implement interventions as approp Involve family in plan Establish resources for help in outpatient care	Ensure patient has resources for help Involve family if approp Ensure patient has resources for food
Education	Continue to educate on depression, factors that contribute to exacerbations Involve family in education Teach new coping skills Educate on meds and side effects Explain food and drug interactions Give nutritional counseling Outline availability of community resources	Ensure that educational materials can be taken home to reinforce teaching Reinforce teaching in outpt tx
Discharge Plan	Develop outpatient tx plan Establish criteria for readmission Determine need for long-term hospitalization	Social worker reviews plan for outpatient tx, living arrangements, insurance, work, activities, finances Transportation home arranged Resources for help established Home health care arranged as approp
Outcomes	____ Patient participates in tx plan ____ Patient demonstrates improvement and stabilization of symptoms ____ Patient understands stabilization of med doses ____ Patient does not harm self ____ Leaves hospital verbalizing understanding of d/c plan, knowledge of living arrangements ____ Verbalizes intention to participate in outpatient tx plan ____ Family demonstrates intention to participate in tx plan ____ Patient able to verbalize medication regimen ____ Verbalizes awareness of symptoms signaling need for more help ____ Verbalizes resources for help Progressing per pathway? Yes _____ No _____ If no, referred to _____	Progressing per pathway? Yes _____ No _____ If no, referred to _____

Nursing Care Plan: DEPRESSION

Nursing Diagnosis #1: Self Esteem Disturbance evidenced by statements of low self-esteem, misinterpreting positive or pleasurable experiences, expressions of shame and guilt, pessimistic outlook related to feelings and thoughts of worthlessness, negative reinforcement, learned helplessness

Client Outcome Criteria:
- Modifies unrealistic negative expectations of self.
- Verbalizes realistic positive aspects about self.
- Practices techniques to increase self-esteem and assertiveness.

Interventions
- Provide emotional support through empathic listening and supportive encouragement. Demonstrate acceptance.
- Encourage the client to identify positive personal aspects.
- Genuinely praise and recognize areas of improvement but avoid false and blanket reassurances.
- Encourage the client to share feelings. Listen to his or her concerns.
- Point out any tendencies to focus on the negative. Challenge this negative thinking. Remind the client of past successes. If the client minimizes these, point out the tendency to devalue past successes.
- Teach assertiveness and effective communication skills by role modeling and identifying situations where these skills can be effective. Point out how standing up for one's beliefs reinforces one's self-esteem.

Nursing Diagnosis #2: Powerlessness evidenced by lack of initiative, indecision, nonachievement of realistic goals, overdependence on others related to decreased motivation; Hopelessness, Chronic Low Self-esteem

Client Outcome Criteria
- Identifies factors that are within the client's control.
- Participates in decisions about his or her care.
- Demonstrates independent thinking on some issues.
- Verbalizes feeling more in control of self and identified situations.

Interventions
- Encourage the client to establish realistic goals and make decisions about own care. If this is too difficult, give the client choices in his or her care and then follow through on the client's decision.
- Help the client break down goals into small, achievable steps.
- Assist the client in setting up a system for monitoring progress.
- Problem solve with the client to identify solutions to situations in which the client feels powerless.
- Explore areas in the client's life that he or she has mastered.
- Identify factors that contribute to the client's sense of powerlessness, and then assist in developing strategies to challenge these.
- Provide positive reinforcement for the client's attempts to make decisions and be more independent.
- Add responsibility to the client gradually.

Nursing Diagnosis #3: High Risk for Violence: Self-directed, evidenced by suicide attempts, self-mutilation, suicide plan, refusal to care for self related to depressed mood, poor impulse control, suicidal ideation, feelings of abandonment

Client Outcome Criteria
- Does not harm self.
- Verbalizes more optimistic view of the future.
- Identifies and uses available resources for assistance.
- Verbalizes any suicidal ideation and contracts to not harm himself or herself.

Interventions
- Make a thorough suicide assessment including the client's past history, determination of a suicide plan, access to a lethal method, and current coping abilities. Ask the client directly, "Have you thought about harming yourself?"
- Talk openly with the client about your concern. Encourage the client to share feelings. However, never promise confidentiality about information the client may share with you.
- Share your concern with other health team members, and seek their input as appropriate.
- Create a safe environment for the suicidal client by removing all potentially harmful objects and implementing suicide precautions per agency policy.
- Determine the client's strengths and coping abilities and reinforce these.
- Identify factors that are overwhelming the client now and problem solve to develop possible solutions.
- Reinforce the client's support systems that are available. Identify other resources available and ensure the client knows how to reach them by having access to phone numbers. Assist the client in contacting family, friends, and therapists.
- Contract with the client to tell someone if suicidal thoughts increase or if he or she is feeling closer to acting on them.

Nursing Diagnosis #4: Spiritual distress evidenced by questioning beliefs and existence of God, Dysfunctional Grieving over a loss with suffering and depression

Client Outcome Criteria
- Demonstrates fewer signs of distress.
- Expresses sense of comfort and support.
- Verbalizes losses and demonstrates beginning the grieving process.

Interventions
- Be accepting and nonjudgmental to encourage expression of the client's beliefs and concerns. Allow expressions of sadness and anger, and reminiscing about past losses.
- Empathize with the client's degree of pain and despair.
- Help the client explore issues and losses.
- Assist the client to problem solve and explore new understanding of concerns.
- Promote spiritual support practices and resources, as appropriate, such as clergy visits and spiritual readings.
- Give permission to discuss spiritual matters if he or she wishes.

apy is indicated for moderate to severe depression. It may take the form of supportive therapy with a psychoeducational approach or cognitive-behavior therapy to attempt to change the underlying thought patterns leading to depressive affect.

Interventions for Hospitalized Clients

The major focus of treatment is to ensure that the client remains safe. It includes keeping the environment free of potentially harmful objects, frequently assessing suicidal thoughts and potential, and observing behavior. Monitoring and assessing the key symptoms, for example, mood, activity, sleep, appetite, and functional status, comprise part of the role. Use rating scales to document the severity of symptoms. Teach the individual about the importance of adequate sleep, hygiene, and regular activities, and encourage exercise and adequate nutrition.

Another major part of inpatient care is to advocate for a complete assessment of the client. Because medications and physical conditions can cause symptoms similar to depression, it is important to rule out an underlying organic cause. A complete assessment also should include information from significant others and careful observation of the individual's behavior. For instance, clients may not always openly discuss depressive feelings but may withdraw socially, stop eating, or appear anxious.

In the case of self-care deficits such as inadequate hygiene, reinforce the client's participation and decisions about the timing, sequence, and approach. Allow the client to perform as many tasks as possible. Because decreased energy and fatigue are common, expect that a client will take longer than usual to complete self-care. Encourage as much independence as possible, along with continued participation in activities, exercise, groups, individual psychotherapy, and compliance with medication, if prescribed.

Interventions for Clients in the Community

Untreated major depression takes a significant toll on clients and families. The ability to work and provide for a family may be severely compromised. Financial losses are common, and individuals may need long-term disability compensation. Clients with chronic depression often have difficulty initiating and completing their usual activities such as paying bills, buying groceries, and making meals. Depressed individuals may skip regular physical, dental, and gynecological exams. Clients who have children may neglect their needs. Families may take on the role of surrogate parent or caretaker in order to manage everyday life.

The nurse's role is to support the family throughout the process and to provide education about the illness and the need for ongoing treatment. Family members need to understand that depression is an illness, much like cardiac, pulmonary, and other chronic physical diseases. The nurse should stress that depression is also associated with risk of suicide. Discuss the medications used in the treatment of depression and their side effects. If severe family conflict is present, refer the family for couples or family therapy. The nurse plays a key role in the management of individuals with depressive symptoms that are long term and unresponsive to treatment and of clients with milder but chronic forms of depression (dysthymia). The former, labeled as "treatment-resistant depression," implies that despite adequate treatment, cognitive-behavior therapy, and several complete medication trials, the symptoms of major depression persist.

Living with depression is usually just as debilitating as surviving other major disorders, such as diabetes or cardiac disease. The major role for the nurse caring for these clients in the community is continuing to encourage them to obtain treatment, while simultaneously assisting them to maintain structure and functional ability in their lives. Monitor clients' symptoms and watch for the onset of suicidal tendencies.

Need for Treatment. Depressive symptoms may resolve partially or leave the individual with less severe chronic depression (dysthymia). Individuals with dysthymia can usually continue to function in their social and occupational roles and may not understand the full impact of depression on their lives. Because they have adjusted to the symptoms, clients may not seek treatment. The nurse should encourage individuals and their families to continue to receive psychiatric care, including psychotherapy and pharmacotherapy.

Support. Ongoing support and empathic understanding are a major nursing intervention for individuals with major depressive disorder living in the community. Clients frequently become hopeless and frustrated with their lack of improvement. Listen to their frustrations, and encourage them to continue treatment and take medications as prescribed. Like clients with severe medical disease, depressed clients find it difficult to engage in basic and necessary activities. Every movement or activity is an effort. Stress the need for regular sleep-wake cycles, and discourage daytime naps. If the sleep disturbance is severe, refer individuals for medication evaluation; sedative-hypnotic medications may be needed for insomnia. Support the use of a daily bedtime regimen and other healthy sleep interventions (see Chapter 25), and instruct clients to avoid caffeine or heavy meals prior to bedtime. Although individuals may have severe fatigue, encourage regular exercise. Exercise promotes physical health and may lead to some improvement in depressive symptoms. Assess and monitor clients' diets to ensure that they have adequate and balanced food intake. At times, nurses may accompany clients to the grocery store, help them make appointments, or lead an exercise group. These direct interventions help individuals initiate activity. Break down daily tasks into small steps so that clients can achieve some success. All of these nursing interventions should be balanced; encourage activity without forcing clients to complete these tasks. If the nurse takes an aggressive stance, clients may feel worse about themselves, further reducing

> ### DSM-IV Diagnostic Criteria for 300.4 Dysthymic Disorder
>
> A. Depressed mood for most of the day, for more days than not, as indicated either by subjective account or observation by others, for at least 2 years.
>   NOTE: In children and adolescents, mood can be irritable, and duration must be at least 1 year.
> B. Presence, while depressed, of two (or more) of the following:
>   (1) poor appetite or overeating
>   (2) insomnia or hypersomnia
>   (3) low energy or fatigue
>   (4) low self-esteem
>   (5) poor concentration or difficulty making decisions
>   (6) feelings of hopelessness.
> C. During the 2-year period (1 year for children or adolescents) of the disturbance, the person has never been without the symptoms in Criteria A and B for more than 2 months at a time.
> D. No Major Depressive Episode has been present during the first 2 years of the disturbance (1 year for children and adolescents); i.e., the disturbance is not better accounted for by chronic Major Depressive Disorder, or Major Depressive Disorder, In Partial Remission.
>   NOTE: There may have been a previous Major Depressive Episode provided there was a full remission (no significant signs or symptoms for 2 months) before development of the Dysthymic Disorder. In addition, after the initial 2 years (1 year in children or adolescents) of Dysthymic Disorder, there may be superimposed episodes of Major Depressive Disorder, in which case both diagnoses may be given when the criteria are met for a Major Depressive Episode.
> E. There has never been a Manic Episode, a Mixed Episode, or a Hypomanic Episode, and criteria have never been met for Cyclothymic Disorder.
> F. The disturbance does not occur exclusively during the course of a chronic Psychotic Disorder, such as Schizophrenia or Delusional Disorder.
> G. The symptoms are not due to the direct physiological effects of a substance (e.g., a drug of abuse, a medication) or a general medical condition (e.g., hypothyroidism).
> H. The symptoms cause clinically significant distress or impairment in social, occupational, or other important areas of functioning.
>
> Specify if:
>   Early Onset: if onset is before age 21 years
>   Late Onset: if onset is age 21 years or older
>
> Specify (for most recent 2 years of Dysthymic Disorder):
>   With Atypical Features
>
> **Source:** Reprinted with permission from the Diagnostic and Statistical Manual of Mental Disorders, Fourth Edition. Copyright 1994 American Psychiatric Association.

their self-esteem. Individuals should be gently encouraged, not chastised or pushed into doing what they see as impossible and formidable.

Maintaining Self-Esteem. One of the most profound effects of major depression is decreased self-esteem. Nursing interventions focus on enhancing self-esteem and promoting social interactions. With prolonged depression, client confidence is reduced. If individuals suffer from self-deprecating thoughts, refer them to a cognitive-behavior therapist. The goal of cognitive-behavior therapy is to reduce the distorted thoughts and enhance self-esteem. Writing in journals and other creative outlets, such as art, poetry, or dance, can engage clients in self-reflection to promote healthy self-esteem. Nursing interventions should also be aimed at helping people develop their social roles and support networks. Clients who are unable to work may be able to volunteer for several hours per week. Another alternative is to encourage individuals with depression to take a continuing-education class. Referral to group therapy may promote interpersonal connection and diminish social withdrawal.

Cognitive-Behavior Therapy

Both cognitive and behavior therapies center more on the here and now than on the past. Often the combination of these two therapies is most helpful in reversing the symptoms of depression. For example, a strategy might be to identify the distorted thoughts that prevent action and then develop behaviors to pursue goals. Although further research is necessary, cognitive-behavior therapy remains an effective treatment for depression; in some studies it has been found to be as effective as antidepressant therapy, although some controversy and mixed results exist.

Cognitive-behavior therapy focuses on developing adaptive actions by reinforcing constructive and positive ones. The process involves changing negative thinking to literally "restructure" thoughts. This is different from telling individuals to think positively. Through a series of techniques, clients directly confront "inappropriate views," thereby changing their behavior. If negative and maladaptive thoughts can be changed, so can the depressive behaviors. For instance, clients with depression may feel worthless and unable to work. The idea of working may be overwhelming and anxiety provoking (see Table 19–5). The cognitive-behavior therapist challenges the thoughts of worthlessness by pointing out examples of their strengths. If clients believe that no one will hire them because they are "worthless," the therapist will point out past successes such as running a profitable business and being the top salesperson in the company. A structured plan to begin a short volunteer job and progressive relaxation to manage the anxiety are behavioral measures to promote the return to work. It is the combination of changing the negative tone and "self-talk," along with following a behavior program with clearly defined short- and long-term goals that leads to change. Nursing interventions might include devising a regular schedule, so that each hour of the day is structured with eating, resting, sleeping, hygiene, and exercise. A short "to do list," specific and simple goals, and steps to achieve them are helpful.

Pharmacologic Treatments

Major Depression. Since their introduction in the 1950s, antidepressant medications have provided countless individuals with undeniable relief; however, some clients respond only partially, and antidepressants have limited ability to prevent recurrence. Despite drug studies demonstrating antidepressant efficacy in 65 to 80% of clients, the placebo response rate in some depression studies is as high as 40%, and even higher in studies of childhood depression (Figure 19–4 a and b). Side effects occur with all of these agents despite recent efforts to develop drugs with different or less bothersome side effects. Nonetheless, for the treatment of depression, antidepressants are clearly indicated, and most individuals respond favorably. Commonly used agents, dosages, and side effects are listed in Table 19–6.

Typically, neuropharmacologic theories of major depression have centered on a disruption in norepinephrine, serotonin, and perhaps dopamine. Although antidepressants may target certain neurotransmitters, the selection of a particular antidepressant has little direct connection to these chemicals. Medications that affect serotonin specifically are not more effective than other antidepressants. Of the major classes of antidepressants, the most common choices for treatment are the newer agents. These include the selective serotonin-reuptake inhibitors (SSRIs: fluoxetine [Prozac], sertraline [Zoloft], and paroxetine [Paxil]), bupropion (Wellbutrin), venlafaxine (Effexor), nefazodone (Serzone), and mirtazapine (Remeron). These agents have become the most common choices because they have few adverse side effects and are unlikely to be toxic in overdose (Figure 19–5). Each antidepressant has an equal chance of being effective; overall, about two-thirds of clients will respond positively. Very few predictors exist to guide medication selection. However, if an individual or a close relative has responded well to a particular medication in the past, that medication is more likely to be effective for the client.

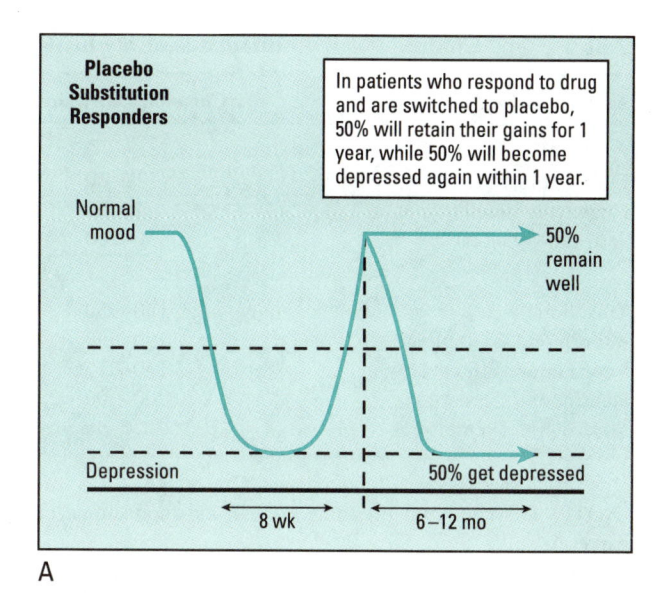

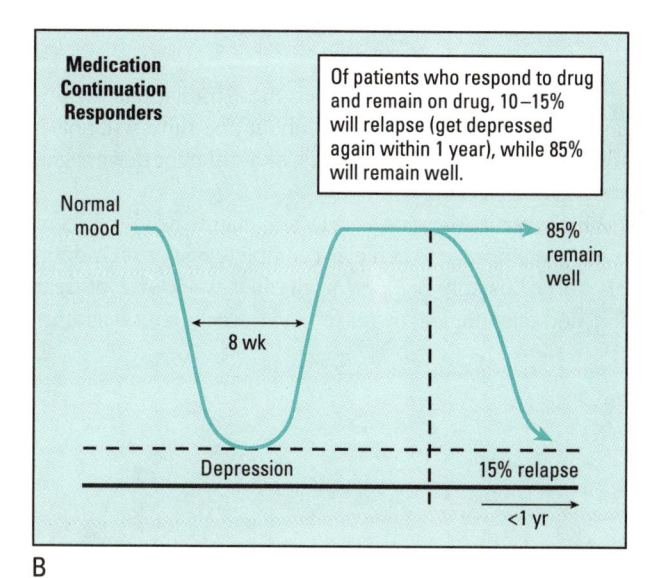

Figure 19–4. (A) Depressed patients who have an initial treatment response to an antidepressant will experience a recurrence at the rate of 50% within 6 to 12 months if their medication is withdrawn and a placebo substituted. (B) Depressed patients who have an initial treatment response to an antidepressant will experience a recurrence only at the rate of 10% to 15% if their medication is continued for a year following recovery. (From Stahl, SM: Essential Psychopharmacology. Cambridge University Press, New York, 1996, p 111.)

Although the newer agents are generally used as the first line of treatment of depression, two classes of medication introduced decades ago are also similarly effective for certain types of depression. They are the tricyclic antidepressants (TCAs) and monoamine oxidase inhibitors (MAOIs) (Figure 19–6). For severe depression or certain depressive subtypes, it is unclear which class of medications is most effective. Both the TCAs and MAOIs may be used for people with treatment-resistant depression who fail multiple medication tri-

TABLE 19–6. Common New Antidepressant Medications, Dosages, and Relative Side Effects

Antidepressant	Common Daily Dose	Anticholinergic	Agitation	Insomnia	Sedation	GI Distress
Selective Serotonin Reuptake Inhibitors						
Fluoxetine (Prozac)	10–80	*	***	***	**	***
Paroxetine (Paxil)	10–50	*	***	***	**	***
Sertraline (Zoloft)	50–200	*	***	***	**	***
Miscellaneous Newer Antidepressants						
Trazodone	150–450	*	**	*	****	*
Bupropion (Wellbutrin)	150–450	*	***	**	*	*
Venlafaxine (Effexor)	150–375	*	***	**	*	***
Nefazodone (Serzone)	200–500	*	*	*	***	***
Mirtazapine (Remeron)	20–35	*	*	*	****	*

* = very low, ** = low, *** = moderate, **** = high

NOTE: Tricyclic antidepressants (TCAs) and monoamine oxidase inhibitors (MAOIs) are used infrequently and are described in Chapter 6.

Source: Adapted from Teicher, MH, Glod, CA, and Cole, CA: Antidepressant drugs and suicidal tendencies. Drug Safety 8:186–212, 1993.

---

als, including the SSRIs. Whereas most individuals will respond to an antidepressant trial, about one-third will not. In those cases, the tricyclics, MAOIs, or a different newer agent may then be selected.

Whichever medication is selected, clients need to receive an adequate dosage to achieve a complete response. Individuals do not usually respond in the first week or 2 of treatment and may not feel better for 2 to 6 weeks after beginning

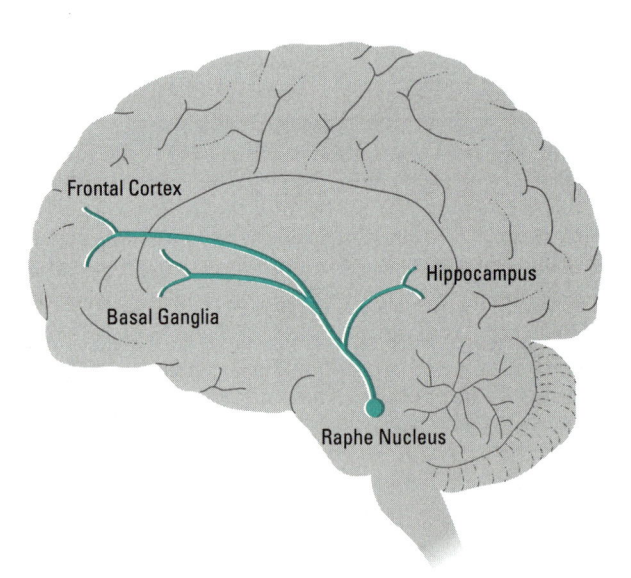

Figure 19–5. SSRIs have their therapeutic action in these key areas of the brain. The cell bodies are located in the raphe nucleus and SSRIs may affect all areas equally by modulating this single area. The antidepressant action of SSRIs is believed to be mediated by their effects on the frontal cortex, where they increase levels of serotonin. Similarly, increased serotonin in the basal ganglia accounts for its therapeutic efficacy in obsessive-compulsive disorder, while SSRIs play a role in panic disorder via their effects on the hippocampus. (Courtesy of Susan Andersen.)

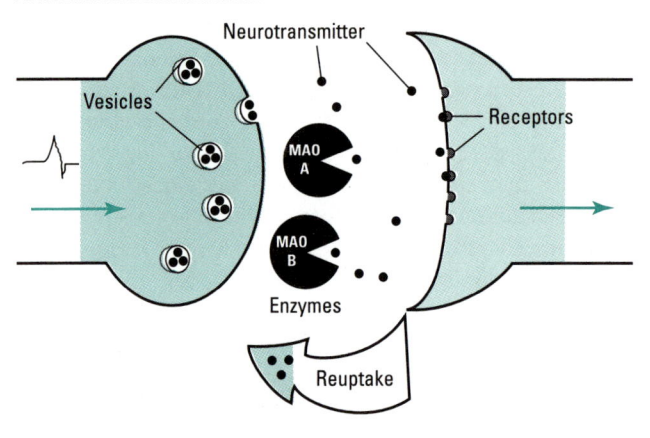

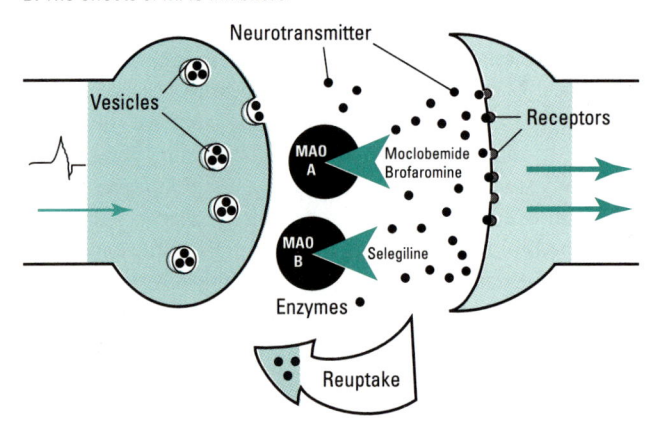

Figure 19–6. The effects of monoamine oxidase inhibitors (MAOIs) on neurotransmission. (A) Normal neurotransmission, with MAO-A and MAO-B partly responsible for keeping synaptic levels of the neurotransmitter low. Arrows indicate strength of neuronal response. (B) Acute treatment with MAOIs (moclobemide, brofaromine, selegiline) results in an increase in synaptic transmitter levels and increased overall response. (Courtesy of Susan Andersen.)

the medication trial. Therefore, it is essential to teach clients and families to wait, sometimes several weeks, to determine whether the medication will be effective. In this key period, noncompliance is likely.

There may be uncomfortable, embarrassing, or potentially dangerous side effects (see Chapter 6). The newer agents, such as fluoxetine or venlafaxine, may cause insomnia, daytime agitation or anxiety, sexual dysfunction (which may become a humiliating and disturbing effect), or occasionally a seizure. Nurses have a key role in monitoring and ensuring individuals achieve therapeutic benefit and experience minimal adverse effects, and in determining whether clients' behaviors are related to increasing depression or an adverse response to antidepressant treatment.

Major Depression with Psychotic Features. Clients suffering from major depression with psychotic features also benefit from pharmacotherapy. Although a small percentage of clients respond to antidepressant treatment alone, the majority require concomitant treatment with both an antidepressant and an antipsychotic agent.

Treatment-resistant Major Depression. For some clients, medication may have partial or no effect, despite several medication trials. Individuals who have received little benefit and remain depressed may need additional or alternative pharmacotherapies. Psychostimulants, such as pemoline (Cylert) or methylphenidate (Ritalin), may be used for these treatment-resistant clients. They are contraindicated in clients with both depression and substance abuse because of the risk of abuse and dependence. Of the psychostimulants, pemoline (Cylert) may be used first because of its lower potential for addiction.

Lithium carbonate, not generally used for treating depression, has shown some effectiveness as an antidepressant. Lithium is sometimes used as an augmentation strategy to boost the antidepressant into working. Either low or therapeutic doses, with therapeutic blood levels of 1.0 mEq/L are used. Lithium augmentation may not take effect for days or weeks. Similarly, adding thyroid hormone or coadministration of two antidepressants may be needed for treatment-resistant depression.

Nonpharmacologic Therapies

Phototherapy. Artificial bright light therapy, *phototherapy*, is used to treat a subtype of major depression, SAD. Several types of phototherapy units have been studied. The most effective are light boxes that deliver a crucial intensity of light, 10,000 lux. Individuals with SAD require about 45 to 60 minutes of daily light exposure during the winter to treat the depressive symptoms. They usually notice a response to phototherapy within a few days or 2 weeks of initiating treatment. Side effects include headache, eyestrain, agitation, and insomnia. Less commonly, phototherapy may be used to treat nonseasonal forms of major depression. Although its action is not well understood, light therapy is thought to work by resetting the body's internal clock to a more stable pattern.

THE CATECHOLAMINE THEORY OF DEPRESSION

Three major neurotransmitters have been implicated in the etiology of major depression: norepinephrine, serotonin, and, to a lesser extent, dopamine. The initial evidence providing a link between these "brain chemicals" and depression arose from research into the pharmacology of antidepressants and their effects. It was first observed that antidepressants blocked the reuptake of norepinephrine into the presynaptic neuron. Blocking reuptake results in increased norepinephrine. Depression, then, was hypothesized to be the result of a deficiency of norepinephrine, known as the "monoamine deficiency hypothesis."* This theory was later extended to include similar effects upon serotonin. The current view, however, is that this theory is oversimplistic and inconsistent with clinical pharmacologic effects. In the popular press, this relatively simple theory continues to be promoted (i.e., depression is due to decreased levels of serotonin or norepinephrine); however, in reality there are major limitations and refutations to this long-standing hypothesis. The major flaw in this theory is that increased levels of norepinephrine and serotonin occur acutely, within hours or days of medication administration. However, the therapeutic effects of antidepressants take weeks to be felt.

*Source: Schildkraut, J: The catecholamine hypothesis: A review of supporting evidence. An J Psychiatry 122:509, 1965.

Electroconvulsive Therapy. Electroconvulsive therapy (ECT) is another effective treatment for mania or depression if pharmacologic treatment fails or if the severity of symptoms demands rapid treatment.[6] It is usually reserved for clients with psychotic depression, treatment-resistant depression, or bipolar disorder, or for pregnant women with mood disorders. Although ECT has been criticized by some, it remains a safe and effective treatment with minimal side effects (memory loss, amnesia, headaches, and risks from anesthesia).

ECT is the induction of a grand mal seizure after the individual has received general anesthesia with partial neuromuscular blockade. Its mechanism of action is unknown. Usually insomnia and fatigue respond initially, followed by improvement in depressed mood and lack of pleasure. Eventually, symptoms of poor concentration, self-esteem, and suicidal ideation resolve. ECT is administered three times per week. The individual receives 6 to 20 treatments initially. Monthly maintenance treatment is less commonly used if symptoms persist. Because of past inhumane treatment with ECT, many individuals need reassurance and an accurate explanation of the process and its potential adverse effects. The major adverse reaction is memory loss. Temporary amnesia may last for the hours surrounding the actual treatment or for some events several months prior to or subsequent to treatment. Long-term pervasive memory loss is rare. Other side effects are minimal, such as heart rate changes, headache, and muscle pain (see Chapter 14).

Nurses have a major role in the care of the individual who receives ECT. Clients should have nothing to eat or drink for 8 hours prior to receiving the treatment. Repeated reminders and regular observation are necessary to prevent accidental fluid intake. Vital signs should be monitored every 15 to 30 minutes immediately after ECT, until they return to baseline. Ideally, medications should not be administered concurrently with ECT. TCAs and other antidepressants raise the seizure threshold, whereas anticonvulsants and benzodiazepines lower the seizure threshold.

Expected Outcomes

For the individual with major depression, improvement will be demonstrated by:
- Adequate sleep duration and continuity
- Adequate nutrition and normalization of weight
- Good concentration and decision making
- The ability to enjoy pleasurable activities
- Absence of suicidal feelings and thoughts
- Absence of depressed mood
- Realistic perception of self and positive self-esteem
- Normalization of physical activity
- An interest in life
- The ability to perform role functions
- An understanding of the nature of depressive disorder and the ability to recognize impending symptoms in the future.

CASE STUDY

Anna C is a 55-year-old woman, admitted to a general hospital for cataract surgery. Prior to admission, she was working as a sales clerk in a bakery. She had raised a family. After her children were grown, she and her husband began having marital difficulties. They separated 7 years ago, and Mrs. C continued her work and maintained her connection with her children.

Although her ophthalmologic surgery was successful, after about 1 week, Anna began complaining of feeling lethargic and not getting much accomplished. She was unable to return to work, despite her improved eyesight; no detectable physical difficulties were present. Food lost its appeal, and she started losing weight. At night she had tremendous difficulty falling asleep and would toss and turn for about 2 hours before falling asleep. She would then sleep only until the early morning and awaken at 4:00 or 5:00 am, unable to fall back to sleep. During the day she had little energy, so that even the simplest things were a chore. It was all she could do to take a shower, and she neglected to wear makeup or get dressed at times. Her contact with the world diminished, and she became more isolated and unproductive. She also stated that she had lost the will to live and felt at times that she would be better off dead.

After about 1 month, Anna met her surgeon for a follow-up appointment. She offered little information about her present state but asked if she could have a letter suggesting she not return to work and receive disability instead. Although she acknowledged that her eyesight had improved, she insisted that she could no longer work. It was then she revealed some of the problems she had functioning, along with her thoughts of death.

Mrs. C was then seen by her primary care nurse practitioner. In addition to her symptoms, she reported a past episode of depression 7 years before, which was treated successfully by doxepin (Sinequan), prescribed by her internist. Although she could not remember the details of the depression, she recalled some similar symptoms. Without consulting her health-care provider, she had decided to decrease and eventually discontinue the doxepin. She was medication-free at the time of assessment, except for eye drops. She denied any problems with alcohol or drugs.

After completing the assessment, the nurse practitioner was concerned about the client's potential for self-harm. She realized that Mrs. C had few supports available and began to devise strategies to help Mrs. C develop them. Some of these included contacting the local self-help association, arranging for her daughter to call frequently and visit, and scheduling phone appointments over the next week with the nurse practitioner. When the client's symptoms persisted at her next office visit 1 week later, she was referred for individual therapy. The therapist focused on her many losses, including her eyesight disability, ongoing separation, and issues of aging. Concurrently, the nurse practitioner began prescribing a new medication, nefazodone, to begin to resolve the client's symptoms. She chose this medication particularly for its sedating effect because Mrs. C complained of insomnia. After several weeks, some of her symptoms were better; she was sleeping and eating better, had more energy, and denied any thoughts of death or suicidal intent. However, because her mood remained somewhat depressed with poor concentration, a subsequent referral was made to a psychiatrist for consultation. With her therapist, she continued to address the issues that persisted and contributed in part to her ongoing depressed mood.

CRITICAL THINKING QUESTIONS

1. What behaviors does Anna manifest that are indicative of major depression?
2. What key characteristics would lead you to recommend hospitalization for this individual?
3. What major life issues might contribute to the development and continuation of depression?
4. Identify the key elements of education for this individual and her family.
5. What are possible long-term interventions to assist her in daily living and functioning?
6. Which theories best explain the behaviors presented?

BIPOLAR DISORDER

Life for the individual with **bipolar** disorder, or manic-depressive illness, is a struggle of ups and downs, mania and depression. This is the typical state of bipolar disorder, called *bipolar I disorder,* although several other types are now recognized. Clear, discrete periods of depression alternate with periods of mania. Mania is characterized by a whole host of symptoms, the most common being a high, elated, or euphoric mood, similar to the "high" experienced by taking illicit drugs. Individuals with mania generally live at an accelerated pace. They are very energetic, with many thoughts and active behaviors. In the depressed phase, the client displays the same behaviors as in major depression. However, certain symptoms may predominate, including hypersomnia, slowed psychomotor activity, and increased appetite. In between the episodes of mania and depression are times when the client is without symptoms or is euthymic, a period of usual or "normal" mood. The length and frequency of these cycles of mania, depression, and **euthymia** vary from individual to individual, yet may follow a characteristic pattern throughout life, for example, mania every summer, depression every winter. An example of how to think about these episodes is shown in Figure 19–7. Imagine the line is euthymia: normal mood and behavior states. A severe dip below this line indicates a depressive episode, which lasts for variable amounts of time. Similarly, the boxes above the line display manic episodes. This charting of episodes can reveal many aspects of the illness and its impact on the individual's ability to function.

Characteristic Behaviors

Mania may begin for no identifiable reason, although some individuals note the onset of symptoms after a major psychosocial stressor. Sometimes a major loss, such as the death of a parent, paradoxically precipitates a manic episode. Environmental factors can also precipitate an episode. Sleep deprivation and travel across time zones have been shown to lead to mania.

No definitive laboratory or physical findings are evident in bipolar disorder or specifically in the manic phase of this disorder. The early signs of mania in any individual are often missed because those with mania feel fine; in fact, they may feel great. People may fail to recognize that their extreme **euphoria** and impulsive and energetic behaviors may get them into trouble.

One young adult was picked up by a store security guard in the middle of the night for filling several shopping carts with excessive amounts of food in order to make his "concoction" for the community. Because he had very little money for this expensive endeavor, he tried to leave the store without paying by covering his cart with paper bags to hide the items. The client's lack of insight and poor judgment are characteristic of someone with mania. Extreme creativity or "off the wall" ideas can be another early clue.

Mania may progress through different stages. In the early stage, sometimes labeled **hypomania**, the symptoms are present to a lesser degree (*hypomania* means "under-mania") with the individual appearing extremely energetic and enthusiastic and more extroverted and assertive than usual. Early clues may be found in faster speech, the expression of creative and expansive ideas, and more productivity than usual. This stage is often a welcome relief from the depressive episode and may be mistaken for remission.

The primary symptom of mania is increased mood or euphoria. Although the individual may seem like the "life of the party," the elation may progress to many different shifts in mood, laughing one minute, crying the next, then angry and aggressive, all within a short span of time. In severe

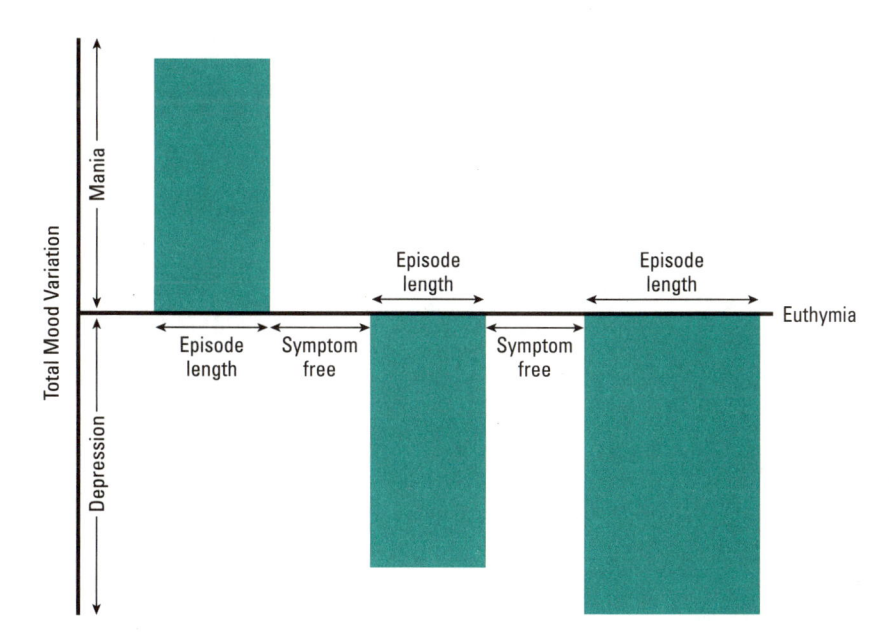

Figure 19–7. Episodes of mania and depression vary in length, intensity, and duration. This figure illustrates a client's mood cycles. The first episode, mania, is followed by euthymia, a period without symptoms. Next, the client experiences a depression, followed by euthymia, and then another more severe and longer episode of depression.

MOODSWING: THE UPS AND DOWNS OF BIPOLAR DISORDER

In the book *Moodswing*, Ronald Fieve, a psychiatrist, describes the periodic surges of depression and mania in his clients.

> Amy, a "Super Mom," has tremendous energy for managing her children, holding down a job, cleaning her house by 7 am, and sending her immaculate kids off to school. Yet there are times when she withdraws, gets physically ill and depressed, and ends up in the hospital.

Clients may describe their cycles and label the mood swings as depressive or manic. They are often aware that others do not understand their disorder, particularly because of the stigma associated with it.

> I believe that depression is terrifying; and elation—its nonidentical twin sister—is even more terrifying, attractive as she may be for the moment. But as she goes higher, mania is even more dangerous than the depths of the depression. However, I'm sure that the thing that is almost as much or more of a menace to the world today is the stupid, almost dogged ignorance of these illnesses; the vast lack of knowledge that they are able to be treated and the seeming ease of the cure, the simplicity of bringing them under control.

Mood swings have also plagued gifted, successful, and artistically oriented people such as Sylvia Plath, Handel, Howard Hughes, Abraham Lincoln, Vincent Van Gogh, and Ernest Hemingway. In fact, creativity may be linked to bipolar disorder. According to Fieve's historical review, Handel wrote the *Messiah* in 6 weeks and Van Gogh reported "furies of painting" when he was without sleep or food for days. Van Gogh's cycles of creativity and mania often led to profound episodes of depression; he would also have times of lucidity indicative of the well-known euthymic periods.

---

mania, or in a special classification called a *mixed state,* the mood may be **dysphoria**. This term refers to irritable and angry affect. Ronald Fieve describes this behavior in *Moodswings*.[14]

In addition to the mood disturbance, a manic episode is characterized by at least three additional symptoms, lasting for at least a week, including exaggerated self-esteem, decreased sleep, and increased speech, energy, and activity (see DSM IV "Criteria for Manic Episode"). These symptoms can be thought of as the opposite to those observed in depression. Individuals may have a string of ideas ("flight of ideas") or **racing thoughts**; each thought is pressured and followed by a whole series of other thoughts. Other manic symptoms include being easily distracted or getting involved in impulsive, potentially dangerous activities. For example, an individual who makes a modest income may spend tens of thousands of dollars on frivolous jewelry, gifts, travel, and gambling during a manic episode, only to be faced with substantial debt after the episode resolves. Another individual may have very high libido (sex drive) and engage in unprotected, cavalier sexual activity with multiple partners and then contract a devastating sexually transmitted disease. Other examples include the manic client who develops an outrageous business scheme or school project that is perceived by friends, superiors, and significant others as extremely unrealistic and nonsensical. These behaviors may also have profound effects on interpersonal relationships. The individual who engages in high-risk sexual behaviors or extreme spending sprees may alienate his or her current partner or loved ones, who now want nothing to do with the client. A manic individual can be extremely aggressive and have a high potential for impulsive, violent acts toward others in the community or hospital staff. Suicide is also a risk. Twenty-five percent of individuals with bipolar disorder who fail to receive treatment will attempt suicide, and 15% will succeed.[15]

Subtypes

Several subtypes of bipolar disorder have been identified (Table 19–7). The individual who cycles between manic, depressive, and euthymic symptoms at different points has bipolar I disorder. Bipolar II disorder is characterized by episodes of major depression that alternate with periods of hypomania and euthymia. To meet the criteria for hypomania, an individual may display the same behaviors as in mania, but to a lesser degree, and without any significant impairment in work, school, interpersonal, or daily functioning. *Cyclothymia,* another subtype of bipolar disorder, is characterized by episodes of hypomania that alternate with mild depressive times (similar to dysthymia) and euthymia. Adolescents may be prone to cyclothymia, and this condition has been associated with the later development of either bipolar I or II disorder. Another subtype, **rapid cycling** bipolar disorder, occurs when the individual suffers from four or more episodes of mania or depression each year, in any order or combination.[3] Rapid cycling may occur as the course of bipolar disorder progresses, leading to more frequent episodes and less interepisode remission. This is one of the most disturbing and disruptive forms of the illness because the client is faced with frequent life-interrupting episodes.

When the symptoms and behaviors overlap between depression and mania, a mixed state may be evident. This state can be very confusing and difficult to understand, for both the client and the nurse, because characteristics of both mania and depression are evident. Also called *dysphoric mania,* mixed states may be more common in adolescents and older adults. Typically the individual is agitated and suffers from insomnia, disturbed appetite, psychotic features, and suicidal ideation.[3] A depressive episode may mistakenly be diagnosed because dysphoric or rapidly shifting moods pre-

DSM-IV Criteria for Manic Episode

A. A distinct period of abnormally and persistently elevated, expansive, or irritable mood, lasting at least 1 week (or any duration if hospitalization is necessary).

B. During the period of mood disturbance, three (or more) of the following symptoms have persisted (four if the mood is only irritable) and have been present to a significant degree:
  (1) inflated self-esteem or grandiosity
  (2) decreased need for sleep (e.g., feels rested after only 3 hours of sleep)
  (3) more talkative than usual or pressured to keep talking
  (4) flight of ideas or subjective experience that thoughts are racing
  (5) distractibility (i.e., attention too easily drawn to unimportant or irrelevant external stimuli)
  (6) increase in goal-directed activity (either socially, at work or school, or sexually) or psychomotor agitation
  (7) excessive involvement in pleasurable activities that have a high potential for painful consequences (e.g., engaging in unrestrained buying sprees, sexual indiscretions, or foolish business investments).

C. The symptoms do not meet criteria for a Mixed Episode

D. The mood disturbance is sufficiently severe to cause marked impairment in occupational functioning or in usual social activities or relationships with others, or to necessitate hospitalization to prevent harm to self or others, or there are psychotic features.

E. The symptoms are not due to the direct physiological effects of a substance (e.g., a drug of abuse, a medication, or other treatment) or a general medical condition (e.g., hyperthyroidism).

NOTE: Manic-like episodes that are clearly caused by somatic antidepressant treatment (e.g., medication, electroconvulsive therapy, light therapy) should not count toward a diagnosis of Bipolar I Disorder.

Source: Reprinted with permission from the Diagnostic and Statistical Manual of Mental Disorders, Fourth Edition. Copyright 1994 American Psychiatric Association.

---

dominate. The characteristic symptoms of manic, depressive, and mixed states are listed in Table 19–8.

Culture, Age, and Gender Features

CULTURE

The prevalence and expression of bipolar disorder does not differ between racial or ethnic groups.[3]

AGE

Adolescents. Clients' development stage may affect how the beginning symptoms of bipolar disorder present. Mania is thought to be relatively rare in prepubertal children. Because of their characteristic moodiness and opposition, adolescents may be difficult to diagnose. If severe, symptoms of bipolar disorder may present as a developmental issue or difficulty with a major life or school transition, such as going off to college. Clues to identifying mania in adolescence are irritable mood or severe mood swings. Depressed adolescents with rapid symptom onset, psychomotor retardation and psychotic features, family history of bipolar disorder, and medication-induced hypomania are at high risk for the development of a manic episode. Thirty percent of individuals with bipolar disorder will begin to show symptoms prior to age 25.[15] Therefore, some adolescents experiencing frequent mood shifts or clear episodes of depression may be prone to developing bipolar disorder.

Elderly. At the other end of the age spectrum, bipolar disorder is often unrecognized in the elderly, despite evidence for the classic symptoms. In primary care settings, depression in older adults is beginning to be recognized more; however, the high energy, mood, and activity seen in mania can be missed. The presence of bipolar disorder raises the high risk of suicide in geriatric clients. In addition, older adults may first present with organic conditions, such as

TABLE 19–7. Characteristics of Bipolar Subtypes

Subtype	Mania	Depression	Hypomania	Dysthymia	Euthymia
Bipolar I	X	X			X
Bipolar II		X	X		X
Bipolar III (Cyclothymia)			X	X	X
Bipolar IV	X*	X			X

*Develops only during antidepressant therapy.

TABLE 19–8. Common Behaviors Evident in the Phases of Bipolar Disorder

Behavior	Mania	Depression	Mixed
Sleep	Decreased	Increased	Either increased or decreased
Appetite	Decreased	Increased	Either increased or decreased
Energy	Increased	Decreased	Either increased or decreased
Activity level	Increased	Decreased	Either increased or decreased
Predominant mood	Euphoric	Depressed	Irritable

dementia, that lead to bipolar symptoms. Twenty percent will have their first episode of the illness after age 50[15]; older adults may present with symptoms of mania despite having no previous history of psychiatric difficulties.

GENDER

Bipolar disorder affects men and women equally, although women may have depression as their first cycle of the illness. Women are more likely than men to be affected by rapid cycling bipolar disorder (see Research Note) and may be at higher risk for an episode of mania or depression after giving birth. Menses may precipitate or worsen an episode.

Etiology

Biological Theories

The leading theory of the pathogenesis of bipolar disorder is the **kindling** hypothesis, borrowed from theories about seizure disorders. Kindling, like the wood used to start and maintain a fire, refers to a process that begins and promotes mood episodes. As seen in Figure 19–8, very brief and minor symptoms start and then build upon each other over time. The client may have mild episodes of depression (dysthymia) or mania that fail to meet the full criteria, are brief, and resolve on their own. Repeated expression of these minor episodes leads to more frequent and severe symptoms that

RESEARCH NOTE

Leibenluft, E: Women with bipolar illness: Clinical and research issues. Am J Psychiatry 153:163–173, 1996.

Findings: Mood disorders such as major depression affect women more commonly than men; however, little is known about gender differences in bipolar illness. The author summarizes the literature on gender effects in the course of bipolar disorder and provides a framework that identifies treatment issues with bipolar women. The course of illness, bipolar subtypes, and effects of the female reproductive cycle and endocrine changes are addressed.

The findings indicate that women are more likely to develop rapid cycling bipolar disorder than men. They may also be at higher risk for experiencing depressive and mixed states rather than manic episodes. The review also suggests that women may be more likely than men to have their first episode of bipolar disorder in their late 40s (from 45 to 49 years). The author raises several possible explanations for these findings. First, the onset of puberty may be a factor in the greater prevalence of women with rapid cycling bipolar disorder. The onset of menses, with its concomitant hormone surges, may precipitate cycles of mania and depression. Second, bipolar disorder may be associated with the cyclic nature of the menstrual cycle. Symptoms of manic and depressive episodes may fluctuate at the same time as different menstrual phases; for instance, mania may occur during the follicular phase each month. Third, women with bipolar disorder are at high risk for postpartum episodes. Mania or depression (as part of bipolar disorder) is more common during the month following delivery than major depression or schizophrenia. Fourth, the course of bipolar disorder may be related to the administration of hormone replacement treatment for postmenopausal women or to hormones administered as birth control agents. Fifth, hypothyroidism is a risk factor for rapid cycling and may differentially affect women. Unfortunately, there is limited research to date to clearly support any definite theories about gender differences in bipolar disorder.

Application to Practice: Similar to major depression, women may be at higher risk for experiencing recurring episodes of depression as part of bipolar disorder. This implicates biological differences, particularly hormonal factors, in the etiology of mood disorders. Major life stressors such as puberty, pregnancy, and menopause may change women's biology and predispose them to developing bipolar disorder. Similarly, mild mood changes that occur naturally during the menstrual cycle may worsen and promote bipolar illness. These are potential risk factors that nurses should include in their health assessment. Furthermore, whereas antidepressants effectively treat depression, they are also known to precipitate manic symptoms. Antidepressants may be useful, but mania and, perhaps, rapid cycling episodes may occur in susceptible women. It is important to warn clients of the potential for antidepressants to induce mania and to carefully assess early manic symptoms.

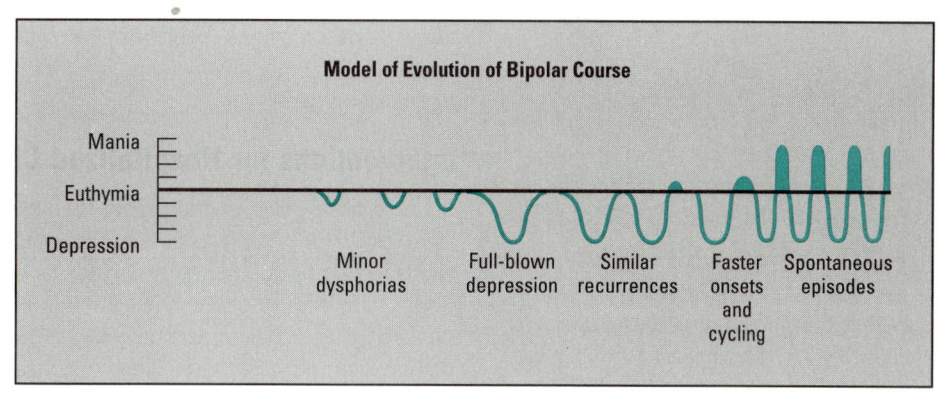

Figure 19–8. Illustrates the concept of kindling. Minor brief mood episodes, for example, of mild depression, become more severe and frequent. These states become "kindled" into major mood episodes of depression and mania. (From Post et al. Br J Psychiatry 149:191–201, 1986.)

finally culminate in a full-blown manic or depressive state. Left untreated, the episodes then continue, forming the basis for bipolar disorder. In the extreme, these states become so frequent and severe that an individual develops rapid cycling bipolar disorder (four or more episodes per year). Treatment is aimed at quelling these episodes; anticonvulsants reduce the kindling process, like throwing water on a fire.

Initial evidence from studies that examined neurotransmitters revealed higher norepinephrine levels during the manic phase of bipolar disorder. Other evidence suggests that the enzyme that degrades neurotransmitters, monoamine oxidase (MAO), is reduced in individuals with bipolar disorder and their relatives. Unfortunately, these studies have not been replicated. Neurotransmitters may also play an important role in the regulation of cortisol; as a result, the hypothalamic-pituitary-adrenal axis may be disrupted in bipolar disorder. Increased levels of cortisol, a hormone produced by this system, have been found, particularly during mixed or rapid cycling states. Increased levels of calcium have also been reported in individuals with bipolar disorder. Although these studies suggest that biology plays a role in the development of mania and depression, no clear-cut explanation has emerged.

Genetic Theories

Poor parenting or defenses against the development of depression were once thought to account for the expression of manic symptoms. Studies of the family transmission of bipolar disorder have since suggested a genetic contribution. First-degree relatives of individuals with bipolar disorder (children, parents, siblings) are about 24 times more likely to develop this condition than others. However, because the environment, including parenting style, culture, and viruses, may have an effect, genetics is only one factor.

Twin studies provide a more convincing basis for establishing the role of heredity. If one identical twin has bipolar disorder, the other has a 69% chance of developing it; in nonidentical twins, the risk is reduced to 19% if one twin is affected.

Complex techniques, such as segregation and linkage analysis, are used to determine how bipolar disorder is inherited and where the "bipolar disorder" chromosome is located on the gene. Although it has been reported that bipolar disorder was found on two chromosomes, chromosome 11 and the long arm of the X chromosome, no definitive results have been replicated. The current view is that manic-depressive illness may affect different genes in different people yet result in a similar clinical picture.

Circadian and Other Rhythm Theories

Circadian rhythm theories suggest that bipolar disorder, like major depression, may result from the system being "less circadian" or out of sync. In addition, bipolar disorder may arise from other disturbances in the body's internal clock. This clock, located in the suprachiasmatic nucleus of the brain, helps regulate various physical and psychological functions such as sleep, activity, and hormones. The internal clock may be running faster than 24 hours in individuals with bipolar disorder. In the "free-running" hypothesis, the circadian rhythms fail to follow a 24-hour pattern or a normal schedule; disturbances in mood, sleep, and activity then result.

The phases of bipolar disorder may also follow a seasonal pattern or recur every several years. Over a century ago, Esquirol and Pinel[10] stated, "maniacal paroxysms . . . generally begin after the summer solstice . . . are continued . . . during the heat of the summer, and commonly terminate toward the end of autumn." This illustrates a pattern lasting longer than a 24-hour or circadian cycle. Clients with the rapid cycling subtype may have moods that follow a certain pattern, for instance, depressive symptoms for several weeks followed by manic symptoms for several weeks.

Prognosis

The prognosis for bipolar disorder is variable. With the introduction of lithium carbonate and other mood stabilizers, many individuals suffer less frequent, less severe episodes of mania and depression. Medications increase periods of euthymia between cycles, although euthymic periods tend to decrease with age.

> I didn't really like the idea of taking medication to "control" my moods. I thought that I might end up feeling dull or "out of it." Instead, it stabilized my moods and kept me from plunging into the depths of depression and soaring into the highs of mania. I've been able to finish school, get engaged, and pursue my interests.

Despite adequate treatment, some clients will have milder or "breakthrough" symptoms. For some, living with bipolar disorder is like living with recurrent episodes of cancer: times of remission alternate with unpredictable symptoms that appear without any clear precipitant. Living with bipolar disorder is similar to riding a roller coaster.

> I can't remember which came first—stopping the Depakote or getting manic. It wasn't the first time this had happened, though. Once I restarted the medication, the mania was controlled, but then I got really depressed. I continued to take the Depakote, but it didn't make any difference. I had to take Prozac for the severe depression, and soon after that I got high again. It seems like I'm on a perpetual cycle sometimes.

Some clients with bipolar disorder achieve remission more rapidly than others. For those who do not, the unpredictable nature of manic and depressive episodes affects their personal, occupational, social, parental, and marital roles and responsibilities. Families and friends frequently do not understand their quick and intense mood shifts. Individuals in the depressed phase of bipolar disorder withdraw from personal and occupational responsibilities. Individuals may get fired for their extreme manic behaviors. Clients with children may demonstrate significant deficits in parenting. Child abuse or neglect is possible. In an attempt to medicate their symptoms, clients may abuse alcohol or illicit drugs.

Planning Care

Nursing care plans must consider clients' developmental stage and level of acceptance of the disorder. Because euphoria associated with mania can be so invigorating and a considerable relief from past depressive states, individuals have difficulty acknowledging their illness. As a result, clients are sometimes resistant to treatment and initially not active participants in planning their care. In extreme states of mania, individuals may need to be committed to an inpatient facility to protect them from harm. Dangerous and assaultive behavior may be a consequence of manic overactivity and excitement. An individualized plan of care should foresee and anticipate the impulsive and unpredictable nature of clients' behavior. Essential elements of the plan include family involvement, obtaining past records, and maintaining safety.

Interventions for Hospitalized Clients

Because manic clients often deny their illness and lack insight into the consequences of their behavior, the nurse needs to point out potentially dangerous behavior to clients. Room schedules or quiet rooms are often necessary for hospitalized clients. These measures are used to decrease stimulation from the environment that may lead to more activity and distractibility. Individuals who are manic need to be observed frequently. Their behavior should be redirected into nondangerous activities. For individuals who run up excessive phone charges and are prone to impulsive shopping sprees, a possible strategy is to have clients relinquish credit cards and limit phone time. This can be accomplished earlier in treatment, when clients can understand that excessive spending is potentially dangerous.

Because the individual with mania lacks the internal controls to limit impulsive and potentially dangerous behavior, it is important to set limits. Use a firm voice to help contain the client's behavior with clear, repeated statements of your expectations. Avoid confrontational statements because they can be inflammatory. When possible, let the client know a given behavior is dangerous and that his or her energy and activity are excessive. Use simple statements with few words because this client is easily distracted.

The individual in a manic state is highly energized, and therefore interventions may be ignored or easily forgotten. Because the manic client may become verbally or physically aggressive when challenged, it is important to keep a safe distance and anticipate impulsive violent acts. Similarly, with the frequent mood shifts and periods of dysphoria, suicidal acts are possible. A careful assessment and ongoing monitoring of suicidal impulses are essential to the treatment plan. Regular activity and a ward schedule are important ways to direct the excessive energy in hospitalized clients. Consistent sleep-wake schedules and adequate sleep duration are important.

Interventions for Clients in the Community

The nurse's chief role is educating clients about the impending signs and symptoms of depression and mania and the need for medication to treat these symptoms. Anticipating shifts in mood and behavior and recognizing impending signs of mania or depression are difficult. For some clients, euphoric moods are difficult to distinguish from "feeling well" or euthymia. The nurse should understand that individuals with bipolar disorder sometimes resist treatment. Because they fear a loss of productivity, feeling dull, or decreased creativity, they may also not want to accept the long-term, recurring nature of the illness. Clients with bipolar disorder "miss" their "highs" and may discontinue their medication.

Compliance. Monitoring compliance is essential for maintaining remission. A study that reviewed the consequences of lithium discontinuation reported that 50% of remitted clients relapsed within 6 months of stopping the medication, with the development of mania more likely than depression.[15] Nurses should ensure that clients obtain regular lithium blood levels. Suggest that levels of mood stabilizers be checked during periods of stress or beginning symptoms. Encourage family or significant others to become involved in the treatment. It is also essential to observe adverse effects to maintain compliance. Stress the importance of medication in controlling symptoms, and suggest ways to manage uncomfortable reactions that interfere with clients' quality of life. Like other pharmacologic treatments, the nurse can suggest medication adjustment, such as changing the timing of the dose. For instance, if medication doses are skipped, propose that all medication be taken at bedtime. Refer the client for psychopharmacologic evaluation if adverse effects are intolerable; alternative pharmacotherapy may enhance compliance. Because medication is a key part of the overall treatment plan, stress that maintenance treatment prevents future episodes.

Family System. Because the key feature is cycling moods, living with bipolar disorder is filled with ups and downs. When individuals are manic, excessive involvement in pleasurable activities can lead to dangerous consequences. Individuals and families may be faced with excessive spending, enormous debt, or potential bankruptcy. Spouses may be confronted with extramarital affairs or a partner who contracted a sexually transmitted disease during a manic episode. Grandiose or bizarre business schemes may lead to unemployment and loss of the their professional reputation. When clients are manic, these extreme behaviors become intolerable, and relationships undergo severe stress. Impulsive and potentially dangerous behaviors have a profound effect on the family that can lead to marital problems or divorce. Clients' loss of control may send the entire family system out of control. Nurses can help families and significant others identify and understand these behaviors. Stress that manic or depressive behaviors are symptoms of an illness. To help them live successfully with bipolar disorder, families should be told that treatment usually controls intense moods and unpredictable behaviors. It is important that families be active participants in long-term treatment planning. They can provide early clues to impending mood switches and can notify the nurse that intervention may be necessary.

Genetic Risk. Because bipolar disorder is inherited, couples may need counseling to make decisions about having children. If the couple decides to have children, the nurse should refer them for expert medication evaluation. A woman's decision to remain on medication during pregnancy is complicated. Manic or depressive states are asso-

---

RESEARCH NOTE

Pollack, LE: Striving for stability with bipolar disorder despite barriers. Arch Psychiatr Nurs 9:122–129, 1995.

Findings: The researcher conducted in-depth interviews with 33 clients with bipolar disorder to determine how they lived with and managed their illness. *Grounded theory,* a qualitative method of research, was used to elicit clients' perceptions, enabling development of a theoretical model of living with bipolar disorder. The author found that the processes of seeking information and self-management to control symptoms and achieve stability continue throughout the course of bipolar disorder. Subjects in this study described several barriers to managing their illness. The most important barrier identified was denial. The clients described denying the initial diagnosis of bipolar disorder, as well as denying the need for medication treatment once remission occurred. The process of denial emerged as a major factor in relapse, rehospitalization, and suicide.

The author also found that clients with bipolar disorder pass through several phases of information seeking and self-management. Initially, clients identify a need for information before pursuing information about bipolar disorder. Once identified, data about the disorder are sought, depending on the individual's level of motivation, desire for stability, concerns about family, and the severity of and pain associated with the illness. At this stage, the client is committed to obtaining information about bipolar disorder. The research suggests that clients then face a "critical juncture in treatment." Several factors interact that allow individuals to manage their illness successfully: Clients identified adequate energy, stability, motivation, support, and access to health-care resources. Self-management was impeded by lack of information, suitable living environments, persistence, cooperation, reliance on others, and compliance with medication.

Application to Practice: This is one of the first studies to document bipolar clients' perceptions of their illness. Seeking information and self-management skills continuously evolved with other factors to either enhance or impede their stability. Nurses can use this knowledge in several ways. When providing education about bipolar disorder, clients may first need to realize that the information is important. After the need is identified, clients may better understand and integrate knowledge. When clients do seek information, this is probably a crucial stage in helping them manage their illness. Nursing interventions should include helping clients access health-care resources, develop adequate support systems, and find suitable living arrangements. Monitoring compliance with medication and encouraging clients to see the consequences of their behavior are other components of successful treatment.

ciated with self-care deficits that may lead to inadequate nutrition and poor fetal development. Then again, little is known about the effects of medication on the developing fetus. The decision to continue medication during pregnancy is based on carefully weighing the advantages of treatment (absence of mania or depression) with the risks of medication (tetratogenic effects). Some couples will choose not to have children because of the risks involved with pharmacotherapy or reemergence of symptoms. Others will decide against having children because of the genetic risk.

Support. For some individuals with bipolar disorder, episodes of mania and depression may become more frequent and severe, with fewer periods of euthymia. Provide support to clients and their families, and refer clients for intensive day treatment if possible. Assess whether rapid cycling bipolar disorder is beginning; ask about suicidal thoughts, and support clients toward meeting small short-term goals such as attending a class or a volunteer job.

Pharmacologic Treatments

Mood Stabilizers. Similar to their use in major depression, antidepressants are indicated for the depressed phase of bipolar disorder. Doses and side effects are similar. However, because mania is a side effect of antidepressant treatment, clients are also maintained on therapeutic levels of a mood stabilizer concurrently.

Lithium Carbonate. The advent of lithium treatment for the prevention and acute treatment of mania marked a major shift in the successful treatment of bipolar disorder. Until lithium's effectiveness was established, antipsychotic medications were the primary medications used. The two major indications for lithium are acute resolution of manic symptoms and prophylaxis (preventive treatment). Lithium effectively quells mania in most individuals; however, the positive effects may not be evident for 1 to 2 weeks. Therefore, until lithium takes effect, short-term use of high-potency benzodiazepines or low-dose antipsychotics is often necessary. For the control of bipolar disorder, lithium decreases both the frequency and duration of cycles of mania and depression.

How lithium works to reduce mania or prevent future mood episodes is poorly understood. Unlike most psychotropic medications that produce effects within neuronal synapses, lithium produces its effects intracellularly, affecting certain enzyme subsystems such as cyclic adenosine monophosphates (cAMP) and phosphatidylinositol biphosphate (PIP_2). These processes in turn alter calcium-mediated intracellular functions to release calcium, affecting many other cellular processes.

For lithium to be effective for bipolar disorder, adequate blood levels are essential. A level of 0.8 to 1.2 mEq/L, measured 12 hours after the last dose, is indicated. Doses then vary from about 600 to 2400 mg or more daily, in order to achieve appropriate levels (Table 19–9). Side effects generally increase with higher doses. Missed doses or noncompliance leads to a rapid decline in therapeutic blood levels

TABLE 19–9. Mood Stabilizers Used in the Treatment of Bipolar Disorder

Mood Stabilizer	Common Daily Dose (mg)
Lithium Carbonate (Eskalith, Lithobid)	600–2400
Carbamazepine (Tegretol)	400–1500
Valproic Acid (Depakote, Depakene)	750–2000
Medications under Investigation	
Clonazepam (Klonopin)	0.5–10
Verapamil (Isoptin)	120–480
Diltiazem (Cardizem)	30–120
Nifedipine (Procardia)	30–120
Lamotrigine (Lamictal)	not established

*Available in capsule, pill, liquid, and sustained-release preparations.

and the potential for rapid emergence of symptoms. The psychiatric nurse has a key role in monitoring compliance and educating clients about the need to continue taking medication. The nurse can recommend taking the dose once daily to help minimize "forgotten" doses. Despite these interventions, some individuals miss their "highs" without realizing the consequences of discontinuing the medication. Side effects, such as mental sluggishness and mood flattening, lead clients to stop or skip their medication.

Although lithium is a major treatment for bipolar disorder, 30 to 50% of people who take it continue to have episodes, receive only partial relief, or cannot tolerate its side effects. In addition, some subtypes such as rapid cycling or mixed states of bipolar disorder are unresponsive to lithium's effects.

Anticonvulsants. Two anticonvulsants are effective for the treatment of bipolar disorder: carbamazepine (Tegretol) and valproic acid (Depakene), also called divalproex (Depakote). They are used to treat acute mania and to prevent future manic and depressive episodes. Their major pharmacologic effects occur by reversing the process of kindling. They act on certain brain areas, such as the temporal lobe, to decrease the frequency and severity of mania and depression. As illustrated in Figure 19–1, the anticonvulsants block the development of bipolar disorder by reducing the process of kindling. These agents block the development of mood episodes like throwing water on a fire. The result is a reduction in the severity and frequency of mania and depressive states.

Clients with certain conditions and subtypes of bipolar disorder respond better to anticonvulsants (see Table 19–10). Carbamazepine and valproic acid are the first choice for individuals with more severe mania, rapid cycling, or mixed states of bipolar disorder. Dosages of each vary according to treatment response, and typical doses are listed in Table 19–9. Although anticonvulsant levels are obtained, there is no direct relationship between therapeutic blood levels and therapeutic effectiveness. After the first several weeks of treatment with carbamazepine, blood levels drop because

TABLE 19–10. Indications for Anticonvulsants as Initial Medication Treatment in Bipolar Disorder

- Lithium unresponsiveness
- Lithium intolerance
- Rapid cycling bipolar disorder
- Dysphoric or mixed states of mania
- Bipolar disorder with psychotic features
- Possible organic basis
- Concurrent alcohol or substance abuse
- Several previous unmedicated episodes
- Client preference

---

the medication metabolizes. Breakthrough symptoms are common at this time. Carbamazepine doses may need to be adjusted to continue the therapeutic response. Higher dosages are necessary to achieve the same effect.

The combination of carbamazepine and valproic acid is used in treatment-resistant cases; if they are ineffective alone, they may be used in combination with lithium to treat bipolar disorders. Recent studies of lamotrigine (Lamictal), another anticonvulsant, suggest some efficacy, although further study is necessary.

Benzodiazepines. Benzodiazepines are given in the treatment of bipolar disorder during the acute phase of mania, while awaiting the effects of lithium or another mood stabilizer. The most common medications are lorazepam (Ativan), used in doses of 1 to 4 mg, and clonazepam (Klonopin), in doses of 1 to 6 mg daily. Clonazepam has a sedating effect, allowing clients more control over their behavior. Studies are underway to determine whether clonazepam is effective in the prevention of future manic and depressive episodes. One recent study found that the combination of lithium plus clonazepam was as effective as lithium and haloperidol, yet no evidence has emerged that either is as effective as other mood stabilizers when used alone.[16] The mechanism of action of benzodiazepines is poorly understood.

Calcium Channel Blockers. Calcium channel blockers may be prescribed for individuals with mania who cannot tolerate lithium or anticonvulsants, are brain damaged, or are pregnant. Little information is available about their use in preventing future episodes of mania or depression, and further studies are needed. Their mechanism of action in bipolar disorder is not known. Verapamil and nifedipine are examples of calcium channel blockers used for treatment-resistant mania. Their investigational doses are listed in Table 19–9.

Antipsychotics. Antipsychotic medications such as haloperidol are usually used either for extreme cases of acute mania or when psychotic symptoms such as hallucinations and grandiose delusions predominate. They are often necessary while awaiting the effects of the mood stabilizer. Antipsychotics are usually used acutely, until the mood stabilizer takes effect, because of the risk of tardive dyskinesia and other side effects.

Client and Family Education

Teaching

Teaching interventions can enhance understanding about the illness, its etiology, and ways to recognize the onset of symptoms. Stress that major depression exacts a greater toll than most physical illnesses on functioning and work productivity. Reinforce the teaching with written information. Books the layperson can read to learn about mood disorders are listed in Box 19–3.

Discuss the medications used in the treatment of mood disorders and their common and potentially dangerous side effects. Because of the prolonged onset of action of antidepressant medications, it may take 4 to 6 weeks for the depressive symptoms to resolve. Careful planning is needed to ensure that the individual remains on the medication. Families and significant others should also be included in the teaching plan. Use the clinical management tips to educate them.

For the client with bipolar disorder, education can focus on the destructive consequences of mania. This may be hard to convey when the individual is actively manic. A client is more receptive to understanding the consequences of unhealthy behaviors when he or she is hypomanic or euthymic. Nursing interventions for clients with bipolar disorder often focus on living with the episodic nature of the illness and adjusting to its impact on daily functioning and goals. Many fear recurrence. Others may express anger at family for "transmitting" the disorder. Because of the genetic association, many are concerned about the decision to have children or the development of bipolar disorder in relatives.

Counseling

Documenting episodes of moods can help clients to anticipate and determine the frequency of either mania or depression. To prevent dangerous consequences, counsel individuals and their families to recognize the beginning symptoms of mania. Certain precipitants can be identified by clients, such as decrease in sleep, medical illness (Table 19–11), and psychosocial stressors. One client in college was encouraged by roommates to stay up late, despite his early

---

Box 19–3. Books for Client and Family Education

Darkness Visible by William Styron
The Good News about Depression by Mark Gold, MD
Feeling Good by David Burns, MD
Winter Blues by Norman Rosenthal, MD
Listening to Prozac by Peter Kramer, MD
Moodswing by Ronald Fieve, MD
An Unquiet Mind by Kay Redfield Jamison, PhD

morning classes. He was able to determine that reduced sleep led to symptoms of mania. Eventually, with help, he was able to request a single room to ensure he would obtain adequate sleep. Other important behavioral suggestions include maintaining a regular schedule, including sleep-wake and rest-activity, and avoiding overactivity or underactivity. Referral to a self-help group, the Manic Depressive–Depressive Association (MDDA), is also helpful.

Expected Outcomes

For the individual with acute mania, improvement will be demonstrated by:
- Adequate sleep duration and continuity
- Adequate nutrition and diet
- Good concentration without distractibility
- Involvement in activities to a natural (nonexcessive) degree
- Absence of suicidal feelings and thoughts
- Absence of manic or dysphoric mood
- Realistic perception of self and positive self-esteem
- Normalization of physical activity
- Absence of participation in activities that lead to dangerous consequences
- The ability to perform role functions
- An understanding of the nature of manic disorder and the ability to recognize impending mood switches.

CASE STUDY

Jim D is an 18-year-old college freshman who planned to major in biology and apply to medical school. In high school he was an outstanding athlete and an A student, whom people described as the "life of the party." He had many friends and worked part-time in a video store. Because of his outstanding academic performance, extroverted personality, and creativity, Jim and his family had high hopes for his success. He was accepted to a prestigious college away from home. At college, Jim would stay up very late or not sleep at all, and then attend early morning classes. Afterwards, he would go running, work out, and party late into the night. Initially, he did well in classes and wrote creative papers; however, his grades began to slip. He began developing bizarre, grandiose business schemes. He would approach strangers to tell them about how his ideas would make them millions. He would also call friends in the middle of the night to tell them about his plans. Other students commented on his excessive ideas and energy.

Jim eventually began to fail his courses and blamed his professors for their inability to recognize his special talents. In an attempt to sleep, he would drink several beers each night, yet obtain little sleep. He also became involved with several different women and engaged in casual and unprotected intercourse. His friends, who previously enjoyed his humor and activities, were growing tired of his endless ideas, excessive talking, and irritability. Jim began to blame his friends for their "seriousness" and

Resources for Clients, Families, and Nurses

Information	Contact
Centers specializing in treatment of depressive disorders	National Foundation for Depressive Illness Box 2257, New York, NY 10116 (212) 268-4260 www.depression.org
Referral to private practitioners	National Mental Health Association 1021 Prince St., Alexandria, VA 22314-2971 (800) 969-6642 www.nmha.org
General assistance to clients with depressive disorders	National Depressive and Manic Depressive Assn. 730 N. Franklin, Suite 501 Chicago, IL 60610 (312) 642-0049
Information on a range of mental illnesses	National Alliance for the Mentally Ill 200 N. Glebe Rd., Suite 1015 Arlington, VA 22203 (800) 950-6264 www.nami.org
Information about national educational programs	Depression/Awareness, Recognition, and Treatment (D/ART) National Institute of Mental Health Room 7C-02, 5600 Fisher Lane Rockville, MD 20857 (301) 443-4513 www.nimh.nih.gov

became annoyed with them. Concerned about his behavior, they suggested he go to the college counseling service, but he refused. Finally, his advisor insisted he obtain an evaluation because he had failed all courses and was in danger of being dismissed from the school.

Jim continued to refuse help. He believed he was the "Messiah" and could perform miracles. He stopped sleeping, eating, and bathing. When his advisor told him he needed a leave of absence, Jim became angry and shouted, "You're just jealous of my powers." Afraid for his safety, his advisor called campus security. Jim was taken to an emergency room for evaluation. While there, he began running into other clients' rooms. When a nurse attempted to redirect him and offer medication, he threatened to punch her. He was then placed into four-point restraints and given haloperidol intramuscularly. For the next hour, Jim talked rapidly and incessantly and proclaimed his special powers.

After he calmed down somewhat, Jim was told that he needed psychiatric hospitalization. He refused to admit himself voluntarily because he needed to "complete God's mission." The psychiatric clinical nurse specialist committed him to the hospital because of his poor control, inability to care for himself, and potentially dangerous behavior. On the inpatient unit, Jim walked into other clients' rooms and talked about being sent by God. He was started on lithium carbonate and haloperidol. After a few days, Jim remained energetic, with racing thoughts, pressured speech, and grandiose ideas. However, he began sleeping 6 hours each night and no longer believed he was sent by God.

His parents arrived after several days. In a family meeting with the primary nurse, psychiatrist, and social worker, they were told that Jim suffered from bipolar disorder that required pharmacotherapy. His parents were shocked by their son's behavior and concerned about how they would convince Jim that he needed medication. They also disclosed that Jim's maternal grandfather displayed similar "eccentric" behaviors. When his mother asked how long Jim needed treatment, the psychiatrist told them it would be "for the rest of his life." His parents were very concerned about Jim's future plans. Together they discussed a discharge plan: He would return home until his symptoms remitted completely, take a leave of absence from school, and try to return to college in several months.

CRITICAL THINKING QUESTIONS

1. What behaviors does Jim display that indicate the manic phase of bipolar disorder?
2. Which of these behaviors can be classified as potentially dangerous?
3. What precipitants, if any, were present?
4. What impact do these behaviors have on Jim's present functioning and future plans?
5. Suggest possible interventions that may be necessary to help this individual.
6. Which communication strategies would be best?
7. How would acute medication treatment differ from chronic treatment?
8. What interventions would help Jim accept his illness and treatment?
9. How would you counsel his family about his occupational and social potential?
10. What factors might contribute to long-term medication compliance?

TABLE 19–11. Organic Conditions That May Present as Major Depression

- Hypokalemia
- Hypercalcemia
- Reserpine-induced reactions
- Steroid psychosis
- Hypothyroidism
- Organic brain syndromes
- Hepatitis
- Cirrhosis
- Infectious mononucleosis
- Postviral infection syndrome
- Cessation of amphetamine or cocaine use
- Carcinoma of the pancreas
- Degenerative diseases of the central nervous system

DIFFERENTIAL DIAGNOSIS[3]

Medical Disorders

- Medications or physical conditions may precipitate mood disorders.
- Symptoms are similar to mood disorders but are excluded from the diagnosis.
- Medical and pharmacologic conditions are considered before making the diagnosis of a mood disorder (see Table 19–12).

Dysthymia

- Depressed mood is present more days than not for at least 2 years (versus daily for 2 weeks in major depression).
- Dysthymia requires the presence of only two (versus four in major depression) additional depressive symptoms, such as increased or decreased appetite, sleep disruption, low energy, poor self-esteem, poor concentration, indecision, or hopelessness.
- It has a slower, more chronic course.
- Symptoms do not remit for more than 2 months.
- Inadequacy or lack of productivity predominates.
- Can co-occur with major depression.

TABLE 19–12. Medical and Pharmacologic Differentials for the Diagnosis of Mania

Medical	Pharmacologic
• Multiple sclerosis	• Antidepressants
• Huntington's disease	• Steroids
• Stroke	• Levodopa
• Head trauma	• Cocaine
• Viral encephalitis	• Phencyclidine (PCP)
• CNS tumor	
• AIDS	
• Hyperthyroidism	

Depressive Disorder Not Otherwise Specified (NOS)

- Adjustment disorders with depressed mood are the most common (see Chapter 26).
- It is often brought on by a specific type of event or stressor such as leaving home, getting married, unemployment, retirement, or breaking up an important romantic or marital relationship.
- Symptoms develop within 3 months of the identified stressor.
- Other examples include a period of regular and severe depressive symptoms that occur premenstrually, episodes involving the five symptoms of depression but lasting for only several days, or episodes that last for 2 weeks but do not include five symptoms.

Psychotic Disorders

- Schizophrenia and other psychotic disorders are commonly misdiagnosed.
- Psychotic symptoms, such as hallucinations, delusions, and paranoia, occur with both mood disorders and schizophrenia and do not differentiate the two illnesses.
- Mood symptoms predominate regardless of psychotic symptoms during the mood disorder. For instance, clients display depressed mood during major depression or euphoria during the manic phase of bipolar disorder.
- Schizophrenia, schizoaffective disorder, and delusional disorder are all characterized by distinct periods of psychotic symptoms that present without prominent mood symptoms.

Alcohol and Substance Abuse and Dependence

- Alcohol or illicit drugs may lead to symptoms of a mood disorder or coexist.
- Alcohol has depressant effects, may lead to abuse and dependence, and complicates treatment (see Chapter 17).
- Marijuana, cocaine, and other substance abuse may precipitate or accompany the presentation of depression or mania.
- Denial of a coexisting abuse or dependence disorder is likely.

Anxiety Disorders

- Mood disorders, particularly major depression, often exist with anxiety disorders.
- Common comorbid anxiety conditions include generalized anxiety, panic disorder, social phobia, PTSD, or obsessive-compulsive disorder.

Personality Disorders

- Personality disorders, especially borderline personality disorder, complicate diagnosis or coexist with depression.
- Borderline personality disorder is characterized by frequent mood shifts, without the other symptoms of depression or mania. Anger is the predominant mood.

Attention-Deficit and Hyperactivity Disorder (ADHD)

- Symptoms begin before age 7.
- ADHD is recognized as a disorder in childhood that may continue in adulthood.
- Sustained disturbances in mood are absent.
- ADHD is characterized by distractibility and inability to pay attention to details or to sustain attention in activities.
- High levels of activity, impulsivity, poor judgment, and distractibility are characteristic of ADHD and mania disorders.
- Mania tends to have a more episodic course, with clear onset and remission of symptoms.
- Mania is characterized by prominent mood disturbances, such as elevated moods.

COMMON NURSING DIAGNOSES

Self Care Deficit, feeding, bathing/hygiene, dressing/grooming, toileting
Violence, risk for, directed at self/others
Coping, individual, ineffective
Hopelessness
Powerlessness
Sleep Pattern Disturbance
Grieving, dysfunctional
Self Esteem disturbance
Social Isolation
Nutrition: altered, less than body requirements
Nutrition: altered, more than body requirements
Nutrition: altered, risk for more than body requirements

SYNOPSIS OF CURRENT RESEARCH

The links between depression and physical illness and the debilitating consequences are the focus of several lines of study. Depression has the most negative effects on functioning, leaving clients more socially and physically disabled than people with hypertension, diabetes, and arthritis. People with major depression are four times more likely to have a heart attack than those without depression. The reasons remain under investigation; depressed clients may be noncompliant with antihypertensive medications, less likely to eat well and reduce their weight, or at higher risk for blood clots.

Research is advancing rapidly on the role of serotonin in mood disorders. Serotonin was proposed to have a major role in the pathogenesis of mood disorders more than 30 years ago. Alterations in serotonin function are most evident in individuals with major depression. Several research studies support a reduction in serotonin levels. Levels of the metabolite of serotonin, 5-HIAA, are reduced in the cerebrospinal fluid of depressed clients.[17] Autopsy studies of depressed individuals have found decreased 5-HIAA levels and decreased serotonin in brain tissue. The substance that makes serotonin, tryptophan, is also diminished in depression. The serotonin reuptake inhibitors, antidepressants that specifically increase serotonin, are effective in treating depressive behaviors. Although these studies indicate that serotonin plays a major role in the development of major depression, its exact mechanism continues to be investigated. Recent theories about the biology of depression suggest that antidepressants may work by correcting an underlying imbalance in neurotransmitters including serotonin and norepinephrine.[7] Antidepressants have been developed recently to target these chemicals, with fewer uncomfortable or dangerous adverse reactions. Several new antidepressants under development may offer alternatives. Other treatments, based on cognitive-behavior theories, have found that correcting distorted thinking patterns alleviates depression. Taken together, the current research on depression suggests that a combination of treatment approaches is necessary to treat symptoms effectively.

Research on bipolar disorder has focused on the need for continued medication treatment to adequately control symptoms. Anticonvulsants have been recently shown to reduce and prevent episodes of mania and depression. Divalproex and carbamazepine represent two effective options to lithium carbonate, with different adverse effects. The therapeutic efficacy of anticonvulsants has generated new theories about the development of bipolar disorder. Minor depressive and manic states may occur, culminate, and eventually lead to major depression or mania. The original states are brief, minor, and usually resolve on their own. Through the process of kindling, mood states become more frequent and severe. Anticonvulsants quell the process. To treat the symptoms of bipolar disorder that fail to respond to mood stabilizers, antihypertensive or antipsychotic medications such as clozapine are under investigation.

Although medications are an essential part of the treatment plan, recent studies have focused on the consequences of bipolar disorder. Earlier age of onset, family history of bipolar disorder, presence of psychotic features, and comorbid substance abuse are associated with a worsened course and prognosis.[18] One group of researchers recently compared bipolar clients with and without comorbid substance abuse. Those with substance abuse recovered more slowly, were more likely to relapse, and were less compliant with medications.[19] Further research is investigating the natural course of bipolar disorder to compare individuals who continue treatment and those who do not.

AREAS FOR FUTURE RESEARCH

- What is the impact of mood disorders on family, friends, and coworkers?
- Why do some individuals with depression respond to placebo whereas others do not?
- What is the impact of education by psychiatric nurses on medication compliance in clients with mood disorders?
- What is the role of antidepressants in treating milder forms of depression and as "mood enhancers" for individuals without clear depressive disorders?
- What is the impact of early identification of mood disorders on long-term outcome?
- What are the first identifiable behaviors of mania or depression, and are any biochemical changes associated with them?
- What is the role of nursing in genetic counseling about mood disorders?
- How can nurses destigmatize the public's view of mania and depression?
- What is the impact of managed care on the treatment of mood disorders?
- What are the most effective components of the role of the psychiatric clinical nurse generalist in successful treatment?
- What is the impact of mania or depression on the individual's quality of life?

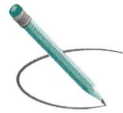

KEY POINTS

- Mood disorders are recurring psychiatric conditions that severely affect personal, occupational, and social functioning.
- Individuals with depression have a 25 to 30% risk of suicide during their lifetime, whereas 15% of those with bipolar disorder take their lives.
- The major mood disorders described in *DSM-IV* include major depression, bipolar disorder, and dysthymia.
- Mood disorders are characterized by disturbances in mood, energy, sleep, appetite, activity, and concentration.
- Major depression and bipolar disorder represent medical illnesses, not personal weaknesses or faulty personality development.
- Biology and heredity play a major role in the development of depression and bipolar disorder; however, no clear-cut explanations have been identified.
- Women are twice as likely as men to suffer from depression, whereas equal gender ratios exist for bipolar disorder.
- Research on the effectiveness of antidepressants in treating depression has supported the involvement of certain neurotransmitters such as serotonin and norepinephrine.
- All antidepressants are equally effective in treating the symptoms of major depression, although each is associated with a potentially different response in the individual client.

- Mood stabilizers such as lithium carbonate and anticonvulsants such as divalproex and carbamazepine effectively treat acute manic states and prevent future episodes of mania and depression. The anticonvulsants are more effective than lithium for more severe forms of bipolar disorder.
- The therapeutic efficacy of anticonvulsants has indicated that the process of "kindling" may explain the development of bipolar disorder.
- Certain instruments (HDRS and BDI) can be helpful in detecting and measuring the severity of depression.
- Left untreated, depression and mania are associated with poor prognosis, suicide, and significant impairment.
- Effective treatment of mood disorders requires a comprehensive approach that includes pharmacotherapy, client and family education, and psychotherapy. Cognitive-behavior therapy has been shown to be particularly effective for major depression.

REFERENCES

1. Styron, W: Darkness Visible. Random House, New York, 1990.
2. Jamison, KR: An Unquiet Mind. Alfred A Knopf, New York, 1995.
3. American Psychiatric Association: Diagnostic and Statistical Manual of Mental Disorders, ed 4. American Psychiatric Association, Washington, DC, 1994.
4. Yehuda, R, Resnick, H, Kahana, B, et al: Persistent hormonal alterations following extreme stress in humans: adaptive or maladaptive? Psychosom Med 55:287, 1993.
5. Beck, AT: Beck Depression Inventory-II (BDI-II). The Psychological Corporation, San Antonio, TX, 1996.
6. Hamilton, M: A rating scale for depression. J Neurol Neurosurg Psychiatry 23:56, 1960.
7. Hyman, SE, and Nestler, EJ: Initiation and adaptation: A paradigm for understanding psychotropic drug action. Am J Psychiatry 153:151, 1996.
8. Siever, LJ, and Davis, KL: Overview: Toward a dysregulation hypothesis of depression. Am J Psychiatry 142:1017, 1985.
9. Hyman, SE, and Nestler, EJ: The Molecular Foundations of Psychiatry. American Psychiatric Press, Washington, DC, 1993.
10. Rosenthal, NE, Sack, DA, and Gillin, C: Seasonal affective disorder: A description of the syndrome and preliminary findings with light therapy. Arch Gen Psychiatry 41:7280, 1984.
11. Teicher, MH, Glod, CA, Harper, D, et al: Locomotor activity rhythms in depressed children and adolescents I: Circadian dysregulation. J Am Acad Child Adolesc Psychiatry 32:760, 1993.
12. Stewart, AL, Hays, RD, Wells, KB, et al: Long-term functioning and well-being associated with physical activity and exercise in patients with chronic conditions in the Medical Outcomes Study. J Clin Epidemiol 47:719, 1994.
13. Blumenthal, SJ, and Kupfer, DJ: Suicide over the Life Cycle: Risk Factors, Assessment, and Treatment of Suicidal Patients. American Psychiatric Press, Washington, DC, 1990.
14. Fieve, R: Moodswing. Bantam Books, New York, 1989.
15. Goodwin, FK, and Jamison, KR: Manic-Depressive Illness. Oxford University Press, New York, 1990.
16. Sach, GS, Weilburg, JB, and Rosenbaum, JF: Clonazepam versus neuroleptics as adjuncts to lithium maintenance. Psychopharmacol Bull 26:137, 1990.
17. Owens, MJ, and Nemeroff, CB: Role of serotonin in the pathophysiology of depression: Focus on the serotonin transporter. Clin Chem 40:288, 1994.
18. Tohen, M, Tsuang, MT, and Goodwin, DC: Prediction of outcome in mania by mood congruent or mood incongruent psychotic features. Am J Psychiatry 149:1580, 1992.
19. Tohen, M, Zarate, C, and Turvey, C: The McLean first episode mania project (abstract). American Psychiatric Association, May 20, 1995.

CHAPTER 20
Anxiety Disorders

CHAPTER 20

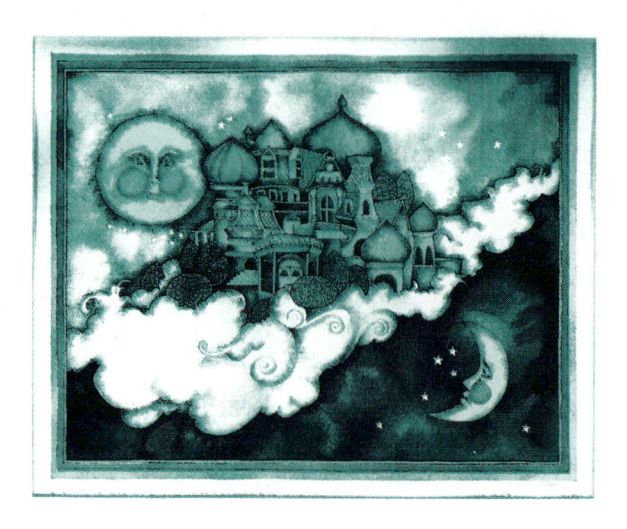

CHAPTER OUTLINE

Generalized Anxiety Disorder
Characteristic Behaviors
Culture, Age, and Gender Features
Etiology
Prognosis
Interventions for Hospitalized Clients
Interventions for Clients in the Community

Panic Disorder with or without Agoraphobia
Characteristic Behaviors
Culture, Age, and Gender Features
Etiology
Prognosis
Interventions for Clients in the Community

Phobias
Characteristic Behaviors
Culture, Age, and Gender Features
Etiology
Interventions for Clients in the Community

Obsessive-Compulsive Disorder (OCD)
Characteristic Behaviors
Diagnostic Aids
Culture, Age, and Gender Features
Etiology
Prognosis
Interventions for Hospitalized Clients
Interventions for Clients in the Community

Differential Diagnosis
Expected Outcomes
Common Nursing Diagnoses
Synopsis of Current Research
Areas for Future Research

Doreen Cawley, RN, MS, CS, ARNP

Anxiety Disorders

LEARNING OBJECTIVES

After completing this chapter, the reader should be able to:

- Recognize the symptoms and behaviors of anxiety disorders.
- Explain and contrast theories of anxiety.
- Implement the nursing process in planning care for the individual with an anxiety disorder.
- Analyze the impact of anxiety on the individual's daily functioning.
- Distinguish between the different anxiety disorders.
- Teach clients and their families about the consequences and management of anxiety disorders.

KEY TERMS

agoraphobia
anxiety
compulsions
obsessions
panic attack
panic disorder
phobia

Anxiety, a normal human emotion, is experienced in varying degrees as a state of emotional or physical uneasiness. Excess anxiety occurs in response to an actual or anticipated situation or as a pathological state.[1] As shown in Table 20–1, anxiety can be conceptualized on a continuum; a mild amount is necessary and can be adaptive, whereas severe anxiety or panic can be debilitating or even disabling. Hildegard Peplau[2] identified three levels of anxiety: mild, moderate, and severe. She suggested that the nurse work with the client, first, to identify the level of anxiety; next, to understand the behaviors associated with it; and finally, to better cope.

Anxiety disorders are common conditions that have disturbances in anxiety as the characteristic feature (Table 20–2). Panic disorder with or without agoraphobia, generalized anxiety disorder (GAD), obsessive-compulsive disorder (OCD), phobias, and posttraumatic stress disorder (PTSD, covered in Chapter 22) are the major anxiety disorders. The most prevalent psychiatric illnesses, anxiety disorders affect up to 25% of the population, and they can strike individuals at any point in their lifetimes. Because symptoms of anxiety can have physical manifestations, distinguishing anxiety or an anxiety disorder from a physical condition can be difficult.

A nursing student who is mildly anxious about the first exam of the semester can illustrate the difference in degrees of anxiety. Mild anxiety creates a "state of heightened arousal and alertness" that enables the student to focus on learning necessary materials. However, told that only a perfect score would be acceptable and that anything less would result in dismissal from the program, that same student's level of anxiety might rise to a less functional moderate range. A telephone call just before the exam, advising that a close family member had been in a serious car accident, could cause that student to experience severe anxiety with emotional and physical symptoms serious enough to reduce the student's ability to function.

Several theorists have studied why some individuals seem to be resilient and cope well with severe levels of anxiety, whereas others decompensate or become physically ill. Several characteristics have been identified in "stress-resistant" people: an *internal locus of control* (feeling that they can exert

TABLE 20–1. Anxiety Continuum

Adaptive	Maladaptive	Pathological
Mild	Moderate	Severe
		Anxiety Disorders
	Phobias	OCD
		GAD
	Panic Disorder	
	Agoraphobia	

Symptoms of Anxiety and Anxiety Disorders

Physiologic: Increased heart rate, elevated BP, palpitations, pain or tightness in chest, difficulty breathing, tightness of neck or back muscles, sweaty palms, trembling, twitching, headache, urinary frequency, nausea and vomiting, diarrhea, sleep disturbances, decreased appetite, sneezing, fatigue, accident proneness, frequent minor illnesses, and poor posture.

Cognitive: Forgetfulness, blocking on important details, rumination, poor judgment, decreased concentration and attention, decreased creativity, decreased productivity, and decreased attention.

Emotional and Affective: Irritability, depression, feelings of worthlessness, helplessness, or hopelessness, angry outbursts, suspiciousness, restlessness, social withdrawal, decreased motivation, crying, critical of self or others, self-deprecation, anhedonia.

TABLE 20–2. Prevalence of Anxiety Disorders

Disorder	Prevalence
Panic disorder	3.5%
Generalized anxiety disorder	6.4%
Simple phobia	11.3%
Social phobia	13.3%
Obsessive-compulsive disorder	2.5%

Source: Data derived from Schatzberg, AF: Overview of anxiety disorders: Prevalence, biology, course, and treatment. J Clin Psych 52:509, 1991; p. 509; and the Diagnostic and Statistical Manual of Mental Disorders, Fourth Edition. Copyright 1994 American Psychiatric Association.

control over events in their lives), a healthy lifestyle, a well-balanced diet, regular exercise patterns, and the use of others for support.[3] Factors that affect an individual's reaction to anxiety-provoking stimuli include genetic constitution, defense mechanisms, coping strategies for stress, and lifestyle factors such as sleep habits, diet, and exercise patterns. Although some of these factors can help an individual maintain balance, others can be harmful and worsen the experience of anxiety.

GENERALIZED ANXIETY DISORDER

Characteristic Behaviors

I always thought I was just a worrier. I'd feel keyed up and unable to relax. At times it would come and go, and at times it would be constant. It could go on for days. I'd worry about what would be a great present for somebody. I just couldn't let something go.

I'd have terrible sleeping problems. There were times when I'd wake up wired in the morning or in the middle of the night. I had trouble concentrating, even reading the newspaper or a novel. Sometimes I'd feel a little lightheaded. My heart would race or pound. And that would make me worry more.

Individuals with generalized anxiety disorder (GAD) have persistent anxiety and worry, lasting at least 6 months and often for a lifetime. Many report that they have been anxious for as long as they can remember. They experience extreme anxiety, much higher than the natural adaptive anxiety discussed previously. This chronic excessive worry is not usually provoked by any specific triggers but seems to have taken on a life of its own. People with GAD tend to anticipate the worst. They worry excessively about health, money, family, or work. Worries are often accompanied by physical symptoms such as muscle tension, nausea, or headache.[4] As shown in *DSM-IV* Diagnostic Criteria for General Anxiety Disorder, the anxiety and worry of GAD are accompanied by at least three other symptoms, such as irritability, muscle tension, restlessness, disturbed sleep, difficulty concentrating, or being easily fatigued. Other somatic manifestations include cold clammy hands, dry mouth, sweating, nausea, urinary frequency, trouble swallowing, and an exaggerated startle response. Physical manifestations of depessive disorders are similar to those of organic problems; accurate diagnosis is difficult.

Diagnostic Criteria for 300.02 Generalized Anxiety Disorder

A. Excessive anxiety and worry (apprehensive expectation), occurring more days than not for at least 6 months, about a number of events or activities (such as work or school performance).

B. The person finds it difficult to control the worry.

C. The anxiety and worry are associated with three (or more) of the following six symptoms (with at least some symptoms present for more days than not for the past 6 months).
   NOTE: Only one item is required in children.
   (1) restlessness or feeling keyed up or on edge
   (2) being easily fatigued
   (3) difficulty concentrating or mind going blank
   (4) irritability
   (5) muscle tension
   (6) sleep disturbance (difficulty falling or staying asleep, or restless unsatisfying sleep)

D. The focus of the anxiety and worry is not confined to features of an Axis I disorder, e.g., the anxiety or worry is not about having a Panic Attack (as in Panic Disorder), being embarrassed in public (as in Social Phobia), being contaminated (as in Obsessive-Compulsive Disorder), being away from home or close relatives (as in Separation Anxiety Disorder), gaining weight (as in Anorexia Nervosa), having multiple physical complaints (as in Somatization Disorder), or having a serious illness (as in Hypochondriasis), and the anxiety and worry do not occur exclusively during Posttraumatic Stress Disorder.

E. The anxiety, worry, or physical symptoms cause clinically significant distress or impairment in social, occupational, or other important areas of functioning.

F. The disturbance is not due to the direct physiological effects of a substance (e.g., a drug of abuse, a medication) or a general medical condition (e.g., hyperthyroidism) and does not occur exclusively during a Mood Disorder, a Psychotic Disorder, or a Pervasive Developmental Disorder.

Source: Reprinted with permission from the Diagnostic and Statistical Manual of Mental Disorders, Fourth Edition. Copyright 1994 American Psychiatric Association.

Culture, Age, and Gender Features

Culture and Gender

Anxiety disorders such as GAD may be expressed somewhat differently, depending upon the culture in which the patient lives.[5,6] For example, in some cultures individuals express anxiety through somatic complaints, whereas elsewhere people have more cognitive symptoms. For this reason it is especially important to assess the cultural context to decide whether treatment is indicated. Generally, the disorder affects twice as many women as men.

Age

Children and Adolescents. Half of adults with GAD report onset in childhood. Children and adolescents tend to worry about school, performance in sports and other activities, or catastrophic events such as earthquakes.[6] They often need reassurance that things will be all right.

Elderly. Studies suggest that anxiety symptoms are significant in adults over age 65. There is accumulating evidence that anxiety disorders often occur for the first time in old age.[7] GAD and major depression often coexist in older adults.

Etiology

Genetic Theories

Studies suggest that a tendency for anxiety may be inherited, which may predispose a child to be more vulnerable to adverse developmental experiences.[8] Twenty percent of first-degree relatives of clients with GAD also have the disorder.

Biological Theories

Research on the biology of GAD points to a dysfunction of γ-aminobutyric acid (GABA) receptors in the central nervous system (CNS). Evidence to support this theory comes from the actions of antianxiety agents such as benzodiazepines on GABA receptors. GABA, the major inhibitory neurotransmitter, acts as a natural antianxiety chemical. It is present in 30% or more of nerve synapses, particularly in the hypothalamus, the substantia nigra, and the globus pallidus. As shown in Figure 20–1, GABA enhances the permeability of certain substances in the CNS, such as chloride. Benzodiazepines, which effectively treat GAD, enhance chloride ion permeability assisted by the presence of GABA.[1] The increased flow of chloride ions into the neuron appears to diminish anxiety.

Prognosis

The course is usually chronic but may fluctuate in severity, worsening during times of high stress.[6] Response to treatment depends on the severity of the disorder and the motivation of the individual to follow treatment recommendations.

Interventions for Hospitalized Clients

To intervene with hospitalized clients with severe anxiety, ask how often these symptoms occur, what helps to alleviate them, how long the symptoms last, and if the individual avoids any activities. Try to meet with them in a quiet, stress-free location. Ask about alcohol and substance abuse that may worsen or complicate symptoms. Advocate for clients to receive a complete physical and blood tests to rule out any organic causes.

Assess suicide risk. Ask clients directly if they have ever had any thoughts or plans about harming themselves, now or in the past. Use the suicide assessment process described in the mood disorders chapter (19). Intervene immediately with any client who admits to having a suicide plan.

Administer standing and as-needed doses of medication, particularly when clients are continuing to have moderate to severe levels of anxiety. Evaluate if and when the medication

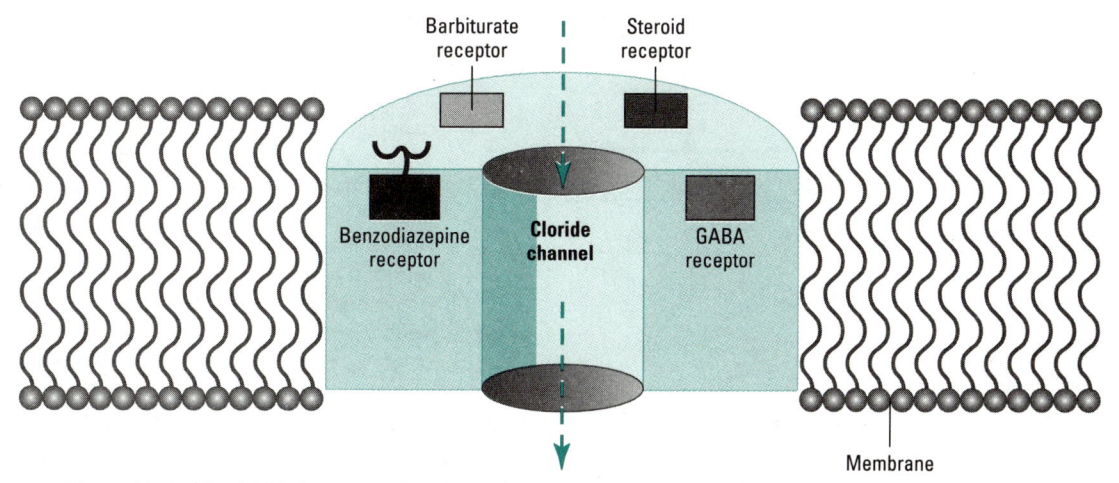

Figure 20–1. The GABA-A receptor. This receptor has multiple binding sites that regulate an inhibitory chloride channel. These sites include a barbiturate site, a steroid receptor, and a benzodiazepine site, where valium and librium have their effects. (Courtesy of Susan L. Andersen, PhD.)

takes effect and the side effects. Teach progressive relaxation and refer clients for cognitive-behavior therapy.

Interventions for Clients in the Community

Cognitive-Behavior Therapy

Cognitive-behavior therapy treats anxiety more effectively than traditional "talk" therapies. Cognitive therapy assumes that thoughts affect behavior. For behavior to change, thoughts must first change. Restructuring techniques involve "self-statement training." The therapist first coaches anxious clients to identify negative self-statements. They then explore the role or influence of the negative statement on self-concept, behavior, and mood. Finally, negative self-statements are replaced with positive ones.

Individuals with GAD may also respond to behavioral therapy techniques such as progressive relaxation, biofeedback, and assertiveness training. Regular use of progressive relaxation (alternate tensing and relaxing of muscles) can reduce physical tension and anxious feelings. The individual is taught the technique and can use it daily, as well as when severe anxiety strikes. Biofeedback, used for more than 20 years, may also be effective. This form of treatment is generally short term, averaging 8 to 12 sessions. Physiological data such as heart rate are displayed to the client, in order to foster insight through learning ways to identify patterns of emotional arousal. Specifically, the biofeedback assists the client in identifying stressors not previously labeled as sources of anxiety. The individual learns to control physiological arousal, thus decreasing anxiety.

Pharmacologic Treatments

Benzodiazepines. The discovery of diazepam (Valium) and its ability to reduce anxiety eventually led to the development of other benzodiazepines. These medications are indicated for the treatment of GAD. Because of the risk of addiction, they should not be prescribed to individuals who are abusing alcohol or drugs. Table 20–3 lists the most common benzodiazepines and their relative equivalency in dosage. Overall, the benzodiazepines are well tolerated but may lead to sedation. Clients should not stop these medications abruptly, because withdrawal symptoms such as worsening anxiety, shaking, and seizures may occur.

Buspirone. Buspirone (Buspar) is a nonaddictive antianxiety agent used to treat GAD. Unlike the benzodiazepines, buspirone may take 2 to 4 weeks to take effect, which may be difficult for the individual with severe anxiety. Instruct clients to continue taking the medication, even if they don't notice an immediate effect.

PANIC DISORDER WITH OR WITHOUT AGORAPHOBIA

Characteristic Behaviors

It started 10 years ago. I was sitting in a seminar in a hotel and this thing came out of the clear blue sky. I felt like I was dying.

For me, a panic attack is almost a violent experience. I feel like I'm losing control in a very extreme way. My heart pounds really hard, things seem unreal, and there's this very strong feeling of impending doom.

DSM-IV Diagnostic Criteria for Panic Attack

NOTE: Panic Attack is not a codable disorder. Code the specific diagnosis in which the Panic Attack occurs (e.g., 300.21 Panic Disorder With Agoraphobia).

A discrete period of intense fear or discomfort, in which four (or more) of the following symptoms developed abruptly and reached a peak within 10 minutes:

(1) palpitations, pounding heart, or accelerated heart rate
(2) sweating
(3) trembling or shaking
(4) sensations of shortness of breath or smothering
(5) feeling of choking
(6) chest pain or discomfort
(7) nausea or abdominal distress
(8) feeling dizzy, unsteady, lightheaded, or faint
(9) derealization (feelings of unreality) or depersonalization (being detached from oneself)
(10) fear of losing control or going crazy
(11) fear of dying
(12) paresthesias (numbness or tingling sensations)
(13) chills or hot flushes

Source: Reprinted with permission from the Diagnostic and Statistical Manual of Mental Disorders, Fourth Edition. Copyright 1994 American Psychiatric Association.

TABLE 20–3. Medications Used to Treat Generalized Anxiety Disorder

Medication (Generic/Trade)	Oral Dosage Equivalency (mg)
Alprazolam (Xanax)	0.5
Chlordiazepoxide (Librium)	10
Clonazepam (Klonopin)	0.25
Clorazepate (Tranxene)	7.5
Diazepam (Valium)	5
Lorazepam (Ativan)	1
Midazolam (Versed)	—
Oxazepam (Serax)	15

Source: Adapted from Teicher, MH: Biology of anxiety. Med Clin North Am 72:791–814, 1988.

> **DSM-IV Diagnostic Criteria for Panic Disorder without and with Agoraphobia**

Diagnostic Criteria for 300.01 Panic Disorder without Agoraphobia

A. Both (1) and (2):
  (1) recurrent unexpected Panic Attacks
  (2) at least one of the attacks has been followed by 1 month (or more) of one (or more) of the following:
    (a) persistent concern about having additional attacks
    (b) worry about the implications of the attack or its consequences (e.g., losing control, having a heart attack, "going crazy")
    (c) a significant change in behavior related to the attacks
B. Absence of Agoraphobia.
C. The Panic Attacks are not due to the direct physiological effects of a substance (e.g., a drug of abuse, a medication) or a general medical condition (e.g., hyperthyroidism).
D. The Panic Attacks are not better accounted for by another mental disorder, such as Social Phobia (e.g., occurring on exposure to feared social situations), Specific Phobia (e.g., on exposure to a specific phobic situation), Obsessive-Compulsive Disorder (e.g., on exposure to dirt in someone with an obsession about contamination), Posttraumatic Stress Disorder (e.g., in response to stimuli associated with a severe stressor), or Separation Anxiety Disorder (e.g., in response to being away from home or close relatives).

Diagnostic Criteria for 300.21 Panic Disorder with Agoraphobia

A. Both (1) and (2):
  (1) recurrent unexpected Panic Attacks
  (2) at least one of the attacks has been followed by 1 month (or more) of one (or more) of the following:
    (a) persistent concern about having additional attacks
    (b) worry about the implications of the attack or its consequences (e.g., losing control, having a heart attack, "going crazy")
    (c) a significant change in behavior related to the attacks
B. The presence of Agoraphobia.
C. The Panic Attacks are not due to the direct physiological effects of a substance (e.g., a drug of abuse, a medication) or a general medical condition (e.g., hyperthyroidism).
D. The Panic Attacks are not better accounted for by another mental disorder, such as Social Phobia (e.g., occurring on exposure to feared social situations), Specific Phobia (e.g., on exposure to a specific phobic situation), Obsessive-Compulsive Disorder (e.g., on exposure to dirt in someone with an obsession about contamination), Posttraumatic Stress Disorder (e.g., in response to stimuli associated with a severe stressor), or Separation Anxiety Disorder (e.g., in response to being away from home or close relatives).

Source: Reprinted with permission from the Diagnostic and Statistical Manual of Mental Disorders, Fourth Edition. Copyright 1994 American Psychiatric Association.

In between attacks there is this dread and anxiety that it's going to happen again. It can be very debilitating, trying to escape those feelings of panic.

At least 16% of adult Americans, or 30 million people, will have a panic attack at some point in their lives.[4] A **panic attack** is a discrete episode of intense fear or discomfort accompanied by at least 4 of 13 symptoms (see *DSM-IV Diagnostic Criteria for Panic Attack*). The attack has a sudden onset and builds rapidly to a peak, usually in 10 minutes or less. It may be accompanied by a sense of impending doom and an urge to escape.[6] Although often unprovoked or unexpected, panic attacks at times may be provoked by a situation, for instance, being in a grocery store or driving. After having a panic attack in a specific place such as a grocery store, clients may avoid that situation or place because they fear having another attack.

Panic disorder is characterized by recurring panic attacks that come out of the blue, along with concern about having more attacks and worry about the consequences of them (see *DSM-IV Diagnostic Criteria for Panic Disorder without and with Agoraphobia*). Clients may also change their behavior and avoid places that trigger the panic reaction. Behavioral changes may signal the development of **agoraphobia**, literally, "fear of the marketplace"; people become afraid of being in any place or situation where escape might be difficult or help unavailable in the event of a panic attack. Some may avoid highways where they previously had panic attacks and be limited to driving short distances from home. Others may not be able to leave home alone unless accompanied by a family member. In severe cases, individuals become housebound.

People with panic disorder do not always present themselves to psychiatric care facilities. Surveys reveal that primary care doctors see more clients with anxiety and depression than with diabetes or asthma. However, most clients are reluctant to discuss their psychiatric symptoms. Nurses working in medical settings may be the first to identify symptoms suggestive of panic disorder or agoraphobia.

Agoraphobia

As shown in the *DSM-IV* Diagnostic Criteria for Agoraphobia, agoraphobia is fear or avoidance of any place or situation where escape might be difficult in the event of a panic attack.[6] Typically, clients are apprehensive about any place where there may be a crowd, such as theaters, malls, grocery stores, or public transportation. Some adapt by using strategies such as sitting on the aisle seat of a theater by the door. However, many gradually restrict their activities to places where they feel safe. Because leaving their homes or even their bedrooms becomes difficult, this illness can be quite disabling. Most people with agoraphobia have panic disorder.

Culture, Age, and Gender Features

Children and Adolescents

Panic disorder is rare in childhood but may emerge in late adolescence. Separation anxiety, a common disorder of childhood, is characterized by excessive fears and worries of harm befalling a parent and extreme anxiety when separated from parents. Children may refuse to attend school, sleep over at others' houses, or go to sleep at night. Physical symptoms such as headaches and stomach aches are common. Separation anxiety in childhood may be associated with the development of panic disorder in adulthood.

TABLE 20–4. Biological Theories of Panic Disorder

Lactate Hypothesis
Respiratory and Carbon Dioxide Hypothesis
Norepinephrine Hypothesis
Serotonin Hypothesis
Adenosine Hypothesis
GABA-Benzodiazepine Hypothesis

Elderly

Panic disorder exists in older adults but usually presents earlier in adulthood. The age of onset is often in the mid-30s.[6]

Etiology

Genetic Theories

Family and twin studies suggest a genetic basis. Panic disorder seems to run in families; 15% of first-degree relatives have this condition.[1] A combination of inheritance and stressors may also explain its etiology. Genetic abnormalities may predispose some individuals to be more vulnerable to stress, which then triggers the disorder. There is an extremely high incidence of distressing life events preceding the first panic attack.[5]

Twin studies demonstrate a higher concordance rate for monozygotic than dizygotic twins, suggesting that genetic factors play a role;[9] if one identical twin is affected, the other has a 31% chance of also having panic disorder. Early studies also reported that a marker for panic disorder existed on chromosome 16q22; however, further work has not sup-

---

DSM-IV Diagnostic Criteria for Agoraphobia

NOTE: Agoraphobia is not a codable disorder. Code the specific disorder in which the Agoraphobia occurs (e.g., 300.21 Panic Disorder With Agoraphobia or 300.22 Agoraphobia Without History of Panic Disorder).

A. Anxiety about being in places or situations from which escape might be difficult (or embarrassing) or in which help may not be available in the event of having an unexpected or situationally predisposed Panic Attack or panic-like symptoms. Agoraphobic fears typically involve characteristic clusters of situations that include being outside the home alone; being in a crowd or standing in a line, being on a bridge, and traveling in a bus, train, or automobile.

NOTE: Consider the diagnosis of Specific Phobia if the avoidance is limited to one or only a few specific situations, or Social Phobia if the avoidance is limited to social situations.

B. The situations are avoided (e.g., travel is restricted) or else are endured with marked distress or with anxiety about having a Panic Attack or panic-like symptoms, or require the presence of a companion.

C. The anxiety or phobic avoidance is not better accounted for by another mental disorder, such as Social Phobia (e.g., avoidance limited to social situations because of fear of embarrassment), Specific Phobia (e.g., avoidance limited to a single situation like elevators), Obsessive-Compulsive Disorder (e.g., avoidance of dirt in someone with an obsession about contamination), Posttraumatic Stress Disorder (e.g., avoidance of stimuli associated with a severe stressor), or Separation Anxiety Disorder (e.g., avoidance of leaving home or relatives).

Source: Reprinted with permission from the Diagnostic and Statistical Manual of Mental Disorders, Fourth Edition. Copyright 1994 American Psychiatric Association.

ported these findings. Although no gene has been identified, current research suggests that panic disorder is inherited.

Biological Theories

Lactate Hypothesis. Table 20–4 lists the common biological theories of panic disorder. Abnormalities in lactate metabolism may explain this disorder. Lactate stimulates respirations, leading to the shortness of breath and hyperventilation commonly seen in panic attacks. The greater the degree of lactate-induced hyperventilation, the higher the likelihood of having a panic attack. In one experiment, intravenous administration of sodium lactate elicited panic attacks in 50 to 70% of individuals with panic disorder.[10]

Respiratory and Carbon Dioxide Hypothesis. Because shortness of breath and choking sensations frequently occur in panic disorder, abnormalities in respiratory function may explain its development. Of the three main theories—panic disorder results from chronic hyperventilation, an oversensitive carbon dioxide system, or a false alarm system for sensing suffocation—none has been proved. One set of studies found that chronic hyperventilation set off myriad physio-

---

Nursing Care Plan: ANXIETY

Nursing Diagnosis #1: Anxiety evidenced by muscle tension, hypervigilance, distractibility, increased vital signs, insomnia related to stress, threat to self-concept, loss

Client Outcome Criteria
- Expresses feeling calmer.
- Identifies factors that trigger anxiety response.
- Verbalizes greater sense of control over stressors.

Interventions
- Interact with the client in a calm manner using a soft voice and reassuring approach. Give simple, concise directions. If the client is panicky, be very directive.
- Reduce distractions and stimuli in the environment to enhance a sense of calmness.
- Listen to the client's concerns and allow expression of feelings.
- Teach relaxation techniques such as deep breathing, muscle relaxation, and calming self-talk.
- Assist the client to identify factors that contribute to anxiety response.
- Defer in-depth teaching or complex discussions until anxiety has diminished.
- Administer antianxiety medications as appropriate.
- Determine factors that increase anxiety such as caffeine, medications, and nicotine, and teach techniques to avoid them.

Nursing Diagnosis #2: Ineffective individual coping evidenced by fear, phobic response to events or objects, irrational thoughts related to phobias, extreme guilt

Client Outcome Criteria
- Demonstrates appropriate coping responses for reducing anxiety to phobias.
- Demonstrates increased ability to think rationally.
- Tolerates feared objects, events.

Interventions
- Understand that phobic responses are irrational and will not be changed by logical explanations.
- Approach the client in a calm, nonauthoritarian manner using a soft voice.
- Listen and acknowledge the client's fears and emotions in a supportive, nonjudgmental manner.
- Assist the client to clarify thoughts and avoid misinterpretations of events.
- Assist the client to develop coping mechanisms to control anxiety response. Work with the client to use these responses. Role play alternate responses.
- Allow the client to have some control over anxiety-provoking situations. Never force the client to do something. If possible, expose the client in very small amounts to the feared object and event while providing support and reassurance.
- When the client is more relaxed, discuss alternative ways to interpret an event. Reinforce any efforts at using these methods. Refer to specific programs for coping with phobias.

Nursing Diagnosis #3: Posttrauma response evidenced by flashbacks, nightmares; increased anxiety symptoms related to traumatic events such as rape, car accident, or war.

Client Outcome Criteria
- Identifies situations that trigger anxiety response.
- Verbalizes ability to control reactions in stressful situations.
- Verbalizes more optimistic response to the future.

Interventions
- Encourage venting feelings of fear, anger, and powerlessness related to traumatic event in a supportive, reassuring environment.
- Explore factors that trigger reminders of the trauma, and increase awareness of how these reminders affect the client.
- Encourage talking about the events of the trauma. Provide a trusting environment without showing judgment or shock during this process.
- Teach relaxation techniques as a way to combat building tension when the client is reliving or exposed to the trauma.
- Encourage the development of new skills and relationships as a way of moving on from the trauma.
- Identify appropriate support group programs based on the client's traumatic event.
- Reassure and reinforce the client of his or her ability to return to a previous level of functioning.
- Assist and support the client with legal and medical issues as appropriate.
- Educate the client on normalcy of reactions to a traumatic event.

logical and behavioral symptoms, primarily panic attacks. Other studies found that 50 to 80% of individuals who inhaled carbon dioxide had panic attacks, suggesting an increased sensitivity of carbon dioxide receptors in the brain. Other researchers propose that individuals with panic disorder can detect impending suffocation very sensitively. In this model, people prone to panic attacks have a "false suffocation alarm."[11] This alarm system is naturally protective, triggering the "fight-or-flight" response to danger, but in panic disorder this alarm goes off at too low a threshold.

Norepinephrine Hypothesis. Increased levels of norepinephrine are associated with physical signs of hyperarousal such as higher heart rates and tachycardia and heart palpitations are commonly seen in panic attacks. Therefore, researchers have explored whether a norepinephrine-related disturbance may provide an explanation for panic disorder. The "noradrenergic dysregulation" theory suggests that the norepinephrine system is either overactive or underactive.

Norepinephrine, a neurotransmitter also involved in the etiology of major depression, is largely produced in one part of the brain, the locus caeruleus, where increased activity is associated with anxiety. Studies have used medications that affect the norepinephrine system to test the reaction of individuals with panic disorder. Yohimbine, a medication that blocks the receptors that norepinephrine binds to, increases anxiety. This blocking suggests that these receptors are very sensitive, in fact, overly sensitive in panic disorder. Another medication, clonidine, with opposite effects on the receptors that norepinephrine binds to, decreases cardiac-related panic effects, suggesting a reduced sensitivity. Because these lines of evidence conflict—that is, oversensitivity and undersensitivity of the receptors that norepinephrine binds to—the model is labeled *dysregulation*. The changes in the receptor sensitivity point to both an increase and decrease in norepinephrine levels, suggesting a more complicated disturbance.

Other support for the norepinephrine dysregulation hypothesis comes from the actions of medications that effectively treat panic disorder. Tricyclic antidepressants (TCAs) decrease activity in the locus caeruleus, thereby affecting norepinephrine levels. More research is needed to fully explain the nature of the disturbance.

Serotonin Hypothesis. Serotonin functioning may also be impaired. A drug that mimics or acts like serotonin, m-CPP, precipitates panic attacks in individuals with panic disorder. Fenfluramine, another medication, increases the release of serotonin and also leads to panic attacks. These results suggest that the serotonin "lookalikes" enhance serotonin, thereby producing panic disorder. The selective serotonin reuptake inhibitors (SSRIs), by affecting the serotonin system, effectively treat panic disorder. There may be an as-yet undefined abnormality in the serotonin system that leads to panic attacks, which is corrected by treatment with SSRIs.

Adenosine Hypothesis. Adenosine dysfunction may also explain panic disorder. Because of the exaggerated anxiety effects due to caffeine, which blocks adenosine receptors, panic disorder may develop because of abnormalities in neuronal systems involving central adenosine receptors. Individuals with a history of panic disorder have an increased sensitivity to the effects of one cup of coffee and are more likely than others to have voluntarily discontinued coffee. In one study, high-dose caffeine exacerbated anxiety in 50 to 70% of clients and triggered attacks in 17%.[1] Adenosine also affects synaptic transmission and releases other neurotransmitters implicated in anxiety, such as norepinephrine, serotonin, and GABA.

GABA-Benzodiazepine Hypothesis. Antianxiety medications such as the benzodiazepines, effective in the treatment of panic disorder, facilitate GABA transmission and decrease anxiety. They act at the GABA-benzodiazepine receptors in the nerve synapse. Hence, disruption in GABA may account for anxiety; however, more research is needed to determine the specific role of GABA in panic disorder.

Limbic System Dysfunction. Decreased blood flow to the hippocampus, part of the limbic system, may help explain the development of panic attacks. The limbic system is responsible for regulating several physiological and emotional functions, including anxiety and arousal. As a result, some researchers have used positron emission tomography (PET) to determine if there are changes in brain functioning. Individuals with panic disorder show a shift (decrease) in blood flow to the left hemisphere, particularly the hippocampus.

Prognosis

Panic attacks typically improve in several weeks with medication and therapy.[4] However, if a person does not seek treatment, the disorder remains. It may continue to worsen with occasional periods of temporary improvement. Fifty percent to 60% of individuals who have panic disorder also develop depression.[6]

Panic disorder can occur with or without agoraphobia. About one-third of those with panic disorder also have agoraphobia. Agoraphobia may develop when treatment is delayed or in more severe cases of the disorder. It usually develops within the first year of having recurrent panic attacks.[6] Less commonly, agoraphobia may develop without panic disorder. In clinical treatment settings, over 90% of those with agoraphobia have panic disorder.

Interventions for Clients in the Community

Clients are rarely hospitalized, and the majority receive treatment in the community; suicide attempts or severe comorbid conditions such as depression may lead to hospitalization. For those with severe agoraphobia, home visits are necessary. The best approach for treating panic disorder with or without agoraphobia is through a combination of behavioral and pharmacologic treatment.[12] Approximately 70 to 90%

> **RESEARCH NOTE**
>
> Schweitzer, P, Nesse, R, Fantone, R, and Curtis, G: Outcomes of group cognitive behavioral training in the treatment of panic disorder and agoraphobia. American Psychiatric Nurses Association 1:83–91, 1995.
>
> **Findings:** These researchers used a comprehensive anxiety management program for groups of 6 to 10 clients. Each group, led by a clinical nurse specialist, met weekly for 2 hours. The objectives were to educate clients about anxiety, cognitive restructuring, and behavioral techniques and to promote successful anxiety-reducing strategies. Daily practice, homework assignments, and individual work in the group resulted in reduced symptoms after 6 weeks of this cognitive-behavior group training. The members reported that the most important aspects were meeting others with the same symptoms, practicing behavioral techniques, and education, particularly about cognitive-behavior strategies.
>
> **Application to Practice:** This study demonstrated the efficacy of a clinical nurse specialist–led group for clients with panic disorder and agoraphobia. Using nursing expertise in education about physical symptoms, medications, cognitive-behavior techniques, and group process skills was a practical, cost-efficient form of treatment. Clients who learn about their condition and practice effective techniques have fewer symptoms. The findings also suggest that early intervention is essential. For instance, individuals with agoraphobia may restrict their activities until it becomes difficult to leave their home or even bedrooms.

benefit from treatment, particularly when it is instituted early in the course of the disorder.

Cognitive-Behavior Therapy

Clients often receive a combination of cognitive restructuring, relaxation training, exposure therapy, and paradoxical intention. In *paradoxical intention,* the therapist instructs the client to hyperventilate or actually bring on a panic attack. By ceasing the struggle to prevent anxiety, the individual gains a sense of control over and tolerance for the discomfort. This promotes a sense of mastery over the threatening symptoms.

Exposure therapy is the main treatment for agoraphobia. Four types of exposure therapy exist: in vivo, systematic desensitization, implosive therapy, and flooding. In vivo therapy involves the client in confronting the feared object or situation, with support from the therapist. *Systematic desensitization* involves progressive-relaxation training, constructing an anxiety hierarchy, and gradual exposure paired with relaxation, in order of increasing difficulty. *Implosive therapy* is the presentation of anxiety-provoking material through imagery in a vivid manner, while the therapist attempts to prevent the client from fleeing the scene. *Flooding,* the most intense of the interventions, is the presentation, either in imagery or in the environment, of the anxiety-provoking stimuli, without relaxation or pause, until the anxiety subsides.

Pharmacologic Interventions

Antidepressants. The SSRIs and, to a lesser extent, the TCAs are effective in reducing the frequency and severity of panic attacks. They may take several weeks to take effect. They are indicated for individuals who have comorbid major depression and, because of their lack of addictive potential, for those with a history of alcohol or substance abuse or dependence. Monitor individuals for response and side effects; because anxiety is a common side effect, the SSRIs may be difficult to tolerate, particularly in the beginning of treatment.

Benzodiazepines. Alprazolam (Xanax) and clonazepam (Klonopin) treat panic attacks effectively. On average, daily doses of 2 to 6 mg of alprazolam are used, although doses as high as 10 mg may be necessary for complete remission. Because of its short-acting effects, alprazolam quickly treats panic anxiety and is given three to five times throughout the day. However, individuals may also experience breakthrough symptoms, anxiety symptoms that occur 3 to 4 hours after the last dose, because the medication is wearing off. Some develop "clock-watching," that is, looking at the clock to decide when to take the next scheduled dose. Clonazepam is longer-acting and usually given in total doses of 1 to 4 mg, twice daily. Because of its longer duration of action, there is less potential for interdose anxiety. Tapering or discontinuing the drug may also be easier. However, clonazepam may lead to more sedation.

PHOBIAS

Characteristic Behaviors

As seen in *DSM-IV* Diagnostic Criteria for Specific Phobia, a specific **phobia** is an irrational fear of a specific object, activity, or event. Examples include fear of flying, crossing bridges, dogs, or snakes. Individuals may have panic attacks or symptoms of severe anxiety when exposed to these situations or objects. Adults with this disorder recognize that the phobia is excessive or unreasonable. Although phobias are common in the general population, they rarely cause enough distress to warrant a diagnosis of a specific phobia. Most people adapt by limiting their exposure to the threatening object or situation.

Social Phobia

Another type of excessive fear is severe social anxiety. Individuals with social phobia markedly fear social or performance situations where embarrassment may occur (see *DSM-*

DSM-IV Diagnostic Criteria for 300.29 Specific Phobia

A. Marked and persistent fear that is excessive or unreasonable, cued by the presence or anticipation of a specific object or situation (e.g., flying, heights, animals, receiving an injection, seeing blood).

B. Exposure to the phobic stimulus almost invariably provokes an immediate anxiety response, which may take the form of a situationally bound or situationally predisposed Panic Attack.
   NOTE: In children, the anxiety may be expressed by crying, tantrums, freezing, or clinging.

C. The person recognizes that the fear is excessive or unreasonable.
   NOTE: In children, this feature may be absent.

D. The phobic situation(s) is avoided or else is endured with intense anxiety or distress.

E. The avoidance, anxious anticipation, or distress in the feared situation(s) interferes significantly with the person's normal routine, occupational (or academic) functioning, or social activities or relationships, or there is marked distress about having the phobia.

F. In individuals under age 18 years, the duration is at least 6 months.

G. The anxiety, Panic Attacks, or phobic avoidance associated with the specific object or situation are not better accounted for by another mental disorder, such as Obsessive-Compulsive Disorder (e.g., fear of dirt in someone with an obsession about contamination), Posttraumatic Stress Disorder (e.g., avoidance of stimuli associated with a severe stressor), Separation Anxiety Disorder (e.g., avoidance of school), Social Phobia (e.g., avoidance of social situations because of fear of embarrassment), Panic Disorder With Agoraphobia, or Agoraphobia Without History of Panic Disorder.

Specify type:
Animal Type
Natural Environment Type (e.g., heights, storms, water)
Blood-Injection-Injury Type
Situational Type (e.g., airplanes, elevators, enclosed places)
Other Type (e.g., phobic avoidance of situations that may lead to choking, vomiting, or contracting an illness; in children, avoidance of loud sounds or costumed characters)

Source: Reprinted with permission from the Diagnostic and Statistical Manual of Mental Disorders, Fourth Edition. Copyright 1994 American Psychiatric Association.

DSM-IV Diagnostic Criteria for 300.23 Social Phobia

A. A marked and persistent fear of one or more social or performance situations in which the person is exposed to unfamiliar people or to possible scrutiny by others. The individual fears that he or she will act in a way (or show anxiety symptoms) that will be humiliating or embarrassing.
   NOTE: In children, there must be evidence of the capacity for age-appropriate social relationships with familiar people and the anxiety must occur in peer settings, not just in interactions with adults.

B. Exposure to the feared social situation almost invariably provokes anxiety, which may take the form of a situationally bound or situationally predisposed Panic Attack.
   NOTE: In children, the anxiety may be expressed by crying, tantrums, freezing, or shrinking from social situations with unfamiliar people.

C. The person recognizes that the fear is excessive or unreasonable.
   NOTE: In children, this feature may be absent.

D. The feared social or performance situations are avoided or else are endured with intense anxiety or distress.

E. The avoidance, anxious anticipation, or distress in the feared social or performance situation(s) interferes significantly with the person's normal routine, occupational (academic) functioning, or social activities or relationships, or there is marked distress about having the phobia.

F. In individuals under age 18 years, the duration is at least 6 months.

G. The fear or avoidance is not due to the direct physiological effects of a substance (e.g., a drug of abuse, a medication) or a general medical condition and is not better accounted for by another mental disorder (e.g., Panic Disorder With or Without Agoraphobia, Separation Anxiety Disorder, Body Dysmorphic Disorder, a Pervasive Developmental Disorder, or Schizoid Personality Disorder).

H. If a general medical condition or another mental disorder is present, the fear in Criterion A is unrelated to it, e.g., the fear is not of Stuttering, trembling in Parkinson's disease, or exhibiting abnormal eating behavior in Anorexia Nervosa or Bulimia Nervosa.

Specify if:
Generalized: if the fears include most social situations (also consider the additional diagnosis of Avoidant Personality Disorder)

Source: Reprinted with permission from the Diagnostic and Statistical Manual of Mental Disorders, Fourth Edition. Copyright 1994 American Psychiatric Association.

IV Diagnostic Criteria for Social Phobia).[6] Some have difficult attending or remaining in social situations, even with a few friends. Others have difficulty eating or speaking in front of others or using public rest rooms. They fear that others see them as weak or stupid; they may have unrealistic concerns about being humiliated. Often these people are very shy. Sometimes they force themselves to attend a social event but worry about it for weeks beforehand. Once in a social setting, they experience severe anxiety and panic attacks. Although they know that their worries are excessive and unreasonable, they cannot control them. Social phobia may also be characterized by poor self-esteem, being easily hurt, difficulty being assertive, poor eye contact, and negative self-evaluation.[6]

Culture, Age, and Gender Features

Age

Children tend to cry, have tantrums, or display "freezing" or clinging behaviors. They may not directly report being fearful. Some phobias are transitory and remit during adolescence.

Gender

Social phobia and specific phobias are generally more common in women, but the gender ratio varies depending on the type of phobia.

Etiology

Genetic Theories

Although the exact rates are unknown, phobias tend to run in families. Twin studies suggest that phobias are accounted for by genetic factors.

Cognitive-Behavior Theories

Learning theorists propose that phobias result from a conditioned response; the person learns to associate the phobic object with a noxious or uncomfortable feeling. Avoidance of the phobia leads to reduced anxiety and reinforces the fear. At times, phobias may arise in response to a traumatic incident.

Interventions for Clients in the Community

Cognitive-Behavior Therapy

Exposure therapy is the main treatment for phobias; systematic desensitization is often used.[13] The therapist first asks the client to create a hierarchy of stressful situations. For example, for individuals with a fear of flying, the following hierarchy might be used:

1. Seeing a picture of a plane
2. Hearing planes overhead
3. Driving past an airport
4. Entering an airport
5. Walking onto a plane
6. Actually flying

At each step, the individual practices relaxation techniques and continues them at home for mastery. As the relaxation response is paired with the stressful trigger—that is, each step in the hierarchy—the client gradually masters and tolerates each step until eventually he or she is able to fly.

Cognitive-restructuring techniques may also be used to help phobic clients confront their fears by changing their negative thoughts and substituting healthier ones.

Pharmacologic Interventions

Medications are not used to treat specific phobias; however, benzodiazepines and certain antidepressants may be effective for social phobia. Clonazepam, monoamine oxidase inhibitors (MAOIs), and perhaps some of the newer antidepressants are used. More research is needed.

OBSESSIVE-COMPULSIVE DISORDER (OCD)

Characteristic Behaviors

I couldn't do anything without rituals. They transcended every aspect of my life. Counting was big for me. When I set my alarm at night, I had to set it to a number that wouldn't add up to a bad number. If my sister was 33 and I was 24, I couldn't leave the TV on channel 33 or 24. I would wash my hair three times as opposed to once because 3 was a good luck number and 1 wasn't. It took me longer to read because I'd count the lines in a paragraph. If I was writing a term paper, I couldn't have a certain number of words on a line if it added up to a bad number.

I was always worried that if I didn't do something my parents were going to die. Or I would worry about harming my parents, which was completely irrational. I couldn't wear anything that said Boston because my parents were from Boston. I couldn't write the word "death" because I was worried that something bad would happen.

Getting dressed in the morning was tough because I had a routine, and if I deviated from that routine, I'd have to get dressed again. I knew the rituals didn't make sense, but I couldn't seem to overcome them until I had therapy.

Twice as common as schizophrenia, OCD was overlooked or misdiagnosed for years. The essential features of OCD are recurrent obsessions or compulsions that are severe enough to be time consuming (for instance, taking more than 1 hour per day), cause marked distress, or lead to significant impairment (see *DSM-IV Diagnostic Criteria for Obsessive-Compulsive Disorder*). **Obsessions** are persistent ideas, thoughts, impulses, or images that are experienced as intrusive and inappropriate and cause marked anxiety or distress.[6] The experience of the intrusive or unpleasant quality of the thought is referred to as *ego dystonic,* that is, uncomfortable or foreign (as opposed to *ego syntonic,* which is experienced as natural or functional). The individual often tries to ignore or suppress

Critical Pathway: Anxiety

Care Needs	First 24 Hours	Days 2–5
Assessment/Evaluations	Past psych hx Medication hx Medical hx Suicide risk Self-care ability Approp legal status Psychiatric eval Nursing assessment	Family interview Social work eval Evals by OT, activity, group rx, PT Continue psych/nursing evals
Diagnostic Tests/Workup	Physical exam by MD/NP Lab tests inc. CBC, drug screen, chem panel, thyroid panel, others as approp ECG, other tests as approp	Review results of evals and lab work Implement interventions based on workup results Psychological testing Implement further medical workup as approp
Treatment	Orient to unit Initial activity orders	Multidisciplinary tx plan developed 1:1 psychotherapy Begin group, OT, PT, activities rx Participate in family sessions as approp
Medications	Order initial doses of approp meds for psych & medical symptoms Establish doses and intervals for prn meds Monitor responses and side effects	Monitor responses & side effects Adjust meds as approp
Safety/Self-care	Establish unit rules r/t suicide, elopement, substance abuse Monitor eating, sleep, self-care	Continue to monitor as per column 1 Begin interventions to enhance sleep
Education	Unit orientation Patient rights	Begin education on anxiety, phobias, medications Impact of workup/test results Educate on coping skills in stress management, insomnia, behavior management of phobias
Discharge Plan	Identify initial concerns	Identify patient/family concerns Identify possible resources/living arrangements
Outcomes	____ Patient assessed by MD and nurse ____ Initial activity orders in place ____ Patient does not harm self Progressing per pathway? Yes ____ No ____ If no, referred to ____	____ Assessments by all disciplines complete ____ Multidisciplinary tx plan implemented ____ Meds adjusted as needed ____ Medical workup complete ____ Patient begins participating in tx plan ____ Patient does not harm self Progressing per pathway? Yes ____ No ____ If no, referred to ____

Care Needs	Days 6–10+	Discharge
Assessment/Evaluations	Ongoing reassessment	
Diagnostic Tests/Workup	Further tests ordered as needed	Follow-up medical care determined & appointments made
Treatment	Continue psychotherapy, group, OT, PT Develop outpatient tx plan	Outpatient tx appointments in place Issues r/t insurance, transportation, work addressed to enhance compliance

Continued on following page

Critical Pathway: Anxiety (*Continued*)

	Days 6–10+	***Discharge***
Medications	Continue to monitor response and adjust doses as needed Consider tapering use of tranquilizers and hypnotics as approp Monitor side effects Determine meds at discharge	Identify discharge meds Ensure access to prescriptions
Safety/Self-care	Continue to monitor for high-risk behaviors Interventions for poor sleep, self-care deficits in place Establish family role in outpatient plan	Ensure resources in place for help Review plan with family Ensure patient has resources for food
Education	Continue education on anxiety Continue education on coping skills, medications, food and drug interactions, nutrition counseling, available community resources Teach stress management Educate on behavioral techniques for phobias	Provide education material to take home Reinforce teaching in outpatient tx
Discharge Plan	Outpatient tx plan developed Criteria for readmission established	Social worker reviews plan for outpatient tx, living arrangements, insurance, finances, activities Discharge transportation arranged Resources for assistance in place Family aware of outpatient tx
Outcomes	____ Patient participating in tx plan ____ Patient sleeping through the night ____ Stabilization of med doses ____ Reduction in use of prn tranquilizers and hypnotics ____ Patient demonstrates improvement and stabilization of symptoms ____ Patient does not harm self ____ Patient demonstrates use of new coping skills and stress management techniques Progressing per pathway? Yes ____ No ____ If no, referred to _____	____ Leaves hospital with understanding of discharge plan, prescriptions ____ Family verbalizes intention to participate in tx plan ____ Patient able to verbalize medication regimen ____ Verbalizes awareness of symptoms signaling need for more help & resources Progressing per pathway? Yes ____ No ____ If no, referred to _____

the obsessive thoughts, which creates a great deal of anxiety, and thus the individual attempts to neutralize the thoughts by repeating behaviors, so-called compulsions. **Compulsions** are behaviors or mental acts designed to prevent or reduce anxiety or distress. A client is aware that the thoughts or behaviors are excessive or unreasonable, but feels compelled to complete them. In fact, attempting to resist a compulsion may lead to a sense of mounting anxiety that is relieved only by yielding to the compulsion.

Many healthy people find themselves involved in certain "checking" behaviors, especially during times of high stress, such as checking to make sure they have their car keys along with them or occasionally rechecking the coffee pot or door lock. This behavior is problematic when it becomes repetitive and time consuming and interferes with daily functioning. Because obsessions or compulsions can displace useful and satisfying behaviors, they can be disruptive and restricting. Many people avoid objects or situations that provoke obsessions or compulsions; for example, clients avoid going out for fear that touching things will result in their contracting a dreaded disease.

According to the National Institute of Mental Health

> **DSM-IV Diagnostic Criteria for 300.3 Obsessive-Compulsive Disorder**
>
> A. Either obsessions or compulsions:
>
>   Obsessions as defined by (1), (2), (3), and (4):
>   (1) recurrent and persistent thoughts, impulses, or images that are experienced, at some time during the disturbance, as intrusive and inappropriate and that cause marked anxiety or distress
>   (2) the thoughts, impulses, or images are not simply excessive worries about real-life problems
>   (3) the person attempts to ignore or suppress such thoughts, impulses, or images, or to neutralize them with some other thought or action
>   (4) the person recognizes that the obsessional thoughts, impulses, or images are a product of his or her own mind (not imposed from without as in thought insertion)
>
>   Compulsions as defined by (1) and (2):
>   (1) repetitive behaviors (e.g., hand washing, ordering, checking) or mental acts (e.g., praying, counting, repeating words silently) that the person feels driven to perform in response to an obsession, or according to rules that must be applied rigidly
>   (2) the behaviors or mental acts are aimed at preventing or reducing distress or preventing some dreaded event or situation: however, these behaviors or mental acts either are not connected in a realistic way with what they are designed to neutralize or prevent or are clearly excessive
>
> B. At some point during the course of the disorder, the person has recognized that the obsessions or compulsions are excessive or unreasonable.
>
>   NOTE: This does not apply to children.
>
> C. The obsessions or compulsions cause marked distress, are time consuming (take more than 1 hour a day), or significantly interfere with the person's normal routine, occupational (or academic) functioning, or usual social activities or relationships.
>
> D. If another Axis I disorder is present, the content of the obsessions or compulsions is not restricted to it (e.g., preoccupation with food in the presence of an Eating Disorder; hair pulling in the presence of Trichotillomania; concern with appearance in the presence of Body Dysmorphic Disorder; preoccupation with drugs in the presence of a Substance Use Disorder; preoccupation with having a serious illness in the presence of Hypochondriasis; preoccupation with sexual urges or fantasies in the presence of a Paraphilia; or guilty ruminations in the presence of Major Depressive Disorder).
>
> E. The disturbance is not due to the direct physiological effects of a substance (e.g., a drug of abuse, a medication) or a general medical condition.
>
> *Specify* if:
> With Poor Insight: if, for most of the time during the current episode, the person does not recognize that the obsessions and compulsions are excessive or unreasonable
>
> **Source:** Reprinted with permission from the Diagnostic and Statistical Manual of Mental Disorders, Fourth Edition. Copyright 1994 American Psychiatric Association.

(NIMH),[4] "The person who suffers from OCD becomes trapped in a pattern of repetitive thoughts and behaviors that are senseless and distressing but extremely difficult to overcome." OCD occurs in a spectrum from mild to severe. If severe and left untreated, people are unable to function at work, school, or home. OCD is often unrecognized and shrouded in secrecy because of shame or embarrassment about symptoms. Many do not seek treatment, or by the time they come to treatment, they have learned to adapt their lives and families' lives around the rituals. Although they may have considerable understanding of the problem, this knowledge is not sufficient to overcome the behaviors.

Diagnostic Aids

Because OCD is often a hidden disorder, rating scales such as the Florida Obsessive-Compulsive are available for its detection (Table 20–5). Nurses can also ask these questions as part of the nursing assessment to screen for OCD. The Yale-Brown Obsession Compulsion Scale (YBOCS)[4] is a clinician-rated instrument that measures the severity of symptoms in three major domains: time spent, interference with life, and stress. Scores range from 0 to 40; on average, clients with OCD have scores around 24.

Culture, Age, and Gender Features

Culture and Gender

OCD is equally common in males and females and in all ethnic groups.[6] It may be more common in individuals from lower socioeconomic groups, in divorced or separated people, and in Catholics. OCD is more common in firstborn than in other children, suggesting that firstborn children may be subjected to higher rates of birth injury or harsher discipline.[14]

Age

Children and Adolescents. One-third of adults with OCD experienced symptoms as children. Children and ad-

> **RESEARCH NOTE**
>
> Baxter, LR, Schwartz, JM, Bergman, KS, et al: Caudate glucose metabolic rate changes with both drug and behavior therapy for obsessive-compulsive disorder. Arch Gen Psychiatry 49:681–689, 1992.
>
> **Findings:** Recent studies suggest that OCD is caused by brain abnormalities, particularly increased blood flow (glucose metabolism) to the caudate nucleus, part of the basal ganglia. These investigators used PET scans to determine cerebral blood flow before and after treatment. They studied two forms of treatment: fluoxetine (Prozac) or behavior therapy. After treatment, clients who responded to both drug and behavior therapy had decreased metabolism to the head of the caudate nucleus. Those who failed to respond to treatment did not show any differences in brain metabolism. The greater the effect of treatment, the greater the reduction in blood flow. Overall, treatment appeared to restore "normal" brain functioning.
>
> **Application to Practice:** This study indicates that abnormalities in glucose metabolism in the head of the caudate nucleus can be corrected by treatment. Regardless of type of treatment—behavioral or medication therapy—brain functioning is restored. Not only does this finding suggest that treatment appears to "heal" the brain, but also it indicates that nonpharmacologic treatment affects brain functioning. These findings may further our understanding about OCD's association with documented brain abnormalities that can be corrected by various forms of treatment. Nurses can educate clients and families that there is an important interaction between the way the brain functions, the appearance of symptoms, and the effects of nonpharmacologic treatments. It also gives hope to individuals with severe psychiatric disorders that research may help to predict treatment response.

olescents present with similar symptoms; however, the obsessions and compulsions may be less likely to be ego dystonic and unpleasant. In these cases, parents often identify behaviors.

Etiology

Genetic Theories

No clear genetic basis has been determined. However, families may have an increased risk of anxiety disorders in general. OCD occurs in families with Tourette's syndrome, as well as trichotillomania (a disorder of repeated hair pulling), suggesting some genetic overlap with these conditions. Although further research is necessary, OCD probably results from nongenetic factors.

Biological Theories

Serotonin Dysfunction. The leading theory is that serotonin plays a central but as yet undefined role in etiology. Researchers have found that the metabolite of serotonin, 5-hydroxyindoleacetic acid (5-HIAA), is both increased and decreased in OCD, suggesting that higher or lower levels of serotonin are present. When given medications that act like serotonin, such as m-CPP, obsessions and compulsions usually worsen, which suggests that increased serotonin may be involved. Medications that affect serotonin such as the SSRIs and clomipramine effectively treat OCD, also pointing to some type of dysfunction in the serotonin system.

Basal Ganglia and Frontal Abnormalities. Imaging studies such as PET scans suggest that clients with OCD have different patterns of brain activity than others. Increased brain flow and cerebral metabolism are present in the basal ganglia, particularly the caudate and orbitofrontal regions of the brain. The basal ganglia–frontal cortex and other systems help regulate thoughts and behaviors; they act like a brake to inhibit certain thoughts and actions. Dysfunction in this pathway is responsible for the unrelenting obsessional thoughts and ritualistic behaviors; when the "brake" fails, unwanted repetitive thoughts and behaviors prevail. If OCD is treated successfully with medication or cognitive-behavior therapy, these regions of the brain return to a normal state.

Prognosis

About 15% of OCD clients show progressive deterioration. Fewer, perhaps 5%, have an episodic course, with minimal to no symptoms between episodes.

OCD often coexists with other psychiatric disorders. Its high rate of comorbidity has recently led to the view that OCD is a series of spectrum disorders, rather than a distinct entity.[15] For example, the spectrum might include the following: OCD with eating disorders, OCD with tics, OCD and psychotic disorders, and OCD with affective disorders, rather than simply OCD alone.

Interventions for Hospitalized Clients

These individuals are usually hospitalized when symptoms become severe and life-threatening, for instance, refusal to eat, suicidal behavior, or a comorbid condition such as major depression. Interventions are aimed at resolving the other disorders and using the following treatments.

Interventions for Clients in the Community

The most effective treatment for both children and adults is a combination of cognitive-behavior therapy and psychopharmacology.[14,16] However, some clients fail to respond or respond only partially and continue to live with debilitating symptoms. If severe symptoms persist, alternative treatments such as psychosurgery may be used.

TABLE 20–5. A Screening Test for Obsessive-Compulsive Disorder

Part A

People who have Obsessive-Compulsive Disorder (OCD) experience recurrent, unpleasant thoughts (obsessions) and feel driven to perform certain acts over and over again (compulsions). Although sufferers usually recognize that the obsessions and compulsions are senseless or excessive, the symptoms of OCD often prove difficult to control without proper treatment. Obsessions and compulsions are not pleasurable; on the contrary, they are a source of distress. The following questions are designed to help people determine if they have symptoms of OCD and could benefit from professional help.

Part A. Please circle YES or NO.

Have you been bothered by unpleasant thoughts or images that repeatedly enter your mind, such as:

1. Concerns with contamination (dirt, germs, chemicals, radiation) or acquiring a serious illness such as AIDS?   Yes   No
2. Overconcern with keeping objects (clothing, groceries, tools) in perfect order or arranged exactly?   Yes   No
3. Images of death or other horrible events?   Yes   No
4. Personally unacceptable religious or sexual thoughts?   Yes   No

Have you worried a lot about terrible things happening, such as:

5. Fire, burglary, or flooding the house?   Yes   No
6. Accidentally hitting a pedestrian with your car or letting it roll down the hill?   Yes   No
7. Spreading an illness (giving someone AIDS)?   Yes   No
8. Losing something valuable?   Yes   No
9. Harm coming to a loved one because you weren't careful enough?   Yes   No

Have you worried about acting on an unwanted and senseless urge or impulse, such as:

10. Physically harming a loved one, pushing a stranger in front of a bus, steering your car into oncoming traffic, inapproprite sexual contact; or poisoning dinner guests?   Yes   No

Have you felt driven to perform certain acts over and over again, such as:

11. Excessive or ritualized washing, cleaning, or grooming?   Yes   No
12. Checking light switches, water faucets, the stove, door locks, or emergency brake?   Yes   No
13. Counting; arranging; evening-up behaviors (making sure socks are at same height)?   Yes   No
14. Collecting useless objects or inspecting the garbage before it is thrown out?   Yes   No
15. Repeating routine actions (in/out of chair, going through doorway, relighting cigarette a certain number of times or until it feels *just right*?   Yes   No
16. Need to touch objects or people?   Yes   No
17. Unnecessary rereading or rewriting; reopening envelopes before they are mailed?   Yes   No
18. Examining your body for signs of illness?   Yes   No
19. Avoiding colors ("red" means blood), number ("13" is unlucky), or names (those that start with "D" signify death) that are associated with dreaded events or unpleasant thoughts?   Yes   No
20. Needing to "confess" or repeatedly asking for reassurance that you said or did something correctly?   Yes   No

If you answered Yes to 2 *or more* of the above questions, please continue with Part B on the next page.

Part B

The following questions refer to the repeated thoughts, images, urges, or behaviors identified in Part A. Consider your experience during the past 30 days when selecting an answer. Circle the most appropriate number from 0 to 4.

	0	1	3	3	4
1. On average, how much *time* is occupied by these thoughts or behaviors each day?	None	Mild (less than 1 hour)	Moderate (1 to 3 hours)	Severe (3 to 8 hours)	Extreme (more than 8 hours)
2. How much *distress* do they cause you?	0 None	1 Mild	2 Moderate	3 Severe	4 Extreme (disabling)
3. How hard is it for you to *control* them?	0 Complete control	1 Much control	2 Moderate control	3 Little control	4 No control
4. How much do they cause you to *avoid* doing anything, going any place, or being with anyone?	0 No avoidance	1 Occasional avoidance	2 Moderate avoidance	3 Frequent and extensive	4 Extreme (housebound)

Continued on following page

TABLE 20–5. A Screening Test for Obsessive-Compulsive Disorder (*Continued*)

Part B

	0	1	2	3	4
5. How much do they *interfere* with school, work or your social or family life?	None	Slight interference	Definitely interferes with functioning	Much Interference	Extreme (disabling)

Sum on Part B (Add items 1 to 5): _____

Scoring: If you answered Yes to 2 or more of questions in Part A *and* scored 5 or more on Part B, you may wish to contact your physician, a mental health professional, or a patient advocacy group (such as the Obsessive Compulsive Foundation, Inc.) to obtain more information on OCD and its treatment. Remember, a high score on this questionnaire does not necessarily mean you have OCD—only an evaluation by an experienced clinician can make this determination.

Source: © Wayne K. Goodman, MD, 1994, Florida Obsessive-Compulsive Inventory (FOCI), Department of Psychiatry Specialty Clinics, University of Florida, Gainesville. Adapted with permission.

RESEARCH NOTE

Swedo, SE, Leonard, HL, Mittleman, BB, Allen, AJ, et al: Identification of children with pediatric autoimmune neuropsychiatric disorders associated with streptococcal infections by a marker associated with rheumatic fever. Am J Psychiatry 154:110–112, 1997.

Findings: Some children appear to develop OCD after exposure to streptococcal infections. In this report, the research team investigated the biological basis to this form of OCD. They identified a biological marker, an antibody, in the affected children, suggesting that a strep-induced form of OCD may be an autoimmune response triggered by antibodies. The antibodies produced to fight off the infection instead attack the basal ganglia of the brain, leading to symptoms of OCD such as hoarding, checking, and ritualistic handwashing. This team labeled these types of obsessive-compulsive disorder PANDAS, pediatric autoimmune neuropsychiatric disorders and associated disorders. Compared to healthy children, 85% of those with PANDAS have the identifiable antibody, D8/17.

Application to Practice: These preliminary results are the first to identify a biological marker for a psychiatric disorder. Long-term, this marker may help to screen children at risk for developing disorders such as OCD. Identification of the antibody may also help prevent the development of this severe chronic disorder. These results also provide more information about the etiology of anxiety disorders, suggesting that biology and environment interact to lead to the expression of symptoms. If biological markers such as D8/17 can be identified, then both pharmacologic and nonpharmacologic treatments can be used to correct the underlying biology. For example, these researchers are testing whether plasma treatments effectively eliminate the antibodies, thereby treating the immunological response and symptoms of OCD.

Cognitive-Behavior Interventions

In addition to the common cognitive-behavior techniques listed previously, clients respond to one particular method, "exposure and response prevention" therapy. This technique exposes them to whatever usually triggers the problem, which helps them forgo the usual ritual. Relaxation exercises are also used to increase their tolerance for uncomfortable or anxiety-provoking situations. The client is asked to gradually extend the time between the trigger and giving in to the ritual. The goal is to eventually decrease or extinguish the compulsive behaviors.

Antidepressants

The most successful antidepressants are those that strongly affect serotonergic functioning. Clomipramine, a TCA, has been used successfully for many years to treat both obsessions and compulsions. More recently, the SSRIs, fluvoxamine, fluoxetine, sertraline, and paroxetine, have also been effective; about 50 to 70% seem to respond to medication treatment. Higher doses than those used to treat depression are common. For instance, doses of 80 mg or more of fluoxetine are necessary to treat OCD. Response is often protracted, taking 8 to 12 weeks or longer. If an individual fails to respond to one agent, another medication may work. Certain augmentation strategies and combinations of drugs may be necessary if nonresponse continues.[17] For instance, clonazepam, a benzodiazepine, may be used in combination with an SSRI.

Other Treatment

Electroconvulsive therapy (ECT) and neurosurgery may be necessary for treatment-resistant clients, for example, those with severe symptoms who do not respond to several medication or behavior therapies. Neurosurgical techniques such as cingulotomy and capsulotomy disconnect pathways in the

Clinical Management Tips for Clients with Anxiety Disorders

Communication Techniques
- Use a calm, nonjudgmental tone.
- Reassure clients that treatment helps to reduce anxiety.
- Convey a tolerant, patient approach.
- Find a quiet, nondisturbing environment to engage the client.
- Reduce distractions such as noise and harsh lights.
- Avoid long, detailed explanations, particularly while the client is extremely anxious.

Client and Family Education
- Educate the client about the physiological reaction of the body to stress, including increased heart rate and breathing, tremors, and sweaty palms.
- Teach self-help skills such as assertiveness, relaxation therapy, and stress reduction techniques and their benefits.
- For those who are prescribed benzodiazepines, stress the need for compliance and the adverse effects of discontinuation, including seizures.
- For those who are prescribed SSRIs, educate about the side effects and risks.
- Provide written material to reinforce teaching.
- Teach about the etiology of anxiety disorders, stressing that the client is not to blame.
- Discuss the effects and duration of pharmacologic and nonpharmacologic treatment.

Ways to Reduce Anxiety and Promote Mental Health
- Encourage use of stress management techniques.
- Eliminate alcohol, caffeine, cigarettes, and other stimulating substances.
- Stress the need for a well-balanced diet.
- Encourage good sleep hygiene and the need for about 8 hours of sleep per night.
- Encourage exercise: at least 20 minutes of aerobic exercise 3 times per week.
- Teach and practice relaxation and breathing exercises.
- Teach and encourage assertiveness techniques.
- Practice cognitive-behavior techniques.
- Refer to a self-help anxiety group to promote support and socialization.
- Determine past successful coping strategies.
- Help the client increase self-awareness of thoughts that provoke anxiety or panic.
- Help the client problem solve.
- Monitor response to medications.
- Differentiate between side effects of anxiety and anxious symptoms in clients receiving SSRIs.
- Observe for changes in behavior that herald worsening anxiety.
- Monitor for severe anxiety escalating to self-harm or aggressive behaviors.
- Provide regular contact and staff time to discuss anxieties and fears.

---

brain, leading to symptom reduction. These techniques are described in the Chapter 14.

DIFFERENTIAL DIAGNOSIS[6]

Medical Disorders
- Medications or physical conditions may precipitate anxiety disorders.
- Symptoms are similar to anxiety disorders but are excluded from the diagnosis.
- Endocrine, cardiac, thyroid, or respiratory conditions commonly cause anxiety symptoms.
- Medical and pharmacologic conditions are considered before making the diagnosis of an anxiety disorder; medical conditions are listed in Table 20–6.

Major Depression
- Depressed mood is present daily for 2 weeks.
- Diagnosis requires the presence of four additional depressive symptoms, such as increased or decreased appetite, sleep disruption, low energy, poor self-esteem, poor concentration, indecision, or hopelessness.
- Can co-occur with anxiety disorders, particularly panic disorder and OCD.

Alcohol and Substance Abuse and Dependence
- Alcohol or illicit drugs may lead to symptoms of an anxiety disorder or coexist with it.
- Alcohol can lead to anxiety, abuse, and dependence and complicates treatment (see Chapter 17).
- Alcohol or substances may be used to self-medicate anxiety symptoms.
- Denial of a coexisting abuse or dependence disorder is likely.

Personality Disorders
- Personality disorders, especially borderline personality disorder, complicate diagnosis or coexist with anxiety disorders.
- Borderline personality disorder is characterized by frequent mood shifts without the other symptoms of depression or mania. Anger is the predominant mood.

TABLE 20-6. Common Medical Conditions Causing Anxiety Symptoms

Endocrine

Hyperthyroidism
Hypoparathyroidism
Hypoglycemia
Pheochromocytoma
Thyrotoxicosis
Thyroiditis
Cushing's disease
Endocrine neoplasias

Cardiovascular

Congestive heart failure
Pulmonary emboli
Arrhythmia
Tachycardia
Angina pectoris
Myocardial infarction

Respiratory

Chronic obstructive pulmonary disease
Pneumonia
Hyperventilation
Pneumothorax
Hypoxia

Intoxication with Substances

Cocaine
Amphetamines
Caffeine
Marijuana

Withdrawal from Alcohol, Sedative-Hypnotics, CNS Depressants

Thyroid preparations
Sympathomimetics
Xanthine derivatives
Antipsychotic medications
Theophylline

Metabolic

Vitamin B_2 deficiency
Porphyria
Metabolic acidosis
Infectious diseases

Neurological

Neoplasms
Encephalitis and CNS infections
Vestibular dysfunctions
Partial complex seizures
Alzheimer's disease
Huntington's disease
Transient ischemic attacks
Postconcussion syndrome
Parkinson's disease

Posttraumatic Stress Disorder (PTSD)

- Anxious mood and panic attacks may occur, but only in response to reminders or thoughts of a traumatic event.
- PTSD is characterized by three sets of behaviors: hyperarousal, reexperiencing symptoms, and avoidance behaviors.
- Requires the presence of an extremely stressful event, beyond most people's experience.

EXPECTED OUTCOMES

For the individual with an anxiety disorder, improvement will be demonstrated by:
- Absence of physical tension and symptoms
- Normalization of anxiety-provoking thoughts
- Decrease in worry and fear
- Ability to socialize and participate in daily life activities
- Absence of suicidal feelings and thoughts
- Reduction in anxious mood
- Realistic perception of self and positive self-esteem
- Ability to perform role functions
- Identification of anxiety-provoking thoughts
- Effective use of coping strategies
- Understanding of the nature of the anxiety disorder and ability to recognize impending symptoms in the future.

COMMON NURSING DIAGNOSES

Powerlessness
Hopelessness
Coping, individual, ineffective
Family Coping: ineffective, compromised
Anxiety
Fear
Social Isolation
Self Care Deficit, feeding, bathing/hygiene, dressing/grooming, toileting
Role Performance, altered
Violence, risk for, directed at self/others

SYNOPSIS OF CURRENT RESEARCH

The focus of recent research is the etiology of anxiety disorders and tests of specific treatments. Most research has been done on panic disorder and OCD. Panic disorder is thought to arise from a combination of factors: genetic, biological, and early life experiences, particularly traumatic separations. Studies on the effectiveness of cognitive-behavior therapy and medications indicate that the combination—for instance, imipramine plus desensitization techniques or alprazolam plus cognitive restructuring—is more effective than either alone. Studies are currently underway to compare the efficacy of the newer SSRIs and cognitive-behavior therapy. Researchers are also exploring whether new antidepressants such as venlafaxine and nefazodone alleviate symptoms of panic disorder.

Of all the anxiety disorders, OCD appears to be a definable neuropsychiatric condition. OCD either results from serotonin or brain abnormalities. The selective effectiveness of SSRIs and clomipramine, medications that affect serotonin to a high degree, led to theories about serotonin dysfunction. Although both increased and decreased levels of serotonin have been reported, recent studies suggest that clients with OCD have an overactive serotonin system. The other leading theory, abnormalities in the orbital frontal lobes and basal ganglia (particularly the caudate), is one of the most reproducible findings in psychiatric illness. Clients have increased activity in the brain circuit of these areas, leading to more obsessional thinking and an inability to "turn off" the uncomfortable thoughts. One study found that when individuals with OCD were exposed to a stimulus that provoked their obsessions—for example, a "contaminated" glove—their brain activity dramatically increased in frontal lobes and the caudate. Behavior therapy or pharmacotherapy reversed the excess brain activity to these affected regions. The serotonin and brain abnormalities may be related; serotonin may stimulate the frontal lobes, leading to the observed increase in brain activity and blood flow and the development of unrelenting obsessions and compulsions.

AREAS FOR FUTURE RESEARCH

- How do hormones influence the higher prevalence of anxiety disorders in females?
- Do cultural factors underlie the gender differences in the incidence of anxiety disorders?
- What alterations in circadian rhythms, if any, predispose an individual to develop an anxiety disorder?
- How do education and regular use of various techniques such as relaxation exercises, therapeutic touch, and guided imagery affect outcome?
- How do the newer antidepressant drugs affect anxiety disorders?
- What symptoms in childhood predict a severe anxiety disorder later in life?
- Is pharmacotherapy effective for children and the elderly who have anxiety disorders?

CASE STUDY

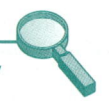

Tammie S was a 24-year-old single woman who contacted the outpatient psychiatric clinic at her doctor's request. She had been in the emergency room the previous day, fearing that she was having a heart attack. Her presenting complaint was daily "attacks" for the past 3 weeks consisting of 10 to 15 minutes of dizziness, shortness of breath, palpitations, tingling and numbness in her arms, and sweaty palms. She stated that the attacks came on for no apparent reason and could happen "anywhere" (at home or work, or while shopping or driving). Over the past week she had been avoiding going to the grocery store or driving for fear of an attack. When asked if there were any stressors in her life, she replied, "Not really . . . I started a new job 2 months ago, but I like it. My boyfriend and I moved 2 months ago. I worry about him because he has only one kidney and may need dialysis. My sister-in-law died suddenly 2 weeks ago. I seem to be handling it all right."

A nurse practitioner (NP) interviewed the client in the outpatient clinic. She confirmed that a complete physical exam with electrocardiogram and lab tests had ruled out any medical reason for the symptoms. The NP discussed the symptoms of panic attacks and explained that panic disorder was a common anxiety disorder, particularly in women. Tammie was initially very nervous about hearing that she had a "psychiatric problem." They discussed her fears, in particular, her fear of "being crazy." They also discussed the possibilities for treatment, including referral to a psychotherapist specializing in cognitive-behavior therapy to help her control her thoughts and severe panic anxiety. When they reviewed medication options, Tammie reacted strongly, saying she "didn't need drugs." The NP explained that the combination of therapy and medications would probably be the most beneficial. She also told her to avoid caffeine and alcohol and begin a regular exercise pattern. In addition, the NP shared her concern about all the recent changes in Tammie's life. Tammie began to realize that the recent stressors may have also contributed to her anxiety attacks. Tammie refused medication treatment and decided to seek out a therapist in the community, try to make some lifestyle changes, and develop other ways to cope with her symptoms.

CRITICAL THINKING QUESTIONS

1. What measures could the nurse have taken during the interview to make Tammie more comfortable about discussing her symptoms?
2. What, if any, factors or life events could have contributed to panic attacks at this time in Tammie's life?
3. Identify the key elements of education for this individual, her boyfriend, and her family.
4. What factors suggest that cognitive-behavior therapy and medication are indicated?
5. Which theories best explain the behaviors presented?
6. What are possible long-term interventions to assist Tammie in daily living and overall quality of life?

CASE STUDY

Amy had always been a meticulously neat and orderly person. As a student, she had her homework done days before the due date but went over and over the project, changing answers. After college she married, at age 22, and soon had a son, Allan. After 2 years of marriage, she and her husband were having communication and companionship difficulties. They began divorce proceedings, and a very difficult custody battle over Allan ensued. Amy found that she began to have intrusive thoughts and worries that something would happen to Allan, such as his lunch would be poisoned at the babysitter's, or he would be kidnapped by a burglar. Seemingly unrelated to the issues involving Allan, she also began to find that more of her time was occupied by rituals, especially in the morning. Specifically, she put all of the items in her closet, drawers, and kitchen cabinets in order. If interrupted, she had to start again from the beginning, for fear that she might have forgotten one crucial step. Once everything was in order, she began a checking process of all lights, electrical appliances, and door locks. Even then, she feared she had forgotten something important as soon as she started out the door. At that point she felt compelled to check again from the beginning. These repetitive behaviors were time consuming, taking hours, and often left Amy exhausted. Her only relief was at work. There she was distracted temporarily by answering the phone and talking to customers. However, she began calling her babysitter several times a day to check on her son.

Amy's family first spoke to their primary care provider about her unusual behavior. They worried that it would be an issue in the custody hearing and asked if she could receive any help. They also noted that Amy's grandfather had had similar behaviors.

Amy finally sought treatment at a community mental health clinic. The nurse told her that OCD was a common condition that affected 1 in every 50 people. They discussed ways to treat the disorder: medication and behavior therapy. Amy worked with a cognitive-behavior therapist to break the repetitive thoughts of harm to her son and her checking behaviors. The nurse encouraged stress management through diet, sleep, exercise, and relaxation techniques.

In spite of her willingness to practice cognitive-behavior techniques, Amy's anxiety increased with the approach of the custody hearing. She felt increasingly depressed and hopeless. She began taking fluvoxamine 50 mg daily and increased it to the maximum dose in a couple of weeks. The nurse told Amy that it would possibly take weeks to have some effect, and slowly they noticed that her obsessions and compulsions began to diminish. After about 4 weeks of pharmacotherapy, and with continued cognitive-behavior therapy, she reported some improvement in symptoms. However, only 3 months later did her behaviors markedly diminish. She remained in treatment to cope with the recent stressors and some mild symptoms.

CRITICAL THINKING QUESTIONS

1. What behaviors did Amy exhibit during her school years that may have suggested a tendency toward OCD?
2. How would the nurse use diagnostic aids to support the diagnosis of OCD?
3. What is the major difference between the thoughts and worries Amy experienced and paranoid fears experienced by a person with a psychotic disorder like schizophrenia?
4. Explain the mechanism of action of fluvoxamine and its biological effects on OCD.
5. What factors indicate cognitive-behavior therapy and medication?
6. Identify behaviors suggesting that Amy is responding to treatment.
7. What are possible long-term interventions to help Amy cope with recent stressors, raising her son, and managing symptoms?

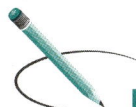

KEY POINTS

- Anxiety can exist on different levels from mild to severe; it can be adaptive or maladaptive.
- Anxiety disorders are the most prevalent of known psychiatric illnesses, are common in all cultures, and affect twice as many women as men.
- Anxiety disorders include panic disorder, agoraphobia, obsessive-compulsive disorder (OCD), generalized anxiety disorder (GAD), and phobia.
- Research on the biology of anxiety disorder points to a dysfunction of GABA receptors in the CNS.
- Biological theories of panic disorder include disturbances in lactate, the respiratory system, norepinephrine, serotonin, adenosine, and GABA.
- There is growing evidence for a genetic predisposition for the development of anxiety disorders.
- Research on the effectiveness of certain drugs in treating anxiety disorders has supported the involvement of certain neurotransmitters, such as GABA, norepinephrine, dopamine, and serotonin.
- A thorough assessment is crucial to rule out medical conditions that can mimic anxiety disorders.
- Diagnostic aids such as the Florida Obsessive-Compulsive Inventory (FOCI) and the Yale-Brown Obsessive-Compulsive Scale (Y-BOCS) can be useful to screen for symptoms and assess treatment response in children and adults.
- OCD results from abnormalities in serotonin and the brain, specifically the basal ganglia and the orbital frontal cortex.
- There is a high comorbidity of anxiety disorders with other psychiatric disorders, especially depression.
- Individuals with anxiety disorders sometimes self-medicate with alcohol, cannabis, or other substances and may develop comorbid substance-abuse problems.
- Nursing care strategies are designed to help the individual accept anxiety as a normal occurrence, gain increased self-awareness, and learn and apply self-help or stress management techniques to reduce anxiety and foster a sense of mastery over one's life.
- A combination of cognitive-behavior therapy and pharmacotherapy is often used to treat anxiety disorders.
- The benzodiazepines and antidepressants are effective for treatment of anxiety disorders.
- Certain characteristics have been identified in more stress-resistant persons: an internal locus of control, a

healthy lifestyle, a well-balanced diet, regular exercise, and a good support network.

REFERENCES

1. Teicher, M: Biology of anxiety. Med Clin North Am 72:791, 1988.
2. Peplau, HE: Anxiety, self, and hallucinations. In O'Toole, AW, and Welt, SR (eds): Interpersonal Theory in Nursing Practice. Springer Publishing Co Inc, New York, 1989.
3. Flannery, RB: From victim to survivor: A stress management approach in the treatment of learned helplessness. In Psychological Trauma. American Psychiatric Association, Washington, DC, 1987, p 217.
4. National Institute of Mental Health: Pamphlets: Anxiety Disorders (No. 943879), Panic Disorder (No. 933508), Understanding Panic Disorder (No. 933509), Obsessive-Compulsive Disorder (No. 943755), U.S. Government Printing Office, Washington, DC, 1994.
5. Laraia, MT: Biological correlates of panic disorder with agoraphobia: Practice perspectives for nurses. Arch Psychiat Nurs 5:373, 1991.
6. American Psychiatric Association: The Diagnostic and Statistical Manual of Mental Disorders, ed 4. American Psychiatric Association, Washington, DC, 1994, p 393.
7. Sheikh, JI: Anxiety disorders and their treatment. Clin Geriatr Med 8:411, 1992.
8. Rosenbaun, JF: Evaluation and management of the treatment-resistant anxiety disorder patient. Paper presented at American Psychiatric Association meeting, May 27, Washington, DC, 1992.
9. Torgersen, S: Twin studies in panic disorder. In Ballenger, J, and Liss, AR (eds): Neurobiology of Panic Disorder. New York, 1990, p 51.
10. Pohl, R, Yeragani, VK, Balon, R, et al: Isoproterenol-induced panic attacks. Biol Psychiatry 24:891, 1988.
11. Klein, DF: False suffocation alarms, spontaneous panics, and related conditions: An integrative hypothesis. Arch Gen Psychiatry 50:306, 1993.
12. Barlow, D: Cognitive-behavior approaches to panic disorder and social phobia. Paper presented at American Psychological Association Meeting, May 27, Washington, DC, 1992.
13. Humphrey, J: Stress in the Nursing Profession. Charles Thereus, IL, 1988.
14. Schwab, JJ: Obsessive-compulsive disorder: Recent advances. Clinical Advances in the Treatment of Psychiatric Disorders 9:111, 1995.
15. Hollander, E, and Wong, C: Developments in the treatment of obsessive-compulsive disorder. Primary Psychiatry 1995.
16. Greist, JH, et al: Efficacy and tolerability of serotonin transport inhibitors in obsessive-compulsive disorder. Arch Gen Psychiatry 52:53, 1995.
17. Rasmussen, S: The treatment of obsessional depression. Lecture given on March 22, Tyngsboro, MA, 1995.

CHAPTER 21
Somatoform Disorders

CHAPTER 21

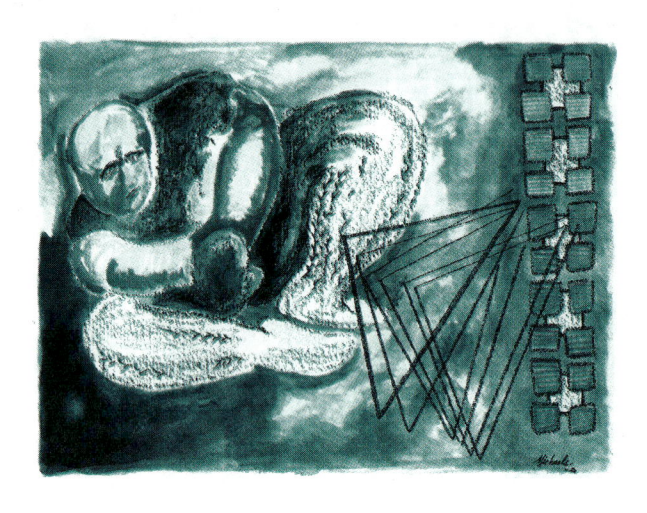

CHAPTER OUTLINE

Somatization
Definition
Characteristic Behaviors
Culture, Age, and Gender Features
Etiology
Prognosis
Assessment
Planning Care
Interventions for Hospitalized Clients
Interventions for Clients in the Community
Expected Outcomes
Differential Diagnosis

Undifferentiated Somatoform Disorder

Conversion Disorder
Characteristic Behaviors
Culture, Age, and Gender Features
Etiology
Assessment
Planning Care
Interventions for Hospitalized Clients
Interventions for Clients in the Community
Expected Outcomes

Pain Disorder
Characteristic Behaviors
Etiology
Assessment
Planning Care
Intervention for Hospitalized Clients
Intervention for Clients in the Community
Expected Outcomes

Hypochondriasis
Characteristic Behaviors
Culture, Age, and Gender Features
Etiology
Prognosis
Assessment
Planning Care
Interventions for Clients in the Community
Expected Outcomes

Body Dysmorphic Disorder
Characteristic Behaviors
Culture, Age, and Gender Features
Etiology
Assessment

Stephanie Stockard Spelic, MSN, RN, CS, CPC, LMHP

Somatoform Disorders

Planning Care
Interventions for Clients in the Community
Expected Outcomes
Somatoform Disorder Not Otherwise Specified
Expected Outcomes
Common Nursing Diagnoses
Synopsis of Current Research
Areas for Future Research

LEARNING OBJECTIVES

After completing this chapter, the reader should be able to:

- Describe the symptoms and behaviors of the somatoform disorders.
- Explain the theories of the somatization process.
- Discuss the process of somatosensory amplification.
- Identify common cultural and gender features of individual somatoform disorders.
- Use the nursing process in planning and delivering care for clients with a somatoform disorder.
- Describe common comorbid psychiatric disorders found with somatoform disorder.
- Identify ethical and care issues related to the identification of somatoform disorder.

KEY TERMS

conversion
hypochondriasis
la belle indifference
primary gain
secondary gain
somatization
somatosensory amplification

There's nothing wrong with my brain, I'm not some kind of nutcracker, you know. You're darn right I feel depressed, but that's because I've traveled from doctor to doctor feeling absolutely miserable, and nobody seems to be able to find out what's causing all these problems I have. My body aches constantly. It's agony to move and my stomach is always hurting, not to mention a lump the size of a golf ball in my throat. I feel dizzy and exhausted all the time so I can't exercise or even go anywhere because I'm afraid I'll collapse and hurt myself even more.

Nobody really understands how much I've suffered, and I sure don't get any sympathy from my husband—huh! Him! I could be on death's door and he'd just move me out of the way so he could go play golf. We went to the Mayo Clinic even, and they couldn't figure out what was wrong with me. Said I was the most puzzling case they'd ever had. Do you know what my husband did the whole time I was in agony and having all these tests and procedures? He played golf.

Doctors just pat you on the head and tell you that you need another tranquilizer. They don't realize that I feel so awful and can't do anything at all, even be sociable. My neighbors never stop over and my two daughters are married and have kids. They're too busy to call unless they want to borrow money or ask me to babysit.

SOMATIZATION

The common denominator in the seven specific diagnoses in the category of somatoform disorders is that the client presents with physical symptoms, such as headache, gastrointestinal distress, or pain, that seem to suggest impaired physical health. However, the physical symptoms cannot be explained by a medical condition, substance abuse, or mental disorder (such as panic disorder). In short, the symptoms are medically unexplainable yet intense enough to cause significant distress or impairment in social, occupational, or other areas of functioning.[1]

The unification of mind and body is an ancient concept. Aristotle wrote about the effects of the emotions upon the body. In the early 1900s, Sigmund Freud began to formulate the idea that anxiety could be demonstrated in various "neuroses" or in mental and emotional illnesses, such as conversion hysteria, that included physical symptoms.

As the twentieth century progressed, researchers began to develop the concept of psychosomatic illness (*psycho* meaning "mind," *soma* meaning "body"), that is, illness that may be caused or exacerbated by the individual's emotional state. Also, as science advanced, more diagnostic equipment and tests became available to differentiate and confirm medical conditions.

Definition

Somatoform is defined as the use of physical symptoms to express emotional problems and psychosocial stress.[2] **Somatization** may be due to many factors, but it is not considered a psychiatric (somatoform) disorder unless behaviors meet certain criteria.

Characteristic Behaviors

At the far end of the continuum of somatization are somatoform disorders. They may be viewed as behavioral expressions of emotion (e.g., loneliness, fear, or anxiety) or emotional needs (e.g., attention, recognition, and belonging) or as cognitive responses: learned behaviors or coping styles that permit needs to be met. Table 21–1 compares criteria for the somatoform disorders.

Somatization disorder was previously known as hysteria or Briquet's syndrome. Its main feature is a pattern of multiple, recurring, and significant physical complaints. The significance of the complaint is judged by whether it is treated medically (e.g., with medication) or is causing significant impairment in an individual's social, occupational, or other roles.

Somatic symptoms often begin before age 30 and occur over a period of several years. Clients with somatization disorder most often present to a general practitioner. Their complaints usually involve more than one organ system and have existed over many years *without* development of physical signs or structural abnormalities that would be present in an advancing, chronic medical condition. There are also no laboratory findings or diagnostic tests that suggest any medical condition. See Table 21–1 for other diagnostic criteria and prevalence, cultural and gender factors, and familial patterns.

Culture, Age, and Gender Features

Golding and colleagues[3] found that more women than men were diagnosed with somatization disorder, but that men were less often perceived by physicians as having unexplained symptoms. Both men and women presented with common symptoms, either pseudoneurological or gastrointestinal. Accompanying diagnoses for women with somatization disorder were major depression or anxiety disorders, whereas accompanying diagnoses for men were alcohol abuse and anxiety disorders.

Etiology

Roberts[4] reviewed several theories of the causes of somatization, including neurobiological, psychological, individuality, perceptual-cognitive, and environmental factors.

Neurobiological Theories

Somatization may be related to the manner in which the central nervous system (CNS) regulates incoming sensory information. There may be either too little inhibition of sensory input, causing an amplified awareness of somatic symptoms, or too much inhibition of sensory input, which may cause a decrease in associating feelings with bodily responses.

Another theory holds that some individuals may have deficient communication between brain hemispheres and thus are unable to express their emotions directly (*alexithymia*); they therefore present physical instead of emotional symptoms. Clients who somatize or have somatoform disorders tend to lack insight into their feelings and have little ability to verbally communicate psychological distress.

Psychological and Psychosocial Theories

Personality and psychological factors have also been implicated. Rodin[5] believed the physical symptoms develop from the individual's inadequate sense of self, related to a lack of empathic and nurturing relationships. Indeed, much research in this area suggests emotional or physical neglect, illness of family members, and sexual or physical abuse as factors in somatoform disorders. Rosen and colleagues[2] suggested that sociocultural or family factors may be involved. For example, if physical symptoms provide relief from unwanted responsibilities, this behavior may become a learned coping style.

Somatization may be viewed as a way of experiencing and communicating somatic distress in response to psychosocial stress, which causes the client to seek medical help.[6] Bass and Benjamin[7] view somatization as a process in which the focus on physical symptoms is "inappropriate" and there is a denial of psychosocial problems. The client's symptoms may permit avoidance of responsibilities (**primary gain**) and caring responses from others (**secondary gain**). Other theorists[8] view somatization as a continuum in which high levels of somatic symptoms signal a greater degree of distress, disability, and maladaptive illness behavior.

Another psychological view of the somatization process finds a representation of inner emotional conflicts of which the client is unaware. For example, an individual is unable to connect a constant, gnawing abdominal pain with unconscious fears that his or her spouse will leave. The client may be completely unaware that those fears of abandonment relate to childhood losses and are manifest in physical symptoms.

Adaptation Theory

Viewed from Roy's adaptation-conceptual framework for nursing,[9] somatoform disorders encompass both adaptation problems and coping problems. The client's physical symptoms are attempts to adapt to a particular stimulus, stressor, or life situation. Although the client's coping mechanisms may have been effective initially, they begin to significantly interfere with, rather than augment, adaptive functioning. The regulator mechanism described by Roy is the autonomic nervous system that prepares the individual for coping by approach, attack, or flight. The autonomic responses in the client with a somatoform disorder may actually increase the focus on bodily symptoms and the belief that one is "sick."

TABLE 21–1. DSM-IV Comparison of Somatoform Disorders

Diagnostic Criteria	Somatization Disorder	Undifferentiated Somatoform Disorder	Conversion Disorder	Pain Disorder	Hypochondriasis	Body Dysmorphic Disorder	Somatoform Disorder (NOS) (not otherwise specified)
Significantly impaired social occupational or other role function	Yes	Yes	Yes	Yes	Yes	Yes	Not necessary for diagnosis
Symptoms have been present 6 months or longer	Yes	Yes	No	Acute: No Chronic: Yes	Yes	No	No
After full medical investigation, symptoms cannot be explained by known general medical condition or direct effects of substance (e.g., drug abuse or medication)	Yes	Yes	Yes (or explained by culturally sanctioned behavior)	Yes (unless a medical condition is associated with pain)	Yes	Yes	Yes
Psychological stressors or conflicts appear to be related to the onset or exacerbation of symptoms or deficits	Not necessary for diagnosis	Not necessary for diagnosis	Yes	Yes	Not necessary for diagnosis	Not necessary for diagnosis	Not necessary for diagnosis
The production of symptoms is not intentional or feigned	Yes	Yes	Yes	Yes	Not necessary for diagnosis	Not necessary for diagnosis	Not necessary for diagnosis
Prevalence of Disorders (Based on U.S. Studies)	Est. 0.2–2%, Women <0.2%, Men	No statistics available	Estimated 11 to 300/100,000 general population; 1–3% outpatient referrals	Common (10–15% of all adults have disability due to back pain alone)	General population, unknown In medical practice, 4–9%	No reliable statistics, but thought to be more common than previously believed	No data

Continued on following page

TABLE 21–1. DSM-IV Comparison of Somatoform Disorders (Continued)

Diagnostic Criteria	Somatization Disorder	Undifferentiated Somatoform Disorder	Conversion Disorder	Pain Disorder	Hypochondriasis	Body Dysmorphic Disorder	Somatoform Disorder (NOS) (not otherwise specified)
Cultural and Gender Features	Wide variations in cultural symptoms. Frequency derived from U.S. studies, but higher rates of diagnosis in Greek and Puerto Rican men indicate culture affects prevalence in men vs. women.	Highest frequency of symptoms found in young women of low socioeconomic status, but the disorder may occur to an individual of any age, gender, or sociocultural group	More common in 1. rural population 2. low socioeconomic group 3. those less educated in medical/psychological concepts 4. those in developing countries 5. ages 10–35 6. more common in women; est. women: men 2:1–10:1	Varies according to ethnic/cultural group; may occur at any age; women experience certain chronic pain conditions (headaches and musculoskeletal pain) more frequently than men	Equally common in men and women; cultural factors may play a role	No data	No data
Familial Patterns	10–20% in 1st-degree female biological relatives of women with this disorder; male relatives have higher rates of antisocial individuality disorder and substance-related disorders; genetic and environmental factors contribute to risk	No data	Data suggest more frequent in relatives; increased risk in monozygotic twins reported	Depression, alcohol dependence, and chronic pain may be seen more often in 1st-degree biological relatives	Serious childhood illness and disease of close family member; death of close individual; anxiety or depression may contribute	No data	No data

Source: Adapted from the Diagnostic and Statistical Manual of Mental Disorders, Fourth Edition. Copyright 1994 American Psychiatric Association.

> ### DSM-IV Criteria for Somatization and Undifferentiated Somatoform Disorder
>
> **Diagnostic Criteria for 300.81 Somatization Disorder**
>
> A. A history of many physical complaints beginning before age 30 years that occur over a period of several years and result in treatment being sought or significant impairment in social, occupational, or other important areas of functioning.
>
> B. Each of the following criteria must have been met, with individual symptoms occurring at any time during the course of the disturbance:
> (1) four pain symptoms: a history of pain related to at least four different sites or functions (e.g., head, abdomen, back, joints, extremities, chest, rectum, during menstruation, during sexual intercourse, or during urination)
> (2) two gastrointestinal symptoms: a history of at least two gastrointestinal symptoms other than pain (e.g., nausea, bloating, vomiting other than during pregnancy, diarrhea, or intolerance of several different foods)
> (3) one sexual symptom: a history of at least one sexual or reproductive symptom other than pain (e.g., sexual indifference, erectile or ejaculatory dysfunction, irregular menses, excessive menstrual bleeding, vomiting throughout pregnancy)
> (4) one pseudoneurological symptom: a history of at least one symptom or deficit suggesting a neurological condition not limited to pain (conversion symptoms such as impaired coordination or balance, paralysis or localized weakness, difficulty swallowing or lump in throat, aphonia, urinary retention, hallucinations, loss of touch or pain sensation, double vision, blindness, deafness, seizures; dissociative symptoms such as amnesia; or loss of consciousness other than fainting)
>
> C. Either (1) or (2):
> (1) after appropriate investigation, each of the symptoms in Criterion B cannot be fully explained by a known general medical condition or the direct effects of a substance (e.g., a drug of abuse, a medication)
> (2) when there is a related general medical condition, the physical complaints or resulting social or occupational impairment are in excess of what would be expected from the history, physical examination, or laboratory findings
>
> D. The symptoms are not intentionally produced or feigned (as in Factitious Disorder or Malingering)
>
> **Diagnostic Criteria for 300.81 Undifferentiated Somatoform Disorder**
>
> A. One or more physical complaints (e.g., fatigue, loss of appetite, gastrointestinal or urinary complaints)
>
> B. Either (1) or (2):
> (1) after appropriate investigation, the symptoms cannot be fully explained by a known general medical condition or the direct effects of a substance (e.g., a drug of abuse, a medication)
> (2) when there is a related general medical condition, the physical complaints or resulting social or occupational impairment is in excess of what would be expected from the history, physical examination, or laboratory findings.
>
> C. The symptoms cause clinically significant distress or impairment in social, occupational, or other important areas of functioning.
>
> D. The duration of the disturbance is at least 6 months.
>
> E. The disturbance is not better accounted for by another mental disorder (e.g., another Somatoform Disorder, Sexual Dysfunction, Mood Disorder, Anxiety Disorder, Sleep Disorder, or Psychotic Disorder).
>
> F. The symptom is not intentionally produced or feigned (as in Factitious Disorder or Malingering).
>
> **Source:** Adapted from the Diagnostic and Statistical Manual of Mental Disorders, Fourth Edition. Copyright 1994 American Psychiatric Association.

Cognitive-Perceptual Theory

Another theory about the cause of somatization is the concept of **somatosensory amplification**, which Barsky and colleagues[10] defined as "the tendency to experience somatic sensation as intense, noxious, and disturbing." They postulate that amplification requires three elements. First, the individual is in a state of hypervigilance (as in family or cultural attention to anxiety or fear) or has heightened attention to bodily sensation (as in family or cultural attention to bodily symptoms, or physical disease in a family member). Second, amplification is displayed as the individual selects and focuses on what seem to be relatively mild and infrequent bodily sensations. Finally, amplification involves the individual's disposition or tendency to react to somatic sensation with feelings and thoughts that intensify them and make them more frightening and disturbing.

For example, a nursing student is studying gastrointestinal disorders. The act of reading and hearing about these disorders heightens awareness of bodily sensations (element 1). Because the student is so aware of this topic and is also somewhat anxious and hypervigilant (as students may be), he or she then may become aware of occasional minor aching in the colon (element 2). The student then becomes concerned that he or she has colitis and is even more anxious, stimulating the autonomic nervous system, which then causes cramping, gastrointestinal distress, and diarrhea. The student's "diagnosis" of colitis may then be "confirmed," and fear and concern increase (element 3).

Amplification is not limited to sensations that are symptomatic of disease. It can also encompass other stimuli, such as noise or sensation. Barsky and colleagues[10] define *amplification* as both a state and a trait. A *trait* is a feature of an individual that is characteristic of that individual and is stable over time. For example, being organized or being "hyper" are traits. Traits can be learned from childhood experiences or can be constitutional, in other words, the way an individual is "wired" at birth. Both experience and constitution may work together, as will be seen in the etiologies of some somatoform disorders.

Amplification also refers to the degree to which sensations are amplified at a given time. Factors such as mood, circumstance, and level of arousal influence *state* amplification. Somatic amplification plays a role in those functional (no medical cause) symptoms seen in somatoform disorders, as well as in depression that is masked by somatic symptoms.

Clients who presented to a medical clinic with upper respiratory infections (URIs) were asked to report on the amount of distress caused by their symptoms and their levels of anxiety, depression, hostility, and amplification.[12] The severity of the clients' symptoms was compared to an objective checklist of doctors' ratings of disease severity. Results showed that amplification was closely associated with depression, anxiety, and hostility, in that these feelings may make people feel sicker overall.[13] A tendency to amplify makes the client focus on localized symptoms and report them as more severe than the objective measures.

Multifactorial Theory

Any number of connections between body and mind, such as genetic predisposition, genetic vulnerability, neurochemical balances, biochemical factors, and the effects of stress (such as abuse or neglect), may combine to produce physical or mental illness.

Prognosis

The prognosis for somatization disorder is not optimistic if the client is not properly diagnosed and treated. Beginning before age 30 and over a period of years, the symptoms form a behavioral pattern and coping mechanism. With proper diagnosis and treatment, especially in cases of comorbid disorders such as depression or alcohol abuse, the client may be able to return to a productive life.

Assessment

Signs of somatization disorder may be observed as early as adolescence, when physical symptoms become the coping behavior for emotional stress. A combination of the pain and gastrointestinal or neurological symptoms described by the *DSM-IV* may be presented as an ongoing behavior pattern, for example, visits to the school nurse or frequent "sick days." Look for a pattern of illness or missed school or work days.

Clients with somatization disorder present in the medical setting rather than the psychiatric setting because of their conviction that the problems are medical and unrelated to any emotions or psychosocial stress. Nursing assessment of this client begins with reviewing the client's current complaints and history of illnesses. Because clients with this disorder typically are "inconsistent historians," medical records should be checked for objective evidence when possible.

Cater[11] hypothesized a possible overlap of somatization disorder and chronic candidiasis syndrome and noted that some clients with somatization disorder had decreased symptomatology with treatment for chronic candidiasis.

The client may present the physical symptoms in a very dramatic or colorful way or may be very demanding, angry, or hostile. It is not uncommon to hear the client give an exhaustive account of tests, diagnostic studies, treatments, and medications that have been tried to no avail, often coming into the clinic with notebooks, charts, and old records detailing previous ailments and treatments. The client may be negative toward all previous health-care providers for failing to discover and treat what he or she believes to be a serious medical condition. The client may have previously been told "it's all in your head" and react defensively toward all health-care professionals.

The client should receive a thorough medical evaluation. If possible, avoid repeating recently performed tests that had negative results. Rather than relying on the client's recollection, the previous health-care data and documented results should be obtained. Following this evaluation, if no organic cause can be found, or if there is some general medical condition unrelated to the client's concerns, the diagnosis of somatization disorder would be considered. In such diagnosing, it is important to be specific.

- Assess for any history of physical, sexual, or emotional abuse.
  - Were you ever mistreated (hit, kicked, punched) by your parents or adults caring for you?
  - Have you ever been sexually abused, molested, raped, or assaulted? Describe what you mean. (Be sure to ask both male and female clients.)
- Assess for recent life stressors.
  - Have you been under stress recently?
  - Has anyone close to you been ill or died?
  - Have you ever lost a child?
  - Tell me about your job.

- Assess for coexisting depression, suicide ideation, and drug or alcohol use.
    - Have you felt down or sad lately?
    - Is it harder to do your usual activities?
    - Do you ever feel hopeless?
    - Have you ever felt like hurting yourself?
    - What medications or drugs have you taken (or) what have you done to relieve your physical symptoms?
    - Do you find that alcohol relieves your symptoms at times?

In assessing primary and secondary gain, the nurse might say, "Tell me how these physical symptoms have interfered with your life." The client with a somatization disorder will usually report problems in relationships and role function: "My husband and I never have sex," "I've missed a lot of work," or "I can't work." The client may also be on disability.

The client should be asked, "What kind of response do you get from your family and significant others when you are ill?" The client may say that initially there was concern but now he or she is ignored: "People don't realize what I'm going through" or "They don't believe I'm ill."

The nurse will also encounter defense mechanisms such as denial of any feelings or emotional distress, displacement by focusing and refocusing on the somatic symptoms, and projection of blame to past or present health-care providers.

These clients often elicit negative or frustrated responses from health-care providers. Nurses often feel these clients are "just lazy" or "complainers" and resent caring for them when "really sick clients need care." Understanding that the client with somatization disorder is, in fact, ill and will benefit from treatment will help the nurse remain empathic and objective.

Planning Care

Clients with somatoform disorder may have several related nursing diagnoses. Most evident is the sensory or perceptual alteration that may be related to repressed anxiety, psychological stress, unmet dependency needs, and low self-esteem. Because clients often alienate family and friends by their chronic focus on their physical symptoms, social isolation and impaired social interaction diagnoses may be appropriate. The nurse may also recognize self-care deficits, as the clients' physical symptoms interfere with their ability to function.

Interventions for Hospitalized Clients

Somatization disorder is a chronic disorder. By the time the diagnosis is made, often only after the client experiences a major depression, the somatizing behavior is a well-entrenched pattern of feeling, behaving, and relating to others. In acute episodes of somatization disorder, the client either requires hospitalization for severe physical symptoms (which will then have no organic basis) or progresses to severe depression and requires acute psychiatric hospitalization. In either case, psychopharmacologic intervention with antidepressants is initiated to relieve the depression.

Nursing interventions with the client with somatization disorder should begin with the recognition that the goal is to focus less on physical symptoms and to improve the client's ability to function. Because this client tends to have little insight into emotional feelings and issues, the nurse will be more helpful by offering a relationship that is ongoing and focuses on the client as an individual, rather than as a collection of physical symptoms. The nurse who understands that the client meets emotional needs with symptoms will not become frustrated at not "curing" the client's symptoms.

Table 21–2 lists specific interventions and rationales that apply to the client with somatization disorder.

Interventions for Clients in the Community

If a client seen in the general medical setting is diagnosed with somatization disorder, the client should be referred for psychiatric care, including antidepressant medication and psychotherapy. Typically, the client will reject this referral because of the conviction that the problem is physical. A clear explanation of the disorder, emphasizing that the symptoms are real but have no organic basis, is necessary. Explain that this is a way the client learned to cope with distressing situations and feelings that was useful at times but is no longer helping the client feel better.

Unnecessary tests, while reassuring to health-care providers, should be avoided if possible. Clients may easily develop sensitivities to tests and medications or develop dependency on medications.

Clients will most likely respond in one of several ways:

1. Rejecting the information entirely and finding a new doctor
2. Agreeing to take antidepressants if it makes them feel better, but refusing psychiatric care
3. Agreeing to see the psychiatrist and become involved in therapy.

In either of the last two situations, the nurse can provide consistent, supportive contact with clients as the clinic nurse, home health nurse, or advanced practice psychiatric nurse.

In the community, clients may be willing to join support groups that are specific to issues in their lives, and the nurse should make such referrals specifically. For example, if during the assessment, the nurse realizes that a client is married to an alcoholic, Al-Anon would be a helpful referral. Not only would it give the client information and support but also it might be a more acceptable resource. The client would not require great insight into how feelings might be connected to physical symptoms but would learn that an alcoholic spouse makes many people feel distress, anxiety, and hurt, and these feelings become more recognizable and acceptable to the client.

TABLE 21–2. Nursing Interventions and Rationales in Somatization Disorder

Intervention	Rationale
Continuously monitor medical assessments, lab findings, and other reports to assure absence of organic illness.	Maintains safe and adequate client care.
Recognize that physical symptoms are real to the client, and provide a means for meeting emotional needs.	Denying the client's symptoms or perceptions prevents development of a therapeutic relationship and increases defensiveness.
Establish an ongoing, trusting relationship with the client.	Concern for the client as an individual rather than symptoms allows formation of trust.
Encourage expression of feelings, and relate them to stressors and symptoms.	Increases client's awareness of link between physical symptoms and emotional stressors.
Avoid focusing on the physical symptoms, disabilities, or impairment unless the client needs assistance.	Focusing on somatic complaints reinforces and interferes with relating them to psychological causes.
Observe and record the frequency and intensity of somatic complaints and related events.	Provides a baseline for evaluation of outcomes.
Teach clients about the relationship of mind and body, anxiety and stressors, and basic body function.	Increases client's knowledge of the relationship of health and illness to psychological issues.
Teach coping skills such as relaxation techniques, meditation, and exercise.	Provides reduction in anxiety and physical symptoms. Also can decrease need for medication.
Use nondefensive, matter-of-fact approach in dealing with hostile, manipulative, or angry behavior.	Allows client to see that angry feelings are acceptable and can be discussed without rejection of the individual. Neutralizes power struggles.
Set limits on using physical symptoms to manipulate the nurse or others, but remain accepting of the client.	Protects others from manipulative behavior, and limits allow nurse-client relationship to remain therapeutic.
Assist the client to identify needs that are met by the physical symptoms, and formulate more adaptive coping behaviors such as assertive communication.	Helps clients become aware of their emotional needs and their unhealthy coping through somatic symptoms. Assertive communication assists in meeting client's emotional needs in a healthier manner.
Establish gradual increase in social interaction by involvement with friends, support groups (e.g., CoDependents Anonymous, or Al-Anon), and educational programs. Require participation in therapeutic and community groups.	Lessens the client's focus on self and symptoms and enhances social interaction. Starting with one goal and building provides success without an overwhelming threat.
Refer clients needing psychiatric, alcohol, or drug abuse treatment to appropriate resources.	Depression and alcohol and drug abuse often complicate, contribute to, and result from the chronic physical symptoms.
Act as client advocate in protecting client from treatments or tests that are unnecessary for diagnosis and management of disorders.	Prevents clients from being inappropriately treated or actually harmed by repetitive, exploratory tests or fraudulent treatments.
Monitor response to medication using both physical and behavioral assessment. Monitor appropriate use of medication and occurrence of side effects.	Medication for anxiety or depression should result in decrease of symptoms and improved mood. Helps prevent misuse of medication to relieve somatic symptoms or pain.

Expected Outcomes

With proper diagnosis, psychopharmacologic treatment, and ongoing support or therapy, the nurse should expect gradual improvement in the client's ability to cope with work, school, parenting, and increased socialization. The client's ability to connect feelings to physical symptoms will vary greatly, depending on how much insight develops. The client will most likely continue to experience physical symptoms when stressed but may be able to spend less time thinking about the symptoms, complaining about them, and visiting health-care providers. Destructive coping behaviors such as abuse of alcohol, prescription drugs, or illegal drugs should be absent, which will dramatically improve the client's sense of well-being and feelings of control.

Differential Diagnosis

The somatization process with presenting physical symptoms permits the individual to gratify needs such as relief from grief, loneliness, or sadness by interaction with "caring" professionals. Common accompaniments to the somatization process are mood disorders (depression), anxiety, and panic disorders.[1] Adequate treatment of these disorders is essential in relieving the client's distress and decreasing the frequency of somatic symptoms.

Remember that the symptoms, including pain, are real and allow the client to defend against feelings that may be unconscious. Therefore, the symptoms can be viewed as a coping mechanism. The somatoform disorders should be viewed as extreme, maladaptive functioning on a continuum of the somatization process.

> ### CASE STUDY
>
> Patricia was a 19-year-old college student who had been treated as an inpatient for drug abuse and depression. Over the course of her outpatient therapy, she revealed a long history of childhood physical and sexual abuse. A chaotic and violent home life provided minimal nurturing and caring. Patricia recalled that as a child she would deliberately jump off the garage roof or fall off her bicycle in the hope of injuring herself enough to require medical attention, particularly when she needed a respite from her family. Indeed, as a child she had been hospitalized several times for various broken bones and minor surgeries (unrelated to the abuse). Patricia remembered a sense of comfort and feeling of well-being, despite the injuries associated with her hospitalizations, because of the caring nurses and the attention from her family.
>
> ### CRITICAL THINKING QUESTIONS
>
> 1. What was the primary gain that Patricia accomplished by injuring herself?
> 2. Explain how health-care workers provided secondary gain for Patricia, and discuss your individual response to the situation.

UNDIFFERENTIATED SOMATOFORM DISORDER

This diagnosis may be given if the client's symptoms, similar to somatization disorder, do not completely meet the criteria for somatization disorder or other somatoform disorders (see *DSM-IV* Diagnostic Criteria). Like the other disorders, there appears to be no known medical cause, and the symptom(s) must cause significant distress or impairment of function for at least 6 months.

Such complaints may be limited to one such as nausea or vomiting (not due to anorexia), chronic fatigue, or weakness. Usually however, there are several symptoms. The etiologic factors and nursing processes are similar to somatization disorder.[1]

CONVERSION DISORDER

Characteristic Behaviors

In another type of somatoform disorder, conversion disorder, there is a loss or change in bodily function that cannot be traced to any organic cause and seems to be related to psychological stressors.

The term **conversion** comes from the idea that the individual uses the somatic symptom in an unconscious manner to reduce or repress a psychological conflict that creates anxiety. The somatic symptom provides relief from the intolerable anxiety. This is termed *primary gain*. The individual might also receive secondary gain by avoiding responsibilities or from attracting concern and attention.

Psychological factors must be present in order for the diagnosis to be made, and such stressors are clearly evident in the client's history (see DSM-IV Diagnostic Criteria. Unlike other disorders, such as malingering or factitious disorder, in which the client *consciously* feigns or produces symptoms of illness, a person with conversion disorder remains unaware that the symptom is a response to anxiety and is not consciously aware of being anxious. The conversion symptom is the client's defense against anxiety. The client may also project an attitude of **la belle indifference,** a seeming unconcern or lack of distress about being suddenly unble to walk or move an arm.

The most common symptom is a disorder of movement, perhaps inability to walk, stand, or move an arm. Researchers[12] found that 71% of clients with conversion disorder presented with CNS symptoms. Conversion paralysis of a limb is common. Other conversion symptoms may take the form of blindness, deafness, or difficulty swallowing. The disorder may have the symptom of sensory deficit, such as loss of touch or pain sensation. If the only symptom is pain or a sexual dysfunction, conversion disorder is not diagnosed.

Typically the conversion symptoms do not follow usual anatomical pathways and always occur within the voluntary portion of the nervous system. However, careful medical workups must be done to rule out organic conditions, many of which also present with a confusing symptomatology.

Culture, Age, and Gender Features

Women are overrepresented in this disorder, in estimates that vary from 2 to 1 to 10 to 1.[1] Rather than being more prevalent in any age group, conversion disorder appears throughout the life span, from childhood to old age. Individuals with this disorder tend to be less educated, less medically sophisticated, and of lower socioeconomic status.

Etiology

Stevens,[13] in discussing clients with conversion disorder, noted their consistent lack of meaningful relationships. As in the somatization disorder, it is important to explore how the behavior meets emotional needs and how it has been shaped by environmental reinforcement.

Conversion disorder may take many forms within its diagnostic criteria. For example, a client with continuous belching was later found to be an adult incest survivor.[14]

> **DSM-IV Diagnostic Criteria for 300.11 Conversion Disorder**
>
> A. One or more symptoms or deficits affecting voluntary motor or sensory function that suggest a neurological or other general medical condition.
>
> B. Psychological factors are judged to be associated with the symptom or deficit because the initiation or exacerbation of the symptom or deficit is preceded by conflicts or other stressors.
>
> C. The symptom or deficit is not intentionally produced or feigned (as in Factitious Disorder of Malingering).
>
> D. The symptom or deficit cannot, after appropriate investigation, be fully explained by a general medical condition, or by the direct effects of a substance, or as a culturally sanctioned behavior or experience.
>
> E. The symptom or deficit causes clinically significant distress or impairment in social, occupational, or other important areas of functioning or warrants medical evaluation.
>
> F. The symptom or deficit is not limited to pain or sexual dysfunction, does not occur exclusively during the course of Somatization Disorder, and is not better accounted for by another mental disorder.
>
> *Specify* type of symptom or deficit:
> With Motor Symptom or Deficit
> With Sensory Symptom or Deficit
> With Seizures or Convulsions
> With Mixed Presentation
>
> **Source:** Reprinted with permission from the Diagnostic and Statistical Manual of Mental Disorders, Fourth Edition. Copyright 1994 American Psychiatric Association.

Many incest survivors and others experiencing oral sexual abuse report swallowing, gagging, or belching problems.

Other forms of conversion disorder have been diagnosed in cases of hyperemesis gravidarum (severe vomiting during pregnancy),[15] psychogenic stuttering,[16] and war-related posttraumatic stress disorder.[17]

Assessment

In assessing the client with conversion disorder, the nurse finds symptoms that affect voluntary motor (paralysis, seizure) or sensory activity (blindness, paresthesia) or symptoms that suggest a medical condition. The client is not "faking" the symptoms or feigning the illness, yet there is no medical or laboratory evidence suggesting disease. The client is not consciously aware of the emotions or anxiety that has caused the symptoms.

In the client's history, periods of high stress or conflict are evident, for example, a breakup of a relationship, a new job, or entry into college or the armed services. Sometimes this information is obtained only from a family interview. The onset of the symptoms has been sudden and acute, and the client often seems unconcerned about this serious sudden incapacitation (la belle indifference). The symptoms also result in a relatively acute impairment of social, role, or occupational functioning.

Planning Care

A nursing diagnosis that powerfully illustrates the client's needs is impaired communication. The client's physical symptoms of paralysis, blindness, and so forth communicate somatically what the client cannot verbalize. Another nursing diagnosis for the client who has conversion disorder is ineffective individual coping related to severe repressed anxiety and helplessness. The client is also at high risk for individual identity disturbance because of an inability to connect emotions with the physical symptoms. This lack of insight into feelings impairs the client's ability to understand himself or herself and also impairs relationships with others.

Interventions for Hospitalized Clients

At the outset, engage the client in the plan of care. Any medical reason for the disorder should be ruled out. Begin by introducing the client to the idea that emotions are powerful enough to affect our bodies. Validate with the client that this is the way some people deal with stress when they are overwhelmed. Do not deny that the symptoms are real to the client, and avoid "blaming" the client for the illness. A relationship that is supportive and consistent should focus on helping the client recognize that feelings are acceptable, even negative feelings.

In the acute phase, the focus should be on assisting the client to identify recent stressors or conflicts and begin to connect the feelings created by the situations. Minimize attention to physical symptoms, except to ensure the client's safety and well-being (e.g., a client with conversion blindness will need assistance in walking). In the acute phase, the client will benefit from tricyclic antidepressants (TCAs) or selective serotonin reuptake inhibitors (SSRIs) that relieve the depression and anxiety of which the client is not aware.

Because of the acute onset of this disorder, the client will seek immediate medical attention; therefore, the crisis can be resolved readily and the client returned to physical functioning within 1 to 2 weeks. However, the client will need continued care following this phase to avoid repeating the situation.

Supportive one-to-one therapy provides an accepting atmosphere for the client to learn about and discuss feelings and how these feelings affect the body. Because most clients have difficulty expressing emotions, assertiveness training on first an individual basis and then a group basis should be instituted.

Interventions for Clients in the Community

In the community, clients should be encouraged to join appropriate support groups that deal with the conflicts that brought on the symptoms, for example, bereavement groups or codependency groups.

Expected Outcomes

Within 1 or 2 weeks of psychiatric care, the client's incapacitation should subside. The client will be able to resume a usual level of occupational or role function within 1 month; however, if these areas are the source of the stressors, the client may need longer to change jobs, move, or make changes in family relationships. Changes that will create less stress should be part of the discussion in the one-to-one relationship, and monitoring the client's level of function should be ongoing. With immediate intervention, continued support, and use of antidepressants, if indicated, there should be no recurrence of the disorder.

CASE STUDY

Marlene J was a 57-year-old housewife who was diagnosed with conversion disorder, depression, and panic disorder following her admission to the general hospital for paralysis of both legs and total inability to walk. After exhaustive studies had revealed no organic basis for the paralysis, she was admitted to the inpatient psychiatric unit, where she began meeting with the nurse therapist. When she learned there was no organic illness, her symptoms began to abate. She also began talking with the nurse who identified that the precipitating event for the stress was overwhelming responsibility for family members, such as caring for her 90-year-old father-in-law who was recuperating from a hip replacement. She was also caring for children of two of her children who were going through divorces, and she had concerns about her husband's health and impending retirement.

The nurse helped Marlene identify feelings of anger and resentment about her current situation and discussed the reality of the burdens she had shouldered. Marlene was unable to say "no" to family members or ask others for help, because a "strong" individual such as herself should be able to handle it. She even acknowledged the message of her "paralyzed" legs to her family: "I won't take one more step for you!"

The next step was to begin to change the situation at home. The care of her father-in-law was turned over to his daughter, and before leaving the hospital, Marlene met with her two children and discussed the amount of child care she could manage. She was quite frightened at confronting her family and telling them she could not and would not "do" for them because it was more than she could handle, but she was very pleased and relieved at their supportive response.

Marlene was discharged to outpatient therapy, which continued with the same nurse therapist. In exploration of her difficulties in expressing hurt and anger, Marlene revealed a previous episode of major depression as a young wife, an English war bride with two small children, isolated from friends and family in a new country. Prior to this, she had also survived the bombing of London during World War II, in which both her parents had died. Marlene had seldom discussed the feelings of loss and abandonment created by early life experiences and developed the attitude "just be strong and get through it," which, the nurse pointed out, she had done quite well, but that this approach did not work in every situation.

Throughout the outpatient sessions, which lasted about 3 years (gradually decreasing from once a week to once a month or every 6 weeks), Marlene was able to connect current stressors to feelings of anxiety and fear of rejection, both in her current life situation and stemming from traumatic losses in her childhood. She continued with her TCA that had been initiated at the time of diagnosis (amitriptyline 25 mg) but decreased the dosage over 2 years. She also participated in a women's therapy group that taught assertiveness skills and self-esteem building.

She was able to communicate concerns to her husband about his health and her fears of his dying and abandoning her. With her adult children, she set limits on their expectations of her and was able to be more realistic about her expectations of herself. She was again able to enjoy her homemaking and crafts and church activities.

CRITICAL THINKING QUESTIONS

1. What stressors preceded the onset of Marlene's conversion disorder?
2. What nonverbal communication did Marlene's symptoms express for her?
3. How might Marlene's early life experiences have influenced her difficulties in expressing negative emotions?

PAIN DISORDER

Characteristic Behaviors

The single presenting symptom in this disorder is that of pain (see *DSM-IV* Diagnostic Criteria). Pain disorder may be diagnosed solely in relation to psychological factors, in which case there are no or minimal general medical conditions present, or it can be diagnosed in association with both psychological and medical conditions, in which case the pain exceeds what would be expected and is influenced by psychological factors.

As previously discussed with somatoform disorders, the client does not associate pain with psychological factors or stress or "deliberately" lie about the pain in order to gain attention or avoid responsibilities. The pain is not "all in your head," as the client may have been told, but is felt in the body and intensely enough to cause significant disruption of the client's life.

Etiology

Biological Theories

People have varying thresholds of pain and responses to pain. What causes one individual to stop moving when experiencing pain may be ignored by another individual. Neu-

DSM-IV Diagnostic Criteria for Pain Disorder

Diagnostic Criteria for Pain Disorder

A. Pain in one or more anatomical sites is the predominant focus of the clinical presentation and is of sufficient severity to warrant clinical attention.

B. The pain causes clinically significant distress or impairment in social, occupational, or other important areas of functioning.

C. Psychological factors are judged to have an important role in the onset, severity, exacerbation, or maintenance of the pain.

D. The symptom or deficit is not intentionally produced or feigned (as in Factitious Disorder or Malingering).

E. The pain is not better accounted for by a Mood, Anxiety, or Psychotic Disorder and does not meet criteria for Dyspareunia.

Code as follows:
307.80 Pain Disorder Associated with Psychological Factors: psychological factors are judged to have the major role in the onset, severity, exacerbation, or maintenance of the pain. (If a general medical condition is present, it does not have a major role in the onset, severity, exacerbation, or maintenance of the pain). This type of Pain Disorder is not diagnosed if criteria are also met for Somatization Disorder.

Specify if:
Acute: duration of less than 6 months
Chronic: duration of 6 months or longer
307.89 Pain Disorder Associated With Both Psychological Factors and a General Medical Condition: both psychological factors and a general medical condition are judged to have important roles in the onset, severity, exacerbation, or maintenance of the pain. The associated general medical condition or anatomical site of the pain (see below) is coded on Axis III.

Specify if:
Acute: duration of less than 6 months
Chronic: duration of 6 months or longer

Note: The following is not considered to be a mental disorder and is included here to facilitate differential diagnosis.

Pain Disorder Associated With a General Medical Condition: a general medical condition has a major role in the onset, severity, exacerbation, or maintenance of the pain. (If psychological factors are present, they are not judged to have a major role in the onset, severity, exacerbation, or maintenance of the pain.) The diagnostic code for the pain is selected based on the associated general medical condition if one has been established or on the anatomical location of the pain if the underlying general medical condition is not yet clearly established—for example, low back (724.2), sciatic (724.3), pelvic (625.9), headache (784.0), facial (784.0), chest (786.50), joint (719.4), bone (733.90), abdominal (789.0), breast (611.71), renal (788.0), ear (388.70), eye (379.91), throat (784.1), tooth (525.9), and urinary (788.0).

Source: Reprinted with permission from the Diagnostic and Statistical Manual of Mental Disorders, Fourth Edition. Copyright 1994 American Psychiatric Association.

---

robiological theories[4] referred to earlier in the chapter play a role in pain disorder. The CNS may provide too little inhibition of sensory input, causing an amplified awareness of pain. Factors in the CNS may also cause a decrease in associating feelings of emotional distress with somatic pain.

Comorbid Disorders

Research of chronic pain has uncovered a close association with other mental disorders, such as depression, anxiety, and panic disorder. As noted in Table 21-1, 10 to 15% of adults suffer from disabling chronic back pain alone. A study[18] of men with chronic low back pain (CLBP) showed that they (1) had significantly more lifetime somatic complaints (besides pain) than did the control group, (2) the range in severity of pain was wide, and (3) major depression and alcohol dependence were clearly present in men with a higher frequency of pain symptoms.

Other researchers[19] studied pain experienced by 28 men in a cardiology clinic population who experienced noncardiac chest pain (NCCP). Sixty-eight percent of the clients were found to have a diagnosable mental disorder such as panic disorder, major depression, or anxiety disorder. The presence of these other disorders emphasizes the connection of psychological stress with somatic pain.

Sociocultural Theories

Walker and colleagues[20] compared women who received laparoscopies for chronic pelvic pain with women who received laparoscopies for nonpainful gynecological conditions. Their findings supported those of other studies[21] that found women with chronic pelvic pain had a significantly higher prevalence of childhood sexual abuse. Nearly all severely abused women in the study had chronic pelvic pain and were also significantly more likely to have multiple medically unexplained symptoms and lifetime histories of drug abuse and panic disorder. Walker and colleagues[20] theorized that these clients perceived themselves as having little control over their lives and a sense of personal powerlessness because of early life circumstances. Their pain and somatic symptoms were a safe way of expressing chronic distress and obtaining support from health-care professionals and family.

A more recent study[22] disputed the connection between chronic pain and abuse but did find childhood sexual abuse to be a predictor of anxiety and depression, and childhood physical abuse was a predictor of anxiety and somatization.

The history of abuse or experience of depression or anxiety does not diminish the reality of pain symptoms but demonstrates the impact of life experiences upon a client's perception of pain. The pain becomes a way of communicating emotional distress.

Assessment

The client presents with a chronic history of pain that has interfered with role function. The nurse should:
- Assess if complete medical testing reveals no organic reason for the pain.
- Determine if there is a medical condition present and if the pain seems extreme for that condition.
- Carefully note the location, intensity, site, and frequency of the pain.
- Elicit from the client life situations that have occurred before or during the onset of or increase in the pain.
- Assess the client for symptoms of depression, suicidal thoughts or actions, and drug or alcohol abuse.
- Assess ways the client has attempted to alleviate the pain (e.g., exercise, relaxation, alcohol, or prescription drugs).

Planning Care

The most prominent nursing diagnosis is chronic pain related to severe repressed anxiety, low self-esteem, or unmet dependency needs. The repression of feelings manifests itself in the complaints of pain, feelings of physical pain, social withdrawal, and seeking of help from health-care providers. Often worn down by pain, clients accept the specialized assistance of a pain clinic that offers physical therapy, medication, relaxation, and psychological counseling. Other clients, however, may refuse a clinic, insisting there is only a physical cause for the pain and placing their confidence in medical treatment and psychopharmacologic relief through use or abuse of narcotics, barbiturates, or antianxiety medications.

As indicated in the research, repression of early abuse, which is kept out of awareness by expression in the symptoms of pain, fulfills the client's need to avoid painful emotional feelings on a conscious level and results in actual somatic pain.

Planning must also take into account the degree of disability or physical function that is caused by the pain. Disuse of limbs because of pain, for example, could result in wasting of muscle tissue, weakness, and atrophy if immediate intervention does not occur.

Interventions for Hospitalized Clients

Interventions and rationales for pain disorder are similar to those for the client with somatization disorder. Comfort measures such as massage, warm packs, or warm baths can be helpful, but the nurse should avoid creating secondary gain and reinforcing the complaints. Give attention to the client when the focus is not on the pain. In therapy sessions, the client might be given limited time to discuss pain, and the rest of the session might be devoted to communicating feelings and connecting them to bodily symptoms.

Antidepressants to alleviate the depression that underlies the pain are helpful, and client education is necessary. Clients should be discouraged from taking medications such as narcotics, barbiturates, and benzodiazepine anxiolytics because of their addictive potential. Immediate referral should be made for the client who has already developed an alcohol or drug dependency.

Clients experiencing pain disorder should be assisted to identify alternative methods of coping with stress, particularly to avoid maladaptive responses such as alcohol or drug use. Such techniques as biofeedback, guided imagery, breathing exercises, listening to music, reading, or working on hobbies can provide distraction. Give positive reinforcement to clients when they use these other methods of dealing with the pain.

At the heart of intervention is the establishment of trust with the nurse, so that the client feels safe in discussing negative or emotionally painful feelings. The ability to connect painful emotions with the physical pain is usually gradually achieved through psychotherapy or pain clinic treatment.

Interventions for Clients in the Community

Community resources such as groups for adult children of alcoholics, incest survivors, families who have experienced the suicide of a family member, or grief groups can be of immense support to the client in learning about how life events have contributed and prolonged his or her current symptoms of pain. These groups also offer social support and acceptance for the client.

Expected Outcomes

A decrease in the intensity and frequency of pain symptoms will indicate the effectiveness of interventions. The client will be able to verbalize with varying degrees of insight an understanding of the relationship between pain and emotional distress. Behaviorally, the client's level of function should improve (over 1 to 2 years of regular therapy or clinic treatment), and the client should be able to use more adaptive coping mechanisms such as group support, biofeedback, or relaxation techniques. The nurse must remember that this pattern developed over a lifetime and that behavioral changes occur gradually.

CASE STUDY

Bill Z was a 46-year-old auto worker who was admitted to the psychiatric inpatient unit with the diagnosis of major depression with suicide ideation. Bill had been married 28 years and had two sons. He had grown increasingly despondent, lost interest in his usual activities, and had greatly increased his beer drinking (a cultural norm for his workplace and friends). Another cultural norm was "macho" activities such as hunting, fishing, and working on cars. Displays of emotion by men in Bill's culture were viewed as "weak," and emotions were dealt with by alcohol use.

Bill had been seen frequently over the years by his family physician for chronic abdominal pain and severe low back pain. No physical reason for the abdominal pain could be detected, despite numerous tests. Four years ago surgery had been performed on his back for a herniated disc with relief for about 1 year but with a return of pain. His job did require physical work and standing, and he was about 40 lb overweight, mostly in the abdomen. Despite his complaints of severe back pain, some of which could be job and weight related, he refused to go on disability because of his strong work ethic. About 3 years ago, Bill's youngest son and his son's wife had been killed in a car accident by a driver high on drugs. Bill's wife felt he had been unable to grieve this loss over the years and had turned to alcohol for relief.

Bill was seen by a nurse therapist frequently during his inpatient stay to help him connect his feelings to his physical pain and to provide careful monitoring of suicidal thoughts and profound depression. A contract to discuss suicidal thoughts or to call if experiencing them was agreed upon by Bill, the nurse, and his psychiatrist. Supportive acceptance of whatever feelings he could discuss was also a goal, although his ability to express those feelings was restricted.

Bill at times stated that the sessions were a "waste of time," did nothing to help his back and abdominal pain, and that talking about his son's death "wouldn't bring him back" yet he attended each therapy session. When he was discharged and follow-up outpatient therapy was recommended, Bill protested but followed through conscientiously, took his antidepressant medication, and maintained alcohol abstinence.

Over 3 years, Bill was seen by the nurse, intensely during the first 18 months and then every 6 weeks. During this time, Bill's abdominal and back pain would ebb and flow, unrelated to any physical stress, but often clearly related to "anniversary" days of his son's death, a funeral, or a visit to his son's grave.

Throughout therapy, Bill expressed doubt that his pain could be related to his anger and grief. He revealed intense and painful loss in his childhood. His father, an alcoholic, had a severe bleeding ulcer for many years and suffered from intense pain. When Bill was 12, his father shot himself in the home after his pain and depression became unbearable. Bill was unable to recognize any connection.

Bill seemed to find relief in merely talking with the nurse, and conferences with his wife revealed she saw him as "better" and more able to do things after a session. In fact, she would urge him to see the nurse when she believed he was "too down."

Bill's nursing diagnosis was Dysfunctional Grieving related to multiple traumatic loss of significant others resulting in suicidal thoughts, depression, somatic pain, and alcohol abuse.

Bill followed through with therapy conscientiously but liked to have the control of scheduling his next meeting with the thought that he wouldn't "need to talk" as time passed. His intense depression lifted rapidly with his discontinuance of alcohol and use of antidepressants. Although suicidal assessment regularly continued throughout his therapy because of the degree of his feelings of hopelessness, he was able to work, be involved in hobbies, and socialize within 6 months of his hospitalization. Later, the marriage of his other son and his becoming a grandfather were positive and very meaningful events for Bill. Although he continued to have periods of both abdominal and low back pain, it did not interfere with his functioning and activities. He reported occasional bouts of depression but continued with his antidepressants and usual activities.

CRITICAL THINKING QUESTIONS

1. What maladaptive responses did Bill use to manage his pain?
2. Identify and discuss gender and cultural factors that may interfere with a client's ability to discuss feelings. Examine your own cultural and gender beliefs about pain.
3. Why do you think Bill continued with his therapy sessions despite protesting that talking didn't help?

HYPOCHONDRIASIS

Characteristic Behaviors

Although the term *hypochondriac* may be used casually when people seem too worried about their health, hypochondriasis is a very specific diagnosis, as the criteria of the *DSM-IV* indicates.

In **hypochondriasis**, people are preoccupied, for at least 6 months, with the fear or belief that they have a serious disease based on individual misinterpretation of bodily symptoms. As in other somatoform disorders, to receive a diagnosis of hypochondriasis, the preoccupation with this belief must significantly interfere with the individual's role or functioning.

The preoccupation in hypochondriasis may be with small physical problems such as a cough or cut; with usual physical functioning such as heartbeat, peristalsis, or sweating; or with vague physical complaints such as "burning feet" or "weak heart." These symptoms are then attributed to some suspected disease, and the client becomes very concerned and focuses on them. The symptoms may involve one or several body systems, one or several organs, or concerns about a specific disease such as cancer or AIDS.

Often, people with hypochondriasis become alarmed by reading or hearing about certain diseases, by knowing someone with a specific disease, or simply by focusing on their own body functions. Despite tests and reassurances, hypochondriacal clients' fears are not allayed. One study found that hypochondriacal clients "were more likely to feel that their health problems had not been thoroughly evaluated or explained than were other nonhypochondriacal clients" and

DSM-IV Diagnostic Criteria for 300.7 Hypochondriasis

A. Preoccupation with fears of having, or the idea that one has, a serious disease based on the individual's misinterpretation of bodily symptoms.

B. The preoccupation persists despite appropriate medical evaluation and reassurance.

C. The belief in Criterion A is not of delusional intensity (as in Delusional Disorder, Somatic Type) and is not restricted to a circumscribed concern about appearance (as in Body Dysmorphic Disorder).

D. The preoccupation causes clinically significant distress or impairment in social, occupational, or other important areas of functioning.

E. The duration of the disturbance is at least 6 months.

F. The preoccupation is not better accounted for by Generalized Anxiety Disorder, Obsessive-Compulsive Disorder, Panic Disorder, a Major Depressive Episode, Separation Anxiety, or another Somatoform Disorder.

Specify if:
With Poor Insight: if, for most of the time during the current episode, the individual does not recognize that the concern about having a serious illness is excessive or unreasonable.

Source: Reprinted with permission from the Diagnostic and Statistical Manual of Mental Disorders, Fourth Edition. Copyright 1994 American Psychiatric Association.

---

did not feel their physicians were concerned about their health problems.[23]

Culture, Age, and Gender Features

Nurses can encounter clients with hypochondriasis in any general medical setting. The psychiatric setting is generally the last place these clients are found because they are convinced that their problems are medical. This disorder is equally common in women and men.

The diagnosis of hypochondriasis will rule out the possibility of delusional or psychotic thinking. If the nurse encounters delusions or hallucinations in the client, referral for psychiatric treatment should be made.

Etiology

Biological Theory

Although no actual biological mechanism has been identified as causing hypochondriasis, there are a number of theories or perspectives from which to view this disorder. Several researchers and practitioners[24–26] have presented case studies in which hypochondriasis is seen as a form of obsessive-compulsive disorder (OCD). Research into OCD has shown changes in the basal ganglia area of the brain.[27] All of the clients in two studies of hypochondriasis[24,25] were treated successfully with clomipramine, a drug used for OCD, suggesting a relationship between the disorders.

Perceptual-Cognitive Theory

Barsky and Wyshak[28] view hypochondriasis as a disorder of perception and cognition that leads to amplification of benign symptoms and misattribution of these symptoms to serious disease. Hypochondriacs may experience bodily sensations more intensely (just as people have varying thresholds of pain) and become more upset or disturbed than other people.

Because of the intensity or disruption caused by a normal sensation, the hypochondriac then misinterprets the symptoms and misattributes it to disease rather than, for example, overwork or lack of sleep or exercise. A stomachache may be attributed to an ulcer, rather than to eating rich foods, or a bruise misinterpreted as evidence of a blood disorder. Then the individual becomes more anxious and more vigilant and therefore has heightened symptoms. First, perception is narrowed to look for more "evidence" of disease, and then sensory input that disconfirms the individual's beliefs is ignored. Finally, increased anxiety creates its own set of bodily symptoms (e.g., gastric distress, pounding heart, and sweaty palms) that are normal but also ascribed to serious "disease."

Psychological Theory

Starcevic[25] theorized that the individual with hypochondriasis perceives an excessive threat to the self, creating overwhelming anxiety and feelings of individual vulnerability and insecurity. In hypochondriasis, this fear becomes translated into attempts to create self-control, with the focus on the bodily self. This need for control causes the search for unquestionable "proof" of the absence of disease as well as "perfect reassurance" from the health-care provider. However, because of the mistrust this vulnerable individual feels, there is never enough reassurance, causing the endless and repeated rounds of medical testing.

As in severe levels of anxiety, the individual with hypochondriasis may find any ambiguity or uncertainty as another threat, and thus a threat to control. Body sensations that are vague or unexpected then create greater anxiety and greater need for control, exhibited in excessive preoccupation and worry.[25]

Sociocultural and Environmental Factors

In a follow-up study of hypochondriasis,[29] researchers studied the attitudes of 91 clients, 58 of whom met the criteria for hypochondriasis. They found that hypochondriacal clients tended to be younger and of significantly lower socio-

> **RESEARCH NOTE**
>
> **Stern, R, and Fernandez, M: Group cognitive and behavioural treatment for hypochondriasis. Br Medical Journal, 303, 1229–1131, 1991.**
>
> **Findings:** Recognizing the need for treatment of clients with hypochondriasis because of the amount of time and health resources they use, the authors designed a treatment program based on cognitive educational therapy. Realizing that most clients with hypochondriasis are resistive to the idea of psychiatric treatment because they believe that they have a yet-to-be discovered illness, the authors decided to approach the treatment from the concept of *stress*. The concepts of stress and stress management are widely known and accepted by the public, and the aim was to intervene in hypochondriacal behavior using the cognitive educational method.
>
> The cognitive and behavioral hypothesis outlines three mechanisms that act in preoccupation with illness. Initially, there is an increase in autonomic arousal that the clients interprets as an indication that he or she is unwell. Next, the client focuses on some normal variation in bodily function and then begins an obsessive checking behavior.
>
> Clients were recruited by referral from hospital staff physicians and fulfilled the criteria for hypochondriasis. There were six clients selected, three men and three women, ranging in age from 35 to 55 years. Clients had experienced symptoms from 7 to 28 years, with the mean being 12 years. As the authors noted, the clients had huge medical files that reflected their heavy use of health services.
>
> Six months prior to treatment, the clients were asked to complete scales measuring anxiety and depression and also a scale designed to measure the amount of time spent thinking about illness. Treatment occurred in the general hospital setting, in 1 ½-hour sessions over 9 weeks. Clients were educated about how symptoms arose and how to cope with stress. Symptoms were acknowledged and treatment was aimed at helping to explain them satisfactorily to the client. Education about hypochondriasis and relaxation exercises were taught, taped, and practiced at home. Clients recorded symptoms in diaries that were then shared in group. Clients looked at how they sought reassurance and how it provided only short-term relief. Aspects of depression were presented and applied to each client's situation.
>
> By the end of the sessions, although client scores on assessment tools did not significantly change, there was behavioral change in the form of decreased visits to the doctor and decreased amounts of time spent thinking about the illness. Moreover, on a 6-month follow-up, these improvements remained.
>
> In conclusion, the researchers suggest that further studies with larger populations could prove useful. They also note the medical community's difficulty in regarding the illness from other than a physical viewpoint and feelings of frustration about earlier lack of treatment for a hypochondriacal client.
>
> **Application to Practice:** This cognitive educational approach can be used by nurses who have experience in group therapeutic education. Psychiatric nurses who have background in not only group dynamics, but also stress and stress management are in a position to offer this intervention and to design research studies that evaluate the efficacy of this approach. Nurses in medical settings can be helpful in identifying clients who seem to demonstrate symptoms of hypochondriasis and referring them for treatment. Hospitals in many areas offer wellness programs that emphasize stress management, and the opportunity exists for specific groups to assist clients with hypochondriasis.

economic position than other clients. The hypochondriacal clients more often reported having parents with marital problems, being sexually abused, and being victims of violence. These clients also had less often confided in others about being victimized by violence. The hypochondriacal group reported more sickness as children and more days of school missed for health reasons but did not differ from the nonhypochondriacal group in experience of serious illness or in family concerns about illness.

Prognosis

Studies by Noyes and colleagues[23] showed that physicians easily recognized hypochondriasis but rarely diagnosed it because they felt their duty was mainly to rule out medical disease, not to identify a psychiatric illness. Certainly a medical illness can coexist with hypochondriasis about other physical symptoms. If the diagnosis is overlooked or ignored as "not medical," the pattern continues, and the prognosis for the client is poor.

This disorder is chronic, reflecting the client's lifetime pattern of thinking and behavior. However, with proper diagnosis, psychopharmacologic treatment for the accompanying depression, and cognitive and supportive therapy, symptoms should decrease and functioning improve.

Assessment

The client will present with a variety of physical symptoms, yet, as in other somatoform disorders, there is no evidence of disease causing the symptoms. If there is a concurrent medical condition, the hypochondriasis centers around symptoms that are benign or unrelated to the identified medical condition. Hypochondriacal clients may keep notes on their symptoms, tests, and other examinations. They may have researched and read a great deal about various medications and treatments.

These clients use their physical symptoms as a way to relate to others and, because of this overfocus on self, become lonely and isolated as people tire of their chronic complaints. Relationships in their lives tend to be distant and very few. They have often alienated family members by their complaints or use of physical symptoms to manipulate others into meeting their needs for attention. They typically have little insight into their feelings and the effects of illness-focused behavior on others.

The client's symptoms should be thoroughly investigated through complete medical testing; however, there will be no evidence of disease related to the symptoms. The nurse should assess the site, intensity, frequency, and times of occurrence of the symptoms. The nurse should listen for indications of loneliness ("No one ever calls to invite us out anymore") and indications of disruption or stress in the family ("My husband is gone all the time at work" or "My children never call me."). Ask the client to describe his or her usual routine, any recent stressors or disruptions, and usual coping methods.

As with other somatoform disorders, assess for symptoms of depression and use or abuse of alcohol and drugs. Drug abuse may take the form of overdosing on vitamins, aspirin, laxatives, or other common over-the-counter preparations. Some clients even create their own medications through "natural" methods and may be harming themselves through overuse of certain ingredients. Asking clients what seems to give them relief may elicit this information.

Assess what the symptoms achieve for the client (primary gain). Do they relieve the client of care of the children or home? Do they allow the client to avoid work? The basic purpose served by the symptoms is to keep anxiety out of consciousness, so it is unlikely the client will report feelings of anxiety or depression. The nurse should therefore be observant for behavioral and verbal cues when exploring the client's social history.

Planning Care

The difficulty with planning care for clients with hypochondriasis arises from their need to keep anxiety and distress out of consciousness, thus resulting in the disorder. They lack insight into their feelings and the way hypocondriacal behavior affects others. Nursing diagnoses include anxiety related to fear of having a serious disease, resulting in overfocus on bodily symptoms and excessive seeking of health-care treatments and reassurance. Another diagnosis may be impaired adjustment related to feelings of helplessness, fears of assuming responsibilities, and low self-esteem, resulting in overfocus on physical concerns. Personal identity disturbance also exists related to inaccurate beliefs about the self, physical symptoms that cannot be validated, frustration, and anxiety resulting in impaired role functioning, self-doubt, and social isolation.

Interventions for Clients in the Community

Therapeutic intervention in hypochondriasis has not been studied in depth. There are different opinions as to whether it is a single diagnosis or part of other disorders such as depression or anxiety disorders. Intervention is difficult because the client lacks insight into the feelings underlying the physical symptoms and therefore sees no need to alter behavior.

Do not give clients reinforcement for the physical symptoms by providing useless medical or diagnostic treatment, and avoid lengthy discussion of physical concerns. Be alert to the possibility that the side effects of repeated tests and examinations could induce actual illness.

Nurses should listen carefully to the client's concerns and express interest in the client as an individual, rather than as a recital of symptoms. Consistently connect the concerns to anxiety: "These physical symptoms must make you feel very anxious. Do you find the more you think of them, the worse you feel?" Teach the client about the relationship between the mind and the body, that is, that thinking affects how we feel physically. Expect the client to initially reject any relationship of this idea to his or her situation.

An ongoing relationship with clients in which they can feel accepted by the nurse and not viewed as "a complainer" or "problem client" (as has probably been the case) is very important. A nurse who understands that hypochondriasis is a way of expressing psychic pain and anxiety will be able to avoid seeing the client in a negative and nonconstructive manner. Ford and colleagues[30] suggest that the approach to take is "management rather than cure."

Cognitive therapy addresses the hypochondriac's automatic dysfunctional thinking and misattribution of body stimuli. Behavioral therapy may be used to decide which cues trigger anxiety in the client and then to expose the client to the feared situation repeatedly to extinguish an anxiety response.[31] Compulsive checking rituals (e.g., taking one's blood pressure, pulse, or temperature repeatedly) and compulsive seeking of inappropriate reassurance about health should be discouraged.

Some clients may be able to understand the relationship of stress to their symptoms, and they will use relaxation techniques and behavioral interventions. Nurses should also emphasize the importance of medication when other disorders are being treated and discuss frankly with the client the frequent coexistence of depression and anxiety with the physical concerns.

Pharmacologic interventions that have been helpful are the antidepressants such as fluoxetine (Prozac) and clomipramine (Anafranil). In studies of the use of fluoxetine on hypochondriacs who did not meet criteria for major depression,[32] it was found that fear of disease or belief that one had a disease decreased, but bodily preoccupation did not change, although clients were less likely to interpret body sensations negatively. Fluoxetine has also been helpful in treating clients with both hypochondriasis and OCD.[24]

Supportive discussion with family members should be directed at educating them about the client's disorder and involving them in sessions to discuss their views of the client's behavior and improvement. Support and encourage the family members to avoid a blaming attitude and to discuss their own feelings of anger and frustration with the client's behavior. The distancing of the client from family members that generally occurs can be identified, and specific behaviors begun to draw the client closer to significant others. For example, a husband who has hypochondriasis will be asked to agree not to discuss any health-related problems between 7 pm and 10 pm while he and his wife attend a movie she's wanted to see.

Expected Outcomes

While insight is desirable, it is unlikely. The client may develop gradual awareness of the connection of feelings and physical symptoms if a trusting, ongoing relationship is established. With treatment of any comorbid depression or anxiety disorder, particularly with antidepressants, the nurse can expect to see a decrease in the time the client spends thinking about the symptoms or illness and a decrease in health-care visits.

Clients who are willing to remain in individual therapy and participate in supportive or educational group therapy are likely to experience a diminished sense of isolation, increased ability to communicate with significant others, and identifiable improvements in role function. The client should show a decrease in acute symptoms within a month, but over the years will likely experience exacerbations of somatic concerns that are traceable to life stressors. Leave the door open for clients to return to therapy or group as needed.

CASE STUDY

Francine R was a 55-year-old married woman who was initially diagnosed with major depression, hospitalized, treated with an antidepressant (imipramine 25 mg qid) and an antianxiety medication (clonazepam 0.5 mg prn q 6 hr), and released to outpatient care. She had one son who had recently left home for the Army. Although she had two medical conditions that required care but did not impair function, she focused on unrelated vague physical symptoms. Gastrointestinal distress was a "sure sign" of cancer, and pain of any sort was certain to be a "tumor." All of these other conditions had been ruled out.

In Francine's outpatient sessions, the nurse therapist worked to build a trusting relationship and learned about Francine's life as an only child of two very emotionally distant parents. Her retired husband had built a social life with his church that excluded her because of her constant physical complaints. She missed her son, yet constantly complained about his behavior and ingratitude. She felt lonely and isolated from neighbors and friends, and it was readily apparent that her somatic complaints drove people away.

One evening the nurse therapist overheard Francine regaling a complete stranger with stories of her ailments. In the next session, the nurse therapist related her observations to Francine, who could not see how this type of behavior drove people away and even denied doing this.

Because of Francine's lack of insight, the goal of therapy was to provide support for her painful feelings of isolation and loneliness, which she was able to express. The nurse therapist continued to draw her attention to the relationship of her feelings to her physical symptoms and how her physical complaints might affect her relationships with others in a gently confrontational way over 3 years. The outpatient sessions began on a weekly basis and decreased to every 3 months the last year.

Francine agreed to attend a community support group for panic and anxiety, and her husband attended the meetings with her.

Because Francine had experienced major depression she accepted treatment with a tricyclic antidepressant, which was decreased over the last year of treatment to a low maintenance dose. The antidepressant was very helpful in relieving Francine's feelings of fatigue and hopelessness. She was more able to do household tasks and work on a genealogy project she had started prior to her severe depression.

Clonazepam, an antianxiety medication, had been prescribed initially when she was severely depressed and her physical concerns were intense and disabling. This medication, because of its addictive properties, was decreased gradually and discontinued within the first 6 months of treatment because Francine began to view it as the solution to any distress.

Francine also willingly involved herself in a women's self-esteem group. Initially, the other women listened politely. Over the 12-week period, several confronted her about her focus on her physical complaints and her general negativity. Francine's response was to withdraw from the group, complain of being "picked on," and refuse to work through feelings about the group's feedback.

A positive dimension of Francine's treatment dealt with her spiritual and religious beliefs. She discussed with the nurse therapist how her faith was helpful to her when she felt overwhelmed with her physical disabilities, both those that had an organic basis and the symptoms of the hypochondriasis. Francine was encouraged to use prayer to ease her concerns, which she found helpful when she felt neglected and lonely at home.

At the time of her discharge from therapy, Francine remained on 25 mg of imipramine twice a day. She had resumed cooking and cleaning, and through her genealogy project had increased her contact with relatives across the country with whom she maintained correspondence. She had made efforts to be neighborly by offering plants from her garden and hosting a baby shower for a niece. Her relationship with her husband remained distant but cordial, and she had increased her contact with her son by more letter writing and a trip to visit him.

CRITICAL THINKING QUESTIONS

1. Describe what your individual response would be to Francine's behavior.

2. Why did the nurse therapist limit Francine's discussion of her physical symptoms?
3. Describe the connection between Francine's early life experiences and her use of physical symptoms to express distress in her current life.

BODY DYSMORPHIC DISORDER

Characteristic Behaviors

Body dysmorphic disorder (BDD), earlier known as *dysmorphophobia*, is a chronic, disabling condition in which the individual is preoccupied with a perceived defect in appearance. This defect may be imagined or, if present, is so minor that the individual's concerns are out of proportion.

This focus is not just sensitivity but a preoccupation. The client spends so much time thinking about, checking, or trying to change or avoid his or her appearance that there is impairment in social, occupational, or other function.

Typical concerns focus on imagined or minor flaws of the face or head: wrinkles, complexion tone, markings such as freckles or scars, excessive or thinning hair, or asymmetry of the face, eyes, ears, or nose.[1] Other parts or aspects of the body may also be the focus of concern: breasts, genitals, body size, and shape. Anorexia nervosa or extreme weight loss is not included in this disorder. Clients describe feeling tormented by their supposed defect or may refuse to even discuss it, referring only to their generalized "ugly" appearance.

Individuals with the disorder may spend inordinate amounts of time checking their "defect" in mirrors or reflective surfaces (e.g., store windows) and carefully avoid reflections of their appearance. Often, extreme grooming rituals involve hair, makeup, and skin, and compulsive face picking may be present. Some clients believe their "defective" part will malfunction or be easily damaged.

Culture, Age, and Gender Features

Although no hard data exist, this disorder is thought to be more common than previously believed. The earliest occurrence of body dysmorphic disorder is in the teen years, so that nurses working with adolescents should be alert to excessive preoccupation with appearance (see *DSM-IV Diagnostic Criteria*). Nurses who work in settings where plastic surgery is performed may also encounter individuals with these symptoms. Community health nurses may even encounter clients who have withdrawn into their homes. Nurses in outpatient mental health centers or crisis centers may find clients brought in by concerned family members when the disorder has caused serious impairment.

The onset of BDD is often in adolescence, a time when most individuals are exquisitely sensitive to their physical appearance. It may be sudden or gradual, and symptoms may increase or decrease in intensity over time.

> **DSM-IV Diagnostic Criteria for 300.7 Body Dysmorphic Disorder**
>
> A. Preoccupation with an imagined defect in appearance. If a slight physical anomaly is present, the individual's concern is markedly excessive.
>
> B. The preoccupation causes clinically significant distress or impairment in social, occupational, or other important areas of functioning.
>
> C. The preoccupation is not better accounted for by another mental disorder (e.g., dissatisfaction with body shape and size in Anorexia Nervosa).
>
> **Source:** Reprinted with permission from the Diagnostic and Statistical Manual of Mental Disorders, Fourth Edition. Copyright 1994 American Psychiatric Association.

Etiology

There are a number of theories about the causes of body dysmorphic disorder. Most likely, many factors are contributory.

Neurobiological Theory

The high **comorbidity** of BDD with OCD suggested in Hollander and colleagues'[33] study supports a neurobiological influence. OCD has been associated with cortical and subcortical brain anomalies, neurological damage, and a response to SSRI antidepressants. Body dysmorphic disorder has also responded favorably to treatment with SSRIs, no matter how little insight the client may have about the disorder.[34]

Psychological Theory

Psychological factors include insecurity, low self-esteem, and shame. Narcissistic preoccupation with the self and isolation may also be part of the client's personality. The "defect" causes the client to feel ashamed and to withdraw, thus intensifying the client's difficulty in functioning.

Other psychiatric disorders are frequently present. A review of 50 clients diagnosed with BDD[35] found that 39 had coexisting OCD. Thirty-four had depression and 30 suffered from anxiety disorders. Family members also had high rates of these disorders.

Although no research addresses social factors, the strong influence of society's values about appearance would seem to contribute to body dysmorphic disorder. Young, thin, and pretty with large breasts is the ideal look for women, whereas men are expected to be tall, handsome, strong, and lean. Many movie stars, actors, and models have expensive and well-publicized plastic surgeries. At the same time, advertising bombards us with unrealistic standards of physical beauty.

Assessment

The preoccupation with appearance that overtakes the client's life leaves little time for normal activities. The shame and disgust clients feel about their "defective" appearance causes many to withdraw and become housebound.[33]

There is no evidence of psychotic or delusional thinking in this disorder, although clients' insight varies widely. Many can state, "I know it's not that bad" or "I know it's ridiculous" and realize their concerns are exaggerated, but this insight does not alleviate the worry. Researchers disagree about the existence of a psychotic subtype of BDD, but delusional thinking about the body in a psychotic state would be considered a somatic delusion, not BDD.[34]

Clients with BDD may undergo extensive plastic surgery to correct these imagined defects. Body contouring, liposuction, breast augmentation, rhinoplasty, and other procedures may all be done on the same individual.

No physical findings are evident in this disorder, unless the preoccupation is with some actual physical "flaw" such as freckles or a receding chin. Behaviorally, the client may only casually mention the "flaw" when seeking treatment for other medical problems. If the client enters counseling, it is likely to be for feelings of low self-esteem, isolation, or loneliness, rather than to seek help for the preoccupation with the imagined physical flaw. The client may feel too much shame about the "defect" to even mention it in therapy. Socially, the client may be isolated and withdrawn, perhaps even unable to work because of fears that others will notice this humiliating flaw. Withdrawal from family and marital relationships may be the catalyst that causes either family members or the client to seek help.

The client's verbal communication about appearance should be assessed by asking, "How do you feel in general about your body or appearance? Is there any part of your physical appearance that concerns or upsets you?"

When the diagnosis of body dysmorphic disorder has been made, ascertain the focus of the client's concern. The nurse should assess its level of interference with the client's abilities in marital, family, social, and occupational areas. Assess grooming or cleansing rituals that might irritate the skin or other body parts and cause infection.

Assess the client's level of depression and the existence of any suicidal thoughts. Ask how the client has tried to manage the distressing feelings about appearance, such as alcohol or drugs.

Planning Care

The client should be referred for psychiatric care if assessed in the general medical setting. Nursing diagnoses would primarily include:
- Perceptual alterations related to anxiety about physical appearance and chronic low self-esteem and shame, resulting in distorted view of physical features.
- Personal identity disturbance related to feelings of helplessness and fear; identity confusion resulting in intense preoccupation with imagined physical defects and altered role performance.

Interventions for Clients in the Community

With the diagnosis of body dysmorphic disorder, immediate attention to the client's sense of depression and isolation is important. SSRIs have been documented in research literature as effective.[34,35] Education about the medication should highlight the relief of anxiety and depression, the importance of taking the medication long enough to experience relief (2 to 3 weeks), and the need to continue the medication.

The client should be encouraged to participate in individual therapy to alleviate feelings of isolation and shame. In this context, the client experiences a sense of acceptance and understanding from the nurse.

Because of the chronic nature of this disorder, the client should be encouraged to maintain both psychopharmacologic and psychotherapeutic treatment. Encourage the client to participate in group therapy to reduce feelings of social isolation and of being unacceptable.

Educate significant others along with the client so that they understand and support the client's therapeutic efforts. The intense preoccupation with self strains family relationships and has prompted one woman to divorce her husband with BDD, calling it "the selfish disease."[34] When presented with neurobiological findings, the client and family may be more able to view the disorder objectively rather than as a "deliberately" destructive behavior.

Expected Outcomes

This disorder tends to be chronic, although management of stress and anxiety through individual, group, and psychopharmacologic measures can relieve severe interference with functioning. The client should be able to resume work or school following 2 weeks to a month of effective antidepressant therapy.

The client's preoccupation with appearance will likely intensify with stress, which can be modified with stress management techniques. With successful experience in socializing and working, the client's self-esteem should show some improvement, marked by less preoccupation with the physical and social self.

SOMATOFORM DISORDER NOT OTHERWISE SPECIFIED (NOS)

This category is for disorders that do not meet criteria for other somatoform disorders (see *DSM-IV* Diagnostic Criteria). Somatoform symptoms are present but not to the extent or intensity of other somatoform disorders. An example of disorders in this category is pseudocyesis, the false belief that one is pregnant with actual physical symptoms of pregnancy

> ### DSM-IV 300.81 Somatoform Disorder Not Otherwise Specified (NOS)
>
> This category includes disorders with somatoform symptoms that do not meet the criteria for any specific Somatoform Disorder. Examples include:
>
> 1. Pseudocyesis: a false belief of being pregnant that is associated with objective signs of pregnancy, which may include abdominal enlargement (although the umbilicus does not become everted), reduced menstrual flow, amenorrhea, subjective sensation of fetal movement, nausea, breast engorgement and secretions, and labor pains at the expected date of delivery. Endocrine changes may be present, but the syndrome cannot be explained by a general medical condition that causes endocrine changes (e.g., a hormone-secreting tumor).
>
> 2. A disorder involving nonpsychotic hypochondriacal symptoms of less than 6 months' duration.
>
> 3. A disorder involving unexplained physical complaints (e.g., fatigue or body weakness) of less than 6 months' duration that are not due to another mental disorder.
>
> **Source:** Reprinted with permission from the Diagnostic and Statistical Manual of Mental Disorders, Fourth Edition. Copyright 1994 American Psychiatric Association.

such as decreased or absent menstrual flow, enlarged abdomen, nausea, or breast enlargement. No medical reason for the changes can be found. This category also includes nonpsychotic hypochondria symptoms of less than 6 months' duration and unexplained physical complaints for less than 6 months that are not due to other physical or mental disorders.[1]

Expected Outcomes

For the individual with somatoform disorder, improvement will be demonstrated by:
- Decreased somatic complaints.
- Fewer pain symptoms.
- Less time spent thinking about symptoms.
- Fewer visits to health-care providers.
- Absence of destructive coping methods, such as alcohol or narcotics abuse.
- Increased ability to perform activities of daily living.
- Improved ability to perform role functions (work, school, parenting, social).
- Enhanced ability to verbalize feelings.
- Increased ability to relate physical symptoms to emotional causes or stressors.
- Improved ability to use stress management techniques.
- Realistic perception of bodily functions and body image.

COMMON NURSING DIAGNOSES

- Coping, individual, ineffective
- Communication, impaired verbal
- Pain, chronic
- Personal Identity Disturbance
- Grieving, dysfunctional
- Body Image Disturbance
- Self Esteem disturbance
- Social Isolation
- Social Interaction, impaired
- Sensory/Perceptual Alterations (specify): visual, auditory, kinesthetic, gustatory, tactile, olfactory
- Self Care Deficit, feeding, bathing/hygiene, dressing/grooming, toileting
- Knowledge Deficit (specify)

SYNOPSIS OF CURRENT RESEARCH

Researchers have found a significant connection between somatoform disorders and early childhood physical and mental abuse and neglect. Of the 99 women Pribor and colleagues[36] studied who met the criteria for somatization disorder, they found a higher prevalence of sexual, physical, and emotional abuse than in the total study population. More than 90% of the women with somatization disorder reported some type of abuse.

Other researchers[37] studied the influence of early life experiences on 234 clients who were categorized as somatizers. The findings indicated that these clients experienced more childhood physical illnesses, were more often exposed to chronic illness in a parent, or had lost a parent by death or separation before age 17. The researchers postulated from their data that childhood illness allowed an escape from conditions of neglect or abuse and permitted the child to receive much-needed attention. A pattern began of somatic, care-eliciting responses that met emotional needs or at least lessened exposure to hostility. This hypothesis accounts for the lack of insight into the connection between physical symptoms and emotional needs. The client has developed the symptoms as a defense and a way to meet needs, and an automatic pattern of relating emerged in which the feelings and needs are out of awareness, but gratification is found in attention to physical symptoms.

Livingston[38] studied parents with somatization disorder and their children. He found that these children, compared to other children of parents without the disorder, were significantly more likely to have a psychiatric diagnosis, to have more than one psychiatric diagnosis, and to be diagnosed with overanxious disorder. These children also presented with more medically unexplained symptoms, more maltreatment, and more previous hospitalizations.

Guze and colleagues[39] also found the disorder to be present in first-degree female relatives of women with somatization disorder; increased antisocial individuality disorder was present in first-degree male relatives of clients with somatization disorder.

AREAS FOR FUTURE RESEARCH

- Research in the area of neurobiological regulation of incoming sensory information with regard to the body's physical state could delineate differences in individual experience.
- Studies of how sensory information is processed in various parts of the brain may reveal differences in gender and age.
- Study of sociocultural factors may reveal vulnerable populations for somatoform disorders and provide implications for prevention.
- Nurses in the community are in a position to develop ongoing relationships with clients with somatoform disorders and to study the effects of interpersonal and social factors in the course of illness.
- Nurses in medical settings have the opportunity to research client use of health-care resources and explore patterns of use and the economic impact on the system.
- Research comparing various treatment modalities or combinations of treatment modalities for specific disorders is very sparse. Continued study in this area could develop protocols for treatment of specific disorders.

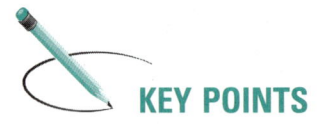

Clinical Management Tips: Somatoform Disorders

- Avoid reinforcing the somatic symptoms by focusing on the pain or other somatic symptom.
- Always ask the client what is going on emotionally when he or she is complaining of somatic symptom.
- Reflect back to the client the feeling that you see displayed (e.g., "You must have felt very lonely during that time" when the client describes a situation involving physical symptoms).
- Avoid assumptions that all somatic complaints are invalid. The client may have a legitimate physical complaint that requires attention.
- Do frequent self-assessment for personal responses to the client's concerns.
- Avoid a punitive attitude. Give physical care that is required with the same gentle approach you would use with any client and the same attitude of concern.
- Involve the client in his or her care as much as possible through teaching about his or her own personal responses to stress and physical manifestations of the stress.
- Limit time spent discussing physical concerns. Seek out the client and direct positive attention at times when physical symptoms are not the focus of concern.
- Recognize the value of supportive therapy that increases the client's functional level rather than aim for "cure."

KEY POINTS

- Anxiety and internal emotional distress can be out of an individual's conscious awareness and can result in physical symptoms of distress, including pain.
- Certain individuals, because of neurobiological makeup, may be more vulnerable to heightened awareness of physical sensations.
- Early childhood and continuing life experiences may lend themselves to the development of a pattern of automatically and unconsciously translating negative emotions into physical symptoms.
- In the theory of somatosensory amplification, individuals may possess both "trait" amplification (being born with the neurobiological tendency to amplify physical sensation) and "state" amplification, which is any given moment that the individual's physical awareness is aroused.
- Somatoform disorders are diagnosed when behavior patterns interfere with the individual's ability to function and are generally chronic, ongoing patterns of behavior. They are more severe and extreme than the occasional "somatizing" that occurs with stress.
- Clients with somatoform disorders truly experience suffering even though there is no "organic" reason for their symptoms.
- Depression, alcohol dependency, anxiety, and personality disorders often accompany somatoform disorders and require appropriate treatment.
- It is essential that clients with these disorders receive a medical (psychiatric) diagnosis to initiate appropriate treatment and prevent the continuance of inappropriate or unnecessary medical treatment.
- The development of a trusting, ongoing relationship with the nurse allows the client to learn about the diagnosis and the connection of mind and body, to develop some understanding of the relationship between feelings and symptoms, and to have a safe environment in which to explore the painful emotions causing the symptoms.
- The nurse must advocate for clients to protect them from unnecessary or potentially harmful treatment in their search for a "cure."
- Antidepressant medication, stress management techniques, biofeedback, group support, and socialization skills all contribute to the client's improved ability to function.
- Clients with somatoform disorders are likely to experience exacerbation of symptoms when stressed. Education and intervention can lessen the intensity of the response.

REFERENCES

1. American Psychiatric Association: Diagnostic and Statistical Manual of Mental Disorders, ed 4. American Psychiatric Association, Washington, DC, 1994.
2. Rosen, G, Kleinman, A, and Katon, A: Somatization in family practice: A biopsychosocial approach. J Fam Pract 14:493, 1982.
3. Golding, JM, Smith, R, and Kashner, TM: Does somatization occur in men? Arch Gen Psychiatry 48:231, 1991.
4. Roberts, SJ: Somatization in primary care. Nurse Pract 5:47, 1994.
5. Rodin, G: Somatization and the self: Psychotherapeutic issues. Am J Psychother 38:257, 1984.
6. Lipowski ZJ: Somatization: The concept and its clinical application. Am J Psychiatry 145:1358, 1988.
7. Bass, C, and Benjamin, S: The management of chronic somatization: Br J Psychiatry 162:472, 1993.
8. Katon, W, Lin, E, VonKorff, M, Russo, J, Lipscomb, P, and Bush, T: Somatization: A spectrum of severity. Am J Psychiatry 148:34, 1991.
9. Roy, SC: Adaptation: A conceptual framework. Nurs Outlook 1:42, 1970.
10. Barsky, AJ, Goodson, JD, Lane, RS, and Cleary, PD: The amplification of somatic symptoms. Psychosom Med 50:510, 1988.
11. Cater, RE: Somatization disorder and chronic candidiasis syndrome: A possible overlap. Med Hypotheses 35:126, 1991.
12. Tomasson, K, Ken, D, and Coryell, W: Somatization and conversion disorders: Comorbidity and demographics at presentation. Acta Psychiatr Scand 84:288, 1991.
13. Stevens, C: Lorazepam in the treatment of acute conversion disorder. Hosp Comm Psychiat 41:1255, 1990.
14. Hendricks-Matthews, M: Conversion disorder in an adult incest survivor. J Fam Pract 3:298, 1991.
15. El-Mallakh, RS, Liebowitz, NR, and Hale, MS: Hyperemesis gravidarum as conversion disorder. J Nerv Men Dis 178:655, 1990.
16. Mahr, G, and Leith, W: Psychogenic stuttering of adult onset. J Speech Hear Res 35:283, 1992.
17. Daie, N, and Witztum, E: Short-term strategic treatment in traumatic conversion reactions. Am J Psychother 45:335, 1991.
18. Bacon, NMK, Bacon, SF, Hampton, Atkinson, J, Slater, MA, Patterson, TL, Grant, I, and Garfin, SR: Somatization symptoms in chronic low back pain patients. Psychosom Med 56:118, 1994.
19. Alexander, PJ, Prabhu, SGS, Krishnamoorthy, ES, and Halkatti, PC: Mental disorders in patients with noncardiac chest pain. Acta Psychiat Scand 89:291, 1994.
20. Walker, EA, Katon, WJ, Hansomn, J, Harrop-Griffiths, J, Holm, L, Jones, ML, Hickok, L, and Jemelka, RP: Medical and psychiatric symptoms in women with childhood sexual abuse. Psychosom Med 54:658, 1992.
21. Reiter, RC, Shakerin, LR, Gambone, JC, and Milburn, A: Correlation between sexual abuse and somatization in women with somatic and nonsomatic chronic pelvic pain. Am J Obstet Gynecol 165:104, 1991.
22. Walling, MK, O'Hara, MW, Reeter, RC, Milburn, AK, Lilley, G, and Vincent, SD: Abuse history and chronic pain in women: II. A multivariate analysis of abuse and psychological morbidity. Obstet Gynecol 84:200, 1994.
23. Noyes, R, Kathol, RG, Fisher, M, Phillips, M, Suelzer, MT, and Holt, CS: The validity of DSM-IIIR hypochondriasis. Arch Gen Psychiatry 50:961, 1993.
24. Fallon, BA, Javitch, JA, Hollander, E, and Leibowitz, MR: Hypochondriasis and obsessive compulsive disorder: Overlaps in diagnoses and treatment. J Clin Psychiatry 52:457, 1991.
25. Starcevic, V: Relationship between hypochondriasis and obsessive compulsive personality disorder: Close relatives separated by nosological schemes? Am J Psychother 44:340, 1990.
26. Stone, AB: Treatment of hypochondriasis with clomipramine (letter). J Clin Psychiatry 54:200, 1993.
27. Rapport, JL: The biology of obsession and compulsions. Sci Am 3:83, 1989.
28. Barsky, AJ, and Wyshak, G: Hypochondriasis and somatosensory amplification. Br J Psychiatry 157:404, 1990.
29. Barsky, AJ, Wool, C, Barnett, MC, and Cleary, PD: Histories of childhood trauma in adult hypochondriacal patients. Am J Psychiatry 151:397, 1994.
30. Ford, CV, Katon, WJ, and Lipkin, M: Managing somatization and hypochondriasis. Client Care 30:31, 1993.
31. Fallon, BA, Klein, BW, and Liebowitz, MR: Hypochondriasis: Treatment strategies. Psychol Ann 23:374, 1993.
32. Fallon, BA, Liebowitz, Salmon, E, Schnerer, FR, Jusino, C, Hollander, E, and Klein, D: Fluoxetine for hypochondriacal patients without major depression. J Clin Psychopharmacol 13:438, 1993.
33. Hollander, E, Cohen, LJ, and Simeon, D: Body dysmorphic disorder. Psychiatr Annuals 23:359, 1993.
34. McElroy, SL, Phillips, KA, Keck, PE, Hudson, JL, and Pope, HG: Body dysmorphic disorder: Does it have a psychotic subtype? J Clin Psychiatry 54:389, 1993.
35. Katon, W, Ries, RK, and Kleinman, A: The prevalence of somatization in primary care. Compr Psychiatry 25:208, 1984.
36. Pribor, EF, Yutzy, SH, Dean, JT, and Wetzel, RD: Briquet's syndrome, dissociation and abuse. Am J Psychiatry 150:1507, 1993.
37. Craig, TKJ, Boardman, AP, Mills, K, Daly-Jones, O, and Drake, H: The South London somatization study: I. Longitudinal course and influence of early life experience. Br J Psychiatry 163:579, 1993.
38. Livingston, R: Children of people with somatization disorder. J Am Acad Child Adolesc Psychiatry 32:536, 1993.
39. Guze, SB, Cloninger, R, Martin, RL, and Clayton, PJ: A follow-up and family study of Briquet's syndrome, Br J Psychiatry 149:17, 1986.

CHAPTER 22

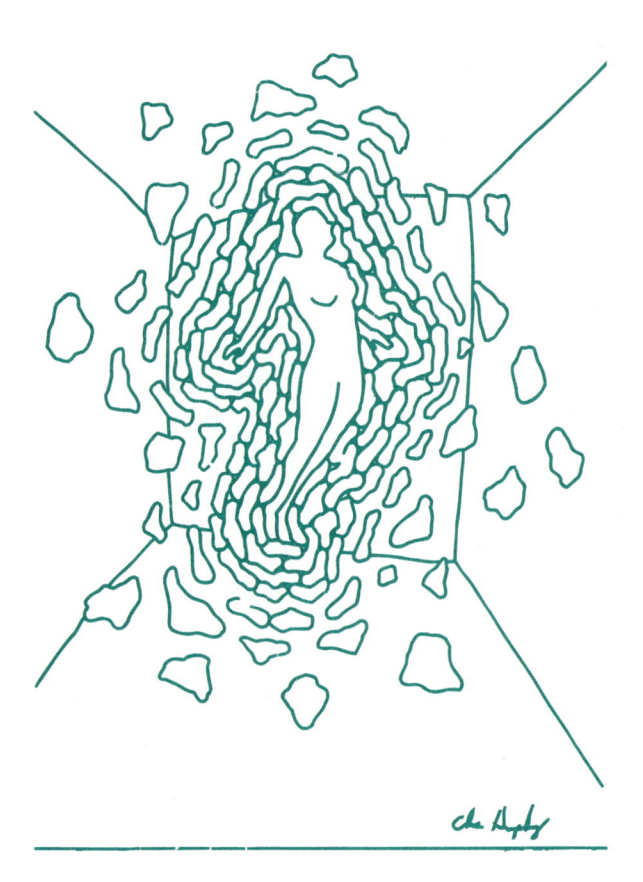

CHAPTER OUTLINE

Posttraumatic Stress Disorder (PTSD)
 Characteristic Behaviors
Dissociative Disorders
 Characteristic Behaviors
Risk Factors
Prevalence
Culture, Age, and Gender Features
Etiology
Prognosis
Planning Care
Interventions for Hospitalized Clients
Interventions for Clients in the Community
Client and Family Education
Expected Outcomes
Differential Diagnosis
Common Nursing Diagnoses
Synopsis of Current Research
Areas for Future Research

LEARNING OBJECTIVES

After completing this chapter, the reader should be able to:

- List the prominent characteristics of posttraumatic stress disorder (PTSD) and dissociative disorders.
- Recognize traumatic events that may lead to PTSD or dissociative disorders.
- Explain the potential neurobiological effects of trauma.
- Identify the physical and psychological sequelae of PTSD and dissociative disorders.
- Analyze the impact of PTSD and dissociative disorders on daily functioning.
- Implement the nursing process in planning care for the individual with PTSD or a dissociative disorder.
- Educate others and develop community programs addressing the potential effects of extreme stress.

KEY TERMS

depersonalization
dissociation
flashbacks
fugue
hyperarousal

hypervigilance
numbing
opioid
startle response

Carol A. Glod, RN, CS, PhD

Posttraumatic Stress and Dissociative Disorders

Stress is a natural part of life. Mild forms of stress can motivate people to change, deal with everyday issues, or seek help for major life problems. However, in its severe forms, stress may create a substantial burden on the individual. Such trauma may come from child abuse or neglect, domestic violence, natural disasters, or warfare. Extreme stress can lead to severe enduring reactions, including posttraumatic stress disorder (PTSD) and dissociative disorders.

PTSD is a set of reactions to an extreme stressor. These reactions include intense fear, helplessness, or horror that leads individuals to relive the trauma.[1] Individuals with PTSD develop three groups of symptoms: intrusive reexperiencing of the trauma, **hyperarousal**, and avoidance behaviors. Symptoms can develop acutely, within the first 3 months of exposure to the stress, or chronically, several years later.

I don't like to talk about being in "Nam" (Vietnam). In fact, I don't like to think about it, hear about it, or be reminded of it. My counselor suggested that I should go to a group with other Vets to talk about the experience, but I thought: no way. Why would I want to talk about it? You see the thing was—nobody expected how bad it would be. I was only 19 and kinda messed up to begin with. I was doing a little pot before I left and not sure about what I really wanted to do with my life. Then I got drafted, and my parents thought being in the army would straighten me out. Straighten me out! No way—it just messed me up. The things I saw, the things I was made to do. You wouldn't believe them. I saw a buddy of mine get blown up right beside me. One minute he was there, the next he was in a million pieces. For the first few weeks I was just numblike. I was like a zombie. Then all of a sudden, after we went through some nasty fighting, it all came back. I still can't get that picture of him out of my mind. I don't want to think about it, but it just keeps coming back, like it haunts me. I don't think I'll ever let it go. Sometimes, I'll be walking along the street and a car will backfire. Then I'll jump a mile and automatically that image of my buddy all blown up comes back. Sometimes it'll just come up for no reason at all. He's also in my dreams. It's that same bad scene, bad dream, all the time. I wake up screaming and crying. The only thing that helps me a little is booze. It takes some of the pain away, but only temporarily. I used to do a lot of drugs, but I kicked that habit. I was into some heavy stuff, heroin and all, when I was in the war. It was really bad when I came back too.

Dissociation, literally, dis-association, refers to feeling detached from usual experiences, "cut off," in a dreamlike state, or unable to remember things. Most frequently it occurs to individuals who have experienced something so traumatic that they "split off" from personal experiences. Although dissociation can occur in PTSD, it is the hallmark of dissociative disorders such as dissociative amnesia, dissociative **fugue**, dissociative identity disorder (formerly called *multiple personality disorder*), **depersonalization** disorder, and dissociative disorder not otherwise specified.[1] The underlying feature in each disorder is the presence of dissociation.

I just woke up and there I was, in the middle of the bridge. I could see that my car was parked down at the foot of the bridge, but I didn't even remember driving there. I was really feeling out of it. When I looked at my watch, I realized that several hours had gone by. It was the middle of the night. The last thing I remembered was feeling kinda detached, like I was in a dream, and the world was just moving on without me. It was like the world around me wasn't real. I felt like I was outside my own body, watching myself. I knew who I was and that I was in the middle of the bridge in my hometown, but I had no idea what had happened and why I was there. It almost seemed like I was going to commit suicide. I didn't feel suicidal when I woke up, though. And that's exactly how it was: It was like I was in a dream, remembering only parts of it and then I woke up, but I wasn't in bed. I was really scared. I think these "spells" have been happening more often. They've also been going on at work. One day I went to my job dressed in these really strange clothes with crayons in my purse. Crayons! I haven't used crayons in years. I did find some really bad, childlike drawings in the trash, but couldn't figure out exactly how they got there. No one else was around, but I don't remember doing them. I'm starting to think that I'm going crazy. It's not right to forget things you've done. It's pretty dangerous too—like that time I woke up on the bridge.

Abused people, combat veterans, Holocaust survivors, prisoners of war, and individuals who were involved in or witnessed extremely dangerous events such as bombings,

TABLE 22–1. Traumatic Events That May Lead to the Development of Posttraumatic Stress Disorder and Dissociative Disorders

- Military combat
- Bombings or war
- Kidnapping
- Mugging or robbery
- Physical, sexual (e.g., rape), or psychological abuse
- Terrorist attack
- Prisoner-of-war or concentration-camp experience
- Torture
- Natural or manmade disasters
- Witnessing violence (domestic, criminal)
- Severe automobile accidents
- Seeing dead body or body parts
- Serious injury or death of family member or a close friend
- Diagnosis of a life-threatening disease in self or child
- Unexpected death of family member or a close friend

drive-by shootings, and earthquakes commonly develop PTSD or a dissociative disorder (Table 22–1). These extremely stressful events are the primary causes of PTSD. Dissociative disorders frequently are associated with severe trauma, but not always. *Stress* or *trauma*, terms used commonly to describe a variety of experiences, differ from the impact leading to PTSD or dissociative disorders. Stress may be acute or chronic and negative (such as loss, death, or separations) or positive (such as moving, marriage, or birth of a child). In PTSD and dissociative disorders, the events are extremely stressful, life threatening, and beyond most individuals' usual experience. For instance, although the loss of a parent is stressful and can have severe consequences, witnessing the shooting of a parent while in imminent danger of death is the kind of trauma that leads to PTSD or a dissociative disorder.

POSTTRAUMATIC STRESS DISORDER (PTSD)

Characteristic Behaviors

A severely stressful event should alert nurses to the potential for a client to develop significant psychological, physical, or behavioral disruption. A more recent stress, such as medical illness, separation, or birth of a child, may precipitate memories of past traumas. A physical assault on an adult may call up memories of past childhood abuse or domestic violence. As a child, one client had watched and heard bombing raids over Europe during World War II and witnessed significant death and destruction. He sought treatment after watching a fireworks demonstration that got out of control, injured and maimed several people, and subsequently set a building on fire. The sound of the fireworks and the sight of physical destruction and injury to others were reminiscent of the events he witnessed as a child. Although fireworks displays had always bothered him, it wasn't until this terrible situation that he began having severe **flashbacks** and nightmares of the earlier experience.

In addition to exposure to a severe stressor, individuals with PTSD display symptoms in three major areas: intrusive reexperiencing of the traumatic event, hyperarousal, and avoidance and **numbing** of responsiveness (see *DSM-IV* Diagnostic Criteria). The trauma may be reexperienced in the form of disturbing flashbacks (acting or feeling as if the event were actually happening), intrusive recollections, or nightmares.[1] Individuals feel like the trauma is actually happening again. Hyperarousal may be experienced as increased pulse, sleep disruption, and difficulty concentrating. Individuals frequently avoid things that remind them of the trauma. Avoidance may also lead to feeling numb or to periods of dissociation.

Physical signs may be elicited in situations that are reminiscent of the trauma. For instance, a woman raped in an elevator develops autonomic hyperarousal, such as increased pulse, fearfulness, and sweating, while in elevators. She may avoid thoughts or feelings associated with the trauma, have difficulty remembering the event, or be detached or numb. Along with avoiding elevators or buildings with elevators, she may seek out treatment for hypertension and cardiac complaints. Increased arousal may be evident in sleep disruption, angry outbursts, trouble concentrating, **hypervigilance** (close attention to and anticipation of approaching danger), or being easily startled (**startle response**).

In general, these behaviors occur within 4 weeks of the traumatic event and persist for at least 1 month.[1] If these behaviors continue for 1 to 3 months, the individual has acute PTSD, whereas if they remain for more than 3 months, the individual is suffering from chronic PTSD. Sometimes, PTSD emerges months or years after the initial trauma, and thus PTSD, with delayed onset, may be evident if the onset occurs after 6 months.[1]

DISSOCIATIVE DISORDERS

Characteristic Behaviors

Dissociative experiences include periods of forgetfulness, memory loss for past stressful events, feeling disconnected from daily events, or severe identity confusion or distinctly different personality states. One of the key features of dissociative disorders is memory impairment, beyond usual forgetfulness, usually for something personal and important. The response may be impaired consciousness, memory, identity, or perceptions of the environment.[1] The Dissociative Experience Scale (DES, Table 22–2) has been used in several studies to measure lapses in memory, déjà vu expe-

> ### DSM Diagnostic Criteria for 309.81 Posttraumatic Stress Disorder
>
> A. The person has been exposed to a traumatic event in which both of the following were present:
>   (1) the person experienced, witnessed, or was confronted with an event or events that involved actual or threatened death or serious injury, or a threat to the physical integrity of self or others
>   (2) the person's response involved intense fear, helplessness, or horror.
>   NOTE: In children, this may be expressed instead by disorganized or agitated behavior.
>
> B. The traumatic event is persistently reexperienced in one (or more) of the following ways:
>   (1) recurrent and intrusive distressing recollections of the event, including images, thoughts, or perceptions
>   NOTE: In young children, repetitive play may occur in which themes or aspects of the trauma are expressed.
>   (2) recurrent distressing dreams of the event
>   NOTE: In children, there may be frightening dreams without recognizable content.
>   (3) acting or feeling as if the traumatic event were recurring (includes a sense of reliving the experience, illusions, hallucinations, and dissociative flashback episodes, including those that occur on awakening or when intoxicated).
>   NOTE: In young children, trauma-specific reenactment may occur.
>   (4) intense psychological distress at exposure to internal or external cues that symbolize or resemble an aspect of the traumatic event
>   (5) physiological reactivity on exposure to internal or external cues that symbolize or resemble an aspect of the traumatic event
>
> C. Persistent avoidance of stimuli associated with the trauma and numbing of general responsiveness (not present before the trauma), as indicated by three (or more) of the following:
>   (1) efforts to avoid thoughts, feelings, or conversations associated with the trauma
>   (2) efforts to avoid activities, places, or people that arouse recollections of the trauma
>   (3) inability to recall an important aspect of the trauma
>   (4) markedly diminished interest or participation in significant activities
>   (5) feeling of detachment or estrangement from others
>   (6) restricted range of affect (e.g., unable to have loving feelings)
>   (7) sense of a foreshortened future (e.g., does not expect to have a career, marriage, children, or a normal life span)
>
> D. Persistent symptoms of increased arousal (not present before the trauma), as indicated by two (or more) of the following:
>   (1) difficulty falling or staying asleep
>   (2) irritability or outbursts of anger
>   (3) difficulty concentrating
>   (4) hypervigilance
>   (5) exaggerated startle response
>
> E. Duration of the disturbance (symptoms in Criteria B, C, and D) is more than 1 month.
>
> F. The disturbance causes clinically significant distress or impairment in social, occupational, or other important areas of functioning.
>
> Specify if:
>   **Acute:** if duration of symptoms is less than 3 months
>   **Chronic:** if duration of symptoms is 3 months or more
>
> Specify if:
>   **With Delayed Onset:** if onset of symptoms is at least 6 months after the stressor
>
> **Source:** Reprinted with permission from the Diagnostic and Statistical Manual of Mental Disorders, Fourth Edition. Copyright 1994 American Psychiatric Association.

riences (an unfamiliar place seems familiar), and other behaviors suggestive of dissociation.[2]

Dissociative Amnesia

In dissociative amnesia, clients have difficulty remembering past periods of time (see *DSM-IV Diagnostic Criteria*). The memory loss goes beyond usual forgetfulness. There may be defined gaps in memory for years or for self-destructive, violent, or suicidal episodes. Traumatic events such as physical or sexual abuse frequently account for the memory impairment. Most individuals with dissociative amnesia cannot remember a period of months or years or the first few hours of a very disturbing event, or they have only partial recall for the event. A common example is an individual who has no memory of childhood.

Dissociative Fugue

Dissociative fugue, which is relatively uncommon, is confusion about one's personal identity and inability to remember one's past (see *DSM-IV Diagnostic Criteria*). Fugue states

TABLE 22–2. The Dissociative Experience Scale (DES)

I.D. Number Code _____

This questionnaire consists of 28 questions about experiences you may have had in your daily life. We are interested in how often you have had these experiences. It is important, however, that your answers show how often these experiences happen to you when you are not under the influence of alcohol or drugs. To answer the questions, please determine to what degree the experience described in the question applies to you and mark the line with a vertical slash at the appropriate place, as shown in the example below.

Example:
0% |————————\————————| 100%

1. Some people have the experience of driving a car and suddenly realizing that they don't remember what has happened during all or part of the trip. Mark the line to show what percentage of the time this happens to you.
0% |————————————————| 100%

2. Some people find that sometimes they are listening to someone talk and they suddenly realize that they did not hear part or all of what was just said. Mark the line to show what percentage of the times this happens to you.
0% |————————————————| 100%

3. Some people have the experience of finding themselves in a place and having no idea how they got there. Mark the line to show what percentage of the time this happens to you.
0% |————————————————| 100%

4. Some people have the experience of finding themselves dressed in clothes that they don't remember putting on. Mark the line to show what percentage of the time this happens to you.
0% |————————————————| 100%

5. Some people have the experience of finding new things among their belongings that they do not remember buying. Mark the line to show what percentage of the time this happens to you.
0% |————————————————| 100%

6. Some people sometimes find that they are approached by people that they do not know who call them by another name or insist that they have met them before. Mark the line to show what percentage of the time this happens to you.
0% |————————————————| 100%

7. Some people sometimes have the experience of feeling as though they are standing next to themselves or watching themselves do something and they actually see themselves as though they were looking at another person. Mark the line to show what percentage of the time this happens to you.
0% |————————————————| 100%

8. Some people are told that they sometimes do not recognize friends or family members. Mark the line to show what percentage of the time this happens to you.
0% |————————————————| 100%

9. Some people find that they have no memory for some important events in their lives (for example, a wedding or graduation). Mark the line to show what percentage of the important events in your life you have no memory for.
0% |————————————————| 100%

10. Some people have the experience of being accused of lying when they do not think that they have lied. Mark the line to show what percentage of the time this happens to you.
0% |————————————————| 100%

11. Some people have the experience of looking in a mirror and not recognizing themselves. Mark the line to show what percentage of the time this happens to you.
0% |————————————————| 100%

12. Some people sometimes have the experience of feeling that other people, objects, and the world around them are not real. Mark the line to show what percentage of the time this happens to you.
0% |————————————————| 100%

13. Some people sometimes have the experience of feeling that their body does not seem to belong to them. Mark the line to show what percentage of the time this happens to you.
0% |————————————————| 100%

14. Some people have the experience of sometimes remembering a past event so vividly that they feel as if they were reliving that event. Mark the line to show what percentage of the time this happens to you.
0% |————————————————| 100%

15. Some people have the experience of not being sure whether things that they remember happening really did happen or whether they just dreamed them. Mark the line to show what percentage of the time this happens to you.
0% |————————————————| 100%

16. Some people have the experience of being in a familiar place but finding it strange and unfamiliar. Mark the line to show what percentage of the time this happens to you.
0% |————————————————| 100%

17. Some people find that when they are watching television or a movie they become so absorbed in the story that they are unaware of other events happening around them. Mark the line to show what percentage of the time this happens to you.
0% |————————————————| 100%

18. Some people sometimes find that they become so involved in a fantasy or daydream that it feels as though it were really happening to them. Mark the line to show what percentage of the time this happens to you.
0% |————————————————| 100%

19. Some people find that they sometimes are able to ignore pain. Mark the line to show what percentage of the time this happens to you.
0% |————————————————| 100%

Continued on following page

TABLE 22–2. The Dissociative Experience Scale (DES) (*Continued*)

20. Some people find that they sometimes sit staring off into space, thinking of nothing, and are not aware of the passage of time. Mark the line to show what percentage of the time this happens to you.
    0% |—————————————————| 100%

21. Some people sometimes find that when they are alone they talk out loud to themselves. Mark the line to show what percentage of the time this happens to you.
    0% |—————————————————| 100%

22. Some people find that in one situation they may act so differently compared to another situation that they feel almost as if they were two different people. Mark the line to show what percentage of the time this happens to you.
    0% |—————————————————| 100%

23. Some people sometimes find that in certain situations they are able to do things with amazing ease and spontaneity that would usually be difficult for them (for example, sports, work, social situations, etc.). Mark the line to show what percentage of the time this happens to you.
    0% |—————————————————| 100%

24. Some people sometimes find that they cannot remember whether they have done something or have just thought about doing that thing (for example, not knowing whether they have just mailed a letter or have just thought about mailing it). Mark the line to show what percentage of the time this happens to you.
    0% |—————————————————| 100%

25. Some people sometimes find evidence that they have done things that they do not remember doing. Mark the line to show what percentage of the time this happens to you.
    0% |—————————————————| 100%

26. Some people sometimes find writings, drawings, or notes among their belongings that they must have done, but cannot remember doing. Mark the line to show what percentage of the time this happens to you.
    0% |—————————————————| 100%

27. Some people sometimes find that they hear voices inside their head that tell them to do things or comment on things that they are doing. Mark the line to show what percentage of the time this happens to you.
    0% |—————————————————| 100%

28. Some people sometimes feel as if they are looking at the world through a fog so that people and objects appear far away or unclear. Mark the line to show what percentage of the time this happens to you.
    0% |—————————————————| 100%

To score the DES, measure each 100 mm line, add the 28 items, and divide by 28. A score greater than or equal to 15 suggests dissociation. Note: This is an example only and is not drawn to scale.

Source: Bernstein, EM, and Putnam, FW: Development, reliability, and validity of a dissociation scale. Journal of Nervous and Mental Disease 174:727–735. Copyright Williams & Wilkins, 1986.

---

are characterized by sudden unexpected travel away from home or work and amnesia for the client's identity or past.[1] Individuals with this disorder may even take on new identities; however, they act and behave as if nothing were different.

Depersonalization Disorder

Depersonalization disorder is characterized by episodes of depersonalization, times of feeling detached or numb, or acting as if in a dream or a movie (see *DSM-IV* Diagnostic Criteria). Sometimes people describe this phenomenon as "being outside of my body, as if I were watching myself." Although these experiences may occur commonly in very mild forms, for the individual with depersonalization disorder, symptoms interfere with relationships, memory, and occupational functioning.

Dissociative Identity Disorder

Severe identity disruption, in the form of two or more distinct personalities that take control over behavior, may occur in dissociative identity disorder (see *DSM-IV* Diagnostic Criteria). Individuals with dissociative identity disorder describe very different personalities, with distinct histories, ages, gender, names, and mood styles such as angry, depressed, or domineering. Sometimes referred to as "alters," that is, alter personalities, these states may also be characterized by different physical ailments or disorders, visual problems (needing glasses or not), pain tolerance, or electroencephalogram (EEG) patterns. Memory lapses are common. The presence of "voices," *auditory hallucinations,* may represent different personality states. Most individuals with dissociative identity disorder have histories of severe childhood abuse.

RISK FACTORS

Although it is unclear who develops PTSD or a dissociative disorder, several factors increase the risk. Sometimes, having a child can precipitate previous memories of abuse and trigger symptoms. Some women have reported the development of PTSD behaviors after their children reached the age at which they were abused. Certain populations are also at risk: civilians of countries with civil unrest or war, homeless per-

> ### DSM-IV Diagnostic Criteria for Dissociative Amnesia, Fugue, Identity Disorder, and Depersonalization Disorder
>
> **Diagnostic Criteria for 300.12 Dissociative Amnesia**
>
> A. The predominant disturbance is one or more episodes of inability to recall important personal information, usually of a traumatic or stressful nature, that is too extensive to be explained by ordinary forgetfulness.
>
> B. The disturbance does not occur exclusively during the course of Dissociative Identity Disorder, Dissociative Fugue, Posttraumatic Stress Disorder, Acute Stress Disorder, or Somatization Disorder and is not due to the direct physiological effects of a substance (e.g., a drug of abuse, a medication) or a neurological or other general medical condition (e.g., Amnestic Disorder Due to Head Trauma).
>
> C. The symptoms cause clinically significant distress or impairment in social, occupational, or other important areas of functioning.
>
> **Diagnostic Criteria for 300.13 Fugue**
>
> A. The predominant disturbance is sudden, unexpected travel away from home or one's customary place of work, with inability to recall one's past.
>
> B. Confusion about personal identity or assumption of a new identity (partial or complete).
>
> C. The disturbance does not occur exclusively during the course of Dissociative Identity Disorder and is not due to the direct physiological effects of a substance (e.g., a drug of abuse, a medication) or a general medical condition (e.g., temporal lobe epilepsy).
>
> D. The symptoms cause clinically significant distress or impairment in social, occupational, or other important areas of functioning.
>
> **Diagnostic Criteria for 300.6 Depersonalization Disorder**
>
> A. Persistent or recurrent experiences of feeling detached from, and as if one is an outside observer of, one's mental processes or body (e.g., feeling like one is in a dream).
>
> B. During the depersonalization experience, reality testing remains intact.
>
> C. The depersonalization causes clinically significant distress or impairment in social, occupational, or other important areas of functioning.
>
> D. The depersonalization experience does not occur exclusively during the course of another mental disorder, such as Schizophrenia, Panic Disorder, Acute Stress Disorder, or another Dissociative Disorder, and is not due to the direct physiological effects of a substance (e.g., a drug of abuse, a medication) or a general medical condition (e.g., temporal lobe epilepsy).
>
> **Diagnostic Criteria for 300.14 Dissociative Identity Disorder**
>
> A. The presence of two or more distinct identities or personality states (each with its own relatively enduring pattern of perceiving, relating to, and thinking about the environment and self).
>
> B. At least two of these identities or personality states recurrently take control of the person's behavior.
>
> C. Inability to recall important personal information that is too extensive to be explained by ordinary forgetfulness.
>
> D. The disturbance is not due to the direct physiological effects of a substance (e.g., blackouts or chaotic behavior during Alcohol Intoxication) or a general medical condition (e.g., complex partial seizures).
>
> NOTE: In children, the symptoms are not attributable to imaginary playmates or other fantasy play.
>
> **Source:** Adapted from the Diagnostic and Statistical Manual of Mental Disorders, Fourth Edition. Copyright 1994 American Psychiatric Association.

sons, those with substance abuse, and those in certain professions, such as rescue workers. Health-care personnel, firefighters, and police officers showed symptoms of PTSD after the Oklahoma City bombing. Emergency rooms may be one practice setting where the presence of an extreme stressor and its response can be detected.

Stress and trauma care are integral parts of nursing, and several nurse theorists and scientists have used the stress-adaptation framework as a basis for their work. One of the major roles for nursing is to assist in the early identification of those predisposed to developing PTSD or a dissociative disorder and to routinely assess the presence of recent or lifetime stressors. The predictors of who will develop these disorders are not known. Furthermore, not every individual who is exposed to a very traumatic event will display symptoms. Factors such as severity, duration, and proximity to the stressful event are likely to affect the risk. Some individuals suffer no discernible effects (so-called resiliency), whereas others develop depression, difficulties in interpersonal relationships, or physical problems. Clients with PTSD

> **RESEARCH NOTE**
>
> Teicher, MH, Glod, CA, Surrey, J, and Swett, C, Jr: Early childhood abuse and limbic system ratings in adult psychiatric outpatients. J Neuropsychiatry Neurosci 5:301–306, 1993.
>
> **Findings:** Several studies have suggested that extreme stress in the form of physical, sexual, or psychological abuse is associated with deleterious effects on brain development. In this study, the authors evaluated the association between childhood physical and sexual abuse and limbic system dysfunction in more than 250 adult outpatients who presented for psychiatric assessment. These investigators looked at individuals with and without abuse histories and scores derived from a self-report instrument, the limbic system checklist-33 (LSCL-33), which evaluated four broad areas of physical and psychological dysfunction related to changes in the limbic system: somatic, sensory, behavioral, and memory symptoms. The participants rated these symptoms as occurring "never," "sometimes," and "often." Clients who experienced either physical or sexual abuse had higher LSCL-33 scores, suggesting that severe childhood abuse was associated with more neurologic-like symptoms. Those who acknowledged both physical and sexual abuse had LSCL-33 scores 110% greater than those who denied abuse. These researchers also found that abuse before age 18 was associated with greater limbic system dysfunction than abuse experienced after age 18.
>
> **Application to Practice:** This study provides nurses with a different approach to understanding the effects of severe trauma on neurobiological symptoms. Physical and sexual abuse during early childhood may lead to physical as well as psychological symptoms in adults. Severe forms of abuse may affect the development of the brain, particularly the limbic system, responsible for regulating mood, heart rate, memory, and aggressive behavior. This study suggests that childhood abuse may lead to the development of somatic complaints, memory problems, sensory distortions, and dissociative experiences. In clients with PTSD or dissociative disorders, these symptoms may predominate and signal the need for further neurological evaluation. As providers of primary prevention, nurses need to be actively involved in educating clients about the potential consequences of abuse and raising public awareness about the effects of trauma on brain functioning. The results of this study also suggest that early intervention is necessary for children who have been exposed to physical and sexual abuse, to prevent long-term biological and psychological problems.

or dissociative disorders can also have substantial unexplained medical complaints and as a result are frequent consumers of health care.

PREVALENCE

The prevalence of PTSD ranges from 1 to 14%. It may be more likely to occur in countries with severe violence, torture, or war.[1] PTSD is more likely in individuals with childhood abuse who then suffer a subsequent trauma. For instance, PTSD is more common in war veterans who reported a history of childhood abuse than in those without previous abuse.[3] The exact rates of dissociative disorders are unknown; however, their prevalence has increased in recent years, perhaps because of greater awareness of their existence.[1]

CULTURE, AGE, AND GENDER FEATURES

Culture

As noted before, individuals from countries with social unrest and civil conflict may be more prone to developing these conditions.

Dissociation is not necessarily a psychiatric disorder. In some cultures, trancelike states are common and should be distinguished from dissociative disorders. For instance, Western Pacific cultures describe *amok* (periods of dissociation followed by aggression), and residents of the Arctic display *pibloktoq* (dissociative episodes of excitement followed by seizures and coma). Navajos display "frenzy" witchcraft, and individuals from Honduras and Nicaragua describe *grisi siknis*.[1] These episodes involve trancelike states, high activity levels, and purposeless running, with amnesia for the events.

Age

Children may also develop PTSD or dissociative disorders, although the diagnosis is more difficult to make, and different features may predominate. For instance, in place of traditional flashbacks, children may demonstrate or "reenact" the traumatic event in their play. Children frequently display a sense of foreshortened future, leading them to believe that they will not become adults. Agitation, sleep disturbance, and nightmares of monsters or of abuse are also common in youngsters.

Gender

PTSD affects both males and females at any age. Dissociative identity disorder is generally diagnosed more in the United States, suggesting that perhaps it is culture specific, with females receiving the diagnosis three to nine times more often.[1]

ETIOLOGY

Neuropharmacologic Theories

Very little is known about the etiology of dissociative disorders, and until recently the biological basis of posttraumatic disorders was largely neglected. Unlike other major psychiatric disorders that implicate neuropharmacologic mechanisms in the development of the condition, abnormalities in neurotransmitter regulation have been more difficult to pinpoint in PTSD. Some studies have found elevated levels of norepinephrine and epinephrine, whereas others have reported normal levels.[4,5] However, when levels of norepinephrine and epinephrine are measured in individuals with PTSD under stressful conditions, they are increased.[6] The receptors associated with these neurotransmitters are reduced, presumably in response to increased levels of norepinephrine and epinephrine. Increased levels of norepinephrine and epinephrine are probably reflected in the elevated BP and pulse observed in clients with PTSD. Individuals with PTSD have autonomic hyperarousal, manifested by increased BP and pulse, and some intermittent sympathetic nervous system hyperfunction. As a result, individuals may display hyperarousal, sleep deprivation, poor concentration, and irritability, making it difficult for them to function effectively.

Other neurotransmitters may be implicated in the pathogenesis of PTSD. Although limited information is available, PTSD may be associated with low amounts of serotonin. Reduced serotonin levels have been found in animals that were subjected to traumatic conditions. Low serotonin levels may produce symptoms of hyperarousal and mood changes. Antidepressant medications that increase levels of serotonin, selective serotonin reuptake inhibitors (SSRIs), have been shown to reduce symptoms of PTSD.

Endogenous Opioid Theory

The body's biological reaction to severe stress may be activation of the endogenous **opioid** system. Endogenous opioids act like natural narcotics to help soothe or dull the senses in individuals with PTSD. Under extremely stressful conditions, the body releases opioids, which decrease the emotional responses to extreme stress such as fear, helplessness, and anxiety. This theory may explain why individuals with trauma histories tend to hurt themselves or subject themselves to other traumatic situations (repetition of the trauma). The desire to reengage in these behaviors is linked to release of endogenous opioids. In essence, traumatized individuals may "seek" further trauma to release opioids to "self-medicate" their discomfort, fear, and PTSD reactions. Opioid release may provide a form of analgesia to deal with these overwhelming feelings. In an experiment to test this theory, van der Kolk asked war veterans to watch a violent war movie (*Platoon*).[7] He found that the internal opioid system was activated during the stressful scenes. Thus, the body's biological reaction to experiencing similar stressful events (combat scenes) led to the release of opioids to help individuals reduce their psychological response. It is similar to taking narcotic medications to "dull the pain."

Stimulation of endogenous opioids may also explain the co-occurrence of PTSD and alcohol or substance abuse. During the Vietnam War, some combat veterans abused illicit substances, particularly heroin, perhaps in an attempt to cope with the atrocities of war by helping the body's physiological adaptation to extreme stress. Like endogenous opioids, illicit substances such as heroin may provide the necessary "analgesia" for extreme emotional responses. The result is to inhibit emotional pain and reduce fear and panic.

Neuroendocrine Theory

In recent years, a stress hormone, cortisol, has been implicated in the etiology of PTSD. The amount of cortisol released may vary, depending on whether the individual is subjected to extreme stress acutely or chronically. Under acute conditions, increased amounts of cortisol are secreted. In chronic states, however, such as PTSD, individuals show decreased cortisol output.[8] After chronic exposure to stress, the endocrine system, working on a feedback signal, senses the initial outpouring of cortisol and "resets" the system to lower levels. This change is similar to turning down the thermostat when too much heat is produced.

In addition, clients with PTSD show a response opposite that of depressed individuals to the dexamethasone suppression test (DST). In this test, individuals are given a synthetic steroid, dexamethasone, to examine the function of their endocrine systems. In response to dexamethasone, individuals with depression continue to produce cortisol, so-called nonsuppression (see Chapter 19). In response to the administration of dexamethasone, those with PTSD set their systems lower, so-called enhanced suppression of cortisol on the DST.[8] Instead of nonsuppression, individuals with PTSD produce even less cortisol than individuals with no psychiatric disorders.

Neurodevelopmental and Neurobiological Theories

PTSD and dissociative disorders provide a clear example of how environment and severe stress lead to definable neurobiological consequences. An intriguing recent theory is that extreme stress, particularly in the form of physical, sexual, or psychological abuse, is associated with deleterious effects on brain development, particularly reduced hippocampal size and abnormalities in the limbic system.[9-11] Studies of physically, sexually, and psychologically abused children found more neurological problems such as increased EEG abnormalities in the frontal and temporal lobes.[11] Combat veterans and sexually abused women have smaller hippocampui, and the greater the hippocampal shrinkage, the more dissociative symptoms clients experience.[9,12] These changes in the limbic system may result in behaviors commonly observed in PTSD and dissociative disorders: memory lapses, dissociation, difficulty controlling emotions, hyperarousal symptoms such as increased heart rate, and neuropsychological problems. In addition to psychological effects, severe trauma may lead to definable changes in the brain's morphology and functioning.

> **RESEARCH NOTE**
>
> Bremner, JD, Randall, P, Scott, TM, Bronen, RA, Seibyl, JP, Southwick, SM, Delaney, RC, McCarthy, G, Charney, DS, and Innis, RB: MRI-based measurement of hippocampal volume in patients with combat-related posttraumatic stress disorder. Am J Psychiatry 152:973–981, 1995.
>
> **Findings:** The hippocampus plays an important role in memory, and damage to the hippocampus has been associated with short-term memory problems. Memory loss and dissociation is prominent in clients with PTSD. This study examined structural brain changes in PTSD and dissociation, specifically hippocampal changes in Vietnam veterans with a history of combat-related PTSD via magnetic resonance imaging (MRI) techniques. They found that clients with PTSD had an 8% shrinkage in the right hippocampus compared with volunteers without PTSD. A smaller shrinkage in left hippocampal volume (4%) was also found in the PTSD individuals. Smaller size of the right hippocampus was associated with more deficits in short-term memory, commonly seen in PTSD. The researchers concluded that the changes in the hippocampus were due to the effects of exposure to severely traumatic war and combat events. They hypothesized that the shrinkage in the hippocampus may have resulted from high levels of stress hormones such as glucocorticoids, which are produced in response to severe trauma. The outpouring of glucocorticoids may lead to brain cell destruction, particularly in the right hippocampus.
>
> **Application to Practice:** The hippocampus, part of the limbic system, is in part responsible for memory. The left hippocampus is thought to be involved in verbal memory, whereas the right hippocampus plays a role in visual memory. The findings in this study suggest that shrinkage of the right hippocampus may occur secondary to PTSD and result in memory deficits, particularly for visuospatial performance. Clients with PTSD may not be able to learn or recall information because of these memory deficits. Nurses should advocate for clients receiving information and education in different ways, such as written forms. Individuals with PTSD may also need frequent reinforcement of new information. Education for families can include similar strategies to help clients deal with these problems. This study also suggests that clients with PTSD need vocational rehabilitation that acknowledges memory deficits.

Two nurse researchers proposed another theory, the information processing of trauma (IPT) model, to explain the effects of PTSD on the brain.[13] In this model, the limbic system, responsible for encoding information, is overwhelmed during severe trauma such as child abuse. Therefore, the usual ways in which information is experienced, filtered, and related to memory retrieval and recall is impaired. The result is that traumatized individuals then have difficulty with basic processes: eating, sleeping, attachment, affect, sex, and aggression.[13] According to this model, trauma impedes the development of the information processing necessary for healthy interpersonal relationships and ideas of trust, blame, and control.

Repetition and Family Influences Theory

According to the theory of transgenerational abuse, those with a history of suffering or witnessing childhood physical or sexual abuse may tend to repeat the abusive behavior in adulthood (see Chapter 31). This repetition over generations has been called the "cycle of violence." Another part of this theory is revictimization, the traumatized client's tendency to be reexposed to other forms of trauma in the future. In this model, individuals subjected to severe trauma are less able to protect themselves from future traumatic events.

PROGNOSIS

PTSD and dissociative disorders tend to have a chronic, fluctuating course, often associated with other problems, including substance abuse and mood disorders. Often individuals use illicit substances or alcohol to escape or to enhance numbing from the emotional pain. Social support, family history, childhood experiences, personality style, and other disorders may influence recovery. Dissociative fugue usually lasts for a single episode, for hours to days.[1]

PLANNING CARE

Effective treatment depends on assessing the degree of distress experienced by the individual. Those with PTSD or a dissociative disorder with concomitant substance or alcohol abuse, mood disorder, or other conditions need immediate, intensive treatment to treat the substance or alcohol abuse first. Individuals who are already numb and who have difficulty remaining connected put themselves at further risk by engaging in these self-destructive behaviors. Sustained periods of dissociation or persistent reexperiencing of the trauma may prevent clients from functioning successfully in school or work and from meeting the usual daily demands. If the symptoms are severe or the client is actively planning suicide, hospitalization or intensive outpatient treatment is necessary. Medications may help with severe mood changes, anxiety, and depression.

Clients require individual psychotherapy to overcome the

effects of trauma on their current functioning. They need a consistent empathic approach to help them tolerate the intense memories and emotional pain. Treatment focuses on helping clients acknowledge the intensely traumatic event without experiencing it over and over again. Although it may be cognitive-behavioral, supportive, or another form, it is usually a long-term process. Both individual and group therapy are useful to decrease denial, enhance trust, cope with loss and guilt, modulate anger, and enhance recognition of overwhelming feelings. The ultimate goal is to improve functioning and interpersonal relationships.

Because little research has been conducted on the effectiveness of various treatments, it is unclear which interventions are most helpful. Constant assessment and reevaluation may be necessary in that individuals with PTSD may experience intrusive recollections at one time, whereas avoidance behaviors and dissociation may predominate at another point. Those with dissociative disorders first need to learn how to control their detachment and "spacing out." In the case of comorbidity, the initial treatment may be aimed primarily at resolving the other condition. For instance, antidepressant medication may be needed for severe depression. The overall goal of treatment is to help clients control their emotional responses, develop more connectedness, and, if severe trauma has occurred, let go of the haunting memories to become more engaged in the present.

Clients may avoid regular medical, dental, and gynecological care and need referral to providers sensitive to their needs. Because of fear, their basic health-care needs may go unmet for years. The treatment plan should encompass interventions for physical and psychological needs.

INTERVENTIONS FOR HOSPITALIZED CLIENTS

Address basic safety issues first, such as suicidal and dangerous behavior. Use the Clinical Management Tips listed in the table. Clients with PTSD or dissociative disorders are more likely to hurt themselves than others and may display self-destructive behaviors such as minor cutting (often on their wrists) or cigarette burns. Although these actions may seem suicidal, they are done to diminish dissociation and become more connected to reality. Clients need to understand this process and develop more effective coping mechanisms. When dissociation becomes severe, other interventions such as grounding techniques with familiar items can be employed. For example, one client used a stuffed animal and pictures of her horse to remember her current life on a farm. Simple, reorienting, reassuring statements can also help to prevent suicidal ideation, danger to others, and self-care inabilities. For the individual who has been recently exposed to trauma, the emphasis should be on promoting adaptation and security.

Try to develop a trusting relationship. An essential component of communicating with individuals with PTSD or dissociative disorders is to convey a sense of respect, acceptance of their distress, and belief in the clients' reactions. They may be fearful and distrustful. These clients require specialized care, particularly if they suffer from dissociative identity disorder. The alternative identity may be that of a child, unable to cope with adult demands and expectations. Communicating with clients who assume children's identities entails taking into account their "developmental levels" at the time.

A major intervention is to reconnect individuals with their existing support systems or to develop new ones. Involvement in healthy, secure relationships is the goal. Whatever the nature of the trauma, generally promote independence and the clients' highest level of functioning. Encourage individuals with PTSD or a dissociative disorder to restart activities that provide a sense of mastery. Success in personal endeavors such as hobbies can enhance self-esteem and diminish detachment.

The benefits of talking directly about the stressful events are unclear, and some studies have found that discussing it immediately may lead to more harm. Simply "uncovering" the traumatic memories is not enough. The safest approach is to direct the client to discuss the details of the trauma with an experienced psychotherapist.

Another major issue in communication is countertransference. Because of the nature and severity of their trauma and trauma response, these clients can evoke strong feelings of anger, sadness, or even disgust in health-care providers. Working with them may be draining, time-consuming, and difficult, particularly on inpatient units that specialize in their care. The first step in managing countertransference reactions is to identify them and then make an opportunity to discuss and process them with a skilled supervisor.

Group therapy, which promotes connectedness to others, can help these clients even on a short-term basis. Most of the documented evidence on the effectiveness of group therapy has been with combat veterans with PTSD, but the emerging data suggest this type of therapy may be especially helpful in decreasing maladaptive behaviors and their effects on relationships. For example, several weeks of group therapy for adolescents who had witnessed severe violence (drive-by shootings, gangs who murder) helped to decrease their isolation and allowed them to discuss the effects of trauma on their lives and develop alternative coping mechanisms.[14] Many of the teenagers had not received any attention from health-care providers (except emergency medical care), and most had not discussed the incident with anyone, despite profound consequences such as depression, social withdrawal, and sleep disruption.

INTERVENTIONS FOR CLIENTS IN THE COMMUNITY

Long-term community-based treatment is necessary for PTSD and most dissociative disorders. A balanced treatment approach that combines adequate health care, individual ther-

Clinical Management Tips for Clients with PTSD and Dissociative Disorders

Effective Communication Strategies
- Use a consistent, supportive approach to begin to develop trust and reduce fear.
- Strive to convey an empathic, respectful, concerned approach in each interaction.
- Avoid excessive probing into the details of trauma; redirect the client to discuss goals and strategies.
- Avoid simplistic reassurances such as "things will get better soon."
- Carefully word statements to avoid blaming the client for past events; empathize with physical and emotional pain.
- For clients with dissociative personality states, maintain a calm, consistent approach.

Ways to Reduce or Prevent Violence to Self or Others
- Provide and monitor a safe environment for the client in the hospital or in the community.
- Frequently reassure clients that they are safe and will receive help.
- Ask about any suicidal thoughts or plans.
- Set firm, unambiguous limits on aggressive or impulsive behaviors.
- Provide and help the client maintain a low-stimulus environment, free of dangerous objects.

Ways to Promote Physical and Psychological Health
- Focus on concrete short-term goals such as developing a plan to manage daily demands.
- Acknowledge and allow the client to verbalize anxiety and fears.
- Encourage the client to seek and remain in individual and possibly group psychotherapy.
- If concurrent substance or alcohol abuse is present, refer the client to appropriate self-help groups such as AA or NA.
- Encourage the client to be as independent as possible.
- Point out any small improvement in symptoms.
- Let individuals know when behaviors put them at risk for further trauma.
- Do not allow clients with PTSD to focus only on trauma; gently redirect them to the feelings or lack of feelings (dissociation, numbing) that have resulted.
- Refer the client for medication assessment if sleep disturbance, dissociation, hyperarousal, or depression is moderate to severe.
- Assess social and family support.
- Assess and reevaluate depression.
- Encourage moderate exercise and healthy activity patterns.
- Monitor fluctuations in behaviors such as avoidance or reexperiencing symptoms.
- Jointly establish with the client daily structure and long-term goals.
- Help the client identify physical, environmental, and emotional triggers that precede a flashback or reexperiencing of the traumatic event.
- During periods of dissociation, use familiar objects to gently reorient the client to promote concentration and focus on the present.
- Help identify precipitants to dissociation.
- To minimize fear, hyperarousal, and avoidance, prepare the client in advance for any procedures or appointments.
- Allow client to vent frustrations about the need for long-term treatment.
- Encourage self-care and reinforce new coping strategies learned in psychotherapy to deal with memories of the traumatic event.
- Carefully assess the response to medications, particularly those that may lead to side effects of anxiety (SSRIs) or addiction (benzodiazepines).
- Encourage the client to write frequently in a journal to manage reactions and feelings.

Client and Family Education
- Educate clients and families about the need for long-term psychiatric treatment.
- For the noncompliant client, encourage restarting treatment, perhaps with another provider or clinic.
- Educate about the impact of untreated PTSD and dissociative disorders on the individual's functional ability.
- Teach clients that the trauma is a past event and not their fault.
- Tell the client and family to report any worsening symptoms or suicidal thoughts.
- Educate about the detrimental effects of alcohol and substance use, including depression and sleep disruption.
- Help the client and family identify community resources.

Source: Adapted from Gorman, LM, et al: Davis's Manual of Psychological Nursing. Copyright FA Davis, 1996.

apy, group or family therapy, treatment for substance abuse (if present), and pharmacotherapy will probably be most effective. However, symptoms such as avoidance and numbing may prevent individuals from engaging in treatment. Progress by "fits and starts" is common, because these individuals have substantial difficulty remaining in treatment. The intense personal relationships that are part of therapy may be too overwhelming, or clients may be unable to confront the trauma. Treatment noncompliance leads to being haunted by the past and unable to fully engage in the present; clients reexperience the trauma, and dissociation persists. Nurses need to encourage these clients to try to remain in treatment. An effective approach is persistent, gentle reminders that long-term treatment is necessary and can help.

Treatment must occur in the context of a safe and trusting relationship. The initial phase of treatment focuses on helping the individual achieve stability. The overall goal is symptom reduction and continued safety. Simple short-term goals include attending individual and group therapy sessions and becoming actively involved in self-help groups to stop drinking or using drugs, if substance abuse is present. Medications may quell some of the symptoms and relieve distress but frequently provide only partial or temporary benefit.

Because PTSD and dissociative disorders have significant effects on family, occupational, and social relationships, ongoing treatment needs to address the client's relationships to others. Although adequate social support and reintegration into a community or occupation are important, everyday demands of work and interpersonal relationships are overwhelming for these clients, who may restrict work activities and involvement with others to avoid symptoms and reminders of the trauma. Daily events such as going to the grocery store may cause fear and avoidance.

Clients may become chronically suicidal or aggressive, sometimes even with ongoing treatment. Their states of reactivity to the environment may lead to extreme impulsivity. For instance, a sexually abused woman may strike a male friend or coworker who reminds her of her father. The usual thought process that puts the brake on these aggressive and impulsive actions does not work. Clients frequently fail to understand that their reactions are an exaggerated response related to past traumatic events. In fact, they often cannot figure out what has made them upset. These destructive behaviors may destroy relationships. Alcohol and substance abuse is common at this point to escape the pain and to self-medicate symptoms. If clients remain in this pattern chronically, psychotherapy and other treatments are much less effective. In long-term therapy, clients learn that substance abuse is an ineffective solution, that these "all or nothing" reactions are common, and that a middle ground is healthier.

Once some stability is achieved, the goal is to integrate the trauma into the individual's life. If dissociation is prominent, the objective is being fully in touch with the environment. The focus of treatment is on developing alternative coping strategies to remain in touch with the world and to take responsibility for actions.

Those with dissociative identity disorder need several years of treatment to integrate the different personalities. Learning to tolerate previously hidden memories is part of their integration and recovery process. Ideally, clients learn that the trauma was an event that occurred at a point in time, and the "reliving" of the traumatic situation can be put in the past. At this time, healthier relationships with family and friends can be strengthened, and volunteer or occupational functioning can be established. Cognitive-behavior therapy can help clients "practice" encounters with reminders of the trauma, regain control over their emotions, and reduce exaggerated responses. The goal is to help clients take charge of lives that are out of control and to see that the world is a manageable place.

Cognitive-Behavior Treatment

Emerging evidence suggests that adults and children with PTSD or dissociative disorders may benefit from cognitive-behavior intervention and that some cognitive-behavior techniques are more successful than supportive counseling. Cognitive-behavior therapy has also been used in group therapy, with benefit noted in rape trauma survivors. Much of the basis for cognitive-behavior therapy is centered on psychoeducation, exposure to situations reminiscent of the trauma, progressive relaxation, and cognitive restructuring to develop alternative ways of coping. For instance, for the individual with PTSD secondary to rape, cognitive restructuring might involve ways to prevent rape or to find a healthy way out of the rape flashback when it reoccurs.

Eye Movement Desensitization and Reprocessing. One of the most promising new cognitive-behavior treatments used for PTSD is eye-movement desensitization and reprocessing (EMDR). This therapy was developed to help individuals decrease the near-constant experiencing of traumatic memories, particularly nightmares and flashbacks. EMDR is a structured, client-centered model that attempts to integrate intrapsychic, cognitive-behavior, body-oriented, and interactional approaches.[15] In this procedure, which is carried out by a trained clinician, the client generates trauma memories while relating physical and emotional states. As the individual concentrates on these states, a particular form of eye movements (side-to-side saccadic movements) are induced. EMDR appears to rapidly relieve traumatic stress, although its mechanism is not well understood. It is theorized that the client reprocesses information to allow dysfunctional information to be more adaptively resolved, leading to increased insight and functioning.[15] More recent studies question whether the specific eye movements used in EMDR are necessary for the treatment to be effective. Further research is needed to understand how EMDR works to relieve symptoms.

Therapeutic Exposure

Exposure techniques are also used in the treatment of PTSD and dissociation. This approach uses direct contact with reminders of the trauma under carefully controlled conditions, guided by a psychotherapist. Because individuals may avoid events or thoughts reminiscent of the trauma, exposure therapy is necessary to overcome avoidance and integrate the event as a past experience. The goal of this treatment is to learn to tolerate memories and reminders of the traumatic event. One particular type of exposure treatment, image habituation training (IHT), instructs clients to generate and record verbal descriptions of the trauma.[16] They are then instructed to continue to listen to the tape at home while visualizing the described traumatic event. In some initial but preliminary results, many of the clients with PTSD showed moderate to great improvement, which lasted more than 6 months.[16,17] Other forms of exposure techniques have used "helicopter ride therapy" for combat veterans with PTSD or "model muggings" to help victims of assaults. Exposure techniques may be more helpful in reducing intrusive recollections of the traumatic event.

Hypnosis

Hypnosis is a controversial treatment. Proponents note that it allows controlled access to repressed trauma memories, can positively restructure them, and may help clients face and bear a traumatic experience.[18] If successful, these techniques can be taught to the individual so that self-hypnosis can continue. The goal of hypnosis may be to "recover" repressed memories of trauma or to reconnect feelings to traumatic events. Hypnosis has been one of the main treatments used for dissociative disorders, although further study is necessary to determine its effectiveness.

Pharmacologic Treatments

Antidepressants. Several antidepressant medications have been used to treat PTSD with some effectiveness; however, little information is available on their use in dissociative disorders. Tricyclic antidepressants (TCAs), monoamine oxidase inhibitors (MAOIs), some of the selective serotonin reuptake inhibitors (SSRIs), and perhaps other antidepressants are indicated for clients with PTSD, particularly those clients who also suffer from depression. A recent study found that fluoxetine (Prozac) was effective in relieving symptoms of PTSD secondary to combat or childhood abuse.[19] Antidepressants may diminish hyperarousal, startle responses, panic symptoms, intrusive recollections, and sleep problems. Their mechanism of action centers on restoring levels of neurotransmitters. TCAs and MAOIs tend to increase levels of norepinephrine and serotonin. SSRIs such as fluoxetine, sertraline, and paroxetine increase levels of serotonin. Because PTSD is associated with norepinephrine and serotonin dysfunction, antidepressants may treat symptoms by increasing serotonin and possibly norepinephrine levels. Clients with PTSD commonly experience side effects of antidepressants, and therefore lower doses are often necessary, especially initially.

Mood Stabilizers. Little is known about the effects of mood stabilizers on PTSD, and these agents have yet to be studied in individuals with dissociative disorders. Because of the mood fluctuations that commonly occur in PTSD, lithium carbonate, carbamazepine (Tegretol), or valproic acid (Depakote) may be effective. Carbamazepine and valproic acid may be more effective treatments because they are also anticonvulsants and reduce dissociative and numbing behaviors, intrusive symptoms, and aggression. Their mechanism of action is unknown and needs further study.

> **RESEARCH NOTE**
>
> Moyers, F: Oklahoma City bombing: Exacerbation of symptoms in veterans with PTSD. Arch Psychiatr Nurs 10:55–59, 1996.
>
> **Findings:** One of the key aspects of PTSD is reexperiencing the traumatic event through flashbacks, nightmares, and feelings and thoughts that are reminiscent of the trauma. These symptoms can be triggered by everyday experiences or by other severe stressors. This study examined the reactions of 15 World War II, Korean War, and Vietnam veterans who attended support groups to the Oklahoma City bombing. Clients who had witnessed severe bombings and destruction during combat appeared to be most affected. Two-thirds of the veterans experienced worsening of their PTSD symptoms after watching news accounts of the bombing. Uncomfortable memories of the war, nightmares, and hyperarousal symptoms such as increased heart rate, sweating, and difficulty sleeping worsened. One veteran reported flashbacks and seeing faces of war victims during media coverage of the bombing. Others reported that they were reminded of being called "baby killers" after witnessing the effects of the Oklahoma City bombing on children.
>
> **Application to Practice:** Exposure to severe stressors later in life can affect individuals with PTSD and dissociative disorders by activating and worsening symptoms, particularly reexperiencing behaviors. The findings suggest that stimuli that are reminders of the original trauma led to an exacerbation of symptoms in individuals with PTSD. The extensive media coverage appeared to have a profound effect on veterans, particularly those who had witnessed bombings. Nurses need to be aware of how severe stress, in various forms, affects individuals with PTSD and dissociative disorders. This experience may lead to being "retraumatized." For instance, children who have witnessed drive-by shootings that have injured or killed friends and family may reexperience the trauma if continually exposed to reminders of it. Nurses can play a major role in helping clients identify potential triggers, such as news accounts of related types of events. In this way, worsening of symptoms may be avoided.

Antihypertensives. Individuals with PTSD may respond to antihypertensive medications such as propranolol or clonidine. Propranolol may reduce intrusive recollections, especially nightmares, as well as sleep disturbance, hyperarousal, startle responses, and aggression. These two agents affect the receptors that norepinephrine binds to, which may explain their mechanism of action.

Anxiolytics. Benzodiazepines such as clonazepam and alprazolam as well as buspirone may reduce startle responses, hyperarousal, and anxiety. Clonazepam may be useful in treating dissociation in PTSD or dissociation disorders, although there has been little formal research on anxiolytics in clients with these disorders. Benzodiazepines effectively reduce anxiety and fear; however, these medications are contraindicated in clients with present or past histories of substance abuse.

CLIENT AND FAMILY EDUCATION

Clients may think they are "going crazy," and their families and friends may be surprised by their behaviors. Education about the illness, its etiology, ways to recognize the onset of symptoms, and the need for continued treatment is an important intervention. Emphasize that substance abuse, anxiety, and depressive behaviors may frequently coexist. Successful outcomes are generally associated with continued treatment, abstinence from illicit substances and alcohol, and active participation in treatment.

Education can also help clients understand the link between traumatic events and related thoughts and feelings. A cognitive understanding of their behaviors can lessen and regulate overwhelming emotions. Explain the value of identifying the events that trigger memories of the stressor to reduce feelings that the traumatic event is happening again.

The impact of severe trauma or dissociation on family members may suggest that family or couples therapy is necessary. Because reduced libido or avoidance of a healthy sexual relationship is a common consequence of incest or rape, specific psychoeducational groups have been developed to assist partners of abuse survivors. Helping the individual and the family sort out their most important psychological and health-care needs is essential for preventing long-term difficulties.

EXPECTED OUTCOMES

For the individual with PTSD or a dissociative disorder, improvement will be demonstrated by the ability to:
- Remain safe, and not engage in self-destructive or mutilating behaviors.
- Avoid or abstain from alcohol or drugs.
- Understand and recognize the presence of dissociative and PTSD-related behaviors.
- Begin to develop healthy interpersonal interactions to promote growth and self-esteem.
- Use techniques to manage or prevent dissociation.
- Demonstrate adequate sleep and activity patterns.
- Become more motivated and establish short-term goals.
- Have a basic understanding of the illness and ways to manage it.
- Recognize the impact of behavior on relationships.
- Identify impending symptoms of dissociation and stressors that precipitate their onset.
- Demonstrate diminished fear, anxiety, and depression, or show appropriate expression of affect.
- Continue to follow a medication regimen as prescribed (if indicated).

DIFFERENTIAL DIAGNOSIS

Medical Disorders
- Medications or physical conditions may precipitate symptoms of PTSD or dissociation.
- Symptoms are similar but are excluded from the diagnosis.
- Medical conditions should be ruled out, especially seizure disorders, stroke, head injury, and delirium.

Acute Stress Disorder
- It occurs acutely after exposure to an extreme stressor.
- The symptoms are the same as PTSD.
- The duration is shorter than PTSD; symptoms occur for 2 to 30 days.
- It frequently progresses to PTSD.

Adjustment Disorders
- They are often brought on by a mild or moderate stressor such as leaving home, getting married, unemployment, retirement, or breaking up an important romantic or marital relationship.
- The symptoms are minor and resolve quickly.
- Functioning is slightly but not grossly impaired.
- PTSD and dissociative disorders are characterized by exposure to severe stress leading to lasting symptoms.

Psychotic Disorders
- Schizophrenia and other psychotic disorders may be misdiagnosed.
- Schizophrenia, schizoaffective disorder, and delusional disorder are all characterized by distinct periods of psychotic symptoms.
- Psychotic symptoms such as hallucinations, delusions, and paranoia are absent in PTSD and dissociative disorders.
- Dissociative identity disorder is often characterized by personality states with "voices" that "talk" to one another and resemble hallucinations.

Alcohol and Substance Abuse and Dependence

- Alcohol or illicit drugs may lead to symptoms or coexist.
- Alcohol has depressant effects, may lead to abuse and dependence, and complicates treatment (see Chapter 17).
- Marijuana, cocaine, and other substance abuse may precipitate or accompany the presentation of hyperarousal or dissociation.
- Denial of a coexisting abuse or dependence disorder is likely.

Obsessive-Compulsive Disorder (OCD)

- OCD is characterized by repetitive intrusive thoughts and behaviors, for example, "sex is dirty."
- Obsessive thoughts do not usually involve a severe stressor, and dissociation is absent.
- PTSD is characterized by thoughts, dreams, and memories of being abused.
- Dissociative disorders are not characterized by obsessions; feeling cut off from usual experiences predominates.

Personality Disorders

- Personality disorders, especially borderline personality disorder, complicate the diagnosis or coexist.
- Borderline personality disorder is characterized by frequent mood shifts, without the other symptoms of depression or mania. Anger is the predominant mood.

COMMON NURSING DIAGNOSES

- Fear
- Coping, individual, ineffective
- Powerlessness
- Self Care Deficit, feeding, bathing/hygiene, dressing/grooming, toileting
- Injury, risk for
- Self-Mutilation, risk for
- Sleep Pattern Disturbance
- Social Interaction, impaired
- Anxiety
- Self Esteem disturbance
- Personal Identity Disturbance
- Sexuality Patterns, altered
- Rape-Trauma Syndrome
- Role Performance, altered

SYNOPSIS OF CURRENT RESEARCH

Recent studies have begun to examine the neurobiological and neurodevelopmental effects of PTSD. An emerging body of evidence suggests that PTSD is associated with an effect different from and opposite to that of major depression, particularly in the hypothalamic-pituitary-adrenal axis.[8] Individuals with PTSD have lower levels of a stress hormone, whereas those with major depression have higher levels. Several investigators have found differences between PTSD clients and those without trauma, particularly in limbic system dysfunction.[9-12] Magnetic resonance imaging (MRI) of individuals with PTSD has found reduced hippocampal size, particularly on the right side.[12] In a similar study, Vietnam veterans who were exposed to intense combat and subsequently developed PTSD also had smaller hippocampi than combat veterans without PTSD.[20] Other investigators found that women with a history of severe childhood sexual abuse had smaller hippocampi than those without abuse.[9] These researchers also found that women who had smaller hippocampi reported more dissociative symptoms on the DES. Taken together, these studies suggest that severe forms of trauma such as sexual abuse and combat may affect the brain and, in particular, lead to destruction of cells located in the hippocampus. Disruption in the hippocampus may be a biological correlate of symptoms observed in individuals with PTSD, including being easily startled, hyperarousal, mood lability, dissociative episodes, and loss of memory.

Other studies have explored the effects of PTSD and dissociation on functioning. Ross and colleagues reported that sleep disturbance is the hallmark of PTSD yet found conflicting results in sleep studies of traumatized individuals.[21] For instance, when PTSD clients were studied in the sleep laboratory for overnight examination of their sleep, no significant abnormalities were found. One hypothesis is that the sleep of PTSD clients may be improved when they are in a safe place, being watched and monitored by a technician.

Sleep of physically and sexually abused children has also been studied. Abused children took longer to fall asleep and had more activity during the night than both depressed and normal children.[22]

AREAS FOR FUTURE RESEARCH

- Who is at greatest risk for developing PTSD after exposure to a traumatic event?
- Which forms of treatment are most effective for PTSD?
- Are there differential responses to treatment in PTSD versus dissociative disorders?
- What are the most important early interventions to help someone exposed to trauma?
- What are the differences in trauma response in individuals with medical injury (for example, burns, head injury) versus those witnessing or experiencing severe violent acts?
- Is family therapy an effective technique for individuals with PTSD or dissociative disorders, particularly if abuse or battering has occurred?
- What medications most effectively diminish dissociation?
- Are medications effective for children with PTSD and dissociative disorders, and do they prevent long-term symptoms?

CASE STUDY

Susan is a 32-year-old divorced woman who presented to the emergency room with stomach pain and sleep disturbance. Her medical workup was negative except for mild anemia, despite several scars on her wrists and recent bruises. She said she was having "a hard time" and eventually revealed that she was being beaten by her boyfriend. She also related that from ages 11 to 17 she had an incestuous relationship with her father. Susan married her first boyfriend at age 17, while pregnant, to "get out of the home." She subsequently miscarried and was divorced after just 1 year of marriage. Afterwards, in order to pay her bills, she worked as a prostitute and began abusing alcohol and heroin for several years, until she met a man who offered to pay her rent and support her. He would frequently call her names, put her down, and physically abused her for years. She also became pregnant and miscarried once again.

She described being unable to sleep at night because of the fear that she would be hurt either by her boyfriend or by an unknown intruder. She would awaken during the night with nightmares of her father and frequently blocked the door with furniture to allay her anxiety and to improve her ability to sleep. She denied using illicit drugs for the last 2 years and said she had been attending Narcotics Anonymous (NA) to cope with her addiction. Susan did admit to several drinks each week, particularly after fights with her boyfriend. Recently her sister married, and at the wedding she saw her father, with whom she had not had any contact for years. After this event, flashbacks of her sexual abuse began, and she remembered how he would sexually molest her when she was in the bathroom. Over the next several weeks, it was becoming increasingly difficult to venture out of the house, yet she realized that her current situation was unhealthy. Her mood appeared very depressed and anxious.

Some of the initial interventions focused on Susan's safety. She agreed to go to a shelter that provided apartments for battered women, with an address that would be unknown to her boyfriend. She was referred to an outpatient clinic for further assessment and individual psychotherapy, and one that also had groups for incest survivors and treatment for substance abuse. At first, Susan seemed overwhelmed and admitted that she couldn't understand how this was happening to her, especially since she really loved her boyfriend. Although she was ambivalent, she followed through with the plan to go to the shelter and begin treatment. As she left the emergency room, she asked if there was a way to help her finish her high school degree in order to find a good job. She commented that she had never had a "real job" but always wanted one. The staff felt hopeful about her strengths but were unsure if she would be able to follow through and face the major changes she needed to make.

At the shelter, the nurse worked with Susan to develop short-term goals. These included remaining safe, attending group and individual psychotherapy, starting a volunteer job, enrolling in classes to get her high school degree, continuing at NA, and developing her resume. The nurse also referred her for a psychopharmacology evaluation, and she began a trial of fluoxetine (Prozac). She spent several weeks at the shelter and frequently stated her love for her boyfriend even though he had physically abused her. The nurse and the other residents helped Susan realize that this was a common feeling at this stage. The nurse also helped Susan confront the reality of the situation: If she returned to her boyfriend, her life would be in danger and her self-esteem, substance and alcohol abuse, depression, and post-traumatic symptoms would worsen. The nurse also kept encouraging her to participate in a volunteer job at a day care center, groups at the shelter, NA and Alcoholics Anonymous (AA) meetings, and individual therapy. Susan was given support and encouragement to follow through on these goals. Although she remained ambivalent about returning to her boyfriend, she was able to move out of the shelter and into a safe apartment. She began working part-time as a home health aide, with the goal of becoming more independent and self-sufficient. Her self-esteem remained low, she had difficulty sleeping, and she was fearful of her surroundings, but her flashbacks and depression had diminished. The nurse spoke with Susan about how recovery from trauma was a long-term process, that her symptoms would probably wax and wane for years, and how she needed to work on these issues in individual and group psychotherapy. Together they devised a long-term plan for her to afford ongoing therapy and how to manage it in her new schedule.

CRITICAL THINKING QUESTIONS

1. What behaviors does Susan manifest that are indicative of PTSD?
2. What key characteristics would lead you to recommend hospitalization for this individual?
3. Which theories best explain the behaviors presented?
4. Explain the mechanism by which fluoxetine reduces post-traumatic symptoms.
5. How does a nurse convince a client that living in a shelter is the best course of action?
6. What major life issues contribute to the development and continuation of PTSD?
7. Identify the key elements of education for this individual and her family.
8. Identify behaviors that show that Susan is responding to treatment.
9. What are the most appropriate long-term interventions to assist her in daily living and functioning?
10. How can the nurse maximize the client's compliance with treatment?

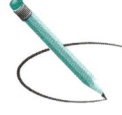

KEY POINTS

- Trauma and stress affect each individual differently; however, extreme forms of stress can lead to discrete disorders such as PTSD and dissociative disorders.
- PTSD emerges acutely or chronically after exposure to severe stress, such as incest, rape, war, torture, or other events beyond most individuals' usual experience. Dissociative disorders may occur in response to this type of stress.
- PTSD is characterized by symptoms in three major areas: intrusive reexperiencing of the traumatic event, hyperarousal, and avoidance behaviors. The intrusive reexper-

iencing of the event leads to reliving the past through flashbacks, intrusive thoughts, and nightmares of the trauma. Hyperarousal may be experienced as increased pulse or blood pressure, difficulty concentrating, sleep disruption, anger outbursts, being easily startled, or hypervigilance. Avoidance behaviors include feeling numb, having periods of dissociation, and avoiding feelings, thoughts, and places reminiscent of the trauma.

- Dissociative episodes may include periods of forgetfulness, memory loss for past stressful events, feeling disconnected from daily events, severe identity confusion, or distinctly different personality states.
- Five dissociative disorders are recognized currently: dissociative amnesia, dissociative fugue, dissociative identity disorder (formerly termed multiple personality disorder), depersonalization disorder, and dissociative disorder not otherwise specified (NOS).
- The predictors of who will develop PTSD or a dissociative disorder are not known. Factors such as severity, duration, and proximity to the stressful event are likely to affect the risk.
- PTSD may result from disruption in neurotransmitter levels such as increased norepinephrine or low serotonin or increased endogenous opioids. It is also associated with changes in the endocrine and limbic systems.
- PTSD and dissociative disorders tend to have a chronic fluctuating course, often associated with other problems, including substance or alcohol abuse and mood disorders.
- Neuroendocrine studies suggest that in contrast to major depression, PTSD may produce a different biological response. Depressed individuals generally produce excess cortisol, whereas individuals with PTSD produce less cortisol.
- Treatment of PTSD and dissociative disorders frequently takes years and requires a balanced approach that combines adequate health care, individual therapy, group or family therapy, treatment for substance abuse (if present), and pharmacotherapy.
- Treatment noncompliance occurs frequently. Clients with these disorders need consistent reassurance to remain in treatment.
- Education can help clients with PTSD or dissociative disorders understand the link between traumatic events and related thoughts and feelings. Families can learn about the fluctuating and long-term course of the illness, as well as the need for ongoing treatment.
- Antidepressants appear to be the most effective medications for treating PTSD; mood stabilizers, antihypertensives, and benzodiazepines may also be beneficial. Benzodiazepines, particularly clonazepam, may be useful for treating dissociative disorders.
- Certain instruments, such as the DES, can be helpful in detecting and measuring the severity of dissociation.
- Left untreated, PTSD and dissociative disorders are associated with a poor prognosis, alcohol and substance abuse, self-destructive behaviors, and significant impairment.

REFERENCES

1. American Psychiatric Association: Diagnostic and Statistical Manual of Mental Disorders, ed 4. American Psychiatric Association, Washington, DC, 1994.
2. Bernstein, EM, and Putnam, FW: Development, reliability, and validity of a dissociation scale. J Nerv Ment Dis 174:727, 1986.
3. Bremner, JD, et al: Childhood physical abuse and combat-related posttraumatic stress disorder in Vietnam veterans. Am J Psychiatry 150:235, 1993.
4. Kosten, TR, et al: Sustained urinary norepinephrine and epinephrine elevation in posttraumatic stress disorder. Psychoneuroendocrinology 12:13, 1987.
5. Pitman, RK, and Orr, SP: 24-hour urinary cortisol and catecholamine excretion in combat-related post-traumatic stress disorder. Biol Psychiatry 27:245, 1990.
6. Blanchard, ER, et al: Changes in plasma norepinephrine to combat-related stimuli among Vietnam veterans with posttraumatic stress disorder. J Nerv Ment Dis 179:371, 1991.
7. van der Kolk, BA: The body keeps the score: Approaches to the psychobiology of posttraumatic stress disorder. In van der Kolk, BA, McFarlane, AC, and Weisaeth, L (eds): Traumatic Stress: The Effects of Overwhelming Experience on Mind, Body, and Society. The Guilford Press, New York, 1996.
8. Yehuda, R, et al: Persistent hormonal alterations following extreme stress in humans: Adaptive or maladaptive? Psychosom Med 55:287, 1993.
9. Stein, MB, et al: Structural brain changes in PTSD. Annals NY Acad Sci 821:76–82, 1997.
10. Teicher, MH, et al: Early childhood abuse and limbic system ratings in adult psychiatric outpatients. J Neuropsychiatry Clin Neurosci 5:301, 1993.
11. Ito, Y, et al: Increased prevalence of electrophysiological abnormalities in children with psychological, physical and sexual abuse. J Neuropsychiatry Clin Neurosci 5:401, 1993.
12. Bremner, JD, et al: MRI-based measurement of hippocampal volume in patients with combat-related posttraumatic stress disorder. Am J Psychiatry 152:973, 1995.
13. Hartman, CR, and Burgess, AW: Information processing of trauma. Child Abuse Negl 17:47, 1993.
14. Pynoos, R: Neurobiological aspects of trauma. Symposium, Athens, Greece, International Society of Adolescent Psychiatry, 1995.
15. Shapiro, F, Vogelmann-Sine, S, and Sine, LF: Eye movement desensitization and reprocessing: Treating trauma and substance abuse. J Psychoactive Drugs 26:379, 1994.
16. Vaughn, K, and Tarrier, N: The use of image habituation training with post-traumatic stress disorders. Br J Psychiatry 161:658, 1992.
17. Vaughn, K, et al: A trial of eye movement desensitization compared to image habituation training and applied muscle relaxation in post-traumatic stress disorder. J Behav Ther Exp Psychiatry 25:283, 1994.
18. Spiegel, D, and Cardena, E: New uses of hypnosis in the treatment of posttraumatic stress disorder. J Clin Psychiatry 51 (Suppl):39, 1990.
19. van der Kolk, BA, et al: Fluoxetine in posttraumatic stress disorder. J Clin Psychiatry 55:517, 1994.
20. Gurvitz, TV, et al: MRI hippocampal volumes in chronic PTSD. American Psychiatric Association Abstract NR513, 1995.
21. Ross, RJ, et al: Sleep disturbance as the hallmark of posttraumatic stress disorder. Am J Psychiatry 146:697, 1989.
22. Stein, MB, et al: Structural brain changes in PTSD: Does trauma alter neuroanatomy? Ann NY Acad Sci 821:76, 1997.

CHAPTER 23

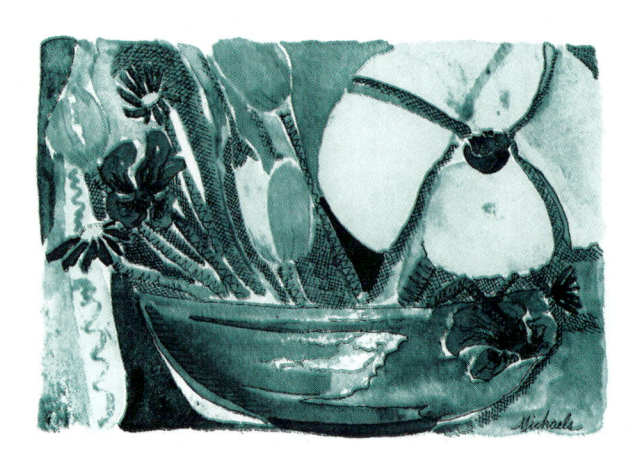

CHAPTER OUTLINE

Normal Sexual Functioning in Men and Women
Sexual Dysfunctions
Characteristic Behaviors
Culture, Age, and Gender Features
Etiology
Prognosis
Planning Care
Interventions for Clients in the Community
Gender Identity Disorder
Characteristic Behaviors
Culture, Age, and Gender Features
Etiology
Prognosis
Interventions for Clients in the Community
Paraphilias
Characteristic Behaviors
Culture, Age, and Gender Features
Etiology
Prognosis
Interventions for Clients in the Community
Client and Family Education
Expected Outcomes
Common Nursing Diagnoses
Synopsis of Current Research
Areas for Future Research

Margery Chisholm, RN, EdD, CS, ABPP
Carol A. Glod, RN, CS, PhD

Sexual and Gender Identity Disorders

LEARNING OBJECTIVES

After completing this chapter, the reader should be able to:

- List the prominent characteristics of sexual and gender identity disorders.
- Describe the different types of gender and identity disorders, and identify symptomatology associated with each.
- Differentiate between gender and identity disorders and other major psychiatric disorders.
- Explain the development of gender and identity disorders.
- Identify the stigma associated with gender and identity in adjustment disorders.
- Analyze the impact of gender and identity disorders on the individual's daily functioning.
- Implement the nursing process in planning care for the individual with a gender and identity disorder.

KEY TERMS

anorgasmia
dyspareunia
libido
paraphilias
premature ejaculation
sexual dysfunctions
sexual response cycle
vaginismus

The sexual and gender identity disorders fall in three broad diagnostic categories: the sexual dysfunctions, paraphilias, and gender identity disorders. These disorders include problems with sexual arousal, functioning, and beliefs about sexual identity. Sexual dysfunctions, the most common disorders, are disturbances in sexual desire (**libido**) and sexual performance that cause substantial distress.[1] Gender identity disorder or *transsexualism* is the desire to be the other sex. The **paraphilias** are less common disorders that involve intense and unusual sexual urges: exhibitionism, fetishism, frotteurism, pedophilia, sexual masochism, sexual sadism, transvestic fetishism, voyeurism, and paraphilia not otherwise specified (NOS).[1] Sexual disorder NOS may consist of sexual disturbances such as severe feelings of sexual inadequacy or distress about one's sexual orientation.

NORMAL SEXUAL FUNCTIONING IN MEN AND WOMEN

Masters and Johnson,[2] two researchers interested in sexual functioning, investigated sexual activity in healthy men and women. They described four stages of the **sexual response cycle**: desire, excitement, orgasm, and resolution. The first, the desire stage, involves sexual wanting and fantasizing about sexual activities. During the excitement stage, men experience increased heart rate and blood pressure and erotic feelings, leading to erection of the penis; in women, the physical and erotic feelings lead to vaginal lubrication. In the next stage, men ejaculate semen from the penis, whereas women experience orgasm, rhythmic contractions

Clinical Management Tips for Individuals with Sexual Dysfunction

- Provide an atmosphere of understanding and openness.
- Determine whether medical, pharmacologic, and substance abuse causes have been investigated.
- Use an accepting, nonjudgmental tone.
- Interact with the client in a safe, private environment.
- Assess client's knowledge of healthy sexual functioning and anatomy.
- Ask about fears and anxieties related to sexual arousal or performance.
- Be accepting of client's concerns about sexual function.
- Explore cultural, social, religious, and parental influences on current beliefs and behaviors.
- Determine whether conflict or tension exists in the client's relationships.
- Include sexual partner in discussions when appropriate.
- Reinforce cognitive-behavior interventions.
- Refer the client and his or her partner for couples or sex therapy.
- Help the client link the stressor, if present, and the development of sexual dysfunction.

of the vaginal muscles. During the last stage, resolution, physiological processes return to the resting state. Generally men are unable to have another erection for a period of time, usually hours, whereas women may be able to have multiple sequential orgasms. Sexual dysfunctions may arise during any of these stages.

SEXUAL DYSFUNCTIONS

Characteristic Behaviors

People with hypoactive sexual desire disorder and sexual aversion disorder have reduced sexual desire, whereas those who have male erectile disorder or female sexual arousal disorder complain of difficulty in becoming sexually aroused. Difficulty in achieving or maintaining orgasms is the hallmark of female and male orgasmic disorders. When men ejaculate prior to intercourse or before their partner wishes, **premature ejaculation** is present. Sexual pain disorders include **dyspareunia**, pain during intercourse, and **vaginismus**, involuntary vaginal muscle spasms. **Sexual dysfunctions** commonly result from medical conditions, medications, or substance abuse.

> *It was a gradual thing, I think. My husband and I used to have a wonderful sexual relationship when we began dating. That was years ago, though. I used to get so turned on. Then we got married, and I guess we just fell into some sort of rut. We'd make love once a week or so, mostly on weekends. Then it got so I just didn't care whether we had intercourse or not. I remember thinking that my lack of desire—what do you call it?—libido, wasn't really there and that was pretty strange. It's now been years since I really had any sexual feelings for my husband or anyone else. And it's been about a year since my husband and I have had sex.*

Beginning Symptoms

Establishing the presence of a disorder requires excluding medical, psychiatric, and pharmacologic causes, as well as alcohol and substance abuse. The sexual assessment guide described in Chapter 11 is often used; examples of specific questions are shown in Table 23–1. Help clients identify sexual fantasies and behavior. Note the onset and course of the dysfunction, and determine the degree of control over problematic behavior. Assess relationships with significant others. Consider age and sexual experience, sexual stimulation, sexual partner, and frequency of sexual activity.

Sexual dysfunctions may be longstanding or occur after a recent stress or in response to a certain situation, such as a new sexual partner. If a stressor is present, identify it. Disruption in sexual functioning can occur during any of the four stages of the sexual response cycle.

Sexual Desire Disorders

Two conditions constitute the sexual desire disorders: hypoactive sexual desire disorder and sexual aversion disorder

TABLE 23–1. Questions for the Assessment of Sexual and Identity Disorders

- How would you describe your sexual relationship?
- Have you noted any changes in sexual desire or functioning?
- Are there any medications that you've recently begun taking?
- Are there any health problems that may be affecting your sexuality?
- Have there been any recent events or stressors that may be affecting your sexuality?
- What problems, if any, do you have about your sexuality?
- How often do you have some form of sexual release, either with or without a partner?
- Are you comfortable with your level of sexual desire and functioning?
- Has there been a change in your sexual thoughts or feelings?
- Has there been a change in your level of sexual arousal?
- Have you been avoiding sexual activity?
- Has there been a change in your frequency of masturbation?
- Have you had any pain or discomfort or other negative feeling during sexual activity?
- What are the most important factors that influence whether you have sex?
- Has there been a change in your ability to have an erection?
- Has there been a change in your ability to experience orgasm?
- Are you able to tell your partner what you find sexually pleasurable?
- Are there any concerns about your sexuality that you haven't mentioned?

Source: Adapted from Segraves, KB, and Segraves, RT: Hypoactive sexual desire disorder: Prevalence and comorbidity in 906 subjects. J Sex Marital Ther 17:55–58, 1991.

(see *DSM-IV* Diagnostic Criteria). Problems in the desire stage characterize hypoactive sexual desire disorder. These individuals feel less sexual; they have reduced sexual desires and fantasies. Intercourse and other sexual activities such as masturbation are of little interest. They spend little or no time thinking about sexual activities and fail to become aroused. Those who have extreme anxiety and avoid sexual activity may develop sexual aversion disorder. In this disorder, a person does not engage in sexual activity with a partner and goes out of his or her way to avoid it. Some fear sex and express no interest in it.

> A couple developed sexual tension and dysfunction after the birth of their first child. Their dysfunction included the wife's lack of sexual desire, depression, and anger and the husband's fears about sexual performance. The wife noted discomfort with a changed body image, whereas the husband was anxious about the new demands and responsibilities associated with parenthood. Because of child care demands, the cou-

> ### DSM-IV Diagnostic Criteria for Hypoactive Sexual Desire Disorder and Sexual Aversion Disorder
>
> **Diagnostic Criteria for 302.71 Hypoactive Sexual Desire Disorder**
>
> A. Persistently or recurrently deficient (or absent) sexual fantasies and desire for sexual activity. The judgment of deficiency or absence is made by the clinician, taking into account factors that affect sexual functioning, such as age and the context of the person's life.
>
> B. The disturbance causes marked distress or interpersonal difficulty.
>
> C. The sexual dysfunction is not better accounted for by another Axis I disorder (except another Sexual Dysfunction) and is not due exclusively to the direct physiological effects of a substance (e.g., a drug of abuse, a medication) or a general medical condition.
>
> *Specify* type:
>   Lifelong Type
>   Acquired Type
> *Specify* type:
>   Generalized Type
>   Situational Type
> *Specify*:
>   Due to Psychological Factors
>   Due to Combined Factors
>
> **Diagnostic Criteria for 302.79 Sexual Aversion Disorder**
>
> A. Persistent or recurrent extreme aversion to, and avoidance of, all (or almost all) genital sexual contact with a sexual partner.
>
> B. The disturbance causes marked distress or interpersonal difficulty.
>
> C. The sexual dysfunction is not better accounted for by another Axis I disorder (except another Sexual Dysfunction).
>
> *Specify* type:
>   Lifelong Type
>   Acquired Type
> *Specify* type:
>   Generalized Type
>   Situational Type
> *Specify*:
>   Due to Psychological Factors
>   Due to Combined Factors
>
> **Source:** Reprinted with permission from the Diagnostic and Statistical Manual of Mental Disorders, Fourth Edition. Copyright 1994 American Psychiatric Association.

ple was fatigued and needed to renegotiate shared tasks. Neither one had time for his or her individual activities. Other issues included religious prohibitions about when to resume sexual relations, and their unresolved feelings of loyalty to their own parents, who visited spontaneously and interrupted their time alone.

Sexual Arousal Disorders

Male erectile disorder and female sexual arousal disorder make up the sexual arousal disorders (see *DSM-IV* Diagnostic Criteria). In these conditions, individuals have difficulties in the excitement phase; they are either unable to attain or unable to maintain the physiological process necessary for sexual activity. Men typically cannot achieve or maintain an erection during intercourse or masturbation. Women cannot become or remain lubricated. For both genders, these difficulties lead to substantial distress and difficulty in relationships.

Orgasm Disorders

Three conditions make up the orgasm disorders: female orgasmic disorder, male orgasmic disorder, and premature ejaculation. Women and men with orgasmic disorder either are unable to have an orgasm or have delayed ones following the usual excitement phase. Sometimes women are able to achieve orgasm during masturbation but not during sexual intercourse, which is referred to as situational **anorgasmia**. Both genders experience substantial distress that interferes with relationships and their ability to experience pleasurable sexual relationships. Premature ejaculation is a mismatch in the orgasm phase; men ejaculate prior to intercourse or before their partner wishes. Premature ejaculation can also occur shortly after penetration. The orgasm disorders can lead to substantial upset and difficulty in relationships.

An older couple presented with several sexual problems; he was having premature ejaculation and she was developing an aversion to sexual activity. Married for 35 years and both in their late 50s, they had seven children, raised them successfully, and were at the stage of life that was supposed to be "their time." Important factors included the wife's postmenopausal vaginal dryness, the husband's fears of increasing his wife's discomfort during intercourse, and years of avoiding intimate and affectionate exchanges because of a busy household. Each had also developed separate interests that did not include the other.

> **DSM-IV Diagnostic Criteria for Female Sexual Arousal, Male Erectile, Female Orgasmic, and Male Orgasmic Disorders and Premature Ejaculation**

Diagnostic Criteria for 302.72 Female Sexual Arousal Disorder

A. Persistent or recurrent inability to attain, or to maintain until completion of the sexual activity, an adequate lubrication-swelling response of sexual excitement.

B. The disturbance causes marked distress or interpersonal difficulty.

C. The sexual dysfunction is not better accounted for by another Axis I disorder (except another Sexual Dysfunction) and is not due exclusively to the direct physiological effects of a substance (e.g., a drug of abuse, a medication) or a general medical condition.

Specify type:
  Lifelong Type
  Acquired Type

Specify type:
  Generalized Type
  Situational Type

Specify:
  Due to Psychological Factors
  Due to Combined Factors

Diagnostic Criteria for 302.72 Male Erectile Disorder

A. Persistent or recurrent inability to attain, or to maintain until completion of the sexual activity, an adequate erection.

B. The disturbance causes marked distress or interpersonal difficulty.

C. The erectile dysfunction is not better accounted for by another Axis I disorder (other than a Sexual Dysfunction) and is not due exclusively to the direct physiological effects of a substance (e.g., a drug of abuse, a medication) or a general medical condition.

Specify type:
  Lifelong Type
  Acquired Type

Specify type:
  Generalized Type
  Situational Type

Specify:
  Due to Psychological Factors
  Due to Combined Factors

Diagnostic Criteria for 302.73 Female Orgasmic Disorder

A. Persistent or recurrent delay in, or absence of, orgasm following a normal sexual excitement phase. Women exhibit wide variability in the type or intensity of stimulation that triggers orgasm. The diagnosis of Female Orgasmic Disorder should be based on the clinician's judgment that the woman's orgasmic capacity is less than would be reasonable for her age, sexual experience, and the adequacy of sexual stimulation she receives.

B. The disturbance causes marked distress or interpersonal difficulty.

C. The orgasmic dysfunction is not better accounted for by another Axis I disorder (except another Sexual Dysfunction) and is not due exclusively to the direct physiological effects of a substance (e.g., a drug of abuse, a medication) or a general medical condition.

Specify type:
  Lifelong Type
  Acquired Type

Specify type:
  Generalized Type
  Situational Type

Specify:
  Due to Psychological Factors
  Due to Combined Factors

Diagnostic Criteria for 302.74 Male Orgasmic Disorder

A. Persistent or recurrent delay in, or absence of, orgasm following a normal sexual excitement phase during sexual activity that the clinician, taking into account the person's age, judges to be adequate in focus, intensity, and duration.

B. The disturbance causes marked distress or interpersonal difficulty.

C. The orgasmic dysfunction is not better accounted for by another Axis I disorder (except another Sexual Dysfunction) and is not due exclusively to the direct physiological effects of a substance (e.g., a drug of abuse, a medication) or a general medical condition.

Specify type:
  Lifelong Type
  Acquired Type

Specify type:
  Generalized Type
  Situational Type

Specify:
  Due to Psychological Factors
  Due to Combined Factors

Continued on following page

Diagnostic Criteria for 302.75 Premature Ejaculation

A. Persistent or recurrent ejaculation with minimal sexual stimulation before, on, or shortly after penetration and before the person wishes it. The clinician must take into account factors that affect duration of the excitement phase, such as age, novelty of the sexual partner or situation, and recent frequency of sexual activity.

B. The disturbance causes marked distress or interpersonal difficulty.

C. The premature ejaculation is not due exclusively to the direct effects of a substance (e.g., withdrawal from opioids).

Specify type:
  Lifelong Type
  Acquired Type
Specify type:
  Generalized Type
  Situational Type
Specify:
  Due to Psychological Factors
  Due to Combined Factors

Source: Reprinted with permission from the Diagnostic and Statistical Manual of Mental Disorders, Fourth Edition. Copyright 1994 American Psychiatric Association.

Sexual Pain Disorders

In these disorders, sexual pain occurs before, during, or after sexual intercourse. In dyspareunia (see *DSM-IV* Diagnostic Criteria), men or women experience genital pain at any stage in the sexual response cycle. Women with vaginismus experience involuntary muscle tightening in the outer third of the vagina. Both conditions interfere significantly with intercourse.

Culture, Age, and Gender Features

Box 23–1 lists the prevalence of sexual and gender identity disorders. Depending on the individual's age, health, gender, and culture, there are wide differences in sexual arousal and function. Ethnic and racial background is an important consideration for the diagnosis. For instance, different cultures may value men's sexual desire and performance over

DSM-IV Diagnostic Criteria for Dyspareunia and Vaginismus

Diagnostic Criteria for 302.76 Dyspareunia

A. Recurrent or persistent genital pain associated with sexual intercourse in either a male or a female.

B. The disturbance causes marked distress or interpersonal difficulty.

C. The disturbance is not caused exclusively by Vaginismus or lack of lubrication, is not better accounted for by another Axis I disorder (except another Sexual Dysfunction), and is not due exclusively to the direct physiological effects of a substance (e.g., a drug of abuse, a medication) or a general medical condition.

Specify type:
  Lifelong Type
  Acquired Type
Specify type:
  Generalized Type
  Situational Type
Specify:
  Due to Psychological Factors
  Due to Combined Factors

Diagnostic Criteria for 306.51 Vaginismus

A. Recurrent or persistent involuntary spasm of the musculature of the outer third of the vagina that interferes with sexual intercourse.

B. The disturbance causes marked distress or interpersonal difficulty.

C. The disturbance is not better accounted for by another Axis I disorder (e.g., Somatization Disorder) and is not due exclusively to the direct physiological effects of a general medical condition.

Specify type:
  Lifelong Type
  Acquired Type
Specify type:
  Generalized Type
  Situational Type
Specify:
  Due to Psychological Factors
  Due to Combined Factors

Source: Reprinted with permission from the Diagnostic and Statistical Manual of Mental Disorders, Fourth Edition. Copyright 1994 American Psychiatric Association.

> **Box 23–1. Prevalence of Sexual and Gender Identity Disorders**
>
> | Disorder | Prevalence |
> |---|---|
> | Sexual dysfunctions | Common |
> | Orgasmic disorder | 5–30% of females |
> | | 4–10% of males |
> | Premature ejaculation | 35% |
> | Gender identity disorders | Rare* |
> | Paraphilias | Rare |
>
> *Affects an estimated 30,000 people.
>
> Source: Reprinted with permission from the Diagnostic and Statistical Manual of Mental Disorders, Fourth Edition. Copyright 1994 American Psychiatric Association.

women's. Cultural or religious beliefs may also influence or inhibit sexual activity.

Etiology

Biological Theories

The most common biological causes are medical or psychiatric conditions, prescribed medications, and alcohol or illicit substances. For instance, diabetes and vascular insufficiency often lead to difficulty in achieving orgasm. Those who, because of medical disorders, experience symptoms that are similar to *DSM-IV* diagnoses are excluded from the mental disorder diagnosis. Therefore, an essential assessment strategy is to determine whether a medication or physical condition may have precipitated the dysfunction. Sexual processes need intact neural and vascular functioning to the genitals. Box 23–2 shows medical conditions that often lead to sexual dysfunction.

Because many medications, such as antihypertensives and steroids, cause decreased libido or problems with orgasm or erection as side effects, symptoms that appear soon after beginning a medication may well be drug induced. As shown in Box 23–3 many medications can lead to reduced sexual desire or functioning, including most antidepressants. Alcohol, cocaine, and opiates often lead to sexual dysfunction. Discontinuing the pharmacologic agent or switching to another medication may resolve symptoms.

If a medical condition is the major factor, sexual dysfunction due to a general medical condition is diagnosed (see *DSM-IV* Diagnostic Criteria). If a medication or illicit substance is the cause, clients are diagnosed with substance-induced sexual dysfunction.

Multicausal Theories of Sexual Dysfunction

Some investigators theorize that these disorders result from a combination of internal, interpersonal, and behavioral factors. In the multicausal model, misinformation or lack of information about sexual relationships may interact with un-

> **Box 23–2. Medical Conditions Associated with Sexual Dysfunctions**
>
> *Female*
> - Menopausal hormone imbalance
> - Atrophic vaginitis
> - Lactation (estrogen)
> - Removal of vulva
> - Vaginal excision and reconstruction
> - Vaginal and urinary tract infections
> - Vaginal scar tissue
> - Episiotomy scar
> - Endometriosis
> - Pelvic infection
> - Uterine prolapse
> - Shortened vagina
> - Oophorectomy
> - Estrogen deficiency
>
> *Male*
> - Renal failure
> - Peripheral neuropathy
> - Peripheral vascular disease
> - Withdrawal from opioids
> - Post–alcohol abstinence
> - Hypogonadal states
> - Testicular disease
> - Post-prostatectomy complications
> - Abnormal testosterone levels
> - Abnormal prolactin level
>
> *Both*
>
> *Neurological*
> - Multiple sclerosis
> - Spinal cord injury
> - Injury to autonomic nervous system
> - Neuropathies
> - Temporal lobe lesions
>
> *Endocrine*
> - Diabetes mellitus
> - Hypothyroidism
> - Hypoadrenocorticism and hyperadrenocorticism
> - Hyperprolactinemia
> - Pituitary dysfunction
>
> *Genitourinary conditions*
> - Urethral infections
> - Genital injury or infection
>
> *Neoplasms*
> - Pelvic cancer
> - Radiotherapy of pelvis
>
> *Gastrointestinal conditions*
> - Crohn's disease
> - Irritable bowel syndrome
>
> Source: Adapted from Levine, 1995; and the Diagnostic and Statistical Manual of Mental Disorders, Fourth Edition. Copyright 1994 American Psychiatric Association.

> **Box 23–3. Medications and Substances that Lead to Sexual Dysfunction**
>
> **Illicit Substances**
> Alcohol
> Opiates
> Cocaine
>
> **Antidepressants**
> Tricyclic antidepressants (TCAs)
> Monoamine oxidase inhibitors (MAOIs)
> Selective serotonin reuptake inhibitors (SSRIs)
> Trazodone
> Venlafaxine
>
> **Antipsychotics**
> Thioridazine
> Chlorpromazine
> Fluphenazine
> Clozapine
>
> **Antihypertensives**
> Thiazide diuretics
> Methyldopa
> Clonidine
> Beta-blockers
> Guanethidine
>
> **Others**
> Cimetidine
> Steroids
> Estrogen
> Chemotherapy
> Antihistamines

conscious guilt and anxiety about intercourse, lack of communication about sexual feelings and preferences, and *performance anxiety,* fears of behaving inadequately during sex. The combination of these factors leads to problems with sexual arousal or performance.[3]

Prognosis

Most individuals with sexual dysfunctions develop problems after a major stressor, during times of psychosocial distress, or while having interpersonal difficulties.[1] The course typically waxes and wanes, depending on these factors. Less common are dysfunctions that begin in adolescence and have a chronic course.

Planning Care

The most important factors in determining treatment are clients' concerns about their symptoms and an accurate diagnosis of the primary conditions and secondary problems. For those with sexual dysfunctions, shame and humiliation are common. Most clients have difficulty openly discussing their symptoms. Assess clients' quality of life and the role the disorders play. For those who fulfill the full criteria for a sexual dysfunction, a complete physical and psychiatric evaluation is necessary. Once a physiological cause is excluded, treatment takes place in the community setting. Use the clinical management tips to facilitate care.

Interventions for Clients in the Community

Cognitive-Behavior Therapy

Cognitive-behavior therapy is the mainstay of treatment for sexual and gender identity disorders. It attempts to change the individual's thoughts and uses practice exercises to improve sexual activities.

Sexual Arousal Disorders. Sexual arousal disorders are more effectively treated when both partners engage in treatment. One of the most useful is a behavioral technique called *sensate focus*. The purpose is to use behavioral assignments to reduce anxiety during sexual activity. Clients and their partners concentrate on pleasurable feelings without any sexual activity. Nongenital and tender caressing is encouraged instead. In the next stage, they progress to pleasurable sexual activities involving the genitals but without intercourse. After the clients' anxieties have diminished substantially, penetration and intercourse is "allowed."

Another effective treatment for male sexual arousal disorder is a vacuum device. Connected to a vacuum pump, this device is a plastic cylinder with an opening. Blood is drawn into the penis and a tension ring is moved from the cylinder to the base of the penis to maintain an erection.[4]

Orgasmic Disorders. For women and men with orgasmic disorders, a systematic behavior program is effective. *Directed masturbation* is a set of techniques aimed at helping individuals explore and become more comfortable with their bodies.[5] They are instructed to begin to masturbate, exploring the muscles associated with orgasm. Women are encouraged to use visual exploration and devices such as vibrators. During the physical stimulation, clients are taught to use sexual fantasies to promote orgasm. Once mastered, clients and their partners practice the stimulating behaviors. Specific sexual positions may be recommended.

Premature Ejaculation. Behavioral techniques such as the start-stop technique are useful for premature ejaculation. In these exercises, the client's partner strokes his penis while he experiences pleasurable feelings. When he feels the urge to ejaculate, his partner stops the stimulation. This is repeated at least four times before ejaculation.

Sexual Pain Disorders. Systematic desensitization is the most effective technique for sexual pain disorders. Very gradual physical stimulation is introduced, progressing to penile stimulation and penetration.

Couples and Sexual Therapy

Couples and sexual therapy, the most common treatments for sexual dysfunctions, attempt to improve communication

Diagnostic Criteria for Sexual Dysfunction due to a General Medical Condition and Substance-Induced Sexual Dysfunction

Diagnostic Criteria for Sexual Dysfunction Due to . . . [Indicate the General Medical Condition]

A. Clinically significant sexual dysfunction that results in marked distress or interpersonal difficulty predominates in the clinical picture.

B. There is evidence from the history, physical examination, or laboratory findings that the sexual dysfunction is fully explained by the direct physiological effects of a general medical condition.

C. The disturbance is not better accounted for by another mental disorder (e.g., Major Depressive Disorder).

Select code and term based on the predominant sexual dysfunction:

625.8 Female Hypoactive Sexual Desire Disorder Due to . . . *[Indicate the General Medical Condition]*: if deficient or absent sexual desire is the predominant feature

608.89 Male Hypoactive Sexual Desire Disorder Due to . . . *[Indicate the General Medical Condition]*: if deficient or absent sexual desire is the predominant feature

607.84 Male Erectile Disorder Due to . . . *[Indicate the General Medical Condition]*: if male erectile dysfunction is the predominant feature

625.0 Female Dyspareunia Due to . . . *[Indicate the General Medical Condition]*: if pain associated with intercourse is the predominant feature

608.89 Male Dyspareunia Due to . . . *[Indicate the General Medical Condition]*: if pain associated with intercourse is the predominant feature

625.8 Other Female Sexual Dysfunction Due to . . . *[indicate the General Medical Condition]*: if some other feature is predominant (e.g., Orgasmic Disorder) or no feature predominates

608.89 Other Male Sexual Dysfunction Due to . . . *[Indicate the General Medical Condition]*: if some other feature is predominant (e.g., Orgasmic Disorder) or no feature predominates

Coding Note: Include the name of the general medical condition on Axis I, e.g., 607.84 Male Erectile Disorder Due to Diabetes Mellitus; also code the general medical condition on Axis III (see Appendix G for codes).

Diagnostic Criteria for Substance-Induced Sexual Dysfunction

A. Clinically significant sexual dysfunction that results in marked distress or interpersonal difficulty predominates in the clinical picture.

B. There is evidence from the history, physical examination, or laboratory findings that the sexual dysfunction is fully explained by substance use as manifested by either (1) or (2):
   (1) the symptoms in Criterion A developed during, or within a month of, Substance Intoxication
   (2) medication use is etiologically related to the disturbance

C. The disturbance is not better accounted for by a Sexual Dysfunction that is not substance induced. Evidence that the symptoms are better accounted for by a Sexual Dysfunction that is not substance induced might include the following: the symptoms precede the onset of the substance use or dependence (or medication use); the symptoms persist for a substantial period of time (e.g., about a month) after the cessation of intoxication, or are substantially in excess of what would be expected given the type or amount of the substance used or the duration of use; or there is other evidence that suggests the existence of an independent non-substance-induced Sexual Dysfunction (e.g., a history of recurrent non-substance-related episodes).

NOTE: This diagnosis should be made instead of a diagnosis of Substance Intoxication only when the sexual dysfunction is in excess of that usually associated with the intoxication syndrome and when the dysfunction is sufficiently severe to warrant independent clinical attention.

Code [Specific Substance]—Induced Sexual Dysfunction: (291.8 Alcohol; 292.89 Amphetamine [or Amphetamine-Like Substance]; 292.89 Cocaine; 292.89 Opioid; 292.89 Sedative, Hypnotic, or Anxiolytic; 292.89 Other [or Unknown] Substance)

Specify if:
With Impaired Desire
With Impaired Arousal
With Impaired Orgasm
With Sexual Pain

Specify if:
With Onset During Intoxication: if the criteria are met for Intoxication with the substance and the symptoms develop during the intoxication syndrome

Source: Reprinted with permission from the Diagnostic and Statistical Manual of Mental Disorders, Fourth Edition. Copyright 1994 American Psychiatric Association.

between partners and solve underlying problems in the relationship. The specific strategies and practice exercises used are outlined in Chapter 11. An effective treatment for many sexual dysfunctions is a combination of cognitive-behavior therapy and couples therapy.

Pharmacologic Interventions

Sexual Arousal Disorders. Pharmacologic interventions for sexual arousal disorders include penile injections and oral and topical medications, although their mechanism of action is not well understood. Yohimbine, thought to be an aphrodisiac, may be an effective oral medication for both men and women. Testosterone, once used with both men and women, is generally not effective and has masculine effects, such as facial hair, in women.

Erectile Disorders. For individuals with erectile dysfunction, the combination of papaverine, a muscle relaxant, and phentolamine, an α-adrenergic blocker, may successfully produce erection. However, undesirable side effects, including painful and sustained erections, may result. Topical medications such as nitroglycerin patches and minoxidil have shown some preliminary effectiveness. These topical agents appear to work by directly relaxing muscles in the penis.

GENDER IDENTITY DISORDER

Characteristic Behaviors

Beginning Symptoms

Symptoms can be identified in childhood. Although there is a normal "tomboy" stage for girls, and boys may play house and experiment with female activities, children and adolescents who display gender confusion consistently act like and believe that they are of the opposite sex. Children may also explicitly state the desire to become the opposite sex and identify with role models of the opposite sex.

Adults may first present in search of medical or surgical ways to alter their sex, such as requests for steroid hormones or sex reassignment surgery. Women may buy binding clothing to restrict their breasts, and men may wear makeup. Less commonly, some individuals present as transsexuals and portray themselves as the opposite sex.

These individuals feel extremely uncomfortable with their gender. They state that they want to be the opposite sex and strongly prefer clothing and activities associated with the opposite sex. The desire to become the opposite sex is established by adolescence and persists into adulthood.[1] These individuals are different from individuals with transvestic fetishism, so-called cross dressing. In gender identity disorders, individuals feel "male" when they have female attributes, or "female" when they have male physical characteristics.

Ever since I was young, I wanted to be a boy. I mean, I felt like a boy. I did boy things—played outside a lot, was a tomboy, was very interested in contact sports, and I even dressed like a boy. My physical characteristics were that of a girl. I remember telling my parents that I never wanted to have breasts because I wanted to look more like a boy. They really flipped out. I stopped telling them anything about it after that. I always have felt trapped—I'm a man on the inside and a woman on the outside.

Individuals often pass as the other sex, want to be treated like the other sex, and believe that they have the typical feelings and reactions of the other sex.[1] Children experience similar feelings; they also wear clothing of the opposite sex, participate in "make believe" play as the other sex, play games of the other sex, and prefer playmates of the other sex. Many find that their gender is uncomfortable, distressing, and inappropriate. Some believe that they or their genitals are physically disgusting. Because they are so distressed with their gender, adults frequently present for sex reassignment surgery (see *DSM-IV* Diagnostic Criteria for Gender Identity Disorder).

Culture, Age, and Gender Features

Individuals with gender identity disorder may report the onset of symptoms in childhood. Children establish their gender identity by age 3; however, parents of children with these disorders may observe that their children continue to be interested in opposite-sex activities into childhood or adolescence. Sexual orientation does not appear to strongly influence gender identity disorder; thus, expressing homosexual feelings is not related to this disorder. Individuals with gender identity disorder show a strong desire to become the opposite sex and request sex-reassignment surgery. Others show more gender confusion and are more ambivalent about surgery; these individuals typically develop symptoms later in adulthood.

These disorders affect men more often than women.

Etiology

Biological Theories

The cause of gender identity disorder is unknown. It may result from abnormalities in the temporal lobe. Preliminary findings suggest that some individuals have temporal lobe epilepsy or electroencephalograph abnormalities.[6] Further study is necessary to support these theories.

Learning Theories

Learning theorists suggest that gender identity disorder results from the failure to identify with same-sex individuals during childhood. Some children may receive minimal or inconsistent reinforcement for identifying with same-sex role models such as a parent. For instance, girls may be strongly encouraged to be "tomboys," act like their fathers, dress like boys, and refrain from playing with dolls. They then expe-

> ### DSM-IV Diagnostic Criteria for Gender Identity Disorder
>
> **A.** A strong and persistent cross-gender identification (not merely a desire for any perceived cultural advantages of being the other sex).
> In children, the disturbance is manifested by four (or more) of the following:
> (1) repeatedly stated desire to be, or insistence that he or she is, the other sex
> (2) in boys, preference for cross-dressing or simulating female attire; in girls, insistence on wearing only stereotypical masculine clothing
> (3) strong and persistent preferences for cross-sex roles in make-believe play or persistent fantasies of being the other sex
> (4) intense desire to participate in the stereotypical games and pastimes of the other sex
> (5) strong preference for playmates of the other sex
>
> In adolescents and adults, the disturbance is manifested by symptoms such as a stated desire to be the other sex, frequent passing as the other sex, desire to live or be treated as the other sex, or the conviction that he or she has the typical feelings and reactions of the other sex.
>
> **B.** Persistent discomfort with his or her sex or sense of inappropriateness in the gender role of that sex.
> In children, the disturbance is manifested by any of the following: in boys, assertion that his penis or testes are disgusting or will disappear or assertion that it would be better not to have a penis, or aversion toward rough-and-tumble play and rejection of male stereotypical toys, games, and activities; in girls, rejection of urinating in a sitting position, assertion that she has or will grow a penis, or assertion that she does not want to grow breasts or menstruate, or marked aversion toward normative feminine clothing.
>
> In adolescents and adults, the disturbance is manifested by symptoms such as preoccupation with getting rid of primary and secondary sex characteristics (e.g., request for hormones, surgery, or other procedures to physically alter sexual characteristics to simulate the other sex) or belief that he or she was born the wrong sex.
>
> **C.** The disturbance is not concurrent with a physical intersex condition.
>
> **D.** The disturbance causes clinically significant distress or impairment in social, occupational, or other important areas of functioning.
>
> *Code* based on current age
> 302.6 Gender Identity Disorder in Children
> 302.85 Gender Identity Disorder in Adolescents or Adults
>
> *Specify* if (for sexually mature individuals):
> Sexually Attracted to Males
> Sexually Attracted to Females
> Sexually Attracted to Both
> Sexually Attracted to Neither
>
> **Source:** Reprinted with permission from the Diagnostic and Statistical Manual of Mental Disorders, Fourth Edition. Copyright 1994 American Psychiatric Association.

rience gender confusion and begin to identify with opposite-sex individuals, which gets reinforced directly or indirectly.

Prognosis

Most children's symptoms will not continue into adulthood, whereas adults who develop gender identity disorder tend to have a chronic course.

Interventions for Clients in the Community

The most common intervention is individual psychotherapy with a supportive or cognitive-behavior approach. Treatment may involve identifying, practicing, and developing behaviors of the desired sex. The treatment may also focus on clarifying the wish and need for actual change in physical manifestations of the desired sex. Therapists educate clients about the course of hormone treatment to change sexual characteristics and the use of surgery. For those who do receive sex-reassignment surgery and subsequent hormone therapy, psychotherapy can help to monitor and assess adjustment.

PARAPHILIAS

Characteristic Behaviors

Beginning Symptoms

The initial symptoms of paraphilias sometimes begin in adolescence. Teenagers may become aroused by contact with objects such as women's undergarments or shoes or by observing others disrobing. Sexual activity may occasionally include behaviors suggestive of one of the paraphilias. Minimal distress may be present initially. These thoughts, however, progress to a set of defined behaviors in adulthood that are pervasive and compelling, indicating the full expression of the paraphilia. These people develop urges and fantasies underlying the behaviors that are exclusive and strongly preferred.

Recurrent sexual urges and fantasies about nonhuman or nonconsenting partners predominate. Usually clients have acted on or are very distressed by these urges for at least 6 months. Exhibitionism, frotteurism, voyeurism, pedophilia, fetishism, transvestic fetishism, sexual masochism or sadism,

Diagnostic Criteria for Exhibitionism, Fetishism, Frotteurism, Pedophilia, Sexual Masochism, Sexual Sadism, Transvestic Fetishism, and Voyeurism

Diagnostic Criteria for 302.4 Exhibitionism

A. Over a period of at least 6 months, recurrent, intense, sexually arousing fantasies, sexual urges, or behaviors involving the exposure of one's genitals to an unsuspecting stranger.

B. The fantasies, sexual urges, or behaviors cause clinically significant distress or impairment in social, occupational, or other important areas of functioning.

Diagnostic Criteria for 302.81 Fetishism

A. Over a period of at least 6 months, recurrent, intense sexually arousing fantasies, sexual urges, or behaviors involving the use of nonliving objects (e.g., female undergarments).

B. The fantasies, sexual urges, or behaviors cause clinically significant distress or impairment in social, occupational, or other important areas of functioning.

C. The fetish objects are not limited to articles of female clothing used in cross-dressing (as in Transvestic Fetishism) or devices designed for the purpose of tactile genital stimulation (e.g., a vibrator).

Diagnostic Criteria for 302.89 Frotteurism

A. Over a period of at least 6 months, recurrent, intense sexually arousing fantasies, sexual urges, or behaviors involving touching and rubbing against a nonconsenting person.

B. The fantasies, sexual urges, or behaviors cause clinically significant distress or impairment in social, occupational, or other important areas of functioning.

Diagnostic Criteria for 302.2 Pedophilia

A. Over a period of at least 6 months, recurrent, intense sexually arousing fantasies, sexual urges, or behaviors involving sexual activity with a prepubescent child or children (generally age 13 years or younger).

B. The fantasies, sexual urges, or behaviors cause clinically significant distress or impairment in social, occupational, or other important areas of functioning.

C. The person is at least age 16 years and at least 5 years older than the child or children in Criterion A.

NOTE: Do not include an individual in late adolescence involved in an ongoing sexual relationship with a 12- or 13-year-old.

Specify if:
  Sexually Attracted to Males
  Sexually Attracted to Females
  Sexually Attracted to Both

Specify if:
  Limited to Incest

Specify type:
  Exclusive Type (attracted only to children)
  Nonexclusive Type

Diagnostic Criteria for 302.83 Sexual Masochism

A. Over a period of at least 6 months, recurrent, intense sexually arousing fantasies, sexual urges, or behaviors involving the act (real, not simulated) of being humiliated, beaten, bound, or otherwise made to suffer.

B. The fantasies, sexual urges, or behaviors cause clinically significant distress or impairment in social, occupational, or other important areas of functioning.

Diagnostic Criteria for 302.84 Sexual Sadism

A. Over a period of at least 6 months, recurrent, intense sexually arousing fantasies, sexual urges, or behaviors involving acts (real, not simulated) in which the psychological or physical suffering (including humiliation) of the victim is sexually exciting to the person.

B. The fantasies, sexual urges, or behaviors cause clinically significant distress or impairment in social, occupational, or other important areas of functioning.

Diagnostic Criteria for 302.3 Transvestic Fetishism

A. Over a period of at least 6 months, in a heterosexual male, recurrent, intense sexually arousing fantasies, sexual urges, or behaviors involving cross-dressing.

B. The fantasies, sexual urges, or behaviors cause clinically significant distress or impairment in social, occupational, or other important areas of functioning.

Specify if:
  With Gender Dysphoria: if the person has persistent discomfort with gender role or identity

Diagnostic Criteria for 302.82 Voyeurism

A. Over a period of at least 6 months, recurrent, intense sexually arousing fantasies, sexual urges, or behaviors involving the act of observing an unsuspecting person who is naked, in the process of disrobing, or engaging in sexual activity.

B. The fantasies, sexual urges, or behaviors cause clinically significant distress or impairment in social, occupational, or other important areas of functioning.

Source: Reprinted with permission from the Diagnostic and Statistical Manual of Mental Disorders, Fourth Edition. Copyright 1994 American Psychiatric Association.

and paraphilia NOS constitute the paraphilias (see *DSM-IV* Diagnostic Criteria). Other sexual urges that fall into paraphilia NOS include sexual arousal with corpses (necrophilia) or feces (coprophilia).

Most individuals with paraphilias experience unusual fantasies and urges nearly every day; some may have symptoms of multiple paraphilias. *Exhibitionism* is exposing one's genitals to an unsuspecting stranger. In *frotteurism*, individuals are sexually aroused by rubbing up against a stranger. Observing an unsuspecting individual naked, while disrobing, or during sexual activity is called *voyeurism*. *Pedophilia* involves sexual attraction to prepubescent children. Examples of sexual urges and fantasies about nonhuman objects include *fetishism*, sexual urges toward apparel such as women's undergarments, and *transvestic fetishism*, becoming sexually aroused while cross-dressing. *Sexual masochism* involves sexual excitement from being bound, beaten, or hurt, whereas *sexual sadism* involves sexual arousal from causing psychological or physical suffering.

> As far as I can remember I was attracted to young boys. Even seeing boys would turn me on. I guess it started when I was a teenager, but the feelings have been really strong ever since then. I fantasize about intercourse with them. I know this must sound disgusting—I used to be disgusted by it, too. I don't understand why I have these feelings, I just know that I do. I've never actually had sex with a child, but I have with teenage boys. One of them threatened to beat me up afterwards. That's when I decided I better get some help.

Culture, Age, and Gender Features

Paraphilias affect men more often than women. About half of those with the disorder are married.[1]

Etiology

Biological Theories

Some studies implicate abnormalities in the limbic system, which is partly responsible for controlling sexual and aggressive impulses, particularly the temporal lobe. Temporal lobe epilepsy and temporal lobe tumors have been found in violent sex offenders with paraphilias.[7] Some evidence for this theory also comes from animal studies in which limbic system abnormalites are associated with increased sexual behaviors.

Learning Theories

Learning theories may also explain the development of these disorders. Certain sexual behaviors may begin in childhood and are reinforced, culminating in a paraphilia. For instance, a male adolescent who engages in sexual play with a young male child may begin to fantasize and develop distinct sexual desires to have intercourse with children. The sexual fantasies toward children strengthen and eventually develop into pedophilia.

RESEARCH NOTE

Kafka, MP, and Prentky, R: Fluoxetine treatment of nonparaphilic sexual addictions and paraphilias in men. J Clin Psychiatry 53:351–358, 1992.

Findings: Disruption of the neurotransmitter serotonin may be related to the development of paraphilias. These investigators examined the effectiveness of fluoxetine (Prozac) in these disorders. Sixteen men with paraphilias and sexual addictive behaviors were treated for 12 weeks. Most of the participants also had comorbid mood disorders such as major depression or dysthymia. Fluoxetine significantly reduced paraphilic behaviors after 4 weeks of treatment. The medication failed to affect nonparaphilic sexual behaviors. Along with improvement in their depressive symptoms, disturbing sexual fantasies and urges decreased, whereas healthy sexual functioning was preserved. These findings suggest that abnormalities in serotonergic functioning are present in clients with paraphilic and sexual addictive behavior. Specifically, decreased serotonin neurotransmission may be enhanced by treatment with fluoxetine and lead to improved mood and sexual functioning.

Application to Practice: Clients with paraphilias can be very difficult to treat. This study suggests that fluoxetine, given for 4 to 12 weeks, reduces these behaviors. These results also suggest that paraphilias have a biological origin and that medication reverses abnormalities in the serotonin system. Nurses can refer clients with disturbing sexual urges and fantasies for psychopharmacologic evaluation.

Prognosis

Paraphilias emerge by early adulthood, tend to be chronic, and may abate in older adulthood. Symptoms may fluctuate in intensity, particularly during times of psychosocial stress.

Interventions for Clients in the Community

Cognitive-Behavior Therapy

Individuals with a paraphilia need psychotherapy, and a referral to a cognitive-behavior therapist may be the most beneficial. *Aversive conditioning* is sometimes used to treat paraphilias. In combination with another behavior method, *covert sensitization*, individuals are exposed to noxious odors or anxiety-provoking scenes during sexual fantasies; they begin to associate the unpleasant experiences with the paraphilia. Limited success has been reported.

Pharmacologic Interventions

Antiandrogen agents such as Depo-Provera are useful in the treatment of individuals with paraphilias, particularly sex offenders. They are given orally or intramuscularly in long-acting preparations to decrease libido and break the individual's pattern of sexual urges and actions. These medications are most effective in those with a high sex drive who do not have antisocial personality disorder. They do not specifically reduce inappropriate sexual behaviors.

New research suggests that selective serotonin-reuptake inhibitors (SSRIs) such as fluoxetine are effective treatments, particularly for voyeurism, exhibitionism, pedophilia, and frotteurism. These agents may work by decreasing sexual urges and inhibiting orgasm, but their mechanism of action is poorly understood. More research is needed to determine their effectiveness and dosage range.[8]

CLIENT AND FAMILY EDUCATION

For individuals, their sexual partners, and their families, having a sexual or gender identity disorder is often fraught with humiliation and shame. As a result, these disorders are hidden and not openly discussed. Include the following in education:
- Convey that these behaviors are symptoms of a disorder, the way chest pain and shortness of breath reflect cardiac disorders.
- Inform clients and families that they are not alone; for those with sexual dysfunctions, these behaviors are a common occurrence.
- Explain the various etiologies for sexual dysfunctions.
- Educate men and women about the healthy sexual response cycle.
- Tell them that sexual desire and activity are normal.
- Teach that homosexual relationships are not abnormal and do not reflect psychiatric problems.
- Investigate the clients' fears and anxieties about expressing their symptoms.
- Teach parents that whereas some identification with the opposite sex is part of normal child development, children's repeated desires to be the opposite sex should be evaluated.
- Refer clients, when necessary, for further assessment to clinicians who specialize in the treatment of sexual disorders.
- Convey acceptance and openness about sexual difficulties and unusual sexual behaviors when discussing clients' sexual concerns.

EXPECTED OUTCOMES

For the individual with a sexual or gender identity disorder, improvement will be demonstrated by:
- Recognizing that behaviors reflect a sexual or gender identity disorder.
- Devising short- and long-term goals to promote healthy sexual behaviors.
- Identifying pressures or stressors, if present, that contribute to unhealthy sexual behaviors.
- Engaging in healthy, satisfying sexual activity.
- Avoiding medication, alcohol, or illicit substances that contribute to sexual dysfunction.
- Openly discussing problems with sexuality or gender identity.
- Substituting more effective ways of relating to promote healthy sexual functioning.

COMMON NURSING DIAGNOSES

- Sexual Dysfunction
- Sexuality Patterns, altered
- Coping, individual, ineffective
- Social Isolation
- Anxiety
- Powerlessness

SYNOPSIS OF CURRENT RESEARCH

Compared to other major psychiatric disorders, very little research has been done on the sexual and identity disorders. Current research is focused on demonstrating the effectiveness of sexual therapy, particularly cognitive-behavior therapy, in the treatment of the specific sexual dysfunctions. Preliminary research also suggests that the SSRIs such as fluoxetine and sertraline may be useful for treating premature ejaculation and the paraphilias. Studies to understand the etiology of sexual and gender identity disorders are also underway. In particular, serotonin dysregulation and limbic system dysfunction may be implicated in the pathogenesis of paraphilias.

Another major area of study is the link between sexual dysfunction and medications, particularly antidepressants. Antidepressants may cause hypoactive sexual desire, anorgasmia, and difficulties with ejaculation. Differentiating medication-induced sexual dysfunction, worsening psychiatric disorders such as depression, and underlying sexual dysfunction is currently being investigated. Systematic treatment of medication-induced sexual dysfunction with medications such as yohimbine, cyproheptadine, or bethanechol is also under investigation.

AREAS FOR FUTURE RESEARCH

- What is the impact of sexual and gender identity disorders on family, friends, and coworkers?
- What is the impact on treatment compliance of nurses' education of clients with sexual and gender identity disorders?
- What is the effect of early identification of sexual and gender identity disorders on long-term outcome?

- What are the first identifiable behaviors of gender identity disorder, and are any biochemical changes associated with them?
- How can nurses destigmatize the public's view of sexual and gender identity disorders?
- What are the most effective components of the role of the psychiatric clinical nurse generalist in successful treatment?
- What is the impact of a sexual and gender identity disorder on an individual's quality of life?
- What is the relationship between criminal behavior and pedophilia?
- How do SSRIs work to treat paraphilias?
- What is the long-term outcome associated with cognitive-behavior treatment of sexual and gender identity disorders?

CASE STUDY

Larry R is a 43-year-old married man who was seen for hypertension at a medical clinic. During the routine nursing assessment, Larry related that he was having problems with his sexual performance over the last "few years." He was ashamed and embarrassed when he conveyed these problems, reluctantly answering further questions about his sexual relationship. He noted that he and his wife had "drifted apart." He also noted that his sex drive continued to be strong, in fact, stronger than his wife's libido. When asked directly, he acknowledged ejaculating early, usually as he and his wife began intercourse.

The nurse then asked if she could speak to his wife and continued the assessment with the couple. Although Larry had a strong sex drive, his wife had not been aware of this. The frequency of intercourse had dropped to once per month for the last 2 to 3 years. During the first years of their marriage, intercourse occurred two to three times each week. Both he and his wife denied any problems with alcohol or substance abuse. He also denied any problems with depressed mood, sleep or appetite disturbance, or other symptoms of depression. The only medication he was taking was hydrochlorothiazide for hypertension.

The nurse taught Larry and his wife that sexual dysfunctions are common disorders. She also informed them that a more complete evaluation was necessary to determine the nature of the disruption. She taught them that problems with ejaculation could be related to alcohol, drugs, or underlying medical problems. In the absence of those factors, stress or relationship issues could contribute to sexual dysfunction. The nurse suggested that the sexual disruption be investigated further during the visit with his nurse practitioner. Larry and his wife agreed. The nurse practitioner discovered that his sexual desire was healthy and tentatively diagnosed Larry with premature ejaculation. No medical evidence suggested an organic etiology. Because the antihypertensive might have been contributing to his dysfunction, he began taking a different medication.

After 2 weeks, Larry and his wife returned to the clinic. His blood pressure remained in the normal range; however, his difficulties with premature ejaculation continued. The couple was referred to a psychotherapist who specialized in the treatment of sexual disorders.

During the sex therapy, Larry and his wife were taught, with some success, specific behavioral techniques to tolerate high levels of excitement without Larry's ejaculating. Both were initially reluctant to try the exercises. They also watched videotapes that instructed them on how to perform these exercises. In particular, they focused on techniques that promoted sexual arousal and control of premature ejaculation. With practice, some of the exercises were effective, and the couple reported increased satisfaction with their sexual relationship. Larry continued to be concerned that his desire for intercourse was greater than his wife's. His wife was concerned about the "emotional distance" between them. They continued with the therapist to address these issues and other communication problems in their marriage.

CRITICAL THINKING QUESTIONS

1. What are the most important physical conditions and medications to consider in the client with a sexual dysfunction?
2. What psychiatric diagnoses could contribute to sexual dysfunction?
3. What measures could the nurse have taken to reduce Larry's discomfort about relating his symptoms?
4. Explain the mechanism by which behavior therapy reduces sexual dysfunction.
5. Develop a care plan, including short- and long-term goals, for Larry's sexual relationship.
6. Identify behaviors that indicate Larry is responding to treatment.
7. Design a teaching plan for the couple to maintain healthy sexual functioning.

KEY POINTS

- The sexual and gender identity disorders include three broad diagnostic categories: the sexual dysfunctions, paraphilias, and gender identity disorders.
- Sexual dysfunctions are the most common disorders; they involve disturbances in sexual desire (libido) and sexual performance that cause substantial distress.
- The paraphilias are less common disorders that involve intense and unusual sexual urges; they include exhibitionism, fetishism, frotteurism, pedophilia, sexual masochism, sexual sadism, transvestic fetishism, voyeurism, and paraphilia not otherwise specified (NOS).
- Individuals with gender identity disorders feel extremely uncomfortable with their gender, want to be the opposite sex, and engage in activities associated with the opposite sex.
- Masters and Johnson described four stages of the healthy sexual response cycle: desire, excitement, orgasm, and resolution. Disruption can occur in any of these stages.

- Most individuals with sexual dysfunctions develop problems after a major stressor, during times of psychosocial distress, or while having interpersonal difficulties.
- Medications, alcohol, illicit substances, and medical and psychiatric conditions may contribute to sexual dysfunction.
- The etiology of paraphilias and gender identity disorder is poorly understood. Some studies implicate abnormalities in the limbic system in individuals with paraphilias or gender identity disorder.
- Cognitive-behavior therapy is the mainstay of treatment for sexual and gender identity disorders. Cognitive-behavior therapy attempts to change the individual's thoughts and uses practice exercises to improve sexual activities.
- Couples and sexual therapy, alone or in combination with cognitive-behavior therapy, is often used to treat sexual dysfunctions.
- One of the most important nursing interventions is to convey acceptance and openness about sexual difficulties and unusual sexual behaviors in discussions of sexual concerns.

REFERENCES

1. American Psychiatric Association: Diagnostic and Statistical Manual of Mental Disorders, ed 4. American Psychiatric Association, Washington, DC, 1994.
2. Masters, WH, and Johnson, VE: Human Sexual Inadequacy. Little, Brown & Company, Boston, 1970.
3. Kaplan, HS: The New Sex Therapy: Active Treatment of Sexual Dysfunctions. Brunner/Mazel Inc, New York, 1974.
4. Turner, LA, et al: External vacuum devices in the treatment of erectile dysfunction: A one-year study of sexual and psychosocial impact. J Sex Marital Ther 17:81, 1991.
5. LoPiccolo, J, and Stock, WE: Treatment of sexual dysfunction. J Consult Clin Psychol 54:158, 1986.
6. Hoenig, J: Etiology of transsexualism. In Steiner, BW (ed): Gender Dysphoria: Development, Research, Management. Plenum Publishing Corp, New York, 1985, pp 33–73.
7. Bradford, JMW, and McLean, D: Sexual offenders, violence, and testosterone: A clinical study. Can J Psychiatry 29:335, 1984.
8. Perilstein, RD, Lippeer, S, and Friedman, LJ: Three cases of paraphilias responsive to fluoxetine treatment. J Clin Psychiatry 52:169, 1991.

CHAPTER 24

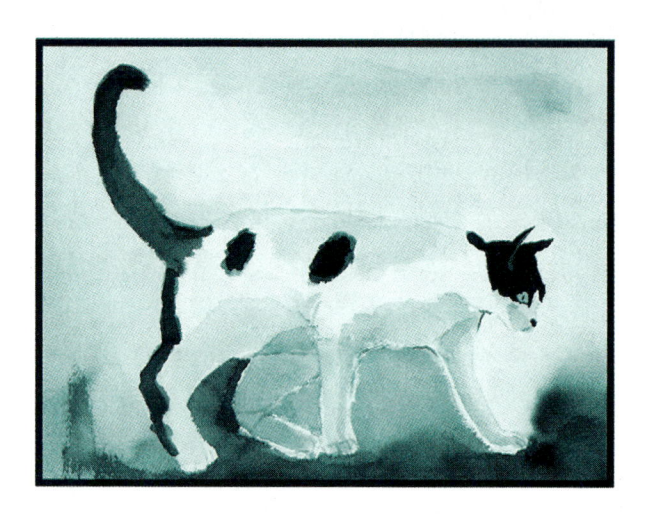

CHAPTER OUTLINE

Characteristic Behaviors
Culture, Age, and Gender Features
Culture
Age and Gender
Etiology
Neurobiological Factors
Genetic Factors
Prognosis
Assessment
Anorexia Nervosa
Bulimia Nervosa
Planning Care
How to Determine an Effective Treatment Strategy
When to Refer
Interventions for Hospitalized Clients
Effective Communication Strategies
Milieu Therapy
Cognitive-Behavior Approaches
Behavior and Interpersonal Therapies
Pharmacologic Treatments
Interventions for Clients in the Community
Expected Outcomes
Differential Diagnosis
Anorexia Nervosa
Bulimia Nervosa
Comorbidity
Common Nursing Diagnoses
Areas for Future Research

Barbara E. Wolfe, RN, CS, PhD

Eating Disorders

LEARNING OBJECTIVES

After completing this chapter, the reader should be able to:

- Describe and differentiate between diagnostic categories: anorexia nervosa, bulimia nervosa, and eating disorder not otherwise specified.
- Identify populations at risk for the development of eating disorders.
- Explain etiologic factors that may contribute to the development of an eating disorder.
- Describe areas of assessment for individuals with or suspected of having an eating disorder.
- Recognize differential and comorbid diagnoses to be considered for a person presenting with eating disorder symptomatology.
- Specify interventions used in acute and chronic care.
- Discuss expected client outcomes and factors influencing outcome.
- Summarize current psychobiological advances in the area of eating disorder research, and cite examples of areas in need of further investigation.

KEY TERMS

amenorrhea
anorexia nervosa
binge eating disorder
bulimia nervosa
lanugo
Russell's sign

Eating disorders are psychiatric illnesses with substantial psychosocial and biological consequences. Although many affected individuals initially appear to function normally, these disorders can cause significant emotional and physical turmoil. This chapter provides an overview of the diagnostic and clinical characteristics of the eating disorders anorexia nervosa and bulimia nervosa. In addition, the more recently identified provisional *Diagnostic and Statistical Manual of Mental Disorders, Fourth Edition (DSM-IV)*[1] diagnostic category of binge eating disorder is discussed.

Both anorexia nervosa and bulimia nervosa are characterized by altered eating patterns and disturbances in body image. Symptoms of **anorexia nervosa** include preoccupation with body shape and weight, refusal to maintain body weight in a normal range for age and height, and, in women, **amenorrhea** for three consecutive menstrual cycles (see *DSM-IV* Diagnostic Criteria). Preoccupations usually center on an intense fear of gaining weight and excessive concern with dietary intake. For example, people with anorexia nervosa are often absorbed with calories and the fat content of meals and exhibit distorted perception of their body shapes, commonly overestimating the size of their stomachs or hips.

DSM-IV Diagnostic Criteria for 307.1 Anorexia Nervosa

A. Refusal to maintain body weight at or above a minimally normal weight for age and height (e.g., weight loss leading to maintenance of body weight less than 85% of that expected; or failure to make expected weight gain during period of growth, leading to body weight less than 85% of that expected).

B. Intense fear of gaining weight or becoming fat, even though underweight.

C. Disturbance in the way in which one's body weight or shape is experienced, undue influence of body weight or shape on self-evaluation, or denial of the seriousness of the current low body weight.

D. In postmenarcheal females, amenorrhea, i.e., the absence of at least three consecutive menstrual cycles. (A woman is considered to have amenorrhea if her periods occur only following hormone, e.g., estrogen, administration.)

Specify type:
  Restricting Type: during the current episode of Anorexia Nervosa, the person has not regularly engaged in binge-eating or purging behavior (i.e., self-induced vomiting or the misuse of laxatives, diuretics, or enemas)
  Binge-Eating/Purging Type: during the current episode of Anorexia Nervosa, the person has regularly engaged in binge-eating or purging behavior (i.e., self-induced vomiting or the misuse of laxatives, diuretics, or enemas)

Source: Reprinted with permission from the Diagnostic and Statistical Manual of Mental Disorders, Fourth Edition. Copyright 1994 American Psychiatric Association.

> **DSM-IV Diagnostic Criteria for 307.51 Bulimia Nervosa**
>
> A. Recurrent episodes of binge eating. An episode of binge eating is characterized by both of the following:
>   (1) eating, in a discrete period of time (e.g., within any 2-hour period), an amount of food that is definitely larger than most people would eat during a similar period of time and under similar circumstances
>   (2) a sense of lack of control over eating during the episode (e.g., a feeling that one cannot stop eating or control what or how much one is eating)
> B. Recurrent inappropriate compensatory behavior in order to prevent weight gain, such as self-induced vomiting; misuse of laxatives, diuretics, enemas, or other medications; fasting; or excessive exercise.
> C. The binge eating and inappropriate compensatory behaviors both occur, on average, at least twice a week for 3 months.
> D. Self-evaluation is unduly influenced by body shape and weight.
> E. The disturbance does not occur exclusively during episodes of Anorexia Nervosa.
>
> *Specify* type:
>   Purging Type: during the current episode of Bulimia Nervosa, the person has regularly engaged in self-induced vomiting or the misuse of laxatives, diuretics, or enemas
>   Nonpurging Type: during the current episode of Bulimia Nervosa, the person has used other inappropriate compensatory behaviors, such as fasting or excessive exercise, but has not engaged in self-induced vomiting or the misuse of laxatives, diuretics, or enemas
>
> **Source:** Reprinted with permission from the Diagnostic and Statistical Manual of Mental Disorders, Fourth Edition. Copyright 1994 American Psychiatric Association.

Bulimia nervosa is a disorder characterized by regular binge eating episodes and the use of compensatory behaviors to prevent weight gain (see *DSM-IV* Diagnostic Criteria). Binge eating is the consumption of 1500 to 3000 calories or more of food in 15 minutes to 2 hours. The binge episode typically includes high-carbohydrate foods such as breads and pastries. Because of their feelings of shame and embarrassment, binge eaters frequently hide their eating. The behaviors they engage in to prevent weight gain include self-induced vomiting and abuse of laxatives, diuretics, and syrup of ipecac. Clients may try to increase their metabolism by exercising excessively and abusing stimulants like caffeine and diet pills.

A third *DSM-IV* diagnostic category, Eating Disorder Not Otherwise Specified (EDNOS), is useful for classifying clients who do not meet all of the diagnostic criteria for bulimia or anorexia. For example, EDNOS may apply to people who meet all of the criteria for bulimia nervosa but have binge eating episodes once a week. Another example is people who fulfill the criteria for anorexia nervosa except that they have

> **DSM-IV Research Criteria for Binge-Eating Disorder**
>
> A. Recurrent episodes of binge eating. An episode of binge eating is characterized by both of the following:
>   (1) eating, in a discrete period of time (e.g., within any 2-hour period), an amount of food that is definitely larger than most people would eat in a similar period of time under similar circumstances
>   (2) a sense of lack of control over eating during the episode (e.g., a feeling that one cannot stop eating or control what or how much one is eating)
> B. The binge-eating episodes are associated with three (or more) of the following:
>   (1) eating much more rapidly than normal
>   (2) eating until feeling uncomfortably full
>   (3) eating large amounts of food when not feeling physically hungry
>   (4) eating alone because of being embarrassed by how much one is eating
>   (5) feeling disgusted with oneself, depressed, or very guilty after overeating
> C. Marked distress regarding binge eating is present.
> D. The binge eating occurs, on average, at least 2 days a week for 6 months.
>   NOTE: The method of determining frequency differs from that used for Bulimia Nervosa; future research should address whether the preferred method of setting a frequency threshold is counting the number of days on which binges occur or counting the number of episodes of binge eating.
> E. The binge eating is not associated with the regular use of inappropriate compensatory behaviors (e.g., purging, fasting, excessive exercise) and does not occur exclusively during the course of Anorexia Nervosa or Bulimia Nervosa.
>
> **Source:** Reprinted with permission from the Diagnostic and Statistical Manual of Mental Disorders, Fourth Edition. Copyright 1994 American Psychiatric Association.

a menstrual cycle every other month. EDNOS may also be used to describe individuals who do not exhibit symptoms of anorexia or bulimia but have other behaviors that suggest psychopathological eating behavior, for example, regularly chewing and spitting out food.

Recent research has focused on a potential fourth eating disorder, **binge eating disorder** (BED; see *DSM-IV* Diagnostic Criteria). Initial studies suggest that women are more likely than men to be affected. Because of its proposed status, those who meet BED criteria are now classified under the *DSM-IV* diagnostic category EDNOS.

Characteristic Behaviors

Early clues suggesting a possible eating disorder include changes in usual eating patterns, regular dieting, skipping meals, and fasting behavior. Ritualized eating-related behavior, such as cutting food into tiny pieces and weighing themselves after meals, are common. In addition, characteristics of perfectionism are often present.

Clients usually present for treatment several months or years after the onset of the illness. Their reasons for seeking help are typically parental concerns regarding weight loss or their discovery of bingeing and purging behavior; significant coexisting illnesses such as depression, impulsivity, or substance abuse; medical problems; or serious disruptions in social functioning such as absence from school because of the amount of time consumed by symptomatology.

Dieting is common among adolescent girls and young women. It is also the most prominent precipitating factor in the development of an eating disorder. Although not everyone who diets develops an eating disorder, in susceptible individuals dieting in the presence of etiologic vulnerabilities may lead to preoccupation with body shape and weight.

Social activities during adolescence like gymnastics, wrestling, crew, and ballet emphasize and sometimes require a certain body shape and weight. Early adolescence, a period when normal biological and physiological changes happen, is when initial eating disorder symptomatology typically occurs. The extent to which physiological changes associated with puberty contribute to the onset of eating disorder symptoms remains unknown.

Because early signs can often be detected, it is important to emphasize assessment by school nurses and community health nurses. Common to both bulimia nervosa and anorexia nervosa is a preoccupation with body shape, weight, and appearance, as well as compensatory behaviors such as excessive exercising to prevent weight gain. Routine trips to the bathroom immediately after eating may indicate self-induced vomiting. Some clients steal food, laxatives, or body image–related items, although this behavior seems targeted at items that support, or are driven by, eating disorder symptomatology.

Physical signs may include significant weight loss or weight fluctuations. Client's parotid glands may be swollen, a sign thought to be related to binge eating activity. Calluses and abrasions on the knuckles, known as **Russell's sign**, are the result of friction from the teeth during self-induced vomiting.

Culture, Age, and Gender Features
CULTURE

Few studies have examined the prevalence of eating disorders among various cultures. Anorexia nervosa and bulimia nervosa appear to be less prevalent in developing nations than in industrialized countries. Sociocultural values relating body weight and perceived attractiveness may, in part, explain the diverse prevalence rates across cultures. For example, higher body weights are considered attractive and preferable in some cultures, whereas in many industrialized nations thinness is idealized.

AGE AND GENDER

Eating disorders affect an estimated 1 to 5% of young women and a smaller number of young men.

Anorexia Nervosa

The age of onset for anorexia nervosa is typically during adolescence.[2] Women are approximately 10 times more likely to be affected by anorexia nervosa than men.

Bulimia Nervosa

The average age of onset of bulimia nervosa is during late adolescence, although symptoms may appear in much younger people or in adulthood. Like anorexia nervosa, it is more prevalent in women than men, with less than 10% of all cases in males. It appears to affect an estimated 1 to 2% of young adult women.[3,4]

Binge Eating Disorder

Preliminary findings suggest that the age of onset of BED is usually during early adulthood, with a reported prevalence rate ranging from 2% (community sample) to 30% (sample obtained from weight loss programs).[5]

Etiology

Several etiologic theories have been proposed to explain the development of an eating disorder. Sociocultural theories have focused on values concerning body weight; for example, a paradoxical association has been noted in industrialized countries between the increasing cultural and social value of thinness and the trend for women to have higher body weights than previously.

Family systems theories have centered on the role of the eating symptomatology in decreasing or avoiding familial conflict caused by marital discord, diffused or inappropriate boundaries among family members, and rigid or demanding standards. For some clients, the eating disorder may be an attempt to maintain control within a chaotic family environment. Also related to family theories are family members' attitudes toward body images and food.

Developmental psychological theories have focused on clients' difficulties with autonomy and identity. Psychodynamic perspectives now center on clients' desire to suppress or avoid psychological and physiological maturation; previous psychodynamic theories suggested a fear of oral impregnation or desire for pregnancy as the etiologic bases for anorexia nervosa and bulimia nervosa, respectively.

Difficulties with developmental psychological tasks and psychodynamic conflicts may occur simultaneously with biological developments such as puberty. Some psychological theories speculate that inability to integrate the rapid bodily changes of puberty predisposes people to developmental and psychodynamic impediments. Although each of these perspectives offers a unique contribution to an etiologic understanding, a combination of several factors is more likely to cause eating disorders.

NEUROBIOLOGICAL FACTORS

Biology, environment, psychology, and behavior are not mutually exclusive. Behavior can influence biology, which can, in turn, influence behavior. An example is the fight-or-flight response to an environmental stimulus. For nursing assessment, care planning, intervention, and evaluation, an awareness of the biobehavioral interface is important.

Anorexia Nervosa

Clinical studies suggest that clients with anorexia nervosa have decreased activity in central nervous system (CNS) pathways that involve the neurotransmitter norepinephrine (NE). The significance of this finding is confounded by the nutritional and low-weight status of clients, which can also influence NE functioning. Besides nutrition and body weight, comorbid depressive pathology may influence neurotransmitter regulation in individuals with anorexia nervosa because decreased CNS NE activity has been observed in some subgroups of patients with depression.

The neurotransmitter dopamine may play a role in anorexia nervosa. Because dopamine-agonist drugs in animal and clinical studies cause an anorexic effect, excessive dopaminergic function is hypothesized as a cause. Clinical studies of clients with anorexia nervosa suggest that decreased dopamine function may be related to extent of weight loss.[6,7]

Preclinical and clinical studies also suggest a role for the neurotransmitter serotonin in the regulation of eating behavior. Normal serotonin function is thought to inhibit feeding behavior.[8] Disturbances in serotonin function have been reported in weight-recovered individuals with anorexia[9]; however, as with dopamine, the extent to which nutrition and weight influence these changes remains uncertain.

Peptides may also be involved in altered eating patterns in anorexia nervosa, although much of this research has been conducted in animals. Neuropeptide Y stimulates feeding

TABLE 24–1. General Associations between Neurochemicals and Eating Behavior

	Effect on Eating
Monoamine neurotransmitters	
Dopamine	↑ And ↓ feeding
Norepinephrine	↑ Feeding
Serotonin	↑ Satiety, ↓ feeding
Peptides	
Neuropeptide Y	↑ Feeding
Cholecystokinin	↓ Feeding

behavior. Inhibition of neuropeptide Y regulation may, in turn, decrease eating behavior. Another peptide, cholecystokinin (CCK), inhibits eating behavior. Excessive stimulation of CCK activity might contribute to decreased appetite in anorexia nervosa. Table 24–1 summarizes some of these neurobiological influences on eating behavior.

Bulimia Nervosa

Serotonin is thought to be implicated in the psychopathology of bulimia nervosa. Preclinical and clinical research suggests that CNS serotonin concentrated in the hypothalamus is involved in the regulation of satiety—how full a person feels after a meal—and mood. Binge eating may reflect an impaired satiety response. In that more than half of clients with bulimia nervosa have current or past histories of major depressive disorders, serotonergic regulation of mood may also be impaired. Initial studies in individuals with bulimia nervosa suggest impairment of CNS serotonin function may be associated with increased symptom severity.[10]

The reason for altered serotonin function is poorly understood, although genetic predisposition, altered function at the presynaptic or postsynaptic neuron sites, or nutritional intake may be responsible. The influence of nutritional intake on neurotransmitter function is interesting, given the chaotic eating patterns observed in the bulimic population. Clients often restrict food intake by dieting between binge episodes. Certain restrictions in dietary intake may reduce the quantity of the essential amino acid tryptophan (the precursor to serotonin synthesis in the CNS) available to cross the blood-brain barrier in order to convert into serotonin.[11] Thus, dieting has the potential for influencing brain chemistry. For some individuals, binging and purging symptoms decrease in response to antidepressant medications that enhance CNS serotonin function, suggesting a role for serotonin in bulimia nervosa.

Peptides, which contribute to normal regulation of eating behavior, may also be important. CCK, for example, is normally released in the intestines after a meal and inhibits feeding behavior. Clinical studies suggest that individuals with bulimia nervosa have reduced CCK secretion. Alterations in the regulation of neuropeptide Y may lead to excessive stim-

> **RESEARCH NOTE**
>
> Jimerson, DC, Lesem, MD, Kaye, WH, and Brewerton, TD: Low serotonin and dopamine metabolite concentrations in cerebrospinal fluid from bulimic patients with frequent binge episodes. Arch Gen Psychiatry 49:132–138, 1992.
>
> **Findings:** To follow up on models proposing a role for several neurotransmitters in the regulation of eating behavior, the investigators examined whether 29 hospitalized patients with bulimia nervosa had the same serotonin, dopamine, and norepinephrine function as 17 healthy volunteers. The patients included 18 individuals in a low binge frequency (LBF) group and 11 individuals in a high binge frequency (HBF) group. The HBF individuals had an average of three binge eating episodes per day. The study measured lumbar cerebrospinal fluid (CSF) for concentrations of 5-hydroxyindoleacetic acid (5-HIAA), homovanillic acid (HVA), and 3-methoxy-4-hydroxyphenylglycol (MHPG), the serotonin, dopamine, and norepinephrine neurotransmitter metabolites (by-products), respectively. CSF concentrations of neurotransmitter metabolites provide an index of central nervous system activity.
>
> CSF concentrations of 5-HIAA, HVA, and MHPG were not significantly different in the total patient group and the healthy volunteer group. The same measures were not significantly different in patients with and without a history of major depression. When analyzed based on symptom severity, the HBF group had significantly lower concentrations of CSF 5-HIAA and HVA than both the LBF group and control group. CSF concentrations of MHPG did not differ significantly between client subgroups. CSF concentrations of 5-HIAA and HVA were inversely correlated with frequency of binge eating episodes, whereas MHPG concentrations did not show a relationship with frequency of binge eating episodes.
>
> The results of this study suggest that serotonin and dopamine may play a role in the regulation of eating behavior.
>
> The authors speculate that blunted serotonin regulation may contribute to decreased satiety, and blunted dopamine activity may be related to altered hedonic response to food. Thus, for some individuals, blunted neurotransmitter regulation may decrease the ability to receive neurosignaling for fullness or satiety as well as possibly contribute to food cravings, leading to increased binge eating episodes. The observation of different CSF 5-HIAA and HVA concentrations between the HBF and LBF groups suggests an association with binge frequency. However, the question of which occurred first (the binge eating or altered neurotransmitter regulation) in the HBF group is in need of further research.
>
> **Application to Practice:** Clients often request etiologic information including biological correlates. This investigation suggests that neurotransmitter alterations are more apparent in individuals who have significant symptom severity in terms of binge eating episodes. Although results suggest a role of serotonin and dopamine in the disorder, it is not clear to what extent these alterations are markers for the illness or a consequence of illness-related factors such as altered nutrition. It is important for the client to understand that this finding may have several possible explanations, and that binge eating behavior is likely to be the result of a multitude of interrelated factors rather than a single entity.
>
> The results of this study may help in explaining the clinically observed therapeutic effect of serotonin-enhancing antidepressants in decreasing binge frequency in clients with bulimia nervosa. Observation of decreased CSF serotonin function supports the clinical use of pharmacologic agents targeted at the serotonin system.

ulation of feeding behavior, as reflected by binge eating episodes.

GENETIC FACTORS

Monozygotic (identical) twins have significantly higher concordance rates for anorexia nervosa than dizygotic (fraternal) twins, which suggests a genetic predisposition.[12] Although few twin studies in individuals with bulimia nervosa suggest a higher concordance of the illness in monozygotic twins,[13] the morbid risk for bulimia nervosa in relatives of individuals with the illness (referred to as *proband*) is estimated to be as high as 10%, providing evidence in support of a genetic predisposition.[14]

Prognosis

Recovery rates from an eating disorder are quite variable. Follow-up studies in bulimia nervosa suggest that many clients experience an initial substantial improvement in their symptoms. Although few long-term follow-up studies have been done, clinical and investigational observations suggest a significant risk for relapse in this population.

Anorexia nervosa has an estimated mortality rate of up to 10%. Fatalities are usually a consequence of starvation or metabolic instability associated with altered electrolytes. Additionally, psychiatric comorbidity such as depression can lead to greater suicide risk. Although some people recover after a single episode, many have recurring symptoms and experience the illness as a chronic condition lasting several years.

Assessment

Tables 24–2, 24–3, and 24–4 highlight key areas of a comprehensive assessment.

TABLE 24–2. Comprehensive Assessment of Eating Disorders

Family History. Assessment of the family can provide clues to potential environmental stressors and genetic vulnerability to the development of an eating disorder. A genogram* is helpful in identifying medical illnesses and psychopathology in first-degree and extended family members. It may provide insight into familial attitudes toward food and body weight expectations and perceptions. Similarly, it can point to potential familial medical illnesses that, if present, may further compromise health in the presence of altered eating patterns. For instance, binge-eating episodes and fasting states can have life-threatening consequences in the individual with diabetes.

It is helpful to get a description of the client's relationship with parents, significant others, and siblings. Identifying sibling positions and significant changes in family structure, including birth of sibling or parental divorce, helps in understanding family stress and discord. Family cultural values, boundaries, and perceptions of food, body shape, and weight may define the meaning of food for the family system and help in defining the meaning of the eating disorder symptoms.

Social-Developmental History. Childhood, adolescent, and adult experiences are important areas for social and developmental assessment. Assessment of social activities includes degree of social isolation and alcohol and drug use. Many individuals with bulimia nervosa report a history of alcohol and substance abuse. Type, frequency, age of use, and last use should be noted. In addition, assess for alcohol-related episodes of extended periods of drinking, blackouts, loss of consciousness, and inability to stop drinking. Establish whether any of the substance-abuse episodes were suicide attempts. Developmental assessment includes consideration of the ability to master particular developmental tasks such as individuation and identity. For some individuals, difficulties with individuation may manifest as symptoms of neediness, dependency, or fears of abandonment. Negligible sense of self-worth, low self-esteem, and little self-confidence are common. Assessment of trauma may also provide insights regarding impaired social or developmental functioning.

Mental Status. Because of the high incidence of depressive disorders in this population, careful attention to mood and affect is warranted. Assess suicidal tendencies, thoughts, plans, and recent attempt(s). The mental status examination should also include assessment of appearance, psychomotor behavior, degree of orientation, short- and long-term memory, fund of knowledge, general appearance, and speech. Assessment of reliability, judgment, and insight assists in determining interventions and treatment strategies. Insight regarding the illness is more limited during the earlier phases of the disorder.

Medical Status. Eating disorders are associated with serious medical complications (see Table 24–4). Cardiovascular symptoms, most notably bradycardia (pulse <60 beats per minute) are primarily related to dehydration. ECG abnormalities may result from electrolyte imbalances, whereas myocarditis has been associated with abuse of syrup of ipecac. Dental erosion is thought to be a consequence of the presence of stomach acid following self-induced vomiting. Fine hair growth on the facial area or trunk of the body, known as **lanugo**, may occur in individuals with anorexia nervosa. Signs of poor nutrition may also include brittle hair and dry skin.

Hypercortisolism is exhibited in individuals with anorexia nervosa, resulting from excessive production of cortisol and a decrease in its metabolism. Low levels of triiodothyronine (T3) in anorexia nervosa are most likely related to starvation and may contribute to impaired thermal regulation. Generally individuals with anorexia nervosa do not display other signs indicative of hypothyroidism. Although leukopenia does not generally lead to increased risk of infection in anorexia nervosa, osteoporosis may contribute to increased risk for fractures. Metabolic rate is generally reduced in anorexia nervosa and, together with decreased fat stores, may contribute to cold intolerance. Hyperamylasemia and salivary or parotid gland enlargement are thought to result from hyperstimulation of the parotid gland through binge-eating episodes.

Significant self-induced vomiting and diuretic abuse can result in metabolic alkalosis, whereas laxative abuse is associated with metabolic acidosis. Long-term laxative abuse can result in impaired peristalsis. Stomach acid associated with vomiting can lead to esophagitis.

Collecting information about concurrent medical conditions is important. For example, the combination of an eating disorder and diabetes poses several potential risks. Fasting behavior in the individual with anorexia nervosa and diabetes risks decreased blood glucose levels. The individual with bulimia nervosa and diabetes is at risk for blood sugar complications and for potential insulin abuse (in insulin-dependent diabetes) as a means to prevent weight gain.

For clients taking medications, note the type, dose, route, frequency, and response for assessment of drug interactions, efficacy, and side effects. The time of drug administration in reference to self-induced vomiting provides information on drug absorption and availability.

Persons with an eating disorder may find it difficult to become pregnant, given the irregularity of menstrual cycles. Poor nutritional intake in individuals with anorexia and bulimia nervosa may pose potential risks to the fetus, although there is limited research on this topic. Of possible birth complications, low birth weights in infants is a more consistent finding in clinical studies and case reports at this time, although studies are few in number.[†]

Sources: *McGoldrick, M, and Gerson, R: Genograms in Family Assessment. WW Norton & Co Inc, New York, 1985.
[†]Franko, DL, and Walton, BE. Pregnancy and eating disorders: A review and clinical implications. Int J Eat Disord 13:41, 1993.

TABLE 24-3. Assessing Social History in Individuals with Eating Disorders

- How many close friends do you have?
- How many times a week do you socialize with others?
- How much time do you spend engaged in eating-related symptoms (e.g., binge eating, purging, preoccupation with pursuit for thinness) at the exclusion of other social activities?
- Do you avoid social situations that involve food for fear of losing control or embarrassing yourself in front of others?
- Are you able to work or go to school?
- Does your occupational history revolve around food service employment, and if so, to what extent has this been difficult for you?
- Is your recreation limited to activities emphasizing food or body shape and weight (e.g., cooking, cheerleading, modeling, gymnastics, wrestling)?

TABLE 24-4. Medical Complications of Anorexia Nervosa and Bulimia Nervosa

	Anorexia Nervosa	*Bulimia Nervosa*
Cardiovascular	Bradycardia Hypotension ECG abnormalities Mitral valve prolapse	Bradycardia Hypotension ECG abnormalities Myocarditis (ipecac)
Dental		Enamel erosion
Dermatologic	Brittle hair & nails Dry skin Hair loss Lanugo	Russell's sign
Endocrine	Amenorrhea Hypoglycemia Cold intolerance ↓ LH, FSH, estradiol ↑ Cortisol ↓ T3	Irregular menses Hypoglycemia
Fluid & Electrolyte	Dehydration (↑ BUN)	↑ Dehydration (BUN) Alkalosis (vomiting) Acidosis (laxatives) ↓ K⁺
Gastrointestinal	↓ Motility Constipation	↓ Motility Constipation Esophagitis Hyperamylasemia Salivary-parotid gland hypertrophy
Hematologic	Anemia Leukopenia	Anemia
Metabolic	Osteoporosis ↑ Cholesterol ↑ LFTs	

Note: Frequency of complications is variable across diverse client groups.
Source: Casper, RC: The pathophysiology of anorexia nervosa and bulimia nervosa. Ann Rev Nutr 6:299, 1986; Pomeroy, C, and Mitchell, JE: Medical complications and management of eating disorders. Psychiatr Annals 19:488, 1989.

ANOREXIA NERVOSA

The cardinal feature of anorexia nervosa is a body weight less than 85% of that normally expected for age and height. For example, Leonna is age 18 and 67 inches tall (170.2 cm), and she weighs 105 lbs (47.6 kg). The expected body weight for age and height (as obtained from a standard insurance chart)[15] is 137 lb (62.1 kg). Therefore, she is currently at 76.7% of her expected body weight (47.6 kg/62.1 kg × 100). Another common way of expressing relative body weight is body mass index (weight/height² [kg/m²]). Because low-weight individuals often dress in layers of clothing, they often do not look as thin as they are. Measurement of body weight is obtained without clothes; height is evaluated without shoes (Figure 24-1).

The client's attitude toward weight and weight gain is important for distinguishing the individual who meets the criteria for anorexia nervosa from one who is experiencing a low-weight episode secondary to a major depressive illness. Areas to assess include desired amount of weight loss, current satisfaction with body weight and shape, degree of preoccupation with body weight and shape, and insight into the medical consequences of low-weight episodes. The Diagnostic Survey for Eating Disorders (DSED),[16] the Eating Attitudes Test (EAT),[17] and the Eating Disorders Inventory (EDI)[18] can elicit this information. Some of these questionnaires ask, for example, how satisfied the individual is with aspects of body shape, what types of compensatory behaviors are used, and the extent of preoccupation with food and related rituals (for example, counting calories). A nutritional history may provide insight into attitudes toward eating and identify meal patterns, nutritional deprivation, and estimates of caloric intake.

Determining the diagnostic subtype requires assessing for the presence of binge eating episodes and purging behavior.

In addition, information about the history and regularity of the client's menstrual cycle is key to diagnosing amenorrhea.

BULIMIA NERVOSA

The eating patterns in people with bulimia nervosa are chaotic. The perception of what a binge is varies from person to person. Two saltine crackers might be perceived as a binge by someone with anorexia nervosa–restricting type; someone with bulimia nervosa may describe a binge as eating half

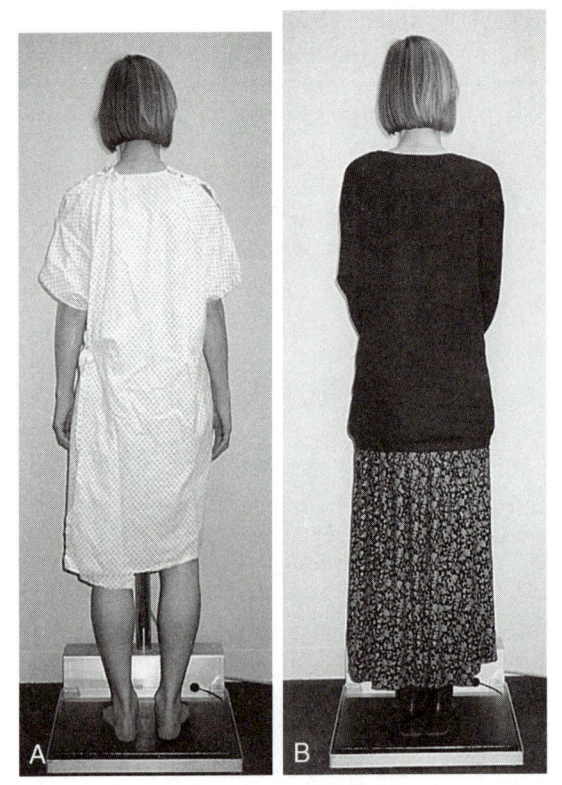

Figure 24–1. In a healthy individual, body weight is 120 lb in an examination gown (*A*) compared with 124 lb in street clothes (*B*). This difference will be much larger in clients who are trying to conceal their weight or body shape through excessive clothing.

a gallon of ice cream, two full-size bags of cookies, and two liters of cola in 20 minutes. Many of these individuals no longer know what a normal meal is.

Information about the frequency, amount, and type of food consumed during a binge episode, the time frame of the episode, and whether the person experiences a lack of control over the eating is important for determining whether an individual meets diagnostic criteria for bulimia nervosa (see Figure 24–2). For some individuals, severity of binge eating varies with the season or environment. For instance, symptoms may be exacerbated in winter or at school.

Information about compensatory behaviors aimed at preventing weight gain is important. Ask the client a general, nonleading question, such as "People do many things to avoid gaining weight; what types do you do?" Ask about previous compensatory behaviors that no longer work, such as self-induced vomiting with or without mechanical stimulation. As with anorexia nervosa, questions about body weight, body perceptions, and eating attitudes are relevant. Someone with bulimia nervosa is usually within a normal weight range for age and height (differentiating the diagnosis from anorexia nervosa) but experiences wide fluctuations in weight. It is not uncommon for an individual with bulimia nervosa to have a history of anorexia nervosa.

In addition to assessment of current and past core symptoms, collect information regarding past psychiatric illness and treatment. Knowing the client's previous types of treatment, focus, and behavioral response, including the type and name of any psychotropic medication taken, duration of use, frequency, dose, and side effects, helps in planning future interventions.

Planning Care

HOW TO DETERMINE AN EFFECTIVE TREATMENT STRATEGY

Treatment strategies are influenced by many factors, such as severity of symptoms, previous treatment history, response to previous treatments, medical stability, comorbidity, motivation, insight, and social support. In general, less invasive treatments are preferred as a first-line intervention unless the client's condition dictates otherwise. Such strategies generally include insight-oriented, behavior, cognitive-behavior, and interpersonal approaches in individual, group, or family therapy settings. The type of therapy is determined by the client's presentation, capacities, and needs. For example, in-

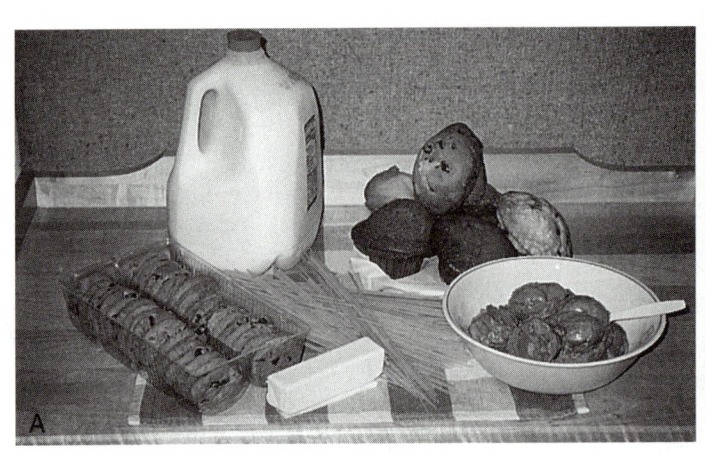

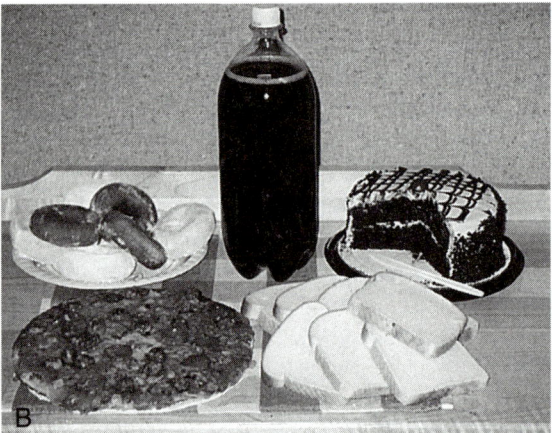

Figure 24–2. Binge episodes typically include foods that are sweet or have a high fat content. These photographs (*A*, *B*) show a typical binge episode, costing $15.00 to $20.00.

dividuals with limited psychological insight or inability to identify emotional states, a characteristic of *alexithymia*, may not do as well in traditional insight-oriented therapy. Pharmacologic intervention is also an option. In some instances, antidepressants may be used before or along with another form of treatment in clients with bulimia nervosa and comorbid depression.

When deciding whether a treatment is efficacious, consider several factors. What are the identified short- and long-term outcomes? Are these outcomes reasonable, given the client's capabilities? Has the client had a long enough trial of the selected treatment? Has there been any improvement? Has the symptomatology been exacerbated? Is the client compliant with the selected treatment modality, and if not, why? Is the client engaged in treatment decisions? Are there identifiable obstacles to the treatment modality such as stigma associated with psychotherapy, cost, or side effects of medications? Is the therapy focused on the client's immediate needs, or is a shift in focus needed?

WHEN TO REFER

Inpatient hospitalization is considered when the client exhibits severe comorbidity, such as depression, or poses a threat to self or others. Hospitalization may also be needed if the client exhibits substance abuse requiring detoxification, is medically compromised, or presents with persistent symptoms refractory to less invasive treatments.

The least restrictive environment is preferred as long as it does not jeopardize clients' health and safety. Day treatment programs are particularly useful for clients who require structure, but not to the extent of hospitalization, or who are moving from an inpatient setting to a less restrictive environment. For individuals who need less structure and are not medically compromised, outpatient therapy may be appropriate.

Interventions for Hospitalized Clients

Acute interventions for the hospitalized individual with an eating disorder are directed at keeping the person safe and medically stable. Additional interventions depend on the degree of comorbidity and medical stability and the length of stay in the hospital. Strategies to assist with the primary goal of safety and stability include effective communication, milieu therapy, behavior intervention, and, when indicated, medication.

EFFECTIVE COMMUNICATION STRATEGIES

Admission to a hospital can be frightening, particularly under circumstances beyond the client's control, as in involuntary admission. Many clients feel abandoned and betrayed by family members or friends and direct their anger and frustrations at the hospital staff. However, establishing a rapport with clients is essential. Create an environment where clients feel safe to share thoughts and experiences without being judged. In the following vignette, the client is revealing her history of purging behavior to the nurse:

Client: Well, I make myself throw up . . . you know . . . I just do it. . . . I wish it would stop, but it doesn't.

Nurse: You know that's not good for you. There are a lot of complications that can happen. What do you do to self-induce vomiting?

Client: I just make myself do it.

A more therapeutic response is:

Nurse: That sounds hard. It seems as though you don't want to be throwing up.

Client: No, I wish I could stop. Sometimes it gets bad . . . if I can't just do it, I'll resort to other things.

Nurse: Tell me more about what you might do.

Client: Well, . . . you'll think it's crazy, . . . but I'll use my fingers or a toothbrush . . . [pause of silence] . . . sometimes if that doesn't work . . . I'll take the stuff they give you in the emergency room to make you throw up.

Effective communication skills influence how much information the client discloses. In the example, the individual stopped sharing information when her description of symptoms was translated into medical jargon and judged as dysfunctional. The client is probably already aware of this likely reaction and is embarrassed. Further confrontation before rapport has been established only limits the amount of information that will be shared. The nurse's response suggests that the client can readily "control" her illness, which is analogous to asking the person with schizophrenia to stop hallucinating. In the second example, the nurse was able to elicit a history of abuse of syrup of ipecac that otherwise might not have been revealed. This additional information may lead to further evaluation, including an electrocardiogram, because abuse of syrup of ipecac can influence cardiac functioning.

Communication that puts the client at ease is important but needs to occur within appropriate boundaries. For example, a hospitalized client might request the nurse's home telephone number because the nurse is "easy to talk with." Blurring the boundaries between professional and personal relationships with the nurse can be detrimental to the client. Inappropriate or diffuse boundaries may have contributed to the client's hospitalization in the first place. Dependency and manipulative behavior are likely to be decreased by maintaining appropriate boundaries in the context of a professional relationship. Establishment and maintenance of appropriate boundaries provide positive role modeling for the client. Clinicians also have to be aware of their own perceptions of body weight and shape and how they may influence interactions with these clients.

Clients need to know the treatment plan and the staff and unit expectations. Clear communication can reduce the risk of conflict, particularly in the presence of manipulative behavior. It is helpful to provide some clients with a unit schedule and a copy of any behavioral agreements made. Behavioral agreements, also referred to as *contracts*, are written agreements between the client and the treatment team that clearly identify what is expected of patients and the privileges that will be granted for maintaining such expectations. Written contracts can be particularly useful for individuals who display manipulative behaviors because contracts can provide clear, direct, and consistent communication with all members of a treatment team.

MILIEU THERAPY

Inpatient units often use a privilege system associated with treatment progress. Privileges reinforce desirable behaviors. At the time of admission, a chart outlining the expectations for each level of the program is provided to the client. For the client with anorexia nervosa, medical and nutritional stabilization is the entry-level goal. Activities are limited to the unit, and visits are restricted. Meals, planned by a nutritionist, are monitored by the staff. The client is given a designated amount of time to complete meals, followed by at least a 1-hour observation period because the client may exercise to prevent weight gain. During this period, bathroom visits are monitored, particularly if self-induced vomiting is suspected. At the final level, the client maintains normal eating patterns, stable medical condition, and a normal weight for age and height. Privileges include unsupervised bathroom visits, unrestricted activities and visitations, planning meals, eating meals unsupervised, and having meals off the unit. Unit activities introduced at various levels of the privilege system include community meetings, family group therapy, stress management, and recreational therapy. Exercise activities are closely supervised, given the potential compensatory use to prevent weight gain.

For the individual with bulimia nervosa, the entry level of the privilege system is directed at interrupting and decreasing binge eating episodes and purging behavior. This level, as for the client with anorexia nervosa, is associated with unit and visitation restrictions as well as meal supervision. During the level progression, the client keeps a dietary log noting the type and amount of food consumed, time and place, and associated thoughts and feelings (Fig. 24–3). The food diary provides both client and clinician with information regarding behavioral and emotional precipitating factors. Increased privileges are introduced as the individual progresses through each level. The goal of the final level is to maintain and reinforce normal eating patterns, medical stability, and decreased or interrupted binge and purge behavior.

COGNITIVE-BEHAVIOR APPROACHES

Cognitive-behavior strategies are aimed at reducing symptoms and restructuring the belief system that perpetuates the illness. Cognitive-behavior therapy (CBT) is usually conducted by a therapist on an outpatient basis, although some strategies may be adopted for inpatient settings. Interventions, particularly for bulimia nervosa, include planning problem-solving strategies for times when the individual is most likely to be at risk for binging or purging behavior. Restructuring the distorted belief system regarding body image and food preoccupation is facilitated by client education, journal recordings, and dietary logs. As shown in the research note, the dietary log allows the client to begin to identify "at risk" periods, as well as to self-monitor eating patterns. Although the dietary log is frequently helpful in bulimia nervosa, it is generally not used in anorexia nervosa, given the already excessive preoccupation with food in this patient group.

BEHAVIOR AND INTERPERSONAL THERAPIES

In addition to CBT, other therapy approaches include behavior therapy and interpersonal therapy (IPT).[19] Unlike CBT, behavior therapy uses behavior interventions alone. It is directed at extinguishing targeted behaviors, namely, the symptoms of the disorder. In contrast, IPT is directed at interpersonal difficulties rather than the eating disorder symptomatology.

DIETARY LOG for ___/___/___ Mo Day Yr

Location	Meal*	Time	Duration	Antecedents	Amount of Food & Beverage	Responses

* B = breakfast, L = lunch, D = dinner, S = snack, BE = binge episode

Figure 24–3. Dietary Log.

> **RESEARCH NOTE**
>
> Fairburn, CG, Norman, PA, Welch, SL, O'Connor, ME, Doll, HA, and Peveler, RC: A prospective study of outcome in bulimia nervosa and the long-term effects of three psychological treatments. Arch Gen Psychiatry 52:304–312, 1992.
>
> **Findings:** The authors compared the long-term effects of cognitive-behavior therapy (CBT), behavior therapy (BT), and focal interpersonal therapy (IPT) in a combined group of 91 individuals with bulimia nervosa from two separate treatment trials. CBT used cognitive restructuring and behavioral interventions designed at interrupting eating disorder symptomatology. IPT centered on interpersonal issues, unlike other treatments that predominantly focus on the eating disorder and core symptoms. BT employed behavioral procedures alone, targeted at interrupting eating disorder symptomatology. Treatments were administered over 18 weeks in 19 therapy sessions. Participants were interviewed, on average, 5.8 years following treatment. At follow-up, 46% of the participants continued to have a *DSM-IV* eating disorder. This included predominantly the diagnosis of EDNOS (24%), followed by bulimia nervosa (19%). Fewer individuals met criteria for anorexia nervosa (3%) at follow-up.
>
> Treatment type did not predict which individuals met criteria for bulimia nervosa or anorexia nervosa at follow-up. Overall, however, clients who received CBT or IPT showed significant improvement compared to those individuals who received BT.
>
> **Application to Practice:** As suggested by the authors, effects of BT may be short-lived in comparison to CBT and IPT. Individuals who are engaged in strictly a BT approach may be at greater risk for relapse during the 5-year posttreatment period. This points to the importance of assessment for current related symptomatology in individuals reporting a past history of an eating disorder. Interventions that not only redirect the behavior but also assist clients in changing the way they view themselves and food may have a lasting beneficial impact.

PHARMACOLOGIC TREATMENTS

In some situations, pharmacologic agents can be therapeutic, although medications in conjunction with other treatment modalities are likely to be associated with a better outcome than drug intervention alone.

Anorexia Nervosa

Pharmacologic intervention is generally not the primary intervention in anorexia nervosa.[20] Antidepressant medication may be considered, but depressive symptoms may be a consequence of malnutrition that will remit upon weight restoration.

Bulimia Nervosa

Antidepressant medications that may decrease binging and purging behavior include tricyclic antidepressants (TCAs), monoamine oxidase inhibitors (MAOIs), and selective serotonin reuptake inhibitors (SSRIs).[21] Antidepressant treatment may be indicated for depressive comorbidity, anxiety, and obsessive symptoms. Treatment with MAOIs requires strict adherence to dietary restrictions that may be problematic for the client. Also, because weight gain is a potential side effect, noncompliance may occur. Insufficient response to pharmacologic intervention may result from drug loss during self-induced vomiting, and clients should be encouraged not to purge after taking medications to allow for adequate absorption.

Interventions for Clients in the Community

Eating disorders are often a chronic or recurring condition, and in the course of treatment a client may require several different types of structured environments. To facilitate the transition between treatments, communication among the person's health-care providers is essential. Although symptoms may improve, many individuals do not abstain from binge eating or purging behaviors for an extended time. Monitoring the client's medical and nutritional status continues beyond the hospital, where the focus shifts to identifying and understanding what factors support the client's illness. Because long-term abstinence is difficult, a more appropriate goal may be a decreased frequency. Community support groups for both client and family members are often helpful.

Expected Outcomes

For the client with an eating disorder, improvement will be demonstrated by:
- Long-term outcomes that include:
  - maintaining stable body weight in a normal weight range
  - maintaining normal eating patterns
  - showing marked decrease in preoccupation with appearance
  - engaging in activities reflecting healthy self-esteem
  - effectively implementing adaptive coping strategies.
- Short-term or acute outcomes such as:
  - vital signs within normal limits and normal blood chemistries
  - adequate hydration, weight gain, and increased caloric intake for anorexia nervosa
  - decreased binge and purge episodes for bulimia nervosa
  - verbalization of positive self-esteem
  - descriptions of nutritional requirements
  - identification of high-risk situations for relapse
  - demonstration of decreased preoccupation with body shape and weight.

Both short- and long-term client outcomes depend on many factors including severity of symptoms, comorbidity, motivation, and insight.

Differential Diagnosis

ANOREXIA NERVOSA

Weight loss may be a symptom of a serious medical illness, such as AIDS, Crohn's disease, or cancer, or of other psychiatric disorders, including major depression. These illnesses are not associated with the distorted body perceptions and fear of weight gain that are diagnostic of eating disorders.

Also consider other psychiatric conditions. Fear of eating in public may be related to a social phobia. Erratic eating patterns may occur in schizophrenia, whereas ritualistic eating along with non-eating-related obsessions or compulsions suggests obsessive-compulsive disorder (OCD). Preoccupation with body shape and weight is a key feature of body dysmorphic disorder (BDD).

BULIMIA NERVOSA

Rarely, patients with some neurological illnesses, such as Kleine-Levin syndrome, may exhibit a ravenous appetite. Depressive disorders may also be associated with increased appetite. Binge eating episodes are also described as an impulsive characteristic in borderline personality disorder. The diagnosis of EDNOS should be considered for a client who shows compulsive overeating.

COMORBIDITY

People with an eating disorder often exhibit comorbid psychiatric illnesses, most commonly mood, anxiety, and substance-use disorders.[22–24] Estimates of personality disorders are quite varied, with a greater likelihood of avoidant disorder and OCD in anorexia nervosa, and of borderline personality disorder in bulimia nervosa.[25]

Common Nursing Diagnoses

Many NANDA nursing diagnoses[26] are applicable to clients with eating disorders (Table 24–5). Body image disturbance applies to individuals with anorexia nervosa as well as bulimia nervosa. The diagnosis of Altered Nutrition: More than body requirements can likewise be applied to individuals with bulimia nervosa and to those who meet the *DSM-IV* proposed criteria for BED (but are currently diagnosed as EDNOS). Comorbid psychopathology may

---

TABLE 24–5. NANDA Nursing Diagnoses Related to Eating Disorders

Activity and Rest
- Fatigue
- Body Image Disturbance
- Coping, individual, ineffective
- Fear (related to weight gain)
- Self Esteem, chronic low
- Self Esteem disturbance

Elimination
- Bowel Incontinence (associated with laxative abuse)
- Constipation

Food and Fluid
- Fluid Volume Deficit, risk for

Fluid Volume Deficit
- Nutrition: altered, less than body requirements
- Nutrition: altered, risk for more than body requirements
- Oral Mucous Membrane, altered

Neurosensory
- Sensory/Perceptual Alterations: gustatory

Safety
- Injury, risk for (related to osteoporosis in anorexia)
- Skin Integrity, impaired
- Skin Integrity, impaired: risk for

Related to Eating Disorders
- Social Interaction, impaired
- Family Coping: ineffective, compromised
- Family Coping: ineffective, disabling
- Family Coping: potential for growth
- Family Processes, altered
- Social Isolation

Teaching and Learning
- Knowledge Deficit (related to nutrition, stress management, medications)

Source: Doenges, ME, and Moorhouse, MS: Nurse's Pocket Guide: Nursing Diagnoses with Interventions, ed 5. FA Davis Co, Philadelphia, 1996.

TABLE 24–6. NANDA Nursing Diagnoses for Consideration with Psychiatric Comorbidity in Eating Disorders

Activity/Rest
- Fatigue (depressive disorder)
- Sleep Pattern Disturbance (depressive disorder)

Ego Integrity
- Anxiety
- Hopelessness (depressive disorder)

Safety
- Violence, risk for, directed at self (depressive disorder)
- Self-Mutilation, risk for (borderline personality disorder)

Teaching and Learning
- Noncompliance
- Therapeutic Regimen: (individuals) ineffective management

Source: Doenges, ME, and Moorhouse, MS: Nurse's Pocket Guide: Nursing Diagnoses with Interventions, ed 5. FA Davis Co, Philadelphia, 1996.

Nursing Care Plan: ACUTE CARE FOR THE CLIENT WITH ANOREXIA NERVOSA

Nursing Diagnosis #1: Nutrition: altered, less than body requirements

Goals:
- Stabilized weight loss, followed by progressive gain toward goal weight
- Well-balanced dietary intake
- Normalized laboratory findings
- Behaviors that support normalization of weight and nutritional status

Nursing Interventions:
- Establish range for weight outcome with treatment team and client
- Establish daily caloric regimen for weight stabilization and eventual weight gain in collaboration with nutritionist
- Establish structure surrounding meals (e.g., length of meal), exercise patterns, and bathroom routines
- Assess understanding of nutritional needs
- Record intake and output
- Collect daily a.m. weight
- Monitor vital signs, including orthostatic BP
- Review laboratory results and report abnormal values to the primary clinician
- Monitor meals
- Observe for at least 1 hour after meals
- Accompany to BR if self-induced vomiting suspected
- Explore feelings associated with eating behavior
- Refocus efforts directed at food preoccupation (e.g., calorie counting)
- Administer nutritional supplements as ordered
- Provide small, frequent snacks
- Provide positive feedback for improved eating behavior
- Provide opportunities for feeling a sense of control (e.g., allow to choose from a selection of snack offerings)

Measurable Outcomes:
- Weight stabilizes with subsequent attainment of goal weight. Body weight is at least 85% of expected body weight for age and height
- Maintains adequate dietary intake as evidenced by caloric intake and food selection choices
- Laboratory findings and vital signs are within normal limits
- Engages in regular meal patterns (e.g., scheduled times)
- Verbalizes an initial understanding of nutritional needs and awareness of illness

Nursing Diagnosis #2: Fluid volume deficit, risk for

Goals:
- Maintenance of adequate fluid volume and electrolyte balance
- Normalized serum electrolyte laboratory findings
- Behaviors that support adequate hydration

Nursing Interventions:
- Monitor intake and output
- Record daily weight
- Encourage fluid intake of 2000-3000 cc qd
- Assess condition of mucous membranes and skin turgor
- Monitor orthostatic BP qd or more frequently if indicated, e.g., complaints of vertigo
- Accompany to BR if self-induced vomiting suspected
- Review laboratory results and report abnormal values to primary clinician
- Provide teaching on fluid intake needs and skin care
- Provide teaching regarding gradual position changes to avoid orthostatic hypotension
- Explore feelings and/or fears associated with increased fluid intake
- Promote oral hygiene

Measurable Outcomes:
- Maintains normal weight for age and height
- Laboratory findings and vital signs are within normal limits
- Adequate daily fluid intake
- Verbalizes importance of adequate fluid intake
- Demonstrates increased responsibility for adequate hydration by adhering to daily fluid intake regimen

---

present additional characteristics for consideration (Table 24–6).

Nursing care plans highlight nursing diagnoses, goals, interventions, and desired outcomes for clients with anorexia nervosa and bulimia nervosa. Different diagnoses are presented to illustrate their use, although several of the diagnoses may be applicable to both disorders.

Areas for Future Research

- Dimensions of treatment response need to be defined.
- Relapse prevention strategies ought to be developed.
- Studies of the interface between biological and behavioral correlates must be undertaken.
- Controlled studies of long-term outcomes are needed.
- Comparative studies should include recovered and active illness groups.
- Predictors of response to different treatment modalities are needed.
- Additional intervention studies expanding the range of current strategies (for example, nutritional intervention) must be undertaken.

CASE STUDY

Franny, a 21-year-old single, white, attractive woman, appearing younger than her stated age, was admitted to an inpatient psychiatric unit. Her chief complaint was "I've been feeling pretty depressed . . . all I do is cry . . . I can't seem to get along with my family... last week I OD'ed." She was admitted to the unit after a medical admission, where she received a gastric lavage for an overdose of antidepressant medication and alcohol. Franny described a 4-year history of binge eating and purging (via self-induced vomiting and laxative abuse), which she said has recently felt "out of control." Her most recent binge episodes included "about 12 chocolate chip cookies, a bag of bagels, a box of doughnuts, and a jug of soda." She currently experiences 15 binge episodes per week and 15 episodes of self-induced vomiting (occurring within 15 minutes of binging) per week, and she takes 2 laxative tablets every day. She reports recently worsened symptomatology and increased conflict with her parents regarding academic progress. Although Franny is a solid B student, in the process of completing her senior year of college, she describes her grades as "unacceptable" to her parents. Additionally, she describes feeling depressed and worthless about her weight, adding that her parents are "continually telling me I could afford to shed 10 to 20 lb." At the time of admission, her weight was 105% of expected body weight for age and height; BP, 90/70; P, 70; T, 98.6°F. Serum electrolytes were within normal limits. Her menstrual cycle was regular, although she reported a history of amenorrhea.

Mental status examination revealed neurovegetative signs: increased weight and appetite (5 to 7 lb weight fluctuation in the past week), decreased energy and libido, and difficulty falling asleep. Her mood was dysphoric, with notable feelings of guilt, worthlessness, anxiousness, and episodic irritability. Psychomotor functioning was slowed. She displayed no evidence of psychosis. Although her concentration was poor, her thought processes were logical and coherent.

Community-Based Care Plan for the Client with Bulimia Nervosa

Nursing Diagnosis #1: Body image disturbances/Self esteem disturbances

Goals:
- Decreased emphasis of body shape and weight on self-evaluation and self-worth
- Increased sense of control in internal and external environment
- Behaviors that support positive self-image

Nursing Interventions:
- Develop therapeutic relationship with initial emphasis on listening and positive feedback
- Assess motivation for change
- Assess how client views self and perception of how viewed by others
- Assess family dynamics for interactions that may perpetuate distorted body image and self esteem
- Allow for the expression of fears concerning body image
- Provide reality testing regarding grossly distorted perceptions of body image while acknowledging that perceptions currently feel real to the client
- Explore both positive and negative aspects of self
- Explore means of self-evaluation other than through body shape or weight
- Encourage individuality rather than comparisons of self to others
- Encourage involvement in decision-making and problem-solving activities

Measurable Outcomes:
- Acknowledges negative self-evaluation
- Identifies areas other than body shape and weight as defining characteristics of self
- Verbalizes positive aspects of self
- Demonstrates ability to make decisions
- Engages in treatment activities facilitating change in body image and self esteem

Nursing Diagnosis #2. Coping, Individual, ineffective (related to eating behavior)

Goals:
- Identify ineffective and/or maladaptive behaviors
- Identify antecedents and consequences of ineffective coping
- Increase use of adaptive coping mechanisms

Nursing Interventions:
- Establish therapeutic relationship
- Assess degree of insight and motivation for change
- Assess current functioning capacities
- Assess impact of illness on functional activities (e.g., socialization)
- Assess previous use, effect, and types of coping skills
- Explore fears associated with gaining weight
- Explore sense of control regarding environment
- Use food diary to record eating behavior and associated activities
- Assist in identifying common precipitants to binge eating episodes and consequences of compensatory behaviors
- Assist in identifying "at risk" situations that may trigger or facilitate a binge eating episode
- Assist in developing a list of alternative activities designed to interrupt or delay binge eating.
- Use role playing to teach and model problem-solving skills related to identifying and planning for "at risk" situations
- Role play situations involving expression of emotions (e.g., anger), confrontation, and/or situations where others are feared to be disappointed
- Encourage use of new coping mechanism
- Provide positive feedback for use of new and functional coping skills

Measurable Outcomes:
- Identify and verbalize maladaptive behaviors and consequences
- Identify and verbalize "at risk" situations for maladaptive behaviors
- Verbalize alternative coping strategies

Critical Pathway: Anorexia Nervosa

Care Needs	1st 24 hours	Days 2–5
Assessment/Evaluations	Past psych hx Medication hx Medical hx Suicide risk Self-care ability Appropriate legal status Psychiatric eval Nursing eval	Family interview Social work eval Evals by activities, OT, PT, group rx, others Continue psych and nursing evals
Diagnostic Tests/Workup	Physical exam by MD, NP Lab tests inc CBC, kidney and liver functions, electrolytes, hormone levels, cardiac enzymes, albumen, drug screen, others as approp	Review results of labs and evals Implement interventions based on workup Psychological testing Further workup as approp
Treatment	Orient to unit Initial activity orders	Develop multidisciplinary tx plan 1:1 psychotherapy Begin group rx Begin OT, PT, activity therapies Participate in family sessions as approp
Medications	Order initial doses of meds for psych & medical symptoms Monitor responses & side effects	Monitor responses & side effects Adjust doses as needed
Safety/Self-care	Establish unit rules r/t suicide risk, elopement, substance abuse Closely monitor for eating, exercise, elimination behaviors If dehydrated, establish fluid intake Establish baseline weight Monitor self-care ability	Continue to monitor & intervene per column 1 Implement changes in diet/fluids as approp Establish schedule r/t mealtime, exercise, elimination Establish weighing schedule
Education	Unit orientation Patient rights	Begin education on eating disorders, meds, nutrition program, hazards of poor nutrition Educate on coping skills for anxiety
Discharge Plan	Identify initial concerns	Identify pat/family concerns Identify possible resources, living arrangements
Outcomes	____ Patient assessed by MD/Nurse ____ Initial activity orders in place ____ Patient does not harm self ____ Remains stable medically	____ Assessments completed by all disciplines ____ Medical workup complete & tx plan implemented ____ Multidisciplinary tx plan implemented ____ Patient does not harm self and remains stable medically ____ Patient begins participating in tx plan ____ Meds adjusted as approp
	Progressing per pathway? Yes ____ No ____ If no, referred to _____	Progressing per pathway? Yes ____ No ____ If no, referred to _____

Care Needs	Days 6–15+	Discharge
Assessment/Evaluations	Reassessment ongoing	
Diagnostic Tests/Workup	All results available Further workup as needed	Establish follow-up medical care and make appointments

Continued on following page

Critical Pathway: Anorexia Nervosa (Continued)

Care Needs	Days 6–15+	Discharge
Treatment	Continue implementing tx plan Develop outpatient plan	Ensure outpatient tx appointments in place Establish issues r/t insurance, transportation, activities to enhance compliance
Medications	Continue to monitor Establish outpatient regimen	Ensure medication regimen established Ensure access to prescriptions
Safety/Self-care	Continue to monitor & intervene as in days 1–5 Establish family involvement in nutrition plan Continue nutrition interventions based on weight and patient response Develop discharge plan inc needs for home health, home equipment, family assistance Establish family cooperation in inpatient and outpatient tx plan	Ensure equipment, home health follow-up arrangements in place Ensure assistance available for family
Education	Continue patient/fam education on eating disorders, nutrition program, medications, food/drug interactions Educate as needed on specialized needs, e.g., central lines, enteral feedings if present Educate on coping skills for anxiety Suggest community resources	Ensure educational materials available to take home Reinforce teaching in outpatient tx
Discharge Plan	Develop outpatient tx plan Address discharge home versus need for placement Establish readmission criteria	Social worker reviews dc plan for outpatient tx, living arrangements, finances, etc. Arrange discharge transportation Ensure resources for assistance in place
Outcomes	____ Patient participating in tx plan ____ Patient demonstrating improvement and stabilization of symptoms ____ Patient has appropriate weight gain ____ Family involved in tx plan ____ Patient does not harm self ____ Patient remains stable medically Progressing per pathway? Yes ____ No ____ If no, referred to _____	____ Patient leaves hospital with intention of participating in outpatient tx plan ____ Family demonstrates plan to comply with tx plan ____ Patient verbalizes awareness of when to call for help & resources ____ Patient leaves hospital with understanding of outpatient plan, meds, home health needs Progressing per pathway? Yes ____ No ____ If no, referred to _____

Franny recently moved out of her dormitory suite after feeling embarrassed about the bulimia and betrayed by her friends, who threatened to call the police after discovering her stealing food at a grocery store and who requested a visit from the dormitory counselor because of her eating behavior, excessive drinking, and depressed mood. She also reported that it has been increasingly difficult to attend class and complete class assignments.

Franny's history included six brief outpatient therapies ranging from four visits to weekly visits over a 6-month period. She was recently prescribed an antidepressant agent by her primary care clinician, who was concerned about her depression. She had a history of regular cocaine use and episodic use of marijuana.

CRITICAL THINKING QUESTIONS

1. What behavior clues did Franny exhibit during the few months preceding hospitalization?
2. Outline potential etiologic factors contributing to Franny's binge eating episodes and depressed mood.
3. Outline a level system to use as part of Franny's milieu therapy.
4. Develop a care plan, including short-term and long-term goals, for Franny's inpatient stay.
5. Identify behaviors that would indicate that Franny is responding to the treatment.
6. Describe considerations for the use of antidepressant medications with Franny.

7. Design a teaching plan to prepare Franny for discharge from the hospital.

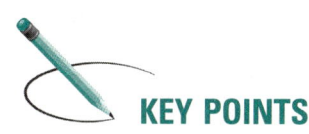

KEY POINTS

- Eating disorders described in the *DSM-IV* include anorexia nervosa, bulimia nervosa, eating disorders not otherwise specified, and the proposed category of binge eating disorder.
- Women are more likely to be affected by an eating disorder than men.
- Several neurobiological chemicals may play a role in eating behaviors, particularly with regard to regulating food intake and satiety signals.
- Eating disorders are often chronic illnesses with significant psychosocial and medical consequences.
- A thorough assessment is crucial to rule out other medical and psychiatric conditions that can mimic core symptoms of eating disorders.
- Self-rated questionnaires, including the DSED, can be particularly helpful in eliciting historical and current information about eating behaviors and related experiences.
- There is a high comorbidity of eating disorders with other psychiatric illnesses, especially depression.
- Cognitive-behavior strategies are commonly used in the treatment of eating disorders.
- Antidepressant medications, particularly TCAs and SSRIs, have been shown to reduce the frequency of binge eating episodes in bulimia nervosa.

REFERENCES

1. American Psychiatric Association: Diagnostic and Statistical Manual of Mental Disorders, ed 4. American Psychiatric Association, Washington, DC, 1994.
2. Lucas, AR, et al: 50-year trends in the incidence of anorexia nervosa in Rochester, MN: A population-based study. Am J Psychiatry 148:917, 1991.
3. Schotte, DE, and Stunkard, AJ: Bulimia vs bulimic behaviors on a college campus. JAMA 258:1213, 1987.
4. Fairburn, CG, and Beglin, SJ: Studies of the epidemiology of bulimia nervosa. Am J Psychiatry 147:401, 1990.
5. Spitzer, RL, et al: Binge eating disorder: A multisite field trial of the diagnostic criteria. Int J Eat Disord 11:191, 1992.
6. Kaye, WH, et al: Abnormalities in CNS monoamine metabolism in anorexia nervosa. Arch Gen Psychiatry 41:350, 1984.
7. Gerner, RH, et al: CSF neurochemistry of women with anorexia nervosa and normal women. Am J Psychiatry 141:1441, 1984.
8. Blundell, JE: Serotonin and appetite. Neuropharmacology 23:1537, 1984.
9. Kaye, WH, et al: Altered serotonin activity in anorexia nervosa after long-term weight restoration: Does elevated cerebrospinal fluid 5-hydroxyindoleacetic acid level correlate with rigid and obsessive behavior? Arch Gen Psychiatry 48:556, 1991.
10. Jimerson, DC, et al: Low serotonin and dopamine metabolite concentrations in cerebrospinal fluid from bulimic patients with frequent binge episodes. Arch Gen Psychiatry 49:132, 1992.
11. Fernstrom, JD: Dietary amino acids and brain function. J Am Diet Assoc 94:71, 1994.
12. Walters, EE, and Kendler, KS: Anorexia nervosa and anorexic-like syndromes in a population-based female twin sample. Am J Psychiatry 152:64, 1995.
13. Kendler, KS, et al: The genetic epidemiology of bulimia nervosa. Am J Psychiatry 148:1627, 1991.
14. Kassett, JA, et al: Psychiatric disorders in the first-degree relatives of probands with bulimia nervosa. Am J Psychiatry 146:1468, 1989.
15. Society of Actuaries and Association of Life Insurance Medical Directors of America: Build Study. Society of Actuaries, Chicago, 1979.
16. Johnson, C: Initial consultation for patients with bulimia and anorexia nervosa. In Garner, DM, and Garfinkel, PE (eds): Handbook of Psychotherapy for Anorexia Nervosa and Bulimia. The Guilford Press, New York, 1985, p 19.
17. Garner, DM, et al: The Eating Attitudes Test: Psychometric features and clinical correlates. Psychol Med 12:871, 1982.
18. Garner, DM: Eating Disorder Inventory-2 Professional Manual. Psychological Assessment Resources, Odessa, FL, 1991.
19. Fairburn, CG, et al: A prospective study of outcome in bulimia nervosa and the long-term effects of three psychological treatments. Arch Gen Psychiatry 52:304, 1995.
20. American Psychiatric Association: Practice guidelines for eating disorders. Am J Psychiatry 150:207, 1993.
21. Jimerson, DC, et al: Medications in the treatment of eating disorders. Psychiatry Clin North Am 19(4):739, 1996.
22. Braun, DL, Sunday, SR, and Halmi, KA: Psychiatric comorbidity in patients with eating disorders. Psychol Med 24:859, 1994.
23. Brewerton, TD, et al: Comorbidity of axis I psychiatric disorders in bulimia nervosa. J Clin Psychiatry 56:77, 1995.
24. Holderness, CC, Brooks-Gunn, J, and Warren, MP: Co-morbidity of eating disorders and substance abuse review of the literature. Int J Eat Disorders 16:1, 1994.
25. Skodol, AE, et al: Comorbidity of *DSM-III-R* eating disorders and personality disorders. Int J Eat Disord 14:403, 1993.
26. Doenges, ME, and Moorhouse, MF: Nurse's Pocket Guide: Nursing Diagnoses with Interventions, ed 5. F A Davis Co, Philadelphia, 1996.

CHAPTER 25

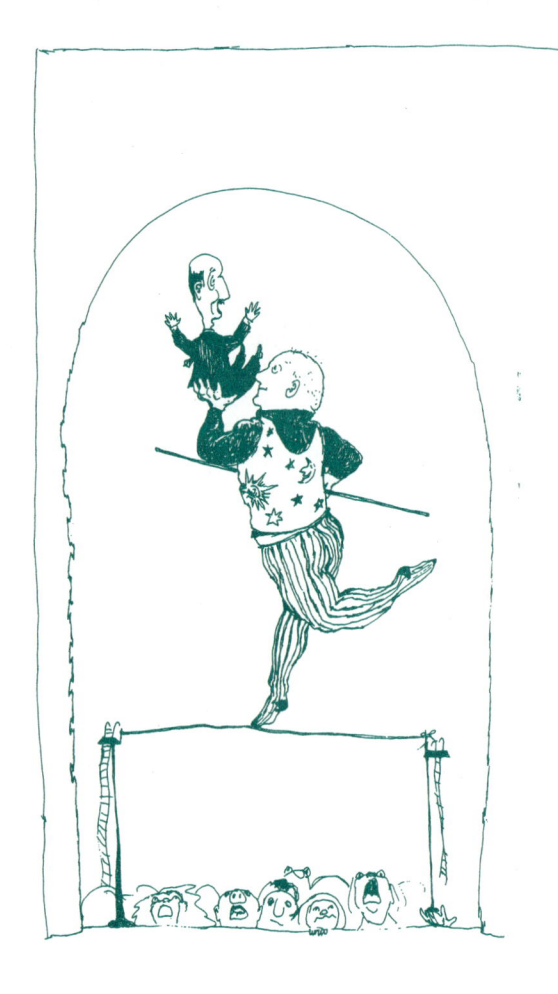

CHAPTER OUTLINE

Normal Sleep-Wake Patterns
  Culture, Age, and Gender Features
Primary Insomnia
  Characteristic Behaviors
  Etiology
Primary Hypersomnia
  Characteristic Behaviors
  Etiology
Breathing-Related Sleep Disorders
  Characteristic Behaviors
  Etiology
Narcolepsy
  Characteristic Behaviors
  Etiology
Circadian Rhythm Sleep Disorder
  Characteristic Behaviors
  Etiology
Dyssomnia Not Otherwise Specified (NOS)
  Characteristic Behaviors
Parasomnias
  Characteristic Behaviors
  Etiology
Sleep Disorders Due to Medical and Psychiatric Disorders
Prognosis
Planning Care
Interventions for Hospitalized Clients
Interventions for Clients in the Community
Client and Family Education
Expected Outcomes
Differential Diagnosis
Common Nursing Diagnoses
Synopsis of Current Research
Areas for Future Research

Carol A. Glod, RN, CS, PhD

Sleep Disorders

LEARNING OBJECTIVES

After completing this chapter, the reader should be able to:

- Recognize the primary sleep disorders and list their prominent characteristics.
- Explain normative sleep patterns, basic sleep stages, and sleep hygiene.
- Identify the health and psychological sequelae of sleep disorders.
- Analyze the impact of sleep disorders on the individual's daily functioning.
- Implement the nursing process in planning care for the individual with a sleep disorder.
- Develop a teaching plan for individuals and communities to promote healthy sleep patterns.

KEY TERMS

central sleep apnea (CSA)
CPAP
delayed sleep phase disorder
dyssomnia
hypersomnia
insomnia
narcolepsy
obstructive sleep apnea (OSA)
parasomnia
phase-advanced sleep pattern
rapid eye movement (REM) sleep
sleep diary
sleep hygiene

The sleep-wake cycle is a basic human process, necessary for sustaining life and restoring health. Sleep may also serve a particularly significant role in fostering brain development during infancy. Primary sleep disorders are definable conditions associated with many daytime impairments that affect nearly 50 million adults in the United States. They are diagnosable states that differ from occasional sleep difficulties or sleep problems related to environmental conditions such as noisy surroundings. In any specialty, and particularly in the hospital, nurses play a key role in maintaining and monitoring sleep.

NORMAL SLEEP-WAKE PATTERNS

The sleep-wake cycle follows a 24-hour or *circadian* pattern. Sleep is a cyclical process with 90-minute cycles that repeat four to five times a night.[1] Each 90-minute cycle is characterized by specific stages of sleep, distinguishable by changes in an electroencephalogram (EEG) pattern. As seen in Table 25–1, sleep progresses from stage 1 (the transitional stage) into stage 2 (light sleep), and then stages 3 and 4 ("slow wave" or "deep sleep"). The cycle is completed with **rapid eye movement (REM) sleep**, which is characterized by actual eye movements, a general decrease in muscle tone (*atonia*), and dreaming.

Throughout the life cycle, the pattern of sleep stages evolves. The newborn lacks the 24-hour sleep pattern at birth and spends approximately two-thirds of the day sleeping. Although REM sleep predominates early in life, it accounts for only about 20% of sleep during the adult years.[1] Total sleep duration decreases with age, and older adults experience a decline of deep sleep (stages 3 and 4) because sleep becomes increasingly fragmented.

Circadian rhythmicity is known to play a major role in

TABLE 25–1. Characteristics of Sleep Stages in Normal Adults

NREM (Non–Rapid Eye Movement) Sleep

Stage 1. A transitional stage of wakefulness into sleep, lasting only a few minutes. Drowsiness and slowing of eye and muscle movements accompany this stage. Easy awakening is possible. A common sign of severely disrupted sleep is increased stage 1 sleep.

Stage 2. A stage of light sleep, lasting about 10–25 minutes, when muscles further relax. On the electroencephalograph (EEG), sleep spindles emerge.

Stage 3. A stage of deep sleep, lasting from a few minutes to 30–40 minutes. The EEG wave patterns display slow wave activity. Vital signs and physical activity decrease.

Stage 4. The final stage of NREM sleep, characterized by slow wave patterns on the EEG. Another stage of deep sleep, lasting 20–40 minutes. Body functioning and activity are at lowest level. Sleep disruption is characterized by decreased stages 3 and 4 sleep.

REM (Rapid Eye Movement) Sleep

Completes the 90-minute cycle of sleep. Bursts of rapid eye movements, dreaming, and lack of muscle tone. REM sleep lasts 5–30 minutes and predominates in the last third of the night's sleep, when body temperature is lowest. The EEG is characterized by "sawtooth," i.e., notched-shaped, waves.

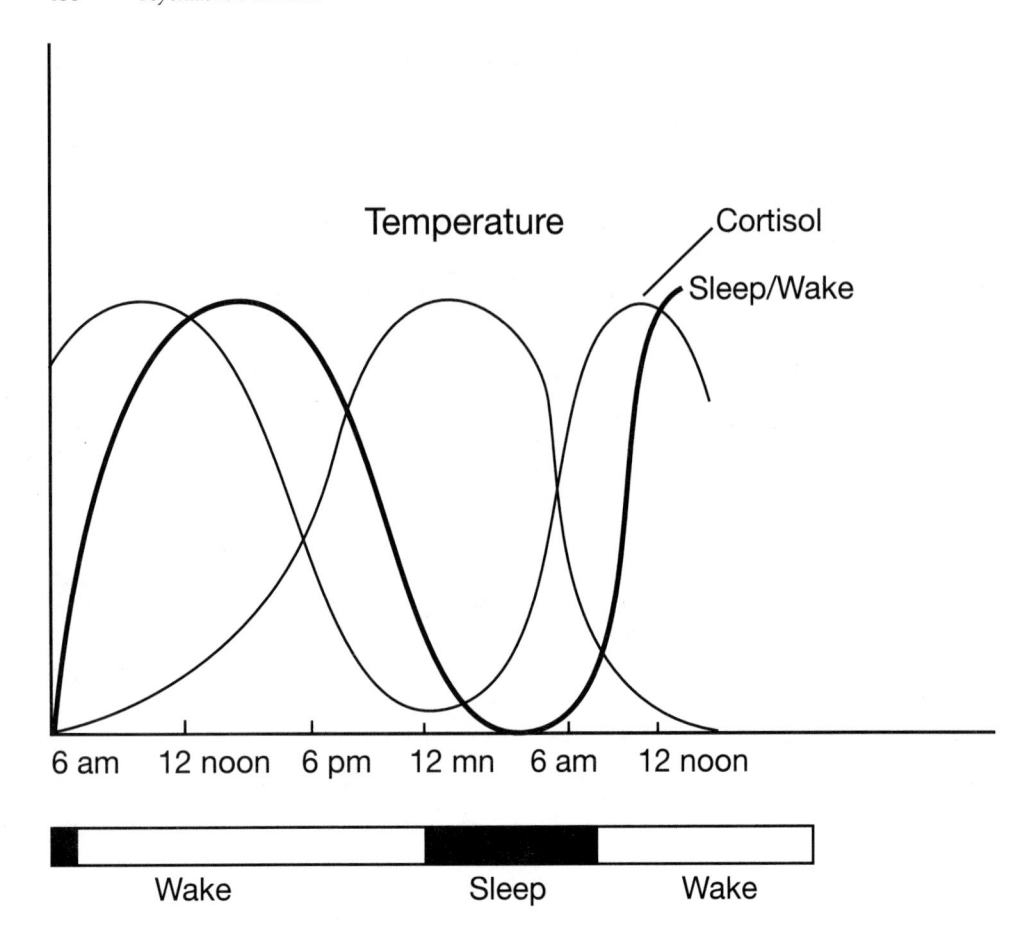

Figure 25-1. Physiologic processes follow a circadian (24-hour) pattern along with the sleep/wake pattern. Serum cortisol reaches its low point at sleep onset and increases before morning awakening, while temperature reaches its peak at midnight and low point at noon.

sleep onset, stages, and onset of REM sleep. Several physiological parameters that follow a circadian rhythm are displayed in Figure 25-1. Body temperature, which also follows a circadian pattern, has been shown to coincide (synchronize) with the sleep cycle.[2] REM sleep is most likely to occur when body temperature is lowest, generally in the early morning hours.[2] Hormones, growth hormone, prolactin, and luteinizing hormone also have sleep-dependent secretion rhythms, and *melatonin* is released at night around the time of sleep onset (see About Melatonin). Serum cortisol generally reaches its low point at sleep onset and increases before morning awakening.

People vary in the amount of sleep they need. So-called short sleepers require less sleep each night and fall asleep without difficulty; for light sleepers, noise, light interruptions, stress, anxiety, worry, and other environmental effects lead to **insomnia** or other sleep complaints. Light sleepers' problems are distinguished from primary sleep disorders by their duration and severity. Although temporary sleep disruption that resolves with minor intervention may develop into a disorder, it is not usually a primary sleep disorder. For example, insomnia that occurs during hospitalization or before a major job interview and then resolves is situational sleep disruption in response to an uncomfortable or stressful situation; severe insomnia or hypersomnia that significantly interferes with functioning and lasts at least 1 month indicates a primary sleep disorder.

Some individuals may recognize that they have difficulty sleeping, whereas others may notice only that they fail to feel rested after a night's sleep. Still others may have daytime problems, such as feeling sleepy, that they don't recognize as a sleep disorder. Complaints of not feeling rested may be the first suggestion of a sleep disorder. Other clues may be hidden: poor job performance, excessive daytime sleepiness, or the use of large amounts of stimulants such as caffeine. Beginning symptoms may also emerge because of work schedules or travel. For instance, shift work and jet lag are two common states associated with circadian schedule changes, resulting in sleep disruption.

Primary sleep disorders are divided into two categories, the dyssomnias and parasomnias, whereas secondary sleep disorders are caused by medical or psychiatric illness, medications, or substance abuse. **Dyssomnia** is characterized by difficulty in initiating or maintaining sleep or by excessive sleep; included are primary insomnia, primary hypersomnia, narcolepsy, breathing-related sleep disorder, circadian rhythm sleep disorder, and dyssomnias not otherwise specified (NOS). **Parasomnia** is characterized by abnormal behaviors or physiological events linked to sleep, certain sleep stages, or sleep-wake transitions. The parasomnias include nightmare disorder, sleep terror disorder, sleepwalking disorder, and parasomnia not otherwise specified (NOS). Table 25-2 lists the primary sleep disorders, their prevalence, and the major sleep complaints associated with each disorder.

Although sleep disruption is evident in every primary sleep disorder, clients are diagnosed by a full set of criteria. The *DSM-IV* Diagnostic Criteria for the primary sleep disorders are listed in the diagnostic box.

Culture, Age, and Gender Features

Culture

Very little research has been done on cultural differences in the expression of sleep disorders, although such differences probably do exist. Up to 60% of workers on night shifts have a significant sleep distrubance.

Age

Newborns spend about half of their sleep time in REM sleep.[1] Infants sleep about 18 hours daily, which tapers off to about 10 hours per night in childhood and to about 8 hours in adulthood.

Nightmares are common during childhood; 10 to 50% of children 3 to 5 years old have disturbing nightmares.[3] Although adolescents were once thought to require less sleep, researchers have found that increased sleep may be necessary during the teenage years to ensure optimal daytime performance and facilitate learning.[4] **Delayed sleep phase disorder** (see Fig. 25–2) is more common in adolescents (up to 7%).

ABOUT MELATONIN

Melatonin comes in two forms, endogenous and exogenous. Endogenous melatonin is a hormone occurring naturally in the body, made by the pineal gland. Melatonin is secreted in large amounts at night, coinciding with the beginning of sleep, and its production is suppressed in the morning; light from the sun signals the pineal gland to stop releasing melatonin. As a result, release of endogenous melatonin follows a circadian pattern. Disruption in melatonin secretion has been linked to primary sleep disorders, such as insomnia, and circadian rhythm sleep disorders, such as jet lag and shift-work sleep problems.

Exogenous melatonin is available in tablet form in health food stores and some pharmacies. This substance treats primary insomnia and circadian rhythm sleep disorders by resetting the body's internal clock. For individuals with insomnia, the timing or amount of melatonin secretion may be disrupted. For those with circadian rhythm disorders, the timing of melatonin is out of sync with other processes such as sleep-wake patterns, temperature, and hormone release that follow a 24-hour pattern. Very little research is available on the use of exogenous melatonin; however, preliminary studies suggest that it may be effective for certain forms of sleep disruption.

TABLE 25–2. Primary Sleep Disorders, Prevalence Rates, and Common Sleep Complaints

	Prevalence	Primary Sleep Complaint
Dyssomnias		
• Primary insomnia	30–40%	Difficulty falling or staying asleep
• Primary hypersomnia	Unknown	Excessive sleep during the night or day
• Narcolepsy	0.02–0.16%	Brief, irresistible attacks of refreshing sleep
• Breathing-related sleep disorder		Excessive sleepiness or insomnia
Obstructive sleep apnea	1–10%	Sleepiness or insomnia due to airway blockage or snoring
Central sleep apnea	Unknown	Sleepiness or insomnia due to cardiac or neurological conditions that affect breathing
• Circadian rhythm sleep disorder		
Delayed sleep phase type	7%*	Difficulty falling asleep and late awakening
Shift work type	70%†	Sleepiness during the major wake period and insomnia during the major sleep period because of changing shifts or night-shift work
Jet lag type	Unknown	Daytime sleepiness and nighttime alertness after travel across more than one time zone
• Dyssomnia not otherwise specified	Unknown	Insomnia or hypersomnia; could result from environmental conditions, sleep deprivation, or leg movements
Parasomnias		
• Nightmare disorder	Unknown	
• Sleep terror disorder	Unknown	
• Sleepwalking disorder	1–5%	
• Parasomnia not otherwise specified	Unknown	

*Of adolescents.
†Of night-shift workers.
Source: Adapted from the Diagnostic and Statistical Manual of Mental Disorders, Fourth Edition. Copyright 1994 American Psychiatric Association.

> **DSM-IV Diagnostic Criteria for Primary Insomnia, Primary Hypersomnia, Narcolepsy, Breathing-Related Sleep Disorder, Circadian Rhythm Sleep Disorder, Nightmare Disorder, Sleep Terror Disorder, Sleepwalking Disorder, Insomnia Related to an Axis I or II Disorder, Hypersomnia Related to an Axis I or II Disorder, Sleep Disorder due to a General Medical Condition, and Substance Induced Sleep Disorder**

Diagnostic Criteria for 307.42 Primary Insomnia

A. The predominant complaint is difficulty initiating or maintaining sleep, or nonrestorative sleep, for at least 1 month.

B. The sleep disturbance (or associated daytime fatigue) causes clinically significant distress or impairment in social, occupational, or other important areas of functioning.

C. The sleep disturbance does not occur exclusively during the course of Narcolepsy, Breathing-Related Sleep Disorder, Circadian Rhythm Sleep Disorder, or a Parasomnia.

D. The disturbance does not occur exclusively during the course of another mental disorder (e.g., Major Depressive Disorder, Generalized Anxiety Disorder, a delirium).

E. The disturbance is not due to the direct physiological effects of a substance (e.g., a drug of abuse, a medication) or a general medical condition.

Diagnostic Criteria for 307.44 Primary Hypersomnia

A. The predominant complaint is excessive sleepiness for at least 1 month (or less if recurrent) as evidenced by either prolonged sleep episodes or daytime sleep episodes that occur almost daily.

B. The excessive sleepiness causes clinically significant distress or impairment in social, occupational, or other important areas of functioning.

C. The excessive sleepiness is not better accounted for by insomnia and does not occur exclusively during the course of another Sleep Disorder (e.g., Narcolepsy, Breathing-Related Sleep Disorder, Circadian Rhythm Sleep Disorder, or a Parasomnia) and cannot be accounted for by an inadequate amount of sleep.

D. The disturbance does not occur exclusively during the course of another mental disorder.

E. The disturbance is not due to the direct physiological effects of a substance (e.g., a drug of abuse, a medication) or a general medical condition.

Specify if:
  Recurrent: if there are periods of excessive sleepiness that last at least 3 days occurring several times a year for at least 2 years

Diagnostic Criteria for 347 Narcolepsy

A. Irresistible attacks of refreshing sleep that occur daily over at least 3 months.

B. The presence of one or both of the following:
  (1) cataplexy (i.e., brief episodes of sudden bilateral loss of muscle tone, most often in association with intense emotion)
  (2) recurrent intrusions of elements of rapid eye movement (REM) sleep into the transition between sleep and wakefulness, as manifested by either hypnopompic or hypnagogic hallucinations or sleep paralysis at the beginning or end of sleep episodes

C. The disturbance is not due to the direct physiological effects of a substance (e.g., a drug of abuse, a medication) or another general medical condition.

Diagnostic Criteria for 780.59 Breathing-Related Sleep Disorder

A. Sleep disruption, leading to excessive sleepiness or insomnia, that is judged to be due to a sleep-related breathing condition (e.g., obstructive or central sleep apnea syndrome or central alveolar hypoventilation syndrome).

B. The disturbance is not better accounted for by another mental disorder and is not due to the direct physiological effects of a substance (e.g., a drug of abuse, a medication) or another general medical condition (other than a breathing-related disorder).

CODING NOTE: Also code sleep-related breathing disorder on Axis III.

Diagnostic Criteria for 307.45 Circadian Rhythm Sleep Disorder

A. A persistent or recurrent pattern of sleep disruption leading to excessive sleepiness or insomnia that is due to a mismatch between the sleep-wake schedule required by a person's environment and his or her circadian sleep-wake pattern.

B. The sleep disturbance causes clinically significant distress or impairment in social, occupational, or other important areas of functioning.

C. The disturbance does not occur exclusively during the course of another Sleep Disorder or other mental disorder.

D. The disturbance is not due to the direct physiological effects of a substance (e.g., a drug of abuse, a medication) or a general medical condition.

Continued on following page

Specify type:

Delayed Sleep Phase Type: a persistent pattern of late sleep onset and late awakening times, with an inability to fall asleep and awaken at a desired earlier time

Jet Lag Type: sleepiness and alertness that occur at an inappropriate time of day relative to local time, occurring after repeated travel across more than one time zone

Shift Work Type: insomnia during the major sleep period or excessive sleepiness during the major awake period associated with night shift work or frequently changing shift work

Unspecified Type

Diagnostic Criteria for 307.47 Nightmare Disorder

A. Repeated awakenings from the major sleep period or naps with detailed recall of extended and extremely frightening dreams, usually involving threats to survival, security, or self-esteem. The awakenings generally occur during the second half of the sleep period.

B. On awakening from the frightening dreams, the person rapidly becomes oriented and alert (in contrast to the confusion and disorientation seen in Sleep Terror Disorder and some forms of epilepsy).

C. The dream experience, or the sleep disturbance resulting from the awakening, causes clinically significant distress or impairment in social, occupational, or other important areas of functioning.

D. The nightmares do not occur exclusively during the course of another mental disorder (e.g., a delirium, Posttraumatic Stress Disorder) and are not due to the direct physiological effects of a substance (e.g., a drug of abuse, a medication) or a general medical condition.

Diagnostic Criteria for 307.46 Sleep Terror Disorder

A. Recurrent episodes of abrupt awakening from sleep, usually occurring during the first third of the major sleep episode and beginning with a panicky scream.

B. Intense fear and signs of autonomic arousal, such as tachycardia, rapid breathing, and sweating, during each episode.

C. Relative unresponsiveness to efforts of others to comfort the person during the episode.

D. No detailed dream is recalled and there is amnesia for the episode.

E. The episodes cause clinically significant distress or impairment in social, occupational, or other important areas of functioning.

F. The disturbance is not due to the direct physiological effects of a substance (e.g., a drug of abuse, a medication) or a general medical condition.

Diagnostic Criteria for 307.46 Sleepwalking Disorder

A. Repeated episodes of rising from bed during sleep and walking about, usually occurring during the first third of the major sleep episode.

B. While sleepwalking, the person has a blank, staring face, is relatively unresponsive to the efforts of others to communicate with him or her, and can be awakened only with great difficulty.

C. On awakening (either from the sleepwalking episode or the next morning), the person has amnesia for the episode.

D. Within several minutes after awakening from the sleepwalking episode, there is no impairment of mental activity or behavior (although there may initially be a short period of confusion or disorientation).

E. The sleepwalking causes clinically significant distress or impairment in social, occupational, or other important areas of functioning.

F. The disturbance is not due to the direct physiological effects of a substance (e.g., a drug of abuse, a medication) or a general medical condition.

Diagnostic Criteria for 307.42 Insomnia Related to . . . [Indicate the Axis I or Axis II disorder]

A. The predominant complaint is difficulty initiating or maintaining sleep, or nonrestorative sleep, for at least 1 month that is associated with daytime fatigue or impaired daytime functioning.

B. The sleep disturbance (or daytime sequelae) causes clinically significant distress or impairment in social, occupational, or other important areas of functioning.

C. The insomnia is judged to be related to another Axis I or Axis II disorder (e.g., Major Depressive Disorder, Generalized Anxiety Disorder, Adjustment Disorder With Anxiety), but is sufficiently severe to warrant independent clinical attention.

D. The disturbance is not better accounted for by another Sleep Disorder (e.g., Narcolepsy. Breathing-Related Sleep Disorder, a Parasomnia).

E. The disturbance is not due to the direct physiological effects of a substance (e.g., a drug of abuse, a medication) or a general medical condition.

Diagnostic Criteria for 307.44 Hypersomnia Related to . . . [Indicate the Axis I or Axis II disorder]

A. The predominant complaint is excessive sleepiness for at least 1 month as evidenced by either prolonged sleep episodes or daytime sleep episodes that occur almost daily.

B. The excessive sleepiness causes clinically significant distress or impairment in social, occupational, or other important areas of functioning.

Continued on following page

C. The hypersomnia is judged to be related to another Axis I or Axis II disorder (e.g., Major Depressive Disorder, Dysthymic Disorder), but is sufficiently severe to warrant independent clinical attention.

D. The disturbance is not better accounted for by another Sleep Disorder (e.g., Narcolepsy. Breathing-Related Sleep Disorder, a Parasomnia) or by an inadequate amount of sleep.

E. The disturbance is not due to the direct physiological effects of a substance (e.g., a drug of abuse, a medication) or a general medical condition.

Diagnostic Criteria for 780.xx Sleep Disorder Due to . . . [Indicate the General Medical Condition]

A. A prominent disturbance in sleep that is sufficiently severe to warrant independent clinical attention.

B. There is evidence from the history, physical examination, or laboratory findings that the sleep disturbance is the direct physiological consequence of a general medical condition.

C. The disturbance is not better accounted for by another mental disorder (e.g., an Adjustment Disorder in which the stressor is a serious medical illness).

D. The disturbance does not occur exclusively during the course of a delirium.

E. The disturbance does not meet the criteria for Breathing-Related Sleep Disorder or Narcolepsy.

F. The sleep disturbance causes clinically significant distress or impairment in social, occupational, or other important areas of functioning.

Specify type:
  .52 Insomnia Type: if the predominant sleep disturbance is insomnia
  .54 Hypersomnia Type: if the predominant sleep disturbance is hypersomnia
  .59 Parasomnia Type: if the predominant sleep disturbance is a Parasomnia
  .59 Mixed Type: if more than one sleep disturbance is present and none predominates
  CODING NOTE: Include the name of the general medical condition on Axis I, e.g., 780.52 Sleep Disorder Due to Chronic Obstructive Pulmonary Disease, Insomnia Type; also code the general medical condition on Axis III (see Appendix G for codes).

Diagnostic Criteria for Substance-Induced Sleep Disorder

A. A prominent disturbance in sleep that is sufficiently severe to warrant independent clinical attention.

B. There is evidence from the history, physical examination, or laboratory findings of either (1) or (2):
  (1) the symptoms in Criterion A developed during, or within a month of, Substance Intoxication or Withdrawal
  (2) medication use is etiologically related to the sleep disturbance

C. The disturbance is not better accounted for by a Sleep Disorder that is not substance induced. Evidence that the symptoms are better accounted for by a Sleep Disorder that is not substance induced might include the following: the symptoms precede the onset of the substance use (or medication use); the symptoms persist for a substantial period of time (e.g., about a month) after the cessation of acute withdrawal or severe intoxication, or are substantially in excess of what would be expected given the type or amount of the substance used or the duration of use; or there is other evidence that suggests the existence of an independent non-substance-induced Sleep Disorder (e.g., a history of recurrent non-substance-related episodes).

D. The disturbance does not occur exclusively during the course of a delirium.

E. The sleep disturbance causes clinically significant distress or impairment in social, occupational, or other important areas of functioning.
  NOTE: This diagnosis should be made instead of a diagnosis of Substance Intoxication or Substance Withdrawal only when the sleep symptoms are in excess of those usually associated with the intoxication or withdrawal syndrome and when the symptoms are sufficiently severe to warrant independent clinical attention.

Code [Specific Substance]-Induced Sleep Disorder:
  (291.8 Alcohol; 292.89 Amphetamine; 292.89 Caffeine; 292.89 Cocaine; 292.89 Opioid; 292.89 Sedative, Hypnotic, or Anxiolytic; 292.89 Other [or Unknown] Substance)

Specify type:
  Insomnia Type: if the predominant sleep disturbance is insomnia
  Hypersomnia Type: if the predominant sleep disturbance is hypersomnia
  Parasomnia Type: if the predominant sleep disturbance is a Parasomnia
  Mixed Type: if more than one sleep disturbance is present and none predominates

Specify if (see table on p. 177 [*DSM-IV*] for applicability by substance)
  With Onset During Intoxication: if the criteria are met for Intoxication with the substance and the symptoms develop during the intoxication syndrome
  With Onset During Withdrawal: if criteria are met for Withdrawal from the substance and the symptoms develop during, or shortly after, a withdrawal syndrome

Source: Reprinted with permission from the Diagnostic and Statistical Manual of Mental Disorders, Fourth Edition. Copyright 1994 American Psychiatric Association.

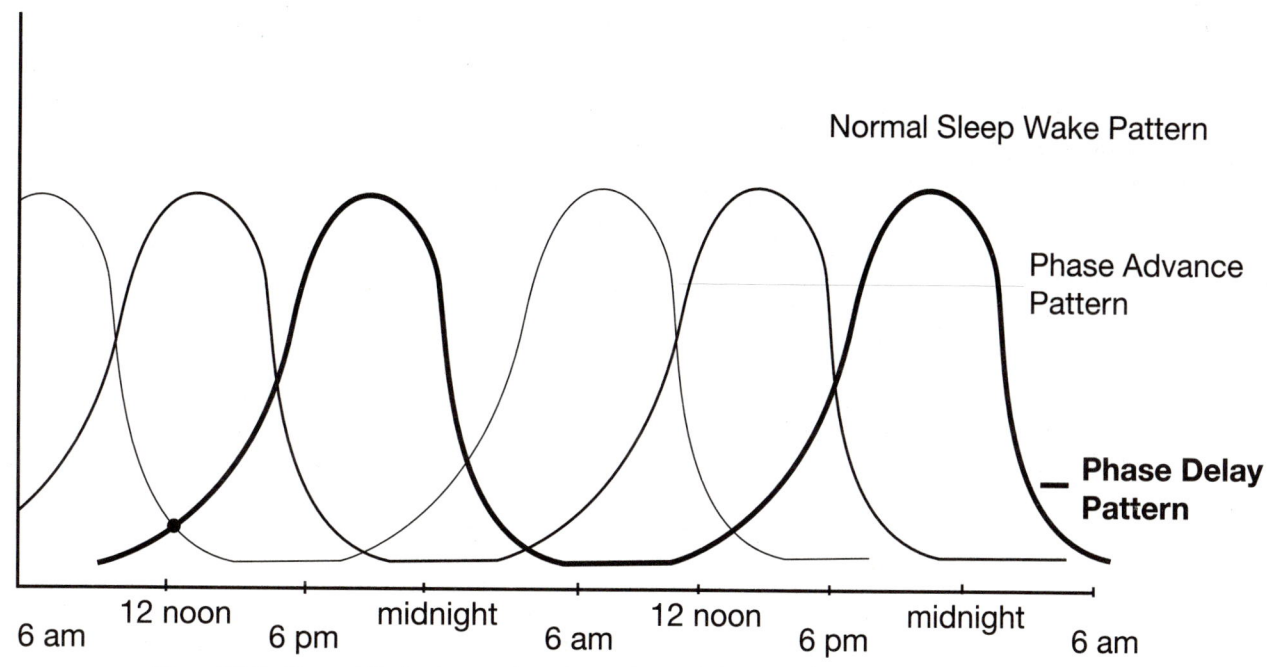

Figure 25-2. Phase-shifts in sleep cycles; phase-advanced sleep patterns have an earlier sleep onset and offset, while phase-delayed patterns have a later onset and wakening.

Older adults may present with the greatest sleep disturbances. About 50% of elders experience poor sleep or report insomnia, and up to 94% of those institutionalized have sedative-hypnotic medications prescribed for sleep disruption.[5] Older adults manifest differences in the sleep-wake and rest-activity schedules, in part because of age-related changes in their internal body clocks. As seen in Figure 25-2, the circadian sleep cycle becomes "phase-advanced" in the elderly; that is, they tend to go to bed early (about 7:00 pm) and to wake early (about 3:00 am). They may have a typical **phase-advanced sleep pattern** and obtain an adequate amount of sleep but believe they have insomnia. Older adults also tend to have less of the deep stages (stages 3 and 4) of sleep, wake more frequently, and thus may have more light sleep (stage 1). Daytime naps are also more common in this age group. As women age, their sleep becomes more phase-advanced than that of men, with increased daytime fatigue and sleepiness.

Gender

Although insomnia and most primary sleep disorders affect both genders equally, men have eight times the risk for obstructive sleep apnea. Women generally develop sleep apnea after menopause.[3]

PRIMARY INSOMNIA

Characteristic Behaviors

Primary insomnia consists of difficulty, for at least 1 month, in falling or staying asleep, leading to impairment in social, occupational, or school performance.[3] Environmental factors, noise, light, temperature, stressful life situations, hospitalization, and irregular sleep-wake schedules may contribute to insomnia. Individuals with primary insomnia may experience depression, irritability, or drowsiness during the day. Ongoing insomnia is associated with a greater risk for major depression and suicide.

I never was a good sleeper, especially as I've gotten older. In college I had weird sleep habits compared to my friends. I'd sleep a few hours during the day and stay up all night. That was easy to do since the library was open all night. Now it takes me hours to fall asleep. It doesn't matter what I do; I never fall asleep before 1:00 am. I also wake up really early in the morning. Overall, I probably sleep only 4 or 5 hours at the most. My father had the same problems. I barely function during the day, but I push myself to do things. I have a pretty good job, but I'm worried that I might get fired. Sometimes I walk around in a daze and can't really concentrate. To help me fall asleep, I might have a drink or two. Alcohol is the only thing that works. I don't think I'll ever sleep good.

Etiology

The cause of primary insomnia is unknown. One proposed theory is that some individuals have a strong arousal drive; that is, their alertness drive is much greater than their sleep drive. The most common cause of insomnia is psychological, social, or medical stress. Less commonly, a history of "light" sleep in the early adult years develops into insomnia. Sleep in this disorder is characterized by a longer period of time needed to fall asleep, frequent awakenings, increased stage

1 sleep, decreased stages 3 and 4 sleep, and extreme muscle tension.

PRIMARY HYPERSOMNIA

Characteristic Behaviors

Primary **hypersomnia** is characterized by excess sleep, with long sleep periods during the night or significant daytime sleeping, for at least 1 month.[3] Individuals with this disorder sleep continuously but fail to feel rested. Because of "sleep drunkenness," periods of prolonged confusion and difficulty waking, waking in the morning is usually difficult. Primary hypersomnia often coexists with major depression.

Etiology

The cause of primary hypersomnia is unknown.

BREATHING-RELATED SLEEP DISORDERS

Characteristic Behaviors

Breathing-related sleep disorders such as **obstructive sleep apnea (OSA)** and **central sleep apnea (CSA)** are characterized by frequent nighttime arousals and daytime sleepiness. Excessive sleepiness during the day is the most common presenting complaint. During OSA, the upper airway becomes partially or totally obstructed, causing the individual to stop breathing for as long as 90 seconds, resulting in brief "mini-awakenings." Cardiac arrhythmias, obesity, hypertension, and impotence are associated conditions. A prominent symptom of OSA is loud snoring, comparable to the noise when airplanes take off. Individuals with apnea are essentially gasping for breath. Because they are asleep, they fail to notice their snoring or gasping. Family members often report the client's loud snoring, complain of sleep disruption secondary to their bed partner's snoring, and describe apneic individuals as restless sleepers. In both disorders, irritability, sleepiness, or fatigue may occur during the day. Although individuals with CSA stop breathing, they do not have blocked airways. Cardiac or neurological conditions are the most common causes of CSA. In the morning, individuals with breathing-related sleep disorders may complain of serious headaches and "sleep drunkenness."

> *At first I thought that my husband was having an affair. He would work late, come home, and fall asleep while watching television. He never seemed to do too much and we had no sex life. I tried to sign us up for an adult education class, but he refused to go. He said he was too tired; that was always his excuse. I began to wonder what was wrong with me. Our marriage was nonexistent. I thought he was depressed. I spoke with some friends of mine, and they suggested that he see a psychiatrist. After receiving a full evaluation, my husband was told that he needed to spend the night in a sleep disorders clinic, being continuously monitored. Later, when we met with the sleep disorders specialists, we found out that he had a sleep disorder called sleep apnea, in which daytime sleepiness was a common feature. They asked me if he snored a lot during the night; he snored so loud I couldn't fall asleep sometimes. Snoring was his way of trying to clear his breathing, and that's why he wasn't getting a good night's sleep. That's also why he was so sleepy and uninvolved with me. Now he has to use a special device at night to keep his airway open in order to sleep.*

Etiology

Genetic Theories

No precise family pattern or gene has been discovered; however, sleep apnea tends to run in families, suggesting a genetic basis.

Physiological Theories

OSA results from collapsed airways during sleep and blocked breathing. The blocked breathing may be caused or exacerbated by obesity or by a structural abnormality in the jaw, uvula, tonsils, or other tissues in the throat. Apneic events, periods of not breathing lasting longer than 10 seconds, and *hypopneas*, periods of reduced airflow, lead to reduced oxygen availability. These impairments result in short sleep periods, frequent wakenings, increased amounts of stage 1 sleep, and decreased amounts of deep sleep (stages 3 and 4) and REM sleep. Clients do not feel rested because of the frequent awakenings and lack of deep sleep.

NARCOLEPSY

Characteristic Behaviors

Narcolepsy is characterized by short periods of irresistible sleepiness daily, lasting at least 3 months. These sudden urges to sleep or "sleep attacks" occur several times throughout the day. Clients relate that even brief periods of sleep (5 to 15 minutes) relieve their fatigue; they often feel "refreshed" after a few minutes of sleep. Narcolepsy can be accompanied by *cataplexy*, sudden attacks of muscle weakness or collapse, sometimes triggered by strong emotional situations, and nighttime sleep disruption. While falling asleep or waking up, clients may experience *hallucinations*, such as hearing a name being called, or *sleep paralysis*, temporary muscle paralysis lasting a few seconds. Sleep during the night may be shortened or broken up into short periods. Some individuals with narcolepsy do not have any nocturnal sleep disruption.

Etiology

Genetic Theories

Narcolepsy appears to have a strong genetic link. Studies show that nearly all individuals with narcolepsy have two leukocyte antigens, DQw6 and DQw1. These and other family studies reveal that about 5 to 15% of first-degree relatives of those with narcolepsy have the disorder, whereas 25 to 50% have a related sleep disorder such as primary hypersomnia.[3]

Physiological Theories

Although the exact etiology is unknown, abnormal manifestations of REM sleep occur; individuals fall quickly into REM sleep during the day. The rapid onset of REM sleep leads to the key feature of narcolepsy, that is, excessive sleep attacks during the day. During the night, sleep is broken up into periods leading to insomnia, which may cause a greater likelihood of daytime sleep attacks.

CIRCADIAN RHYTHM SLEEP DISORDER

Characteristic Behaviors

Circadian rhythm sleep disorder is characterized by either insomnia or hypersomnia. Clients' sleep cycles are mismatched with their internal 24-hour sleep-wake pattern. In delayed sleep phase type, individuals tend to have very late sleep onset and are sometimes referred to as night owls. School, career, and other usual demands become problematic because the wake time is significantly later. In jet lag and shift-work subtypes, sleepiness occurs during the wake time, and alertness occurs during sleep periods. In jet lag type, the sleep-wake changes result from traveling to a new time zone. Eastbound travel is usually more difficult to adjust to than westbound flights. Shift-work type disorders arise from the sleep-wake cycle changes from rotating shifts or working the night shift. These workers usually sleep less and have more frequent sleep disturbances. Adjustments to sleep are more tolerable when switching from day to evening or from evening to night shifts, rather than the reverse.

Regardless of the subtype, circadian rhythm sleep disorders result in physical and emotional problems. Memory, concentration, and physical abilities may be compromised, leading to poor work performance. Irritability, anxiety, and depression affect interpersonal relationships. Left untreated, these behaviors may progress to more severe impairment or psychiatric disorders.

Etiology

Circadian Rhythm Theories

Circadian rhythm sleep disorders have a disrupted 24-hour pattern; the sleep-wake cycle is out of sync with environmental sleep patterns and other rhythms. Exactly why this maladjustment occurs is unknown; however, several studies suggest that the sleep-wake rhythm and body temperature rhythm are mismatched. The sleep and temperature cycles, driven by an internal body clock, begin to run at different times, just like two clocks that keep different time. The mismatch between the sleep and temperature rhythms occurs during frequent shift changes or after traveling to different time zones. The discord between the two rhythms interferes with daytime and nighttime functioning. For instance, shift workers often notice feeling sleepy in the middle of the night and alert during the day when they need to sleep.

DYSSOMNIA NOT OTHERWISE SPECIFIED (NOS)

Characteristic Behaviors

Dyssomnia NOS comprises two major disorders: *restless legs syndrome* and *nocturnal myoclonus*. Both conditions feature abnormal leg movements during sleep. Restless legs syndrome is characterized by uncomfortable feelings such as motor restlessness that make individuals feel like moving their legs. The leg movements usually begin prior to sleep onset and keep clients from falling asleep. Restless leg syndrome may also lead to waking in the middle of the night.

In nocturnal myoclonus, involuntary movements of the legs occur during sleep. These leg jerks emerge during stage 1 sleep and later abate during stages 3 and 4 and REM sleep. The leg jerks occur rhythmically every 20 to 60 seconds and may be so severe that the bed partner is kicked and bruised. Although clients may awaken briefly, they frequently fail to notice or remember the leg movements.

PARASOMNIAS

Characteristic Behaviors

The most common parasomnias are nightmare disorder, sleep terror disorder, and sleepwalking disorder. Nightmare disorder is characterized by severe nightmares that awaken the individual during sleep or naps. The content of the frightening dreams may be threats to survival, security, or self-esteem.[3]

The main feature of sleep terror disorder is periods of abrupt wakening that occur during the first third of the night, accompanied by screaming, crying, intense fear, and autonomic arousal. The client is difficult to awaken from these sleep terrors and frequently is unaware of them. Sleep terror disorder and sleepwalking disorder often co-occur.

Sleepwalking disorder is characterized by rising up in bed or walking around. During sleepwalking, individuals generally have a blank look and are unresponsive. Once awake, they may be confused initially and have little recall for the event.[3]

The first thing that I noticed was that my wife would be sound asleep and in the middle of the night she would sit up. Then I noticed her walking around while she was sleeping. One night, she was sound asleep, walked around, ate a lot of food, and left the kitchen a mess. In the morning, she accused me of making the mess! I told her that I had seen her walking during the night, but she denied it. One night, I tried to wake her up while she was sleepwalking. I wanted to prove to her that she was sleepwalking, but I couldn't wake her at all. I later found out that my wife had episodes of sleepwalking as a child. I finally insisted that she get some help after she walked out in the middle of the night in her nightgown in the middle of the winter. I was really scared. She could have been raped or died of exposure.

Etiology

Although little is known about the precise etiology of parasomnias, sleepwalking and sleep terrors tend to run in families, which suggests a genetic pattern.

SLEEP DISORDERS DUE TO MEDICAL AND PSYCHIATRIC DISORDERS

Severe sleep complaints that are primarily associated with psychiatric disorders such as major depression, the manic phase of bipolar disorder, or posttraumatic stress disorder are classified as sleep disorders related to another mental disorder. Physical illness that directly affects sleep is referred to as sleep disorder due to a general medical condition. For instance, individuals with chronic pain may have substantial difficulty falling or staying asleep. Illicit or prescribed drugs and alcohol can also cause sleep disruption, either by use or by discontinuation. In this case, substance-induced sleep disorder is diagnosed.

Distinguishing among Primary Sleep Disorders

Insomnia, excessive daytime sleepiness, and other sleep complaints are common to several primary sleep disorders. Distinguishing among the sleep disorders can be difficult, even for the trained sleep disorders specialist. Each primary sleep disorder has a set of defined criteria that can be elicited from the client and family and through sleep studies such as *polysomnography*. Table 25–3 lists the common distinguishing features of the dyssomnias and parasomnias.

PROGNOSIS

With proper diagnosis, sleep disorders can be managed successfully. Sleep schedules, environmental manipulation, and nonpharmacologic treatments such as phototherapy can promote healthy sleep-wake patterns. Misdiagnosed or left untreated, however, sleep disorders are associated with high rates of morbidity and mortality.

The consequences of sleep disorders include difficult and even life-threatening situations. For instance, individuals with sleep apnea or narcolepsy may fall asleep while driving, children or adults who sleepwalk may wake to find themselves outdoors or in places they don't recognize, and individuals with primary insomnia commonly develop major depression. If not treated, these conditions lead to substantial use of health-care resources and possibly death. Nurses are often among the first health-care providers to suspect underlying sleep disorders and refer affected individuals for further evaluation.

PLANNING CARE

In planning care, assess any other factors that might contribute to the sleep disorder before recommending treatment. If the individual does fulfill the criteria for a primary sleep disorder, an evaluation by a sleep disorders specialist and a polysomnographic study are generally indicated. The nature and severity of the primary sleep condition dictate choice of treatment. Many individuals with sleep disorders benefit from nonpharmacologic treatments such as sleep hygiene techniques, behavioral therapy, or phototherapy. Individuals with sleep apnea need devices that open the airway.

For some severe sleep disorders, pharmacologic treatments are carefully instituted. Treating sleep disorders with sedative-hypnotics may be useful for some but lead to severe negative consequences in others. For instance, sedatives may effectively treat primary insomnia but worsen sleep apnea.

Evaluation of Sleep Disruption

Several key questions are asked to ascertain the nature of the individual's sleep and the potential for a sleep disorder (Table 25–4). If the answer to any of the questions is yes, assess whether the sleep disturbance is a consequence of an underlying medical, psychiatric, or medication-related problem. Determine the amount of alcohol, caffeine, illicit substances, or medications that may be directly causing sleep impairment. Table 25–5 lists the methods sleep experts use to fully assess the nature and severity of a potential problem. Figure 25–3 shows a common method of measuring sleep, polysomnography; Figure 25–4 shows a sleep disorders specialist reviewing recordings obtained from polysomnography.

INTERVENTIONS FOR HOSPITALIZED CLIENTS

Although individuals with primary sleep disorders are not usually hospitalized, hospitalization for medical illness disrupts an individual's internal body clock and daily patterns,

TABLE 25–3. Distinguishing among Primary Sleep Disorders

Sleep Apnea	Narcolepsy	Primary Insomnia	Primary Hypersomnia	Circadian Rhythm Sleep Disorder	Nightmare Disorder	Sleep Terror Disorder	Sleepwalking Disorder
Excessive daytime sleepiness	Excessive daytime sleepiness ("sleep attacks")	Difficulty initiating or maintaining sleep	Excessive nighttime sleepiness	Sleep schedule conflict	Nighttime awakening (complete)	Nighttime awakening (partial)	Rising from bed or walking
Heavy loud snoring	Cataplexy	Daytime fatigue	Excessive daytime sleepiness	Excessive sleepiness	Extremely frightening dreams that occur later in night	Screaming, crying	Blank, staring face
Intervals of breathing cessation	Sleep paralysis			Insomnia	Fearfulness	Arise in first third of night	No memory for event
Awaking feeling unrefreshed	Hallucinations				Mild autonomic hyperarousal	Fearfulness	Unresponsive during event
Morning headaches						Autonomic hyperarousal	
Unrefreshing daytime sleep						Lack of dream recall	

489

TABLE 25-4. Assessment Questions for the Evaluation of Sleep-Wake Pattern Disruption

- Do you fall asleep too early?
- Do you awaken frequently or sleep too much?
- Do you snore or does your bed partner complain about your snoring?
- Do you feel restless or do your legs twitch at night?
- Do you frequently walk or talk in your sleep?
- Do you ever find that you have apparently eaten during the night, but don't remember?
- Do you suddenly lose control of your muscles when startled or overcome with strong emotion?
- Are you frequently awakened by nightmares?
- Are you ever awakened gasping for breath or unable to breathe?
- When falling asleep or waking, do you ever feel unable to move?
- Do you ever experience vivid, dreamlike hallucinations, even though you know you're awake?

Source: Adapted with permission from the McLean Hospital Sleep Disorders Center, Belmont, MA.

commonly leading to sleep disruption. Sleep problems may result directly from a medical condition or medication or, indirectly, from noise, light, interruptions, lack of familiarity with surroundings, fears, new routines, and separation from family. Left untreated, sleep disruption has profound consequences; clients take longer to recover, are hospitalized longer, deteriorate, and may develop other physical or psychological problems. Early intervention is key. Use the clinical management tips to promote healthy sleep-wake patterns in the hospital.

INTERVENTIONS FOR CLIENTS IN THE COMMUNITY

Most individuals with sleep disorders live in the community. Long-term disruption may lead to a whole host of occupational, interpersonal, psychiatric, and medical problems. The primary nursing role is to complete a full assessment and to encourage clients to receive evaluation and treatment from a trained sleep disorders specialist. After the nature of the sleep disruption is diagnosed, help clients initiate and make lifestyle changes to enhance healthy sleep-wake patterns. Reinforce good **sleep hygiene** practices. Stress the need for a long-term weight management and exercise program. Point out the importance of daily compliance with treatment to avoid problems at school or work, feelings of failure, poor academic or job performance, or unemployment.

Refer individuals who develop comorbid major depression or an anxiety disorder for psychotherapy and pharmacotherapy. Continuously assess medication, alcohol, and substance use. Emphasize the need to avoid alcohol or substances that seem to promote sleep, and teach them that these agents instead exacerbate sleep problems. If alcohol or substance abuse is severe, refer clients to Alcoholics Anonymous or other self-help groups or for evaluation of substance abuse.

TABLE 25-5. Methods for Evaluating Sleep Disorders

Sleep Diaries

Detailed daily reports of sleeping and waking times that clients complete for at least several days. More detailed diaries may record each 15-minute period during the day and night as either a sleep or wake period. Sleep diaries can help determine subjective and, possibly, long-term daily sleep-wake patterns. An example of a sleep diary is shown in Table 25-7.

History, Physical Exam, Detailed Sleep Disorders Assessment

The evaluation is usually performed by a sleep disorders clinician to ascertain diagnosis. Careful questioning about the individual's sleep can begin to distinguish whether the sleep disruption is due to a primary sleep disorder or to a medication, substance abuse, medical condition, or psychiatric disorder.

Polysomnography (PSG)

Overnight sleep studies in a sleep laboratory while electroencephalogram (EEG) brain waves, eye movements, and muscle movements are continuously monitored. Figure 25-3 shows a client receiving a sleep study; Figure 25-4 shows a sleep disorders specialist monitoring sleep recordings. The exact timing and duration of sleep stages, the amount of time it takes the individual to fall asleep (sleep onset latency), how long any nighttime wakenings are, and the total number of minutes of sleep time (sleep duration) are noted. To diagnose possible airway obstruction, oral or nasal airflow measurement, respiratory effort, and other measures may also be used. Newer methods include portable (home-based) ambulatory PSG, which provides similar evaluation as in a sleep center.

Multiple sleep latency test (MSLT)

Daytime sleep studies to monitor clients for sleep attacks while they are given the opportunity to sleep in a quiet, dimly lit room. Narcolepsy is diagnosed if the individual cannot resist sleeping two or more times during this procedure.

Actigraphy

An emerging method to assess daily activity and nighttime sleep patterns naturally. Individuals wear small, wristwatch-sized devices that measure movement on their wrists (Figure 25-5). Although somewhat less reliable than PSG, the activity derived from these monitors can estimate sleep disruption and assess the circadian pattern of sleep-wake.* These devices are worn continuously for several days in the individual's usual environment. A sample actigraph recording is presented in Figure 25-6.

*Teicher, MH: Actigraphy and motion analysis: New tools for psychiatry. Harv Rev Psychiatry 3:18, 1995.

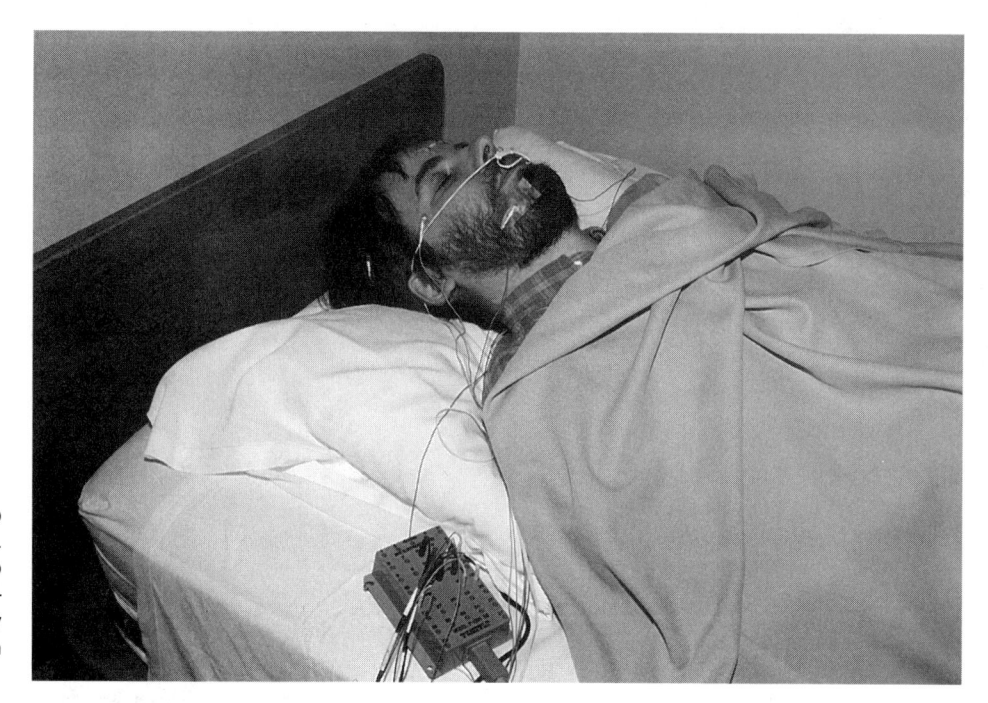

Figure 25–3. A simulated sleep study using polysomnography. The client is sleeping in a sleep laboratory with EEG and monitoring of eye, muscle, and respiratory movements. (Courtesy of Kenneth Hanrahan, McLean Hospital.)

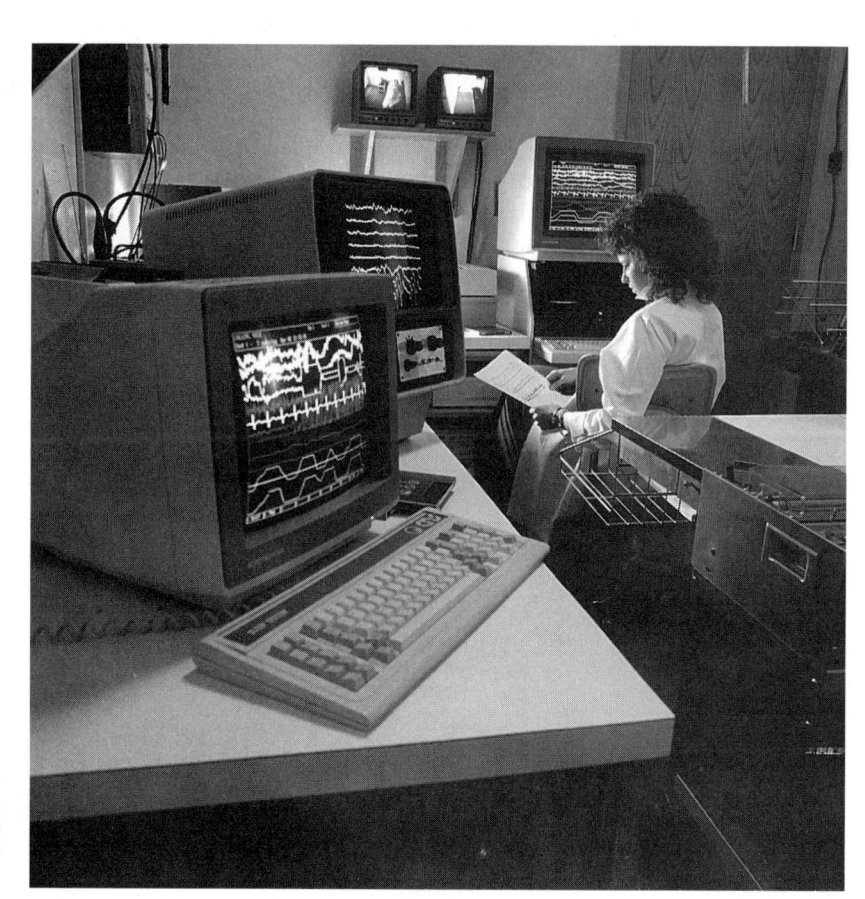

Figure 25–4. A sleep disorders specialist examining the brain wave patterns, movements, eye movements, and respirations of a client being studied in a sleep clinic. (Courtesy of Kenneth Hanrahan, McLean Hospital.)

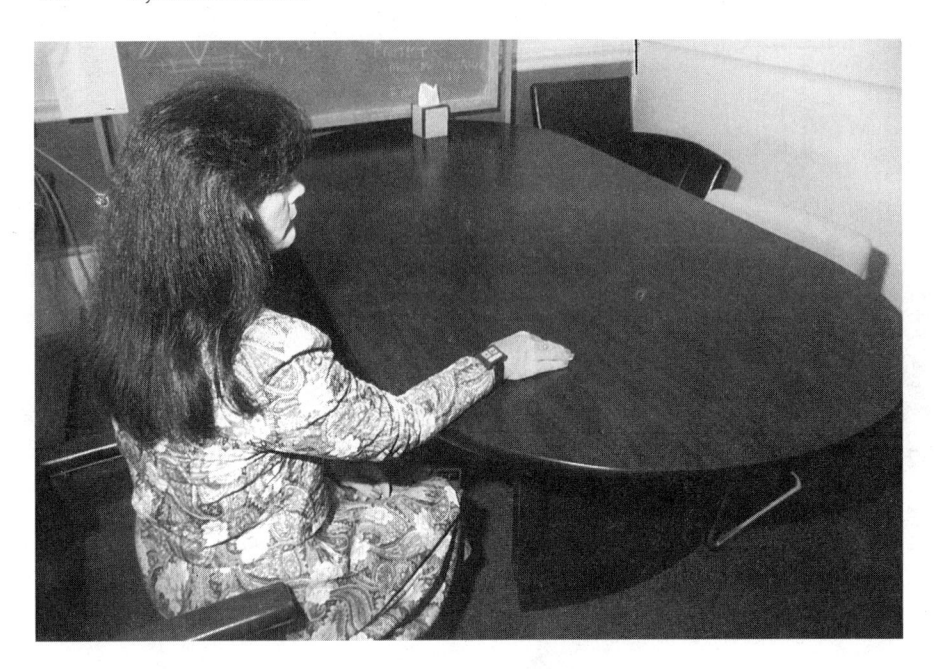

Figure 25-5. An actigraph, a device used to measure levels of activity during the day and night.

Behavioral and Other Nonpharmacologic Treatments

The major nursing role in the treatment of sleep disorders is behavior management. Individuals with either diagnosed sleep conditions or transient insomnia may benefit from learning basic sleep hygiene, which includes environmental manipulation, adjustments to facilitate sleep, and avoidance of behaviors that disrupt sleep (see Clinical Management Tips). Progressive relaxation, another useful technique, consists of having the client systematically tense and relax key muscles, with intense concentration. Sleep hygiene and behavioral measures are most useful in primary insomnia, however, and provide little benefit in sleep apnea, nocturnal myoclonus, or narcolepsy.

Obstructive Sleep Apnea

A major nursing intervention for clients with OSA is a weight loss program. Reducing caloric intake and beginning a regular exercise program can help. Reducing or eliminating alcohol, particularly before bedtime, is essential. Some individuals with OSA have physical problems, such as a specific upper airway abnormality, nasal obstruction, or enlarged tonsils or adenoids, and require surgery. If no airway obstructions are found, a common treatment for OSA and also for CSA is continuous positive airway pressure (**CPAP**; Figure 25-7). CPAP works by applying ongoing "pressure" to keep the upper airway open; it has been described as a "pneumatic splint."[6] It is a safe, effective, and noninvasive procedure, it requires long-term nightly use, and the ma-

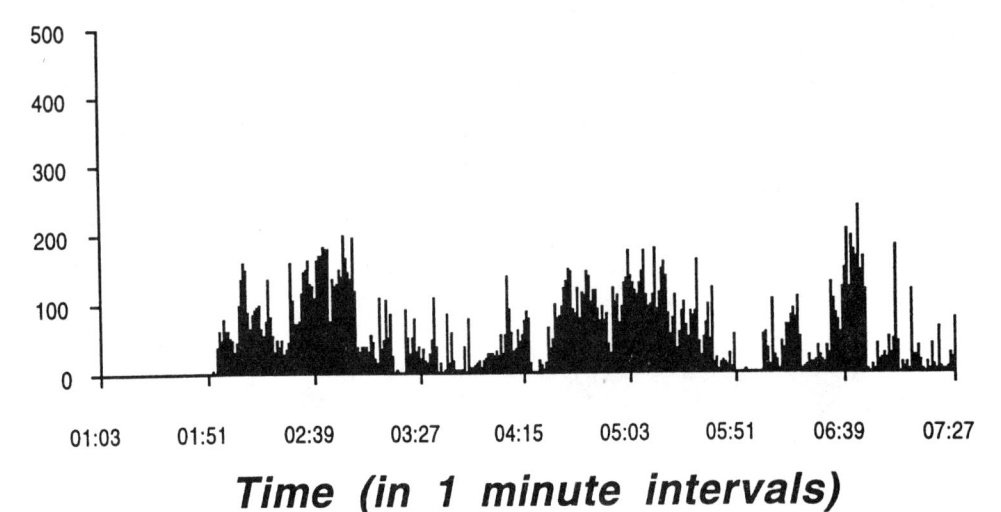

Figure 25-6. A sample actigraph recording of a client with a sleep disorder, "sleeping" from 1:50 am to 7:27 am. The higher the lines, the more movement is present. Note the large amounts of movement that occur.

Time (in 1 minute intervals)

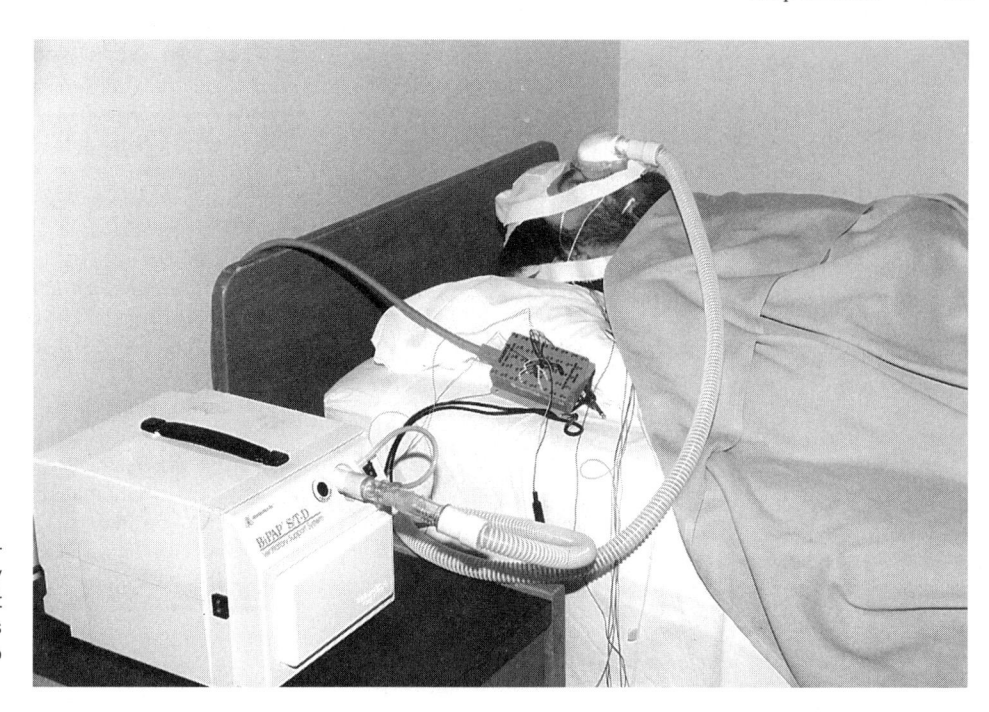

Figure 25-7. A client being administered continuous airway pressure as a nighttime treatment for sleep apnea. The client wears the device throughout the night to maintain an open airway.

chine is noisy. Dental appliances, used to increase airway space and position the jaw and tongue, are simple, quiet, and effective in persons who cannot tolerate CPAP.

Circadian Rhythm Sleep Disorders

For those with circadian rhythm sleep disorders, progressive relaxation combined with phototherapy may be effective. Phototherapy or exposure to intense (10,000 lux) artificial light sources may help "reset" the body's internal clock. For individuals with a phase-advanced sleep cycle, the delivery of light in the late afternoon or early evening may help shift the sleep pattern later, whereas those who are phase-delayed generally benefit from morning light and nighttime progressive relaxation. Similarly, phototherapy, timed at key points during travel or shift work, can successfully treat sleep disruption and daytime fatigue. For instance, encourage individuals who work night shifts to avoid bright light exposure, wear sunglasses when leaving work, and receive phototherapy prior to or during the night shift.

Parasomnias

Parasomnias, if severe and continuous, require treatment. Psychotherapy alone or in combination with antidepressant therapy may be useful for nightmare disorder, sleep terrors, and sleepwalking. Environmental manipulation is also important for sleepwalking disorder. To protect clients, instruct them to lock windows and doors, put an alarm on the outside door, and cover windows with heavy drapes.

Melatonin. Melatonin, in doses of 2 to 5 mg at bedtime, is sometimes used to treat insomnia. Similar doses are used to treat jet lag; however, the timing of melatonin administration is based on the type and length of travel. Melatonin is generally not effective for time-zone transitions of less than 4 hours or trips of less than 4 days in the new time zone. For instance, when traveling eastward, 2 to 5 mg of melatonin are taken on the departure day at about 7 pm and then at the "new" bedtime for 4 consecutive days. For westward travel, 2 to 5 mg are taken at the "new" bedtime for 4 nights. The timing of doses is essential to reset the body's clock.

Side effects of melatonin include sedation, decreased alertness, headache, and, infrequently, nausea. Although contraindications have not been established, it probably should be avoided in pregnant and lactating women. Because melatonin does not require a prescription and is not regulated, the actual quantity in each capsule or pill varies.

Sedative-Hypnotics. Sedative-hypnotics such as benzodiazepines are not the first choice for treating most sleep disorders. Although potent, giving effective relief from nighttime insomnia, these agents are best used only for the short-term relief of insomnia (several days to 2 weeks on average). The most common sedative-hypnotics and adult dosages are listed in Table 25-6. Some agents such as oxazepam may be used to treat insomnia and anxiety; however, "hangover effects" such as daytime sedation may present problems. Newer agents such as midazolam, triazolam, and zolpidem potently treat difficulty in falling asleep and are very rapidly eliminated from the body, leading to little or no sedation.

Persistent sleep disruption is usually a sign of a major sleep, medical, or psychiatric condition, and until the underlying disorder is accurately diagnosed and treated, sedative-hypnotics may cause more harm than good. For instance, sedatives prescribed to individuals with undiagnosed sleep apnea may impair the normal arousal process that oc-

> **RESEARCH NOTE**
>
> Haimov, I, Lavie, P, Laudon, M, Herer, P, Vigder, C, and Zisapel N: Melatonin replacement therapy in elderly insomniacs. Sleep 7:598–603, 1995.
>
> **Findings:** Alterations in melatonin release often occur in elderly individuals with insomnia. In this study, the researchers tested the effects of melatonin on the sleep of older adults with insomnia. The investigators compared a 2-mg dose of melatonin, one in sustained-release form, another in standard form, with placebo taken 2 hours before bedtime. The standard formulation of 2 mg of melatonin had the greatest effect on helping elders fall asleep. The sustained-release preparation had the greatest effect on problems staying asleep; clients were able to remain asleep with fewer awakenings. The positive effects of melatonin continued for months, without higher doses. Older adults reported that their sleep worsened shortly after the melatonin was discontinued.
>
> **Application to Practice:** Insomnia can have profound effects on ability to function and is associated with increases in psychiatric and medical disorders. Elderly individuals are often very sensitive to standard medications, such as sedative-hypnotics, commonly used to treat insomnia. Melatonin provides another alternative to promote sleep. It probably works by shifting the sleep-wake pattern rather than by providing sedation. This study suggests that melatonin is an effective and safe treatment for insomnia that is characterized by difficulty either falling asleep or staying asleep.

TABLE 25–6. Sedative-Hypnotic Medications Used in the Treatment of Insomnia

Flurazepam (Dalmane), 15–30 mg. Used to reduce frequent nighttime awakenings; produces daytime sedation.
Midazolam (Versed), 7.5–15 mg. Used to induce sleep; very rapidly eliminated.
Oxazepam (Serax), 15–30 mg. Slow absorption; used to sustain sleep and as an anxiolytic.
Quazepam (Doral), 7.5–15 mg. Used to induce sleep and reduce nighttime awakenings; may produce daytime sedation.
Temazepam (Restoril), 10–20 mg. Used to induce sleep; rapidly eliminated from body.
Triazolam (Halcion), 0.125–0.25 mg. Used to induce sleep; very rapidly eliminated; associated with daytime sedation and rebound insomnia.
Zolpidem (Ambien), 5–10 mg. Used to induce sleep; very rapidly eliminated, no daytime sedation.

curs with suppressed breathing. These agents should be avoided in older adults with a typical phase-advanced sleep pattern, such as sleeping from 7:00 pm to 3:00 am, because they have already slept several hours. Sedative-hypnotics may also increase sedation in the elderly because of their slowed metabolism and increase their risk of falls and fractures.

Psychostimulants. Psychostimulants are the primary treatment for narcolepsy. These agents promote wakefulness because of their "stimulating" properties. Pemoline, dextroamphetamine, and methylphenidate are used in frequent daily doses, titrated to maintain daytime alertness. However, individuals with the potential for substance or alcohol abuse should not be prescribed these stimulants because of their abuse potential.

Antidepressants. Antidepressants, particularly tricyclic antidepressants (TCAs), are sometimes used to promote sleep in clients with primary insomnia and major depression. Some of the newer agents such as the selective serotonin reuptake inhibitors (SSRIs) may contribute to insomnia, and their use should be carefully assessed. More research is needed on the effectiveness of antidepressants in primary sleep disorders.

CLIENT AND FAMILY EDUCATION

Teaching interventions can enhance understanding about healthy sleep-wake patterns, sleep disorders and their etiologies, and factors that enhance or disrupt sleep. Focus on ways to adjust to the effects on daily functioning and goals. Explain that individuals with sleep disorders cannot control their symptoms with willpower. Documenting the exact sleep-wake pattern and disruptions with a **sleep diary** (Table 25–7) can help clients identify the sleep disturbance and anticipate the frequency of parasomnias such as nightmares, sleep terrors, and sleepwalking.

An important part of educating the client and family is helping them identify factors that precipitate or aggravate symptoms and detract from adequate sleep hygiene (Table 25–8). Warn clients and families that certain medications, caffeine, and illicit substances can worsen sleep. Teach them that exercise and maintaining adequate weight and nutrition promotes sleep. Stress compliance with treatment; even brief periods of noncompliance may lead to reemergence of symptoms. For some, referral to self-help groups such as those for narcolepsy is also helpful.

EXPECTED OUTCOMES

For the individual with a primary sleep disorder, improvement will demonstrated by:
- Maintaining a regular sleep-wake schedule.
- Obtaining an adequate amount of sleep, without excessive daytime sleepiness.
- Avoiding activities and substances that interfere with sleep.
- Understanding the course and consequences of an untreated sleep disorder.
- Initiating and maintaining lifestyle changes to enhance healthy sleep-wake patterns.

> **RESEARCH NOTE**
>
> Rogers, AE, Caruso, CC, and Aldrich, MS: Reliability of sleep diaries for assessment of sleep-wake patterns. Nurs Res 42:368–372, 1993.
>
> **Findings:** In this study, the authors compared two methods of sleep assessment, the sleep diary and home-based polysomnography (PSG), to see if sleep diaries were an accurate way of obtaining data on sleep-wake patterns. Fifty individuals completed the study; 25 clients with narcolepsy and 25 healthy normal volunteers. The participants were asked to record any sleep period greater than 15 minutes during the day or night for 24 hours, while being monitored simultaneously with PSG. The information on sleep and wake time derived from sleep diaries was in very good agreement with information from PSG. However, the clients with narcolepsy were less accurate in reporting their daytime sleep-wake periods than the normal volunteers.
>
> **Application to Practice:** Sleep diaries can be used clinically to assess the frequency and severity of sleep disturbances. They are a simple and inexpensive method to quantify and document sleep disruption. When administered before and after treatment, they can also be used to evaluate the effectiveness of an intervention. Diaries also actively engage clients in assessing and monitoring their own symptoms by promoting self-management.
>
> Sleep diaries may be slightly less useful for individuals who have difficulty reporting their own levels of sleepiness or alertness. By design, sleep diaries are subjective reports. These methods could be used as a screening tool to determine if more expensive and sensitive testing is necessary.

TABLE 25–7. Sleep Diary Used in the Assessment of Sleep

Instructions. Please fill out the following for every day for at least 1 to 2 weeks. Complete the form when you first wake up; otherwise the information may not be accurate.

Day/date:_____
What time did you go to bed last night? _____ (hour)
_____ (min) _____ AM or _____ PM
How long did it take to fall asleep? _____ (hours)
_____ (min)
How many times did you wake during the night? _____
How long were you awake after falling asleep?
_____ (hours) _____ (min)
What time did you wake up? _____ (hour)
_____ (min) _____ AM or _____ PM
What time did you get up out of bed? _____ (hours)
_____ (min)
How long did you sleep last night? _____ (hours)
_____ (min)
How rested do you feel now? _____ very
_____ somewhat _____ a little _____ not at all

TABLE 25–8. Recommendations for Adequate Sleep Hygiene

Environment
Provide adequate, comfortable temperature (not too hot or too cold).
Ensure absence of light (from lamps, windows, clocks, etc.).
Reduce and eliminate noise.
Remove television from the bedroom and avoid watching TV or listening to the radio in bed.
Avoid other activities, other than sleeping or sex, in bed.
Avoid working in bed and set a reasonable limit for finishing work prior to bedtime.
Avoid serious discussions or arguments prior to bedtime.
Avoid working on potentially upsetting things prior to bed (e.g., bills).
Do not make late night phone calls.
Exercise in the morning, or several hours prior to bed.
Obtain about one-half hour of sunlight shortly after arising.
Make the bedroom and bed as comfortable as possible.
Protect bedtime and sleep from disruptions.
Minimize effects from bed partner with sleep disruption (snoring, different bedtime, movement).
Take a hot bath within 2 hours of sleep time to enhance sleep.
Drink a small amount of a warm drink (noncaffeinated), e.g., milk, to help promote sleep.

Substances
Avoid alcohol, particularly at night.
Avoid caffeine.
Avoid over-the-counter medications that cause sleep problems.

Bedtime Routine
Establish a regular pattern prior to bed (brush teeth, change clothes, etc.).
Set regular bedtime and rise times—even on weekends!
Avoid naps.
Determine your individual amount of sleep duration (6–10 hours for adults).
Don't sacrifice sleep, especially several nights in a row; avoid accumulating a sleep debt.
If insomnia, daytime sleepiness, movements during sleep, or falling asleep quickly continues, consult a clinician or sleep disorders expert.

- Taking medication, if prescribed, as instructed.
- Complying with treatment consistently.

DIFFERENTIAL DIAGNOSIS

Sleep Disorder due to a General Medical Condition

- A physical condition may precipitate sleep disruption; common medical problems are listed in Table 25–9.
- Organic causes are ruled out before making the diagnosis of any sleep disorder.

TABLE 25–9. Medical Conditions Associated with Sleep Disruption

Fibromyalgia
Cystic fibrosis
Head injury
Migraine headaches
Huntington's chorea
Tourette's syndrome
Alzheimer's disease
Cancer
Arthritis
Chronic fatigue syndrome
Hyperthyroidism
Menopause
Allergies
AIDS
Pain secondary to a medical condition

- Most medical conditions decrease sleep duration, reduce stages 3 and 4 sleep, and increase awakenings during the night.
- Severe sleep disturbances directly related to the physical disorder are diagnosed as sleep disorder due to a medical condition; subtypes are insomnia, hypersomnia, parasomnia, or mixed type, depending on the major sleep complaint.

Substance-Induced Sleep Disorder

- Many medications have insomnia or sedation as a side effect.
- Sleep disturbances that appear soon after beginning a medication are often drug induced.
- Antidepressants, antihypertensives, antihistamines, corticosteroids, stimulants, sedative-hypnotics, cholinergic agents, and over-the-counter cold preparations lead to sleep problems.
- Discontinuing or switching the medication may resolve the sleep disturbance.
- Severe sleep disturbance related to a necessary medication is diagnosed as substance-induced sleep disorder; subtypes are insomnia, hypersomnia, parasomnia, or mixed type.
- Alcohol, caffeine, and illicit substances and withdrawal from these drugs cause sleep disturbances.
- Alcohol, initially sedating, leads to wakefulness and vivid dreams in the latter part of the night because of reduced stages 3 and 4 sleep.
- Alcohol withdrawal causes difficulty in remaining asleep and an increase in vivid dreams.
- Caffeine, amphetamines, and cocaine commonly lead to insomnia during acute use and to hypersomnia during withdrawal.
- Opioids cause hypersomnia initially and insomnia chronically.

Mood Disorders

- Mood disorders often have sleep disruption as a chief complaint, for instance, insomnia occurs during mania.
- Major depression is characterized by either insomnia or hypersomnia, whereas the manic phase of severe sleep problems that co-occur with other symptoms of a mood disorder, last at least 1 month, need intervention, and are out of proportion to the other symptoms are diagnosed as insomnia or hypersomnia related to another mental disorder.

Anxiety Disorders

- Sleep disorders often exist with anxiety disorders.
- Worry and nervousness commonly lead to sleep disruption.
- Primary insomnia occurs in generalized anxiety, panic disorder, and posttraumatic stress disorder.

COMMON NURSING DIAGNOSES

- Sleep Pattern Disturbance
- Role Performance, altered
- Fatigue
- Breathing Pattern, ineffective
- Adjustment, impaired

SYNOPSIS OF CURRENT RESEARCH

Much of the current basic (animal) research focuses on developing an understanding of the purpose of sleep, sleep stages, REM sleep, and why sleep-wake patterns change throughout the life cycle. The research is beginning to challenge previously held notions about sleep throughout development. For example, one group of researchers has found that the need for sleep does not decrease in adolescence; however, the actual sleep duration does.[7] What this implies is that teens receive much less sleep than required, in part because of delayed bedtimes. Furthering this research, this group studied young adults in their freshman year of college, determining that delayed bedtimes were associated with less than optimal overall sleep duration.[7] They found that students who went to bed earlier achieved sufficient sleep to perform adequately.[7]

Another important area of research is focused on the overlap between sleep disorders and psychiatric disorders. About 80% of psychiatric illness has insomnia as part of the presenting symptomatology. The reason for the overlap is unclear. Theories about the pathophysiology of affective illness have proposed a disruption in circadian rhythms ("phase-advance" or "desynchronization" hypotheses). Extending this further, research is underway to investigate the sleep and activity patterns of persons with physical and sexual abuse histories, with the theory that trauma may affect the circadian rhythms governing these basic processes.[8] Nurse investigators are also studying the relationship between sleep and pregnancy, sleep deprivation as a treatment for depres-

> **Clinical Management Tips for Hospitalized Clients with Temporary Sleep Disturbance**

Client and Family Teaching
- Teach clients and families good sleep hygiene.
- Help clients pinpoint periods of peak alertness or intense drowsiness.
- Stress the importance of maintaining a regular sleep-wake schedule.
- Emphasize the need to avoid overactivity or underactivity.

Ways to Promote Sleep
- Assess whether pain, medication, or anxiety is leading to sleep disruption.
- Provide a calm, quiet environment.
- Establish the client's baseline sleep pattern.
- Ask the client what factors interfere with sleep in the new environment.
- Reestablish a bedtime routine similar to client's prehospitalization routine.
- Individualize care to mimic the client's baseline sleep-wake pattern.
- Discourage daytime naps.
- If possible, encourage client to sit up in a chair during the day.
- Teach progressive muscle relaxation.
- Plan nursing care activities to minimize nighttime interruptions and increase sleep periods.
- Provide appropriate daytime stimulation.
- Promote bright surroundings during the day and dark environment during the night.
- Inform all members of the treatment team of the client's sleep-wake schedule and post on the door.
- Provide adequate room temperature, avoiding extremely hot or cold environment.
- Encourage the client's use of personal clothing and bedding.
- Use soothing music or relaxation tapes.
- Encourage participation in daily activities as tolerated.
- Use sedative-hypnotics when other interventions have failed or for severe insomnia.

sion, sleep in children after cardiac surgery, and gender differences in sleep problems.

AREAS FOR FUTURE RESEARCH

- What is the prevalence of sleep disorders in individuals with psychiatric disorders?
- What are the most effective nursing interventions to help with insomnia in acute medical and surgical settings?
- What is the relationship between circadian temperature and hormonal rhythms and persistent insomnia?
- What is the purpose of REM sleep?
- What effect do a daily schedule and regular sleep-wake times have on sleep?
- What are the effects of the hospital environment and lack of light exposure on recovery from medical illness?
- What are the financial and personal "costs" of undiagnosed sleep disorders?
- What is the quality of life of persons with chronic insomnia?
- What are the most effective nonpharmacologic treatments for insomnia and daytime sleepiness?
- What other uses exist for melatonin?

CASE STUDY

Bert B is a 50-year-old salesman who visited his primary care provider because of "not feeling rested" and daytime sleepiness. His major reason for seeking treatment was that he was so fatigued he nearly fell asleep at the wheel. Because driving is an essential part of his job, he was very concerned about his ability to drive safely. Bert completed some basic health assessment questionnaires, a physical examination, and blood work and was given an assessment by the nurse. The evaluation revealed an obese man who drank two to three "highballs" on the weekend but otherwise showed no significant abnormal results. He was taking no medication.

Bert noted he had gained 20 pounds over the past year, in part because of his work schedule and frequent business dinners. He had begun to notice that he felt sleepy during the day but attributed it to stress and pressures within his company to produce more sales. As a result, he had had little time for his family, leisure activities, or the weekly golf game he used to play. He also noted that he sometimes naps in his car between appointments to obtain more rest.

When asked about his sleep patterns, Bert stated that he fell asleep without any difficulty, at 9:30 pm and slept to 5:30 am, later on weekends. He often ate his dinner, watched television in bed, and fell asleep shortly thereafter. He knew he should lose weight but hadn't been able to stick to a diet and had no exercise regime. His sexual relationship had waned over recent months. When asked if his wife has noticed any difficulty with his sleep, he revealed that she sometimes sleeps in another room because his snoring is so loud.

The nurse referred Bert to a sleep disorders clinic for further evaluation. The results of polysomnography revealed that he was having more than 30 apneic episodes per night, and he was diagnosed with OSA. The nurse discussed the purpose of CPAP therapy with Bert and his wife, explaining that its major purpose was to keep his airway open and promote sleep. She also listened to Bert's concerns about wearing the device each night and the effect it would have on his relationship. The nurse explained that the apneic events led to times when Bert stopped breathing and that his snoring was a sign that he wasn't getting enough air and gave them both educational materials about sleep apnea. She also told them that this treatment should improve his sleep, lessen his daytime sleepiness, and lead to his feeling more rested.

Along with suggesting that he avoid alcohol and caffeine, she devised a schedule for Bert to decrease his intake of these substances. She also recommended golf and an exercise and weight program.

Two weeks later, Bert noted improvement in his nighttime sleep, particularly during the nights he used the CPAP device. He complained that the machine was noisy, especially to his wife, so he did not use the device consistently each night. He had significantly decreased his alcohol and caffeine intake. His weight remained constant. He had not played golf because of his busy work schedule and did not follow through on an exercise or weight program. The nurse emphasized that these measures would help his overall well-being and that weight loss would promote sleep and decrease the apneic periods. She stressed the need for continued nightly use of the CPAP device and suggested that his wife go to bed first, before the machine was turned on. Bert agreed to try these suggestions and seemed to better understand the need for treatment.

CRITICAL THINKING QUESTIONS

1. What behavioral clues did Bert exhibit during the few months preceding the onset of the sleepiness?
2. What measures could Bert use to promote healthy sleep-wake patterns?
3. How might alcohol worsen Bert's condition?
4. What additional information or procedures would be helpful to promote sleep?
5. Develop a care plan, including short- and long-term goals for Bert's sleep complaints.
6. Identify behaviors that indicate that Bert is responding to treatment.
7. Design a teaching plan to assist Bert in developing healthy sleep and activity patterns.

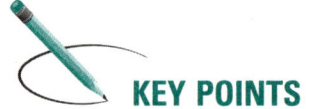

KEY POINTS

- Primary sleep disorders are definable conditions that differ from occasional sleep problems or sleep disruption related to psychiatric, medical, and substance-abuse disorders.
- Primary sleep disorders are divided into two categories: dyssomnias and parasomnias. The dyssomnias include primary insomnia, primary hypersomnia, breathing-related sleep disorders such as obstructive sleep apnea, narcolepsy, and circadian rhythm sleep disorder. Parasomnias include nightmare disorder, sleep terror disorder, and sleepwalking disorder.
- Misdiagnosed or left untreated, sleep disorders are associated with high rates of morbidity and mortality.
- Sleep complaints can include difficulty in initiating or maintaining sleep, oversleeping, daytime sleepiness or naps, and unusual behaviors that occur during sleep.
- Sleep-wake patterns change with age; sleep duration decreases during adolescence and drops in late adulthood. Changes in the timing of sleep occur developmentally; adolescents tend to go to bed later and awaken later (phase-delay pattern), whereas older adults tend to go to bed earlier and wake up early (phase-advance pattern).
- Sleep disturbances are commonly caused by general medical or psychiatric conditions. Alcohol, caffeine, illicit substances, or medications may also cause sleep impairment or worsen a preexisting condition.
- Sleep schedules, environmental manipulation, and non-pharmacologic treatments such as progressive relaxation and phototherapy are useful treatments for some primary sleep disorders.
- Sedative-hypnotic medications are reserved for severe sleep disorders and are generally used for short-term relief.
- The major nursing role in the treatment of primary sleep disorders is behavioral management. The techniques include teaching sleep hygiene, progressive relaxation, and weight management.
- Melatonin is a naturally occurring hormone produced at night by the pineal gland in the brain. It is used to treat primary insomnia and circadian rhythm sleep disorders and works by resetting the body's internal clock.
- Client and family teaching should focus on ways to promote healthy sleep-wake patterns, factors that enhance or disrupt sleep, sleep disorders and their treatment, and the consequences of noncompliance.

REFERENCES

1. Carskadon, MA, and Dement, WC: Normal human sleep: An overview. In Kryger, MH, Roth, T, and Dement, WC (eds): Principles and Practice of Sleep Medicine, ed 2. WB Saunders, Philadelphia, 1994.
2. Cziesler, CA, et al: Human sleep: Its duration and organization depend on its circadian phase. Science 210:1264, 1980.
3. American Psychiatric Association: Diagnostic and Statistical Manual of Mental Disorders, ed 4. American Psychiatric Association, Washington, DC, 1994.
4. Carskadon, MA: Patterns of sleep and sleepiness in adolescents. Pediatrics 17:5, 1990.
5. National Commission on Sleep Disorders Research: Wake Up America, A National Sleep Alert. US Department of Health and Human Services, Washington, DC, 1993.
6. Sullivan, CE, and Gruensetin, RR: Continuous positive airway pressure in sleep-disordered breathing. In Kryger, MH, Roth, T, and Dement, WC (eds): Principles and Practice of Sleep Medicine, ed 2. WB Saunders, Philadelphia, 1994.
7. Carskadon, MA, Vieira, C, and Acebo, C: Association between puberty and delayed phase preference. Sleep 16:258, 1993.
8. Glod, CA. Circadian dysregulation and abused individuals: A proposed theoretical model for practice and research. Arch Psychiatr Nurs 6:347, 1992.

CHAPTER 26
Adjustment Disorders

CHAPTER 26

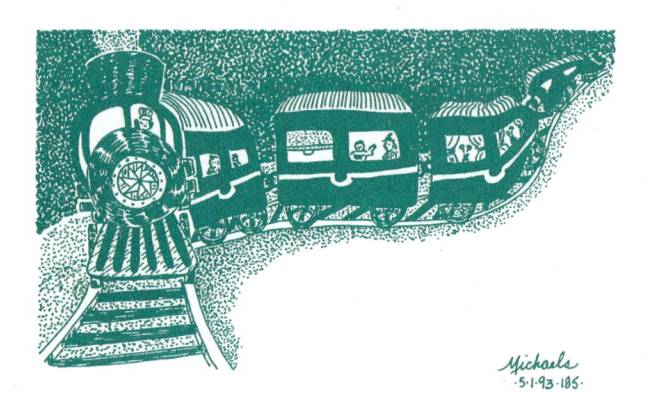

CHAPTER OUTLINE

Characteristic Behaviors
  Beginning Symptoms
Culture, Age, and Gender Features
Etiology
  Stress-Adaptation Theories
  Neuropharmacologic Theories
Prognosis
Planning Care
Interventions for Clients in the Community
  Interventions for Chronic Adjustment Disorders
  Cognitive-Behavior Therapy
  Pharmacologic Interventions
Client and Family Education
Expected Outcomes
Differential Diagnosis
  Mood Disorders
  Posttraumatic Stress Disorder (PTSD) and Acute Stress Disorder
  Bereavement
Common Nursing Diagnoses
Synopsis of Current Research
Areas for Future Research

LEARNING OBJECTIVES

After completing this chapter, the reader should be able to:

- List the prominent characteristics of adjustment disorders.
- Describe the different types of adjustment disorders and identify symptomatology associated with each.
- Differentiate between adjustment disorders and other major psychiatric disorders.
- Explain the development of adjustment disorders.
- Identify the personal and psychological sequelae of adjustment disorders.
- Analyze the impact of adjustment disorders on the individual's daily functioning.
- Implement the nursing process in planning care for the individual with an adjustment disorder.

KEY TERMS

adjustment
coping
stressor

Carol A. Glod, RN, CS, PhD

Adjustment Disorders

Adjustment disorders occur in response to a precipitating **stressor,** an event leading to marked distress and impairment. As seen in *DSM-IV* Diagnostic Criteria for Adjustment Disorders, these events range from losses such as separations, unemployment, divorce, and miscarriage to the diagnosis of an acute or chronic illness; they include circumstances surrounding developmental events such as leaving home and going to college. The reaction is manifested by significant impairment in social or occupational functioning or marked psychological distress.[1] Changes in mood and behavior are characteristic of these disorders. Most clinicians consider adjustment disorders to be mild conditions commonly treated in the community with counseling or psychotherapy. The diagnosis is made after major psychiatric conditions such as mood and anxiety disorders are ruled out.

> *I couldn't believe it—one day I was fine, teaching class, and the next day I thought, "Oh no, I'm going to die." I'd been having some stomach pain and nausea, so I went in for a few tests. The doctors told me it was my gallbladder and recommended that I have surgery right away. I arranged for a substitute teacher to cover my classes and scheduled the surgery. I never had any surgery before. In fact, I've always been pretty healthy. When I woke up after the operation, the surgeon told me that I had cancer. He explained that they removed a mass on my ovaries. I don't even remember what he said after that. I was so shocked. All I could think about was that my mother had died from ovarian cancer when she was 40. Now the same thing was happening to me. I cried for days. I still cry. I sometimes don't want to get out of bed and face the world. I can't stop thinking about what will happen to me. I still have to face chemotherapy and other treatment. I just wasn't prepared for any of this.*

Characteristic Behaviors
BEGINNING SYMPTOMS

Nurses are in a key position to identify those individuals at risk for developing adjustment disorders. The presence of a stressor, with its resulting sequelae of behavioral and emotional responses, indicates an individual at risk. The stressful conditions may be single events, such as ending a significant romantic relationship, or multiple events, such as financial difficulties and marital discord. Similarly, the stressor may be either recurrent in nature, such as seasonal business crises or exacerbations of illness, or continuous, such as living in a crime-ridden environment.[1] It can affect an individual, family, or community; natural disasters such as earthquakes and hurricanes are examples of community adjustment disorders. The stressor may accompany developmental changes when an individual attends college, leaves home, marries, becomes a parent, or retires.[1]

As with most disorders, it is important to assess and identify symptoms early in treatment. An early symptom is marked and extreme distress. Clients may complain of difficulty sleeping and poor concentration, or they may withdraw from life. Individuals with adjustment disorders may feel sad, tense, or on edge. Children and adolescents may display "acting out" behaviors: truancy, lying, stealing, or fighting.

Changes in mood and behavior are common; these individuals feel fearful, nervous, depressed, angry, worried, guilty, or a mixture of these states. The stressor may interfere with their ability to think and concentrate. They may find themselves "staring off into space" or plagued by thoughts about the stressful event; indecision or poor concentration results. Lowered confidence and decreased self-esteem frequently occur. Some experience sleep disruption and have difficulty falling or staying asleep. Others withdraw from the world and have little energy to accomplish things. Difficulties in interpersonal relationships may emerge, including tension, irritability, and frequent arguments.

For clients with adjustment disorders, these feelings and behaviors differ from their usual moods and states and are a direct response to a stressor. Each client has a unique response that may mimic past adjustment reactions. These reactions are maladaptive and interfere with completing work or school assignments. Individuals typically convey substantial psychological distress.

Adjustment usually occurs within 3 to 6 months of the stressor. Behaviors that last less than 6 months represent an acute adjustment disorder, whereas those that persist longer constitute chronic adjustment disorder.[1] For individuals faced with a long-term stressor, the adjustment period is longer. These clients are at high risk for developing worsening problems such as major depression, posttraumatic stress disorder (PTSD), and alcohol or substance abuse.

Depending on the specific behaviors, adjustment disorders are subtyped into categories (Table 26–1). Individuals who exhibit depressed mood, tearfulness, or feelings of hopelessness in response to a stressor suffer from adjustment disorder with depressed mood, whereas those who experi-

> **DSM-IV Diagnostic Criteria for Adjustment Disorders**
>
> A. The development of emotional or behavioral symptoms in response to an identifiable stressor(s) occurring within 3 months of the onset of the stressor(s).
> B. These symptoms or behaviors are clinically significant as evidenced by either of the following:
>   (1) marked distress that is in excess of what would be expected from exposure to the stressor
>   (2) significant impairment in social or occupational (academic) functioning
> C. The stress-related disturbance does not meet the criteria for another specific Axis I disorder and is not merely an exacerbation of a preexisting Axis I or Axis II disorder.
> D. The symptoms do not represent Bereavement.
> E. Once the stressor (or its consequences) has terminated, the symptoms do not persist for more than an additional 6 months.
>
> *Specify* if:
>   **Acute:** if the disturbance lasts less than 6 months
>   **Chronic:** if the disturbance lasts for 6 months or longer
>
> Adjustment Disorders are coded based on the subtype, which is selected according to the predominant symptoms. The specific stressor(s) can be specified on Axis IV.
>   309.0   With Depressed Mood
>   309.24 With Anxiety
>   309.28 With Mixed Anxiety and Depressed Mood
>   309.3   With Disturbance of Conduct
>   309.4   With Mixed Disturbance of Emotions and Conduct
>   309.9   Unspecified
>
> **Source:** Reprinted with permission from the Diagnostic and Statistical Manual of Mental Disorders, Fourth Edition. Copyright 1994 American Psychiatric Association.

TABLE 26–1. Axis IV: Psychosocial and Environmental Problems

> **Problems with Primary Support Group.** Death of a family member; health problems in family; disruption of family by separation, divorce, or estrangement; removal from the home; remarriage of parent; sexual or physical abuse; parental overprotection; neglect of child; inadequate discipline; discord with siblings; birth of a sibling.
>
> **Problems Related to the Social Environment.** Death or loss of friend; inadequate social support; living alone; difficulty with acculturation; discrimination; adjustment to life-cycle transition (such as retirement).
>
> **Educational Problems.** Illiteracy; academic problems; discord with teachers or classmates; inadequate school environment.
>
> **Occupational Problems.** Unemployment; threat of job loss; stressful work schedule; difficult work conditions; job dissatisfaction; job change; discord with boss or coworkers.
>
> **Housing Problems.** Homelessness; inadequate housing; unsafe neighborhood; discord with neighbors or landlord.
>
> **Economic Problems.** Extreme poverty; inadequate finances; insufficient welfare support.
>
> **Problems with Access to Health-Care Services.** Inadequate health-care services; transportation to health-care facilities unavailable; inadequate health insurance.
>
> **Problems Related to Interaction with the Legal System or Crime.** Arrest; incarceration; litigation; victim of crime.
>
> **Other Psychosocial and Environmental Problems.** Exposure to disasters, war, other hostilities; discord with nonfamily caregivers such as counselor, social worker, or physician; unavailability of social service agencies.

Source: Adapted from the Diagnostic and Statistical Manual of Mental Disorders, Fourth Edition. Copyright 1994 American Psychiatric Association.

ence nervousness, worry, or jitteriness have adjustment disorder with anxious mood.[1] When the predominant behaviors involve violation of the rights of others or of age-appropriate societal norms, adjustment disorder with disturbance of conduct is present. A combination of behaviors, such as both conduct and mood disruption, represents adjustment disorder with mixed disturbance of emotions and conduct. If nonspecific behaviors such as somatic complaints, social withdrawal, or difficulties in school or work performance predominate, adjustment disorder not otherwise specified (NOS) is present.

I knew that my wife had Alzheimer's disease, but I thought I'd be able to take care of her. We had planned our retirement carefully and decided to move to Florida. Well, we had a few happy years there. Her memory got so bad so fast; then she started wandering around the apartment all hours of the night. I finally had no choice—I had to place her in a nursing home. It nearly killed me to do it. Because it was so hard to say goodbye, I had my daughter-in-law take her to the nursing home. I can't bring myself to visit her. Everyone keeps telling me that it was the right thing to do because I couldn't take care of her anymore. I feel terribly guilty. Life just isn't the same anymore. I don't really do much. I just feel, "Why bother?" I walk around the apartment and remember all the things that we used to do together. I look at her clothes and other things and wonder how she's doing. I worry about her a lot and I worry about myself now too. Sometimes thoughts about her just go around and around in my head—I can't really read or concentrate on much. So much for retirement.

TABLE 26–2. Prevalence of Adjustment Disorders

Disorder	Prevalence
Adjustment disorder	5–20%*

*Of individuals treated in outpatient mental health settings.
Source: Adapted from the Diagnostic and Statistical Manual of Mental Disorders, Fourth Edition. Copyright 1994 American Psychiatric Association.

Culture, Age, and Gender Features

Adjustment disorders are some of the most common psychiatric conditions (Table 26–2). Because nearly everyone will be faced with a situational stress that produces a psychological response, these disorders affect both males and females of any age. Individuals subject to more disadvantaged or deprived circumstances may be at higher risk for developing an adjustment disorder.[1]

Culture

To judge whether an individual's response is maladaptive, knowledge of his or her personal and cultural background is necessary. An important characteristic is how the stressor is perceived and the meaning the client derives from it. An overwhelming stress may have little effect on one person, whereas a relatively minor one may have a profound effect on someone else. For instance, someone who has invested many years in a career and is suddenly laid off probably has derived from the job a large part of his or her sense of self and reason for living. Another individual may see unemployment as a way to reevaluate career ideas and an opportunity to return to school.

Age

Children may manifest the disorder through fears of separation or through conduct disturbances.

Etiology

STRESS-ADAPTATION THEORIES

The major etiologic theory proposes that a maladaptive coping response occurs as a reaction to the stressor and then leads to an "excessive" psychological response or distress (literally *dis-stress*), difficulty in interpersonal relationships, and poorer vocational functioning. Much of this theory is derived from the work of Lazarus,[2] who studied individuals' coping responses to various events. **Coping** is those behaviors and psychological reactions that occur in response to a threat. Lazarus proposed that the function of coping was to regulate problem-solving or adaptive behaviors. Callista Roy,[3] basing some of her work on these psychological theories, was the first nursing theorist to incorporate coping into a consolidated theoretical framework for nursing. Extending this work to coping with various illnesses, another nurse, Jean Johnson,[4] has been a pioneer in investigating the coping response to surgery, hysterectomy, colposcopy, and other surgical procedures. For instance, she found that preparation for surgery was beneficial prior to stressful surgical procedures because it promoted more effective coping.

NEUROPHARMACOLOGIC THEORIES

Little is known about the neuropharmacologic or genetic basis of adjustment disorders. What is known, however, is that acute stressors lead to dysfunction in the hypothalamic-pituitary-adrenal (HPA) axis. In contrast to chronic stress disorders, acute stress in both animals and humans results in the release of stress hormones. These corticosteroids aid the body's physiological and perhaps psychological response to stress (see Chapter 22).

Prognosis

Once identified, the course of illness is usually limited to weeks or months. However, chronic stressors, such as ongoing medical illness or chronic marital stress, may have a longer course. Some people may be at risk for suicide because of the nature and severity of their responses. Left untreated, these disorders may progress to mood and anxiety disorders.

Planning Care

Some individuals with adjustment disorders may be unaware of their reaction and its severity. Therefore, the first step in determining an effective treatment strategy is a complete evaluation. Adjustment disorders can be difficult to assess, particularly in medical settings or in the absence of a long-term relationship. Ask clients to describe the stressors to assess their level of distress. Because the reaction to the stressor represents a major change, obtain information about their baseline moods and behaviors. Ask how their current feelings and actions differ from usual ones. Information from significant others or school or business colleagues may help determine problems with social or occupational functioning. Ask family members and friends about changes in clients' mood and behaviors; establish whether they are currently different from their baselines.

Identify symptoms and help individuals understand their reactions to the stressors; ask about the presence of depressed mood, anxiety, crying, hopelessness, and anger. Evaluate any physical complaints such as headaches, backaches, or fatigue. Determine whether social withdrawal or work or school difficulty is a problem. After these symptoms are established, refer individuals to therapy, counseling, or self-help groups. Employee assistance programs (EAP) or school counseling services may be the most appropriate resources for those who are confronting an occupational or school stress. If suicidal ideation develops, more severe

> **Clinical Management Tips for the Individual with an Adjustment Disorder**
>
> *Effective Communication Strategies*
> - Use supportive statements such as "We'll find a way to help you with this."
> - Avoid overly simplistic statements such as "Everything will be fine."
> - Maintain a calm, comforting attitude.
>
> *Ways to Promote Healthy Coping*
> - Help the client identify the precipitating stressor.
> - Review ways the client has coped with stressful situations in the past.
> - Encourage journal writing to express feelings.
> - Ask about angry feelings and behaviors.
> - Provide regular contact with consistent staff.
> - Reinforce positive behavior and effective coping strategies.
> - Foster the expression of feelings through art, music, and other creative outlets.
> - Help the client begin or maintain a regular exercise program.
> - Encourage participation in self-help and support groups.
> - Encourage structure; jointly devise a daily plan.
> - Avoid anxiolytic medications; use them only for short-term relief of severe anxiety or insomnia.
> - Develop or encourage use of existing support systems.
> - Refer the client to appropriate social services and programs such as food stamps, school organizations, and shelters, if appropriate.
> - Help the client make decisions about incorporating the change or loss into his or her lifestyle.
> - Encourage the use of religious and spiritual beliefs to cope with the stressor.
>
> *Ways to Prevent Worsening Symptoms*
> - Observe the client's behavior frequently.
> - Carefully evaluate the presence of suicidal thoughts.
> - Encourage the client to verbally express feelings of sadness, loss, and nervousness.
> - Assess alcohol and drug use; encourage the client to avoid substances.
> - Avoid reinforcing dependent behaviors.
> - Continually evaluate behaviors and feelings; refer for further assessment if symptoms worsen.
> - Encourage the client to discuss how the stressful event will affect his or her life in the future.
> - Refer the client for short-term psychotherapy or cognitive-behavior therapy.
> - Encourage as much independence as possible.
> - Develop ways for the individual to resume work or school.
>
> *Client and Family Teaching*
> - Teach the client that adjustment disorders are usually short term.
> - Help the client identify resources within the community such as school, neighborhood, or church organizations.
> - Teach the client the benefits of progressive relaxation and other behavioral techniques.
> - Stress the need to avoid using drugs or alcohol, which may worsen the situation.
>
> **Source:** Adapted from Gorman, LM, et al: Davis's Manual of Psychosocial Nursing. FA Davis Co., Philadelphia, 1996.

problems may exist; refer them to a mental health professional.

Because the response is distressful and uncomfortable, complete an alcohol and drug evaluation. Clients commonly "self-medicate" with substances to cope with the stressor, leading to the potential for substance abuse or dependence. Ask family and friends about any changes in alcohol or drug use.

Interventions for Clients in the Community

Most individuals with adjustment disorders do not need psychiatric hospitalization. However, these disorders commonly occur in acute medical-surgical units, emergency rooms, and community clinics. The first step is to establish a trusting relationship to allow individuals time to express their feelings. Listening is a key intervention; allow clients time to express feelings and build rapport. Encourage clients to talk about their lifestyles prior to the disorder. Use supportive remarks to encourage them to disclose the events leading to their disorder. Promote regular one-to-one interactions and participation in groups. Use the clinical management techniques listed.

These clients can usually meet their daily obligations. To return to baseline functioning, they have to enhance their problem-solving skills and develop alternative coping strategies. Begin with helping them identify possible options to deal with their stressors. Review coping mechanisms that helped them deal with past stressors. Discuss the benefits and consequences of each option. Help clients select the most appropriate options and evaluate the responses. If possible, refer clients for short-term psychotherapy to systematically implement more adaptive coping.

Encourage socialization and help clients develop a support system or use existing ones. Help them devise regular schedules to structure each hour of their days. Refer them to appropriate self-help or support groups: disease-oriented groups such as multiple sclerosis, cancer, and chronic pain support groups; family support groups such as Alzheimer's support groups; or those that address a specific concern such as infertility, menopause, witnessing community or domestic violence, and transitioning into a nursing home. These groups can provide support, empathy, and practical suggestions from others who are coping with the same stressor.

Another strategy is to develop short-term support groups. For example, a utilization review nurse noted that many women experienced emotional, social, and occupational dysfunction after a hysterectomy. She began a short-term group to focus on the impact of hysterectomy upon their lives and to develop ways to minimize distress and promote more effective adaptation. The result was that women were able to share their experiences, derive support from one another, and suggest effective coping strategies to deal with the hysterectomy.

INTERVENTIONS FOR CHRONIC ADJUSTMENT DISORDERS

Most individuals who develop an adjustment disorder in response to a single event successfully cope with the stressor and resume functioning. By contrast, those exposed to a continuous or recurrent stressor may require long-term treatment; ongoing or recurring medical conditions or having a family member with a long-term illness such as Alzheimer's disease may lead to chronic adjustment disorder. An important treatment is ongoing support, teaching, and reinforcement of new coping mechanisms. Regular psychotherapy, individually or in a group, is essential.

Help clients devise a long-term plan to deal with the stressor. Teach and reinforce cognitive-behavior techniques. Encourage continued participation in self-help or support groups. Promote long-term sources of social support, including friends, family, neighbors, organized leisure groups, and religious activities. Stress the need for exercising regularly, maintaining nutrition, and obtaining adequate sleep and rest. Give reassurance and positive feedback when clients follow through successfully.

For individuals with a chronic adjustment disorder, hopelessness may become pervasive. Monitor for worsening symptoms suggestive of a more severe psychiatric disorder. Regularly assess alcohol and drug use. Ask about any suicidal thoughts or plans. Help clients reduce other forms of stress in their lives. For instance, for families caring for individuals with long-term illnesses, suggest respite care or day treatment, so that the families can take a break. Refer them to a financial advisor or to social service agencies if money is a major issue.

> **RESEARCH NOTE**
>
> **Sharts-Hopko, NC, Regan-Kubinski, MJ, Lincoln, PS, and Heverly, MA:** Problem-focused coping in HIV-infected mothers in relation to self-efficacy, uncertainty, social support, and psychological distress. Image J Nurs Sch 28:107–111, 1996.
>
> **Findings:** Women are increasingly becoming infected with HIV, yet there is very little information on how they cope with HIV and AIDS. This study investigated 41 HIV-infected mothers and their children to determine their level of coping and factors that influenced adaptation to the virus. The researchers found that women who coped better had higher levels of self-efficacy; they were better able to meet challenges associated with the infection and more confident. Participants who were better able to meet illness-related problems also had less psychological distress. Women whose children had HIV symptoms that lasted longer used fewer problem-solving coping strategies to deal with the stressor. Overall, the investigators found that women who used more adaptive coping mechanisms dealt with the infection better and showed less distress, particularly if their children had a short duration of HIV-related symptoms.
>
> **Application to Practice:** This study suggests that some women cope successfully with the uncertainty and threat of death secondary to HIV. Women with higher levels of self-efficacy appear to cope better. Women with lower levels of self-efficacy are probably at higher risk for maladaptive coping. Having a child with chronic symptoms may also lead to more psychological distress and maladaptive coping. Nursing interventions should target high-risk women with HIV to help them cope more effectively. Women with HIV can be taught that they can meet their parental responsibilities and deal with fatigue and other HIV-related symptoms. They can also be encouraged to participate in activities that enhance self-esteem, such as support groups, work, or volunteer opportunities. After individuals believe that they can meet their responsibilities and feel confident, their overall levels of coping should improve.

COGNITIVE-BEHAVIOR THERAPY

Cognitive-behavior therapy, provided individually or in a group, is a primary treatment. The overall goal is helping the individual effectively cope with disturbing thoughts, moods, and behaviors, promoting more effective functioning, and reducing impairment. Progressive relaxation, self-hypnosis, and desensitization are behavioral interventions aimed at dealing with emotional disruption, particularly if significant worry or anxiety predominates. Cognitive restructuring is very effective for managing unhealthy thoughts and providing alternative reactions to the stressor. Cognitive-behavior therapy is indicated for difficulty initiating or maintaining sleep, if insomnia is present. The strategies include establishing rapport and constructing a plan to deal with the situation, depending on the specific event and the client's resources. The therapist often draws on the client's resources and engages family and community supports. Often a combination of supportive and cognitive-behavior techniques effectively promotes adaptation to the stressor. Whether individual or group therapy is provided, these interventions are usually short-term.

PHARMACOLOGIC INTERVENTIONS

Overall, pharmacologic treatment is best avoided. Antidepressants are not usually indicated because the symptoms of major depression are absent and the presenting behaviors are time limited. If mood or behavioral consequences are severe, however, temporary, short-term, and careful use of certain medications such as benzodiazepines is sometimes indicated. Low doses of anxiolytics may be prescribed for severe anxiety. Sedative-hypnotics may be used for temporary relief of insomnia. Ideally, other measures, particularly individual psychotherapy and cognitive-behavior techniques, are tried before pharmacotherapy.

Client and Family Education

Client and family education is extremely important. Teaching interventions can enhance their understanding about the disorder and the negative effects of the stressor on their lives. Inform clients and families that their reactions are common and natural responses to a stressful event. Help them recognize and identify specific feelings and behaviors. Encourage maintaining or finding a relationship with a psychotherapist to learn more effective ways to cope with the situation. Teach them that adjustment disorders are time-limited and usually resolve within a few weeks or months. Support previously learned coping strategies that are effective and new ways to manage the stressor. Reinforce the need to avoid alcohol and drugs, and educate them about the potential problems that can arise because of substance abuse, such as sleep disruption, depression, and anxiety. Stress the need to report any suicidal thoughts that arise.

I spent many restless nights worrying about Teresa. If alcoholism produces insomnia for its victims, the family also battles this sleeplessness. I dreaded the late-night or early-morning telephone call lest it bring some new note of trouble and disappointment. I became obsessed with Terry's impact on our family gatherings, her children, her siblings, her employers, and her landlords, and her constant encounters with the police, emergency rooms, and treatment and detox centers. It pained me to feel the resentment of my other children, who understandably wondered if a parent so obsessed with one child had any time or concern left for them. Sometimes I tried to pull away from Terry, even when she may have most needed me, because I wanted the others to see that I wasn't totally absorbed in their sister.[5]

GEORGE McGOVERN

Expected Outcomes

For the client with an adjustment disorder, improvement will be demonstrated by:

- Beginning to recognize the impact of his or her response on relationships and occupational functioning.
- Devising short- and long-term goals to promote adaptive behaviors.
- Not engaging in self-destructive or suicidal actions.
- Identifying sources of continuing community support to facilitate coping.
- Avoiding self-medication with alcohol or illicit substances.
- Sustaining good concentration and decision-making abilities.
- Developing ways to perform role functions.
- Substituting more effective ways of relating to promote healthy adaptation.

Differential Diagnosis
MOOD DISORDERS

- Differential diagnosis is difficult because symptoms commonly overlap.
- Adjustment disorders can be distinguished from mood and anxiety disorders by the presence of a stressor; adjustment disorder *requires* the presence of a precipitating stressor.
- They also differ in the number and severity of symptoms that emerge acutely.
- In mood disorders such as major depression, a stressor may or may not be present; mood changes co-occur with many other symptoms, such as decreased appetite, sleep disruption, low energy, poor self-esteem, poor concentration, indecision, hopelessness, and thoughts of death.

POSTTRAUMATIC STRESS DISORDER (PTSD) AND ACUTE STRESS DISORDER

- PTSD and acute stress disorders are difficult to discern.
- In PTSD and acute stress disorder, the stressor is *extreme* and beyond a psychosocial stressor: Rape, torture, and life-threatening events are examples.
- Stress disorders include symptoms of reexperiencing the trauma, such as flashbacks, hyperarousal, and numbing.
- Adjustment disorders involve fewer and less severe symptoms that occur in response to mild, moderate, or severe psychosocial stressors.

BEREAVEMENT

- The disorders are differentiated by experiencing the death of a significant individual and certain symptoms.
- Bereavement involves the death of a loved one.
- Common symptoms include severe grief, guilt, worthlessness, decreased activity, and suicidal ideation.
- Adjustment disorder occurs in response to a wide range of psychosocial stressors, without guilt, suicidal ideation, and other reactions seen in bereavement.
- If the bereavement response is severe and prolonged, adjustment disorder may develop.

Common Nursing Diagnoses

- Coping, individual, ineffective
- Adjustment, impaired
- Communication, impaired verbal
- Hopelessness
- Powerlessness
- Sleep Pattern Disturbance
- Social Isolation
- Social Interaction, impaired
- Self Esteem disturbance
- Anxiety

Synopsis of Current Research

Over the past 5 years, more than 400 articles in the nursing literature investigated coping or psychological adaptation. Clearly, nurses remain a major force in studying the effects of adjustment to psychosocial stressors. This research has explored coping resources in the context of many medical and psychiatric disorders, conditions such as miscarriage and pregnancy, immigrant and migrant groups, caregiver stress, and the effects of developmental stress on special populations such as children and older adults.

To measure coping in clinical and nonclinical populations, nurse researchers[6] at Emory University tested a new instrument, the Cognitive Adaptation to Stressful Events Scale (CASE), with more than 200 pregnant women and subsequently during the postpartum period. This scale uses a cognitive model of adaptation to events, with particular emphasis on the meaning and mastery of the stressors. Another group[7] tested a commonly used scale, the Ways of Coping Questionnaire, with clients who have multiple sclerosis or spinal cord injury. They found that the individuals with long-term chronic illness used different coping strategies than did individuals without any illness.

Another substantial line of nursing research has investigated specific coping mechanisms, such as hope, social support, or uncertainty in different clinical samples. Marden and Rice[8] found that abused women's hope was an effective coping strategy; they used hope to deal with the conflict between their internal beliefs and the external reality of battering. Nichols[9] investigated social support networks of 20 adolescents with cancer by using the Norbeck Social Support Questionnaire (NSSQ). Overall, this researcher found that teenagers used and received a wide range of support from family, friends, and professionals, and they were highly satisfied with the support. Other studies have found that uncertainty associated with life-threatening illnesses influences coping and adaptation pervasively.[10]

Areas for Future Research

- What is the relationship between having an adjustment disorder and the subsequent development of major depression or PTSD?
- What are the most important behaviors that predict the development of an adjustment disorder?
- What are the most important nursing interventions that promote healthy adjustment to recurrent or chronic medical illness?
- What is the prevalence of adjustment disorders in immigrant groups?
- What communities are at highest risk for adjustment disorders?
- What can the nurse do to prevent adjustment disorders?

CASE STUDY

Gladys is an 89-year-old widow who immigrated from Poland 70 years ago. After managing a farm and living independently for all of her life, she was placed into a nursing home after she fell unexpectedly from her bed at home. Although she had cataracts and was legally blind, she was in relatively good health, and no detectable medical illnesses seemed to contribute to her fall. She related that she became tangled in her sheets during the night, fell out of bed, and was "too weak" to get up. The police broke down her door, sent a rescue team, and after a brief hospitalization, she was diagnosed with torn ligaments and severe contusions and lacerations, without head trauma. Gladys was placed into a rehabilitation hospital because of her inability to take care of herself and need to recover from her injuries.

Gladys arrived at the rehabilitation hospital at 10:00 pm, 2 to 3 hours after her usual bedtime. She was placed into a double room, asked to change, but went to bed in her clothes. Several days later, her daughter realized that, in the chaos, her mother had not been oriented to the placement, the hospital's routine, or the location of her belongings. As a result, she failed to brush her teeth, often slept in her clothes, and began eating very little. The regimented routine was totally foreign to Gladys because she had managed independently and had lived alone for several years. She did not engage in any group activities or conversation with her roommate. She complained that the staff was never around, that she often could not understand their language, and that the emergency room nurses took better care of her. In addition, she found the food intolerable ("like dog food"), because it was very different from her usual ethnic foods and unlike the fresh vegetables and fruit she had raised as a farmer. When the social worker asked how she liked being there, she replied, "I hate it," and turned away.

One of the nurses began to talk with Gladys each day to get to know her and to develop a trusting relationship. She asked about the things she liked to do and what led to her hospitalization. In establishing the relationship, the nurse used a janitor who knew some Polish to learn the language and to get the client to converse with someone else. She discovered that Gladys had been very active and independent most of her life, but that her cataracts severely limited her eyesight. She arranged for an ophthalmology consultation to assess whether surgery was possible. The nurse also found out that Gladys had been very active in her church; she arranged for some church members and the priest to visit her regularly.

The nurse also allowed Gladys to reminisce about her past and her love of dancing. She discovered that she had been an excellent cook. She arranged for her daughter to bring in tapes of Polish music to listen and sing along to. Eventually, the nurse devised a brief exercise program that Gladys performed with the music. Her daughter also brought in ethnic foods that Gladys liked. Although the nurse encouraged her to talk about her feelings, Gladys tended to keep them to herself, consistent with her past coping style. Despite encouragement to join other groups at the rehabilitation hospital, she socialized little, but did seek out her "friend," the janitor.

CRITICAL THINKING QUESTIONS

1. What behavioral clues suggested that Gladys had difficulty adjusting to placement?
2. What measures could the nurse or family employ to decrease her maladaptive behavior and promote more effective functioning?
3. What cultural considerations should be employed to help Gladys?
4. Explain the relationship between Gladys's background and her reaction to placement.
5. Develop a care plan, including short- and long-term goals for her rehabilitation.
6. Identify behaviors that indicate she is responding to treatment.
7. Select the most appropriate therapeutic approaches for treating Gladys as an outpatient.
8. Design a teaching plan to assist the family in caring for Gladys when she is discharged.

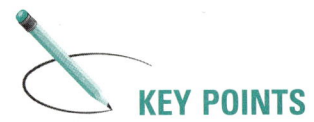

KEY POINTS

- Adjustment disorders occur in response to a precipitating stressor and are manifested by the development of significant impairment in social or occupational functioning or marked psychological distress.
- Depending on the specific behaviors, adjustment disorders are subtyped into certain categories; the most common are adjustment disorder with depressed mood and adjustment disorder with anxious mood.
- The reaction to the stressor is time limited and acute, beginning within 3 months of the onset of the precipitant and lasting perhaps several months.
- Adjustment disorders are some of the most common psychiatric conditions.
- Children may manifest adjustment disorders through fears of separation or through conduct disturbances.
- Left untreated, these disorders may progress to more severe mood and anxiety disorders such as major depression and PTSD.
- The major etiologic theory of adjustment disorders is that a maladaptive coping response occurs as a reaction to the stressor.
- Most individuals with adjustment disorders do not need psychiatric hospitalization. However, these disorders commonly occur in acute medical-surgical units, emergency rooms, and community clinics.
- Individual and group psychotherapy, particularly supportive and cognitive-behavior therapy, are the most effective treatments for adjustment disorders. The major intervention involves helping the client discover and develop effective coping strategies to promote optimal functioning.
- Self-help and support groups provide support, empathy, and practical suggestions from others who are coping with the stressor.
- Pharmacologic treatment is usually avoided in the individual with an adjustment disorder.
- Individuals exposed to continuous or recurrent stressors who then develop these adjustment disorders require long-term treatment.

REFERENCES

1. American Psychiatric Association: Diagnostic and Statistical Manual of Mental Disorders, ed 4. American Psychiatric Association, Washington, DC, 1994.
2. Lazarus, RS: Psychological Stress and the Coping Process. McGraw-Hill, Inc, New York, 1966.
3. Roy, C, and Andrews, HA: The Roy Adaptation Model. Appleton & Lange, Stamford, CT, 1991.
4. Johnson, JE: Coping with surgery. In Werley, HH, and Fitzpatrick, JJ (eds): Annual Review of Nursing Research (vol 2). Springer Publishing, New York, 1984, pp 107–132.
5. McGovern, G: Terry: My Daughter's Life-and-Death Struggle with Alcoholism. Villard, New York, 1996, pp 193–194.
6. Affonso, DD, et al: Cognitive adaptation to stressful events during pregnancy and postpartum: Development and testing of the CASE instrument. Nurs Res 43:338, 1994.
7. Wineman, NM, Durand, EJ, and McCulloch, BJ: Examination of the factor structure of the Ways of Coping Questionnaire with clinical populations. Nurs Res 43:268, 1994.
8. Marden, MO, and Rice, MJ: The use of hope as a coping mechanism in abused women. J Holist Nurs 13:70, 1995.
9. Nichols, ML: Social support and coping in young adolescents with cancer. Pediatr Nurs 21:235–240, 1995.
10. Mast, ME: Adult uncertainty in illness: A critical review of research. Sch Inq Nurs Pract 9:3, 1995.

CHAPTER 27
Personality Disorders

CHAPTER 27

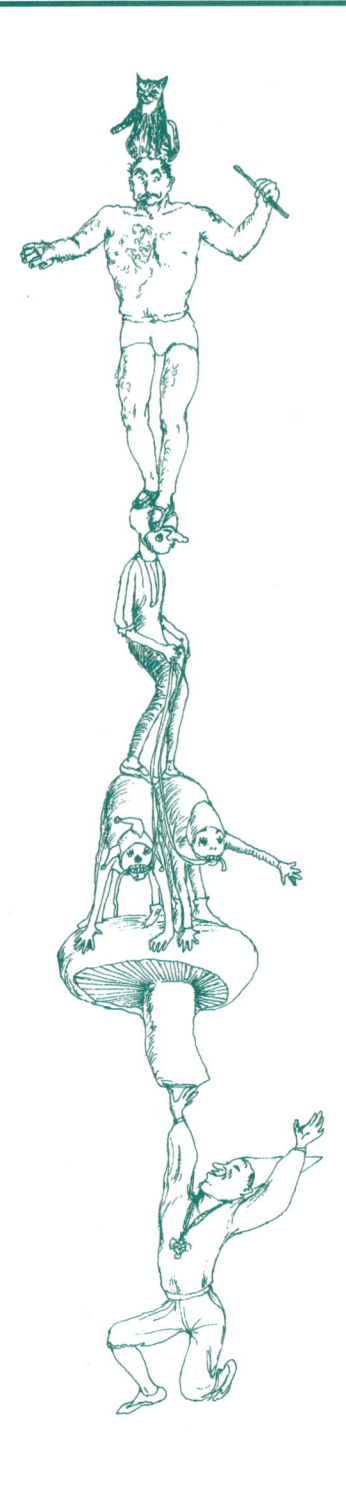

CHAPTER OUTLINE

Cluster A Personality Disorders
  Characteristic Behaviors
  Culture, Age, and Gender Features
  Etiology
  Prognosis
  Planning Care
  Interventions for Hospitalized Clients
  Interventions for Clients in the Community

Cluster B Personality Disorders
  Characteristic Behaviors
  Culture, Age, and Gender Features
  Etiology
  Prognosis
  Interventions for Hospitalized Clients
  Interventions for Clients in the Community

Cluster C Personality Disorders
  Characteristic Behaviors
  Culture, Age, and Gender Features
  Etiology
  Prognosis
  Interventions for Clients in the Community

Expected Outcomes
Differential Diagnosis
Common Nursing Diagnoses
Client and Family Education
Synopsis of Current Research
Areas for Future Research

LEARNING OBJECTIVES

After completing this chapter, the reader should be able to:

- List the prominent characteristics of personality disorders.
- Differentiate among personality disorders and understand their consequences.
- Explain the developmental and biological theories about the etiology of personality disorders.
- Identify the personal and psychological sequelae of personality disorders.
- Analyze the impact of personality disorders on the individual's daily functioning.
- Implement the nursing process in planning care for the individual with a personality disorder.

Carol A. Glod, RN, CS, PhD

Personality Disorders

KEY TERMS

antisocial
avoidant
borderline
dependent
histrionic
narcissistic
obsessive-compulsive personality disorder
paranoid
schizoid
schizotypal

Personality disorders are lasting patterns that result in significant social and occupational impairment. This pattern of inner experience and behavior goes beyond usual personality traits and is pervasive in two of the following areas: cognition, affect, interpersonal relationships, and impulse control.[1] Whatever the personality characteristics, the pattern is more than just a particular personality style. Ten different disorders are now recognized in three groups (Table 27–1). As shown in Table 27–2, personality disorders are generally uncommon.

All of the personality disorders consist of enduring patterns of relating, usually beginning in adolescence or early adulthood, that pervade nearly every area of the individual's life. A key feature is that the behaviors remain stable across different life situations, regardless of recent events or stressful circumstances. The clients with such a disorder may exhibit exacerbation of the condition during stressful events such as a medical illness. Personality disorders frequently coexist with major psychiatric disorders such as mood, anxiety, and substance-abuse disorders.

Some personality disorders may have identifiable precursors in childhood. For instance, some children who exhibit extreme shyness, social withdrawal, and fear of strangers may go on to develop avoidant personality. In contrast, children who exhibit truancy, aggression, deceitfulness, or theft suggestive of conduct disorder may eventually demonstrate antisocial behaviors. Isolation, poor peer relationships, and poor school performance during childhood may be precursors for schizoid personality. The addition of odd or eccentric behaviors, peculiar thoughts and language, and bizarre fantasies may lead to the development of schizotypal personality. If chronic physical illness or separation anxiety disorder is present in childhood, dependent personality disorder may result. Despite these possible predictors, personality disorders generally do not become evident until adolescence or early adulthood.

Although the onset of personality disorders is developmentally based and the course of behaviors is relatively stable over time, certain situations may bring them to the attention of others. A recent stress or loss, medical illness, or change in health status may exacerbate the personality disorder. Repeated difficulties in social, romantic, or occupational relationships may bring to light that an inner pattern of relating is at issue. In extreme situations, a suicide gesture or attempt may be the "signal" that an underlying maladaptive pattern has progressed to severe consequences.

Personality traits may be exaggerated during a medical illness, and certain personality disorders may become more pronounced during assessment or treatment for a major mental illness. The individual may present with behaviors characteristic of dysthymia, major depression, eating disorders, or substance-abuse disorders yet also possess a personality disorder. For instance, an individual with major depression may show little initiative and self-care deficits. If further investigation reveals a lifelong pattern of an inability to be alone, to make decisions, or to assume responsibility, the individual may have dependent personality disorder. However, if these behaviors were observed only during the depressive episode, they are related to the mood disorder because they are not stable or pervasive over several years.

Because personality disorders have profound effects on interpersonal relationships, families and significant others can provide essential information. Individuals close to the client may be the first to notice pervasive unhealthy behaviors. For instance, families may recognize the lack of stability in relationships seen in borderline personality or the lack of regard for others apparent in narcissistic personality. A family history of psychiatric disorders is also helpful in differential diagnosis. A family history of schizophrenia may suggest the presence of one of the cluster A personality disorders.

CLUSTER A PERSONALITY DISORDERS

Characteristic Behaviors

Each personality disorder has distinct features. General diagnostic criteria include an enduring pattern of inner experience and behavior, across different personal and social situations, of long duration (since adolescence or early adulthood), leading to significant distress or impairment, mani-

TABLE 27–1. DSM-IV Categories of Personality Disorders

Cluster A: Odd, Eccentric
Paranoid Personality Disorder
Distrustful, suspicious, lacks trust in others, bears grudges, accuses others of harm or plots.
Schizoid Personality Disorder
Detached from others, a "loner," little to no sexual intimacy, little involvement in activities, lacks close friends, cold or aloof.
Schizotypal Personality Disorder
Ideas of reference, odd beliefs, behavior, and speech, suspicious, inappropriate affect, lacks close friends.

Cluster B: Dramatic, Emotional, Erratic
Antisocial Personality Disorder
Lies, disregards and violates the rights of others, impulsive, aggressive, irresponsible.
Borderline Personality Disorder
Frequent mood changes, intense anger, suicidal, sees the world as good or bad, impulsive, feels empty, fears abandonment.
Histrionic Personality Disorder
Seeks attention, uses provocative behavior, easily suggestible, dramatic, flamboyant.
Narcissistic Personality Disorder
Arrogant, needs admiration, entitled, exploitative, grandiose, lacks empathy, preoccupied with power, beauty, or love.

Cluster C: Anxious, Fearful
Avoidant Personality Disorder
Avoids others and activities, fears rejection, feels inhibited and inept.
Dependent Personality Disorder
Passive, indecisive, fears loss of approval, has difficulty doing things alone, fails to assume responsibility.
Obsessive-Compulsive Personality Disorder
Perfectionistic, controlling, inflexible, overconscientious, stubborn, miserly.

Source: Adapted from the Diagnostic and Statistic Manual of Mental Disorders, Fourth Edition. Copyright 1994 American Psychiatric Association.

TABLE 27–2. Prevalence of Personality Disorders

Personality Disorder	Prevalence
Paranoid	0.5–2.5%
Schizotypal	3%
Schizoid	Unknown
Antisocial	3%*
Borderline	2%
Histrionic	2–3%
Narcissistic	<1%
Dependent	Unknown
Avoidant	1%
Obsessive-compulsive	1%

*Of males.
Source: Adapted from the Diagnostic and Statistical Manual of Mental Disorders, Fourth Edition. Copyright 1994 American Psychiatric Association.

---

fested in at least two of the following areas: cognition, affect, interpersonal functioning, and impulse control.[1]

Individuals who tend to be odd or eccentric make up cluster A. This group consists of paranoid, schizotypal, and schizoid personality disorders (see *DSM-IV* Diagnostic Criteria).

Paranoid Personality Disorder

Individuals with **paranoid** personality disorder are suspicious and mistrustful. They believe that others are plotting harm or talking about them behind their backs. Forming intimate relationships is difficult for them because they are so "on guard" and fear that others will hurt them. They may find "evidence" that confirms their suspicions and hold grudges against others. As a result, they have difficulty maintaining jobs and have few close relationships. Sometimes individuals with this disorder are aloof and removed, whereas others are very angry and aggressive.

I just knew that those people were going to cheat me. I could tell by the way they looked at me. I bet they thought I didn't notice them looking at me and talking about me. I don't know what they want from me.

Schizoid Personality Disorder

These individuals lack social and close relationships and have difficulty relating to others. They are usually isolated and, although they may work, hold jobs that require little or no contact with others. They are very isolated, usually do not marry, and have little interest in activities. Clients with **schizoid** personality disorder are loners who tend to be detached, show little emotion, and are indifferent to praise or criticism. They often appear to be emotionally cold or flat.

I don't understand why my son spends all day at his computer. He's been like that for years. He never had many friends in childhood, but in college he really withdrew from others. At first, I thought he was really into his studying for his degree in computer science. He doesn't have any friends, and he hasn't had a date or gone out to see a movie for years. I can understand being interested in computers, but he has no social life. He doesn't seem to mind having no friends, and he doesn't understand why I'm so worried about him. It's not like he's depressed or anything—he's just aloof and apathetic about things. I guess you'd call him a "loner." He's got nobody but me. What will happen to him as he gets older?

DSM-IV Diagnostic Criteria for Paranoid, Schizotypal, and Schizoid Personality Disorders

Diagnostic Criteria for 301.0 Paranoid Personality Disorder

A. A pervasive distrust and suspiciousness of others such that their motives are interpreted as malevolent, beginning by early adulthood and present in a variety of contexts, as indicated by four (or more) of the following:
   (1) suspects, without sufficient basis, that others are exploiting, harming, or deceiving him or her
   (2) is preoccupied with unjustified doubts about the loyalty or trustworthiness of friends or associates
   (3) is reluctant to confide in others because of unwarranted fear that the information will be used maliciously against him or her
   (4) reads hidden demeaning or threatening meanings into benign remarks or events
   (5) persistently bears grudges, i.e., is unforgiving of insults, injuries, or slights
   (6) perceives attacks on his or her character or reputation that are not apparent to others and is quick to react angrily or to counterattack
   (7) has recurrent suspicions, without justification, regarding fidelity of spouse or sexual partner

B. Does not occur exclusively during the course of Schizophrenia, a Mood Disorder With Psychotic Features, or another Psychotic Disorder and is not due to the direct physiological effects of a general medical condition.

NOTE: If criteria are met prior to the onset of Schizophrenia, add "Premorbid," e.g., "Paranoid Personality Disorder (Premorbid)."

Diagnostic Criteria for 301.22 Schizotypal Personality Disorder

A. A pervasive pattern of social and interpersonal deficits marked by acute discomfort with, and reduced capacity for, close relationships as well as by cognitive or perceptual distortions and eccentricities of behavior, beginning by early adulthood and present in a variety of contexts, as indicated by five (or more) of the following:
   (1) ideas of reference (excluding delusions of reference)
   (2) odd beliefs or magical thinking that influences behavior and is inconsistent with subcultural norms (e.g., superstitiousness, belief in clairvoyance, telepathy, or "sixth sense"; in children and adolescents, bizarre fantasies or preoccupations)
   (3) unusual perceptual experiences, including bodily illusions
   (4) odd thinking and speech (e.g., vague, circumstantial, metaphorical, overelaborate, or stereotyped)
   (5) suspiciousness or paranoid ideation
   (6) inappropriate or constricted affect
   (7) behavior or appearance that is odd, eccentric, or peculiar
   (8) lack of close friends or confidants other than first-degree relatives
   (9) excessive social anxiety that does not diminish with familiarity and tends to be associated with paranoid fears rather than negative judgments about self

B. Does not occur exclusively during the course of Schizophrenia, a Mood Disorder With Psychotic Features, another Psychotic Disorder, or a Pervasive Developmental Disorder.

NOTE: If criteria are met prior to the onset of Schizophrenia, add "Premorbid," e.g., "Schizotypal Personality Disorder (Premorbid)."

Diagnostic Criteria for 301.20 Schizoid Personality Disorder.

A. A pervasive pattern of detachment from social relationships and a restricted range of expression of emotions in interpersonal settings, beginning by early adulthood and present in a variety of contexts, as indicated by four (or more) of the following:
   (1) neither desires nor enjoys close relationships, including being part of a family
   (2) almost always chooses solitary activities
   (3) has little, if any, interest in having sexual experiences with another person
   (4) takes pleasure in few, if any, activities
   (5) lacks close friends or confidants other than first-degree relatives
   (6) appears indifferent to the praise or criticism of others
   (7) shows emotional coldness, detachment, or flattened affectivity

B. Does not occur exclusively during the course of Schizophrenia, a Mood Disorder With Psychotic Features, another Psychotic Disorder, or a Pervasive Developmental Disorder and is not due to the direct physiological effects of a general medical condition.

NOTE: If criteria are met prior to the onset of Schizophrenia, add "Premorbid," e.g., "Schizoid Personality Disorder (Premorbid)."

Source: Reprinted with permission from the Diagnostic and Statistical Manual of Mental Disorders, Fourth Edition. Copyright 1994 American Psychiatric Association.

Schizotypal Personality Disorder

Odd and peculiar speech, thoughts, and behaviors characterize **schizotypal** personality disorder. Ideas of reference, unusual beliefs, and clairvoyant experiences occur. These individuals are suspicious, lack friends, and display inappropriate affect. For instance, they may believe they can predict the future, dress oddly, and laugh when discussing serious matters. Their behavior frequently appears eccentric and out of the ordinary. They may talk to themselves in public or point to others for no reason. Some clients with schizotypal personality disorder display behaviors that seem like a milder, nonpsychotic state of schizophrenia.

> *Crazy—that's what people think of me. Hey, I live my life the way I want. I live on the streets and dress in whatever I can find. I don't need nobody, and I don't need nobody telling me what I can and can't do.*

Culture, Age, and Gender Features

Culture

An individual's cultural background and beliefs, seemingly odd or different from other cultures, do not represent a personality disorder. Different cultures value certain personality characteristics, and behaviors that reflect the usual habits, customs, or styles of a culture do not constitute a personality disorder. For instance, paranoid personality disorder may be confused with guarded or defensive behaviors displayed by immigrants or migrants or by religious beliefs and rituals (voodoo, speaking in tongues, shamanism, mind reading, magical beliefs, and sixth sense).[1]

Age

Children and adolescents are not usually diagnosed with personality disorders; dramatic or unusual behaviors may reflect a specific developmental stage. Personality disorders may begin in adolescence and develop a persistent stable pattern; the enduring pattern is solidified by early adulthood. Some individuals with personality disorders do not come to clinical attention until later in life, after the loss of a spouse or job.[1]

Gender

Gender differences in the cluster A personality disorders need further investigation. Schizotypal personality may be more common in males.

Etiology

Biologic Theories

There have been few studies on the neuropharmacologic or biological basis of personality disorders, in part because of traditional theoretical notions about their development. It is difficult to conclude that one specific biological abnormality is the source. Personality disorders develop according to a complicated interplay of environmental, genetic, and biological factors.

Biology plays an important role in schizotypal personality disorder; increased dopamine levels may explain its development. Research shows that increased levels of homovanillic acid (HVA), a metabolite of dopamine, in clients with schizotypal personality correlates with a higher number of psychotic symptoms displayed.[2,3] As in schizophrenia, more neuropsychological abnormalities, increased attentional and informational processing impairment, and eye movement abnormalities have been reported in individuals with schizotypal personality disorder.[2,4] These preliminary findings suggest that higher levels of dopamine and neuropsychological problems may reflect a biological basis for this condition.

Genetic

The clustering of certain personality disorders is evident in biological relatives; however, the exact role of genetic factors is unknown. Schizophrenia and cluster A personality disorders run in the same family, suggesting that they are inherited in some complex way. Individuals with paranoid, schizoid, or schizotypal personality disorders have an increased prevalence of schizophrenia in first-degree biological relatives.[5]

Twin and adoptive studies on personality disorders have revealed that certain personality traits, particularly fearfulness and shyness, may be inherited and continue long-term.[6] Another interesting study compared twins reared apart. Examining scores on a personality questionnaire, researchers found that about 50% of personality could be attributed to genetic factors.[7] As seen in Table 27-3, 11 personality traits were found to possess a genetic component. For instance,

TABLE 27-3. Personality Traits with a Genetic Contribution

Social potency: forcefulness, decisiveness vs. indecision
Achievement
Well-being: confidence, optimistic vs. pessimism
Social closeness
Stress reaction: nervousness, reactive vs. being less reactive
Alienation: feeling mistreated, unlucky vs. feeling one is treated fairly
Aggression
Traditionalism: following rules and standards, disciplined, religious vs. rebellious, nonquestioning behaviors
Harm avoidance: preferring safety and tedium vs. risk-taking behavior
Control: cautious, sensible vs. impulsive, spontaneous
Absorption: vivid imagination, fantasy vs. nonimaginative, reality-based reactions

Source: Adapted from Tellegren, A, et al: Personality similarity in twins reared apart and together. J Pers Soc Psychol 54:1031–1039, 1988.

one trait that may be inherited is well-being, a tendency to be either confident and optimistic or pessimistic. Another trait, stress reaction, a person's tendency toward being nervous and reactive to the environment or not, also appears to be inherited.

Psychoanalytic-Developmental Theories

Psychoanalytic and developmental theorists believe that parenting and environmental influences shape personality, and that personality is formed as the result of an interaction between the child's temperament and parenting and childhood experiences. In the extreme, these factors may lead to personality disorders. Problems in early childhood and in the parent's response may arrest normal development and lead to behaviors that become enduring personality patterns and disorders.

Cluster A personality disorders may arise from specific poor parenting experiences. For instance, paranoid personality may arise from childhood experiences of extreme parental rage or humiliation. The child may become suspicious of others and fear harm, leading to more pervasive paranoid patterns of relating to others. Children with cold, unavailable, and neglectful parents may view relationships as unimportant or not worth pursuing and develop schizoid personality disorder.

Prognosis

By definition, personality disorders are pervasive and affect the individual's long-term functioning. Cluster A personalities generally remain stable into older adulthood. The presence of a major Axis I psychiatric disorder such as mood disorder, substance abuse, or anxiety disorder, in combination with a personality disorder, is associated with poorer prognosis and a more deleterious course.

Planning Care

Referral for the treatment of a personality disorder is usually necessary when it impairs relationships or daily functioning. If another psychiatric disorder or substance abuse is the primary concern, then treatment for it takes precedence. If the individual is suicidal, immediate safety concerns need to be addressed. Hospitalization may be indicated. The individual may also need to be admitted for treatment of an Axis I psychiatric disorder such as mood disorder.

Because personality disorders are long-standing, long-term treatment is usually required. The client will need to be an active and willing participant in the lengthy and, at times, uncomfortable process to make substantive change. The client with a personality disorder frequently avoids getting help despite others' encouragement.

A complete assessment that includes a detailed evaluation of past and present psychiatric behaviors, health, and medication history is essential to rule out contributions from organic factors. Information should be obtained from both client and family. An electroencephalograph (EEG) or brain imaging study may be necessary to fully determine the nature of the presenting behaviors. A culturally sensitive evaluation will take into account whether the behaviors are consistent with cultural norms, such as superstition or magical thinking.

Interventions for Hospitalized Clients

Individuals with personality disorders are a challenge because their personality characteristics may be unpleasant and arouse strong feelings in providers. Maintaining a respectful, caring attitude can be difficult, even for the most experienced nurse. In acute situations, such as emergency rooms and medical-surgical units, the underlying personality dynamics may not be understood or recognized, and clients may be difficult to relate to. For example, clients with cluster A personality disorders may avoid eye contact and display odd communication patterns. If clients are hospitalized for another psychiatric disorder, apply the interventions that are appropriate for that condition. For example, if they are hospitalized for depression, use the interventions outlined for depressed clients.

Interventions for Clients in the Community

These individuals rarely seek psychiatric treatment. Because of the unusually eccentric and isolating nature of their problems, they avoid relationships. Strive to establish trust and rapport; however, this may be impossible except after years of consistent contact. Try to engage a trusted family member, if possible. Be honest and open, and attempt to react nondefensively to clients' paranoid or odd accusations. Ignore or gently confront peculiar beliefs and behaviors. Convey a caring and interested attitude, and be a role model for healthy relationships. Suggest cognitive-behavior therapy to encourage social skills and interactions.

Pharmacologic Treatment

Because personality disorders have traditionally been grounded in psychoanalytic-developmental theories, few studies on pharmacotherapy exist. However, individuals with personality disorders may be some of the most frequent users of medications. When assessing these clients, determine whether medications actually treat the underlying personality disorder or provide symptomatic relief. The most systematic study to date has focused on schizotypal and borderline personality disorders.

Schizotypal Personality Disorder. The antipsychotic agents haloperidol and thiothixene have been shown to reduce transient episodes of psychosis, odd communication, illusions, phobic anxiety, and ideas of reference. Antipsychotics may reduce symptoms through their effects on dopamine; more research is needed. Low doses of antipsy-

DSM-IV Diagnostic Criteria for Antisocial, Borderline, Histrionic, and Narcissistic Personality Disorders

Diagnostic Criteria for 301.7 Antisocial Personality Disorder

A. There is a pervasive pattern of disregard for and violation of the rights of others occurring since age 15 years, as indicated by three (or more) of the following:
 (1) failure to conform to social norms with respect to lawful behaviors as indicated by repeatedly performing acts that are grounds for arrest
 (2) deceitfulness, as indicated by repeated lying, use of aliases, or conning others for personal profit or pleasure
 (3) impulsivity or failure to plan ahead
 (4) irritability and aggressiveness, as indicated by repeated physical fights or assaults
 (5) reckless disregard for safety of self or others
 (6) consistent irresponsibility, as indicated by repeated failure to sustain consistent work behavior or honor financial obligations
 (7) lack of remorse, as indicated by being indifferent to or rationalizing having hurt, mistreated, or stolen from another

B. The individual is at least age 18 years.

C. There is evidence of Conduct Disorder with onset before age 15 years.

D. The occurrence of antisocial behavior is not exclusively during the course of Schizophrenia or a Manic Episode.

Diagnostic Criteria for 301.83 Borderline Personality Disorder

A pervasive pattern of instability of interpersonal relationships, self-image, and affects, and marked impulsivity beginning by early adulthood and present in a variety of contexts, as indicated by five (or more) of the following:
 (1) frantic efforts to avoid real or imagined abandonment.
 NOTE: Do not include suicidal or self-mutilating behavior covered in Criterion 5.
 (2) a pattern of unstable and intense interpersonal relationships characterized by alternating between extremes of idealization and devaluation
 (3) identity disturbance: markedly and persistently unstable self-image or sense of self
 (4) impulsivity in at least two areas that are potentially self-damaging (e.g., spending, sex, substance abuse, reckless driving, binge eating).
 Note: Do not include suicidal or self-mutilating behavior covered in Criterion 5.
 (5) recurrent suicidal behavior, gestures, or threats, or self-mutilating behavior
 (6) affective instability due to a marked reactivity of mood (e.g., intense episodic dysphoria, irritability, or anxiety usually lasting a few hours and only rarely more than a few days)
 (7) chronic feelings of emptiness
 (8) inappropriate, intense anger or difficulty controlling anger (e.g., frequent displays of temper, constant anger, recurrent physical fights)
 (9) transient, stress-related paranoid ideation or severe dissociative symptoms

Diagnostic Criteria for 301.50 Histrionic Personality Disorder

A pervasive pattern of excessive emotionality and attention seeking, beginning by early adulthood and present in a variety of contexts, as indicated by five (or more) of the following:
 (1) is uncomfortable in situations in which he or she is not the center of attention
 (2) interaction with others is often characterized by inappropriate sexually seductive or provocative behavior
 (3) displays rapidly shifting and shallow expression of emotions
 (4) consistently uses physical appearance to draw attention to self
 (5) has a style of speech that is excessively impressionistic and lacking in detail
 (6) shows self-dramatization, theatricality, and exaggerated expression of emotion
 (7) is suggestible, i.e., easily influenced by others or circumstances
 (8) considers relationships to be more intimate than they actually are

Diagnostic Criteria for 301.81 Narcissistic Personality Disorder

A pervasive pattern of grandiosity (in fantasy or behavior), need for admiration, and lack of empathy, beginning by early adulthood and present in a variety of contexts, as indicated by five (or more) of the following:
 (1) has a grandiose sense of self-importance (e.g., exaggerates achievements and talents, expects to be recognized as superior without commensurate achievements)
 (2) is preoccupied with fantasies of unlimited success, power, brilliance, beauty, or ideal love
 (3) believes that he or she is "special" and unique and can only be understood by, or should associate with, other special or high-status people (or institutions)
 (4) requires excessive admiration
 (5) has a sense of entitlement, i.e., unreasonable expectations of especially favorable treatment or automatic compliance with his or her expectations
 (6) is interpersonally exploitative, i.e., takes advantage of others to achieve his or her own ends
 (7) lacks empathy: is unwilling to recognize or identify with the feelings and needs of others
 (8) is often envious of others or believes that others are envious of him or her
 (9) shows arrogant, haughty behaviors or attitudes

Source: Reprinted with permission from the Diagnostic and Statistical Manual of Mental Disorders, Fourth Edition. Copyright 1994 American Psychiatric Association.

chotic medications may be useful in treating the behaviors associated with schizotypal personality; because of the limited amount of information available, however, they should be used cautiously. A short-term trial might be of benefit, with careful assessment of efficacy and regular observation for the development of side effects, including tardive dyskinesia.

CLUSTER B PERSONALITY DISORDERS

Characteristic Behaviors

Tendencies to be dramatic, emotional, or erratic form cluster B personality disorders, the antisocial, borderline, histrionic, and narcissistic personality disorders (see *DSM-IV* Diagnostic Criteria).

Antisocial Personality Disorder

Individuals with **antisocial** personality disorder have a long-standing pattern of lack of concern for and violation of the rights of others. They display socially irresponsible behaviors including lying, stealing, physical fights, disregard for safety of others, and behaviors that result in reckless actions or breaking the law. Clients with antisocial personality disorder often do not feel remorseful over the harm or pain they cause. They may blame others and fail to take responsibility for their actions. As children, they often displayed conduct problems such as truancy, assaults, cruelty to animals, fire-setting, stealing, and substance abuse.

I tried to raise my son to know right and wrong. Even when he was little, he didn't seem right. He had a cat that he used to hurt—I don't even like to remember the things he'd do. He started stealing from us; he'd just take money out of my wallet and then deny it. Then he progressed to stealing from others, running away, and then he became a junkie. I never raised him to be that way.

Borderline Personality Disorder

Borderline personality is one of the most disruptive disorders; it is characterized by unstable and intense interpersonal relationships. The hallmark of borderline personality disorder is manipulative, demanding, needy, and angry behavior (see The Hemophiliacs of Emotion). These individuals are unable to form secure relationships with others and frantically avoid real or imagined loss or abandonment. When threatened with some type of interpersonal separation, clients shift from admiring, liking, and even loving the other individual to devaluing and hating them.

This fluctuation of good and bad views of the world and of relationships is termed *splitting*. For instance, they may see the staff or their families as good or bad or may shift in their perceptions, idealizing nurses one moment and demeaning them the next. Clients with borderline personality disorder are often angry, rageful, and vindictive. Mood shifts, impulsive eating or spending, and acts of physical harm are common. Repeated suicidal threats and actions emerge. For instance, they may repeatedly threaten to overdose or cut their wrists.

Nobody cares about me. I'm just unlovable. Sometimes I think that my husband wishes I was dead. There's just no point to living—I could kill myself at any time. I have plenty of pills, and I've planned to overdose many times. In the past I would

---

THE HEMOPHILIACS OF EMOTION

In the book, *I Hate You—Don't Leave Me: Understanding the Borderline Personality*, the authors describe and interview individuals with borderline personality disorder. They describe them as "hemophiliacs of emotion" because they "lack the clotting mechanism" that regulates feelings, causing them to "emotionally bleed to death." For them, life is a set of emotional roller coaster rides. Those affected have chaotic, baffling, reactive, impulsive, and self-destructive lives. Instead of seeing the world as ambiguous and filled with shades of gray, individuals with borderline personality disorder see it as black and white; other people are worshiped one minute and devalued the next. Because they fear abandonment, clinging behavior results; because they fear engulfment, rejecting behaviors result.

> Usually I'm okay . . . But there's another side that takes over and controls me. I'm a good mother. But my other side makes me a whore; it makes me act crazy!

Many have had negative childhood experiences including sexual abuse and neglect. Therapists and other health-care providers who try to help these clients may feel they "have a tiger by the tail." One message from a client, "I hate you—don't leave me!" describes borderline personality disorder. Interactions with these clients are stormy and changable, just like their underlying emotions and behaviors. They may frequently threaten suicide, often in response to what they see as a rejection or loss. They may also lose themselves in dissociative states: periods of detachment from themselves and reality. Self-mutilation such as wrist cutting or overdosing may result.

> Gloria tells her husband Alex that she is forlorn and depressed. She says she plans to kill herself but forbids him from seeking help for her. In this situation, Alex is confronted with two messages: 1, Gloria's overt message, which essentially states, "if you care about me, you will respect my wishes and not challenge my autonomy to control my own destiny and die, if I choose," and 2, the opposite message, conveyed in the very act of announcing her intentions, which says, "For God's sake, if you care about me, help me, and don't let me die."

Kreisman, JJ, and Strauss, H: I Hate You—Don't Leave Me: Understanding The Borderline Personality. Avon Books, New York, 1989.

> *slit my wrists a little, and I have scars from all the cutting. My husband threatened to leave me a few times. If he did leave, he'd be sorry. I started screaming at him the other day. I was really out of control, but I was so mad I couldn't help it. At first I told him to leave. Then I told him I couldn't live without him. Sometimes I really love him and think he's the greatest man on earth; other times he's a jerk. I don't really understand myself very well. One minute I'm furious, like I could kill someone, the next I'm scared, and the next I'm depressed. I think that's what led to my getting fired from a few jobs. They just wanted someone who was quiet, complacent, and a good little girl. So I was a little outspoken—I have a right to my opinions. Things just got too hard for them to handle.*

Clinical Management Tips for the Manipulative Client

Effective Communication Strategies
- Maintain an honest, respectful, and nonretaliatory stance.
- Avoid labeling the client as manipulative; establish a pattern of behavior that can be changed.
- Avoid ultimatums or control struggles.
- Encourage putting feelings into words rather than actions.
- Offer empathic statements.
- Confront the client who tries to undermine other clients' treatment.
- Monitor your own reactions to avoid becoming defensive.
- Discuss neutral and less emotionally charged topics.
- Encourage control over daily decisions.

Ways to Promote Healthy Interactions and Functioning
- Set clear, realistic expectations.
- Determine the goal behind manipulative behaviors.
- Engage clients in developing their treatment plans.
- Schedule regular talks with consistent staff if possible.
- Provide feedback about observations of manipulations using clear behavioral examples.
- Give positive reinforcement for appropriate behavior.
- Encourage as much independence as the client can tolerate.
- Use supervision and consultation with other staff.
- Avoid collusion with "splitting" behaviors.
- Help the client identify triggers for manipulative behaviors.
- Review the client's behaviors with interdisciplinary staff to promote consistency.

Client and Family Education
- Inform clients about which behaviors are unacceptable and give rationale.
- Discuss alternate ways that the client can deal with situations and feelings.
- Teach about the benefits of participation in activities such as exercise, journal writing, and activity groups.
- Teach families to avoid collusion with "splitting" behaviors.

Ways to Reduce or Prevent Violence to Self or Others
- Confront verbal and physical threats of harm.
- Use "time outs," periods of time that the client can think about his or her behavior before discussing it further.
- Set limits on unacceptable, dangerous, or inappropriate behaviors.
- Give the client options for behaving.
- Develop a written contract with the client about acceptable and appropriate behaviors.
- Describe the consequences for potentially dangerous behavior and enforce any consequences that have been reviewed.
- Point out that the behaviors are undermining the client's care.

Histrionic Personality Disorder

These individuals are nearly always seeking attention. They draw notice to themselves through their dramatic speech, flamboyant dress, or sexually provocative behaviors. At times, they may portray themselves as victim or princess.[1] Their feelings are often excessive, shallow, changeable, and short-lived. Their flair for the dramatic pervades all situations and relationships. Clients with **histrionic** personality disorder want desperately to be noticed and liked. Underneath the facade, however, are feelings of insecurity, low self-esteem, and inadequacy.

> *My daughter has always had to be the "life of the party." She needed the spotlight; in fact, she was a very good actress in her high school play. But she never seems to have close friends. Other people get turned off by her flair and need for attention. She describes them as her "dear" friends, when they don't want to have much to do with her. I don't think she realizes her effect on them.*

Narcissistic Personality Disorder

This disorder consists of an extreme sense of arrogance, entitlement, and self-importance. Individuals exaggerate their abilities, need to be admired excessively, and believe they have high status, in response to underlying low self-esteem. They frequently use other individuals for their own needs. Clients with **narcissistic** personality disorder are driven by their "self-love" and take advantage of others or fail to have empathy for them. They focus almost exclusively on themselves and their own needs.

> *I have been married three times; women just can't seem to understand me. They don't appreciate my unique style and status. In fact, they didn't appreciate that I was the best thing that ever to happened to them. Who needs them anyway? I was just wasting my time with them.*

Culture, Age, and Gender Features

Age

Antisocial personality disorder is not diagnosed until after age 18; conduct disorder in childhood usually precedes its development. Antisocial and borderline personality disorder may be less common in older adults.

Gender

Antisocial personality disorder is more commonly seen in men, whereas borderline and histrionic personality disorders are more common in women.[1] It remains unclear whether this reflects true gender differences, or whether particular traits or behaviors are associated with gender stereotypes. Of those diagnosed with borderline personality disorder, 75% are female, whereas with narcissistic personality, 50 to 75% are male.[1]

Etiology

Biological Theories

An important biological study compared serotonergic functioning in major depression personality disorders. Because borderline personality is most commonly associated with impulsive aggression, researchers hypothesized a psychobiological basis in this condition. Specifically, they suggested that reduced serotonin may lead to borderline personality disorder. In a complicated test of the serotonin system, an agent that enhances serotonin release (fenfluramine) was given to individuals, and serotonin activity was measured indirectly. Reduced serotonergic functioning was found in some of the clients with personality disorders, particularly those with impulsive and aggressive behaviors.[8] In the depressed group, only those individuals with aggressive suicidal behaviors had decreased serotonin. Thus, reduced serotonin may be a major explanation for the development of borderline personality disorder.

Preliminary studies have also found cholinergic dysfunction and increased norepinephrine in individuals with borderline personality disorder. In particular, increased norepinephrine was associated with irritability and hostility, commonly observed in borderline personality disorder.[9]

Genetic Theories

Antisocial personality disorder is more common among first-degree biological relatives with the disorder, with a greater risk of developing the disorder if the relative is female.[1] Children of parents with antisocial personality disorder, whether adopted or biological, are also at increased risk, suggesting that both environmental and genetic factors play a role. Borderline personality disorder is about five times more common in first-degree biological relatives.[1] No specific data are available on the influence of heredity on the other cluster B personality disorders.

Psychoanalytic-Developmental Theories

Cluster B personality disorders may also develop because of specific parental failures early in childhood. Borderline per-

---

Clinical Management Tips for the Dependent Client

Effective Communication Strategies
- Convey a sense of optimism about the client's abilities.
- Use a patient, nonaggressive tone.
- Set limits on negative remarks that lessen self-confidence.
- Avoid making decisions or taking-over behaviors.
- Devise short- and long-term goals; state them in understandable language.

Ways to Encourage More Independent Functioning
- Strongly encourage the client's self-care and hygiene activities.
- Promote participation in activities that encourage accomplishment.
- Engage the client in treatment planning.
- Give several choices to promote independent decision making.
- Encourage participation in assertiveness training.
- Role model taking responsibility for decisions and actions.
- Directly outline what behaviors the client is expected to do and what will be done for him or her.
- Set limits on behavior that attempts to engage others in doing things for the client.
- Explore the underlying feelings of inadequacy, shame, anxiety, and fear.
- Reinforce the client's attempts at more independent behaviors.
- Give positive feedback for healthy independent behaviors.
- Identify healthy supports for the client.
- Point out that the behaviors are undermining the client's care.
- Help the client identify triggers for dependent behaviors.
- Set limits on childlike or whiny behavior.

Client and Family Education
- Teach problem-solving skills.
- Emphasize the client's strengths.
- Teach families to avoid "taking over" and making decisions for clients.
- Review the importance of focusing on behavioral change.

---

sonality has been the most extensively studied; it may result from the parents' difficulty in managing the young child's attempts to separate, or the parents may aggravate the child's anger or neglect the child's feelings.[10,11] The child fails to develop healthy intimate relationships or a healthy sense of self.

Individuals with antisocial personality disorder may have parents with antisocial personality and substance-abuse disorders that led them to ignore the needs of their children, who then develop antisocial personality disorder and ignore the needs of others. Histrionic personality disorder may arise from difficult childhood experiences from ages 3 to 5 years. For instance, parents may strongly encourage dramatic and sexually provocative behaviors that continue to develop into exaggerated fantasies and attention-seeking behaviors. Narcissistic personality disorder may be due to extremely critical or neglectful experiences in early childhood.

Childhood Abuse and Trauma Theories

Driven in part by the feminist movement and an increasing understanding of women's development and psychology, another theory of borderline personality disorder is the influence of severe physical or sexual abuse in childhood. Pioneering work by Herman, Perry, and van der Kolk[12] revealed that 81% of clients with borderline personality reported a history of childhood trauma. Since then, several studies have documented high rates of abuse in individuals with borderline personality disorder and suggested an overlap between this disorder and posttraumatic stress disorder (PTSD). In fact, several clinical features are evident in both conditions: affective instability, impulsivity, difficulty in relationships, dissociation, and a tendency toward substance abuse. Although the distinction between borderline personality and PTSD is blurred, severe trauma in the form of physical and sexual abuse during early development may lead to borderline personality disorder. Many unanswered questions remain: whether PTSD and borderline personality disorder are distinct disorders, variations of the same disorder, or influenced by the development of the other.

Prognosis

Borderline and antisocial personality disorders may remit over time, waning in later life. Clients with borderline personality disorder often engage in self-destructive behavior, leading perhaps to higher mortality due to suicide. Antisocial behaviors may result in criminal behavior and subsequent incarceration.

Interventions for Hospitalized Clients

Develop a treatment plan that encourages appropriate expression of feelings and independence. To prevent regression and dependency and to enhance control over behavior, promote self-reliance. Regular, consistently scheduled contact with staff can be invaluable in avoiding overreliance on others and in reinforcing treatment. These talks should focus on short- and long-term goals, as well as assessing the client's needs. Group therapy can take the form of specific "here and now" interventions or center on the effects and consequences of behavior. Confrontation from other clients can be particularly effective in enhancing their understanding of behavior's impact on relationships and in helping to develop healthier ways of relating. Exploration of trauma memories

---

Clinical Management Tips for the Angry Client

- Firmly and calmly instruct the client to stop angry behavior.
- Avoid touching the client.
- Maintain a calm, respectful, and patient approach.
- Offer staff talks in a quiet, undisturbed place; avoid letting the client express anger publicly.
- Treat the client with respect and try not to react angrily or defensively.
- Avoid ultimatums or control struggles.
- Avoid arguments and criticism.

Ways to Promote Healthy and Appropriate Expression of Feelings

- Identify triggers to angry remarks and behaviors.
- Focus on discussing feelings when the client is in control.
- Role model appropriate responses and help the client practice these skills.
- Focus on the client's ability to cope with anger in healthier ways.
- Discern what other feelings, such as anxiety, fear, depression, or guilt, may underlie the anger.
- Set limits on excessive complaining or degrading remarks.
- Encourage the client to accept responsibility and avoid blaming others for anger.
- Engage the client in developing treatment plans.
- Use written contracts to reinforce healthy behavior.
- Teach assertiveness training.
- Problem solve other ways to manage angry situations.
- Explore and clarify any false assumptions underlying the client's anger.

Ways to Prevent Aggression

- Monitor anger for escalation into aggressive behaviors.
- Maintain a safe environment for the client and others.
- Encourage exercise and relaxation techniques to redirect anger.
- Promote participation in activities such as art, journal writing, and music.
- Offer medication if appropriate.
- Be on guard for impulsive angry behaviors.
- Set limits on unacceptable, dangerous, or inappropriate behaviors.
- Give positive reinforcement for appropriate behavior.
- Allow the client time to control behavior before discussing anger.
- Tell the client that you want to help him or her maintain control.
- Assess whether paranoid or psychotic behavior is present.

or upsetting childhood experiences is generally best dealt with in long-term treatment. Maintain the focus on what, if anything, precipitated the difficulties. The majority of work, however, will occur in long-term group or individual day programs to address the pervasive and enduring personality patterns.

Pay attention to one's reactions to these clients. Borderline personality disorder, often a pejorative label, evokes negative feelings such as anger and dislike in providers. The client may become intensely attached to a nurse, or the nurse may become the target of extreme, unstable feelings. Antisocial personality may conjure up images of criminals or "deadbeats," whereas dependent personality is associated with reactions of extreme neediness. The client may have extreme fears of abandonment that become aroused in treatment relationships.

The individual with borderline personality disorder may need frequent, brief hospitalizations for stabilization. The hospital milieu is also subject to splitting; the client may see it as safe and helpful at one point and dangerous and unfavorable the next. One technique is to anticipate shifts in perception, knowing that the "love" or "good" that the individual is currently expressing may quickly turn to anger and hate. If the client engages in extreme emotions or views, avoid collusion. Clarify the realities of the situation. For instance, if the client states that a particular nurse or doctor is "the most caring, understanding individual, and the only one capable of helping," point out that although the caregiver is certainly competent, there are other capable staff. Collaborating with a peer or supervisor or suggesting a consultation may also help manage these behaviors.

An essential component of milieu therapy is to assess suicide potential, especially in those with borderline personality disorder. Take any suicidal behavior or threats seriously. A daily "contract," in essence an agreement about not acting on suicidal impulses, should be devised. As part of the contract, develop very specific short-term goals with the client, such as daily self-care activities, regular schedules, attending group and individual therapy sessions, and making phone calls for discharge planning. Along with these actions, support positive and appropriate behavior; focus on healthy behaviors. Encourage the client to put feelings into words rather than act out feelings, particularly self-destructively. If dangerous behavior does result, clarify it for the client. For instance, the individual who ingests several pills, such as benzodiazepines, may believe this dose is not lethal; however, this behavior could have grave consequences like sedation and vomiting, with possible aspiration, or ataxia and dizziness, falling, and a severe head injury or coma.

Interventions for Clients in the Community

One of the major challenges in providing care for clients with personality disorders is the pervasiveness of their unhealthy behaviors. They may be particularly difficult to work with long-term. The mainstay of treatment is ongoing individual and possibly group psychotherapy. For change to occur, several years of intense treatment is often necessary, which requires a commitment from both therapist and client. For some clients, rehospitalization is necessary, and a major role for nursing is case management of individuals with personality disorders. Part of this role entails advocating for clients when hospitalization or acute day treatment is necessary. Some of these clients are frequent and active users of healthcare resources and as a result may be denied adequate treatment. For instance, some insurers have determined that hospitalization is not effective for those with borderline personality disorder, yet a serious suicide threat or attempt requires intensive treatment.

Because the behaviors are enduring, these individuals may drift in and out of treatment or reject help. One part of long-term treatment includes helping clients develop an understanding of the effects of their behaviors on relationships, occupational functioning, and overall quality of life and well-being. As clients with a personality disorder age, there is some suggestion that the features wane, although further study is necessary.

Specific interventions for antisocial, borderline, histrionic, and narcissistic personality disorders are complicated. The most important factor is to remain objective, accept the client's difficulties, and avoid developing a relationship in which feelings of anger, disgust, or neglect predominate. Remain aware that relationships have been problematic for these clients. Try not to react with dislike or retaliate. Keep in mind that individuals with dramatic, emotional personality disorders frequently have low self-esteem underlying their patterns of relating. Suggest individual psychotherapy to help change unhealthy personality patterns. For individuals with borderline personality disorder, recommend time-limited and cognitive-behavior strategies. If manipulation or anger predominates, use the clinical management tips later in this chapter. Unfortunately, no specific interventions are effective for antisocial personality disorder.

Individuals with personality disorders may lie or display manipulative or other destructive behaviors. Those with narcissistic personality may try to take advantage of other clients or staff. One important aspect of nursing care is to confront and set limits on these behaviors.

Cognitive-Behavior Treatment

Of the most promising therapies for personality disorders, especially borderline personality, is individual and group cognitive-behavior therapy (CBT). Therapists use a particular type of CBT called *dialectical behavior therapy*. Developed by Marsha Linehan,[13] dialectical behavioral therapy is a comprehensive long-term treatment approach that uses specific techniques to diminish destructive behaviors and improve interpersonal relationships. This treatment is based on the theory that those with borderline personality disorder lack certain interpersonal, emotion-regulation, distress-tolerance, and self-regulation skills, and that personal and environmental factors reinforce ineffective behaviors.

Using both individual and group psychotherapy modalities, the therapy follows a manual of techniques that target a hierarchy of dysfunctional behaviors specific to the individual. Individual therapy focuses on motivation and the behaviors since the last session, whereas group therapy teaches how to regulate emotions and behaviors and acceptance skills (distress tolerance and mindfulness skills). Dialectical behavior therapy has been found to be more effective than other psychotherapies such as supportive or psychodynamic in reducing suicidal episodes and behaviors such as noncompliance that interfere with treatment and hospitalization days.[13] A recent study found that dialectical behavior therapy was better than "treatment as usual" in reducing anger and improving social and overall adjustment.[14]

Pharmacologic Treatment

Borderline Personality Disorder. Virtually every class of psychiatric medication has been tried in the treatment of borderline personality disorder, with varying success, including tricyclic antidepressants (TCAs) monoamine oxidase inhibitors (MAOIs), and selective serotonin reuptake inhibitors (SSRIs). Most success has been achieved in reducing comorbid major depression or the depression that is experienced as part of mood instability. MAOIs, with their required diet and medication restrictions, may provide the most benefit overall.[15] In addition to reducing depressive symptoms, they may also reduce impulsive and suicidal behaviors. Fluoxetine appears to reduce hostility and possibility impulsive aggression, whereas TCAs have been associated with worsening behaviors, particularly impulsivity or hostility, in some. Lithium carbonate does not appear to be effective in treating symptoms of borderline personality disorder.

Carbamazepine may reduce mood instability and impulsive behaviors in clients with borderline personality disorder; however, it may lead to depression. It has been shown to increase "reflective delay," the ability to think before acting, thereby inhibiting impulsivity. Similarly, low-dose antipsychotics are helpful in decreasing impulsivity, aggression, and hostility, yet may promote depression. Stimulants and benzodiazepines have received little study. While these agents may lead to improvement, potential addiction and "disinhibition" (sudden behavioral dyscontrol and acts of severe aggression) have been observed with alprazolam.[16] As a result, these medications are generally avoided in individuals with borderline personality.

Table 27–4 shows how clients with borderline personality disorder may have "black-and-white responses" to medication.[15] Instead of a clear, predictable response, some unwanted and uncomfortable reactions might occur.

RESEARCH NOTE

Stein, KF: Affect instability in adults with a borderline personality disorder. Arch Psychiatr Nurs 10:32–40, 1996.

Findings: Affect instability is commonly observed in individuals with borderline personality disorder. Moods can change rapidly and frequently, even over the course of a day; however, little is known about the specific moods and pattern of these fluctuations. This study compared affect instability in clients with borderline personality to clients with anorexia nervosa and to asymptomatic volunteers. Each participant wore a pager for about 1 week, which signaled them 10 times each day to complete a mood questionnaire. Individuals with borderline personality disorder experienced more unstable sad, anxious, and bored moods than asymptomatic volunteers. Those with borderline personality reported more instability in surprised-aroused affects than clients with anorexia nervosa. The borderline personality participants displayed more short-term fluctuations in moods, which occurred over the course of a few hours rather than days. This study indicates that while everyone experiences some shifts in mood, individuals with borderline personality disorder show dramatic and frequent mood changes, suggesting affect instability.

Application to Practice: Ups and downs in moods occur in everyone; however, individuals with borderline personality disorder have more exaggerated and frequent mood shifts. They mostly experience frequent unpleasant states such as sadness, anxiety, and boredom. These mood changes interfere with their ability to develop and sustain healthy relationships and jobs, contributing to poor functioning. Diaries that detail specific mood fluctuations may help document the intensity of emotions experienced by clients with borderline personality disorder. This method may provide a means for monitoring moods to identify triggers. Clients could be instructed to chart their moods every hour and then identify precipitants. Once identified, nursing interventions could be aimed at altering unpleasant and inappropriate moods. For instance, relaxation methods might be used to reduce anxious and fearful moods.

For instance, antipsychotic medications may lead to worsening depression and impulsive behaviors. Overall, a careful approach to medication treatment is warranted, with specific behaviors targeted and the response to medication evaluated frequently. Combinations of agents, such as carbamazepine and an MAOI or an antipsychotic and an MAOI, may be necessary for some. Further research is necessary to test these combinations.

TABLE 27–4. Black-and-White Responses of Borderline Personality Disorder Patients to Medications

Beneficial Effects	Medication	Negative Effects
Decreased impulsivity	Antipsychotics	Depression
Decreased depression	Tricyclic antidepressants	Increased impulsivity
Decreased anxiety	Benzodiazepines	Aggression
Decreased impulsivity	Carbamazepine	Depression

Source: Courtesy of Dr. Martin Teicher, McLean Hospital, Belmont, MA.

An important consideration in the pharmacotherapy of individuals with personality disorders is that strong interpersonal reactions may arise. Similar to the psychotherapeutic process, clients may develop transference reactions to their medication or their prescriber. Waldinger and Frank[17] found that borderline behaviors were evident during pharmacotherapy. In particular, they noted that individuals idealized or devalued the medication or prescriber, issues of control and manipulation arose, and strong feelings of attachment and abandonment to the medication were evident. This study is a salient reminder that enduring personality behaviors can affect and impede the therapeutic process, regardless of modality.

CLUSTER C PERSONALITY DISORDERS

Characteristic Behaviors

Cluster C is the avoidant, dependent, and obsessive-compulsive personality disorders. Individuals with these disorders often appear anxious or fearful (see *DSM-IV* Diagnostic Criteria).

Avoidant Personality Disorder

Individuals with **avoidant** personality disorder are confronted with extreme anxiety and fear in social and intimate relationships. These reactions reflect their low self-esteem and sensitivity to rejection and criticism from others. Clients with avoidant personality disorder are extremely shy, self-conscious, and awkward. Although they may want to be engaged in relationships, their fears keep them isolated. It is nearly impossible for these individuals to take personal risks or engage in new activities, which leads to an unfulfilling life.

People always said I was a shy kid. They would always announce it, like at a party or family get-together. That really made me quiet. What does a shy child say to that? It's true, though; I never really felt comfortable around other people even though I wanted to be with them. It's not really surprising that I don't go out much.

Dependent Personality Disorder

These people show an overreliance on others for support, reassurance, and love. They may be unable to make decisions and expect their friends and families to make them. Functioning without a partner or spouse may be so difficult that they prefer abusive relationships to being alone. They desperately need to be taken care of and have difficulty making independent decisions. Their overreliance upon others is pervasive; major projects cannot be performed independently, and their fear of being alone is excessive. Clients with **dependent** personality disorder tend to agree with others rather than state a different opinion for fear of losing the relationship. Low self-esteem and self-doubt are common. Major depression and anxiety disorders frequently coexist.

I always do what other people want me to do. I hate to tell them that I disagree or want to do something else because I'm afraid that they'll get mad. My friends tell me that I have low self-esteem and that I have trouble putting myself first. I just really want to be liked by other people. Sometimes I find myself going along with something that I don't believe in; I'll even volunteer to do things that I don't like. I've even dated guys that I don't like so I don't have to be alone. I really think that I do best when I'm in a relationship. I can't stand being alone. My boss tells me that I ask too many questions and that I should focus on doing my work. He also complains that I spend too much time talking to other people. I talk to them so that I do things right. Maybe someday I'll be able to figure things out on my own.

Obsessive-Compulsive Personality Disorder

Extreme rigidity and control are the hallmark of this disorder. Individuals are perfectionistic, overly organized, and pay extreme attention to detail, in an exaggerated and unhealthy way. In relationships, these individuals want to control the lives of others and hold on tightly to what they believe is right. Because their way is always "right," clients with **obsessive-compulsive personality disorder** have tremendous difficulty in work situations and intimate relationships. Key features include an overreliance on rules and order, inflexibility, and stubbornness. They frequently insist that oth-

> ### DSM-IV Diagnostic Criteria for Avoidant, Dependent, and Obsessive-Compulsive Personality Disorders
>
> **Diagnostic Criteria for 301.82 Avoidant Personality Disorder**
>
> A pervasive pattern of social inhibition, feelings of inadequacy, and hypersensitivity to negative evaluation, beginning by early adulthood and present in a variety of contexts, as indicated by four (or more) of the following:
> (1) avoids occupational activities that involve significant interpersonal contact, because of fears of criticism, disapproval, or rejection
> (2) is unwilling to get involved with people unless certain of being liked
> (3) shows restraint within intimate relationships because of the fear of being shamed or ridiculed
> (4) is preoccupied with being criticized or rejected in social situations
> (5) is inhibited in new interpersonal situations because of feelings of inadequacy
> (6) views self as socially inept, personally unappealing, or inferior to others
> (7) is unusually reluctant to take personal risks or to engage in any new activities because they may prove embarrassing
>
> **Diagnostic Criteria for 301.6 Dependent Personality Disorder**
>
> A pervasive and excessive need to be taken care of that leads to submissive and clinging behavior and fears of separation, beginning by early adulthood and present in a variety of contexts, as indicated by five (or more) of the following:
> (1) has difficulty making everyday decisions without an excessive amount of advice and reassurance from others
> (2) needs others to assume responsibility for most major areas of his or her life
> (3) has difficulty expressing disagreement with others because of fear of loss of support or approval
> NOTE: Do not include realistic fears of retribution.
> (4) has difficulty initiating projects or doing things on his or her own (because of a lack of self-confidence in judgment or abilities rather than a lack of motivation or energy)
> (5) goes to excessive lengths to obtain nurturance and support from others, to the point of volunteering to do things that are unpleasant
> (6) feels uncomfortable or helpless when alone because of exaggerated fears of being unable to care for himself or herself
> (7) urgently seeks another relationship as a source of care and support when a close relationship ends
> (8) is unrealistically preoccupied with fears of being left to take care of himself or herself
>
> **Diagnostic Criteria for 301.4 Obsessive-Compulsive Personality Disorder**
>
> A pervasive pattern of preoccupation with orderliness, perfectionism, and mental and interpersonal control, at the expense of flexibility, openness, and efficiency, beginning by early adulthood and present in a variety of contexts, as indicated by four (or more) of the following:
> (1) is preoccupied with details, rules, lists, order, organization, or schedules to the extent that the major point of the activity is lost
> (2) shows perfectionism that interferes with task completion (e.g., is unable to complete a project because his or her own overly strict standards are not met)
> (3) is excessively devoted to work and productivity to the exclusion of leisure activities and friendships (not accounted for by obvious economic necessity)
> (4) is overconscientious, scrupulous, and inflexible about matters of morality, ethics, or values (not accounted for by cultural or religious identification)
> (5) is unable to discard worn-out or worthless objects even when they have no sentimental value
> (6) is reluctant to delegate tasks or to work with others unless they submit to exactly his or her way of doing things
> (7) adopts a miserly spending style toward both self and others; money is viewed as something to be hoarded for future catastrophes
> (8) shows rigidity and stubbornness
>
> **Source:** Reprinted with permission from the Diagnostic and Statistical Manual of Mental Disorders, Fourth Edition. Copyright 1994 American Psychiatric Association.

ers submit to their ideas and plans; power struggles result. Lack of emotion, extreme neatness, and an inability to throw out worthless items is common.

> I've been divorced twice. My ex-wives said I was a "control freak." I just think that there is a place and time for everything. Everything in its place. That's the right way; the way it should be. Like the saying, "Early to bed and early to rise...." It's the same with my boss. I keep telling her how to organize the place and schedule things. If she only realized that my plan is the best way.

Culture, Age, and Gender Features

Culture

Some cultures value religious rituals; these should not be confused with the distinct habits or preoccupations observed in individuals with obsessive-compulsive personality. Immigrants may display shyness and isolation that may be misdiagnosed as avoidant personality disorder. Some ethnic groups value politeness and "passivity" that should not be confused with similar characteristics in dependent personality disorder.

Gender

Dependent personality disorder is more common in women, whereas obsessive-compulsive personality is twice as common in men.[1]

Etiology

Psychoanalytic-Developmental Theories

Little is known about the exact etiology of cluster C personality disorders. They may arise from adverse childhood experiences. Children who are rejected by parents and then later by peers may develop an intense fear of relationships and discomfort in social interactions as seen in avoidant personality disorder. Individuals with dependent personality disorder may have had parents who neglected or deprived them of food and other comforts during infancy. These children then fail to develop healthy independent behavior. Obsessive-compulsive personality disorder may result from excessive parental control and criticism, possibly during toilet training, which leads such children to respond in part with perfectionism, control, and orderliness.

Prognosis

These disorders generally remain stable over time, and the behaviors continue to interfere with daily living.

Interventions for Clients in the Community

These individuals are rarely hospitalized for symptoms of a personality disorder. Cluster C personality disorders, characterized by pervasive anxiety and fear, should be met with a gentle and compassionate attitude. Do not force clients to engage with others or in activities; gently encourage them. Suggest assertiveness or social-skills training as a means of becoming more engaged and comfortable with others. For individuals with avoidant personality disorder, be careful to avoid critical, humiliating, or demeaning comments. They are likely to overreact to even slightly rejecting or disparaging remarks. For clients with dependent personality disorder, encourage their independence and support their ability to make simple decisions as much as possible. Use the clinical management tips later in this chapter. Avoid power struggles with individuals with obsessive-compulsive personality disorder. Refer clients with anxious-fearful personality disorders for individual psychotherapy.

Clients with dependent personality disorder may refuse to make decisions. Ideally, it is better to avoid engaging in struggles or in delivering ultimatums, such as "Do this or else" statements, because control struggles can be a frequent outcome. It is more effective to maintain a calm but firm position and design a treatment plan that anticipates manipulative behavior. Discussion with peers or supervisors may be helpful for devising effective individual interventions, or a formal consultation may be necessary.

Pharmacologic Treatment

Avoidant Personality Disorder. For avoidant personality disorder, only antidepressants and anxiolytics have been studied. The most information is known about the MAOI tranylcypromine and the benzodiazepine alprazolam. Both are effective in reducing anxiety in individuals with avoidant personality disorder, although their mechanism of action is unknown. Alprazolam reduces the fear of saying foolish things and the avoidance of situations requiring interpersonal contact. Some preliminary evidence suggests that the SSRIs, because of their anxiolytic effects, might be useful in reducing avoidant behaviors.

EXPECTED OUTCOMES

For the individual with a personality disorder, improvement will be demonstrated by:
- Recognizing the impact of behavior on relationships.
- Devising short- and long-term goals to promote adaptive behaviors.
- Substituting more effective ways of relating to promote healthy relationships.
- Making a commitment to long-term treatment of the unhealthy behaviors.
- Demonstrating safe behaviors anzd not harming self or others.
- Identifying sources of continuing community support to facilitate coping.

DIFFERENTIAL DIAGNOSIS

Medical Disorders

- Medications or physical conditions, including neurological injuries and endocrine, seizure, and rheumatological disorders, may precipitate personality disorders.
- Symptoms are similar to personality disorders but are excluded from the diagnosis.
- Personality characteristics over the greater part of the individual's lifetime differentiate personality disorders from medical disorders.
- Medical conditions lead to rapid, abrupt personality change, whereas personality disorders are enduring patterns.
- Steroid use or abuse may lead to aggression, hostility, agitation, and labile mood, which could be mistaken for a personality disorder.

Psychotic Disorders

- Psychotic disorders and cluster A personality disorders have similar behaviors.
- Cluster A personality disorders differ from schizophrenia in the type and course of symptoms.
- Delusions and hallucinations are present in schizophrenia but not in paranoid personality disorder.
- Behaviors that define paranoid, schizoid, and schizotypal personality disorder are persistent, unlike the remissions and overall course of schizophrenia.
- Schizotypal personality disorder may precede the development of schizophrenia and may be a premorbid condition.

Mood Disorders

- Personality disorders frequently coexist with mood disorders.
- Borderline personality disorder is commonly observed with dysthymia, major depression, and bipolar disorder.
- Borderline personality disorder precedes the development of a mood disorder and continues after the mood symptoms remit.
- Major depression needs to be distinguished from dependent personality disorder.

Anxiety Disorders

- PTSD, obsessive-compulsive disorder (OCD), and social phobia may overlap with personality disorders.
- Obsessive-compulsive personality disorder and OCD are differentiated by the presence of distinct obsessions (intrusive repetitive thoughts) and compulsions (senseless repetitious behaviors) observed in OCD.
- Avoidant personality and social phobia share common behaviors and may be difficult to distinguish.
- Borderline personality disorder is commonly observed with PTSD.

Alcohol and Substance Abuse

- Substance or alcohol abuse frequently coexists with personality disorders, particularly borderline personality disorder.
- Substance or alcohol abuse or withdrawal may lead to aggression, hostility, agitation, and labile mood, which could be easily mistaken for a personality disorder.
- Symptoms are abrupt during abuse or withdrawal in comparison with the pervasive pattern seen in personality disorders.

Common Nursing Diagnoses

- Communication, impaired verbal
- Noncompliance (with treatment plan)
- Social Isolation
- Social Interaction, impaired
- Personal Identity Disturbance
- Self Esteem disturbance
- Coping, individual, ineffective
- Violence, risk for, directed at self/others
- Anxiety

CLIENT AND FAMILY EDUCATION

A useful technique in working with clients with personality disorders and their families is psychoeducation. Often these individuals have recognized their impairment and have also realized that they are different from those with depression or other severe psychiatric disorders. A carefully devised education plan should include a discussion of the nature of the personality disorder, its consequences, theories about its development, and its pervasiveness. Potential treatment and a plan of care can be discussed and devised with clients as active participants. Teach families that allowing clients some control in their care is an especially salient issue when personality disorders are present. Stress the need for appropriate limits on unacceptable and potentially dangerous behavior. Many of the clinical management tips for manipulative, dependent, and angry clients (see Clinical Management Tips that follow) can be taught to families and friends.

SYNOPSIS OF CURRENT RESEARCH

Some of the research on personality disorders is currently focused on the role of abuse and neglect on the developing child. For instance, because borderline personality disorder is associated with high rates of physical and sexual abuse, investigations are underway to determine why some victims develop the disorder and others do not. Along similar lines, research distinguishing PTSD from borderline personality disorder includes studies to determine whether these are distinct conditions, whether one promotes the development of the other, or whether they are variations of the same disorder. Feminist psychologists are also pursuing whether gender influences moral development; girls have been described as possessing a "different voice," reflective of underlying differences in development.[18] This research could have profound implications for understanding gender differences in the diagnosis of certain personality disorders such as dependent, borderline, and antisocial.

Another research aim is to determine the effects of a personality disorder on families. Because individuals with these disorders have pervasive difficulties, intimate relationships are often the most affected. The role of psychoeducation for families is also being investigated as part of this line of research. Similarly, the effects of Linehan's[13] behavioral approach to the treatment of borderline personality disorder are being investigated. These highly structured techniques have been shown to decrease suicidal behaviors, treatment attrition, and hospitalization and to improve interpersonal functioning in individuals with borderline personality.

Increasing study is aimed at understanding the role of medications in the treatment of personality disorders. Studies are underway to assess the efficacy of antidepressants in borderline, dependent, and avoidant personality disorders; of antipsychotics in paranoid, schizotypal, and schizoid personality disorders; and of benzodiazepines in avoidant personality disorder.

AREAS FOR FUTURE RESEARCH

- What are the most effective nursing interventions for individuals with a specific personality disorder?
- What factors promote long-term positive outcomes, particularly in relationships and occupational functioning?
- What factors explain gender differences in the diagnosis of personality disorders?
- What is the role of childhood physical and sexual abuse in the development of borderline and other personality disorders?
- What inherited temperaments are associated with later development of personality disorder?
- What is the role of nursing in behavioral treatment of personality disorders?
- What identifiable behaviors in adolescence predict personality disorder in adulthood?
- Which treatments or combinations of treatments are most effective for borderline personality disorder?
- What factors promote personality disorders?
- What is the long-term outcome for clients with personality disorders?

CASE STUDY

Susan is a 26-year-old woman who lives with roommates in a major city. She was admitted to the hospital after a roommate found that she had either accidentally or purposely taken extra medication. Upon arrival to the hospital she was sedated, "dopey," and initially unable to participate in the evaluation. Her roommate reported that Susan had been told just several hours earlier that she would need to find another apartment. When asked why the roommates had come to that decision, they replied, "We just couldn't take it anymore. We'd ask her not to borrow our clothing or food, but she would fly off the handle and start smashing things. We could never have friends over because she would always intrude and take over. One minute she'd be caring and your best friend, and the next minute she'd be putting you down. We just don't need it anymore; plus, she never was reliable about her rent and bills." Apparently this behavior was evident from the beginning and continued during the 3 months Susan lived with them. Her actions became so severe that she would stay out late, return intoxicated, and bring home strangers to sleep with.

The medications that arrived with her were an empty bottle of acetaminophen and lorazepam prescribed by her internist. The latter medication had been recently filled; however, about one-third of the bottle was empty. A call to her mother was met with the response, "Oh, so what has she gotten herself into now?" Her mother, who had not seen or heard from her daughter in about 1 year, reported that Susan had been previously hospitalized on a psychiatric unit during her first year in college after a suicide attempt. She apparently stayed only briefly, denied ever being suicidal, and signed out against medical advice. Thereafter, she transferred colleges several times but completed only three courses over several years. Her mother described a series of relationships with men who were "bums," as well as lesbian relationships.

After receiving gastric lavage in the emergency room, Susan was transferred to the admission unit of the psychiatric hospital. She was irritable and uncooperative with the medical resident, saying, "You could care less about me, just get me out of here." The nurse who approached Susan confidently and empathically stated, "We do care and we'd like to help you." However, Susan reacted angrily and threw her pillow at the nurse. She then shouted, "You can't keep me here because I'm fine. Besides, if you really cared you'd give me a gun so I could end it all now."

CRITICAL THINKING QUESTIONS

1. What were the pervasive behavioral clues that Susan exhibited during the years prior to her overdose?
2. What would be the initial plan in caring for her?
3. What would be the most effective ways the nurse could deal with her own reactions to the client?
4. Identify key behaviors suggestive of personality disorders.
5. What other information is essential to provide effective care to Susan?
6. What are the major challenges in developing a relationship with the client?
7. Identify behaviors that would indicate that Susan is responding to treatment.
8. Develop a long-term care plan, including short- and long-term goals for Susan.
9. Design a teaching plan for Susan's roommates and family during and after discharge.

KEY POINTS

- Personality disorders are enduring patterns of relating, usually beginning in adolescence or early adulthood, that are pervasive in nearly every area of the individual's life.
- The ten personality disorders described in *DSM-IV* are clustered into three groups. Cluster A, odd-eccentric disorders, consists of paranoid, schizotypal, and schizoid personality disorders. Cluster B disorders tend to display dramatic, emotional, or erratic features; they include antisocial, borderline, histrionic, and narcissistic personality disorders. Cluster C, anxious and fearful disorders, consists of avoidant, dependent, and obsessive-compulsive personality disorders.
- Personality disorders frequently coexist with major psychiatric disorders such as mood, anxiety, and substance-abuse disorders. The combination is associated with poorer prognosis and a more deleterious course.
- Personality disorders develop from a complicated interplay of environmental, genetic, and biological factors.

- Research on personality disorders has supported reduced serotonergic functioning, particularly in borderline personality disorder clients with impulsive and aggressive behaviors.
- Each personality disorder has distinct features that characterize it. General diagnostic criteria include an enduring pattern of inner experience and behavior, across personal and social situations, of long duration, leading to significant distress or impairment, and affecting cognition, affect, interpersonal functioning, and impulse control.
- Certain personality traits and disorders may be inherited.
- Personality disorders may result from early childhood experiences, including specific parental failures such as neglect and abuse.
- Because personality disorders are long-standing, long-term psychotherapy is usually required. The client will need to be an active and willing participant in order to make substantive change.
- Individuals with personality disorders are a challenge to deal with because their personality characteristics may be unpleasant and arouse strong negative feelings in providers.
- Effective treatment of personality disorders requires a comprehensive approach that includes client and family education, psychotherapy, and possibly pharmacotherapy. CBT has been shown to be particularly effective for borderline personality disorder.

REFERENCES

1. American Psychiatric Association: Diagnostic and Statistical Manual of Mental Disorders, ed 4. American Psychiatric Association, Washington, DC, 1994.
2. Siever, LJ, et al: Plasma homovanillic acid in schizotypal personality disorder. Am J Psychiatry 148:1246, 1991.
3. Siever, LJ, et al: Cerebrospinal fluid homovanillic acid in schizotypal personality disorder. Am J Psychiatry 150:149, 1993.
4. Siever, LJ, Kalus, OF, and Keefe, RSE: The boundaries of schizophrenia. Psychiatr Clin North Am 16:217, 1993.
5. Thaker, G, et al: Psychiatric illness in families of subjects with schizophrenia spectrum personality disorders: High morbidity risks for unspecified functional psychoses and schizophrenia. Am J Psychiatry 150:66, 1993.
6. Kagan, J, et al: Childhood derivatives of inhibition and lack of inhibition to the unfamiliar. Child Dev 59:1580, 1988.
7. Tellegen, A, et al: Personality similarity in twins reared apart and together. J Pers Soc Psychol 54:1031–1039, 1988.
8. Coccaro, EF, et al: Serotonergic studies in patients with affective and personality disorders: Correlates with suicidal and impulsive aggressive behavior. Arch Gen Psychiatry 46:587, 1989.
9. Trestman, RL, et al: The differential biology of impulsivity, suicide, and aggression in depression and in personality disorders. Biol Psychiatry 33:46A, 1993.
10. Mahler, M: The Psychological Birth of the Human Infant. Basic Books, New York, 1975.
11. Kernberg, O: Borderline personality organization. J Personal Disord 15:641, 1967.
12. Herman, JL, Perry, JC, and van der Kolk, BA: Childhood trauma in borderline personality disorder. Am J Psychiatry 146:490, 1989.
13. Linehan, MM: Cognitive-Behavioral Treatment of Borderline Personality Disorder. The Guilford Press, New York, 1993.
14. Linehan, MM, et al: Interpersonal outcome of cognitive behavioral treatment for chronically suicidal borderline patients. Am J Psychiatry 151:1771, 1994.
15. Teicher, MH, and Glod, CA: Pharmacotherapy of borderline personality disorder. Hosp Comm Psychiatry 9:887, 1989.
16. Cowdry, RW, and Gardner, DL: Pharmacotherapy of borderline personality disorder: Alprazolam, carbamazepine, trifluoperazine, and tranylcypromine. Arch Gen Psychiatry 45:111, 1988.
17. Waldinger, RJ, and Frank, AF: Transference and the vicissitudes of medication use by borderline patients. Psychiatry 52:416, 1989.
18. Gilligan, C: In a Different Voice. Harvard University Press, Cambridge, MA, 1982.

CHAPTER 28
Attention-Deficit/Hyperactivity Disorder

CHAPTER 28

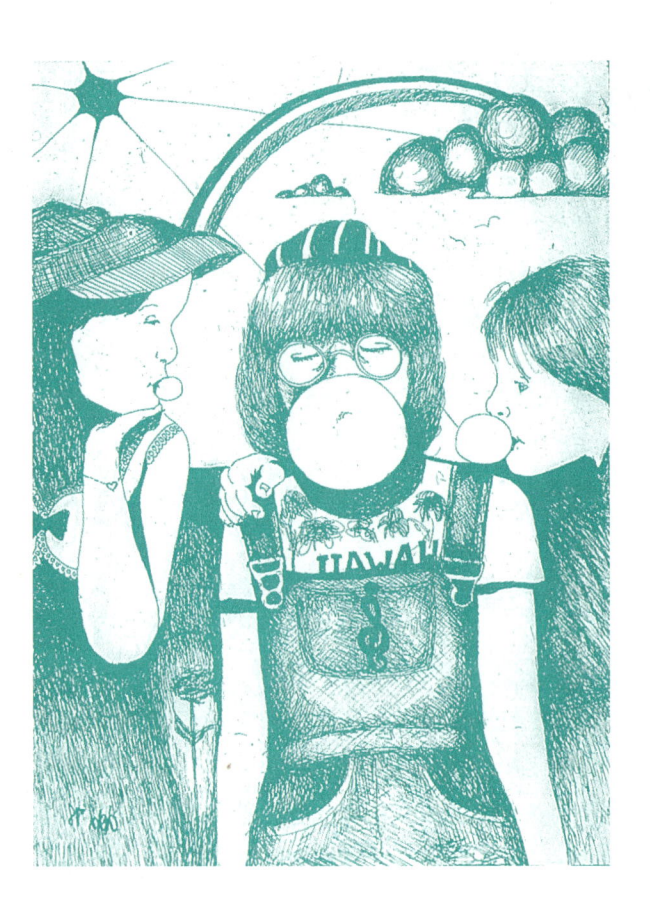

CHAPTER OUTLINE

Characteristic Behaviors
- *Children*
- *Adolescents*
- *Adults*

Culture, Age, and Gender Features
- *Culture*
- *Age*
- *Gender*

Etiology
- *Genetics*
- *Brain Development*
- *Brain Function and Structure*
- *Neurotransmitters in ADHD*

Assessment
- *Clinical Assessment Interview*
- *Assessment Instruments*

Planning Care
- *Role of the Nurse as Resource*
- *Role of the Nurse as Teacher*
- *Role of the Nurse as Leader*
- *Role of the Nurse as Surrogate*
- *Role of the Nurse as Counselor*

Interventions for Hospitalized Clients

Interventions for Clients in the Community
- *Cognitive-Behavior Interventions*
- *Psychopharmacologic Interventions*

Expected Outcomes

Differential Diagnosis
- *Mood*
- *Learning*
- *Traumatic Experiences*
- *Conduct and Oppositional Behaviors*
- *Mental Retardation*
- *Pervasive Developmental Disorders*
- *Tic Disorders*
- *Anxiety*
- *Psychotic Disorder*

Synopsis of Current Research

Areas for Future Research

Ann M. Polcari, RN, CS, PhDc

Attention-Deficit/Hyperactivity Disorder

LEARNING OBJECTIVES

After completing this chapter, the reader should be able to:
- Name the *DSM-IV* criteria for attention-deficit/hyperactivity disorder (ADHD).
- Describe the clinical presentation of ADHD symptoms throughout the life span.
- Understand the impact of ADHD on academic and social functioning for the child, adolescent, and adult.
- Describe the etiology of ADHD symptoms.
- Recognize at least three other psychiatric diagnoses commonly associated with ADHD.
- Describe the assessment interview for psychiatric disorders in children.
- Describe at least two treatment interventions for children with ADHD.

KEY TERMS

acting out
attention-deficit/hyperactivity disorder (ADHD)
cognitive-behavior intervention
conduct disorder
hyperactivity
impulsivity
inattention
play therapy
psychostimulant

A 1990 report to the U.S. Congress, prepared by the National Advisory Mental Health Council, estimated that 12% of American children and adolescents (an estimated 7.5 million) have psychiatric disorders. Of these, fewer than one-fifth receive treatment, which in turn represents an estimated cost of $1.5 billion per year.[1] This cost includes therapeutic care, special educational services, child welfare, and the juvenile-justice system.

Specific disorders identified as having a childhood onset include mental retardation, developmental disorders, elimination disorders, disruptive behavior disorders, and anxiety disorders. Other disorders typically appear in adulthood but are also seen in childhood, such as mood and psychotic disorders. The most commonly diagnosed disorder in childhood is **Attention-Deficit/Hyperactivity Disorder (ADHD)**. Children with ADHD experience difficulty in sustaining attention, ignoring distractions, controlling impulses, and inhibiting behavior. Attention and hyperactivity problems in childhood affect a child's performance at school, at home, and in play situations. For some, the symptoms persist into adolescence and adulthood, affecting relationships and quality of life. In addition, ADHD is associated with a number of other psychiatric problems throughout the life span (Table 28–1).

Diagnosis of attention-deficit and hyperactivity problems takes place in a number of clinical settings. Often a school nurse or a teacher suggests to parents the need for an evaluation. In primary care, the pediatrician or nurse practitioner may diagnosis ADHD and prescribe a stimulant medication. In specialty care, psychologists may uncover problems during testing for school or psychological difficulties. Psychiatric specialists, such as neurologists, psychiatrists, and psychiatric–clinical nurse specialists, can be consulted for diagnosis and prescriptions. In most cases, diagnosis is derived from parent and teacher reports of problematic behaviors, office observation, and behavior rating scales. Clients must meet the criteria listed in the *DSM-IV* Diagnostic Criteria for Attention-Deficit/Hyperactivity Disorder.

Characteristic Behaviors

CHILDREN

ADHD is characterized by a triad of symptoms throughout the life span: inattention, impulsivity, and hyperactivity. To understand the criteria of ADHD, hearing how parents report the symptoms of ADHD for their children is helpful. The children described here, Billy, Janey, Sam, and Sara, exhibit typical inattentive and hyperactive behaviors. **Inattention** includes nine symptoms; six must be present to meet diagnostic criteria.

- Makes careless mistakes. "Billy hates to write. His work is often sloppy and his penmanship is poor. He rushes through tests and gets answers wrong; if he took his time, he would get things right."
- Difficulty sustaining attention. "Janey likes to play cards but after a few minutes gets bored and quits to play with other things."
- Does not seem to listen. "You can call Sam's name ten times before you get his attention, even when he is just looking out the window."

Diagnostic Criteria for Attention-Deficit/Hyperactivity Disorder

A. Either (1) or (2):
  (1) six (or more) of the following symptoms of inattention have persisted for at least 6 months to a degree that is maladaptive and inconsistent with developmental level:
  Inattention
    (a) often fails to give close attention to details or makes careless mistakes in schoolwork, work, or other activities
    (b) often has difficulty sustaining attention in tasks or play activities
    (c) often does not seem to listen when spoken to directly
    (d) often does not follow through on instructions and fails to finish schoolwork, chores, or duties in the workplace (not due to oppositional behavior or failure to understand instructions)
    (e) often has difficulty organizing tasks and activities
    (f) often avoids, dislikes, or is reluctant to engage in tasks that require sustained mental effort (such as schoolwork or homework)
    (g) often loses things necessary for tasks or activities (e.g., toys, school assignments, pencils, books, or tools)
    (h) is often easily distracted by extraneous stimuli
    (i) is often forgetful in daily activities
  (2) six (or more) of the following symptoms of hyperactivity-impulsivity have persisted for at least 6 months to a degree that is maladaptive and inconsistent with developmental level:
  Hyperactivity
    (a) often fidgets with hands or feet or squirms in seat
    (b) often leaves seat in classroom or in other situations in which remaining seated is expected
    (c) often runs about or climbs excessively in situations in which it is inappropriate (in adolescents or adults, may be limited to subjective feelings of restlessness)
    (d) often has difficulty playing or engaging in leisure activities quietly
    (e) is often "on the go" or often acts as if "driven by a motor"
    (f) often talks excessively
  Impulsivity
    (g) often blurts out answers before questions have been completed
    (h) often has difficulty awaiting turn
    (i) often interrupts or intrudes on others (e.g., butts into conversations or games)

B. Some hyperactive-impulsive or inattentive symptoms that caused impairment were present before age 7 years.

C. Some impairment from the symptoms is present in two or more settings (e.g., at school [or work] and at home).

D. There must be clear evidence of clinically significant impairment in social, academic, or occupational functioning.

E. The symptoms do not occur exclusively during the course of a Pervasive Developmental Disorder, Schizophrenia, or other Psychotic Disorder and are not better accounted for by another mental disorder (e.g., Mood Disorder, Anxiety Disorder, Dissociative Disorder, or a Personality Disorder).

Code based on type:
314.01 Attention-Deficit/Hyperactivity Disorder, Combined Type: if both Criteria A1 and A2 are met for the past 6 months
314.00 Attention-Deficit/Hyperactivity Disorder, Predominantly Inattentive Type: if Criterion A1 is met but Criterion A2 is not met for the past 6 months
314.01 Attention-Deficit/Hyperactivity Disorder, Predominantly Hyperactivity-Impulsive Type: if Criterion A2 is met but Criterion A1 is not met for the past 6 months

CODING NOTE: For individuals (especially adolescents and adults) who currently have symptoms that no longer meet full criteria, "In Partial Remission" should be specified.

Source: Reprinted with permission from the Diagnostic and Statistical Manual of Mental Disorders, Fourth Edition. Copyright 1994 American Psychiatric Association.

- Does not follow through on things. "Sara needs you standing over her to finish her homework. She'll do the first few lines, then move on to the next subject, or say she is finished."
- Difficulty organizing. "If you even ask Billy to do more than one thing at a time, he never gets to steps two and three."
- Avoids difficult tasks. "Janey knows how to read, she just hates to now that she has to read book chapters. When the stories were short, like with picture books, she could finish quickly, and they would hold her interest. Now you can't get her to do her reading assignments."
- Loses things. "Sara never remembers to bring home her notebook, and you wouldn't believe how many mittens and hats she loses every winter."
- Distracted. "When Billy is doing homework, it doesn't take much to get him off task—people talking in the next room, a TV on, or even the smell of cooking."

TABLE 28–1. Consequences of ADHD

Short Term
Conduct problems
Poor school performance
Difficulty in relationships
Low confidence
Low self-esteem

Long Term
Conduct problems
Academic or work failure
Conflicts in relationships
Addiction problems
Chronic underachievement
Chronic low self-esteem

- Forgetful. "You can ask Janey to go upstairs, brush her hair, and get her socks for school, and within minutes she is back downstairs, barefoot, carrying a toy."

The criteria for the **hyperactivity-impulsivity** part of the diagnosis has nine symptoms. Six are required to meet the diagnosis.

- Fidgets and squirms. "Billy is always moving, never still. If he is not playing with his hands, touching everything, he is wiggling around in his seat."
- Leaves seat. "It is impossible for Sara to sit through a whole meal, and her teacher is always reporting she's up and down out of her chair, to pick up something, go to the bathroom, or just move around the room."
- Runs and climbs excessively. "Sam has always been a climber. You could catch him on the counters, tables, and even on windowsills. He never just walks; he is always running or hopping, especially when he gets excited."
- Difficulty playing quietly. "Billy is never quiet. Even when he plays Legos for a few minutes, he is humming or noisily crashing the parts into each other."
- Acts as if driven by a motor. "That's Janey, she needs to move all the time. She always wants to be doing something—go, go, go."
- Talks excessively. "Sam never shuts up. He is always commenting on things, telling stories, and all in a rush to get to the next topic."
- Blurts out answers. "Billy's teacher is always reporting that he jumps in with the answer without raising his hand, even when she hasn't called on him."
- Difficulty waiting his turn. "Sam can be very impatient. He always wants to go first, and if he has to wait, he gets fidgety and frustrated. When he jumps ahead in line, he gets all the other children mad at him, and then he feels bad."
- Interrupts or intrudes. "You wouldn't believe how many times I have to say 'wait.' When I'm on the phone or busy, Billy butts in, yanks at my sleeve, or gets so noisy I have to stop what I'm doing."

ADOLESCENTS

ADHD can be harder to describe in adolescence. When asked about inattentive features, an adolescent may deny or make excuses, such as "My teacher flunks everyone," "I can't pay attention when it's so boring," and "If I like a subject, I can do OK." The hyperactive-impulsive features may be best described by asking what the adolescent likes to do for fun. Typical responses are "I'm always on my bike or skateboard, I hate sitting around doing nothing," or "I feel restless; I have to be doing something, not just wasting time." By adolescence, the individual may be able to endorse past childhood symptoms, such as "concentrating on work was always hard for me," "my mother was always reminding me about things," or "I was pretty accident prone, always banging myself up."

ADULTS

Adults often endorse past childhood and present symptoms. They emphasize difficulty with increased expectations and responsibilities, such as "I had to find ways to be organized—calendars, reminder notes—I even tried a tape recorder once," or "I got bored easily my whole life." They may express restlessness and dislike of sedentary activities or desk jobs.[2] Some adults may retain only a few of the ADHD symptoms that cause impairment and can be diagnosed with ADHD, In Partial Remission.[2]

Even though the diagnosis can be first made in adolescence or adulthood, some symptoms that cause impairment must be present before the age of 7. Old school records and report cards are helpful in making a diagnosis. Assess adults for a family history of ADHD, including their own children. Adults may have to question their parents about key ADHD behaviors from childhood. Table 28–2 lists clues to adult ADHD.

Culture, Age, and Gender Features

CULTURE

Although ADHD occurs in various cultures, Western countries are more likely to diagnose it.[2] ADHD has been more

TABLE 28–2 Clues to Adult ADHD

- Underachiever
- Disorganized
- Many simultaneous projects
- Impulsive
- Intolerant of boredom
- Creative
- Seeks high stimulation
- Impatient
- Restless
- Addictive
- Low self-esteem

frequently diagnosed in the United States than in Great Britain. In Great Britain, the child has to be extremely hyperactive and is more likely to be diagnosed with a **conduct disorder** than with ADHD.[3]

AGE

As described in Chapter 4, childhood is a period of complex developmental changes and expectations for each individual. The prevalence of ADHD is 3 to 5% in school-age children[2]; the rates for adolescent and adult populations have not been established. Erikson's[4] theory about the stages of human development provides a structure for evaluating the impact of experiencing ADHD throughout the life span.

Infants and Toddlers

The early tasks for each person are establishing a sense of trust, followed by a sense of self-control.[4] These infancy and toddler years are often the beginning of difficulties for children. Parents often report that the child with ADHD was impossible to potty train, was always into things, and was constantly being told no. Safety issues of climbing out of cribs and onto counters, as well as reckless, daredevil behaviors, led to accidents and trips to the emergency room. Parents report that they could never keep up with the child and often say they feel unsuccessful as parents. The child may be at risk for excessive or punitive discipline from frustrated parents.

Latency Age

By age 5, the child develops a sense of direction and purpose. It is a time of eager learning, cooperative playing, and positively identifying with adults.[4] The hyperactive child might have been in daycare or preschool, where others were able to begin to identify difficulties. These children are at risk for feeling different and experiencing less mastery than peers.

School Age

School age spans ages 6 to 12 and is a time of increasing competency. Children become adept at learning skills and feel the pleasure of completing work and winning recognition from those outside the family.[3] Children with ADHD are at risk for feeling inferior or inadequate at this stage, which can lead to poor self-esteem. This age is most often when a diagnosis of ADHD is first made. Teachers may report that children cannot be still or listen in class. Parents may see that they forget or never finish homework assignments. Whereas other children understand the norms of the classroom, these children are blurting out answers, getting out of their seats, and constantly talking. Peers may reject or fight with them. They have a hard time with socialization.

Adolescence

From ages 12 to 20, adolescents begin to gain a sense of themselves as unique. They form an identify and begin to see their roles in the future. Puberty starts a questioning of the world, linking childhood and the anticipated adult world.[4] They are focused on how they appear in the eyes of others. Adolescents with ADHD may feel particularly vulnerable to seeming different or having a deficit. One adult recalls his adolescence:

> Growing up with undiagnosed [ADHD], I had a bad time. School was hell, my parents were always on my case, I couldn't keep my room clean, and so much other stuff. Everybody blamed me for it all, and I ended up with a lousy self-image and very little self-confidence.[5]

Young Adulthood

Once thought to remit in adulthood, ADHD continues into adulthood for about two-thirds of clients, remitting in old age. The developmental tasks of adulthood can be impacted by the symptoms of ADHD, although most adults develop some compensatory coping. During young adulthood, people seek love and intimacy.[4] The following example illustrates difficulty with intimacy.

> I'm [ADHD] and hyperactive. . . . I've always been drawn to explosive relationships. Not like abusive explosive, but really fast-moving, very intense relationships. What I've found, though, is that those kind of relationships don't last.[5]

This next example illustrates the impact of symptoms on one woman's self-image, relationships, and work.

> I didn't learn that I had [ADHD] until I was 24, about 2 years ago. Prior to that time, I'd always figured that my problem was that I was blond. You know all those jokes they tell about blonds? That's me. I'm forgetful, distractible, impulsive (I used to be a pushover on first dates, unfortunately), impatient, and always interrupting people. After being told for so many years that I was just a typical blond, I'd come to believe it, that there was something genetic or whatever about blonds. I've always been relegated to the dumb blond jobs, and viewed as a dumb blond by men. When I learned about [ADHD], I realized my problem wasn't about being blond, it was about having [ADHD].

Adulthood

Workplace success can be difficult for some people with ADHD. Some frequently change jobs or drift from one career to another. They complain of getting bored and frustrated with routine easily. As people mature through the last stages of life, the idea of leaving an impact on the next generation and attaining wisdom become important.[3] If the sum of their lives is not what was expected, they are at risk for experiencing despair.

GENDER

Gender bias has been a historical problem. The majority of ADHD research has included mostly boys. Even with mixed samples, girls are underrepresented, which does not mean, however, that ADHD is not a significant problem for them. Girls may be less likely to present with ADHD because they tolerate their deficits more easily, perform adequately (but do not excel) in academics, and exhibit fewer disruptive and impulsive behaviors, requiring less adult attention than boys.[6] A national survey in Canada[7] found ADHD rates of adolescents similar for girls and boys. Recent literature suggests that when objective measures are used, such as computer tests and infrared motion analysis, the prevalence of quantifiable ADHD is similar for both boys and girls.[8] The prevalence data are difficult to interpret but suggest that girls with ADHD may be underidentified.

The effects of missing the diagnosis of ADHD in girls are long-term. One study found an overrepresentation of women in adult versus child samples, indicating that problems existed and were not recognized.[9] Girls with attention and activity difficulties in childhood continue with the difficulties into adulthood. They also experience higher rates of major depression, anxiety, and conduct problems.[9]

The trend is gradually changing. One study[10] described trends in diagnosis and stimulant medication treatment from 1975 to 1993 in a public school sample; the gender ratio in 1981 was 1 to 12, female to male, and narrowed to 1 to 6 in 1993.[10] One wonders if the increase in girls treated with medication reflects an increase in perceiving symptoms in girls or is a by-product of a larger nationwide trend in prescribing medication for all childhood behavior problems.[11] Contributing to this controversy is the question of who should diagnose the disturbances: specifically, clinicians in primary family health versus those in a psychiatric specialty. Diagnosis of children with ADHD is complicated by the complexity of symptoms associated with ADHD. Two-thirds of the children referred for psychiatric evaluation have at least one other psychiatric disorder: commonly conduct, learning, anxiety, and mood disorders.[12]

Etiology

At the turn of the century, some children were recognized as having inattention and hyperactivity symptoms, usually along with behavioral disruption. Moral deficiency and biological predetermination were considered the causes for their social misconduct.[3] In 1918, following an epidemic of encephalitis, children who survived had impaired attention, increased activity, and impulsivity, a syndrome referred to as postencephalitic behavior disorder.[3] Based on this observation, over the next decades the leading theory was that brain damage caused behavior disturbances. Early researchers studied the effects of birth trauma, infections, and injuries.[3] Hyperactive behavior was not considered a separate entity but grouped with mental retardation, learning delays, and severe behavior disorders.[3]

Early inferences on etiology were based on clinical observation. During the 1950s, the prevailing view attributed ADHD symptoms to excess stimulation in the brain and an inability to filter out sensory information.[3] Over time, research failed to support this theory. In subsequent decades, studies focused on environmental-factor explanations; popular theories were allergies to food additives, response to refined sugar, response to an overstimulating society, and response to poor parenting.[3] These, too, lacked empirical support.

The diagnosis moved from the minimal brain damage label to hyperkinetic reaction of childhood in 1968 with the second edition of the *Diagnostic and Statistical Manual of Mental Disorders (DSM II)*. Since the 1970s, hyperactivity has been one of the most extensively studied areas, although the focus also moved toward a better understanding of attention and impulse control problems, leading to the diagnostic label of attention deficit disorder (ADD), with or without hyperactivity in the 1980 *DSM-III*.[3] With the 1994 *DSM-IV*, three subtypes are identified: ADHD Predominantly Inattentive Type, ADHD Predominantly Hyperactive-Impulsive Type, or ADHD Combined Type.

To date, no single etiology for ADHD has been identified, although current research is extensive. Discoveries are being made in the areas of genetic transmission, influences during brain development, and alterations in brain function and structure.

GENETICS

ADHD appears to be inherited. Family genetic studies reveal an increased prevalence in family members with ADHD.[13] Parents of hyperactive children are likely to have ADHD symptoms. Twin studies also indicate the inheritability of ADHD. Recent researchers have found a genetic marker for the dopamine transporter gene, which is shown to be associated with the transmission of ADHD in samples of parents and offspring affected with ADHD.

Clinical Management Tips for Clients with ADHD

- Establish a trusting relationship as a foundation for further intervention.
- Provide for the safety needs of the client, such as ensuring no high climbing, rough play, or reckless running.
- Provide low-stimulation situations in which the client is expected to perform cognitive tasks such as written work and listening to directions.
- Allow for periods of gross motor play to expend energy and relieve frustration.
- Provide positive reinforcement through verbal praise and rewards.
- Encourage verbalization of feelings instead of action.
- Encourage positive self-esteem-building activities such as naming positive self-attributes, playing with a peer, and completing a task.

BRAIN DEVELOPMENT

Events during brain maturation, such as injury, severe early malnutrition, and exposure to toxins may explain ADHD development.[14] Children who experienced severe malnutrition in the first year of life scored significantly worse than others on teacher ratings of behaviors such as short attention span, distractibility, and restlessness.[15] Other researchers investigated the role of maternal smoking during pregnancy by comparing families of boys with and without ADHD.[16] They found a significant relationship between maternal smoking and the development of ADHD. Environmental exposure to nicotine or an increase in carboxyhemoglobin in maternal and fetal blood, which causes hypoxia, may damage the brain during development. Exposure to other toxins, such as lead, is associated with ADHD.[14]

BRAIN FUNCTION AND STRUCTURE

In the past 10 years, new ways of viewing the brain have made neuroanatomical and metabolic information about ADHD accessible. Positron-emission tomography (PET) studies mix glucose with a tracer and administer it intravenously to ADHD subjects. Pictures are taken of the brain using the glucose for fuel when concentrating.[17] Studies using magnetic resonance imaging (MRI) have created detailed computer images of the brain. These current breakthroughs in neuroimaging lend support for the two newest theories of ADHD: motivational deficit and disinhibitory psychopathology.

Motivational Deficit Hypothesis

One current model for explaining ADHD is motivational deficit, or an insensitivity to consequences.[3] ADHD children are less likely to respond to the usual things that motivate other children to attend. Support for this view comes from findings in neuroanatomical studies and dopamine pathway studies.

Neuroimaging studies suggest decreased activation of brain reward centers and their corticolimbic regulating circuits.[3] A PET study discovered that brain activity in the striatal regions appears to use less glucose in ADHD children than in normal children.[17] Interestingly, when the **psychostimulant** methylphenidate was given to ADHD children during PET, it increased the flow to the central regions, most significantly to the right and left striatal and posterior periventricular regions.[17]

Using MRI data, other researchers[18] found a significantly smaller right anterior width measurement. This difference suggests a relationship between anterior functioning and ADHD symptoms. A subsequent study[19] found that ADHD children had smaller corpus callosums, which may indicate differences in interhemisphere connection.

The motivational model has appeal for three reasons. It explains the situational variability in attention in ADHD children.[3] It is also consistent with neuroimaging studies that show decreased activation of the brain regions thought to be responsible for reward sensitivity. This model is also consistent with neurotransmitter studies of the dopamine pathways. Barkley[3] writes that:

> deficiencies in dopamine, norepinephrine, or both may be involved in explaining these patterns of brain underactivity—patterns arising in precisely those brain areas in which dopamine and norepinephrine are most involved ... these brain areas are critically involved in incentive or motivational learning and response to reinforcement contingencies.

Disinhibitory Psychopathology Hypothesis

Hyperactive and impulsive behaviors of ADHD can be explained by an underactive inhibition system.[20] This model suggests that the brake on overactivity fails in ADHD. Poor control of motoric responses is a defining characteristic of hyperactive children and may be due to problems in disinhibition.[21] Impulse-control problems are specific to ADHD and can differentiate ADHD from other psychiatric diagnoses.[20]

Deficiency in cortical modulation may be the cause of the problem in inhibiting impulses and actions.[21] Support for this idea comes from previously mentioned neuroimaging studies that found differences in frontal lobe metabolism and size.[17-19]

The disinhibitory psychopathology model[20] has appeal for several reasons. It explains the obvious poor inhibition (or brakes) of motor responses and impulse-control problems experienced in ADHD. It is also consistent with both the neuroimaging and neurotransmitter studies to date.

NEUROTRANSMITTERS IN ADHD

Both hypotheses note the role of neurotransmitters, especially dopamine, in the function of the brain regions studied. The motivational deficit hypothesis recognizes that dopamine pathways help regulate locomotor behavior and incentive learning.[3] The disinhibitory psychopathology hypothesis recognizes the brain systems of behavioral inhibition and behavioral activation as being mediated by neurotransmitters.[20] Disinhibition may indicate a dopamine deficiency.[21]

Studies exploring dopamine and serotonin levels in the brain have relied on measuring the precursors or by-products of neurotransmitters in bodily fluids such as blood, urine, and cerebrospinal fluid.[22] There has not been any consistent disruption, either increases or decreases in the chemicals in those with ADHD.

An indirect way of testing hypotheses about dopamine, norepinephrine, and serotonin has been to test the ADHD individual's response to various medications.[22] Some medications may work by affecting levels of these neurotransmitters. The role of decreased dopamine in the limbic and caudate regions of the brain has been supported by the positive effects of stimulant medication, which acts to enhance dopamine. Tricyclic antidepressants (TCAs), monoamine oxidase inhibitors (MAOIs), and clonidine are also effective and alter the norepinephrine in the serotonergic systems. Serotonin interacts with dopamine; diminished serotonin has been linked to aggression and impulsivity.[12]

Finding a neurobiological explanation for ADHD has scientific appeal. The hypotheses presented take into consideration the mounting neuroimaging data. The majority of neuroanatomical research has been done in the past 10 years, a relatively short amount of time to reach consensus about what the findings indicate. The focus on specific brain regions, using small samples, has been a common limitation of the research. One recent study included a larger sample and examined more brain regions (see Research Note).

Although definitive causes of childhood ADHD have not been determined, clinicians agree that certain factors increase the risk of mental health and behavioral disorders: genetic vulnerability, physical injury or illness, poor prenatal and perinatal care, and environmental stressors such as poverty, malnutrition, and early brain injury. Greater preventive health care for mothers and infants and improvement in the social conditions of children may contribute to the prevention of some childhood psychiatric disturbances. Nurses active in the health policy and advocacy arenas can improve the well-being of children.

Whatever etiology is ultimately supported must take into consideration the subtypes of inattention, impulsivity-hyperactivity, and combined ADHD symptoms. Different subgroups of ADHD may have different sets of causal factors.[20] The existence of associated disorders such as mood, anxiety, conduct, and learning disorders complicates a search for the etiology of ADHD (Table 28–3).

TABLE 28–3. Co-occurrence of ADHD with Psychiatric Disorders in Childhood

Primary Diagnosis	% with Concurrent ADHD
Conduct disorder	30–50%
Mood disorder	15–75%
Anxiety disorder	25%
Learning disorder	10–92%
Tourette's disorder	60%
Mental retardation	3 to 4 times more likely

Adapted with permission from Biederman, J, Newcorn, J, and Sprich, S: Comorbidity of attention deficit hyperactivity disorder with conduct, depressive, anxiety, and other disorders. Am J Psychiatry 148:564–577, 1991.

Assessment

CLINICAL ASSESSMENT INTERVIEW

Assessing a child for ADHD means assessing for all major mental health problems. Nurses must be acquainted with the average life span stages and developmental tasks to assess delayed or deviant symptoms (Table 28–4). Many factors affect a child's or adolescent's mental health, including medical or nutritional deficits, family interactions and resources, social supports or deficits such as poverty, and cultural or community factors. For instance, a child with a hearing impairment may look inattentive. The best information comes from the child, from parents, and, whenever possible, from other caretakers, such as extended family members, daycare providers, and teachers. Before initiating treatment of any kind, obtain extensive background assessment data.

Explore potential problems in as much detail as possible. Include the symptoms, antecedents, and consequences, as well as how the family has attempted to solve the problem. In addition to providing information for planning interventions, this process of problem identification is the first step in clarifying the family's hopes and early goals of treatment.

RESEARCH NOTE

Castellanos, FX, et al: Quantitative brain magnetic resonance imaging in attention-deficit hyperactivity disorder. Arch Gen Psychiatry 53:607–616, 1996.

Findings: This recent MRI neuroanatomical study of ADHD examined differences in 12 subcortical and cortical brain regions in a matched sample of boys, ages 5 to 18, 57 boys with ADHD and 55 controls. They found that subjects with ADHD had significantly smaller total cerebral volume. They also found a reversal in the symmetry in one part of the brain, the caudate. In contrast to normal children, in whom the right caudate is larger than the left, ADHD children had a smaller size difference between the left and right caudate. The following brain areas were significantly smaller for the ADHD subjects: right globus pallidus, right anterior frontal region, and cerebellum. This study confirmed prior research findings of right-sided frontal region and caudate differences.

Application to Practice: Researchers concluded that the findings were consistent with dysfunction of the right prefrontal-striatal systems in ADHD. Identification of an etiology for ADHD will impact all areas of research and practice and benefit ADHD clients.

TABLE 28–4. Key Points of a Child Psychiatric Assessment

- Individual child and family history (both medical and psychiatric)
- Child's developmental history
- Prenatal and perinatal difficulties
- Milestones such as walking, toileting, talking, eating
- Play and socialization history
- Discipline history
- Major events affecting the child—stressors, trauma, abuse
- Support systems to the child

It is important to see the child as part of relationships and systems. During the interview, try to determine the following:

- Why is the family seeking diagnosis or treatment now?
- Is the family in crisis?
- Is there a major precipitant, or is there an accumulation of events and stressors?
- Has there been some external pressure for this referral, such as from a school counselor, court involvement, or a child-protection agency?
- Is the referral a result of change in the family stressors or support systems, such as recent loss, illness, or parent work crisis?

Understanding the child as an individual is vital. What are his or her likes and dislikes, strengths and worries? If they are asked for the positives, as well as problem behaviors, the child and family will not solely focus on a litany of "bad kid" behaviors. Ask for examples of the child's best behaviors and strengths and about the most difficult times. Try to obtain a pattern of what has been tried and has not been helpful, including therapies, medications, and limit-setting techniques. Assess the family's and the child's willingness to try something new.

- Speak with the child or adolescent separately from the parents. Sensitive information about suicidal feelings, physical and sexual abuse, sexuality, smoking, and substance experimentation or use are not often revealed in front of a parent. Ask the child about punishment practices at home. Ask if anyone has touched him or her in a way that was scarey or confusing.
- Children who reveal being hit or hurt at home may be in danger. Nurses, along with other health-care providers, are mandated reporters of suspected physical or sexual abuse or neglect of a minor. The local child-protection agency is responsible for assessing and intervening for the safety of the child after they receive a report. Their work may involve determining that no abuse has occurred, ongoing monitoring of the family, or immediately moving the child to foster care or a relative's home.
- Adolescents are also at risk for abuse outside the home. Ask about relationships with dates and friends. Adolescents may tend to minimize violence from peers, which puts them at risk for injury and exploitation (see Research Note).

ASSESSMENT INSTRUMENTS

Rating scales are an important aid to assessment. Tools have been developed to assess for inattention and hyperactivity. Most list behavioral criteria and ask teachers and parents to rate the child. For instance, the Child Behavior Checklist lists behaviors that identify and categorize the global functioning of the child, including ADHD symptoms.[23] The Connors Rating Scale is the most widely used tool for the study of attention-deficit and hyperactivity problems.[24,25] A 10-item scale was reduced from the 93-question scale by selecting the most frequently identified attention and activity problems, resulting in the Abbreviated Connors Rating Scale (ACRS). The ACRS has a four-point range, with 0 as no problem and 3 as very problematic on the 10 behaviors. It provides a single total score, with high scores suggestive of ADHD. As a screening tool, it is often given to parents and teachers to monitor a child's target behaviors over time. In addition, other instruments are available to aid assessment of psychiatric symptoms in children, adolescents, and adults; some key tools for ADHD are listed in Table 28–5.

Researchers and clinicians have begun to use new objective measures for quantifying ADHD. Inattention can be measured with a computerized test, the *continuous performance test*. There are many versions, but all measure attentiveness through speed and accuracy scores in response to computer-screen cues.[26] To quantify the movement component of ADHD, two devices are used. The *actigraph* is a small computer device worn on the wrist or the waist that records thousands of activity measurements over a number of days. The data demonstrate overall day and night activity,

---

> **RESEARCH NOTE**
>
> Symons, PY, Groer, MW, Kepler-Youngblood, P, and Slater, V: Prevalence and predictors of adolescent dating violence. Journal of Child and Adolescent Psychiatric Nursing, 7:14–23, 1994.
>
> **Findings:** This study examined the relationships among race, parental education, family structure, parental discipline, and family violence exposure, to the dating violence experience. Five hundred sixty-one rural North Carolina adolescents (77% female, 40% black, and 58% white) participated by filling out a questionnaire. Sixty percent of the respondents had experienced violent acts, with 24% reporting extreme violence, such as rape or use of a weapon. A statistical analysis yielded significant difference only for factors of exposure to family violence and family sexual abuse. The factors of race, gender, or religion were not significant. A regression analysis on just the female respondents indicated that only drug and alcohol use predicted an increase in the total abuse score or likelihood of experiencing date violence. Interestingly, adolescents tended not to label violence abusive, denying they were in an abusive relationship although relating abusive and violent events.
>
> **Application to Practice:** This study and others suggest a link between family violence and violence in other relationships. Nurses should routinely ask about abuse from peers. Nurses can identify adolescents at risk due to family history and provide counseling or education about the expectations of a healthy relationship.

TABLE 28–5. Common Instruments for the Measurement of ADHD

Instrument	Description	Obtain by Writing
Child Behavior Checklist: Over 100 questions, including an ADHD subscale	Parent ratings for children or self-report for adolescents	T. Achenbach Univ. Assoc. in Psychiatry 1 South Prospect St. Burlington, VT 05401
Connors Rating Scale: Abbreviated versions have 10 ADHD items	Parent ratings for children or teacher ratings of classroom behaviors	Multi-Health Systems 908 Niagara Falls Blvd. N. Tonowanda, NY 14120
Adolescent and Adult Brown Attention-Deficit Disorder Scales: 40 ADHD items	Self-reports	The Psychological Corp. Harcourt Brace & Co. San Antonio, TX
K-SADS: Semi-structured interview covering major psychiatric disorders (DSM criteria)	Clinical interview with parent and child	Western Psychiatric Institute University of Pittsburgh School of Medicine 3811 O'Hara St. Pittsburgh, PA 15213

Source: Adapted from Scahill, L, and Ort, SI: Selection and use of clinical rating instruments in child psychiatric nursing. J Child Adolesc Psychiatr Nurs 8:33–42, 1995.

minute-to-minute fluctuations in activity, and circadian rhythms. Activity studies have demonstrated that children have overall higher activity levels during the day and night, with few periods of low-level activity. Another device, an infrared motion-analysis system, tracks the vertical and horizontal movement of small circular pieces of reflector tape, placed on a child who is seated performing a task. Figure 28–1 shows a child performing the task. Information on amount and pattern of movement is computer analyzed. Initial studies indicate that boys with ADHD moved, changed position (fidgeted), and were more restless than boys without ADHD. Figure 28–2 illustrates the movement patterns of two children derived from infrared motion analysis. Objective measures like these do not replace parent and teacher observations but add a valuable comparative tool to support or challenge a diagnosis.

Planning Care

In general, interventions with children must be sensitive to their cognitive and developmental level. Use a neutral, calm

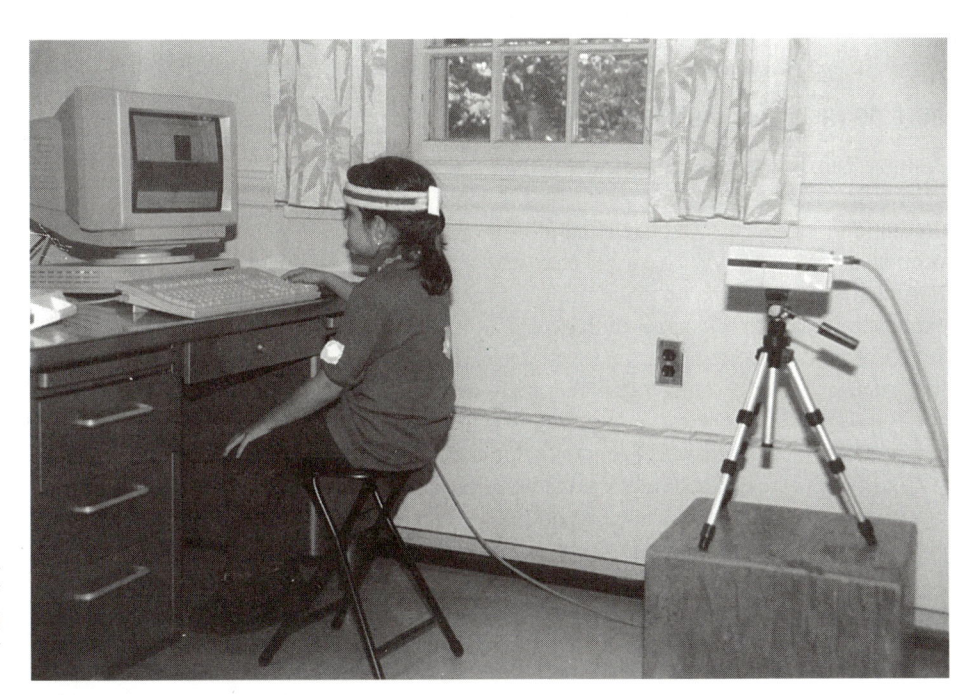

Figure 28–1. The child in this photograph is performing the CPT computer task, while an infrared motion analysis camera records her movements.

Comparison of the Movement Patterns of Two Children

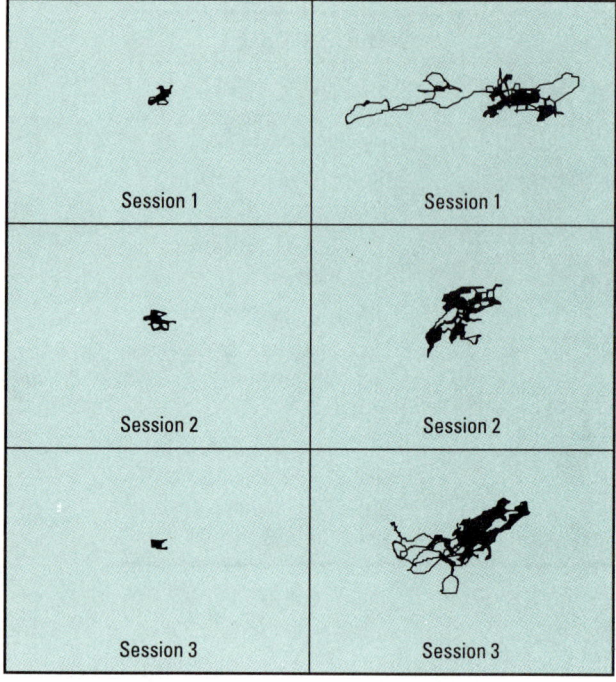

Normal 9-year-old girl   ADHD 9-year-old boy

Figure 28–2. Infrared Motion Analysis. As the child fidgets, the pathway of a reflective marker attached to the head is recorded. These three 5-minute recordings compare a child with normal movement on the left with a child with hyperactivity on the right. The ADHD child moved frequently and covered more area.

tone of voice and concise language because clients are sensitive to tone, cadence, and volume. Establishing trust and an alliance is vital. Peplau's[27] conceptual framework for interpersonal relations applies to the different roles of a nurse working with children. The five roles apply to varied settings, such as home, school, and community.

ROLE OF THE NURSE AS RESOURCE

A nurse can function as a resource person, the source of knowledge and expertise for the client and family,[27] interpreting and clarifying the plan of care. Demonstrate intervention techniques such as sticker charts for positive reinforcement. Be prepared to shift from an age-appropriate explanation for the child to an adult explanation for the parent. Give rationales based on the psychological readiness of the listener.[27] For instance, a mother may ask questions about the stimulant medication prescribed for her child. Assess and offer information pertinent to the mother's concern, such as helpful hints for timing the medication after breakfast to avoid decreased morning appetite. She may not be much interested in the pharmacologic actions of the drug.

ROLE OF THE NURSE AS TEACHER

The role of teacher differs from that of resource person in complexity. Traditional teaching occurs in obtaining permission for treatment, so-called *informed consent*. Give parents who are admitting their child to a facility, releasing confidential records, or initiating a trial of medication crucial information about rights and risks. Obtain the child's assent or verbal agreement before initiating and providing treatment.

As with most teaching, a problem-solving approach is most useful. Families seek services of mental health professionals for a variety of complex, multidimensional problems. The needs and resources available to the client are unique, and solutions are not simple.

ROLE OF THE NURSE AS LEADER

The third role is leader. Families identify the nurse as a leader and seek his or her direction.[27] Develop a leadership style that sets the agenda, goals, and responsibilities for moving forward collaboratively with clients and families. In a mental health treatment setting, there is the risk that families will expect the responsibility for change and improvement in their children's functioning to fall on the shoulders of the counselors or staff. Explain to families that change occurs within the child and family when they are ready and willing. No one can "fix" the situation for them.

ROLE OF THE NURSE AS SURROGATE

The fourth role is as a surrogate. The child may begin to think of the nurse as a substitute figure and react to the nurse based on feelings evoked from a prior relationship.[27] Often the behavior of a nurse, especially in a caretaking role, reminds the client of someone else. The child often views the nurse as a parent figure. Understand one's own reactions, help the child see the similarities and differences between the perceived surrogate and the nurse, and become aware of what feelings the old relationship evokes.[27] It is natural for a child to feel dependent on a nurse who provides positive regard and caring like that of a parent. For example, a 7-year-old girl was always eager to climb on the nurse's lap and kiss her. The feelings of the child toward a person in a caretaking role were appropriate. The blurring of the personal boundaries was not. Careful not to reject the child, the nurse made a game of teaching the girl about physical space, asking her if she was thinking about her mother, in an attempt to help the child connect the behavior with the surrogate confusion.

A child who feels hostile toward his or her mother may "act out" with the nurse. For example, a 13-year-old boy with angry feelings for his mother always challenged the rules of the residential program. Instead of arguing with him, the nurse posted a "struggling sheet" and marked each time he followed a rule without initiating an argument for attending mealtimes, doing homework, and participating in therapy groups. She gave rewards for each five check marks, including extra positive time with his favorite staff member. He was able to engage with the nurses as individuals, instead of struggling for control.

ROLE OF THE NURSE AS COUNSELOR

The final role of the nurse is as counselor. Counseling promotes self-awareness and facilitates self-directed actions in children and families.[27] A therapeutic relationship creates conditions within which children can explore how they feel and what is happening to them. The autonomy and accountability for this role vary, based on the setting and practice level of the nurse. But the therapeutic relationship is the core of psychiatric nursing care for clients and families.

Interventions for Hospitalized Clients

Depending on the severity of symptoms, assessment may lead to hospitalization, outpatient psychotherapy, school and home interventions, or psychopharmacologic intervention. Children with ADHD and related diagnoses may have periods when their symptoms exacerbate, requiring intense intervention. Some are dangerous to themselves or others and require admission to an inpatient psychiatric unit. Frequently the admission takes place after a suicide gesture or attempt, or a major threat or harm to another person. Young children may need admission after a reckless incident, such as attempting to jump out of a window or moving car, setting fires, or having excessive numbers of tantrums that cause bodily harm, such as head banging.

Hospitalization occurs only after less restrictive alternatives such as outpatient intervention, help from extended family, or community resources have been unsuccessful. Child psychiatric hospital units are set up as communities, not as individual rooms. Ideally, this "milieu" environment provides the client with an atmosphere that promotes personal growth and healing. Milieu can refer to inpatient, partial hospitalization, or residential care centers, where the clients live in the setting some or all of the day. All create safe conditions but specialize according to the philosophy of the treatment center. Nurses within a milieu typically establish therapeutic relationships with the children and adolescents, provide client and family education, monitor health needs, plan activities, lead groups, and administer medications.

Interventions for Clients in the Community

Often a timely, brief consultation is all a child and family require. Less commonly, they require longer-term, individual treatment.

Children

Individual therapy with children differs from the traditional talk therapy. It is often less insight-oriented and uses age-appropriate communication strategies, such as **play therapy**. Playing is a natural, healthy part of childhood. Play can also be a therapeutic medium through which nurses can help children. Children can communicate with nurses through action play, fantasy play, or artistic expression, such as drawing. Drawings are often used to understand the thoughts and feelings of children. A simple example is asking children to draw themselves and their families. Children who draw themselves much smaller and on the farthest edge of the page may feel they are not central or equal to other members.

Play can be a corrective experience for the child, using make-believe to redo past anxiety-provoking situations and change the ending.[28] Play can also be used as an educational tool. For instance, a nurse might have the child practice blood-drawing on a doll before doing the actual painful procedure, to help the child anticipate and master the fear. Supervised play groups can increase a child's socialization skills by providing brief successful games involving turn-taking and reciprocity. See Figure 28–3 for an illustration of a small play group.

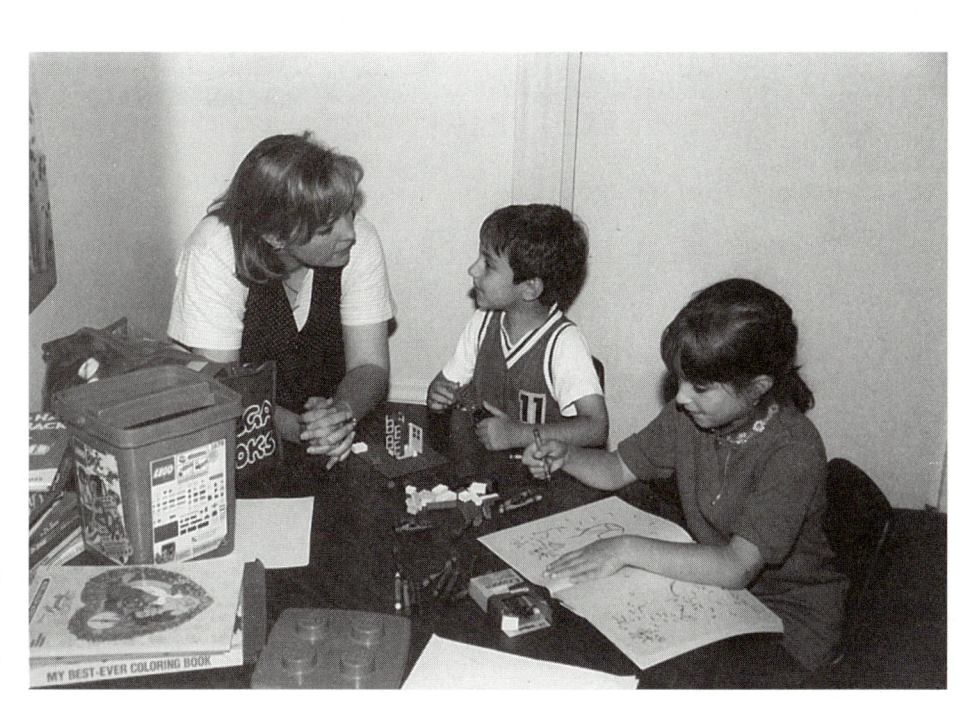

Figure 28–3. Play groups can help a child communicate feelings and increase successful socialization. (Photograph courtesy of Kenneth Hanrahan.)

Adolescents

Young adolescents may also benefit from play settings as opposed to traditional talk therapy. Board games such as checkers and Monopoly, as well as available therapeutic board games, offer an opportunity for enhancing discussion, exploring topics, and increasing self-awareness.[28] With older adolescents, the goals of therapy depend on the primary problem. An adolescent with ADHD and depression may need to focus on self-esteem and expression of feelings. Brief, focused talk therapy may help an adolescent through a difficult transition to a new school or deal with a major loss.

COGNITIVE-BEHAVIOR INTERVENTIONS

Home-based Interventions

Behavior modification helps extinguish negative behaviors and reward positive behaviors. **Cognitive-behavior intervention** focuses on modifying and shaping the child's or adolescent's behavior and thinking. Modeling, positive feedback, rewards, and contingencies are the major techniques. An example of a program for a school-aged child is a positive reinforcement program. At predetermined intervals throughout the day, the child receives positive feedback from adults, either staff, teachers, or parents, depending on the setting. Verbal praise from adults reinforces the positive behavior of meeting goals such as safe behavior, being social to others, and using words to express feelings. The number of times a goal is reached corresponds to a reward or privilege, such as a prize or more play or television time. The Clinical Management Tips for Implementing Behavior Programs offer some suggestions for parents.

Clinical Management Tips for Implementing Behavior Programs

- Pull toward the positive: Give lots of praise when behavior is good and calm neutral consequences when behavior is not good.
- Keep it simple: A program should become part of the routine, not artificial or a burden to the family's schedule.
- Struggle over the safety issues, but let the consequences (such as not earning points) be the limits for the small misbehaviors.
- Give the rewards earned: Consistently follow through on promised rewards; make them easy to do (not too time-consuming or expensive).
- Twice a week make a fresh start on a program, so that a difficult day or two does not set a negative tone for weeks.
- Do not make expectations or rewards "all or nothing": Have levels of what the child can earn so that there will always be some recognition of effort, such as good, very good, or excellent.

Older children and adolescents use cognitive-behavior intervention to identify and practice alternatives to maladaptive coping behaviors. Individuals practice specific interventions, including making lists of antecedents and consequences to behaviors, monitoring mood before and after stressful events, making positive self-statements, rehearsing communication skills, and practicing stress reduction and relaxation techniques. Clients are given "homework" assignments to practice these alternative coping techniques between sessions. For example, a 12-year-old girl with the diagnosis of ADHD and conduct disorder had difficulty in specific areas: following rules, acting out with aggression toward people and objects, not expressing feelings, and not taking responsibility for her grooming and belongings. A child psychiatric nurse set up a cognitive-behavior home-based program that helped her control escalating and acting out behaviors and helped avoid placement in a residential center. Home health aides provided after-school structure and supervision. See Behavioral Home-based Program for the Jones Family for her plan of care.

School-based Interventions

Guidelines and suggestions are helpful to parents. Teach them the basic elements of successful interventions to provide a structured environment with clear and consistent expectations at home and at school. Teachers can help children organize. One strategy is to encourage placing assignments in a multipocket folder. Another is to send home a list to parents of children's expected work for the week. School nurses often notice symptoms and can make referrals, in addition to providing hotline numbers and support groups available to students.

Teach adolescents and adults time-management strategies to help them stay organized, such as calendars, reminder cues, and preplanning techniques. Table 28–6 outlines helpful strategies.

PSYCHOPHARMACOLOGIC INTERVENTIONS

The initiation of drug therapy for a child or adolescent is based on the immediate clinical need. For example, pediatric dosages are based on a range of milligrams per kilogram of the child's body weight, per day. Table 28–7 lists medications that effectively treat ADHD, pediatric dosages, and teaching tips.

Psychostimulants

The stimulants methylphenidate, amphetamine, and pemoline are the most widely used medications to treat ADHD. Amphetamine is approved for age 3 and older, whereas methylphenidate and pemoline are approved for age 6 and older.[29] Despite being stimulants, they calm these children's overactivity and improve attention. Side effects include difficulty sleeping, loss of appetite, headache, rapid heartbeat, and, occasionally, facial tics.[30]

Box 28-1. Behavioral Home-based Program for the Jones Family

Daily Program

Mary will begin a behavioral feedback program negotiated with the home health aide, therapist, and her parents. Mary likes visual cues, so she has agreed to use the posting of smiles and frowns for completing tasks and apples drawn on a tree poster as her points toward a reward. More smiles than frowns equal a green apple drawn on a tree; conversely, more frowns than smiles equal a red "crab" apple drawn on the tree. The home health aides do this daily.

Morning Program

- Wake up with a smile
- Shower
- Eat breakfast
- Brush hair
- Brush teeth
- Take medication
- Manage feelings safely*
- Be on time

Afternoon Program

- Come home with a smile
- Talk about school
- Change into play clothes
- Do homework
- Do something constructive
- Clean up messes; care for own clothes
- Manage feeling safely*
- Use exercise—treadmill, dancing†

*The "manage feelings safely" will help focus Mary's time with the home health aide by labeling her primary problem.
†The exercise point will help Mary develop an alternative to acting out for stress reduction.

Evening Program

Mary's parents, Laura and Tony, will award an evening point (apple) for *safe expression of feelings* from the time the home health aide leaves until bedtime. "Safe" means no physical aggression and good use of time out. Continuing with "apples" allows for continuity with the weekday program. Having the parents focus solely on the *safe expression* behavior helps prioritize the focus of the program.

On the weekends, Saturday will be a day off from the program when Mary will practice being safe and cooperating without the reminders of a program to see how she does. Laura had expressed a need to have a "normal" day of interactions with her daughter. Also, because this is a reward day, the focus can be on positives.

Sunday will begin the new week, and Mary can earn up to three points (apples)—morning, afternoon, and evening for *safe expression of feelings*.

In addition, Laura and Mary have begun a "communication journal" in which they will write back and forth to each other each day, or when they wish. Both agreed not to have this equal any points. Journaling will serve as an alternative expression of feelings and aid in parent-child communication.

Rewards

The arrangements for rewards for positive behavior have been made between Mary and her parents. Both Laura and Mary have agreed on twice-a-week reward times that fit into their routine. The home health aide has agreed to tally the number of points (apples) and make new posters each Tuesday and Friday with Mary.

The Wednesday evening reward for positive points Sunday/Monday/Tuesday (possible 3 per day) will be:

- 7–9 points (apples) = video rental movie with mom
- 5–6 points (apples) = 30-minute late night
- 1–4 points (apples) = 15-minute late night

The Saturday afternoon reward for positive points Wednesday/Thursday/Friday (possible 3 per day) will be negotiated Wednesday and posted as a possible reward to earn:

- 7–9 points (apples) = special event chosen from list
- 5–6 points (apples) = 30-minute late night
- 1–4 points (apples) = 15-minute late night

The range of points and rewards allows for success at different levels of effort.

The following is a list of agreed-upon special events for Mary.

1. Special time with her mother at the hairdresser or movies, baking, arts and crafts projects, visiting favorite relatives, or renting a video.
2. Special time with her father to go fishing or to the beach, or to enjoy Star Trek.
3. Special event with a friend and mom to do an activity.
4. Other special event as arranged.

Mary seems highly motivated by suggestions to spend positive, fun time with her parents. By including the option of a special event with a friend, Mary can be encouraged to have successful supervised interactions with friends.

National concern has been raised about the recent trend of treating school-aged children with stimulants.[11] The frequency of stimulant use has more than doubled since 1990. Parents and teachers may pressure clinicians for an easy fix to behavioral problems. In safe practice, medication treatment is considered after thorough assessment. Cognitive-behavior interventions are usually employed concurrently.

Psychostimulants have the potential to be abused; therefore, they are not prescribed when the individual has a substance-abuse problem. Families must make sure that only the child with ADHD takes the medication.

Antidepressants

The TCAs desipramine and imipramine have been used for treating ADHD.[31] The safety of TCAs for children is in question; several children, 6 to 9 years old, treated with desipramine died.[32] As a result, these medications are usually

TABLE 28-6. Time Management Suggestions for ADHD Adolescents

Suggestions for Organizing
- Fill out a planning schedule on Saturday for the appointments, assignments, and so forth for the upcoming week.
- Check off when you complete something as planned, and write down when you don't.
- Prepare for the morning the night before . . . such as what clothes to wear and what books you'll need for school.

Suggestions for Academics
- Ask teachers for a syllabus for the year, or at least the assignments a month in advance.
- If you know ahead of time the topic for class, read the chapter to become familiar with it: this will help with knowing what notes to take down in class.
- Ask friends to let you photocopy their class notes if you have trouble following your own.
- Ask teachers for help prioritizing what would be important to study for a test, such as a study topic guide.
- Ask teachers for extra time to complete in-class tests.

avoided. When TCAs are used, children need thorough assessment and monitoring of cardiac status including twice-a-year electrocardiograms (ECGs).

A newer treatment for ADHD is bupropion (Wellbutrin), an antidepressant that also reduces overactivity and improves attention.[29] Compared to stimulants, bupropion appears equally effective, without the potential for abuse. Side effects include agitation, insomnia, and dry mouth.

Antihyperhensives

The antihyperhensives clonidine (Catapres) and guanfacine (Tenex) effectively treat ADHD.[31,33] However, they may treat hyperactivity better than inattention. The combination of a stimulant and clonidine may be used for the treatment of ADHD. These medications require monitoring for orthostatic hypotension as the dosage increases. Side effects include sedation, and abrupt cessation may cause nervousness and rebound hypertension.[29]

Expected Outcomes

Expected outcomes for children manifesting inattention and hyperactivity symptoms vary considerably with each individual. Ideally, children will learn to compensate for their difficulties and symptoms resolve. Some children will continue to have difficulties and need medication, therapy, and lifelong adjustments in school and work situations. ADHD is associated with the risk of conduct problems, substance abuse, and mood disorders, making outcomes more difficult to predict. As with any childhood disorder, early detection and intervention improve clinical prospects.

Differential Diagnosis

Misdiagnosis of childhood psychiatric disorders can be a result of developmental, emotional, and social factors. Some children show an immaturity or developmental lag that can be mistaken for a deficit. Others may be seen as inattentive, when actually they have a primary learning difficulty, such as dyslexia, or an expressive problem. Children under a great deal of stress or pressure from life situations can appear overactive and distractible because they focus on their problems, not on schoolwork. Difficulty concentrating occurs in many psychiatric disturbances, primarily major depression. Sad feelings can also indicate depression or poor self-esteem. Depressed mood may be an appropriate reaction to environmental stressors, such as school failure, academic difficulties, or constant frustration with not meeting the expectations of others.

Acting out of negative or disruptive behaviors can be the result of lack of supervision and support at home. It can be an adaptation to family chaos; it is the best way to get attention. In adolescence, acting out does not necessarily denote a psychiatric disorder. Occasional defiance and rule breaking are typically part of the adolescent's struggle to separate from parents. Peer groups can also negatively influence an adolescent's behavior on a temporary basis. Only a pattern of misbehavior that is pervasive and causes impairment indicates a problem, such as Oppositional Defiant Disorder (ODD). ODD is a 6-month pattern of behavior characterized by refusing to comply with adults' requests, being easily annoyed, and blaming others for mistakes.

MOOD

Some children with ADHD have symptoms of irritability and mood lability. Fifteen to 75% of the children diagnosed with a mood disorder also have ADHD.[35] Bipolar symptoms (as described in Chapter 19) usually appear when individuals are in their 20s, but as many as 25% have their first mood episode as adolescents.[36] Although rare, some prepubescent children begin to show mood lability and episodic patterns of depressed and expansive behavior. Increased activity, talkativeness, and impulsivity can appear to be mania in some clients.

Symptoms of poor self-esteem and depressed mood can occur with ADHD, and major depression can occur during both childhood and adolescence. Major depressive disorder in children is usually recurrent and can be associated with a family history of affective disorders.[37] Children or adolescents with depressive symptoms, like adults, may be at risk for suicide. Symptoms such as blaming oneself and hopelessness make the individual vulnerable to impulsive self-destructive thoughts and suicidal behavior. The impulsive

TABLE 28–7. Common Psychopharmacological Treatment of ADHD

Medication	Suggested Pediatric Dosages	Teaching Needs
Stimulants		
methylphenidate (Ritalin)	20–30 mg/day in divided doses;* not to exceed 60 mg/day	• Doses usually given in am. • Give doses before meals to help with decreased appetite. • Avoid doses close to bedtime to help with possible insomnia.
dextroamphetamine (Dexedrine)	20–40 mg/day in divided doses;* not to exceed 60 mg/day	• Monitor for nervousness and increased heart rate. • Alert prescriber at first sign of facial tics.
pemoline (Cylert)	37.5–75 mg/day, in a single am dose; not to exceed 112.5 mg/day	• Give small afternoon dose to help with possible rebound irritability. • Monitor liver function in pemoline users only.
Antidepressants		
imipramine (Tofranil)	50–75 mg in single dose at bedtime;* not to exceed 2.5 mg per kg a day	• Gradually increase dose. • Monitor cardiac status for possible increased BP/pulse, or postural hypotension. • Monitor tricyclic users only with routine ECGs. • Use increased fluids to help with dry mouth and constipation.
bupropion (Wellbutrin)	75–150 mg/day in divided doses* Adult dose is 300 mg/day	
Antihypertensives		
clonidine (Catapres)	0.05–0.3 mg/day in divided doses;* not to exceed 0.01 mg per kg per day Available in 7-day transdermal adhesive patch. 0.05–1 mg (long acting), given once or twice daily*	• Increase gradually based on BP response. • Monitor for BP changes and orthostatic hypotension. • Monitor for sedation. • Avoid sudden discontinuation, which may cause nervousness or a rise in BP.
guanfacine (Tenex)	Adult dose is 3 mg at bedtime	

*Younger children may need lower doses; as with all medications, individual dosages may vary.
Sources: Physicians Desk Reference, ed 50. 1996. Bezchlibnyk-Butler, KZ, and Jeffries, JJ: Clinical Handbook of Psychotropic Drugs, ed 6. Hogrefe & Huber Publications, Toronto, 1996.

nature of ADHD may make them more vulnerable to act before thinking things through.

LEARNING

Ten to 92% of the children with learning deficits also have ADHD.[35] The etiology of learning, communication, and motor skill impairments is thought to be related to the specific area of the brain responsible for the function. Slow maturation or damage may cause neuroanatomical abnormalities.[2] The *DSM-IV* learning disorders include reading disorder, mathematics disorder, and disorder of written expression. For each, poor achievement on standardized tests and interference with academic success must be present.[2]

Learning disorders and ADHD impair academic, social, and self-esteem development, depending on the severity of the impairment and the response from the school, family, and social environments. School nurses are increasingly more involved in the care of children with ADHD; they are taking an active role in identifying and coordinating care for the ADHD child at school.[38]

TRAUMATIC EXPERIENCES

Children and adolescents can experience posttraumatic stress disorder (PTSD) as a consequence of neglect or physical and sexual abuse. The criteria are the same as adult PTSD: There must be exposure to trauma that has threatened death or serious injury and evoked a response of intense fear

> **RESEARCH NOTE**
>
> Glod, CA, and Teicher, MH: Relationship between early abuse, posttraumatic stress disorder, and activity levels in prepubertal children. J Am Acad Child Adolesc Psychiatry 34:1384–1393, 1996.
>
> **Findings:** This study examined the relationship between early abuse, PTSD, ADHD, depression, and activity levels in a sample of 19 abused children (mean age 9.4 years) and 15 controls (mean age 8.3 years). Activity was measured with actigraphs worn continuously for 3 days. The abused children were 10% more active than the controls. Abused children who were experiencing PTSD had activity similar to typical ADHD children. Abuse early in life was associated with current PTSD and hyperactivity, whereas abuse later in life was associated with current activity similar to that seen in typical depressed children.
>
> **Application to Practice:** This study demonstrates an association between ADHD and PTSD, especially in children who have experienced abuse early in life. Hyperactivity, a common symptom of ADHD, also prevails in children with PTSD. It points to the need for early identification and treatment of abused children. Nurses are in a prime position to begin to evaluate these disorders. More objective diagnostic aids may help differentiate symptoms. It also suggests that abuse early in childhood may display overactivity, typically associated with ADHD.

or helplessness.[2] Children may use repetitive play enacting the events or have scary nightmares as part of the usual avoidance and hyperarousal symptoms.[39] Children with ADHD and PTSD can manifest similar overactivity (see the Research Note).

Trauma response has lasting effects on brain chemistry and development, whether the trauma is actively remembered or not.[40] Difficulties modulating emotion, numbing, and hyperalertness to possible environmental dangers affect clients' capacities for positive new experiences and learning more adaptive coping. When this problem is added to the difficulties already experienced by ADHD children, the learning and treatment needs of the individual become quite complex.

CONDUCT AND OPPOSITIONAL BEHAVIORS

Thirty to 50% of children diagnosed with conduct disturbances have concurrent ADHD diagnosis.[35] The diagnosis of conduct disorder identifies a pattern of asocial behaviors that impact school, home, and social relationships. The child or, more commonly, the adolescent, disregards the basic rights of others.[2] Key conduct problems include aggression toward people and animals, bullying, fighting, mugging, deliberate destruction of property, deceitfulness, theft, and serious violations of rules such as truancy and running away.[2]

Oppositional defiant disorder (ODD) is a less severe pattern of disruptive behavior. These children or adolescents have negative, hostile, and defiant behaviors, including often losing their tempers, arguing with adults, deliberately annoying people, and being spiteful or resentful.[2]

Some children with ADHD and conduct disorder develop antisocial personality disorder or mood, anxiety, or substance-abuse disorders.[2] Adults with antisocial personality disorder, in addition to exhibiting a pattern of criminal acts and reckless disregard for others, are impulsive and aggressive.

MENTAL RETARDATION

Children with mental retardation as the primary diagnosis can also experience ADHD symptoms; they are three to four times more likely than children with average intelligence to have ADHD.[35] Mental retardation affects approximately 1% of the general population. It is defined as significant subaverage intellectual functioning with deficits in adaptive functioning, including self-care, communication, and daily living skills.[2] The severity ranges from mild to profound.

The etiology of mental retardation is understood in terms of severity. Mild retardation is typically seen in the children of mentally retarded parents and among individuals with lower socioeconomic status in which inheritance, poverty, and inadequate health care are primary factors.[14] In more severe and profound retardation, 90% have prenatal causes such as genetic chromosomal abnormalities and neurodevelopmental damage secondary to specific infections, physical trauma, and ingestion of toxins. For each individual, the prognosis for function and independent living depends on the severity of symptoms and environmental supports.

PERVASIVE DEVELOPMENTAL DISORDERS

Children with severe developmental impairments, known as pervasive developmental disorder (PDD), also have a higher incidence of ADHD than average children.[20] The most common PDD is autistic disorder. Autistic disorder is characterized by impairments in social interactions, such as no eye contact and no spontaneous play; impairments in communication, for instance, absence or delay of language; and, presence of repetitive stereotypic behaviors, such as hand flapping.[2] In most cases, mental retardation is also present. The etiology of autistic disorder is related to genetic and biological factors, particularly prenatal neurodevelopmental damage.[14]

PDD in young children signals the start of a lifelong chronic course. Specific treatments for language and behavioral components, such as behavior modification and medication, may improve quality of life. These individuals usually require lifelong supervision, either at home with specialized schooling or in long-term treatment centers.

TIC DISORDERS

Tic disorders, such as Tourette's disorder, can occur with ADHD in as many as 60% of the cases.[35] Tics are stereotyped motor movements or vocalizations, such as eye blinking, facial grimacing, grunting, swearing, or repeating sounds or words.[2] Self-consciousness and rejection by peers make this an especially difficult disorder for a child.

ANXIETY

Anxiety disorders, including generalized anxiety disorder, phobias, separation anxiety disorder, and obsessive-compulsive disorder (OCD), occur with ADHD in as many as 25% of the cases.[35] Anxiety in children can be related to a specific event, such as separation from mother; a specific fear, such as snakes; or a specific situation, such as speaking in front of the class. Anxiety disorders are not present unless the child's response is irrational and the fear causes impairment in functioning.[2]

PSYCHOTIC DISORDER

The onset typically occurs between late adolescence and mid-30s[2] and includes disturbances in thinking such as schizophrenia in adults, including delusions, hallucinations, and disorganized speech and actions. Childhood onset is rare and difficult to evaluate because children's symptoms are less obvious, and disorganized speech and behavior are present in other disorders such as ADHD and PDD.[2]

Synopsis of Current Research

Genetic research in ADHD, especially in the areas of mental retardation and PDDs, is identifying markers and chromosomal abnormalities. Prenatal and postnatal influences on brain maturation offer possible etiologic explanations for ADHD. Brain-imaging studies are beginning to identify neuroanatomical abnormalities and examine metabolism in various brain regions.

Research on the efficacy and representativeness of rating-scale measures and objective computerized tools such as actigraphs and motion analysis continues to help with the identification and diagnosis of children with psychiatric disorders. Research into the effects and efficacy of treatments such as psychopharmacology continues. Identifying factors associated with the experiencing of psychiatric difficulties and predicting difficulties tend to be a primary focus for nursing studies, although nurses contribute to all these areas of research.

Areas for Future Research

- What is the role of genetic research in the screening and treatment of ADHD?
- How do brain abnormalities predict treatment response?
- What will the consensus of researchers and clinicians be about the etiology of ADHD?
- What is the efficacy of newer antidepressant and antihypertensive interventions?
- What factors predict long-term persistence of symptoms in adulthood?
- What time-management strategies best help adults manage symptoms of ADHD?

CASE STUDY

Patrick S, a 6-year-old boy, was brought to the emergency room after breaking a wrist while bike riding. This was one of many visits for Patrick, who, according to his mother, is reckless and impulsive. During the emergency room interview, Mrs. S reported a pattern of worsening symptoms over the past year including excessive running and climbing, inability to remain seated, excessive talkativeness, interruption of conversations, inability to wait his turn in games, and constant activity. When the nurse asked about past problems, the mother reported that he was disruptive in kindergarten and did not want to pay attention. Because first grade was starting in a few weeks, and his recklessness was increasing, she wanted to see if anything would help him "settle down." The nurse referred them to a local mental health center for outpatient evaluation.

During the initial family assessment, the following data were obtained. Patrick lived at home with his biological parents, Mary and Carl, both age 24. Carl worked fulltime as a truck driver, while Mary worked parttime as a cashier. Both maternal and paternal grandparents helped out with babysitting and were critical of Patrick's behavior. Family history was mostly without mental health problems, except Carl reported having "attention problems as a kid," which he "outgrew."

Patrick's medical history included occasional ear and throat infections, stitches on his forehead at age 3 from a fall, and multiple ER evaluations for bruises and scrapes on his knees and elbows, with the most serious injury, a fractured wrist, occurring the previous week. Patrick's developmental history was normal, with milestones of walking, toileting, and talking on target for age. Since the age of 3, Patrick had always been curious, daring, and energetic. His parents recalled having to "watch him every minute." They denied any history of physical or sexual abuse. They reported using punishments of taking away toys, making him stay in his room, and occasionally "slapping him on his bottom" for dangerous misbehavior. Both parents described Patrick as a loving child who "tries to be good." Patrick presented as a friendly, smiling child. Although active during the interview, he was able to play briefly with each of the variety of toys in the office. He preferred crashing cars into each other to coloring.

A standard interview screening found that Patrick did not meet the criteria for mood, anxiety, and thought disorders. Using the *DSM-IV* criteria list, the outpatient treatment team determined that Patrick did met the criteria for Attention-Deficit/Hyperactivity Disorder, Predominantly Hyperactive-Impulsive Type.

Treatment team recommendations for Patrick were psychopharmacologic and cognitive-behavior psychoeducation approaches. Patrick was medicated with the stimulant Ritalin (methylphenidate), in gradually increasing doses until the hyperactive symptoms were managed. The nurse clinician worked with Patrick's mother in establishing more structure at home through a bedtime routine and a checklist of necessary activities such as teeth brushing and getting dressed. The nurse clinician provided parent training in using consistent limits, positive feedback, time-out discipline, and clear, concrete instructions with Patrick.

When Patrick began first grade, the teacher also used techniques to structure and organize Patrick's schoolwork and homework. The school nurse administered Patrick's Ritalin at noon daily and was available to assess for further problems in need of referral. These brief, focused interventions stabilized Patrick's symptoms and helped him be more successful in his daily life.

CRITICAL THINKING QUESTIONS

1. What concerns would frequent injuries and emergency room visits raise?
2. If it became apparent that some of the injuries were inflicted by his father, how would that influence your plan of care?
3. What are the family resources and supports?
4. How might Patrick's father's own experience with attention problems affect his understanding and responses?
5. What were the urgent clinical needs that indicated a choice of psychopharmacology intervention now?
6. Identify behaviors that would indicate that Patrick is responding to the treatment.
7. What are long-term goals for Patrick and his family?
8. Design a teaching plan to assist Patrick's family in caring for him.

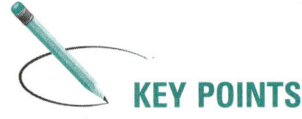

KEY POINTS

- ADHD is diagnosed when children have significant difficulty with inattention, impulsivity, and hyperactivity.
- ADHD children are at risk for poor school performance, rejection by peers, and low self-esteem.
- Adolescents and adults often continue to experience ADHD symptoms and are at risk for difficulties in relationships and work situations.
- The prevalence of ADHD is about 3 to 5% of school-age children.
- ADHD often co-occurs with conduct disorder, mood disorder, anxiety disorder, learning disorder, tic disorder, or mental retardation.
- Many factors affect a child's or adolescent's mental health, including medical or nutritional deficits, family interactions and resources, social supports or deficits such as poverty, and cultural or community factors.
- Disinhibitory psychopathology hypothesis is one explanation for hyperactive and impulsive behaviors. Poor control of motor responses is a defining characteristic of hyperactivity and may be due to an underlying disinhibitory problem in the brain.
- Motivational deficit hypothesis is one explanation for ADHD. Children with ADHD are able to sustain attention in only some situations. Deficits may be due to brain underactivity in the regions that control incentive learning and response.
- Although definitive causes of childhood ADHD have not been determined, clinicians agree that certain factors increase the risk of mental health and behavioral disorders: genetic vulnerability, physical injury or illness, poor prenatal and perinatal care, and environmental stressors such as poverty, malnutrition, and early brain injury.
- Cognitive-behavior interventions focus on modifying and shaping the child's or adolescent's behavior and thinking, with the techniques of modeling, positive feedback, rewards, and contingencies.
- Adolescents and adults find time-management strategies, such as calendars, reminder cues, and preplanning techniques, helpful for staying organized.
- Play therapy is a therapeutic medium through which a child can communicate with the therapist in action play, fantasy play, or artistic expression, such as drawing, instead of words alone.
- Stimulants, such as methylphenidate, amphetamine, and pemoline, are the most widely used medications to treat ADHD. Stimulants calm overactivity and improve attention in ADHD children.

REFERENCES

1. National Institute of Mental Health: National Plan for Research on Child and Adolescent Mental Disorders: A Report Requested by the U.S. Congress. Department of Health and Human Services, Publication No. (ADM) 90–1683. U.S. Government Printing Office, Washington, DC, 1990.
2. American Psychiatric Association: Diagnostic and Statistical Manual of Mental Disorders, ed 4. American Psychiatric Association, Washington, DC, 1994.
3. Barkley, RA: Attention-Deficit Hyperactivity Disorder: A Handbook for Diagnosis and Treatment. The Guilford Press, New York, 1990.
4. Erikson, EH: Childhood and Society. WW Norton & Co Inc, New York, 1963.
5. Hartman, T: ADD Success Stories: A Guide to Fulfillment for Families with Attention Deficit Disorder. Underwood Books, 1995.
6. Berry, C, Shaywitz, S, and Shaywitz, B: Girls with attention deficit disorder: A silent minority? A report on behavioral and cognitive characteristics. Pediatrics 76:801–809, 1985.
7. Szatmari, P, Offord, D, and Boyle, M: Ontario child health study: Prevalence of attention deficit disorder with hyperactivity. J Child Psychol Psychiatry 30:219–230, 1989.
8. Glod, C, Teicher, M, McGreenery, C, Ducsik, M, Anderson, C, Polcari, A, and Becker, S. Gender differences in hyperactivity of elementary school children. Poster presented at the Annual Harvard Medical School Research Day, Department of Psychiatry. March 14, 1996.
9. Biederman, J, Faraone, SV, Spencer, T, Mick, E, and Lapey, KA: Gender differences in a sample of adults with attention deficit hyperactivity disorder. Psychiatry Res 53:13–29, 1994.

10. Safer, DJ, and Krager, JM: The increased rate of stimulant treatment for hyperactive/inattentive students in secondary schools. Pediatrics 94:462–464, 1994.
11. Hancock, L: Ritalin, are we overmedicating our kids? Newsweek, March 18, 1996, 51–56.
12. Cantwell, DP: Attention deficit disorder: A review of the past 10 years. J Am Acad Child Adolesc Psychiatry 35:978–987, 1996.
13. Cook, EH, Stein, MA, Krasowski, MD, Cox, NJ, Olkon, DM, Kieffer, JE, and Leventhal, BL: Association of attention-deficit disorder and the dopamine transporter gene. Am J Hum Genet 56:993–998, 1995.
14. Popper, CW, and Steingard, RJ: Disorders first diagnosed in infancy, childhood, or adolescence. In Hales, RE, Yudofsky, SC, and Talbot, JA (eds): The American Psychiatric Press Textbook of Psychiatry, ed 2. American Psychiatric Press Inc, 729–832, Washington, DC, 1994.
15. Galler, JR, Ramsey, F, Solimano, G, and Lowell, WE: The influence of early malnutrition on subsequent behavioral development, II. Classroom behavior. J Am Acad Child Adolesc Psychiatry 22:16–22, 1983.
16. Milberger, S, Biederman, J, Faraone, SV, Chen, L, and Jones J: Is maternal smoking during pregnancy a risk factor for attention deficit hyperactivity disorder in children? Am J Psychiatry 153:1138–1142, 1996.
17. Lou, HC, Henriksen, L, Bruhn, P, Borner, H, and Nielsen, JB: Striatal dysfunction in attention deficit and hyperkinetic disorder. Arch Neurol 46:48–52, 1989.
18. Hynd, GW, Clikeman, MS, Lorys, AR, Novey, ES, and Eliopulos, D: Brain morphology in developmental dyslexia and attention deficit disorder/hyperactivity. Arch Neurol 47:919–925, 1990.
19. Hynd, GW, Clickeman, MS, Lorys, AR, Novey, ES, Eliopulos, D, and Lyytinen, H: Corpus callosum morphology in attention deficit-hyperactivity disorder: Morphometric analysis of MRI. In Shaywitz, SE, and Shaywitz, BA: Attention Deficit Disorder Comes of Age: Toward the Twenty-First Century. DD Hammill Foundation, Pro-Ed, 245–257, 1992.
20. Hinshaw, SP: Attention Deficits and Hyperactivity in Children. Sage Publications Inc, Newbury Park, CA, 1994.
21. Teicher, MH, Anderson, SL, Navalta, CP, Glod, CA, and Gelbard, HA: Neuropsychiatric disorders of childhood and adolescence. In Yudofsky, SC, and Hales, RE (eds): Textbook of Neuropsychiatry, ed 3. 930–940, 1996.
22. Zametkin, AJ, and Rapoport, JL: Neurobiology of attention deficit disorder with hyperactivity: Where have we come in 50 years? J Am Acad Child Adolesc Psychiatry 26:676–686, 1987.
23. Achenbach, TM: Manual for the Child Behavior Checklist. UVM Dept. Psychiatry, Burlington, VT, 1991.
24. Connors, CK: Symptom patterns in hyperactive, neurotic, and normal children. Child Dev 41:667–682, 1970.
25. Connors, CK: Rating scales for use in drug studies with children. Pharmacology Bulletin. 35–42, 1973.
26. Teicher, MH: Actigraphy and motion analysis: New tools for psychiatry. Harv Rev Psychiatry 3:18–35, 1995.
27. Peplau, H: Interpersonal Relations in Nursing. Putnam, New York, 1952.
28. Worthy, MK: The use of a playroom as a nursing intervention with early adolescent age group. J Child and Adolescent Psychiatric Nursing 7:38–43, 1994.
29. Physicians Desk Reference, Fiftieth Edition. 1996
30. Bezchlibnyk-Butler, KZ, and Jefferies, JJ: Clinical Handbook of Psychotropic Drugs, ed 5. Hogrefe & Huber Publishers, 1995.
31. Kaplan, HI, Sadock, BJ, and Grebb, JA: Synopsis of Psychiatry, ed 7. Williams & Wilkins, Baltimore, 1145–1150, 1994.
32. Elliot, GR, Popper, CW, and Frazier, SH: Tricyclic antidepressants: A risk for 6–9 year olds? J Child and Adolescent Psychopharmacology 1: 105–106, 1990.
33. Hallowell, EM, and Ratey, JJ: Driven to Distraction. Pantheon Books, 201–202, 1994.
34. Biederman, J, Newcorn, J, and Sprich, S: Comorbidity of attention deficit hyperactivity disorder with conduct, depressive, anxiety, and other disorders. Am J Psychiatry 148:564–577, 1991.
35. Strober, M: Bipolar disorder. In Peschel, E, Peschel, R, Howe, CW, and Howe, JW (eds): Neurological Disorders in Children and Adolescents. Jossey-Bass Inc Publ, Old Tappan, NJ, 35–38, 1992.
36. Brent, D: Major depressive disorder. In Peschel, E, Peschel, R, Howe, CW, and Howe, JW (eds): Neurological Disorders in Children and Adolescents. Jossey-Bass Inc Publ, Old Tappan, NJ, 39–44, 1992.
37. Odom, SE, Herrick, C, Holman, C, Crowe, E, and Clements, C: Case management for children with attention deficit hyperactivity disorder. J School Nursing 10:17–21, 1994.
38. Hartman, CR, and Burgess, AW: Information processing of trauma. J Interpersonal Violence 3:443–457, 1988.
39. Burgess, AW, Hartman, CR, and Clements, PT: Biology of memory and childhood trauma. J Psychosocial Nursing 33:16–26, 1995.

UNIT Five

Problems in the Community

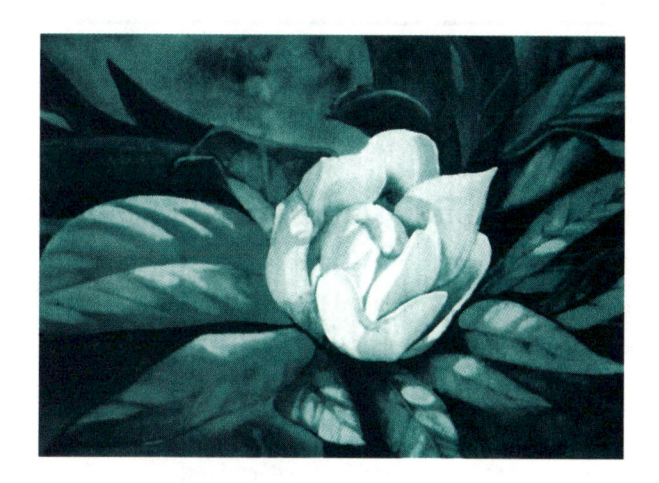

CHAPTER 29
Prolonged Mental Illness: Clients and Their Families in the Community

CHAPTER 30
The Faces of Homelessness

CHAPTER 31
Victims of Abuse

CHAPTER 32
Persons Living with HIV Disease and AIDS

CHAPTER 33
Care of Individuals in Correctional Facilities

CHAPTER 34
Grieving

CHAPTER 29

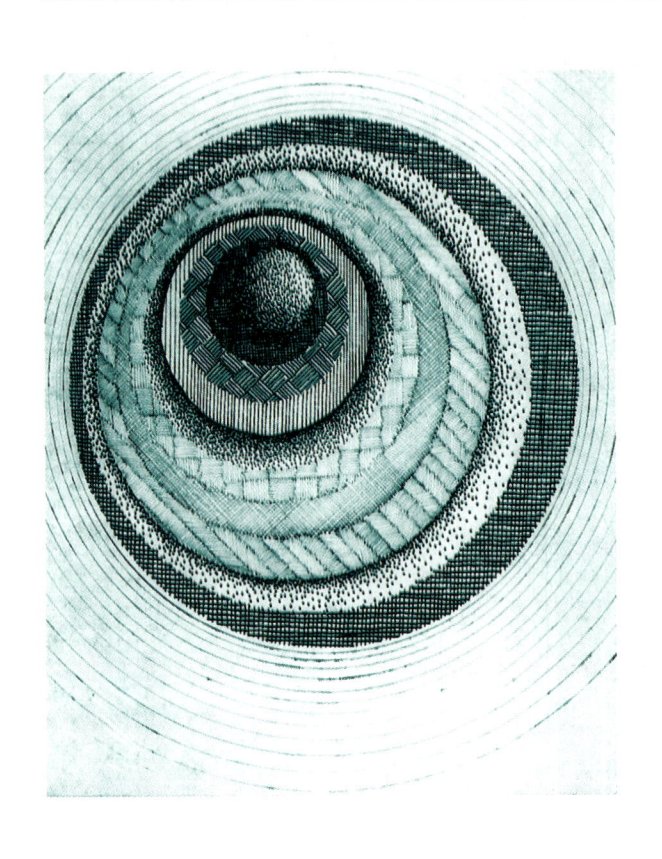

CHAPTER OUTLINE

Characteristics of Prolonged Mental Illness
Concept of Recovery and Nursing Considerations
Impact of Prolonged Mental Illness
Prognosis
Historical Perspectives
   Managed Costs and Rationed Care
   Nursing Process within a Systems Context
Open Systems Model within the Community
   Assessment and Data Collection
   Dilemmas Experienced by Individuals with PMI: Nursing Diagnoses, Outcomes, and Intervention Strategies
   Environments and Support Systems
Models of Treatment and Rehabilitation
   Case Management
   Continuous Treatment Teams
   Residential Care
   Psychosocial Rehabilitation Programs
Evaluating Outcomes
Areas for Future Research

Anne L. Silva, RN, MS, CS
Sonja Stone Peterson, RN, EdD

Prolonged Mental Illness: Clients and Their Families in the Community

LEARNING OBJECTIVES

After completing this chapter, the reader should be able to:

- Describe the characteristics of a prolonged mental illness.
- Discuss the impact of recent economic, social, and scientific forces on individuals experiencing prolonged mental illness.
- Define the term *psychiatric disability*.
- Describe four dilemmas commonly encountered by individuals coping with a prolonged mental illness.
- Identify three types of community resources that assist individuals experiencing a prolonged mental illness.
- Identify essential characteristics of a community support program that help promote health and rehabilitation of individuals experiencing psychiatric disabilities.
- Describe two support groups for family members coping with individuals experiencing a prolonged mental illness.

KEY TERMS

boundary
chronic sorrow
community support
 programs
institutionalization
prolonged mental illness
psychiatric disabilities
psychosocial rehabilitation
revolving door syndrome
stigma

Caring for individuals with prolonged mental illness remains one of the greatest challenges confronting nurses. Clients experiencing this type of long-term illness require frequent evaluation, a respectful, humane approach, and supportive assistance. Nurses must develop empathic understanding of the clients' illness experiences and how they affect individuals, their educational or vocational pursuits, their families, and the community. They need skills in assessing clients' access to health-care programs and in imparting knowledge of **community support programs** available to clients and their families.

CHARACTERISTICS OF PROLONGED MENTAL ILLNESS

A traditional view of illnesses as lasting the duration of clients' lives referred to these illnesses as chronic. The use of the term *chronic* typically reflected progressively worsening symptoms throughout the course of individuals' lives. Bachrach[1] emphasized that labeling illnesses as "chronic" fails to communicate the concept of learning to live with a lifelong disability in which symptom manifestations and remissions occur uniquely among individuals. The term **prolonged mental illness** (PMI) aptly applies to lifelong psychiatric disabilities that

- Interfere with an individual's interpersonal, social, or vocational pursuits.
- May be intermittent or episodic in the manifestation of symptoms but persist over time.
- Require ongoing therapeutic and medical management to minimize symptoms and to optimize an individual's capacity to engage in activities or relationships.

PMI, applicable to a number of psychiatric diagnostic profiles described in the *Diagnostic and Statistical Manual of Mental Illness, Fourth Edition (DSM-IV)*, describes an individual's illness experiences rather than the specifications of any one illness. Although PMI frequently refers to individuals whose illness includes a psychotic component, people with other psychiatric illnesses meeting the previously stated criteria may also be viewed as experiencing PMIs.

CONCEPT OF RECOVERY AND NURSING CONSIDERATIONS

Within the psychiatric rehabilitation literature, the concept of *recovery* has been identified as the mission for mental health services in the 1990s. Anthony[2] describes recovery:

> A deeply personal, unique process of changing one's attitudes, values, feelings, goals, skills, and/or roles. It is a way of living a satisfying, hopeful, and contributing life even with limita-

tions caused by illness. Recovery involves the development of new meaning and purpose in one's life as one grows beyond the catastrophic effects of mental illness. (p 17)

This definition recognizes that, even in the absence of a "cure," people can adapt and evolve beyond their illnesses. Individuals with a PMI can recover, derive meaningful experiences, and enjoy life. The tasks for nurses when collaborating with clients and their families in the rehabilitation process include

- Assisting each person to identify and understand the problems associated with a given illness.
- Helping each person to manage and minimize the problems associated with the illness experience.
- Guiding each person through the process of adaptation that optimizes strengths, abilities, and talents.
- Educating the person in using appropriate resources provided within the community.

IMPACT OF PROLONGED MENTAL ILLNESS

Since 1950, the number of psychiatric state hospital beds per 100,000 of the population has dropped from 339 to 29, in 1994.[3,4] Although the number of hospital beds has decreased, the incidence of mental illness has not. Estimates are that approximately one-third of the homeless in the United States are individuals experiencing PMI. Perhaps even more surprising, according to the National Alliance for the Mentally Ill (NAMI), 30,700 individuals with mental illness are held in U.S. jails because of the inability of the public mental health system to provide adequate community services.[5] Problems related to these two special groups—the homeless and the incarcerated—are discussed later in Chapters 30 and 33.

The pain and suffering, **chronic sorrow**, experienced by individuals with PMI and their families and the effects on the society in general are difficult to appreciate. Table 29–1 shows the prevalence of serious mental illnesses in the United States. The effects on society can also be measured in part by costs: Treatment for individuals experiencing schizophrenia totals $33 billion annually within the United States. A recent analysis[6] estimated the U.S. costs for individuals experiencing depression to be approximately $43.7 billion:

- $12.4 billion, or 28%, constitutes direct costs for medical, psychiatric, and pharmacologic care.
- $7.5 billion, or 17%, comprises mortality costs associated with depression-related suicides.
- $23.8 billion, or 55%, reflects associated costs from individuals' absenteeism and reduced productivity in the workplace because of depression.

PROGNOSIS

Multiple factors (Figure 29–1), such as neurobiophysical, psychosocial, spiritual, cultural, or access and use of resources, influence the outcome of a PMI and its course, remission, and exacerbation. These factors, as well as ongoing scientific advancements in treatment and psychopharmacology, make it difficult to project a long-range prognosis.

Prior to the early 1980s, for example, many individuals were severely disabled by psychosis and unable to cope without highly structured **institutionalization**. Clients required frequent hospitalizations for acute exacerbations of their illnesses and were repeatedly hospitalized, leading to a **revolving door syndrome**. However, because of the development and use of clozapine (Clozaril), many of these individuals today are able to live independently and work within the community. (Chapter 6, focusing on pyschopharmacology, discusses clozapine and other new medications used for clients experiencing PMIs.) Advances in psychopharmacology, coupled with assistance from caregivers, illustrate that individuals and families can be offered realistic hope for the future.

HISTORICAL PERSPECTIVES

Society's views, beliefs, and assumptions about mental illness, as well as historical and political events, have shaped the care and treatment of individuals with mental illnesses. Table 29–2 outlines important markers in mental health care in the United States.

MANAGED COSTS AND RATIONED CARE

Although knowledge about the etiology, treatment, and management of mental illnesses has become more sophisticated and specific, the ability and willingness of society to underwrite such costs is severely compromised.

Economic Forces

For the past 15 years, there has been growing concern about the cost of health care in the United States. In 1965, the

TABLE 29–1. Lifetime Prevalence Rates of Serious Mental Illnesses

Percentage	Type of Illness
0.2–2.0%	Schizophrenia
0.4–1.6%	Bipolar disorders
5.0–25%	Major depressive disorder

Source: Adapted from Reiger, DA, Narrow, W, Rae, D, Manderscheid, RW, Locke, BZ, and Goodwin, FK: The defacto U.S. mental and addictive disorders service system: Epidemiologic catchment area prospective 1-year prevalence rates of disorders and services. Arch Gen Psychiatry 50:85–94, 1993.

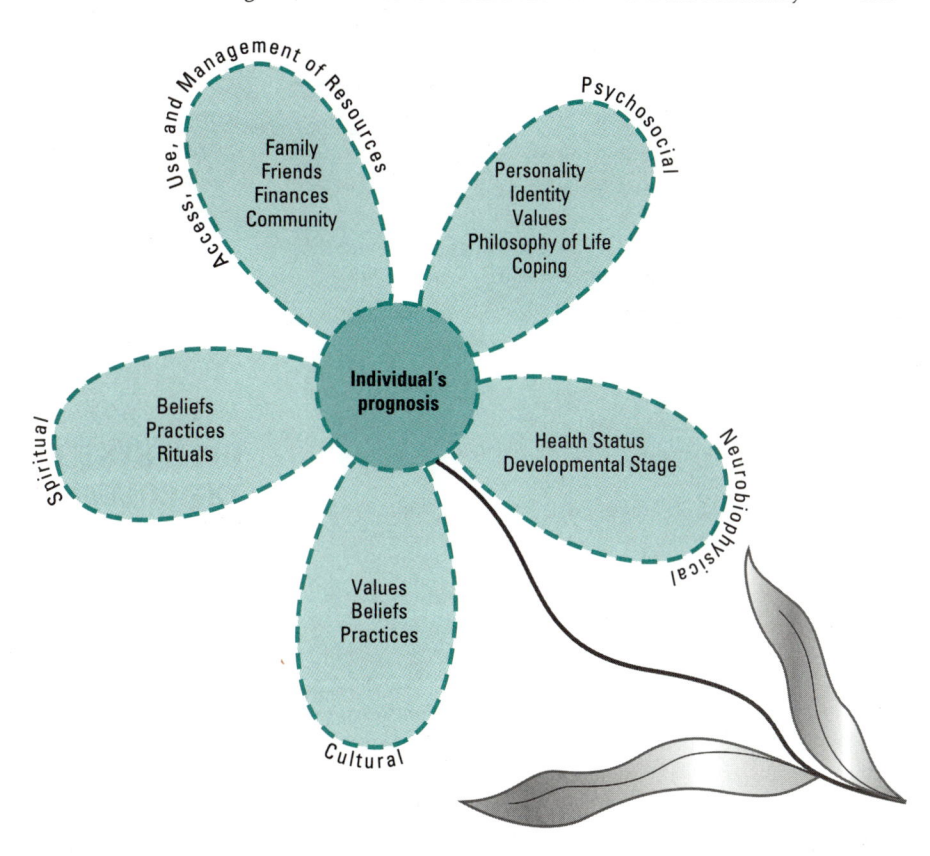

Figure 29–1. Influencing factors on individual's prognosis.

percentage of the U.S. gross national product (GNP) devoted to national health expenditures was 6%. Currently, even with adjustments for inflation, 12% of the GNP is spent on health and illness services.[7] The most expensive health-care cost is hospitalization, and the fastest growing medical expense is mental health and substance-abuse care. Regarding psychiatric illnesses, insurance companies and public mental health agencies alike have attempted to decrease hospitalization frequency and length of stay. However, there has not always been sufficient community or home care services to support fewer and shorter hospitalizations.

Nevertheless, the current economic pressures have provided some positive outcomes. Issues of quality assurance and limited reimbursement for mental health services have caused agencies and clinicians alike to examine the cost effectiveness of specific services and care-delivery structures. Also undergoing financial scrutiny is the utilization of the specific health-care professions. For instance, what level of education and training is needed to provide case management? Are there significant differences in the outcomes of medication groups led by psychiatrists and those led by clinical nurse specialists? There is increasing interest in outcome-focused research to identify the most successful and cost-effective treatment interventions and service delivery structures. Given the current economic climate and the continued stigma of PMI, there is concern about the future. In the effort to do more with less, will the care of individuals with PMI be left to untrained and unlicensed staff?

Consumerism

Members of organizations such as NAMI and the Manic Depressive and Depressive Association (MDDA) demand to be treated as active collaborators in the development of health-care policies and treatment programs. Professional associations like the American Psychiatric Nurses Association (APNA), the Society for Education and Research in Psychiatric Nursing (SERPN), and the American Medical Association (AMA) are recognizing the agenda they share with these advocacy groups: a concern for high-quality care with an emphasis on accessible, humane treatment. An example of this shared endeavor within one state is reflected in a series of town meetings and forums sponsored by the Massachusetts Nurses Association (MNA) during the winter of 1996. The public meetings attracted attendees and participants from the MNA, care provider groups, and consumer-advocate organizations, including NAMI.

Improved Psychopharmacologic Agents

The formulation of new medications that are more symptom-specific in their action and have fewer side effects reflects a significant advance in the care and treatment of individuals with PMI. As neurobiologists and psychopharmacologists discover more about the specificity of neurotransmitters, neurochemicals, and receptors, they have been able to develop medications such as clozapine, risperidone, sertraline, valproic acid, and fluoxetine. For many clients, these new

TABLE 29–2. Markers in Mental Health Care

Decade	Achievements
1950s	Introduction of psychotropic medications. Joint Commission on Mental Illness and Health established.
1960s	Deinstitutionalization movement began with the Community Mental Health Centers Act: Authorized federal funds for development of services in local communities.
1970s	National Institute of Mental Health initiated Community Support Program and established Office of Programs for Homeless Mentally Ill. National Alliance for the Mentally Ill (NAMI) established as a grass-roots family organization offering education, support, and advocacy for improved care and treatment of mentally ill.
1980s	Increased interest and activism with consumer focus: Proliferation of NAMI state affiliate groups; NAMI and Manic Depressive and Depressive Association (MDDA) advocated to be treated as active collaborators addressing health-care policy issues, treatment programs.
1990s	Known as the "Decade of the Brain" with research emphasis into mental illnesses as neurobiological illnesses. The Americans with Disabilities Act (ADA) included rights of individuals with psychiatric disabilities. Managed care movement provided continuity of care for clients in transition from one setting to another. Improved psychopharmacologic agents such as clozapine, risperidone, and amisulpiride.

medications provide more effective treatment options than previous generations of medications. Chapter 6 describes a variety of new medications, their respective benefits, intended effects, and side effects.

NURSING PROCESS WITHIN A SYSTEMS CONTEXT

Because rising medical costs will continue to be a major concern for health-care administrators, nurses will often care for individuals with PMI in settings other than inpatient treatment units. Nurses will encounter clients in a variety of settings: employee health clinics, community residences, private apartments and homes, or prenatal care classes. Consequently, nurses will find themselves caring for individuals coping simultaneously with specific health needs and PMI.

The principles of nursing as articulated by Peplau[8] (and described in Chapter 2) apply whether the registered nurse practices in an acute treatment setting, community clinic, or client's home. The nurse assesses and attempts to meet the client's need for help.[9] However, when this process is applied to an individual experiencing PMI and trying to cope with multiple needs while living in the community, the relevance of an open system's perspective becomes apparent (Figure 29–2). The nurse must critically assess exactly how the individual

1. Manages illness symptoms
2. Accesses resources for care
3. Interacts with other health-care professionals contributing to the continuum of care.

OPEN SYSTEMS MODEL WITHIN THE COMMUNITY

Characteristics of an integrated model of nursing process and a system's framework include that

- The nursing process is directed to bring about adaptation and recovery over time.
- The specific circumstances and experiences of the client will determine the configuration and overlap of the components within the model.
- Exchange and influence may occur at every **boundary** interface.
- The interactions of components are dynamic and change over time.
- The extent to which the nursing process includes or limits the components of the model is determined by the role, abilities, and authorization of the nurse.
- Although the nursing process involves input and data from all components, there is a unique dynamic exchange between the nurse and client.
- The assessment and diagnosis of problems are not limited to the client's state.
- The evaluation of change and adaptation provides new input and data that are used to further refine interventions and strategies to promote adaptation.
- The nursing care plan or treatment plan may provide data to all components, strengthening the coordination of care.

The components of the nursing process as presented in Chapter 2 should be used as a framework for assisting clients. These components include data collection via assessment, intervention planning, implementation of strategies, and the evaluation of outcomes within the context of the open systems model previously presented. Complementing this framework are considerations specific to the nursing care of clients with PMI.

ASSESSMENT AND DATA COLLECTION

A comprehensive assessment is the most significant aspect of the nursing process. The accuracy, relevance, and effectiveness of subsequent parts are dependent on a thorough database. When considered within an open systems context,

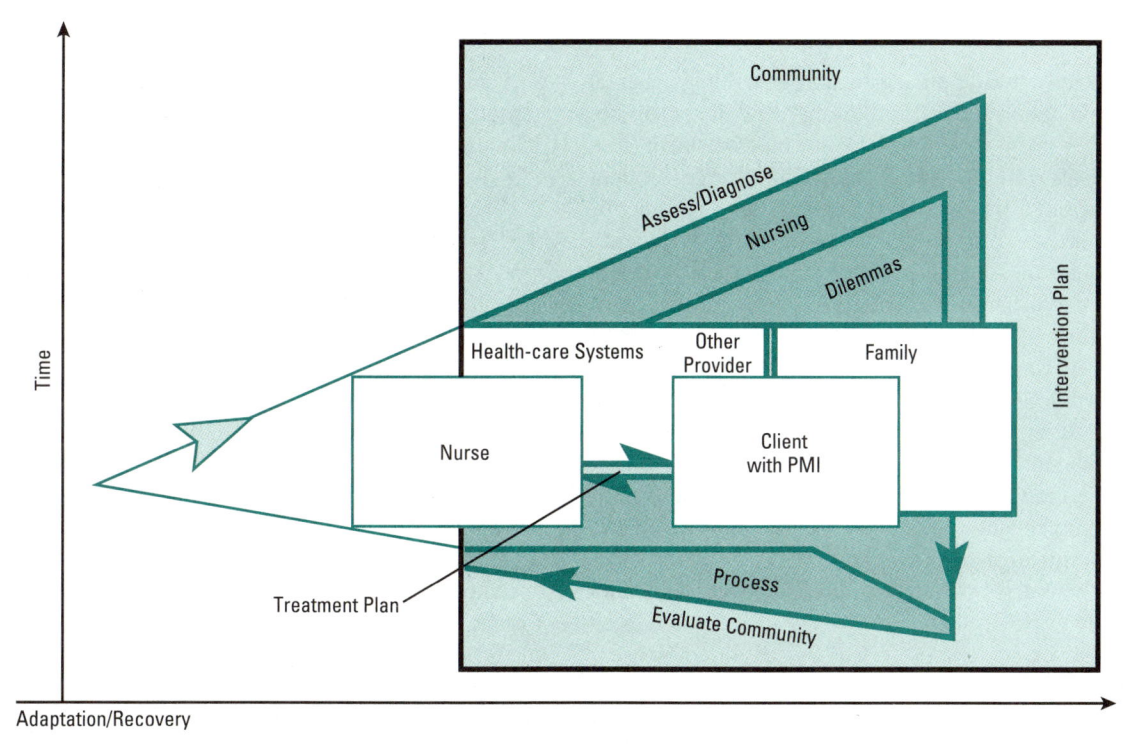

Figure 29–2. Model of the nursing process and systems considerations in the care of a client with PMI.

the assessment phase of the nursing process is not limited to the client. Data should also be gathered about family involvement and resources, other assistive individuals or groups, and accessibility of health-care services and community resources.

Physical Health

Studies[10] over the years have documented the undiagnosed medical problems of individuals with PMI. Whether in the emergency room, private practice setting, or day treatment program, clients' medical problems frequently were neither investigated nor diagnosed; some were mistakenly perceived as attention-seeking behavior, somatization manifestations, or psychotic preoccupations. The problem of diagnosed or overlooked medical problems is complex, because many individuals with PMI do not have optimum health-promoting behaviors or regular access to preventive health care. A safe principle of nursing practice emphasizes a thorough assessment of all physical complaints expressed by clients. Remember, too, that some clients experience altered communication and consequently convey physical complaints indirectly through unclear verbal communication or nonverbal behaviors. The following situation demonstrates the importance of the nurse's attentive listening to a client's communication about physical concerns.

Susan G, a 33-year-old woman with a *DSM-IV* diagnosis of chronic schizophrenia, had resided in a publicly supported group home since she was 20 years old. Susan attended a psychosocial rehabilitation program 5 days a week. One afternoon before the last psychoeducational group began, Susan shouted to the registered nurse who served as leader of the group:

You don't care about me! I have thousands of bees in my butt and you don't hear a word I am saying. All you want me to do is attend those stupid groups all day long. You don't know what it's like. You'll never know. I talk to you, but you don't hear me. I have bees in my butt! I will not go to the groups, never will I go to the groups!

SUSAN G

The astute nurse, perceiving that Susan might have a real physical problem, sought additional information by asking, "Tell me more about the bees in your butt." Susan retorted, "I've had them for weeks and they feel like they're stinging me awfully bad." The nurse continued with an assessment and soon determined that Susan's bowel had possibly prolapsed. A prolapse can cause the intense pain that Susan perceived as being stung by a thousand bees. Susan was taken to a general hospital's emergency room where the physician diagnosed her prolapsed bowel. She then received treatment for her physical complaint.

A holistic approach to clients' care is underscored by the fact that many outpatient treatment centers, as well as insurance companies, require individuals to have physical examinations prior to, or in conjunction with, accessing mental health care services. The case study of Greta J at the end of the chapter provides critical thinking questions that support the value of a thorough assessment of the client by a community mental health center's registered nurse.

Mental Status Examination

The significance and approach for implementing a mental status examination are discussed in Chapter 2. It contributes essential data to a comprehensive client assessment and, when reviewed over time, may demonstrate changes brought about by specific treatments or interventions. The mental status examination also provides an assessment of the individual's ability to function and has implications for determining the immediate level of intervention required to assist the individual.

Sample of Key Questions. Each client needs to be assessed in the following areas so that the mental status examination covers all pertinent data for comprehensive planning and intervention.

- Are the individual's reality testing and judgment sufficient to maintain safety?
- Is the individual able to organize himself or herself sufficiently to carry out self-care and home-care activities of daily living (ADLs)?
- Is the person compromised by distorted sensory perceptions?
- Is the person at risk for self-destructive, aggressive, or impulsive behavior?
- Does the individual have the capacity to problem solve, anticipate outcomes of actions, and make plans?

In general, the more compromised an individual's ego functions, the more likely the client will require medication, external structure, support, and supervision.

History of Prolonged Mental Illness

The adage "He who does not learn from history is doomed to repeat it" is often demonstrated in the lives and treatment interventions of individuals with PMI. Time and effort spent obtaining a comprehensive history from the client, the family, and other health clinicians involved in the client's care help to provide a thorough, up-to-date database. Accurate and current data facilitate the development of the individual's treatment plan, including therapeutic interventions. Complete data gathering ultimately saves time and effort for health-care team members, as well as the clients and their families.

Essential Areas for Inquiry. Important questions to address with clients and families include:

- What circumstances preceded the onset of illness?
- What factors have exacerbated the illness?
- What has helped to improve the individual's health?
- When does the individual believe he or she was functioning optimally?
- Are there specific times of the year, situations, or anniversaries that are especially difficult?
- What has been the course of treatment, including hospitalizations, medications, outpatient programs, and specific treatment team members?
- Have any other family members had any mental illness or similar problems?

Medications

The nurse, client, and family must have a thorough understanding of each prescribed medication. Necessary information provides answers to these questions:

- What is the intended effect of the medication?
- How and when is the medication to be taken?
- What are the potential side effects of the medication?
- What interventions can reduce the side effects?
- What precautionary measures should be exercised while taking the medication?
- What circumstances indicate that the prescribing clinician should be contacted, and how?
- What might be expected if the client decides to discontinue prescribed medication?
- How does the individual obtain the medication?

Because many psychotropic medications have systemic effects, the nurse must ensure that the client is also aware of specific safety precautions and required laboratory tests. Information should include frequency and reason for specific medications. For example, when clozapine is prescribed, a weekly blood test is necessary to monitor white blood cell counts. Because information about medication remains a critical intervention, it is prudent to provide for the client a printed guide or medication information sheet detailing pertinent facts. A sample teaching guide can be found in the chapter focusing on psychopharmacology. Giving the client clear, concise information with individually adapted useful instructions encourages adherence to the prescribed medication regimen. This intervention will serve as a simple reference, reinforcing the client's learning and memory.

Health Risks

Four health risk factors for many individuals with PMI are obesity, substance use, smoking, and neglect of their physical health. Eating, smoking, and the ingestion of alcohol or other nonprescription drugs are often precipitated by boredom or other emotional stressors. Each may provide a sense of soothing or satisfaction or be an attempt at ameliorating distressing symptoms like hallucinations. The behaviors associated with these health problems often occur within a social context or culture that further reinforces the behaviors. Given their specific roles and expertise, nurses may or may not be responsible for implementing a plan to directly address clients' health risks. However, nurses need to assess potential health risks and assist individuals to access the necessary community resources. Although some individuals with PMI have shown lack of awareness of or denied the implications of unprotected sex, Torrey[11] points out that values and cultural beliefs also influence clients' use of condoms with sexual activity.

Family Systems and Social Supports

Increasingly, families, especially mothers, are finding themselves responsible for some aspect of care.[11] Many adult children with PMI return to their parents' homes because they

> **RESEARCH NOTE**
>
> Doornbos, MM: The strength of families coping with serious mental illness. Arch Psychiatr Nurs 10(4): 214–220, 1996.
>
> **Findings:** This study sought to identify variables related to families' stressors, coping, and health when one family member experienced a serious and persistent mental illness. The sample, comprising 85 families, was derived from one midwestern state's support groups, community mental health agency, and public and private psychiatric hospitals. Seventy-three percent of the clients in the sample's families were male, taking medication (96%), and complying (82%) with their medication programs. Survey instruments used to measure variables included: Family Inventory of Life Events and Changes (FILE); Family Crisis Oriented Personal Scales (F-COPES); two scales (cohesion and adaptability), from the Family Adaptability and Cohesion Evaluation Scales (FACES III); Family APGAR for satisfaction with family functioning; and Family Environment Scale (FES) for conflict. Data from sample families were compared to normative families.
>
> This study clearly identified that although families of the mentally ill reported more stressors, they showed more adaptability and at the same time reported less cohesion and less satisfaction. Families also reported significantly less conflict than the normative sample. Several areas of family strengths were revealed in relation to functional abilities. The strengths, reflecting health of the family unit, involved family coping, adaptability, and conflict management. The research demonstrated that the families implemented specific coping and behavioral strategies like seeking social or spiritual support, using community resources, and reframing the presenting problem or situation. The areas where they encountered more difficulty than normative families seemed to be in their affective evaluations, in which they reported feeling less connected or bonded to one another.
>
> **Application to practice:** The research findings provide nurses with insights into families' health, strengths, and limitations related to their abilities to cope with an adult family member experiencing a serious mental illness. Because the families were shown to cope with stressors and deal with conflict in healthy ways, implementation strategies to promote sharing opportunities among multiple families' members may help to maximize existent family strengths. A complete family assessment needs to incorporate questions exploring the family's sense of cohesiveness because interventions may be necessary to facilitate family bonding.

tional aspects of family units and reveals a sense of decreased cohesion in families who are coping with an ill member. A thorough assessment process appreciates the uniqueness of a family system, identifies family strengths, learns cultural and historical factors, and understands the dynamics operating within the family system. Other considerations of family processes are further discussed in Chapter 10. In addition to completing a family genogram (see Chapter 10), ask these key questions to obtain relevant information:

- What financial, health-related, interpersonal, and educational-professional resources are available to the family?
- What past and current monetary stressors, illnesses, losses, interpersonal problems, and educational-professional stressors affect the family?
- What are the religious, political, and cultural influences within the family?
- What are the working assumptions or life philosophies influencing family members? Are their assumptions that (a) people are no good; (b) if you try hard enough, anything is possible; (c) talking about problems does nothing; or (d) people do the best they can?
- What specific individual, maintenance, and task roles do family members play?
- What types of current, short-term, and long-term relationships exist among family members?
- What are the family strengths? Does it have coping skills, adaptive abilities, and conflict management?[10]

Availability and Access to Health Care

Assess the availability of health-care services and community resources for the family. The individual's capacity to access and use these services should also be determined. For example, do not recommend that a client join a support group at a community mental health center during the morning hours that conflicts with the client's schedule at a day treatment program that accepts the insurance and is accessible by public transportation. Some basic questions that address issues of access and availability of health-care services and resources are introduced in Table 29–3.

TABLE 29–3. Nursing Assessment Questions to Identify Health-Care Services and Resources

- Does the individual have health insurance?
- Who are the providers of medical and dental care?
- How does client travel to health-care sites? Does client travel alone or is assistance required?
- How does client contact health-care providers when there is a problem?
- Does the client have routine preventive care or rely on emergency services?
- Is the client able to independently telephone and make an appointment if a need for medical attention is identified or does this need to be facilitated?

are unable to live independently or because the community lacks affordable housing and residential programs.

Assessing a family's strengths and vulnerabilities is a complex undertaking. Doornbos[12] studied families of the seriously and persistently mentally ill to identify their strengths (see Research Note). Her research outlines healthy, func-

Subjective and Objective Data

When carrying out a comprehensive assessment, as well as when evaluating the outcome of a nursing plan, keep in mind that, like the rest of us, individuals with PMI may easily overestimate their abilities. Some may also engage in wishful thinking or experience chronic denial: the persistent belief, in spite of facts, that one's abilities exceed what has been demonstrated. Clients may say, "My problem is not really that bad." Remember that denial functions as a protective coping mechanism that should not be abruptly shattered. Help individuals develop other coping skills or strategies that allow them to view their situation with hope.

In assessing the abilities of a client with PMI, focus on actual accomplishments and strengths rather than on what he or she believes can be accomplished in the future. If an individual tells you that he or she is ready to get a job but has not worked in 2 years, ask what has changed in the client's life that makes the goal of work now possible.

> A clinical nurse specialist with a practice in psychiatric aftercare was asked by a family to assess their son's readiness to live in an independent apartment and work. In reviewing the records, the clinical specialist noted that the client had resided in a halfway house for the past 3 years. Even with supervision, he had had difficulty carrying out self-care and home-care activities. He demonstrated little motivation, often missed his day treatment program, and had difficulty remembering his medication schedule. When the nurse met with him, he acknowledged all of these difficulties but was insistent that in 6 months he would be perfectly able to live independently. When the nurse asked what was going to happen that would allow him to do this, he responded, "In 6 months my clone from the planet Xion is coming to replace me and he has no problems."

This vignette illustrates that the client needs to reside in a supervised setting that provides assistance with ADLs. The client's participation in an independent work program apart from a structured supportive environment is unrealistic at this time.

Another factor that may complicate the assessment process is that an individual's illness experience may be syntonic to his or her lifestyle. The distress, or dystonic experience, may be felt only by those with whom the individual lives and works, and input from family members, friends, or past treatment providers is essential. People who are unable to throw away old newspapers or magazines, for example, are likely not annoyed by the clutter of stacked papers. However, the individual's family members or housemates may be extremely inconvenienced.

DILEMMAS EXPERIENCED BY INDIVIDUALS WITH PMI: NURSING DIAGNOSES, OUTCOMES, AND INTERVENTION STRATEGIES

The use of NANDA-approved nursing diagnoses and corresponding characteristics (Chapter 2) aptly expresses the difficulties experienced by individuals with PMI. NANDA diagnoses are emphasized when coupled with an understanding of the frequent dilemmas and difficulties that individuals with PMI and their families commonly encounter.

Diminished Sense of Control

The ability to use services, supports, and expertise is a hallmark of health and maturity. Working with individuals coping with PMI, nurses consistently find their clients concerned about a diminished sense of control in their everyday lives. Their symptoms may overtake them, they may fear a medication omission, or a life crisis can tip the balance between functioning in the world of reality and again experiencing the terrors of psychosis, homelessness, or hospitalization.

Stressors and Target Symptoms. Clients experiencing PMI, their families, and treatment team members need to be alert to both the stressors that may compromise their coping capacities and the manifestations of any target symptoms that serve as cues to a possible relapse. The more aware and knowledgeable clients are about stressors and target symptoms, the more likely they are to receive timely supports and interventions to prevent further relapse. Individuals, families, treatment providers, and relevant clinical records can all contribute useful information about existent stressors and target symptoms.

With or without PMI, people are all subjected to events in life that cause distress and interfere with their usual adaptive capacities. In addition, many people experience difficulties at certain holidays and times of the year that mark the anniversary of a significant loss or accomplishment. For others, a specific season can be stressful.

Attempting to negotiate any one major life stress is taxing; having to cope with more than one can be overwhelming. For individuals with PMI, orchestrating only one major change or stressor at a time is beneficial. An example of limiting stressors is introducing a new medication before

---

TABLE 29–4. Teaching Clients with PMI and Their Families: Target Symptoms and Coping Strategies

Outcome Goals
Client will participate in seeking help for symptom management.
Family members will participate in development of a plan.

Key Teaching Points
Identify common behaviors, feelings, and moods associated with illness recurrence.
Know key health-care providers and corresponding telephone numbers.
Determine plan for contacting primary health-care provider.
Enlist client's participation if professional intervention is required.
Develop "crisis" plan.

moving the client to a new residence or community program. Introducing only one variable at a time also makes outcomes easier to evaluate.

Depending on the individual and the illness, specific recognized behaviors or beliefs can indicate a possible relapse. The client and family need to be cognizant about target symptoms of the specific PMI and strategies for coping with the symptoms (Table 29–4).

Safety Nets and Strategies to Minimize Loss of Control. The admonition to take care of oneself with sound nutrition, moderate exercise, adequate sleep, positive interpersonal relationships, and minimized stress is emphasized by most health-conscious groups from Alcoholics Anonymous to neighborhood yoga classes. In addition to meeting these basic needs, some specific strategies can assist individuals coping with PMI.

Helping clients remain reality oriented is a major challenge for the nurse. A sad irony of PMI is that the illness symptoms often compromise an individual's judgment and ability to discriminate between consensual reality and perceived experiences. Impaired decision making and poor judgment can result. Therefore, clients with PMI must have trusted individuals to whom they can turn for assistance in reality testing. A trusted friend, family member, nurse, or other caregiver can provide this support. People with PMI need to feel safe, understood, and respected when they seek validation about a belief or behavior, its grounding in reality, and evidence of sound judgment.

For individuals who experience delusions, it may be helpful to refer to these false beliefs as assumptions. This term has less stigma associated with it because we all make assumptions. This approach lends itself to "testing" in that the nurse can examine what data or experiences support an assumption and explore other facts that might better explain the situation.

Managing medications and encouraging compliance are primary interventions for clients with PMI. In helping a person regain a sense of control, often the first intervention is to assess any disruption in the medication management of the illness. Previous difficulty in maintaining a medication schedule calls for external structures that provide cues or help to ensure that omissions do not occur. A medication charting sheet, a prepoured medication cassette that indicates the time and day of a dose, or a watch that beeps when a medication is to be taken can serve as an external reminder. However, the client may need the help of a family member, day treatment staff, or a visiting nurse assistant (VNA) to reestablish a routine. Determine if clients are experiencing any concerns or side effects related to the medication that may increase their reluctance to take it. Such concerns should be actively addressed and, if possible, remedied by the prescribing clinician.

If individuals with PMI experience acute resurgence of target symptoms, advise a consultation with the prescribing clinician. A medication increase or modification could deter an increasingly serious situation. Some clients may have a standing plan specifying the behaviors or beliefs that need to be present to justify a specific PRN (as needed) medication.

Another important strategy for people with PMI is to make sure they have a day's dose of medication readily accessible, including PRN medications. Clients in the community may require assistance in deciding how to organize their medications for quick access.

ENVIRONMENTS AND SUPPORT SYSTEMS

Nightingale[13] was one of the first to speak of the nurse's role in manipulating the environment to optimize the healing forces within the body. Her attention to fresh air, clean water, a quiet atmosphere, and nutritious food continues to be relevant. During the days of extended inpatient hospitalizations, the treatment units were supposed to serve as supportive environments where people could be buffered from overt stresses and daily demands that contributed to their illness. At the same time, clients benefited from human support, education, and interventions aimed at helping them cope with the realities causing their distress.

The environments and support systems of today are different but nonetheless important. Review with clients the available environmental resources and how they may be accessed when a need arises. The plans for clients will vary with their needs and the resources in the community. Frequently used environments and support strategies include:

- Going to a place that has traditionally provided a sense of tranquility or grounding: the individual's room, the ocean, a park, or a garden.
- Making plans with family or friends, especially during weekends and evenings.
- Increasing contact with day treatment programs, social clubs, or residential staff.
- Scheduling an extra therapy appointment.
- Scheduling "check in" telephone appointments with therapists or other care providers to review current mental status, coping strategies, and plans.
- Making use of crisis team services, if necessary.
- Using respite beds or facilities.
- Telephoning paraprofessional or consumer hotlines, such as the Samaritans.
- Seeking admission to an acute psychiatric unit, if the need arises.

Although treatment programs and strategies are aimed at preventing the need for hospitalization, individuals with PMI, their families, and treatment team members need to realize that the use of hospital services is not a failure. In fact, if these services can be accessed before individuals become acutely compromised, timely hospitalizations may minimize exacerbations of clients' mental illnesses and the lengths of hospital stays.

Individuals with PMI, their families, and the various members of the treatment team need to have a collaboratively written treatment plan that addresses the previously discussed information. Equally important is knowledge about whom to contact or where to go, should a crisis occur during business and nonbusiness hours. Anticipate that problems can arise at any time of the day or night, as well as during weekends and holidays.

Sample Plan of Care

This care plan is individualized for a professional woman in her mid-30s experiencing bipolar disorder. Priscilla A is new to the area, having moved from her hometown to take a promising position. She lives alone in her apartment and works as a software engineer in an adjacent city. Priscilla's family lives 1200 miles away; her fiancé lives in another state, a distance of 300 miles. They are all supportive of the client and previously traveled to meet with Priscilla and her new therapist to discuss their concerns and current circumstances.

Priscilla's major concern is that her illness does not interfere with her employment. She and her therapist, a clinical specialist in psychiatric nursing, outlined the following plan based on an assessment of Priscilla's previous hospitalizations and treatment experiences.

Goal. Client will be free from interruption in employment due to mood fluctuations.

Interventions and Strategies to Maintain Euthymic Functioning
- Limit workday to no more than 8 hours.
- Schedule time away from desk to eat lunch.
- Try to take a walk after work to wind down.
- Make plans on weekends to do enjoyable things: read, see movies, cook (things done alone).
- Talk with fiancé at least every other day.
- Plan at least one social activity with a friend or coworker each weekend (things done with others).
- For the next month, maintain weekly therapy appointments.
- Take lithium as scheduled.

Target Symptoms That May Indicate the Beginning of a Manic Phase
- Sleeping less than 6 hours a night.
- Experiencing racing thoughts.
- Believing that Uncle Todd is influencing job performance.
- Drawing numerous connections between unrelated events.
- Not eating.
- Experiencing everything as being funny or a joke.

If Any of the Previous Circumstances Occur
- Take 5 mg of haloperidol (Haldol) stat.
- Contact therapist to review circumstances and develop a further plan.
- Should at any time a family member (or fiancé) be concerned about my health, they will inform me, and we will contact my therapist.

Disorganization of Time and Tasks

The cause and manifestations of problems will vary, depending on the underlying neurobiological illness. However, many individuals with PMI experience a deficit in the skills, memory, or attention required to anticipate situations, prioritize concerns, and develop plans to address these concerns. Such clients may be frequently confused or in a near-constant reactive state that can easily reach crisis proportions. For people who have poor impulse control, the problems are compounded. Common difficulties may include running out of medication, bouncing checks, not opening mail, late charges on unpaid bills, missed appointments, and lack of money to pay for necessities because of impulse buying.

The degree of external structure or support needed is again determined by the extent of the individual's deficits. In some cases, weekly schedules and appointment books can provide a sense of order to an otherwise altered time frame. Getting the client an appointment book is usually not enough. Quite often a client will need help to establish and reinforce the habit of writing down activities and commitments as well as remembering to carry the book. Ideally, the appointment book should also contain a section for telephone numbers and addresses. In this way the client always has the ability to contact people significant to him or her and to the treatment. Many individuals also find a daily "to do" list useful. With education and support as to how these strategies may be used, the person can begin to prioritize and organize the demands of daily life. Not just the harried executive or the clinician benefits from time-management techniques. Such tools, by providing a written record of activities, can also help an individual who is experiencing confusion or memory deficits. This written record documents accomplishments and evaluates progress. The feeling of satisfaction that comes from crossing off tasks completed is not to be underestimated.

For individuals with severe and persistent PMI, more immediate, interactive, and consistent assistance may be required to maintain a sense of organization. Most often these responsibilities fall to family members. Ideally, community treatment programs, the services of case managers, and residential programs are available to help provide some of the direct supervision necessary.

Disenfranchisement and Stigma

Without a collaborative approach by nurses and other health professionals, a sense of disenfranchisement by clients and their families can emerge. Disenfranchisement can reinforce a sense of powerlessness, helplessness, or hopelessness. These normal emotional reactions have the potential of interfering with the development of trust and mutual respect between clients, their families, and health professionals.

Stigma, viewed as a negative perception about an individual or group that deviates in some way from what society values, has been described as the most debilitating handicap for individuals with mental illness.[14] Stigmatization can also extend to family members of mentally ill clients because they may experience altered relationships with extended family members and friends.[15] Two excerpts by family members emphasize their encounters with stigma.

> An adult sister, whose only sibling has had repeated hospitalizations from exacerbations of schizophrenia, reported: "I usually don't tell new acquaintances or talk about my sister with extended family members. They really don't understand. Just like when I went to a recent family gathering. I overheard one of my cousins ask an uncle, 'So where is that crazy Dee? Is she in or out of the hospital again? I hope her sister doesn't catch her craziness.' I really feel labeled along with my ill sister."

> A client, experiencing a 10-year history of bipolar disorder, described stigma as "the worst of all possible reactions. I feel alone, different and conspicuous, especially when my old neighborhood friends make excuses for not inviting me to go to the movies or the beach with them."

Strategies Relevant to Families. Clinical evaluations and treatment plans become compromised by omitting input from clients and their families. Families frequently have experience with their ill members during remissions and exacerbations. They can provide valuable insights about helpful or nonhelpful services and strategies. They can describe the current dilemma and needed interventions and explain why a past course of action was effective or ineffective. This information can be illuminating and pragmatic for nurses and other health team members. Before the implementation of new treatment approaches, involve clients and families by providing treatment-plan rationales and anticipated outcomes to promote participation and compliance. Also outline the process by which further communication and collaboration will be maintained among team members, the client, and family. The communication process needs to include information specifying:

- Name of health team member serving as contact person when questions arise.
- Name of clinician or service available after business hours.
- Frequency of meetings for family, client, and clinician or treatment team.
- Individual responsible for coordinating meetings.

Although there are many benefits to involving the family in an individual's treatment, it can occur only with the individual's consent. Clarify with the person what specific information will be provided to the family. Often the person is struggling with issues of autonomy and independence. In such circumstances, the client may wish certain information to be withheld from the family while other information is shared.

In working with families, a frequent task is helping the family to identify what help is supportive and growth enhancing versus what actions are infantilizing or growth inhibiting. An example might be family members who do not have realistic expectations for an individual to assume responsibility for his or her behavior but rather accommodate and excuse inappropriate behaviors. They may then take the person shopping or plan some fun activity to help the person to feel better. Often the response may originate from a sense of blame, guilt, or an overwhelming desire to make things better. In some instances, it may be because the family dreads the consequences of the individual's not obtaining what is desired. A 32-year-old woman's temper tantrum in the midst of a shopping mall is an incident most of us would like to avoid.

Nurses working with and teaching families and individuals should focus on those essential areas:

- How does the individual's current illness influence or interfere with social behavior?
- What aspects of the individual's personality or level of maturity interfere with social behavior?
- What are realistic expectations concerning the individual's behavior?
- What strategies or responses may be used to help the person be more comfortable in social situations, such as using medication or structuring excursions to avoid sensory overload?
- What has been the family's previous response when the individual has crossed over the threshold of appropriate social behavior?
- Did the response tend to promote the desired outcome?
- Are family members able to be consistent in their responses, or do responses vary among members and promote splitting?
- Are there other options that might provide a more desirable outcome and assist the individual to develop more mature coping skills?

These eight areas can be addressed periodically during formalized family meetings. The community treatment team needs to decide collaboratively, with clients and families, which member of the treatment team will assume the responsibility for leading the meetings.

Often, individuals coping with PMI find themselves removed from their circles of friends. There is the experience of feeling like an outsider. Hospitalizations, the need to modify demanding activities, or the symptoms of the illness disrupt previous life patterns and relationships. Stigma arising from lack of understanding and fear regarding individuals with mental illnesses are recognized as major prejudices faced by clients and families on a daily basis. Comments by family members participating in a "Caring and Sharing" session during a local Alliance for the Mentally Ill meeting illustrate feelings about stigmatization. One elderly father poignantly stated:

> *When my 30-year-old son first got sick 15 years ago, my wife and I told no one. Our neighbors asked us why they hadn't*

seen Rick mowing the lawn, and I would answer, "He's in the hospital for tests," and then I would quickly change the subject. We were afraid to say that Rick was on the psychiatric unit for fear of being alienated from our neighbors.

Need to Belong. To prevent a client's social isolation, plan together ways to initiate and maintain social relationships. The means and the resources used are determined by the social skills of the individual as well as the resources of the community. The client needs to identify a single activity or interest that has brought previous enjoyment or something new to pursue; a corresponding activity should be accessible in the local community. Scholarships may be available for individuals with financial need. In other circumstances, the fee may be lowered if the person is willing to volunteer. As one man with long-standing depression noted: "I know I don't have to be lonely. Any night of the week I can find a contra dance going on in this city. The music, the dancing, and the company all help me feel better."

Having a friend or family member join or attend the first social activity session can be helpful. Within some social or psychiatric rehabilitation programs, it is not uncommon for staff members to attend the first few events with a client. Increasingly, consumer groups are addressing the need for support of members venturing into the community.

Just as it is helpful for individuals with PMI to realize how much they have in common with people free from mental illness, it is also beneficial for clients to learn from the experiences and wisdom of other individuals with PMI. Clients can develop a sense of the universality of their needs, feelings, and difficulties as they share their experiences with others. It is a common experience to hear a person say, "I feel so much better; I thought I was the only one who thought that . . . , felt that . . . , experienced that."

Benefits of peer support include:
- Opportunities to speak candidly with others who have had similar experiences, to ask questions, and to choose the most relevant from the information and suggestions offered.
- Exposure to resources or information beyond one's own frame of reference or knowledge.
- Support for one's efforts to manage an illness and undertake new challenges.
- Opportunities to help others by sharing their own experiences.

A familiar phenomenon observed in peer support groups, in which several members are well engaged in their treatment and recovery, is that the initial denial phase common to new members becomes curtailed. Manny O, a new college graduate recently discharged to his apartment after rehospitalization of 3 weeks, demonstrates the positive influence of a community support group:

Well, yea, it's like I thought it was just who I was, seeing angels and thinking I could heal people. And then I come here, and you've all gone through something like that and have learned about your illness and medications. I had to face that it was my illness too.

MANNY O

Organizations such as NAMI, the NAMI subgroup Siblings and Adult Children of the Mentally Ill (SAC), and MDDA not only provide support, education, and resources for individuals and families but also provide a means for individuals to be socially and politically involved.[11] These organizations welcome the collaborative involvement of professionals. The associations endeavor to educate the public about myths and realities of human beings living with mental illness, the need for and benefits of effective treatment, and the detrimental effects of stigmatization.

Anticipation and Recreation. Many of us are sustained through arduous and mundane routines of everyday life with anticipation of pleasurable diversional activities. Students balance demands of academic and clinical assignments, knowing that an anticipated vacation promises enjoyable pursuits with family or friends. Individuals with PMI experience anticipations. Statements by Tina T, a 38-year-old woman diagnosed with schizophrenia 20 years ago who resides in a supervised group home, acknowledges her need for diversion:

I work hard all week going to my program. Participating in the culinary unit (at a psychosocial club house) makes me tired. I need to go on vacation some weekends every month and for 2 weeks in the summer to my parents' house. You know I really work hard and need a change!

TINA T

The value of planning diversional and engaging recreational activities is as important as planning purposeful and meaningful work opportunities.

A visiting nurse had recently accepted the role of care coordinator for Joseph B, a man with long-standing mood disorder and a borderline personality disorder. Considerable time had been spent assessing the client's needs and arranging services between his day treatment program and his supported work program. Approaches and treatment goals were also coordinated between the client, care coordinator, psychopharmacologist, and family. The nurse was identified as the clinician Joseph should contact if a crisis occurred. The client had been under excessive stress the past several months because his mother, terminally ill with lung cancer, was being cared for at home with hospice assistance.

One afternoon the client telephoned the visiting nurse service, asking to be hospitalized. Joseph explained that he could "no longer cope with the demands" of his new work training program, the responsibilities of his apartment, and the reality of his mother's impending death. "I want to go into the hospital; I can't do all this anymore." After further assessment, the nurse determined that Joseph did not have any source of respite from his responsibilities; however, he did not require hospitalization. Joseph instead needed to find a way to get some distance from his concerns and experience some pleasure. When the nurse saw Joseph the next day, they discussed weekend plans. Joseph decided that he would take a short train trip to a nearby seaside town. The day was to be spent taking in the sights and enjoying lunch. The return trip would be that evening. During the meeting with his care coordinator the following Monday, Joseph enthusiastically relayed how much he enjoyed this excursion, even though he went alone. He agreed to incorporate some type of recreational activities into his weekly schedule.

Disillusionment with Self and Life

When individuals experience an illness that derails them from their anticipated life's path, there is a profound sense of loss for the individual as well as the family. Neugeboren[16] describes his painful sense of loss in a sensitively written memoir about his mentally ill brother, Robert, and their lifelong relationship:

During the weeks that follow Robert's hospitalization, we talk regularly . . . and though sometimes he is angry (at doctors, at me—at life!) and sometimes sad, and sometimes high—and though sometimes I am nearly swept away by grief, from my sense of all that he senses his life has become and not become, I find, strangely enough, real pleasure—as ever—in these talks and in our time together.

J. NEUGEBOREN

Because families learn that a child is likely to have a prolonged mental illness when the individual has reached late adolescence or early adulthood, the information may be difficult to integrate at this later stage in life. Frequently, parents perceive that their son or daughter, who has shown success in high school, is destined for greatness. Family members may attempt to minimize the existence and implications of the illness, preferring to view behaviors and symptoms as a stage or phase of development. However, over time, the reality of the illness becomes evident and the need for treatment cannot be ignored. Individuals and their families need realistic information concerning the causes, treatments, research, anticipated course of the illness, and common human reactions. Eakes's[17] research on chronic sorrow of parents with mentally ill adult children reveals an important area for nursing intervention. Nurses need to first assess parents' feelings that may indicate a normal grief reaction that can recur throughout parents' lives because of their child's enduring mental illness (see Research Note). Family assessment data related to manifestations of chronic sorrow will help determine the need for anticipatory guidance and teaching interventions.

If individuals have had high self-expectations or come from accomplished families, integrating the experience and reality of the mental illness with their sense of identity and

---

RESEARCH NOTE

Eakes, GG: Chronic sorrow: The lived experience of parents of chronically mentally ill individuals. Arch Psychiatr Nurs 10(2): 77–84, 1995.

Findings: This qualitative study focused on parents with an adult child diagnosed with either schizophrenia or bipolar disorder. A convenience sample consisting of ten parents—two mothers and four couples—consented to audiotaped interviews. Data were gathered using the Bruce/Nursing Consortium for Research on Chronic Sorrow (NCRCS) Chronic Questionnaire (Caregiver Version). The research showed that eight of the ten parents experienced chronic sorrow. Chronic sorrow, a normal response, is a recurrent sorrow or sadness that persists over time and can intensify after years following the initial loss or disappointment. The parents' chronic sorrow experience reflected a variety of grief-related feelings first occurring when learning their child's psychiatric diagnosis and then recurring over a prolonged period of time. Parents' feelings included shock, disbelief, anger, sadness, and confusion, with predominant feelings described as confusion, anger, and frustration. The predominant feelings were shown to recur over time. Intensity of parents' grief-related feelings varied. Although multiple trigger events evoked feelings of grief, common triggers were categorized as consistency of caregiving responsibilities that never ended. These responsibilities were described as excessive demands placed on parents' energy or time commitments, lack of respite, and financial burden. Coping mechanisms employed by parents were categorized as interpersonal, emotional, or action oriented. A helpful factor mentioned by parents as they tried to cope with both the initial diagnosis and chronic sorrow experience involved medication provision for their child's symptom management. Health-care professionals were viewed negatively, with parents citing lack of communication or lack of involvement in their child's treatment as nonhelpful factors.

Application to Practice: The study helps to understand the parents' experiences, via first-person accounts, as they live and struggle daily to cope with their adult mentally ill child. Nurses need to realize that coping with caregiving responsibilities and chronic sorrow are part of parents' reality whether the child lives at home or independently. The importance of open communication between parents and health-care professional remains essential to providing assistance and support for the ill children. Nurses are in a position to teach and provide guidance to parents about chronic sorrow as a normal reaction to their loss. This educational approach may help provide a sense of comfort and support for these special parents.

purpose in life is a challenge. At this time, clients and their families reassess their priorities and examine what they truly value. Negotiating an existential crisis within a competitive culture presents a complex task. As one 38-year-old woman, who experienced her first manic episode while establishing her law practice, explained:

> Before, I was concerned with status. I wanted to buy a Lexus and get my house. Now I am more concerned with seeing my friends, enjoying each day, and slowly beginning my career.

Involvement of empathic nurses is essential at a time when individuals mourn the lost sense of their former selves and coexisting possibilities. Enabling clients to bear the realities of loss requires knowledgable support as well as the provision of realistic hope. The ongoing and consistent involvement of sensitive, helping professionals encourages expressions of sadness and grief. As one man explained to the community nurse, "I am more than just biochemical reactions and medications. Sometimes it feels like you are the only one who appreciates what I go through as a person trying to deal with all these changes day in and day out." It is not surprising that while working through this process, clients may experience suicidal thoughts and feelings (Chapter 2 details the nursing process with clients expressing suicidal ideation). Expressions of suicide are serious cues for which individuals, their families, nurses, and the treatment team must cooperatively plan intervention strategies.

The cultural and spiritual community of individuals and their families may also help provide a sense of comfort and belonging. The questions "Why me? Why us?" contribute existential angst and confusion. Individuals may find themselves rethinking previously held assumptions about the purpose and meaning of life. Answers and information provided by medical science alone are insufficient. Spiritual questions and needs may require attention by clergy.

Disadvantaged by Homelessness, Prison, Education, Employment, and Economics

Individuals who experience both homelessness and severe or prolonged mental illness constitute an important group disadvantaged by lack of permanent housing as well as by recognized neurobiological disorders. Statistics show that of the 600,000 individuals homeless on a given night, about 200,000 of them experience a serious mental illness.[18] The presence of homeless mentally ill has become increasingly apparent as they seek temporary protection at bus, train, or airport terminals, parks, cities' heating grates, or overnight shelters. These individuals have little opportunity of independently overcoming homelessness because symptoms of their mental illness, such as poor judgment, lack of motivation, and compromised social skills, interfere with safe adaptation.[18] Also, because their experience with the mental health system has often been negative, they are reluctant to seek assistance. A collaborative working approach is needed at local, state, and national levels to minimize the complex problem of homelessness among the nation's mentally ill.

Another disadvantaged group is individuals with severe and prolonged mental illness who are housed in jails and prisons. Involvement with the legal system may be precipitated by their aberrant behaviors or by their alleged or actual crimes. When these clients end up in correctional institutions, their care is focused on neither treatment nor rehabilitation for their mental illness. Improving care and treatment of forensic clients continues to be a concern and a challenge within our country.

A third disadvantaged group is those facing obstacles related to education or work. Given that many individuals with PMI have sensory distortions that interfere with concentration and the ability to screen, sort, and synthesize information, they are at times handicapped in their abilities to learn and work. Negative illness symptoms such as lack of motivation or poor organization also compromise clients' functional abilities. Add sedation caused by medications, and another obstacle challenges individuals with PMI as they attempt to reintegrate into the world of education and work. Current research illustrates the magnitude of the problem: Kessler[9] estimates that more than 7.2 million people in the United States terminate their education due to early-onset psychiatric disorders. They further note that only a small fraction would later complete either high school or college. These realities not only compromise the workforce but also place a demand on community resources.

Emphasis needs to be placed on modifying the means and methods of assisting individuals with PMI adjust to the demands of the workplace and educational settings. The challenges or obstacles are likely to have an impact on the individual's earning potential and financial status. The realities of lost work days because of reccurrence of symptoms, the time and financial costs of treatment, and the prejudice that may exist on the part of employers, faculty, and peers all take a toll. Anthony's[2] ongoing research conducted at Boston University's Department of Rehabilitation and Counseling has provided data and documentation disproving many of the existent myths regarding the desire and capacity of individuals with PMI to undertake employment.

As seen in Table 29–5, the false assumptions Anthony[2] identified not only have impeded the development of psychiatric rehabilitation but also have biased clinicians toward underestimating the abilities of clients with PMI.

Appreciating the specific strengths and vulnerabilities of each person is crucial to designing plans and strategies that allow the person to optimize talents and potentials. An individual may need to rethink previous life plans and timetables. At this time, package deals often do not work, and the client needs to selectively pick and choose from various options available. For instance, a person who became ill while undertaking graduate studies might confer with academic advisors about the possibilities of decreasing the course load for the next semester, taking a leave of absence, or returning to a previous internship that was less stressful.

Individuals who are more acutely compromised and un-

TABLE 29-5. Myths and Realities about Work and Education

Myths	Realities
• People with psychiatric disabilities have no desire to work	• A statewide Massachusetts survey in 1992 by Rogers, Danley, & Anthony indicated that 70% of individuals with PMI who were unemployed wanted to work and were able to state a preference for a specific type of work.
• People with psychiatric disabilities possess no desire to further their education.	• 62% of individuals with PMI wanted to further their education.
• People with psychiatric disabilities lose jobs because of their inability to perform the job tasks.	• These factors contribute to job loss and work adjustment: getting along with supervisors and coworkers, completing the job, and attendance.

able to return to previous employment or education have to access rehabilitation services and public or community resources to which they are entitled. Although often the social worker or the case manager assists clients in completing forms for Supplemental Security Income (SSI) or Social Security Disability Income (SSDI), part of the nursing assessment should be to determine if other resources exist from which clients may benefit. Individuals with **psychiatric disabilities** are entitled to the same benefits as individuals disabled by physical illnesses, including housing.[19] The local NAMI chapter can often be helpful in providing families and clinicians with listings of resources.[20]

Interestingly, developing countries have higher recovery rates from schizophrenia than the United States.[21] In nonindustrialized societies, each person is known to a community, each person's contributions are needed to get the work done, and in this manner each person is appreciated. In this country, the work available to individuals with PMI is often menial, routine, not highly valued, and without health insurance. The need for training and education that lead to "real jobs," improved wages, and employee benefits such as health insurance, has been identified by mental health consumers and psychiatric rehabilitation professionals alike as a priority.

MODELS OF TREATMENT AND REHABILITATION

Individuals with prolonged mental illness often move between various treatment systems and providers and sometimes become lost in the gaps between these systems. The need to create models and strategies that provide continuity of care for individuals with PMI has been vividly demonstrated by the shortcomings of deinstitutionalization: increased readmission rates to hospitals, increased use of emergency rooms for crisis stabilization, increasing homelessness, and involvement of individuals with PMI in the criminal justice system. Effective mental health care must be focused on and responsive to the needs and realities of individuals and their uniquenesses. It must bridge the gaps that exist and meet the clients where they are, whether that means going to their homes, community programs, or the streets.

The response to these challenges by federal and state agencies has promoted creative innovation. Models of in vivo service-delivery systems actively address the dilemmas and risks faced by individuals with PMI. Effective community models often share basic principles of continuity of care.[22]

- An administrative climate supportive of long-term clients.
- Ready access by clients to the services that they need.
- Provision of a full array of services.
- Flexible program offerings.
- Linkages among agencies serving the client.
- A continuing relationship between client and caregiver.
- Client involvement in service planning.
- Recognition of the cultural factors affecting treatment.

CASE MANAGEMENT

Perhaps one of the first responses to the realization that many individuals with PMI were unable to access traditional clinical services and required assistance beyond the four walls of the consulting room has been the evolution of case management programs. Such programs are often provided and funded by local offices of the state department of mental health. In general, case management programs provide an assessment of a client's needs, the development of a comprehensive service plan, the provision of required services, and the ongoing evaluation of the delivered services and the client's responses to them. As a case manager, one would not just identify the deficits of a client but would also actively help the individual access the resources required. This might entail going with the client to obtain a special needs pass for public transportation or contacting a primary care physician to clarify a prescribed course of treatment.

The term *case management* first appeared with some frequency in professional literature in the late 1970s. Historically, the term has been applied to a variety of different service-delivery systems. As reflected in the literature, variations exist among case managers' education, professional background, responsibilities, functions, caseloads, and capacities to follow clients from one health-care system to another, crossing boundaries between inpatient and outpatient settings. Kanter[23] defined case management as:

a modality of mental health practice that, in coordination with traditional psychiatric focus on biological and psychological functioning, addresses the overall maintenance of the mentally ill person's physical and social environment with the goals of facilitating his or her physical survival, personal growth, community participation, and recovery from or adaptation to mental illness.

Kanter's model argued for a graduate level of education for case managers and recognized the expertise brought to this role by both nursing and social work professionals. It advocated a limited caseload based on acuity and needs of clients. Kanter also addressed the need for a salary reflecting professional status and education.

It has been argued within the profession that nurses are the most qualified to provide case management services to individuals with PMI. As case managers, nurses are able to (a) address concerns related to both physical and mental illnesses, (b) assist clients to access needed care, and (c) actively collaborate with other health-care providers. Zander[24] warned that nurses must assume the role of case managers or there would be a new layer of nonclinical people performing this vital nursing function. In recent years, other models have made use of paraprofessionals and in some cases consumers, acting in roles described as case managers.

Sledge[25] asserts that case management refers to an ambiguous concept lacking a base in a professional discipline, resulting in ongoing uncertainty about its mission, practice, and training. The ambiguity of the term and the diversity of implementation strategies have also contributed to difficulty in determining benefits and cost effectiveness. Following an extensive review of literature on case management, Rubin[26] claimed that even with the plausible hypothesis that case management offers an effective care-providing approach, conclusive claims about its effectiveness have not been empirically demonstrated. Still, psychiatric care settings continue to use a case management approach for their clients.

CONTINUOUS TREATMENT TEAMS

Continuous treatment teams provide an integrated service model in which a mental health team assumes responsibility for an individual with prolonged mental illness "indefinitely . . . no matter where the patient is . . . and no matter what the patient's needs."[27] Typically, a team implements active outreach, client assessment, treatment-service planning, provision of services, referral services, advocacy, and crisis intervention.[28]

The model requires a high degree of collaboration among involved team members as well as a clear understanding of individual accountability. This model additionally requires a high degree of systems linkage, allowing clients to easily make the transition from inpatient to outpatient services as needed. A complicating factor can be the mechanics of funding that may come through multiple sources including medicaid, private insurance, and SSI, depending on the specific services provided.

The following is excerpted from a paper by Guy.[29] It addresses the complexity of her position as a psychiatric nurse with the Bay Cove Community Treatment Team (CTT) in Boston, Massachusetts.

CTT is geared toward the most difficult and treatment-resistant clients of the Department of Mental Health. These clients are usually young, uneducated, unemployed adults with schizophrenia whose substance abuse and legal difficulties result in repeated state hospital psychiatric and detoxification admissions, overuse of emergency rooms, periods of homelessness, recurring contacts with police, and poverty.

CT clinicians are available 24 hours a day, 7 days a week. Whereas the idea in the 60's was to create centers where people would go for treatment, the idea now is to fill the gaps in service by creating a system involving many different resources, that is, residences, crisis beds, respite beds, halfway houses, supervised housing, housing for dual diagnoses, outpatient therapy, vocational training, social and recreational programs, self-help programs, and family programs. CTTs then mobilize utilization of the system by their clients via outreach and community-based service. CTTs serve as a fixed point of responsibility for addressing a wide range of needs: vocational, housing, psychiatric, education, medical health care, family, work, substance abuse, and legal problems.

The client's homes (shelter, street corner, or park bench) and various sites in the community (coffee shops, parks, community centers, AA meetings, grocery stores, courtrooms, and laundromats) become clinical sites. Meetings often take place within the context of helping clients with tasks such as grocery shopping, applying for benefits, and accessing transportation to a job interview. Meeting in these environments emphasizes the client's strengths and abilities rather than pathology and dysfunction, enhances the clinician's awareness of the client's life circumstances, allows the clinician to assess and involve social network members, increases the ability to individualize the treatment plan to client-specific needs, and eliminates the problem of transferring skills from the clinic to the community.[30]

RESIDENTIAL CARE

Residential programs for individuals with PMI are varied and unique. The terms *board and care, halfway house, three-quarter way house, supported apartment program,* and *therapeutic community residence* are commonly used to describe programs that offer housing and some degree of support, supervision, and treatment. Factors that often influence the specifics of a program include whether it is private or state run, reimbursable by insurance, characteristic of a given community, and organized around a particular theoretical framework influencing staff composition, admission criteria, and expectations of residents.

Originally, residential programs were developed to help ease the transitions of individuals from large hospital institutions into the realities of living in a community. Staff assisted clients to learn or relearn skills for self-care, shopping, cooking, and household management. Although some board and care situations offered the bare basics of a room and meals, many programs were based on the principles of a therapeutic community. The forces influencing shorter hospital stays in the late 1970s and 1980s also impacted residential programs. Individuals discharged to community residences tended to be more symptomatic and less knowledgable regarding illness management skills. Programs needed reassessment and redesign to address the pressing needs of their clients.

Programs evolved into a continuum of services. The staffing patterns and activities of a residence would be affected by the acuity of the residents. Some residential programs developed a day program component that offered skills-training classes or groups to address client deficits: symptom management, medication management, leisure skills, stress management, weekend planning, family relationships, and interpersonal skills. Other programs adopted a design in which residents were required to be engaged in activities during the day from 10 am to 3 pm at a site away from the residence. They could attend a day treatment program in the community, participate in a volunteer position, work, or engage in other meaningful activities.

As residents progressed in their abilities to integrate into the community and gained mastery over their illnesses, they could often make the transition to more independent and less costly halfway houses or supported apartment programs. Residents needed to demonstrate more independence and less reliance on staff members. Of major concern were residents' abilities to self-medicate as well as their capacities to access support or resources when necessary. Often this might be beeping the staff member on call to a facility, should a crisis arise.

PSYCHOSOCIAL REHABILITATION PROGRAMS

Although the concept of **psychosocial rehabilitation** is not new, Noorsday and Drake[30] contend that the concept of rehabilitation was first clarified by Williams[31] in 1953 as "that form of therapy which is primarily concerned with assisting the patient to achieve an optimal social role (in the family, on the job, in the general community) within his capacity and potentials."

The first therapeutic social club was founded in 1938 in Great Britain by Joshua Bierer,[32] an Adlerian psychoanalyst and a refugee from Nazi Germany. The main practice of his concept model was socialization, that process by which an individual acquires behavior appropriate to constructive participation in society. His efforts were centered around the belief that the treatment of the mentally ill should be within the natural community. The goals of such clubs were to prepare the individual to adapt to everyday social life and to participate in normal social functions. The use of groups as a therapeutic modality was further supported by the historical reality of World War II and the resulting limited resources and manpower available to hospitals.

Psychiatric Social Clubs

Within the United States, psychiatric social clubs in the 1940s grew from the self-recognized needs of psychiatric patients for support and mutual assistance. Without professional or financial support, clients from Rockland State Hospital, New York, formed a voluntary association that met on the steps of the New York Public Library, We Are Not Alone (WANA).[33] From this group evolved Fountain House, a psychosocial clubhouse program that stressed the importance of former clients, "members," gaining skills that would support independent living and employment.

Fountain House was the first program to recognize the need for community-based treatment that addressed the inadequate socialization and social isolation of individuals with PMI. The initial program had two components, a vocational day program for those who were not yet able to work and an evening program for individuals who were able to maintain employment. During the late 1940s and early 1950s, similar programs were founded by clients experiencing mental illnesses who lived in other major cities.

In the 1950s and 1960s, the benefits of a psychosocial rehabilitation model were recognized in addressing the social deficits experienced by people with PMI, the implications being that in addition to treatment of illness, individuals needed new behaviors and skills to deal with societal demands. In the late 1970s and early 1980s, the National Institute of Mental Health, recognizing the effectiveness of Fountain House in decreasing the rates of rehospitalization, improving the quality of life for its members, and increasing the ability of individuals with PMI to maintain themselves in the community, funded a national training program based on the Fountain House model and principle of psychiatric rehabilitation. The results have been a dramatic increase in the number of these programs, often funded through state departments of mental health.[11]

Although the specific components of a social club may vary, the foundation rests on recognizing members' rights to belong to a place, find meaningful work, develop meaningful relationships, and have a place to return. Psychiatric social clubs provide a niche for every member and are organized around a work-ordered day. Working side by side with staff, most new members initially take part in one of the several work components required to operate the club: snack bar, business office, lunch preparation, housekeeping, and buildings and grounds. For members who are not yet able to engage in these activities, the club provides a social and supportive atmosphere.

At Potter Place, a psychiatric social club located in Waltham, Massachusetts, the atmosphere is one of both pride and acceptance. This Victorian home has been carefully restored and maintained. From the arrangement of potted plants at the reception desk to the details of the wallpaper and woodwork, the building is attractive and comfortable. In this place, members do not shy away from greeting newcomers and asking if they can be of help. The clubhouse focuses on members' strengths and abilities. It is not easy to distinguish staff from members as lunch is prepared and served or as the latest newsletter is composed on the computer.

The majority of psychiatric social clubs have developed educational programs that assist members to improve reading and math skills, complete their high school equivalency diplomas, or pursue other courses within the community. An equally important component of many clubhouses has been transitional employment positions (TEPs) that provide motivated members with opportunities to work in competitive employment settings in industries or businesses. Most placements are part-time and time-limited, typically 20 hours per week for 6 months. Members are paid at least minimum wage by the employer. The selection and training of members for work placements is the responsibility of the clubhouse staff. The support and assistance a member requires to become proficient at a job are also provided by clubhouse staff. Employers are assured that, for whatever reason, should a member be unable to work, a qualified clubhouse member or staff person will fill in. In this manner, employers are guaranteed that work will be completed, and clubhouse members have the opportunity to gain work skills and a degree of competence. From such experience, many members secure independent employment.

TABLE 29–6. Modal Elements of Psychosocial Rehabilitation Programs

1. Culture Base: Rooted in Judeo-Christian and democratic tradition.
2. Community Base: Freeing mental patients from a segregated and isolated role in society.
3. Normalization of Function: Maximizing involvement and participation in natural community activities.
4. Individual Enhancement: Affirming individualism, voluntarism, and freedom of choice.
5. Group Experiences: Using the potentialities of group interactions as the principal vehicle of change.
6. Staff Roles: Emphasizing competency, flexibility, and diversity rather than status and credentials of staff, volunteers, and clients.
7. Planning: Orientation to process rather than to product in program planning.
8. Temporal-existential: Primary attention to here and now rather than past or future.
9. Praxis: Providing varied opportunities for social and self-governance.
10. Rehabilitation Philosophy: Focusing on adaptation beyond illness, development of new meaning and purpose in life.

Source: Adapted from Grob, S: Psychiatric social clubs come of age. Mental Hygiene 54:129, 1970.

Although each psychiatric social club is unique because of the distinctive characteristics of the community in which it is located and the members it serves, modal elements common to successful psychosocial rehabilitation centers have been recognized (Table 29–6). Grob,[33] a professional active in the early days of the Center House psychiatric social club in Boston, noted that these elements were necessary to prevent the original goals and purposes of social club programs from becoming secondary to demands of bureaucratization and economic pressures.

The benefits of psychiatric social clubs and the TEPs are perhaps best addressed by their members. The following is from a speech by an artist and a member of Potter Place who has had schizophrenia for 20 years.

It's been great, is great. 1995 is a year I pushed the envelope and wound up with a whole new package for myself, but I will leave the bad puns. . . . Working Monday through Friday gives me a new feeling about weekends. Maybe a lot of people in the room, certainly in the world, just assume the weekend is naturally great. But for the mentally ill, at least for me and some of my good friends, you can assume nothing. The weekend could be a 72-hour desert between therapy. A weekend in the hospital used to be a long, long, empty time (and boring as hell). Having a 20-hour job has defined my time in a pleasant way. I'm not saying it's easy, no way it's easy, struggling out of bed in the early morning ain't easy. But there is the work time at the job, and then there is free time.

One of my favorite times is Friday morning, about 8:15, and the food truck, known as the "Roach Coach" comes by. I've woken up, at least enough to be there, the weekend is near, and I am looking forward to it, believe me. Ask anyone, the best time to see me is Friday afternoon. So what am I saying, I hate work: Sure, sometimes, everyone does sometimes. I'm also talking about the sense of accomplishment I feel, and I am getting stronger, more durable, learning about the workplace. And I'm making money! Let's not underestimate that, I don't. Do I get along with my boss? Almost never, I mean it feels that way. Ralph said, "You've got to pick up your feet!" Boy, was I angry. Part of my shuffling is a side effect of taking meds for almost 20 years. However, I find myself moving around faster at work. Even if I can't stop some shuffling, I am cruising around at a good speed. I can get quite grouchy when people try to help me. I don't take criticism well, even when it is constructive, but I'm getting better at considering it. 1995 has been a year where I've grown by leaps and bounds. But it is damn hard work. The last thing I want to do is whitewash all this stuff. No sugar coating for sure. But I now see my hard work paying off. After close to a year of working, day in and day out, it's been adding up nicely. And soon it will be a year I have been working. And for me, I never would have thought it. One thing I realized this past Monday, remembered, was how in my job now, it's not only my job, but I am holding the job for Potter Place as a whole. This concept kept me out of a lot of trouble during a few rough days in the beginning of my stint at the florist's. So here I am saying all these great things about the TEPs. No, no one paid me to say all this. It's not all great, there are lots of problems, and lots of hard work ahead, but I am grateful for the opportunity to work.

Training for the Future: Boston University Center for Psychiatric Rehabilitation

A concern often voiced by mental health consumers is that the jobs for which they are trained are outdated and poorly paid. An innovative program designed by the staff of Boston University's Center for Psychiatric Rehabilitation[2] addresses this concern. Training for the Future is the first computer training program for individuals with psychiatric disabilities in a college setting. The program's advantages include:

- Teach marketable and transferable skills.
- Use intellectual abilities that are not affected by the illness.
- Provide instant and objective feedback as to learning and job mastery; prejudice and stigma are less a mediating influence.
- Focus more on data skills and less on interpersonal skills, thereby stressing a strength rather than a deficit for most individuals with PMI.
- Provide training and education in a setting that decreases stigma, increases self-esteem, and promotes normalization.

To be eligible for the program, individuals must be over 18 years old and have experienced a mental illness that has significantly impaired their ability to function in either school or work. Of more importance, individuals must be able and willing to participate in a classroom-based, instructional approach to computers and career planning. They must also be willing to begin work in competitive employment after training.

The program is nonresidential and considered to be full-time. The classroom atmosphere is supportive and interactive with lectures, demonstrations, and a great deal of time to practice, apply, and integrate the skills learned. In addition to the instructor, graduate students provide students with support as it is needed. The goals of Training for the Future focus on:

- Ensuring that each participant develops a high degree of competence in one or more commercial software packages used in business.
- Providing each participant with additional instruction, peer support, and strategies for developing interpersonal skills and good work habits.
- Placing each participant in a worksite internship consistent with his or her skills and career interests. The success of Training for the Future is due, in part, to a broad coalition of support represented on its business advisory council: private foundations, state agencies, the federal government, and some of Boston's largest corporations. The program is the first IBM Disability Job Training Center in New England. Perhaps the greatest drawback to this program is its cost, which is $12,000.

EVALUATING OUTCOMES

In the treatment and recovery of individuals with PMI, how do you measure success? Quite often, studies cite a reduction in the number of hospitalizations, a decrease in the number of hospital days, or a decrease in treatment costs as the criteria for a successful program. Although such statistics are significant, they do not begin to describe the reality of individuals' quality of life, their ability to negotiate the demands of society, or their capacity to support themselves. So, too, in evaluating the results of a specific intervention or program, it is necessary to examine the subjective and objective outcomes from the perspective of the clients as well as the other members of the treatment team. To the professional nurse and other care providers, the use of clozapine may be considered a success because the client's primary symptoms of auditory hallucinations and persecutory delusions may have been ameliorated. However, to the individual, the bedwetting and drooling may dampen the feelings of success. The benefits of the medication may also be questioned by the vocational rehabilitation program staff if the person appears more lethargic and less able to participate in job placement.

Moreover, a person may not be able to specifically and objectively describe the outcome of a given intervention and simply state, "It just makes me feel better." One older man with bipolar illness would predictably groan and complain about how useless group therapy was. Nevertheless, for 4 years he traveled an hour and a half by public transportation, via two subway trains and one bus, to attend the group. He would often observe, "I don't know why I come. I am not a group person! But there is something that makes me feel better—sometimes."

In addition, progress is measured in small and relative increments referred to as goals. For an individual incapacitated by depression or delusional thoughts, to the extent that he or she has not left a supervised residential apartment in 2 months, to be able to attend a Saturday afternoon movie with a family member may be recognized by the family as great progress. However, to outsiders, the progress of attending a movie may be viewed as minuscule. Such small successes deserve to be recognized and celebrated.

For beginning nurses, the fact that individuals with PMI are coping with a recognized disability can be a stark reality.

AREAS FOR FUTURE RESEARCH

- What differences can be observed in treatment compliance between individuals with PMI who take part in regular peer-support groups and those who do not?
- What differences exist regarding quality-of-life issues between individuals with PMI who take part in psychosocial rehabilitation programs and those who do not?
- What components of psychosocial rehabilitation programs do members perceive to be the most helpful?

- How do individuals with PMI perceive services and resources that promote their recovery in comparison to services and resources that prevent relapse?
- What workplace characteristics assist individuals with PMI to maintain their jobs?
- What nursing interventions assist individuals with PMI who are living independently in the community?

CASE STUDY

Mrs. Greta J, an elderly woman with a history of bipolar disorder, poor memory, and confusion, visited the community mental health center for her weekly appointment with the clinical nurse specialist. Greta had been living alone for the past 6 months since the death of her husband. The nurse was concerned about Mrs. J's lethargy and marked confusion after Greta commented, "You said you wanted me to meet me at the clinic in a week. I only saw you yesterday when my husband drove me here for my appointment."

Greta reluctantly revealed to the nurse that she had felt more depressed for the past 6 days and experienced additional stresses within the family during the recent holidays. The nurse realized that both depressed feelings and increased stress could account for the change in Greta's mental status. The nurse asked Greta if her psychiatrist had changed any of her psychotropic medications and was told emphatically, "No, I'm doing just fine with my pills. I certainly don't need any more lithium!" On further questioning, Greta acknowledged that she had not eaten breakfast for fear of being late for the early morning appointment. A container of fruit yogurt was offered to Greta, which she thankfully accepted. Toward the end of the scheduled appointment session, Greta appeared less lethargic and confused, although not as active as usual. As the nurse helped Greta with her coat, they reviewed together the plan they had mutually constructed for continuing the evaluation of Greta's confusion. Greta remarked, "My arm is much better since my doctor gave me that new medicine." On further inquiry by the nurse, Greta revealed that the internist has prescribed Percocet tablets for intermittent elbow pain. The nurse realized that possible side effects of Percocet include drowsiness and confusion.

CRITICAL THINKING QUESTIONS

1. Which of Greta's behaviors suggested to the nurse that the client experienced confusion?
2. What factors contributed to Greta's increased depression?
3. What questions would help the nurse evaluate Greta's confusion and depressed mood?
4. Develop a care plan for Greta, including short- and long-term goals, which will assist with decreasing her confusion.
5. Describe behaviors that would indicate that Greta is feeling less depressed.
6. Identify common intended and side effects of lithium carbonate.
7. Describe the most therapeutic approaches for assisting Greta to continue as an active participant-collaborator in her care.
8. What concerns exist with elderly clients like Greta who are prescribed psychotropic medications?

CASE STUDY

Charles is a 38-year-old man who was diagnosed with bipolar and obsessive-compulsive disorders at the age of 19. He first became ill while in his second year of college. Until age 34, when he was started on clozapine, Charles experienced frequent rehospitalizations and was unable to engage in stable friendships or participate regularly in vocational rehabilitation. Typically, someone or something would disappoint him and he would abruptly terminate his involvement. His current medications also included Carbamazepine (Tegretol), fluoxamine (Prozac), and lorazepam (Ativan) PRN. He was very responsible about taking his medications and getting the necessary laboratory work done.

Charles was fortunate to live in a community that provided tuition for unemployed adults accepted at the regional vocational technical school. He was enrolled in a 2-year program that would lead to a certificate in automotive repair. Charles was doing very well in his classwork and the hands-on component of the program. He had just completed his first year.

Charles has been receiving SSI and SSDI. He lived in a small apartment that his family helped to finance. He met with his psychopharmacologist once a week and saw his psychotherapist twice a week.

CRITICAL THINKING QUESTIONS

1. Given that Charles was actively "ill" between the ages of 17 and 34, what tasks and accomplishments of adulthood are likely to have been affected? What strategies might you suggest to remedy these developmental deficits?
2. Since beginning to take clozapine, Charles gained 60 pounds. He has been concerned about his weight and has asked for help. What strategies or resources would you suggest?
3. What are some of the factors that helped Charles to experience his current successes?
4. What were the benefits of Charles's attendance at the regional vocational technical school?
5. Charles started dating a young woman whom he met through one of his classmates. What issues would you hope his therapist would address with him?
6. Charles has his final exam next week. He is concerned because he has been experiencing religiosity, one of his target symptoms. How would you address this situation with him?
7. Charles is concerned that, when he graduates, he may not be able to handle the demands of a full-time job. What approaches might you suggest?
8. Would you consider Charles to be in a state of recovery, and why or why not?

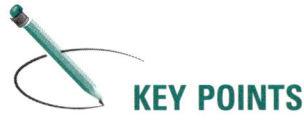

KEY POINTS

- Characteristics of a prolonged mental illness (PMI) are a lifelong process with periods of remission and exacerbation.
- Lifelong mental illnesses reflected in the *DSM-IV* include schizophrenia, bipolar disorders, and major depression.

- Individuals experiencing PMI need to be viewed and treated with respect and hope.
- Planning and implementing strategies for clients with PMI and their families include teaching and providing support. Strategies focus on prescribed medication regimens, effects, expectations if the client discontinues, and whom to contact if symptoms associated with relapse occur.
- A collaborative approach with clients, their families, and health-team members is crucial to effective planning.
- It is helpful to establish with clients realistic short-term outcome goals. Clients can then have the opportunity to experience success and a sense of accomplishment.
- Medication compliance, daily structure, and a supportive environment help maintain a client in the community, minimizing relapse or hospitalization.
- Physical complaints should be thoroughly assessed.
- Stigmatization of clients and their families inhibits the therapeutic process, evoking feelings of alienation and helplessness.
- Groups like NAMI and MDDA, comprised mainly of family members and consumers, have advocated for their active collaboration with health-care providers in the development of health policies and treatment programs for the mentally ill.
- Clients with PMI can be disadvantaged by homelessness, incarceration, lack of education, unemployment, and economics.
- Psychosocial rehabilitation programs and clubhouses provide supportive environments, promote a sense of belonging, assist with skills building, and help with job training for clients with psychiatric disabilities.
- Individuals participating in community programs following a clubhouse model can strengthen abilities, learn new skills, find peer support, and experience a sense of belonging.
- Critical nursing tasks to assist clients during their rehabilitation include helping them understand problems associated with a given disability, guiding them to optimize talents and strengths, and educating them about community resources.
- The concept of recovery rather than cure reflects the capacity for individuals to adapt and evolve beyond their psychiatric disability.

REFERENCES

1. Bachrach, L: Should "the chronic patient" be replaced? Reader response. Hospital and Community Psychiatry 44:817, 1993.
2. Anthony, W: The vocational rehabilitation of people with severe mental illness: Issues and myths. Innovations & Research 3:17, 1994.
3. US Department of Health and Welfare: Patients in mental institutions 1955. (Public Health Service Publication No. 574). US Department of Health and Welfare, Washington, DC, 1956.
4. SAMSHA US Department of Health and Human Services, Survey & Analysis Branch, Center for Mental Health Services: Resident patients in state and county mental hospitals, 1994 survey. US Department of Health and Human Services. Washington, DC, 1994.
5. Torrey, E, et al: Criminalizing the seriously mentally ill. A joint report of the National Alliance for the Mentally Ill and Public Citizens' Health Research Group. National Alliance for the Mentally Ill and Public Citizens' Health Research Group, Arlington, VA, and Washington, DC, 1992, p. 38.
6. Greenberg, P, et al: The economic burden of depression in 1990. J Clin Psychiatry 54:405, 1993.
7. Dorwart, RA: Managed mental health care: Myths and realities in the 1990s. Hospital & Community Psychiatry 41:1087, 1990.
8. Peplau, H: Interpersonal Relations in Nursing. GP Putnam's Sons, New York, 1952.
9. Kessler, RC: Social consequences of psychiatric disorders, I: Educational attainment. Am J Psychiatry 152:1026, 1995.
10. McConnell, S, Inderbitzin, L, and Pollard, W: Primary health care in the CMHC: A role for the nurse practitioner. Hospital & Community Psychiatry 43:72, 1992.
11. Torrey, EF: Surviving Schizophrenia: A Manual for Families, Consumer, and Providers (ed 3). Harper Perennial, New York, 1993.
12. Doornbos, MM: The strength of families coping with serious mental illness. Arch Psychiatr Nurs 10 (4):214–220, 1996.
13. Nightingale, F: Notes on Nursing. Dover Publications Inc, New York, 1969.
14. National Institute on Mental Health: Combating the stigma of mental illness. (DHHS Publication No. ADM 86-1470). U.S. Government Printing Office, Washington, DC, 1986.
15. Lefley, HP: Family burden and family stigma in major mental illness. Am Psychol 44:556–560, 1989.
16. Neugeboren, J: Imagining Robert. William Morrow & Co Inc, New York, 1997.
17. Eakes, GG: Chronic sorrow: The lived experience of parents of chronically mentally ill individuals. Arch Psychiatr Nurs 10 (2):77–84, 1995.
18. Task Force on Homelessness and Severe Mental Illness: Outcasts on Main Street. Interagency Council on the Homeless, Washington, DC, 1992.
19. Cain, L: Obtaining social welfare benefits for persons with serious mental illness. Hospital & Community Psychiatry 44:977, 1993.
20. Woolis, R: When Someone You Love Has a Mental Illness. G P Putnam's Sons, New York, 1992.
21. Sullivan, P: Recovery from schizophrenia: What we can learn from the developing nations. Innovations & Research, 3:7, 1994.
22. Bachrach, L: Continuity of care and approaches to case management for long-term mentally ill patients. Hospital & Community Psychiatry 44:465, 1993.
23. Kanter, J: Clinical case management: Definition, principles, components. Hospital & Community Psychiatry 40:361, 1989.
24. Zander, K: Nursing case management: Strategic management of cost and quality outcomes. JONA 18:231, 1988.
25. Sledge, WH: Case management in psychiatry: An analysis of tasks. Am J Psychiatry 152:1259.
26. Rubin, A: Is case management effective for people with serious mental illness? Health Soc Work 17:238, 1992.
27. Torrey, EF: Continuous treatment teams in the care of the chronically mentally ill. Hospital & Community Psychiatry 37:1243, 1986.
28. Lehman, AF: Strategies for improving services for the chronic mentally ill. Hospital & Community Psychiatry 40:916, 1989.
29. Guy, S: Assertive community treatment of the long-term mentally ill. J Am Psychiatric Nurses Association, in press.
30. Noorsday, DL, and Drake, RE: Case management. In Miller, NS (ed): Treating Coexisting Psychiatric and Addictive Disorders: A Practical Guide. Hazeldenon Publishing & Education, Center City, MN, 1994.
31. Williams, RH: Psychiatric rehabilitation in the hospital. Public Health Rep 11:67, 1953.
32. Bierer, J: A self-governed patients' social club in a public mental hospital. Journal of Mental Science 87:419, 1941.
33. Grob, S: Psychiatric social clubs come of age. Mental Hygiene 54:129, 1970.

CHAPTER 30

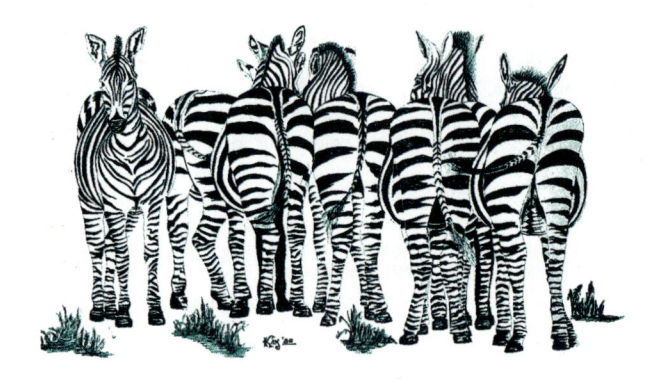

CHAPTER OUTLINE

Defining Homelessness
Historical Perspectives and Related Issues
   Deinstitutionalization and Homelessness
   Economic and Public Policy Factors
Homeless Subgroups and Psychiatric–Mental Health Concerns
   The Homeless Experience and Psychiatric–Mental Health Issues
   Vulnerable Homeless Subgroups
Conceptual Models: The Process of Becoming Homeless
   Social Distress Theory and Homelessness
   Individual Styles of Coping with Social Distress
   Model of the Homelessness Process
Psychiatric–Mental Health Nursing and the Homeless
   Historical Background
   Theoretical Basis for Nursing Practice
   Psychiatric–Mental Health Nursing Intervention Strategies
   Advocacy Role for the Homeless

LEARNING OBJECTIVES

After completing this chapter, the reader should be able to:

- Define homelessness in several ways.
- Discuss historical, socioeconomic, and political perspectives on homelessness in America.
- Explain the process of homelessness using stages and social distress theory.
- Describe key physical, behavioral, affective, cognitive, and cultural aspects that are common in the homeless population.
- Assess and develop nursing intervention strategies that meet the unique and diverse needs of homeless individuals and families.
- Identify ways in which nurses and nursing can advocate for improved conditions and health-care delivery systems for the homeless population.

KEY TERMS

benign homelessness	malignant homelessness
chronic homelessness	marginal homelessness
deindustrialization	new homeless
deinstitutionalization	old homeless
gentrification	recent homelessness
homelessness	social distress theory

Roberta Schweitzer, RN, CS, PhD

The Faces of Homelessness

Within the last two decades, homelessness has become one of this country's major social problems. The number of homeless individuals is larger than it was during the depression years of the 1930s. The homeless population is more heterogeneous and includes men, women, children, adolescents, the elderly, the disabled, and families.[1]

The stereotype of a homeless person as a middle-aged, alcoholic, male vagrant inhabiting the streets of a rundown district in a large city is inaccurate. This group is now joined on the streets by a fast-growing population of families, single women with children, the recently unemployed, adolescent runaways, the mentally ill, and the elderly. These people are subject to high levels of disability and social isolation. Most are poor, but some are not. Many have little education, but some are well educated. African Americans, Latinos, and Native Americans are all overrepresented among the homeless population.[1,2] Due to circumstances frequently beyond their control, they are unable to acquire and maintain permanent housing. As a result, they must live in city streets, subways, parks, public shelters, abandoned cars or buildings, or, when lucky, in crowded and sometimes dangerous single-room-occupancy hotels.

DEFINING HOMELESSNESS

Counting the numbers of those who are homeless is extremely difficult because homelessness can be defined in a variety of ways. General estimates of the homeless population nationwide vary from 360,000 to about 3 million, depending on the area of the country and criteria for defining homelessness.[3] This wide range in estimates applies to a definition of **homelessness** in which people do not have a stable residence or a place where they can sleep and receive mail. Although this definition is technically accurate, it excludes about 7.5 million people who are forced to move in with family members or friends because they lack other housing alternatives.[4,5]

Larew[6] and Youssef, Omokehinde, and Garland,[7] in a sociological definition, see homelessness as a human condition of disaffiliation and detachment. That is, the individual is cut off and estranged from family, community, and peer support and involvement. Bassuck[8] focuses on the intrapsychic nature of homelessness and describes it as more than the lack of a home; it is a metaphor for profound disconnection from other people and social institutions. The Alcohol, Drug Abuse, and Mental Health Administration (ADAMHA) defines the homeless individual as one who lacks adequate shelter, resources, and community ties.[9] ADAMHA estimated that as many as half of the homeless in the United States suffer from alcohol abuse, drug abuse, or mental health problems.[7]

RESEARCH NOTE

Caton, CM, Shrout, PE, Eagle, PF, Opler, LA, Felix, A, and Dominguez, B: Risk factors for homelessness among schizophrenic men: A case-control study. Am J Public Health 84, 265–270, 1994.

Findings: The purpose of the study was to identify risk factors for homelessness among severely mentally ill individuals. Homeless subjects showed significantly higher levels of positive symptoms, higher rates of concurrent diagnosis of drug abuse, and higher rates of antisocial personality disorder.

Homeless subjects experienced greater disorganization in family settings from birth to 18 years and less adequate current family support. Fewer homeless subjects than subjects in the never-homeless comparison group had a long-term therapist. These differences remained when demographic variables were adjusted statistically. Homeless schizophrenic men differed in all three domains investigated: family background, nature of illness, and service use history.

Application to Practice: When clinicians clearly identify risk factors for homelessness, it increases the possibilities for developing preventive intervention strategies. For example, thorough assessment of patterns of substance use, family support, and prior outpatient service use in concert with routine discharge planning can identify those who require additional services and supportive housing. Patients with codisorders can be singled out for intensive case management to improve the successful coordination of mental health and substance-abuse treatment services.

Although risk factors aid in identifying those individuals most vulnerable to homelessness, they do not eliminate the need for all levels of government policymakers to address the chronic shortage of affordable housing for indigent Americans.

Homelessness has also been described using the terms *benign* or *malignant*. **Benign homelessness** describes homelessness of short duration, with minimal effects and a long-lasting resolution. Spending the night in the car, on a vacation, when all the local hotels are filled, would be an example of this category. **Malignant homelessness** refers to long-term or recurrent episodes that create significant hardships for the homeless individual or family.[4]

HISTORICAL PERSPECTIVES AND RELATED ISSUES

Rossi[10] and Kiesler[11] define and explain homelessness through reference to two time periods in American history. They distinguish between the "old" and the "new" homeless. The **old homeless** (those of the 1930s and 1950s) were men, average age 50, white, unmarried, and intermittently employed with about 25% on Social Security. These men were homeless in the sense of not having a permanent residence, but they were seldom without shelter. On the days when they had sufficient income, they stayed in flophouses and cheap hotels. At other times, they were usually able to find a bed in a mission. Few of the old homeless actually had to sleep on the streets. The number of old homeless steadily declined through the 1960s and 1970s and reached a low point by the end of the 1970s.

By the beginning of the 1980s, the **new homeless** had begun to appear, and their numbers have increased rapidly since then. They are shelterless as well as homeless, quite young, disproportionately from minority groups, and die at an average age of 50. They are much poorer than their homeless predecessors, and there are substantial numbers of women and children among them.

Of the major issues that have contributed to the rapidly increasing numbers of new homeless, deinstitutionalization of the chronic mentally ill is certainly one. However, it is now understood to have an important but more indirect significance than originally thought.

DEINSTITUTIONALIZATION AND HOMELESSNESS

The APA's Task Force on the Homeless Mentally Ill reported that 25 to 50% of cases in various samples appeared to have severe or chronic psychiatric illnesses.[12] Bassuk, Rubin, and Lauriat[13] reported that approximately 30% of the homeless have a major mental illness, including schizophrenia and affective disorders such as depression or bipolar disorder. Breakey and colleagues[14] reported that about 12% of the homeless individuals have a dual diagnosis of severe mental illness complicated by substance dependence.

Not all of the homeless have long-term psychiatric disorders, nor do all mentally ill become homeless. However, the combination of psychiatric disorder and poverty often creates a high risk for homelessness and makes housing and financial problems of great concern for clients.[15] Therefore, deinstitutionalization is an important issue in relation to the homeless mentally ill.

Historical Perspective on Deinstitutionalization

Deinstitutionalization, the movement of the chronically mentally ill from long-term facilities to the community, began in the 1950s with the introduction of neuroleptic medications and with the renewed interest in psychosocial rehabilitation. Before deinstitutionalization began, serious chronic mental illness was treated in public mental hospitals that had responsibility for, and control over, numerous aspects of patients' lives, including their shelter, nutrition, medical care, medications, and daily activities. Many public hospitals were substantially overcrowded and understaffed. These hospitals developed a harsh custodialism that led to criticism and devaluation of care in the public mental hospital system.[16]

Deinstitutionalization was spurred by public outrage at conditions in state mental hospitals and shaped by federal legislation in the 1960s that has been likened to a Great Society program for the mentally ill.[17,18] The community mental health movement was intended to promote rehabilitation of the chronically mentally ill and to facilitate their social reintegration.

Instead, there was a shift of the chronically mentally ill population without a concomitant shift of the resources needed for their support. Reports beginning in the late 1960s described precipitous discharges to unprepared or resistant communities.[19] Despite the existence of comprehensive model programs, many of the chronically ill did not receive support services. Group or boarding homes had limited opportunities for community integration and provided a custodial type of care not unlike the state hospital environment.

By 1978, Reich and Siegel[20] described New York's Bowery area as a "psychiatric dumping ground." Bassuk and Gerson[21] referred to central urban districts as "psychiatric ghettos." Residents of these areas depend on a precarious supply of single-unit housing and share a high risk of homelessness because of poverty, isolation, and disability.

The timing of deinstitutionalization coincides with the timing Rossi[10] outlined for the occurrence of the old and new homeless populations. Deinstitutionalization began in the mid-1950s, peaked in the 1960s, and continued into the early 1970s. The number of old homeless was decreasing during the peak of deinstitutionalization, and the number of new homeless began increasing after the peak of deinstitutionalization.

Therefore, additional influences, related more directly to the rise of the new homelessness and resulting psychiatric–mental health issues, need to be addressed. Most informed observers point to economic and public policy factors as core causes of the new homelessness.[10,11,22,23]

ECONOMIC AND PUBLIC POLICY FACTORS

Housing

The availability of affordable low-income housing is decreasing. Over a 15-year period, approximately half of the single-room-occupancy hotels in the United States, more than 1 million rooms, disappeared through urban renewal.[24] McChesney[23] estimated that by 1985 there were roughly 4.7 million low-rent units in the country to accommodate 11.6 million low-income families. In 1983, the Housing Census found that 7 million households lived in crowded conditions.[25] Such conditions are the last stop for those who are subsequently homeless.

A second housing issue is the recessions during the 1980s that resulted in fewer housing starts and placed new homes outside the reach of the middle class. Many of these middle-class individuals had to "buy down" or purchase condominiums converted from former apartment houses, which, in turn, put housing, including rentals, beyond the purchasing power of the poor and the near poor. As a third factor, the Reagan administration eliminated federal subsidies on low-cost housing.[22,26]

Income of the Poor and Near Poor

During the same time that the supply of affordable housing has shrunk, social safety-net programs have been cut also.[27] Inflation and welfare reforms have affected tax policies and reduced welfare real income (such as Aid to Families with Dependent Children). In the 1980s there were also attempts to reduce the number of mentally ill individuals who were receiving Supplemental Security Income (SSI). These purges in benefits (often the sole means of support for the chronically mentally ill), the reduction of affordable housing, and the inability of the chronically mentally ill to advocate for themselves what meager benefits they are entitled to has contributed to the current situation.[28-30]

Similarly, working persons have faced increasing hardships. During the past decade, structural economic changes left many without jobs.[31] A low minimum wage, raised in 1990 for the first time since 1981, left many working families in poverty.[32] Full-time work at the minimum wage of $4.25 per hour left a family of three about $1000 below the poverty line. In July 1997, the 104th Congress passed public law 104-188 to amend the Fair Labor Standards Act of 1993. The minimum hourly wage was increased to $5.15, but this still leaves a family of three near the poverty line.

Health-Care Cost

A third set of economic variables relates to the rapidly increasing cost of health care, which, combined with the large number of uninsured people, puts even routine preventive health care beyond the reach of 25% of the U.S. population.[28] As a result, over the past decade, poor Americans have had to make do with ever-decreasing resources.[32,33] Many uninsured Americans are one major medical expense away from homelessness. For the poorest of the poor, facing decreasing resources and rising housing costs, homelessness was the predictable result.

The Stewart B. McKinney Homeless Assistance Act

In 1987, President Reagan signed the McKinney Homeless Assistance Act into law. It was a landmark event: the first comprehensive federal response to homelessness.[34] Five years earlier, a Reagan administration official had stated publicly that "no one is living on the streets."[35] Against a backdrop of reluctance to acknowledge homelessness as a national crisis, the federal government responded.

The McKinney Act provided, and continues to provide, significant aid to the nation's homeless poor. It created 20 new programs that operate primarily by allocating federal funds to states, local governments, and private, nonprofit organizations. Shelter programs provide funds for the acquisition, rehabilitation, and operation of emergency shelters. Some funds are also available for transitional housing, and modest amounts are available for permanent housing for single homeless adults.

Another group of programs provides funds for health and mental health care for persons in shelters and on the streets. Funded projects include mobile vans and outreach teams. A surplus property program requires federal agencies to make unused property available as facilities for homeless individuals.

Although these programs meet some critical needs, they are grossly inadequate. Most are emergency programs in nature and insufficient to meet the underlying causes of homelessness.[33,36] The McKinney Act receives such low appropriations that most states have only token dollars to respond to the homeless problems. It fails to fully support substantial prevention programs or other needed services, especially for homeless children. In addition, some reform efforts have created ineffective shifts of responsibility between state and local governments.

The process of local governance is one vehicle through which communities can shape services to achieve goals.[37] Although the federal and state governments can promote, encourage, and facilitate this process, it is ultimately the responsibility of local leaders to make it work. An increasing number of organizations and agencies have the specialized goal of helping the homeless across the nation. However, much more needs to be done.

HOMELESS SUBGROUPS AND PSYCHIATRIC–MENTAL HEALTH CONCERNS

Homelessness is much more than not having a place to live. All homeless people suffer from lack of food, appropriate clothing, access to health care and social services (at a reasonable price), educational opportunities, and gainful employment. In addition to these areas of vulnerability, also psychiatric–mental health issues are relevant for homeless individuals. These issues arise from two distinct circumstances of the homeless individual and affect how homelessness is experienced by the individual.

THE HOMELESS EXPERIENCE AND PSYCHIATRIC–MENTAL HEALTH ISSUES

Homelessness and the Chronically Mentally Ill

As discussed previously, some of the homeless have a history of diagnosed major mental illness that often precedes homelessness. Deinstitutionalized chronically mentally ill people often find a lack of community support systems that would make it possible for them to function outside of a hospital.

Homelessness as Psychological Trauma

For other homeless individuals, acute mental distress has been the result of the stressors of homelessness. These stressors, brought on by fears for basic survival and safety, as well as the psychological impact of societal disenfranchisement, create symptoms that meet the *Diagnostic and Statistical Manual of Mental Disorders, Fourth Edition (DSM-IV)* criteria for depression, personality disorder, and anxiety disorders.[3] For example, some common criteria for a diagnosis of major depression are disordered sleep, loss of interest in food and pleasurable activities, poor concentration, psychomotor retardation, feelings of hopelessness and helplessness, and suicidal thoughts. Strasser, Damrosch, and Gaines[38] note that suicide and depression are common in homeless adults and youths.

VULNERABLE HOMELESS SUBGROUPS

Salzman and Curtis[39] note that subgroups of the homeless population are especially vulnerable to the assaults to the self that occur in homelessness: the mentally ill, the physically ill, and children. Other vulnerable subgroups are families with children, single women, single mothers, adolescents, the elderly, and those with substance-abuse problems.

Chronically Mentally Ill

The chronically mentally ill individual lives an impoverished life devoid of even the basic services that were provided at state hospitals.[12] They may become homeless because of their inability to cope with normal activities of life such as maintaining a residence, managing money, obtaining transportation, preparing meals, following medication instructions, and articulating their needs for other basic services. Already unable to deal with these daily demands of life, it becomes almost impossible for these individuals to make a daily search for a place to sleep, eat, rest, and renew themselves—most likely all of these needs will not even be met at the same site.

This lack of day-to-day resources makes it difficult for mentally ill homeless persons to show up for appointments or take required medications, which can result in further decompensation. In other cases, when individuals have family, the family members may have abandoned them because they can no longer cope with the effects of mental illness.

In the period after deinstitutionalization, community mental health centers were supposed to provide inpatient and outpatient care, day care, outreach services, emergency treatment, and educational services, as well as services specifically for children, adolescents, and the elderly. However, for the most part, the community was usually unprepared to support this group of clients because of lack of funding for the centers. Thus, many of the chronically mentally ill received no social or medical support in the community.

Families

The population of homeless families is growing. Since the early 1980s, alarming numbers of families have lost their homes and have turned to emergency shelters or dilapidated welfare hotels for refuge. This change is a consequence of cuts in welfare programs, specifically Aid to Families with Dependent Children (AFDC) and reductions in food-stamp and affordable-housing programs.[40,41] These families are estimated to make up 34% of the overall homeless population and are the fastest-growing subgroup.[42,43] From 79 to 90% of these families are composed of a single adult family member—the mother—and two or three children.

Changes in zoning laws and building codes are making cheap housing a rarity. The problem becomes even more complex if a parent is diagnosed with chronic mental illness or a mental health problem. The remaining 20 to 30% of homeless families are headed by couples who generally have been homeless after the wage earner has lost a higher-wage production job that has been moved to another part of the United States or somewhere overseas.[42,43] In such circumstances, a similar-wage job may be impossible to find, leading the worker to replace the old job with a lower-paying service job.

Women

In the past, most homeless individuals were men over the age of 45. Today, however, most of the homeless are under 40, and the number includes more women.[44] Estimates of the number of women has risen from 3% in 1968[45] to between 25%[46] and 50%.[47,48] A little over one-third of the homeless population is families, the majority of which are headed by a woman with 2 or 3 children, 5 years old or younger. Women also fall into other subgroups of the homeless, including teenagers, elderly, single, divorced, and the chronically mentally ill.[44]

The single-parent women are generally not chronically mentally ill, do not have problems with reality testing, and are not in need of psychotropic medications. Instead, their

> **RESEARCH NOTE**
>
> **Hodnicki, DR, Horner, SD, and Boyle, JS: Women's perspectives on homelessness. Public Health Nursing 9, 257–262, 1992.**
>
> **Findings:** The results of this study provide a new understanding of how some women experience homelessness, as well as the responses they make to solve this problem. The study was conducted by interviewing eight homeless women from a shelter in a southeastern city in a modified ethnographic approach with a semistructured interview to obtain qualitative data. The constant comparison method of analysis identified four central themes that described the women's experience of homelessness: heightened awareness, guarding, identification of needs, and strategies for resolution.
>
> - **Heightened Awareness:** The shelter offered these women temporary respite from the elements and some of their daily needs. However, shelters are filled with a variety of people, some of whom do not follow social rules and regulations well. Thus, although a shelter is better than being on the streets, it is not the safest place. The women's health and safety and that of their children, as well as their daily survival, depended on staying alert and anticipating problems that arose from their circumstance.
> - **Guarding:** This incorporates behaviors that keep self and children safe and sound. The women believed watchfulness and carefulness were necessary because of their vulnerability in the shelter setting. Strategies included recognizing and avoiding unsafe situations while determining ways to meet basic needs and learning to deal with time. They had to become more streetwise to survive. To get inside, out of adverse weather, the women tried to sneak into fast-food restaurants, hide in rest rooms, and so forth to remain obscure and protect their children.
> - **Identification of Needs:** The women saw this as the first step to resolving their homelessness. Also, their children depended on them to solve their problems, and they described how important it was to think of their children's needs first. Their need for identification and planning to resolve homelessness was supported by shelter staff. However, acting on this guidance and advice was often difficult. The women described many frustrations because they encountered many roadblocks and hassles. Identifying health concerns of the women and their children was also important to remaining healthy and moving forward with goals.
> - **Strategies for Resolution:** As the women began to identify needs and possible solutions, they developed strategies to resolve their homelessness. They secured employment when possible and used resources available to them. The women were driven by their vulnerability to engage actively in processes of interaction to solve problems. Often, the women described their time of homelessness as a time of growth. They found inner resources that made them better individuals and better able to deal with their problems. This reporting of a proactive position taken by these women has not been reported elsewhere in the literature.
>
> **Application to Practice:** Although these findings cannot be generalized, nurses may gain insights into homeless women's experiences. One of the most useful findings is that the women were attempting to solve their own problems. Initially, the subjects were all very frightened by the prospects of being homeless. However, as they felt safer, they were better able to function. This points out that the kind of support that was given to the women and the way in which it was given may differ considerably, depending on simply where an individual woman is in her adjustment to homelessness. As she becomes more confident in her abilities to take charge of her life, she must have information, anticipatory guidance, and support from professionals.
>
> Further research needs to be done to better understand this process of recovering from homelessness, because it occurs in various subgroups of homeless individuals and in families.

homelessness has been the result of domestic violence and abuse. Kozol's book, *Rachel and Her Children: Homeless Families in America*,[49] did a great deal to bring to national attention the problem of homeless women and children. Battered women and their children are a significant proportion of occupants of homeless shelters.[49] On an average night, in the shelters that serve primarily families with children, about 50% of women have been involved in domestic violence.[50] The most common problems these women face include lack of money or housing. Women who file domestic-abuse charges may find that they are denied health-insurance coverage or have inflated premiums because of their increased risk for being abused. In New York City's battered women programs, 59% of the women and children seeking shelter were turned away.[50] However, getting into a shelter is often no guarantee of escaping abuse, because most shelters allow only short stays. In New York City, after being sheltered, 31% of abused women return to their batterers, primarily because they could not locate longer-term housing.

Children

Another vulnerable homeless population is children. Beyond the effects of hunger and poor nutrition, increased health problems and inadequate health care, developmental delays and educational underachievement, there are psychological problems: anxiety, depression, and behavioral disturbances such as sleep disorders, hyperaggression, regressive behaviors, inappropriate social interactions with adults, and immature peer interactions.[51]

Bassuk[42] interviewed 156 children of sheltered homeless families and found that approximately two-thirds were preschoolers, 5 years old or younger. The results of her research showed almost half of the preschoolers had severe developmental lags on the Denver Developmental Screening Test in multiple areas tested, including language development, gross motor skills, fine motor coordination, and personal-social development. In addition, the mother in the family was usually depressed and, as a result, spent less time playing, talking, and interacting with the children. Although these children required greater stimulation and more opportunity for interaction, very few were in any kind of daycare or Headstart program that provided it. Significant cuts in social programs during the 1980s decreased the availability of such programs. Also, in many instances, mothers did not take advantage of these opportunities because of lack of information or the severity of their own impairment, which decreased their ability to advocate for their own children.[42,52]

Many of the children do not have the opportunity to attend school. In one study sample of homeless children, 43% had failed a grade, 24% attended special classes, and almost 50% were currently failing.[13,53] Older school-age children find school uncomfortable because they may be ashamed of their family circumstances and are frequently bullied and taunted by peers. These children may express their insecurities by being too aggressive or withdrawn and by having difficulties in school. Also, transferring from shelter to shelter often means transferring from one school to another, creating erratic attendance patterns and added barriers to learning and peer socialization.

In addition to emotional and learning problems, homeless children also suffer from health problems. Using data from the Health Care for the Homeless project, Wright[54] observed that the rate of chronic physical disorders among homeless children was nearly twice that observed among ambulatory children in general. Other researchers have reported immunization delays,[55] lead poisoning,[56] and poor nutritional status[55,56] among homeless children.

Adolescents

Adolescents may be homeless because they have run away from home or have been thrown out by parents. Some have been sexually or physically abused by a relative. In one study, Ihejirika[57] found that 75% of homeless youth had run away at age 14 or younger to escape abuse. In other situations, parents of adolescents who are abusing drugs may feel helpless or threatened and force the teen out of the home to regain control of their lives.

Ihejirika[57] summarizes homeless adolescents as school dropouts with no previous work history and limited marketable job skills. Therefore, they must rely on illegal activities to survive, such as prostitution, pornography, drug dealing, and theft. Often sex is traded for food, shelter, or protection. Adolescents who have run away from home to escape abuse frequently are at high risk for assault, rape, unwanted pregnancy, and sexually transmitted disease.

Substance Abusers

Substance abuse in the homeless population is estimated at rates of 10 to 68%, depending on the study source.[58] According to Fischer and colleagues,[59] alcohol abuse affects 30 to 40% of the homeless, whereas drug abuse affects 10 to 15%. They also found that men were more likely to report problems with alcohol and drugs, whereas women report more problems with mental illness.

Chemical abuse and homelessness are related, but one does not necessarily cause the other. Alcohol and drug abuse can lead to homelessness, or the stresses of homelessness may lead to drug or alcohol use. Chemical dependency, as a dual diagnosis, may compound the challenges of working with the chronically mentally ill homeless individual. For example, a homeless alcoholic may also have schizophrenia,[60] thus necessitating a comprehensive view of physiological and mental processes in the individual. Beyond the physical health risks of drug and alcohol abuse, the combined psychological impact of the hopelessness of a substance problem with the condition of homelessness is overwhelming.

Methods of dealing with chemical dependency in the homeless population have been influenced by current treatment approaches. Earlier in this country's history, public intoxication was a crime, and most homeless alcoholics were taken to drunk tanks at the local police station. In 1971, the Uniform Alcoholism and Intoxication Act encouraged local governments to establish community-based detoxification and alcohol-treatment centers.[58,60] However, substance-abuse treatment programs for the indigent are still quite scarce.[3]

Elderly

An increasing number of elderly are finding themselves at risk for homelessness at a time when the demand for low-income housing is larger than the supply, and the federal allocations for public housing have been severely cut. Those over age 60 are predicted to be the next group hit hard by homelessness.[61] The elderly currently make up a small percentage of the homeless population. Various studies estimate that 6 to 27% of homeless persons are over 60 years old.[58,62] This may be an underestimation because of the high mortality rate among the homeless elderly.[43,63]

The most common mental health problem in this group is organic or alcohol-related dementia, which is manifested by confusion, disorientation, paranoia, and hallucinations.[62] In another study of one shelter population, Lenehan, Mc-

Ginnis, O'Connell, and Hennessey[64] found that 90% of the elderly women exhibited psychiatric symptoms such as hallucinations, paranoia, phobias, and depression. Medical problems such as arthritis, hypertension, diabetes, fractures, pneumonia, and sensory deprivation compound the plight of the homeless elderly.[62] A single medical emergency or tragic incident could place many older persons living near the poverty level at risk for homelessness.

Individuals with Physical Illness

Individuals who are chronically mentally ill or who face the mental health challenges of homelessness also face the obstacles related to physical illness in their daily lives. It is estimated that 41% of the homeless population experiences one or more chronic health conditions,[65] with hypertension present in 40 to 50% of homeless adults. Prevalence rates for tuberculosis are up to 300 times higher than those of the general population.[66] In some populations as many as 20% of the homeless may be HIV positive, particularly among those who turn to prostitution as a means of survival.[67]

Good health is nearly impossible to maintain as the homeless move between soup kitchens and shelters, interspersed with trips to the hospital. Any existing medical conditions are easily exacerbated and difficult to control through "normal" interventions such as diet or medication. The disordered living conditions, exposure to extreme temperatures and the elements, malnutrition, and overcrowding in shelters make it difficult for people dealing with problems such as diabetes, hypertension, or peripheral vascular diseases, as well as mental illness.

CONCEPTUAL MODELS: THE PROCESS OF BECOMING HOMELESS

SOCIAL DISTRESS THEORY AND HOMELESSNESS

The **social distress theory**[39] provides a structure for the phenomenon of homelessness. Social distress theory includes four basic principles.

1. A rapid and unplanned social change that generates a shift in values
2. Development of a conflict between "old" and "new" values
3. Reorganization of social institutions around both sets of values, thereby institutionalizing the conflict and resulting in disability
4. Social distress resulting from the interaction of multiple dysfunctional institutional systems.

Rapid Unplanned Social Change and Development of Values Conflict

The first two principles indicate that rapid and unplanned social change precipitates values shifts, which in turn create a tension or dissonance. This tension is related to needing to decide which values should prevail within a small social system, such as a family, or a larger system, such as the society. Concerning homelessness, significant historical changes in our society should be noted.

These areas of change include deinstitutionalization, which has been discussed previously, deindustrialization, and gentrification. In this context, **deindustrialization** describes the shift in the job market in this country from relatively well-paid manufacturing jobs to lower-paid employment in service industries, like fast-food sales or janitorial work.[43] It stems from changes in the nation's economic and occupational structure.

Inability to pay rent or mortgage is a major contributing factor to homelessness. The term **gentrification** refers to the redevelopment of urban areas with a consequence of losing many low-cost housing units. More affluent members of society move into and rehabilitate areas of cities once inhabited by the poor. Since 1970, more than 1 million single-room occupancy units—half of the supply—have been lost, thus eliminating many low-cost housing alternatives.[43]

Deinstitutionalization, discussed earlier, includes the process of discharging large numbers of mentally ill patients from mental institutions; it occurred when the conditions within these institutions appalled members of society.

Together, changes in these areas have created sets of conflicting values, such as values for free enterprise versus social welfare, and individual rights versus community responsibility.[39] On the one hand, beliefs underlying housing policies in this country are that housing is basic for all citizens. But, at the same time, housing is seen as a commodity to be sold in the marketplace for a profit or as an investment to be protected through zoning laws.

Reorganization of Social Institutions around Both Sets of Values

This conflict in values creates a tension or uncertainty about what we truly believe. When this happens, social institutions cannot enact both sets of values. Social distress may emerge when many conflictual value interactions create a dysfunctional system.

For example, consider the homeless mother's "nightmare" of having to face an appearance in court (because she was evicted), a trip to the hospital (to obtain inoculations for her child), and an appointment with a local landlord (in order to find a new residence) all in the same week.[59]

Resultant Social Distress

Although none of the systems has been designed to produce distress, in conjunction with one another, they do. Implicit in the definition of social distress is that a variety of social forces are combined, thus creating an aversive emotional environment characterized by frustration, irritability, feelings of things being out of control, and helplessness. For the individual experiencing this environment of social distress, there is also an accompanying aversive experience of personal distress.

INDIVIDUAL STYLES OF COPING WITH SOCIAL DISTRESS

Saltzman and Curtis[39] continued development of the social distress theory by examining how individuals cope with social distress. Although the coping mechanisms of denial and dissociation are important, individuals experiencing the social distress generated by interlocking dysfunctional systems deal with it in differing ways, depending on their life situations.

Coping with Social Distress

People who have homes may transform their feelings of discomfort and guilt about the homeless into anger at them. They might deny the homeless person's humanity and blame them for their plight. Victim-blaming feeds a need for the illusion of control in a world that may actually be out of control. Thus, as people become aware of victims, they need to engage in more and more dissociation. By doing so, they turn off feelings of compassion and increasingly dissociate themselves from their own internal processes. This process is called *numbing*.[39] As a result, individuals become psychologically separated from themselves. The numbness interlocks with the larger political-ideological system.

Coping as a Homeless Individual

Everyone copes through dissociation, whether homeless or not. Dissociation in homeless individuals takes on another dimension, however, when people attempt to extricate themselves from a society that denies their humanity. They build "societies outside of societies" where they feel safer and more valued. Furthermore, the homeless individuals deny the humanity of those in the mainstream of society, seeing them as exploitive and oppressive.[39]

This denial can lead to other coping mechanisms that speak to people's psychological needs for control and predictability in their lives. Just as dissociation and victim-blaming allow observers of ongoing victimization to gain a sense of control in a confusing world, individuals who are locked in dysfunctional systems also create ways to direct and control their lives.[68]

Kozinski[68] uses the concept of the "protagonist" to describe people who are able to mobilize their resources in order to sustain and direct their lives. Mobilization may involve physical actions such as building one's own cardboard home as an expression of mastery over the environment. Homeless individuals may also adopt belief systems or ideologies that justify their actions, such as believing that the agencies that provide relief for the homeless are corrupt and that to use their services is to participate in a corrupt system.

Such dissociation strategies are actually attempts to invigorate their "protagonist" selves. Also, people may manipulate reality to raise their self-esteem. For example, they many find positive qualities to being homeless, such as being expert Dumpster divers. The idea of the protagonist self helps explain seemingly bizarre behaviors, such as Dumpster diving, seen in those most oppressed by social distress.[68] The combination of such bizarre behaviors and a chronic mental illness may make understanding the client very difficult. Taken out of context, these can be used to prove that the homeless individual is flawed, lazy, or responsible for his or her own plight. Therefore, the coping mechanisms in this social distress model[39] must be viewed within the person's context in order to understand his or her behavior and dynamics.

MODEL OF THE HOMELESSNESS PROCESS

A conceptual model of the process of becoming homeless developed by Belcher, Scholler-Jacquish, and Drummond[69] can be useful in assessing and intervening with the homeless population. In their study, the authors conducted intensive case study interviews with homeless individuals from a variety of sources within a large city. They identified three stages of homelessness (1) marginal, (2) recent, and (3) chronic.

Marginal Homelessness

Marginal homelessness is exemplified by individuals who live below or slightly above the poverty line. Connection to a home is weak and may be episodic. These people are not often recognized or counted as homeless but frequently use many of the services offered for the homeless community, such as clothing drops and soup kitchens. For this group, one setback can destroy their tenuous network of supports. The majority of these individuals are women. They have greater access to transition shelters, are more likely to be able to stay with friends and relatives, and greater access to welfare assistance than the men.

> Sharon is a 22-year-old woman and a regular at a soup kitchen. She has three children, ages 18 months to 5 years. She has never worked and dropped out of high school when her first child was born. Three years ago, she moved into an apartment with a man who became increasingly assaultive. Sharon is staying with friends on a temporary basis and is not sure how long she will be able to remain. She feels frightened and alone and is not sure where to turn for help.[69]

Recent Homelessness

Individuals in this group have become homeless recently, usually within the previous 9 months. They still identify with the mainstream of their communities rather than with other homeless people. A major characteristic of this group is their hope that they will somehow regain a lost home, job, and social standing and avoid living on the streets.[70] During **re-**

cent homelessness, interactions with family and friends become more negative. Living arrangements with friends and relatives become jeopardized by overcrowding. Frequent problems in this group are depression, substance abuse, low self-esteem, and shame. This group accesses health care on an episodic or emergency basis.

> Bill B is a 42-year-old alcoholic who has never had a steady job. He was married, and his ex-wife lives in the neighborhood. Bill's family home is in the neighborhood, also; however, his brother, who is in charge of the household, refuses to admit Bill to the home. Bill depends almost entirely on temporary welfare checks when he qualifies as disabled. He stays in shelters on an irregular basis. Bill observes, "I am not really homeless, you know, I just don't have a home right now."[69]

Chronic Homelessness

Chronic homelessness is a problem for the person who has been homeless for longer periods (usually more than 1 year and sometimes for many years). The individual accepts his or her life experiences on the streets as normative, is more easily and clearly identifiable as homeless, and is extremely suspicious of members of mainstream society. The individual may drift back and forth between stages 2 and 3, struggling to keep the streets from becoming a permanent home.

> Dan is a 42-year-old man with a long history of alcoholism. He has never married and was thrown out of his family home at age 16. Dan subsequently lived on and off in the streets. Much of his time is spent in jail because of his frequent encounters with the law for minor violations, usually disturbing the peace. Otherwise, Dan wanders the streets. His chronic lung disease is made worse by irregular health care. He resists all encouragement to stop drinking, saying, "What's the use, I'm going to die anyway." Dan is resigned to his life on the streets.[69]

PSYCHIATRIC–MENTAL HEALTH NURSING AND THE HOMELESS

HISTORICAL BACKGROUND

Psychiatric–mental health nursing has historically delivered community mental health care in this country. To a large extent, the concept of mental health came into existence with the Community Mental Health Centers Act of 1963, the first major federal effort to provide comprehensive community-based mental health services to all persons regardless of income.[67] Since that time, nursing interventions have ranged from dealing with the mentally ill by monitoring and administering medications, therapy, and education to a more comprehensive focus on case management, coordinating community services, and reaching out to individuals who are at risk for mental illness, as well as working with the chronically mentally ill. Thus, subgroups of the homeless population that would not traditionally fit into the delivery of mental health services are beginning to receive more attention.

Because homelessness involves so many complex factors, psychiatric–mental health nurses must work collaboratively with many other health-care professionals. Various social, psychological, and physical considerations must be assessed and addressed comprehensively. Nursing, with a holistic approach to practice, based on intervening throughout the entire health-illness continuum, is in a unique position to improve and maintain the homeless individual's physical, mental, and spiritual health, as well as his or her interactions within the community as a whole.

THEORETICAL BASIS FOR NURSING PRACTICE

Nursing theory, such as Peplau's work on the development of nurse-client relationships, offers guidance for formulation of trusting relationships.[71] More recent theory, such as Parse's, can guide the psychiatric–mental health nurse in work with the various subgroups of homeless people.[72] In her human becoming theory, Parse[73] notes that it is clients and not nurses who are the authority figures and decision makers, who choose from options and take responsibility for their actions. The nursing role in this case is to validate the clients' feelings, allow them to express what is important to them, and provide information to make choices. This parallels the process and thinking of the social distress theory and its corollaries discussed previously. Homeless individuals take control of their lives and enhance their self-esteem.

For nurses, the idea of assessing coping mechanisms within a social distress model is especially significant. Nurses value helping people identify their strengths and support the use of these strengths for their clients' advantage. Coping mechanisms that might seem "crazy" can be reframed as behaviors geared at maintaining, or even raising, self-esteem within the extreme conditions of homelessness. For example, Golden[74] describes how women use "crazy behaviors" to protect themselves and to keep others, especially men, away. Reframing unusual coping behaviors helps to change the view that homeless people are helpless, passive creatures, a negative view that can set the stage for public or private policies and actions that devalue the homeless and emphasize their impotence or lack of power. However, remember that the homeless do, in fact, have limited control of the circumstances around them. Although specific acts and thought might be attempts to control their environment, control in the overall sense is out of their hands.

Homelessness has different meanings for different individuals.[75] Also, different populations of homeless are able to withstand their circumstances in different ways, some healthier than others.[74] For example, they may cope through dissociation with excessive drug and alcohol use. Others succumb to depression and learned helplessness, a belief that they cannot influence the course of their own lives. Other indicators of psychological trauma might include social disaffiliation, a persistent reexperiencing of the events leading up to becoming homeless, a general numbing response, or hyperresponsiveness, as in angry outbursts and irritability (all symptoms of posttraumatic stress disorder).

PSYCHIATRIC–MENTAL HEALTH NURSING INTERVENTION STRATEGIES

Nursing interventions with any homeless individuals should consider these stages as a basis for setting realistic mutual goals and plans. The overall goal of psychiatric RNs and advanced-practice psychiatric–mental health nurses is to provide holistic nursing care within a biopsychosocial framework. This care should be aimed at decreasing stressors and promoting emotional and physical health in homeless individuals and families.

Therapeutic relationships may be formed with homeless persons in social support settings such as outreach into missions and shelters as part of mobile emergency teams or working with established programs in shelters, soup kitchens, drop-in centers, transitional housing units, and single-room-occupancy hotels.[76–79] In addition, the homeless with chronic mental or physical illness may be found in inpatient hospital settings during periods of decompensation or relapse. Through case management and by working within a multidisciplinary team, nurses can work with homeless people to address their multiple needs within Caplan's primary prevention model of primary, secondary, and tertiary intervention.[80]

ADVOCACY ROLE FOR THE HOMELESS

Nursing as a profession needs to increase its visibility as an advocate in dealing with the long-term facets of homelessness intertwined within social and political issues in this country. Psychiatric–mental health nurses working with this population can easily become as disheartened or discouraged as the population they serve because of the lack of progress within difficult situations. In addition to the many practical day-to-day difficulties of working with the homeless, it is easy to be drawn into a philosophical and ideological struggle about our values as individuals and as a society regarding human rights and dignity. When faced with such feelings and struggles, the psychiatric–mental health nurse, as a health-care advocate for the homeless, has to to reframe this situation. Instead of feeling helpless or hopeless, the nurse, individually or as part of a group, needs to redirect energy into addressing misconceptions about the homeless and educating the public. Psychiatric–mental health nurses can take a leadership role as advocates of compassion, community responsibility, and social activism to deal with the issues affecting the physical, socioeconomic, and mental health status of the homeless in this country.

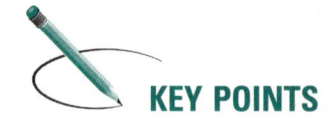

KEY POINTS

- Within the last two decades, homelessness has become one of this country's major social problems.
- The homeless population is a diverse group including men, women, children, adolescents, elderly, disabled, and families.
- Nationwide, the homeless population estimate varies from 360,000 to about 3 million.
- "Old" and "new" groups of the homeless can be distinguished throughout American history.
- The combination of psychiatric disorders and poverty often creates a high risk for homelessness and may increase housing and financial problems; however, the mentally ill do not always become homeless or vice versa.
- Deinstitutionalization, gentrification, and deindustrialization have all contributed to the rising homeless population in the United States.
- Public policy responses from the federal government have only recently acknowledged homelessness as a national crisis, and public policy and funding responses have been limited.
- The Stewart B. McKinney Homeless Assistance Act of 1987 was landmark legislation responding to homelessness in America.
- Numerous agencies and organizations are being developed to deal with the problems of homelessness and the individuals touched by it.
- Homeless individuals and families experience a variety of psychiatric–mental health concerns, from chronic mental illness to varying degrees of psychological trauma resulting from the homeless experience.
- Several subgroups of individuals are especially vulnerable to the experience of homelessness and require more support and advocacy; among them are the very young or old, the physically disabled, women with children, and those having substance-abuse problems.
- Social distress theory is a useful structure for understanding the development of and difficulties associated with homelessness.
- Homeless individuals use a wide array of coping mechanisms, healthy and unhealthy, to cope with homelessness and to gain control and predictability in their lives.
- Belcher and colleagues' stages of homelessness provide a useful way of contextualizing the homeless individual's or family's experiences and status.
- Psychiatric–mental health nurses have a rich history and background of caring for individuals and families in the community, including the homeless.
- Nursing care of the homeless is supported by several nursing theories that provide a framework for addressing

issues that arise from the unique, but basic, concerns of this population.

♦ Psychiatric–mental health nurses have a fundamental role to advocate for homeless individuals and families.

CASE STUDY

Jim was a 47-year-old veteran with schizophrenia who had lived with his mother for 10 years before becoming homeless. When his mother had become ill, Jim took her car and drove to another state. He planned to enter a mission to "find peace" with himself. The car broke down near Tucson, Arizona, and he continued by foot. When the nurse met him at the soup kitchen, he was disheveled, emaciated, talked incessantly about politics, and appeared to be responding to internal stimuli. Jim had open wounds on his neck from sunburn, and his bare feet were lacerated. When the nurse talked to him, he insisted that he did not need help. He was offered new clothes, shoes, and shelter for the night but refused them.

Jim stated that his troubles had begun 20 years ago when he was "exposed to chemicals" that made him "unable to tolerate plastic, soap, and polyester." He claimed he could wear only cotton clothing and shoes without plastic parts. After several daily contacts with the nurse, he agreed to a psychiatric evaluation but refused recommended hospitalization. An interview at a residential treatment facility was arranged, but admission there was refused because he would be required to take antipsychotic medications.

For the next 5 months, he was suspicious of the nurse and intermittently avoided contacts. One day the nurse received a phone call from Jim. He was friendly, but tangential to the nurse: "Come and pick me up." The nurse ultimately deduced that he was being held on a locked psychiatric unit; he had struck a policeman and was considered a danger to others. Although psychotic during the nurse's subsequent hospital visits, he was warm and friendly but unable to accept the need for residential treatment.

CRITICAL THINKING QUESTIONS

1. List areas that should be included in a holistic assessment of Jim's status.
2. Explain his situation according to the social distress theory.
3. Reframe Jim's situation (from his point of view) in an attempt to understand his seemingly bizarre behaviors.
4. Because Jim will not agree to residential treatment, identify some behaviors that would indicate signs of stability or mental health to be used as goals in this situation.
5. Design a plan for optimizing Jim's functioning in a community.

CASE STUDY

Catherine C was a 26-year-old woman who resided at a shelter for homeless families with her husband, Allen, and their children, Steven, 3 years, and Allison, 6 months. The family had been at the shelter for 3 weeks. They had become homeless after Allen lost his job and they were unable to pay their rent. Allen recently found a job, and the family has been saving for the deposit on a new apartment. Usually families are permitted to stay at the shelter for only 2 weeks, but an extension was approved for the C family, because they were progressing toward their goal of a new apartment.

Allen was gone from the shelter from 8 am to 6 pm, during which time Catherine was sole caregiver for the children. Catherine expressed to the shelter staff that she was grateful for the home that was provided during the past 3 weeks but that there were some aspects of shelter life that were really difficult. She said the days were "long" and "I miss the community where I lived. When you are in a shelter, it is very hard on you and your family. Others tell you when to get up and when to go to bed. If I want to take a shower or take a nap with my children, I have to ask permission from the shelter staff. Some of the things I miss the most are keeping the house clean and cooking for my family. I loved our apartment and spending time there with my family. Now, I'm dependent on everyone for everything."

That same day, there was a party for residents of the shelter whose birthdays occurred during that month. The party was organized and donated each month by volunteers. Each person with a birthday was recognized, honored, and presented with a small gift. Catherine enjoyed the party with her children. Near the end of the party, a volunteer asked Catherine to examine a pile of clothes that had just been donated. Catherine went with the volunteer to see whether there were any clothes that she could use. While Catherine was deciding which clothes to select, the volunteers who had organized the party cleaned up the tables and discarded the cupcakes and juice that Catherine had saved to share that evening with her husband. When Catherine returned and saw that the things she saved were not there, she became tearful, loud, and accusatory: "Someone took my plate of cupcakes and juice boxes that I was saving for my husband." When told that the volunteers had cleaned off the tables and probably threw them out, her anger increased. She pointed a finger at the volunteer, "The point is they were mine. No one had a right to touch them." She refused to be consoled by either the shelter staff or the volunteers.

CRITICAL THINKING QUESTIONS

1. Identify the stage of homelessness according to Belcher and colleagues'[69] model of the homeless process.
2. Assess the psychiatric–mental health needs of this family.
3. Develop a care plan with short- and long-term goals for facilitating healthy coping in this family.
4. Identify elements in the shelter setting that negatively affect a family's coping and independence.
5. Design a plan to advocate for homeless families with children in shelter facilities.

CASE STUDY

Rachel stalked into the room. Her eyes were reddened and her clothes in disarray. She wore a wrinkled and translucent nightgown. On her feet, she wore red woolen stockings, at her throat, a crucifix. Over her shoulders was a dark and heavy robe. Nothing I had learned in the past week prepared me for this apparition.

She cried. She wept. She paced left and right and back and forth, pivoting and turning suddenly to face me, glaring straight into my eyes. A sudden halt. She looked up toward the cracked and yellowish ceiling of the room. Her children—two girls, a frightened boy—stared at her, as I did, as her arms reached out—for what? Her hair was gray, a stiff and brushlike Afro.

Angelina was 12 years old, Stephen was 11, and Erica was 9. The youngest child, 11 months, was sitting on the floor. A neighbor's child, 6 years old, sat in my lap and leaned her head against my chest. Her name was Raisin. There were two rooms in the apartment. Rachel disappeared into the second room, and then returned and stood, uneasily, by the door.

Ever since August we been livin' here. The room is either very hot or feezin' cold. When it be hot outside it's hot in here. When it be cold outside we have no heat. We used to live with my aunt but then it got too crowded there so we moved out. We went to welfare and they sent us to the shelter. Then they shipped us to Manhattan. I'm scared of the elevators. Fraid they be stuck. I take the stairs.
ANGIE

Elevator might fall down and you would die.
RAISIN

It's unfair for them to be here in this room. They be yellin'. Lots of times I'm goin' to walk out. Walk out on the street and give it up. No, I don't do it. BCW come to take the children. So I make them stay inside. Once they walk outside that door they are in danger.
RACHEL

I wish someone in New York could help us. Put all of the money that we have together and we buy a building. Two or three rooms for every family with a kitchen. Way it is, you be frightened all the time. I think this world is coming to the end.
ANGIE

This city is rich.
STEPHEN

Surely is.
ANGIE

City and welfare, they got something goin'. Pay $3,000 every month to stay in these here room....
ERICA

I believe the City Hall got something goin' here. Gettin' a cut. They got to be. My children, they be treated like chess pieces. Send all of that money off to Africa? You hear that song? They're not thinking about people starvin' here in the U.S. I was thinkin': Get my kids and all the other children here to sing, "We are the world. We live here too." How come do you care so much for people you can't see? Ain't we the world? Ain't we a piece of it? We are so close they be afraid to see. Give us a shot at something. We are something! Ain't we something? I'm depressed. But we are something! People in America don't want to see.
RACHEL

I saw Mr. Water Bug under my mother's bed. Mr. Rat be livin' with us too.
RAISIN

It's so cold right now you got to use the hot plate. Plug it in so you be warm.... School is bad for me. I feel ashamed. They know we're not the same. My teacher do not treat us all the same. They know which children live in the hotel.
ANGIE

They didn't go to school last week. They didn't have clean clothes. Why? Because the welfare messed my check. It's supposed to come a week ago. It didn't come. I get my check today. I want my kids to go to school. They shouldn't miss a day. How they gonna go to school if they don't got some clothes? I couldn't wash. I didn't have the money to buy food.
RACHEL

Last week a drug addict tried to stab me. With an ice pick. Tried to stab my mother too. Older girls was botherin' us.
ANGIE

Those girls upstairs on the ninth floor, they be bad. They sellin' crack.
RAISIN

This girl I know lives in a room where they sell drugs. One day she asks us do we want a puff. So we said: "No. My mother doesn't let us do it." One day I was walkin' in the hall. This man asked me do I want some stuff. He said: "Do you want some?" I said no and I ran home.
ANGIE

God forgive me, but nobody should have to live like this. Since I came into this place, my kids begun to get away from me.
RACHEL

There's a crucifix on the wall. I ask her: "Do you pray?"

I don't pray! Pray for what? I been prayin' all my life and I'm still here. When I came to this hotel, I still believed in God. I said: "Maybe God can help us to survive." I lost my faith. My hopes. And everything. Ain't nobody—no God, no Jesus—gonna help us in no way. God forgive me. I'm emotional. I'm black. I'm in a blackness. Blackness is around me. In the night I'm scared to sleep. In the morning I'm worn out. I don't eat no breakfast. If I eat, I eat one meal a day. I have ulcers. I stay in this room. I hide. This room is safe to me. I'm afraid to go outside.
RACHEL

CRITICAL THINKING QUESTION

1. Assess the psychiatric–mental health needs of these homeless people.
2. Identify coping behaviors used by these individuals and judge their effectiveness.

3. Identify therapeutic approaches that could be used in building hope in Rachel.
4. Explore how social distress theory applies to this situation.
5. Develop a plan to advocate for women and children based on the social distress theory and nursing theories.

Source: Adapted from Kozel, J: *Rachel and Her Children: Homeless Families in America.* Fawcett Columbine, New York, 1988.

References

1. Seeger, CA: Reflections on working with the homeless. New Dir Ment Health Serv 46:47, 1990.
2. Jahiel, RI: Empirical studies of homeless populations in the 1970s and 1980s. In Jahiel, RI (ed): Homelessness: A Prevention-oriented Approach. The Johns Hopkins University Press, Baltimore, 1992, p 40.
3. Jackson, MP, and McSwane, DZ: Homelessness as a determinant of health. Public Health Nurs 9:185, 1992.
4. Jahiel, RI: The definition and significance of homelessness in the United States. In Jahiel, RI (ed): Homelessness: A Prevention-oriented Approach. The Johns Hopkins University Press, Baltimore, 1992, p 1.
5. Jahiel, RI: Preventive approaches to homelessness. In Jahiel, RI (ed): Homelessness: A Prevention-oriented Approach. The Johns Hopkins University Press, Baltimore, 1992, p 11.
6. Larew, B: Strange strangers: Serving transients. Social Casework 64:107, 1980.
7. Youssef, FA, Omokehinde, RN, and Garland, IM: The homeless and unhealthy: A review and analysis. Issues in Mental Health Nursing 9:317, 1988.
8. Bassuck, C: Addressing the needs of the homeless. Boston Globe Magazine, Nov. 6, 1983, p 12.
9. Levine, I: Homelessness: Its Implications for Mental Health Policy and Practice. Presented at Annual Meeting of the American Psychological Association, 1983.
10. Rossi, PH: The old homelessness and the new homelessness in historical perspective. Am Psychol 45:954, 1990.
11. Kiesler, C: Homelessness and public policy priorities. Am Psychol 46:1245, 1991.
12. Lamb, HR (ed): The Homeless Mentally Ill: A Task Force Report of the American Psychiatric Association. American Psychiatric Association, Washington, DC, 1984.
13. Bassuk, EL, Rubin, L, and Lauriat, A: Characteristics of sheltered homeless families. Am J Public Health 76:1097, 1986.
14. Breakey, WR, Fischer, PJ, Kraner, M, Nestadt, G, Romanoski, AJ, Royall, RM, and Stine, OC: Health and mental health problems of homeless men and women in Baltimore. JAMA 262:1352, 1989.
15. Chafetz, L: Perspectives for psychiatric nurses on homelessness. Issues in Mental Health Nursing 9:325, 1988.
16. Mechanic, D, and Aiken, LH: Improving the care of patients with chronic mental illness. N Engl J Med Dec. 24, 1987, p 1634.
17. Bachrach, LL: A conceptual approach to deinstitutionalization. Hospital and Community Psychiatry 29:126, 1978.
18. Scheper-Hughes, N: Dilemmas in deinstitutionalization: A view from the inner-city. Journal of Operational Psychiatry 12:90, 1981.
19. Chafetz, L, Goldman, HH, and Taube, CA: Deinstitutionalization in the United States. International Journal of Mental Health 11:48, 1983.
20. Reich, R, and Siegel, L: The emergence of the Bowery as a psychiatric dumping ground. Psychiatr Q 50:3, 1978.
21. Bassuk, EL, and Gerson, S: Deinstitutionalization and mental health services. Sci Am 238:46, 1978.
22. Blasi, GL: Social policy and social science research on homelessness. Journal of Social Issues 46:207, 1990.
23. McChesney, KY: Family homelessness: A systematic problem. Journal of Social Issues 46:191, 1990.
24. Mapes, LV: Faulty food and shelter programs draw charge that nobody's home to homelessness. National Journal 9:474, 1985.
25. Institute of Medicine: Homelessness, Health and Human Needs. National Academy Press, Washington, DC, 1988.
26. Carling, PJ: Major mental illness, housing and supports: The promise of community integration. Am Psychol 45:969, 1990.
27. Rossi, P: Down and Out in America. University of Chicago Press, Chicago, 1989.
28. Kiesler, CA: Homelessness and public policy priorities. Am Psychol 46:1245, 1991.
29. Hunter, JK: Nursing and health care for the homeless. State University of New York Press. Albany, NY, 1993.
30. Sosin, MR, and Grossman, S: The etiology of homelessness: A comparison study. Journal of Community Psychology 19:337, 1991.
31. Hopper, K: The ordeal of shelter. Notre Dame Journal of Law and Ethics 4:301, 1989.
32. Barancik: Poverty rate and household income stalemate as rich-poor gap hits post-war high. Center on Budget and Policy Priorities, Washington, DC, 1989.
33. Foscarinis, M: The politics of homelessness: A call to action. Am Psychol 46:1232, 1991.
34. Pear, R: President signs 1 billion dollars in homeless aid. New York Times, 1987, p 1.
35. Hopper, K, and Hamberg, J: The making of America's homeless: From skid row to new poor. In Bratt, RG, Hartman, C, and Meyerson, A (eds): Critical Perspectives on Housing, Temple University Press, Philadelphia, 1986, p 14.
36. Kondratas, A: Ending homeless: Policy challenges. Am Psychol 46:1226, 1991.
37. Vissing, YM: Out of Sight, Out of Mind: Homeless Children and Families in Small-Town America. The University Press of Kentucky, Lexington, 1996.
38. Strasser, JA, Damrosch, S, and Gaines, J: Nutrition and the homeless person. J Community Health Nurs 8:65, 1991.
39. Saltzman, AL, and Curtis, F: Social distress theory and teaching about homelessness: A retrospective analysis. Journal of Social Distress and the Homeless 3:99, 1994.
40. Bassuk, EL: The homelessness problem. Sci Am 251:40, 1984.
41. Bassuk, EL, Rubin, L, and Lauriat, A: Characteristics of sheltered homeless families. Am J Public Health 76:1097, 1986.
42. Bassuk, EL: Who are the homeless families? Characteristics of sheltered mothers and children. Community Ment Health J 26:425, 1990.
43. Dummer, MJ: Care of homeless clients. In Dummer, MJ (ed): Nursing in the Community. Appleton & Lange, Stamford, CT, 1996, p 255.
44. Hodnicki, DR, Horner, SD, and Boyle, S: Women's perspectives on homelessness. Public Health Nurs 9:257, 1992.
45. Bogue, DJ: Skid Row in American Cities. Community and Family Study Center, University of Chicago Press, Chicago, 1963.
46. Bachrach, L: Young adult chronic patients as a concept: Research limitations. Hospital and Community Psychiatry 35:573, 1984.
47. Sebastian, JG: Homelessness: A state of vulnerability. Family and Community Health 8:11, 1985.
48. Slavinsky, AT, and Cousins, A: Homeless women. Nurs Outlook 30:358, 1982.
49. Kozol, J: Rachel and Her Children: Homeless Families in America. Fawcett Columbine, New York, 1988.
50. Zorza, J: Woman battering: A major cause of homelessness. Clearinghouse Review (Special Issue), Aug, 1991.
51. Molnar, J, Rath, W, and Klein, T: Constantly compromised: The impact of homelessness on children. Journal of Social Issues 46:109, 1990.
52. Hirsch, K: Childhood without a home: A new report on the youngest victims. The Boston Phoenix, Jan 21, 1986.
53. Rafferty, M: Standing up for America's homeless. AJN 1614, Dec 1989.
54. Wright, J: The Crisis in Homelessness: Effects on Children and Families. U.S. Government Printing Office, Washington, DC, 1987.
55. Acker, PJ, Freeman, AH, and Dreyer, BP: An assessment of parameters of health care and nutrition in homeless children. American Journal of Disease in Children 141:388, 1987.

56. Gallagher, E: No Place Like Home: A Report on the Tragedy of Homeless Children and Their Families in Massachusetts. Massachusetts Committee for Children and Youth, Boston, 1986.
57. Ihéjirika, M: Young and homeless: A new study in despair. Chicago Sun-Times, June 22, 1993, p 12.
58. Antai-Ontong, D, and Kongable, G (eds): Psychiatric Nursing: Biological and Behavioral Concepts. WB Saunders Company, Philadelphia, 1995.
59. Fischer, PJ, Shapiro, S, Breakey, WR, Anthony, JC, and Kramer, M: Mental health and social characteristics of the homeless: A survey of mission users. Am J Public Health 76:519, 1986.
60. McCarty, D, Angeriou, M, Huebner, RB, and Lubran, B: Alcoholism, drug abuse, and the homeless. Am Psychol 11:1139, 1991.
61. Miller, P, and Herzog, AC: Chronic mental illness and the mentally ill who are homeless. In Varcarolis, EM (ed): Foundations of Psychiatric–Mental Health Nursing, WB Saunders Company, Philadelphia, 1994, p 858.
62. Kutza, EA, and Company Keigher, SM: The elderly "new homeless": An emerging population at risk. Soc Work 36:288, 1991.
63. Damosch, S, and Strasser, JA: The homeless elderly in America. Gerontological Nursing 14:26, 1988.
64. Lenehan, GP, McGinnis, D, O'Connell, D, and Hennessey, M: A nurse's clinic for the homeless. AJN 85:1237, 1985.
65. Wagner, JD, and Menke, EM: Case management of homeless families. Clinical Nurse Specialist 6:65, 1992.
66. Advisory Council for the Elimination of Tuberculosis: Prevention and control of tuberculosis among homeless persons. MMWR 41:13, 1992.
67. Federal Task Force on Homelessness and Severe Mental Illness, National Institutes of Mental Health: Outcasts on Main Street. Interagency Council on the Homeless, Washington, DC, 1992.
68. Kozinski, J: Chance beings. In Giamo, B, and Grunberg (eds): Frames of Reference: Beyond Homelessness. University of Iowa Press, Iowa City, 1992, p 31.
69. Belcher, J, Scholler-Jacquish, A, and Drummond, M: Three stages of homelessness: A conceptual model for social workers in health care. Health Soc Work 16:87, 1991.
70. O'Flaherty, BO: Making Room: The Economics of Homelessness. Harvard University Press, Cambridge, MA, 1996.
71. Forchuk, C: Hildegard E. Peplau: Interpersonal Nursing Theory. Sage Publications Inc, Newbury Park, CA, 1993.
72. Bunting, S: Rosemary Parse: Theory of Human Becoming. Sage Publications Inc, Newbury Park, CA, 1993.
73. Parse, RR: Man-living-health: A theory of nursing. In Riehl-Sisca (ed): Conceptual Models for Nursing Practice. Appleton & Lange, Norwalk, CT, 1989.
74. Golden, S: Single women: The forgotten homeless. City Limits, Jan 12, 1988.
75. Moloney, MM: The meanings of home in the stories of older women. West J Nurs Res 19:166, 1997.
76. Helvie, CO: Students implement community project for the homeless. J Nurs Educ 35:377, 1996.
77. Macness, CL, and Hemphill, JC: Screening clinics for the homeless: Evaluating outcomes. J Community Health Nurs 13:167, 1996.
78. Testani-Dufour, LT, Green, L, and Carter, KF: Establishing outreach health services for homeless persons: An emerging role for nurse mangers. J Community Health Nurs 13:221, 1996.
79. Sibbald, BJ: An oasis of health for poor or homeless people who are HIV-positive. The Canadian Nurse 16, 1996.
80. Caplan, G: Principles of Preventive Psychiatry. Basic Books, New York, 1964.

CHAPTER 31
Victims of Abuse

CHAPTER 31

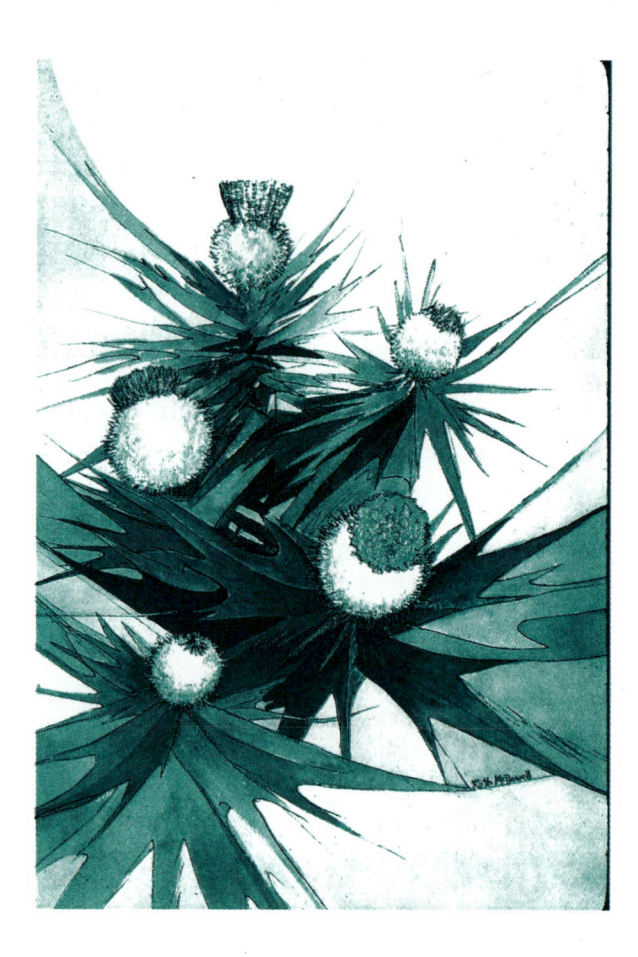

CHAPTER OUTLINE

Prevalence
Types of Abuse
   Physical Abuse
   Sexual Abuse
   Psychological Abuse
   Economic Abuse
Disclosure and Substantiation of Abuse
Components of Abuse
   Perpetrator
   Violence in the Home
   Violence in the Environment
   Survivor
Trauma Responses
Assessment of Abuse
   Indicators
   Abuse-related Symptoms
Key Principles of Treatment
   Maintain Safety
   Empower the Individual
   Report by Mandated Laws
   Minimize Intrusiveness
   Keep No Secrets
   Identify Symptom Clusters
   Know Your Level of Expertise
   Do Not Pathologize
   Do Not Reinforce Perceptions of Shame or Vulnerability
   Be Aware of Possible Cognitive Distortions
Treatment of Abuse Victims
   Individual Psychotherapy
   Group Psychotherapy
   Family, Couples, and Sex Therapy
   Pharmacologic Treatment
   Potential Countertransference

Gail Wangerin, RN, CS, PhD
Carol A. Glod, RN, CS, PhD
Nicole Phillips, RN, BSN

Victims of Abuse

LEARNING OBJECTIVES

After completing this chapter, the reader should be able to:
- List different types of abuse and trauma response.
- Identify warning signs and physical manifestations of abuse.
- Identify situations requiring mandated reporting of abuse.
- Perform an abuse assessment.
- Analyze the key aspects of treatment for the abuse survivor.
- Describe the stages and process of recovery from abuse.
- Describe available treatments and how and where to refer clients.

KEY TERMS

abuse
disclosure
economic abuse
false memories
perpetrator
physical abuse
psychological abuse
sexual abuse
sexual assault
substantiation
survivor
trauma response
violence

Abuse occurs in many settings and across all socioeconomic levels. Abuse risk factors include family dynamics characterized by **violence**. Because research indicates that violence in families may be the product of multigenerational patterns of abuse and neglect,[1,2] abusive family "scripts" and parenting styles that are often difficult to break may be created and perpetuated through succeeding generations. Other factors contributing to risk of abuse include incapacitation of caretakers, substance abuse, and socioeconomic stressors.

Because of their diverse roles and practice arenas, nurses often play a key role in identifying and treating victims of abuse. Nurses have a legal and ethical obligation to recognize and intervene when client safety is compromised because of abuse or risk of abuse. To practice effectively, nurses need to be aware of abuse and subsequent trauma.

Abuse is a traumatic experience. People who have been abused exhibit a wide variety of responses, including dissociative disorders, posttraumatic stress disorder (PTSD), mood disorders, anxiety disorders, substance abuse, and physical responses such as somatization.[3-5] In some cases, victims of abuse display violent or self-injurious behaviors such as risk taking and chaotic lifestyles.[6]

PREVALENCE

Studies on the prevalence of abuse in the general population have produced widely varying results, in part because of the many definitions of abuse, underreporting, and the privacy surrounding family life. According to the U.S. Senate Judicial

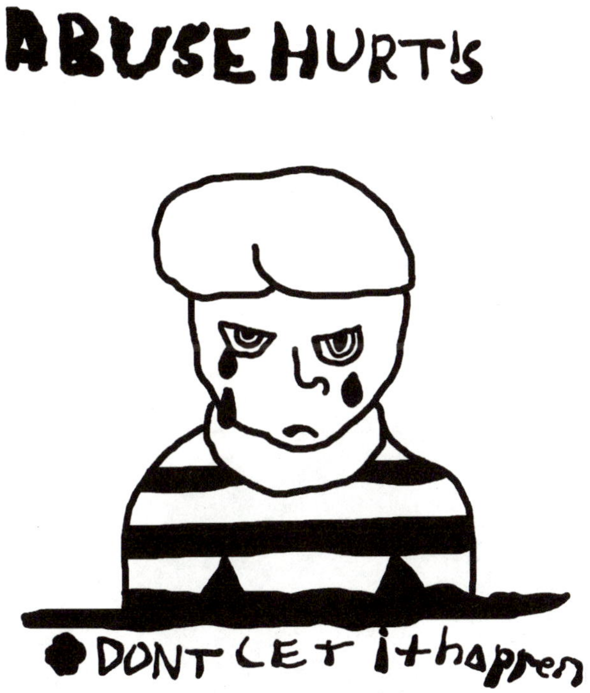

Figure 31–1. Abused children's drawings often depict the effects of trauma. In this drawing, Anthony, from the New School for Child Development, Special Education Division, uses artwork to show his feelings about abuse. Source: US Department of Health and Human Services: A nation's shame: Fatal child abuse and neglect in the United States. A Report of the US Advisory Board on Child Abuse and Neglect, Fifth Report, 1995.

Committee, in 1991 at least 1.1 million assaults, aggravated assaults, murders, and rapes against women were committed in the home and reported to the police. Unreported crimes against women may be more than three times this total.[7] The U.S. House of Representatives issued a report in 1990 that found that 1 of every 20 older Americans, or more than 1.5 million people, may be victims of elder abuse.[7] About 3 million cases of child abuse and neglect were reported in the United States in 1994. Numbers of abused children have maintained steady growth. From 1986 to 1993, physical abuse nearly doubled, sexual abuse more than doubled, and emotional abuse, physical neglect, and emotional neglect increased more than two and one-half times.[8] More than three children die every day from child abuse and neglect. Yet, it is estimated that more than half of child-abuse fatalities are unknown to child protective services. Girls are sexually abused three times more often than boys. Children are consistently vulnerable to sexual abuse from age 3 on. Boys have a greater risk of emotional neglect and serious injury than do girls.[9]

Studies indicate that abuse may be a significant factor affecting mental health. Up to 50% of all clients presenting for outpatient mental health services report a history of abuse.[10] Clients requiring hospitalization report higher rates of traumatic experience.

TYPES OF ABUSE

Abuse is generally categorized as physical, sexual, or psychological. Some groups dedicated to assisting battered women also include economic abuse as a category. The common factor is domination of one individual by another. Figure 31–2 shows the 1995 breakdown of abused children by type of abuse and neglect for 1995. Figure 31–3 depicts victims of abuse by type of abuse and age of victim.

PHYSICAL ABUSE

Physical abuse is defined as subjecting another to untoward physical force. Examples include a young woman describing childhood abuse at the hands of her father. "He would hit us . . . punch us . . . think of things to do to us like put pea beans on the floor and make us kneel on them." Another now-adult client related her experience with her mother: "We were told to stand still . . . if we moved, we got a beating." The battering of adults is also physical abuse and can occur in many settings or circumstances, such as physical abuse within a conflicted marriage and abuse of disabled or dependent adults by caretakers.

SEXUAL ABUSE

Sexual abuse occurs when one person subjects another to inappropriate or unwanted sexual behaviors. Gold[4] defines it as sexual contact between a child age 12 or younger and a person at least 5 years older than the child; sexual contact between an adolescent, ages 13 to 16, and an adult at least 10 years older; and sexual contact between any person under the age of 16 and a person or persons who use physical force. It includes fondling or touching of breasts or genitalia, penetration, or placement of objects in the vagina or rectum.

In practice, many clinicians also include exposure of a child to untoward or age-inappropriate sexual experiences

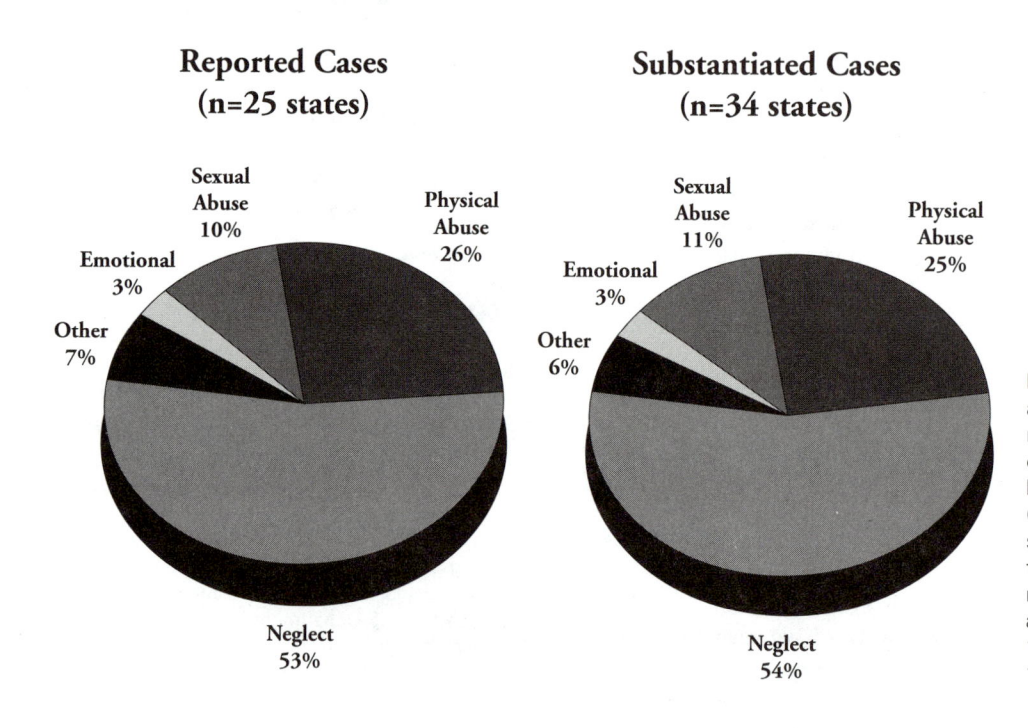

Reported Cases (n=25 states)
- Sexual Abuse 10%
- Physical Abuse 26%
- Emotional 3%
- Other 7%
- Neglect 53%

Substantiated Cases (n=34 states)
- Sexual Abuse 11%
- Physical Abuse 25%
- Emotional 3%
- Other 6%
- Neglect 54%

Figure 31–2. Percentage of child abuse and neglect cases that are reported (left) and the percentage of claims of abuse substantiated by protective service agencies (right). Information is from 25 states. Source: National Committee to Prevent Child Abuse: Current trends in child abuse reporting and fatalities: The results of the 1995 annual fifty state survey, 1996.

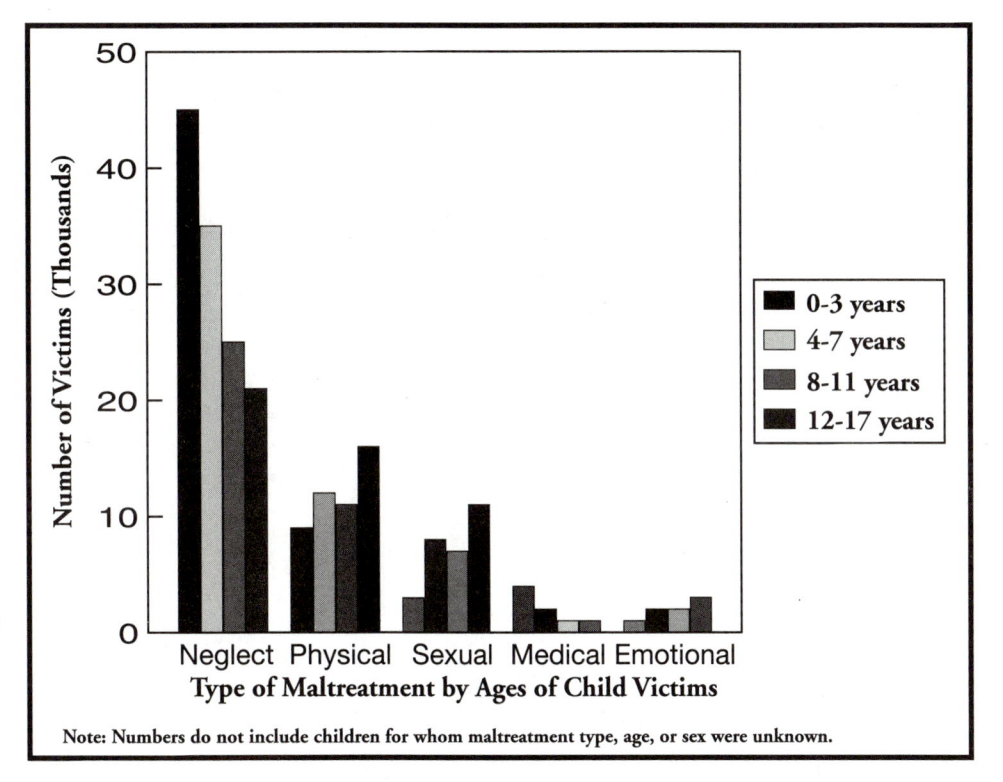

Figure 31–3. Numbers of children affected, by type of maltreatment and age of abuse. Infants are more likely to suffer neglect; teenagers are more likely to be physically or sexually abused. Source: US Department of Health and Human Services, National Center on Child Abuse and Neglect: Child abuse and neglect case-level data 1993: Working paper 1. US Government Printing Office, Washington, DC, 1996.

such as being forced to witness sexual activity or being deliberately exposed to pornographic materials. Rape is clearly a violent and **sexual assault**. Sexual harassment may fall within the realm of sexually abusive acts.

PSYCHOLOGICAL ABUSE

Psychological abuse is more difficult to define and to substantiate. Generally, psychological abuse consists of repeated negative feedback and lack of positive reinforcement: "My father always told me I was a fat pig—a reject," or "I was called stupid and told I would never amount to anything." Adults may be subjected to psychological abuse within conflicted marriages, at the workplace, by caretakers, or by authority figures. *Emotional neglect* includes actions such as chronic or extreme spousal abuse in the child's presence, permitting drug or alcohol use by the child, and refusal or failure to provide needed psychological care.[1] For children, neglect can be a form of psychological abuse.

ECONOMIC ABUSE

Economic abuse pertains, in particular, to people in abusive marriages or relationships. The term specifically refers to the control or withholding of financial resources from the abused partner, who is usually female, by the dominant partner, who is usually male. The underlying dynamic is to limit independence and autonomy and to force the abused partner to remain dependent and submissive, thus precluding escape from the abusive situation. Elders may also be subject to exploitation in which they lose control of their financial resources.

DISCLOSURE AND SUBSTANTIATION OF ABUSE

Disclosure and substantiation refer to the processes of identifying abuse. **Disclosure** means that the abuse victim discloses the fact that abuse has occurred. **Substantiation** means that allegations of abuse have been investigated and evidence suggests that abuse has occurred. Allegations of abuse are unsubstantiated when there is insufficient evidence of actual abuse.

COMPONENTS OF ABUSE

PERPETRATOR

Perpetrator refers to the individual responsible for inflicting abuse on another, specifically sexual abuse.

VIOLENCE IN THE HOME

Violence in the home and in the community has a traumatic effect, particularly on vulnerable individuals such as children or elders. Domestic violence may be either direct or indirect. *Direct victimization* occurs when an individual is subjected

> **RESEARCH NOTE**
>
> **Belluck, P: Woman's killer likely to be her partner, a study finds. New York Times, March 31, 1997, p**
>
> **Findings:** The authors of this study reviewed the files of women murdered in New York City between 1990 and 1994. Of 484 women, nearly half were killed by an "intimate partner," usually a current or former husband or boyfriend. Half of the women were murdered in their own homes, sometimes along with their children or as their children watched. The majority of victims were poor, African American, and between the ages of 21 and 40. Unlike murdered men, they often died as the result of beatings, burnings, and being thrown out of windows.
>
> **Application to Practice:** Domestic violence is a major health-care problem. Nurses can be involved at various levels of care. Primary prevention efforts can be aimed at identifying women and families at risk for violence and murder. Nurses can also get involved in political and community efforts to reduce family violence. Secondary prevention includes early intervention for those at risk. Nurses should evaluate women who present to all health-care settings for possible domestic violence. Battered women are at high risk for being murdered in their own homes by their partners. Attempts to separate from the abuser may put the woman at even higher risk for murder. Similarly, nurses should assess the family status of men with rage or suicide ideation; their violent and self-destructive thoughts may put their partners and children at risk for violence. Tertiary prevention may include efforts to keep women's safety a priority to protect them from potentially murderous partners.

to abuse. *Indirect victimization* occurs when family members witness the abuse of others, such as when children witness parental physical abuse.

Violence in the home has been a long-standing problem. It is not limited by race, age, class, or culture. Often the victim's shame and fear protects the perpetrator. Among the misconceptions and myths that have perpetuated abusive situations are[7]:

- Women battering is only a problem with lower socioeconomic classes.
- Women battering is not a significant problem because most incidents are slaps or punches, not serious injuries.
- Elder abuse is not much of a problem.
- Domestic violence is a private matter; outsiders should not intervene.
- No treatment can change a batterer.
- Only a small percentage of battered women experience symptoms of PTSD.

These views are slowly being dispelled. Consistent reporting, referral, and appropriate counseling will continue to wear away once-accepted societal myths. Some general characteristics of the victim of domestic violence include:

- A passive personality
- Social isolation
- Internalizing blame for the abuse
- Viewing the violence as a survival mechanism
- Demonstrating loyalty to the relationship.[7]

Characteristics of the abuser include:

- Behavior learned in family of origin
- Blaming the victim
- Displacing anger meant for authority figures
- Viewing the victim as a possession
- Unrealistic expectations of the victim
- Forgetting details of the abusive act and using alcohol or drugs.[7]

VIOLENCE IN THE ENVIRONMENT

Environmental violence occurs when an individual is subjected to living in a neighborhood where illegal activities such as drug trafficking, gang fighting, and school violence are endemic. For some, exposure to violence is chronic. Others may be adversely affected by a specific act of random violence. These experiences create a stressful atmosphere that may result in a child's abnormal adjustment, a perception of the world as a threatening and unsafe place, and perpetuation of patterns of abuse and violence.

SURVIVOR

Survivor is a term frequently used to refer to an individual who has been subjected to abuse. The connotation is that victimization can be overcome and transcended. Although the term *victim* suggests vulnerability and impairment, *survivorship* indicates strength and the ability to overcome.

TRAUMA RESPONSES

The core elements of PTSD are described in Chapter 22. The traumatic experience of different forms of abuse may have both immediate and long-lasting effects on an individual's functioning.[6] **Trauma response** symptoms such as hyperarousal, hypervigilance, and a permanently aroused anxiety state may be evident both immediately and years after the event. An individual's sense of self, sense of others, and perceptions of the world may be affected (Box 31–1). Belief systems may be permanently altered in terms of self-esteem, sense of personal security, and ability to trust or relate effectively with others. For some, *emotional constriction* and *numbing* become a survival strategy that affects general functioning and greatly diminishes the overall quality of life.[11] For others, intrusive symptoms produce the same effects.

Box 31–1. Characteristics of Victims

Type of Victim	Characteristics
Child All ages, with greatest risk under age 5 (including infants) and for fatalities under 2 years of age	• Incest generally begins after age 9 years • Self-blame for family conflict • Low self-esteem • Fear of parent or caretaker • Cheating, lying, low achievement in school • Signs of depression, helplessness • One child sometimes singled out in family and labeled as "difficult," product of unwanted pregnancy, reminds the parents of someone they dislike or even themselves, prematurity (inhibited parent-child bonding)
Spouse	• Low self-esteem • Self-blame for batterer's actions • Sense of helplessness to escape abuse • Isolation from family and friends • Views self as subservient to partner • Economic dependence on abuser
Elder	• Over 75 years old • Mentally or physically impaired • Isolated from others

Source: With permission from Gorman, LM, Sultan, DF, and Raines, ML: Davis's Manual of Psychosocial Nursing. FA Davis Co., Philadelphia, 1996.

In addition, because the trauma response sometimes includes somatization, survivors may present at medical facilities for an array of physical complaints. These often-unidentified abuse victims frequently become patients in a broad range of practice settings.

A graphic illustration of the impact of childhood physical, sexual, and psychological abuse is offered by a now-adult female patient.

> Scary . . . very scary. Being abused . . . sexually abused, mentally, physically, takes a toll on somebody's life. (It's being) afraid to go to bed at night because your father's going to come into your room, afraid to get up in the morning because your mother's going to beat you for something you didn't do. I didn't think I was a bad kid. I was just generally afraid to move in the house, period. Anything I did was wrong. I either got pulled by the hair or slapped in the back of the head or grounded for months. Everything I did was wrong. I got thrown out of my house at seven o'clock in the morning after my father went to work and I wasn't allowed to come back home until after he came home at five. I'd have supper and it would start all over again. Be afraid to go to bed, be afraid to take a bath. Basically, it was enough to scare any little kid.

During childhood, this survivor of physical, sexual, and psychological abuse was not offered assistance by her teachers, who ignored her distress; her priest, who did not believe her disclosure; or her school nurse, who later noted, "I thought something was wrong" but did not act on her suspicions. In short, despite her overt indications of distress, this abuse victim was not helped.

ASSESSMENT OF ABUSE

INDICATORS

Individual responses to the trauma of abuse run the gamut from minimal impact to major dysfunction. Among the multiple variables that mediate the response are the nature and duration of the abuse, the age at which the abuse occurred, gender, the perpetrators of the abuse, pretrauma functioning, the context within which the abuse occurred, and the available support system.[5]

There are key indicators that suggest the possibility that abuse has occurred[12] (Table 31–1). Especially when identi-

TABLE 31–1. Warning Signs of Abuse in Children and Adolescents

General Symptoms
- Aggression and oppositional behaviors
- Anxiety
- Clinging behavior
- Decreased attention span
- Hyperactivity
- Nightmares
- Onset of enuresis or encopresis
- Onset of school problems
- Preoccupation
- Psychosomatic complaints
- Regressed behaviors
- Running away
- Sadness, depression
- Sleep disturbance
- Social withdrawal

Symptoms Specific to Sexual Abuse
- Age-inappropriate sexual behaviors
- Escalation of negative behaviors shortly after the abuse or traumatic event
- Excessive masturbation
- Risk-taking behaviors
- Sexual acting out
- Substance abuse

TABLE 31–2. Physical Indications of Abuse

Physical Abuse
- Bruises and welts on face, lips, mouth, torso, back, buttocks, thighs
- Unusual patterns that reflect the shape of the instrument, e.g., belt, wire hanger, hairbrush, hand
- Human bite marks
- Burns
- Cigarette burns
- Immersion burns indicating dunking in a hot liquid
- "Stocking" and "glove" burns on feet and hands
- Doughnut-shaped burns on buttocks and genitalia
- Rope or restraint burns
- Dry burns from iron, hair curler, heater, stove
- Lacerations and abrasions
- Tears in gum tissue due to force-feeding
- Absence of hair
- Hemorrhaging beneath scalp due to vigorous hair pulling
- Fractures
- Head injuries
- Subdural hematomas
- Retinal hemorrhages
- Jaw and nasal fractures
- Fractures caused by twisting or pulling
- Corner fractures of long bones
- Epiphyseal separation
- Periosteal elevation
- Spiral fractures

Sexual Abuse
- Redness, inflammation, bleeding, itching, or injury in genital-anal area
- Torn, stained, or bloody underclothing
- Hematuria, dysuria, or urinary frequency
- Yeast infections
- Vaginal or penile discharge
- Foreign objects in the vagina, urethra, or rectum
- Constipation
- Painful defecation
- Abdominal pain
- Bruising of or bleeding from external genitalia
- Difficulty walking or sitting
- Venereal disease
- Pregnancy

---

fied within a cluster of significant symptoms, they are the building blocks of nursing assessment and provide direction to subsequent treatment planning.

Many clients exhibit one or more symptoms of classic trauma response. *Intrusive trauma* symptomatology includes hyperreactivity, startle responses, explosive or aggressive outbursts, nightmares, flashbacks, reenactment of the trauma, and replication of risk-taking behaviors. These behaviors are often relatively obvious and draw attention to the need for treatment. *Numbing* or *constrictive responses* include emotional constriction, social isolation, anhedonia, and a sense of estrangement. These behaviors do not demand attention and are often missed. Children and adolescents may have varied responses to abusive experiences.

Physical symptoms do not always indicate abuse (Table 31–2). Careful assessment and consideration of all possible causes of these symptoms are essential.

> Laurie G, age 5 years, was referred to the school nurse by her kindergarten teacher after the teacher observed bruises on Laurie's arms. While in the nurse's office, Laurie complained that her back hurt; upon examination, a large red welt was noted. Upon questioning, Laurie became guarded and reticent, avoiding eye contact and stating only, "I've been a good girl."
>
> Her mother stated, "Laurie plays with some rough kids. This must have happened at afterschool daycare." A telephone call to the day-care provider failed to support this explanation; therefore, as a mandated reporter, the nurse filed a report of suspected abuse with the appropriate state child protective agency. The investigating social worker ascertained that Laurie was occasionally left in the care of an older sibling who became punitive if Laurie defied his limit-setting. His attempts to control her physically had led to the bruises and welts. The parents were made aware of the inadvisability of placing their son in charge of his younger siblings. The family was offered counseling around issues of child care and management.

Mandated reporting laws require that the circumstances of such injuries or symptoms be reported and documented to official protection agencies and that social services investigate them.

If the person discloses abuse or an abuse history, determine the impact of abuse on present functioning and the client's resultant clinical needs. Depending on the practice setting, assessment may focus on

- Determining need for mandated reporting and ensuring safety
- Determining need for ongoing, specialized treatment
- Determining patient's needs within the context of ongoing specialized treatment

ABUSE-RELATED SYMPTOMS

Adults demonstrate a broad range of abuse-related symptoms.[6,13] When the abusive experience occurs to adults, the client may exhibit proximate trauma responses. Childhood abuse may be manifested during adult years as a classic delayed PTSD response.[13]

Adults with a history of childhood abuse may demonstrate lifelong patterns of increased anxiety, heightened interpersonal sensitivity, increased anger, paranoid ideation, and sexual dysfunction. Relationship and parenting skills may be impaired. In some cases, memory of the precipitating traumatic event has been compromised, further complicating the clinical presentation. These clients frequently describe memory gaps encompassing years of childhood experience and usually including the precipitating events. It is not unusual for people to describe nightmares, flashbacks, intrusive thoughts, fragmentary memories, and labile emotions. Many individuals who have been traumatized by abuse demonstrate heightened anxiety responses such as hyperreactivity and hypervigilance. Others may present with a general emotional numbing that permeates their relationships and compromises the quality of their lives.

I tried to kill myself because of depression over life in general. I was fed up—sick and tired of being beaten and miserable and taken advantage of. I kept having recurring nightmares about the battering and death threats. Thoughts of the beatings kept popping into my mind almost every morning.... My body took the drugs. I couldn't OD [overdose]. I tried to hang myself in my backyard, but someone pulled into my driveway and rescued me. I found recently I have a lot to live for.[7]

In addition to PTSD symptoms, adults may present with relatively minor adjustment disorders, anxiety disorders, eating disorders, substance abuse, personality disorders, dissociative disorders, major depression, self-injurious behaviors, and ideas of suicide. Physical manifestations may include evidence of past or present physical injuries, anorexia or bulimia, weight fluctuations, dental problems, history of sexually transmitted diseases, and a multitude of physical illnesses.

Assessment directs treatment[12]; the nurse's initial step is to fully assess the situation. General components of assessment include being aware of key indicators, taking as thorough a physical examination as the practice setting allows, screening for past or present abuse and exposure to violence, paying careful attention to the client's mental status, and obtaining data regarding environmental factors. The process of assessment may vary with different practice settings.

Because many adult abuse survivors are not adequately diagnosed, they therefore do not receive optimal treatment. A typical example would be treating a substance-abusing client for substance abuse only, without addressing the underlying trauma issues. A more complex diagnostic problem arises when individuals demonstrate multiple somatic problems that are precipitated, in part, by an unidentified abuse history. Optimal treatment includes addressing both the physical and the psychosocial responses to the abuse.

Sally R, a 47-year-old woman, presented at a diagnostic facility for a colonoscopy to further assess possible irritable bowel syndrome, a common diagnosis in trauma victims. As the procedure progressed, she became increasingly agitated despite having been appropriately medicated to calm her for this somewhat stressful process. Ultimately, the examiner had to stop before completing the procedure.

After the procedure, the nurse asked Sally about the experience. She described herself as being terrified. Only in the context of a therapeutic setting was Sally able to reveal her history of childhood abuse, including anal penetration, and the terror it provoked during the procedure. Unaware of her early abuse history, her medical evaluators were confounded by her obvious fear. Her psychotherapist was uninvolved in her physical treatment. The nurse spoke to both clinicians to coordinate Sally's overall care to preclude another negative experience.

In the past, professionals hesitated to incorporate questions regarding abuse or abuse history into structured assessment interviews. However, these questions are important during a nursing assessment:

1. Are you now or have you ever been physically abused?
2. Are you now or have you ever been sexually abused?
3. Are you now or have you ever been psychologically abused?
4. Are you now or have you ever been exposed to danger or violence?
5. Are you presently safe?

Underscore the clients' personal empowerment and control by noting that they always have the option of not answering any question that is perceived as painful or intrusive. Some may need these terms defined. Some adults may not remember early abuse. Others may be unable to disclose abuse during the assessment phase of treatment. Children, in the presence of abusive parents, may be unable to respond openly to these inquiries. However, nurses can raise these issues, "put them on the table," and pursue them further at subsequent points in treatment, if indicated. Children can be asked such questions when alone; however, do not frighten or put them at further risk.

Do not suggest that clients have been abused based on symptomatic indicators alone. The interpretation of symptoms is best left within the context of ongoing psychotherapy with clinicians well versed in the treatment of abused clients.

False Memories

One phenomenon that has emerged recently is the awareness of false memories. **False memories** refer to confabulations of abuse, recovered memories that describe events that never happened. Controversy continues regarding the possibility of planting "false memories" through inappropriate clinical interventions. Although every allegation of abuse is not necessarily the truth, in order to battle abuse, an environment of openness and acceptance must exist. It is a difficult, but necessary, balance for professionals.

A woman in her mid-30s came to therapy and reported terrifying nightmares, an eating disorder, and difficulties in her interpersonal relationships, especially with men. She claimed to have no idea what caused her symptoms. But soon, with the therapist's help, she recovered some vague memories of sexual abuse occurring at a very early age. As her therapy progressed, the memories became much more graphic and detailed. She remembered that her parents had guests to their home, with whom they forced her to have sex. She

further recalled being tortured and burned with cigarettes when she cried out for help. Her therapist encouraged her to confront the parents with her newly recovered awareness. They respond with vehement and convincing denial.[14]

KEY PRINCIPLES OF TREATMENT

MAINTAIN SAFETY

Above all, consider the client's safety. If abuse is suspected, substantiated, or disclosed, ascertain whether the client is still at risk. If the abuse is occurring at present and the perpetrator has ongoing access to the victim, safety is compromised. In this situation, focus on ensuring safety. If the client is a child, reporting to the appropriate social service agency is usually mandated. The safety of dependent adults, such as elders or developmentally delayed persons, may also be compromised by abuse. Again, often reporting is mandated. Removal from the at-risk situation may be necessary. If the client is a battered spouse, referral to Women's Protective Services or to the appropriate law enforcement agencies may be indicated. In some practice settings, the nurse may take these actions unilaterally; in others, the nurse may function as part of a multidisciplinary team in securing safety.

Nurses can participate in prevention approaches to reduce abuse-related injuries and responses, such as working with local and state coalitions against domestic violence, child abuse, and elder abuse. Another way to minimize the effects of abuse is to ensure that the agency or hospital clearly defines abuse-reporting procedures.

EMPOWER THE INDIVIDUAL

When working with persons who have been subjected to abuse or violence, understand that a key element of the traumatic experience has been *disempowerment*. When individuals have been beaten, molested, or injured, their sense of control over self, over others, and over circumstances may be severely impaired. For some, the sense of disempowerment may be more stressful than the actual abuse. Focus on encouraging their empowerment through collaborative decision making and supporting their autonomy as fully as possible.

REPORT BY MANDATED LAWS

Child abuse is against the law. Each state has an agency that is mandated[15] to receive and to investigate reports of suspected abuse. Reporting is a means of getting help for an individual, a child, or a family. The investigator is responsible for the process of substantiation and proof of abuse. Mandated reporters include police, psychologists, social workers, counselors, teachers, nurses, doctors, and psychiatrists. Mandated reporters make the majority of reports to child protective services (CPS) (Fig. 31–4).

To report a suspected case of child abuse, notify the nearest agency in the state in which the victim resides. The agency will be listed in the telephone directory, usually in the Government Blue Pages under the state's rehabilitative services or children and family services. The local police department can help find the appropriate agencies. See Appendix 6 for resource list.

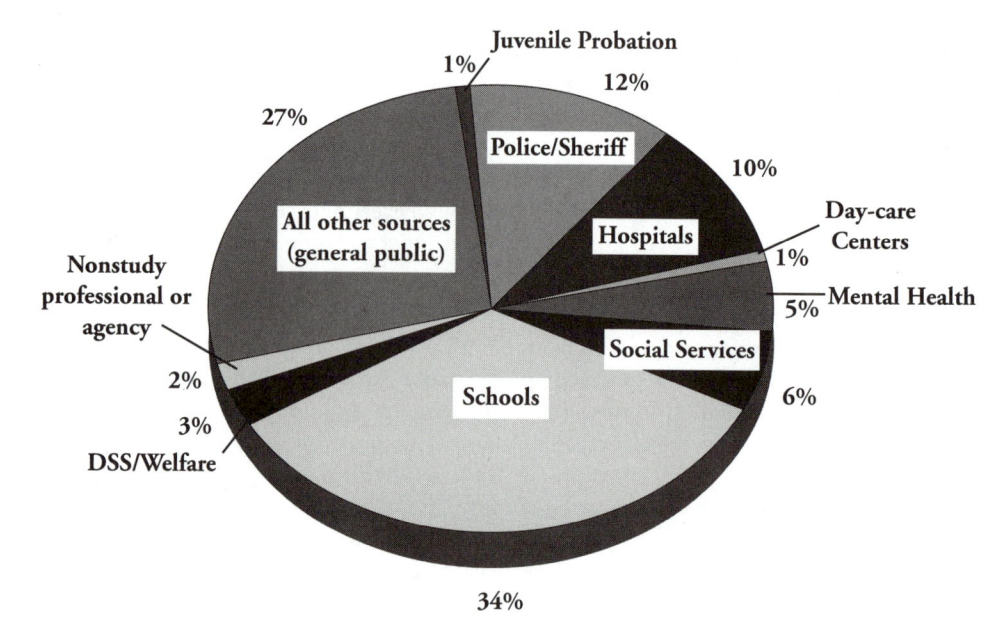

Figure 31–4. Breakdown of who is most likely to suspect and then report abuse. Reports come from both professionals and the general public. Schools are the most common reporters of suspected child abuse, followed by the general public, police, and hospitals. Source: US Department of Health and Human Services: The third national incidence study of child abuse and neglect, 1996.

MINIMIZE INTRUSIVENESS

For many abuse victims, particularly sexual abuse, a key element of the abuse experience has been a sense of *intrusion*. All too often, well-meaning professionals replicate this sense of intrusion by requiring the victim to provide descriptions of the details of abuse or emotional responses. If a physical examination is indicated, either to determine physical injury or to substantiate allegations, the client may see it as a further intrusion. Additionally, inpatients may be subjected to the invasion of privacy and boundaries that is inherent in the hospital setting.

Although it may be necessary to obtain specific information or perform specific procedures, interviews and procedures should be limited to essential information gathering. For some, it may be helpful to "process" or talk about the trauma experience; for others, it may be painful and experienced as a further boundary intrusion. Optimal nursing care is focused on recognizing and minimizing violations of the client's boundaries and privacy.

KEEP NO SECRETS

This caveat specifically applies to the treatment of children and dependent adults who are subject to continuing or present abuse. Abuse victims sometimes disclose and then entreat the professional "not to tell" or offer to share something "only if you won't tell anybody." Because in many cases victims have been threatened by their perpetrators with dire consequences if they disclose, they may be afraid of telling about their abuse.

The conflict between violation of trust and confidentiality and the need to ensure safety can be difficult to negotiate. However, do not keep the "secret"; it is inappropriate and sometimes illegal. Inform abuse victims in a supportive manner that it is necessary to share this information to protect them. Reassure them that all efforts will be made to ensure their safety and well-being. Tell the victims that their disclosure was the "right" or "brave" thing to do and that they should feel positive about taking this difficult step.

IDENTIFY SYMPTOM CLUSTERS

The nurse must realize that one sign or symptom alone is usually not sufficient to indicate a diagnosis of abuse or trauma response. Although incontrovertible physical evidence such as tissue damage following a forceful attack or the presence of a sexually transmitted disease in a young child at times makes the diagnosis clear, more often, assessment is more complex and should be focused on identifying a number of indicators or "symptom clusters."

Molly M, age 29, presented to an outpatient mental health clinic complaining of insomnia, agitation, and a feeling of impending doom. She also noted increasing difficulty managing her daily responsibilities. Upon examination, she described anxiety about the well-being of her 5-year-old daughter that had escalated several times into panic attacks. The initial diagnosis, dysthymia, was suggested by these symptoms. However, further examination revealed that the patient remembered little about her childhood, experienced nightmares in which she was chased and attacked by a faceless man, and had a history of bulimia. She also noted that she thought she may have fragmentary memories of having been molested by a neighbor when she was in kindergarten.

In general, err on the side of caution. Remember that it is possible to inflict damage on innocent families by jumping to conclusions and acting too quickly.

The mother of 4-year-old Tommy S requested treatment for his increasing oppositional behaviors.

> ### RESEARCH NOTE
> **Gary, F, Moorhead, J, and Warren, J: Characteristics of troubled youths in a shelter. Arch Psychiatr Nursing 10:41–48, 1996.**
>
> **Findings:** Adolescents who suffer severe abuse may be unable to disclose the abuse and choose to run away from home to avoid the trauma. In this study, the researchers investigated the characteristics of 78 runaway youths who presented to a shelter in Florida. Based on face-to-face interviews, they found that 67% had been abused, 37% had been sexually abused, and 28% suffered from a combination of sexual, physical, and emotional abuse. When asked about stressful life events, runaway teenagers acknowledged many more stressful experiences than other adolescents. About one-third of youths were living with their parents prior to running away; the remainder were in foster homes, detention centers, residential settings, or hospitals. Sixty-two percent reported alcohol use and 33% used illicit drugs.
>
> **Application to Practice:** Although a direct association between abuse and running away from home cannot be determined from this study, the results suggest that many runaway teenagers have suffered abuse and stressful life events. Adolescence, a time of turmoil and struggle for independence, may be particularly difficult for abuse survivors, who escape by living on the streets and in homeless shelters. Nurses need to devise effective strategies to identify abused children and intervene to stop the cycle of violence. Early intervention is key to prevent teenagers from subjecting themselves to life on the street. Once clients are in shelters, nurses should also target interventions to help them cope with stressful events and avoid unhealthy behaviors such as substance abuse. Because many of these teenagers have a history of abuse, psychiatric referral and treatment is necessary. Interventions may help runaways mitigate other consequences such as delinquency, PTSD, suicide, prostitution, and crime.

Tommy had recently begun to act out aggressively at home and at nursery school. His mother also noted that he had cried out in his sleep and appeared to be having nightmares. Upon further questioning, the mother described her son as having become quite preoccupied with bodily functions. She had observed him masturbating on several occasions. He also complained of pain on defecation. Given the cluster of symptoms, the initial evaluator requested a trauma evaluation for this child to ascertain whether he had been abused. The child was also referred to a pediatrician who was skilled in the treatment of children with possible abuse histories for a complete physical examination.

KNOW YOUR LEVEL OF EXPERTISE

Within the mental health field, effective psychotherapeutic intervention for abuse is considered a specialty area requiring further training. The primary role of most nurses, unless specifically trained in this specialty area, is to provide responsible assessment, triage, crisis intervention, supportive care, and referral to appropriate resources. Often, the client has complex needs that require treatment by a multidisciplinary team working collaboratively to address social, psychological, and physical needs.

DO NOT PATHOLOGIZE

Remember that many victims of abuse are essentially healthy people who have been subjected to traumatic experiences. While they may have symptoms in response to their abuse, these symptoms may be fairly common to those experiencing trauma response. To decrease clients' anxiety, reassure them that their symptoms are not unusual, given the circumstances.

DO NOT REINFORCE PERCEPTIONS OF SHAME OR VULNERABILITY

Although this admonition appears obvious, nurses may inadvertently project their own reactions onto interactions with the abused client. These sometimes unconscious reactions may unintentionally reinforce the client's perceptions of decreased self-worth or lack of personal safety. Reviewing reactions to specific traumas with a supervisor, colleague, or professional support group may help nurses' understanding.

> *It was winter, and for 4½ years of my marriage, the abuse escalated. About the time my son was born, 1½ years into the marriage, the abuse became physical. There were words, fists, threats, silence, and isolation. I lived in constant fear and was always anticipating and trying to avoid the next beating. By the time my daughter was born, it was a nightmare. When she would cry, he constantly threatened that I had better shut her up, and that she had better go to sleep. The baby cried and continued to cry. How could a baby sleep?*

> *I was desperate. I didn't think I wanted to end her life. I only wanted her to be quiet. I'm not sure how sane I was at that point. I have questioned that every year of my imprisonment. I've wondered what role his abuse and the postpartum issues played in my insanity. His threats got severe. Then they got worse and the beatings increased. My wrist was broken. He damaged my right eye. He cracked one of my ribs. Bruises, fear, terror.*

> *All I know was that somehow I focused on the baby. If only I could get her to quiet down. Every whimper from the baby would send me into a panic, trying to calm her to avoid his anger. But I was angry, terrible angry, and knew her crying was annoying him. I was terrified and angry. I gave her some formula, and I put something in it. I thought it would just help to quiet her down. But what I really did was poison her. When I discovered her quiet in the crib and having difficulty breathing, I took her to the hospital. She was very quiet, and I was very scared. I have relived the memories of putting that poison in her bottle over and over again, and the fact that I killed my innocent child.*

> *When I was sentenced to prison, my husband said to me, "You shut her up, and now no one will hear you because you are going to prison."*

BE AWARE OF POSSIBLE COGNITIVE DISTORTIONS

Be aware of the impact a traumatic experience has on thought processes and belief systems. Abusive experiences may have a profound impact on an individual's memories, sense of self, worldview, and perceptual and cognitive processes. Memories may be lost, communication skewed, meanings distorted, and interactions affected. Belief systems may be altered around issues such as personal control, the goodness of others, and the value of existence. Take these alterations of meaning and perception into account in the nursing assessment and the interpretation of behaviors.

TREATMENT OF ABUSE VICTIMS

Most nurses, at one time or another, no matter what their practice settings or clinical specialty areas, provide care to individuals who have been subjected to abuse. For example, children receive health care in pediatrician's offices, emergency rooms, hospitals, schools, and day care facilities as well as mental health facilities. Similarly, adults present for treatment in medical offices, emergency rooms, hospitals, employee assistance programs, substance-abuse treatment programs, and long-term care facilities. In any of these settings, abuse may be a presenting concern or identified later during the course of treatment. Skilled assessment and treatment planning that incorporates an awareness of trauma and abuse symptomatology and appropriate treatment options enhance nursing practice.[16]

> *I had plenty of opportunities to tell people, you know, teachers, doctors, nurses, and neighbors that I was being beaten. Some-*

how, I never thought they'd understand. It was kinda the way that they looked at me. I was ashamed; they never would have believed me. Those types of things didn't happen in our neighborhood. It was almost like I could read their eyes. But I met a nurse in the community clinic; I just felt she'd understand. And she did. I still felt terrible telling her, but I also felt relieved. She understood and just listened.

Although working with traumatized patients may be difficult and draining, it is not without reward. One client related the following:

*I'm not dead. . . . I survived. . . . I am alive and kicking. . . .
I have a life. . . . I have a say in what happens to me.
I have goals . . . and I like being alive.*

Herman[17] conceptualizes the process of trauma recovery in three stages:
- Establishing safety
- Reconstructing the trauma story
- Reconnecting with the world.

A therapeutic relationship focuses on assisting the survivor in the negotiation of these stages. The clinician should adhere to the key principles of ensuring safety and facilitating client empowerment and control through collaborative decision making, recognition and reinforcement of personal efficacy and healthy areas of functioning, and correction of cognitive distortions and altered meanings. The optimal treatment plan often encompasses multiple psychotherapeutic modalities.

INDIVIDUAL PSYCHOTHERAPY

Most clients who have been abused benefit from a course of individual therapy; however, establishing trust within a therapeutic relationship may be difficult. Careful matching of clients to clinicians is important for facilitating trust. For example, a female victim of a male perpetrator may prefer to work with a female clinician.

The primary focus of beginning therapy is stabilization and psychoeducation regarding abuse and trauma response. In adults, this may mean alleviating acute psychiatric symptoms like self-destructive and poor decision-making behaviors. The primary focus with children may be to decrease disruptive behaviors and address concentration problems.

For both children and adults, processing the abuse experience is often an integral part of recovery. This step occurs when the client is ready. For some, it may never be possible to describe, at length, the specifics of their experiences; for others, description, perhaps repeated description, of the abusive experience purges the "unspeakable" events. Individualized treatment recognizes varying needs and facilitates appropriate processing.

In addition to stabilization and processing, psychotherapy focuses on the impact and meaning of the experience on the victim. For many, the therapeutic context provides a safe place to explore the cognitive distortions and alterations in belief systems. Additionally, many adult patients enter treatment only after years of dealing alone with the impact of abuse and its often profound effects on their lives, relationships, and functioning. These issues become an integral part of therapy.

GROUP PSYCHOTHERAPY

For clients who cannot tolerate the intensity of an individual therapeutic relationship, group therapy is an alternative. Group therapy helps to alleviate clients' profound sense of isolation. Some with low self-esteem feel that they do not deserve communication and socialization with others. A positive group experience can facilitate both the processing of abuse and reconnection with the world through building new relationships.[17]

FAMILY, COUPLES, AND SEX THERAPY

Family therapists educate the victim and family members about the pervasive effects of an abuse experience; this process helps manage and alleviate the intensity of trauma response. If the person is still living with the abusive family, the appropriate level of therapeutic intervention may be the family itself. Family therapy is often combined with individual or group therapy; family patterns of interaction also require change.

Survivors may find that their early experiences have an adverse effect on current relationships. For example, sexual dysfunction is a common sequela of early sexual abuse that may need to be addressed both individually and in the context of couples or sex therapy. In addition, the spouse or partner of an abuse survivor may need therapeutic support and psychoeducation about the reactions to abuse.

Parenting skills may also be compromised by an abuse experience. Adults who were inadequately parented may have difficulty parenting their own children. Some may perpetuate the abuse by replicating the abusive parenting they received. Others experience pervasive anxiety as their children approach the age during which they themselves were abused. Many abuse survivors express a strong desire to "change the family script" and provide their own children with a healthy childhood and family experience; however, because of early trauma, they may be unable to accomplish this goal.

Clients abused as adults may become incapacitated, which results in anxiety, resentment, and confusion among other family members. Incorporating family therapy in the overall treatment plan may address these issues.

PHARMACOLOGIC TREATMENT

Pharmacologic treatment for abuse survivors may augment psychotherapy. Pharmacotherapy is considered when PTSD or other psychiatric conditions are diagnosed. At present, no specific drugs are recommended in the treatment of abuse and trauma response.

Generally, pharmacologic treatment addresses specific symptoms. For example, mood alterations in abuse survivors are treated with antidepressants such as the tricyclic antidepressants (TCAs), monoamine oxidase inhibitors (MAOIs), and selective serotonin reuptake inhibitors (SSRIs). Mood stabilizers such as lithium carbonate, carbamazepine (Tegretol), or divalproex (Depakote) may reduce arousal and hyperreactivity.

Clonidine may alleviate chronically heightened anxiety. Disturbed sleep patterns may respond to hypnotics or sedating antidepressants. Benzodiazepines may also offer relief from sympathetic hyperarousal and anxiety. Given the high degree of substance abuse and dependence in abused clients, however, benzodiazepines are usually avoided.

If pharmacotherapy is considered, both the primary clinician and the psychopharmacologist should help empower the client through collaborative decision making. Conceptualizing medication as a tool to be used during trauma recovery may be helpful.[17]

POTENTIAL COUNTERTRANSFERENCE

Mental health professionals have come to acknowledge the difficult countertransference reactions that arise when working with victims of abuse. Clinicians and nurses who work with abuse victims are subject to stress-related burnout, isolation, frustration, and their own feelings of trauma.[18] They may also feel fatigued and overwhelmed.[19] Affective responses such as rage, fear, grief, shame, and survivor guilt are not uncommon.[20] The nurse's own worldview and belief system may be altered; his or her self-image as an effective and compassionate clinician may be challenged.

To maintain well-being and professional effectiveness, try to understand and manage these powerful reactions. Use supervision, peer-support groups, and education to understand and process reactions. In addition, ensure adequate self-care, physical well-being, and involvement in socialization and other nonclinical activities that support a balanced, healthy worldview.

CASE STUDY

Judy S is a 15-year-old who lives with her adoptive mother. Judy's birth parents lost custody of her when she was 7 years old, after years of substantiated abuse. While pregnant with Judy, her birth mother abused alcohol and possibly cocaine; she physically neglected her health and prenatal examinations and contracted gonorrhea. Judy's birth father abandoned the family shortly after her birth, and her mother began living with James, a man who regularly abused drugs. From about age 2 to 3, Judy was sexually abused by James in several different ways. In addition to fondling her genitals, James inserted objects into her rectum. On one occasion, Judy began to bleed profusely from the rectum, and her birth mother took her to an emergency room for evaluation. After an in-depth examination, the nurses and physician suspected abuse and later confirmed the abuse through a detailed physical and psychological evaluation.

After the state Department of Social Services substantiated the sexual abuse, Judy was removed from the home. She was below normal height and weight standards for 3-year-old children. She was placed in several foster homes until she was 7. Little is known about the specifics of those placements. However, Judy does remember "strict" rules at one home; if she accidentally spilled something, she would have to go to her room for hours. She also remembers wetting the bed each night. Her punishment was to sleep on the back porch, sometimes with little heat, for several nights.

When she entered kindergarten, Judy displayed several problem behaviors. She tried to touch the genitals of other children. Once the teacher found her playing with dolls who appeared to be engaged in a sexual act. Sometimes Judy appeared withdrawn. Her report cards noted that she was "in her own world." At other times she was hyperactive; she was unable to stay seated, interrupted the teacher frequently, and squirmed around in her chair. The teacher discussed these behaviors with the school nurse. Together they referred Judy for further evaluation of abuse and treatment of these behavioral problems.

Judy began to develop a relationship with a psychiatric–clinical nurse specialist (CNS) with expertise in problems of childhood. Judy was initially withdrawn and difficult to engage. She did enjoy playing games and slowly began to trust the CNS. Judy then disclosed that her current foster parents were punishing her by hitting her with a belt. She also began to tell the CNS about some of her past sexual abuse and the psychological abuse that occurred in a previous foster home.

The Department of Social Services removed her from the foster family and temporarily placed her in a residential treatment setting. She was then placed with a foster mother, Nancy, who adopted her after the court terminated her birth parents' rights. Judy and Nancy have lived together for several years. As her mother described it, life with Judy has been filled with many "ups and downs." At age 7, Judy was very hyperactive, distractible, and disruptive at home and in school. At times she has been very depressed and suicidal. Over the past 2 years, Judy has appeared to "space out" and lose track of time. Sometimes she gets very angry during these episodes. She also showed other behaviors that reflect PTSD. If she saw the name of her birth mother or someone in her foster families, she would get very upset and quiet. She sometimes acted as if she was being abused again and shouted, "Stop that, don't do that to me." She often awoke in the middle of the night screaming after having nightmares of the trauma. Nancy said that Judy had exquisite "radar"; she could sense slight changes in people's mood and reactions and was "super aware" of her environment.

Judy continued to see the CNS for individual therapy each week. They commonly played games together; the CNS also met with Nancy and Judy to promote their relationship. Despite the severe abusive experiences and trauma response, Judy was an A student. She got along with other children but had difficulty getting close to others and had no best friends. She hoped to be a therapist someday so that she could help other children with emotional and behavioral problems. Judy and her mother cared very much about each other and continued to work on how the abuse affected her ability to relate to and trust other people.

CRITICAL THINKING QUESTIONS

1. What behaviors did Judy display that suggest a trauma response?

2. How did the school nurse and teacher decide to report their suspicions of abuse?
3. Identify Judy's emotional and psychological consequences of abuse.
4. Identify the behaviors that indicate that Judy is responding to treatment.
5. Develop a long-term care plan for Judy and her mother.
6. Devise teaching strategies to help Judy's mother cope with Judy's behaviors.
7. Suggest ways that nurses caring for Judy can deal with their own reactions to the traumatic experience.

KEY POINTS

- Nurses play a key role in identifying and providing treatment to victims of abuse. They have a legal and ethical obligation to recognize and intervene when client safety is compromised because of abuse or risk of abuse.
- People who have been abused exhibit a wide variety of responses, including psychiatric disorders such as PTSD, dissociative disorders, mood disorders, anxiety disorders, substance abuse, or somatization. In some cases, victims of abuse display violent, self-injurious, or risk-taking behaviors and chaotic lifestyles.
- Abuse is categorized as physical, sexual, psychological, or economic. The common factor is domination of one individual by another.
- *Survivor* is a term frequently used to refer to an individual who has been subjected to abuse. Survivorship indicates strength and the ability to overcome.
- Individual responses to abuse vary from minimal impact to major dysfunction. Multiple variables mediate the response, including the nature and duration of the abuse, the age at which the abuse occurred, gender, the perpetrators of the abuse, pretraumatic functioning, the context within which the abuse occurred, and the available support system.
- Many clients exhibit one or more symptoms of classic trauma responses. These symptoms may be either intrusiveness or numbing.
- Nurses carefully assess warning signs and physical signs of abuse. Mandated reporting laws require that the circumstances of such injuries or symptoms be clearly investigated, documented, and, when indicated, reported to the appropriate social service or protective agencies.
- Nursing assessment includes direct questioning about past and present abuse. If the person discloses abuse or an abuse history, determine the impact of abuse on present functioning and the client's resultant clinical needs.
- Key aspects of treatment include maintaining safety, empowering the client, minimizing intrusiveness, avoiding secrets, identifying symptom clusters and cognitive distortions, focusing on health, and dealing with shame.
- The process of recovery from abuse occurs in three stages: establishing safety, reconstructing the trauma story, and reconnecting with the world.
- Abuse survivors often need individual, group, or family psychotherapy. Pharmacotherapy is sometimes used as an adjunct.
- Nurses who work with abuse victims are subject to stress-related burnout, isolation, frustration, and their own feelings of trauma. Difficult countertransference reactions may also arise.

REFERENCES

1. DePanfilis, D, and Salus, M (eds): A Coordinated Response to Child Abuse and Neglect: A Basic Manual. U.S. Department of Health and Human Services. Publication No. (ACF) 92-30362, Washington, DC, 1992.
2. Dodge, K, Bates, J, and Pettot, G: Mechanisms in the cycle of violence. Science 250:1678, 1990.
3. Beitchman, J, et al: A review of the short-term effects of child abuse. Child Abuse Negl 15:537, 1991.
4. Gold, E: Long-term effects of sexual victimization in childhood: An attributional approach. J Consult Clin Psychol 4:471, 1986.
5. Finklehor, D: Early and long-term effects of child sexual abuse: An update. Professional Psychology: Research and Practice 21:325, 1990.
6. Beitchman, J, et al: A review of the long-term effects of child sexual abuse. Child Abuse Negl 16:101, 1992.
7. Roberts, A (ed): Helping Battered Women: New Perspectives and Remedies. Oxford University Press Inc, New York, 1996, pp 67, 74, 235–237.
8. Sedlak, A, and Bradhurst, M (eds): The third national incidence study of child abuse and neglect. U.S. Department of Health and Human Services, Washington, DC, 1996.
9. Daro, D, and Lung, C (eds): Current Trends in Abuse Reporting and Fatalities: The Results of the 1995 Annual Fifty State Survey. National Committee to Prevent Child Abuse, Chicago, April 1994.
10. Bryer, JB, et al: Childhood sexual and physical abuse as factors in adult psychiatric illness. Am J Psychiatry 144:1426–1430, 1987.
11. Hartman, C, and Burgess, A: Information processing of trauma. Journal of Interpersonal Violence 3:4, 1988.
12. Burgess, A, Hartman, C, and Kelley, S: Assessing child abuse: The TRIADS checklist. J Psychosocial Nursing 28:4, 1990.
13. Van der Kolk, B: Traumatic Stress. The Guilford Press, New York, 1996.
14. Yapko, M: Suggestions of Abuse: True and False Memories of Childhood Sexual Trauma. Simon & Schuster, New York, 1994, pp 15, 29.
15. Casey, E: Selected Child Abuse Information and Resources Directory, Working Paper #867. National Committee to Prevent Child Abuse, Chicago, February 1997.
16. Friedman, MJ: Psychobiological and pharmacological approaches to treatment. In Wilson, J, and Raphael, B (eds): International Handbook of Traumatic Stress Syndromes. Plenum Press, New York, 1993, p 785.
17. Herman, JL: Trauma and Recovery. Basic Books, New York, 1992.
18. Hartman, C, and Jackson, H: Rape and the phenomena of countertransference. In Wilson, J, and Indy, J (eds): Countertransference in the Treatment of PTSD. The Guilford Press, New York, 1994.
19. Nader, K: Countertransference in the treatment of acutely traumatized children. In Wilson, J, and Lindy, J (eds): Countertransference in the Treatment of PTSD. The Guilford Press, New York, 1994, pp 179–205.
20. Danieli, Y: Countertransference, trauma and training. In Wilson, J, and Lindy, J (eds): Countertransference in the Treatment of PTSD. The Guilford Press, New York, 1994, pp 368–388.

CHAPTER 32

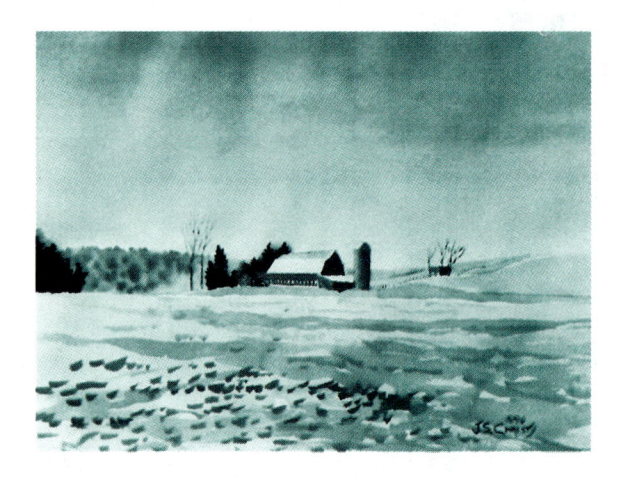

CHAPTER OUTLINE

Mode of Transmission
Epidemiology
  A Mother's Story
  Personal Awareness
Clinical Manifestation and the Spectrum of HIV Diseases
  Early Stage
  Middle Stage
  Late Stage
Neuropsychiatric Testing
Neuropsychological Complications
Other Psychiatric Disorders
Patient Care
  Assessment
  Nursing Diagnosis
  Planning and Therapeutics
  Hope for a Future: Protease Inhibitors
Vulnerable Populations
  The Severely and Persistently Mentally Ill
  Women
  Substance Abusers
Areas for Future Research

LEARNING OBJECTIVES

After completing this chapter, the reader should be able to:

- Explain the epidemiology of human immunodeficiency virus (HIV), and HIV disease.
- Describe the modes of transmission.
- List personal beliefs and values related to caring for clients with HIV disease.
- Describe the clinical manifestation of HIV and three stages in the spectrum of HIV disease.
- Assess the cognitive, behavioral, and emotional impact of HIV disease.
- Apply the patient care process to the client with HIV disease.
- Intervene with vulnerable populations experiencing HIV disease.

George Byron Smith, RNC, MSN, CCM
Debra Ann Danforth, MS, ARNP

Persons Living with HIV Disease and AIDS

KEY TERMS

acquired immunodeficiency syndrome (AIDS)
AIDS-defining illness
AIDS-related dementia
antiretroviral drugs
HIV disease
human immunodeficiency virus (HIV)
mild neurocognitive disorder
protease inhibitor drugs
severely and persistently mentally ill (SPMI)
spectrum of HIV disease

As we move toward the third decade of the **acquired immunodeficiency syndrome** (AIDS), the number of reported cases continues to rise. There are 40,000 new infections each year in this country and 5,000 to 10,000 new infections worldwide every day.

AIDS is the final phase of a chronic, progressive immune function disorder caused by the **human immunodeficiency virus (HIV)**. The CD4 and T lymphocytes are the primary targets for HIV infection because of the virus's affinity for the CD4 surface markers. Because CD4 and T lymphocytes coordinate many important immunologic functions, the virus's attack of these cells results in progressive impairment of the body's immune response. Measures of CD4 and T lymphocytes may be used to guide clinical management and treatment of HIV-infected individuals. Generally, as the CD4 and T lymphocyte counts decrease, the more aggressive prophylaxis and antiretroviral therapies become. However, caution must be used in evaluating the usefulness of a CD4 count in clinical management. Many clients with a CD4 count below 200 remain healthy for many months or years. The CD4 count is only a guide and not an absolute clinical indicator.

The definition of AIDS has continued to change since 1982's original definition, given by the Centers for Disease Control (CDC), which simply defined it as an opportunistic infection in an individual that had no identified medical cause. In 1986, the CDC published a list of specific opportunistic infections that individuals with AIDS might experience. An individual who was HIV positive and had experienced one of the listed opportunistic infections was given a diagnosis of an **AIDS-defining illness**. *Opportunistic infections* are aggressive diseases that would not have occurred in an individual with a healthy, functioning immune system. As HIV progresses, the immune system becomes more compromised and increasingly susceptible to opportunistic infections.

According to Bartlett and Finkbeiner,[1] the problem with this definition of AIDS is that some individuals with HIV infection died without receiving an AIDS-defining diagnosis. Although not a problem for health-care practitioners and medical treatment, this limiting definition was a problem for the purpose of assigning benefits such as disability and clients' eligibility for many social services. In January 1993, the definition of AIDS was revised to include the list of opportunistic infections for an AIDS-defining diagnosis, as well as other common conditions, and a CD4 cell count below 200 (Table 32–1). This definition has improved the benefits and social services for individuals with AIDS.

In the initial stage, an individual is first infected with HIV and is asymptomatic. At the time of initial infection with HIV, some may develop a mononucleosis-like syndrome called an *acute retroviral syndrome*. The mononucleosis-like symptoms are mild and may not be attributed to an HIV infection. The initial infection is followed by a relatively symptom-free period called the clinical latency stage. This period, from infection to the symptomatic stage, averages 8 to 12 years. During this stage, the individual is considered to have **HIV disease.**

During the early symptomatic stage of HIV disease, the individual begins to exhibit symptoms of a weakening immune system. After the immune system is severely weakened, the individual begins to experience opportunistic infections. During this stage, the person is considered to have AIDS.

AIDS, more than any other chronic disease in recent history, is a multidimensional disease that challenges practitioners to call into play their physical, emotional, and social care skills. This chapter explores the neurobiological and biopsychosocial issues that affect the care of HIV-infected individuals.

TABLE 32-1. CDC Conditions in the AIDS Surveillance Case Definition

- Bacterial infection, multiple or recurrent
- Candidiasis of bronchi, trachea, or lung
- Candidiasis, esophageal
- Cervical cancer, invasive
- Coccidioidomycosis, disseminated or extrapulmonary
- Cryptococcosis, extrapulmonary
- Cryptosporidiosis, chronic intestinal
- Cytomegalovirus (CMV) disease (not including liver, spleen, or nodes)
- CMV retinitis and loss of vision
- Encephalopathy
- Herpes simplex, chronic ulcers; or bronchitis, pneumonitis, or esophagitis
- Histoplasmosis, disseminated or extrapulmonary
- Isosporiasis, chronic intestinal
- Kaposi's sarcoma
- Lymphoid interstitial pneumonia or pulmonary lymphoid hyperplasia
- Lymphoma, Burkitt's
- Lymphoma, immunoblastic
- Lymphoma of the brain, primary
- *Mycobacterium avium-intracellulare* complex or *Mycobacterium kansasii*, disseminated or extrapulmonary
- *Mycobacterium*, other species or unidentified species, disseminated or extrapulmonary
- *Pneumocystis carinii* pneumonia
- Pneumonia, recurrent
- Progressive multifocal leukoencephalopathy
- *Salmonella* septicemia, recurrent
- Toxoplasmosis of brain
- Wasting syndrome

Source: Adapted from Centers for Disease Control: Classification system of HIV infection and expanded surveillance case definition for AIDS among adolescents and adults, rev. MMWR 41 (RR-17):1–19, 1993.

MODE OF TRANSMISSION

HIV is spread through exchange of body fluids that contain the virus; it cannot be spread through casual contact. It must have a portal of entry, such as a tear in a mucous membrane or access to the bloodstream, the latter of which can occur in transfusions or by injections with contaminated needles. Another transmission route is from a mother to her unborn child. An HIV-infected individual can transmit HIV to others only a few days after initial infection.

There must be a sufficient amount of the virus introduced through one of these portals of entry into the susceptible host before infection can occur. The duration and frequency of contact, virulence of the virus, quantity of inoculant, and host's immune-defense capabilities all affect whether infection will actually occur after exposure to the virus. Quantity of inoculant or "viral load" in the blood, semen, vaginal secretions, or breast milk is an important variable. Because the viral load for HIV-infected individuals peaks during the first 2 to 6 months after initial infection and again during the late stages of the disease, during these periods, there is a higher risk of transmitting HIV to others.

Certain groups of people are at greater risk for HIV infection. Gay and bisexual males, as well as intravenous drug users, have been hit the hardest in the AIDS epidemic. However, the faces of HIV infection and AIDS are changing. Since 1989, the rate of heterosexual infection with HIV has doubled. For gay and bisexual men, the increase has been 21%; for intravenous drug users, the increase has been 43%.

HIV, like other viruses, affects only specific cells and is an obligate intracellular parasite, characterized by the ability to survive only in a particular set of environmental conditions and only within the host organism. HIV is a fragile virus that can be transmitted from human to human only through infected blood, semen, vaginal secretions, and breast milk. HIV is not spread casually. It cannot be transmitted by kissing, sharing eating utensils, close contact, hugging, or shaking hands with an HIV-positive individual. There is no evidence that the virus can be transmitted through tears, saliva, sweat, respirator droplets, enteric routes, or insect bites.

HIV must use materials from a host cell in order to replicate; it cannot replicate outside the host cell. Its particular host cell is the human CD4 cell (also called T4 cell or T-helper cell), an important part of the human immune system. CD4 cells defend against very primitive invaders such as fungi, yeast, and other viruses. HIV invades CD4 cells and takes over their functions.

The CD4 cells orchestrate the entire immune system. Soon, the CD4 cells are too busy replicating more HIV to perform their own immune function. After the host has been infected with HIV, other immune system components form antibodies to fight the HIV. Detection of these antibodies in several laboratory test is, in most cases, proof positive that the person was exposed to HIV. Such a person is said to be HIV positive.

Because HIV invades those cells that defend against primitive organisms, people living with AIDS (PLWA) commonly suffer from such opportunistic infectious agents as *Candida albicans* (thrush), herpes zoster, and *Pneumocystis carinii* (pneumonia) and such rare cancers as Kaposi's sarcoma and various lymphomas. As mentioned previously, opportunistic infections are diseases that would not have occurred in a healthy individual with a functioning immune system.

EPIDEMIOLOGY

The statistics on HIV and AIDS continue to be staggering. The World Health Organization (WHO) conservatively estimates that 14 million people have been infected by HIV and that by the year 2000, between 30 and 40 million people will have been infected. In the United States, there have been over 200,000 cases of AIDS reported and an additional one million people are believed to be infected with HIV[2]; this accounts for approximately 70% of AIDS cases reported in the world. According to the CDC, among persons between ages 25 and 44, AIDS has rapidly grown from a disease with zero reported deaths in 1980 to being the leading cause of death in men and the fourth leading cause of death in women by 1995. AIDS has become the nation's eighth leading cause of death; it was the ninth leading cause of death in the United States in 1991; tenth in 1990.[3] Also according to the CDC, 1 in 92 American men ages 27 to 39 years old may be HIV infected, 1 in 33 for African-Americans. There is one AIDS-related death every 15 minutes, one AIDS diagnosis every 9 minutes, and someone infected with HIV every 13 minutes. AIDS has become the leading cause of death among all Americans between the ages of 25 and 44. Since the first reported AIDS cases in 1981, the mortality rate was 93%; the mortality rate was down to 63% by June 1996.

HIV infection has become a pandemic affecting every region of the world. HIV is spread worldwide primarily through heterosexual contact, with women accounting for 5 of every 11 new HIV infections in adults.[4] Seventy percent of AIDS cases among U.S. women were among African-American and Hispanic-Latino women; African-American women are 17 times, and Hispanic women 8 times, more likely to have AIDS than are white women.[5] Experts estimate that one-fourth to one-third of children born to HIV-positive mothers may become infected with the virus.

HIV infection is spreading rapidly in the adolescent population, in which AIDS cases have increased by 77% from 1993 to 1995. As of 1995, more than 30,000 HIV-infected adolescents were reported in the United States. Many experts believe there is underreporting of HIV-infected adolescent cases because many states are not required to report them. Since 1988, HIV disease has been the sixth leading cause of death among 15- to 24-year-olds.[6] Given the long latency period between infection with HIV and an AIDS-defining illness, most individuals diagnosed with HIV disease under the age of 30 years were probably infected as adolescents.[7]

Currently, there are an estimated 15,000 to 20,000 HIV-infected infants and children in the United States. In 1985, perinatal HIV transmission accounted for 8520 AIDS cases in children under 13 years of age.[7] By 1989, pediatric AIDS cases had become the eighth leading cause of death in children ages 1 to 4 years. However, approximately 75% of infants exposed to HIV perinatally were not infected. In addition, pediatric HIV occurs disproportionately with impoverished minority populations, which are groups with limited access to health care. For children between birth and 12 years of age, there were 942 pediatric AIDS cases reported in 1993 and 1017 pediatric AIDS cases reported in 1994.[8]

A MOTHERS STORY

HIV and AIDS—What is it? The communicable disease control and health officials might say it is an epidemic of major proportions that must be controlled. The major concern and purpose is that the population as a whole—just a nonhuman, faceless, nameless, nonfeeling statistical fact—must be addressed scientifically.

If only I could erase all else and deal with just this cold, practical scientific approach. No faces—no feelings—no real individuals—no emotions—no pain—no caring—no panic—no love—no rejection—no grief—no frustration—no hate—no guilt—Just cold facts without faces or names. Oh, how much easier to bear; how much easier to bare.

Many have readily chosen either rejection or only this nonhumane approach to HIV and AIDS. Compassionate people, where are you? Can't you see the pain? Why can't you feel what I feel? How can you know the grief? My wonderful son has HIV and AIDS, don't you care? It could easily be your son or daughter, you know. And with the continued spread of the disease, it may yet be. I pray not. No one should have to bear the pain, isolation, indignity, hopelessness, and the fear that this fatal and "socially unacceptable" disease brings. Surely neither my son nor yours deserves such a fate.

As I contemplate the life I've shared with this special son of mine, I am engulfed by both wonderful and painful memories. These thoughts bring forth hearty laughter and happiness, joy, frustration, and tears, but most of all, love. The present and the future never fade. They are with me to give me hope, comfort, to tease, haunt, and terrify. So many of my emotions intermingle and are constantly at war with one another. At times I feel like one huge frustrated time bomb ready to explode from all the feelings that occasionally overwhelm me.

Surely hope is around the corner somewhere. When I really dive deep enough into my rapidly expanding bag of feelings tied up inside, I can usually find hope and peace, but at times

	Clinical Categories		
CD4 + T-Cell Categories	**A** Asymptomatic, Acute HIV, or PGL[a]	**B** Symptomatic, Not A or C Condition	**C**[b] AIDS-Indicator Conditions
1. >500/μL	A1	B1	C1
2. 200–499/μL	A2	B2	C2
3. <200/μL AIDS-indicator T-cell count	A3	B3	C3

**Shaded area indicates an AIDS-defining diagnosis.

[a]PGL-Persistent generalized lymphadenopathy.
[b]Clinical conditions in category C are listed in Table 1.

Figure 32–1. 1993 Revised Classification System of HIV Infection and Expanded Surveillance Case Definition of AIDS Among Adolescents and Adults. (From Centers for Disease Control (1992). 1993 Revised classification system of HIV infection and expanded surveillance case definition for AIDS among adolescents and adults. Morbidity and Mortality Weekly Report, 41 (RR-17), 1–19.)

it is a monumental struggle to maintain calm spirit in the midst of such terminal uncertainty. What parent can ever be the same after experiencing the threat of losing a child of any age? Nature never intended for parents to cope with such a prospect.[9]

PERSONAL AWARENESS

It is imperative that health-care providers recognize their own responses to HIV disease. Personal discomfort can interfere with effective assessment and treatment of HIV-positive clients. Understanding and taking responsibility for one's feelings, thoughts, and behaviors are essential to effective communication and professional practice. Understanding the self will facilitate self-awareness. To be effective, practitioners must examine their own values, prejudices, and belief systems related to:

- Sexual orientation and homophobia
- Heterosexist biases
- Sexual behaviors
- Diminished cognitive capacity
- Death and dying
- Pain and suffering
- Substance abuse and IV drug use

Health-care practitioners who work with HIV-positive individuals may experience conscious or unconscious countertransference. The combination of sex, drugs, and serious medical illness or death as a result of HIV infection may arouse an irrational reaction if countertransference issues have not been adequately addressed.

CLINICAL MANIFESTATION AND THE SPECTRUM OF HIV DISEASES

Because symptoms of HIV infection can go from none for many years to death from an AIDS-related opportunistic infection, HIV-positive persons are referred to as being on a continuum of HIV infection, the **spectrum of HIV disease.** As shown in Figure 32–1, it ranges from an asymptomatic stage to severe immunodeficiency and associated serious secondary infections and neoplasms.[10,11] Problems requiring psychiatric–mental health care interventions can affect individuals at all points on the HIV spectrum.

The HIV-infected client experiences significant psychosocial distress at each stage of the illness, but specific stressors vary as the disease progresses. Many clients experience mild to severe emotional responses at times of crisis and transition or under the burden of chronic stress. The healthcare practitioner has a vital role in assisting the client to adapt to and cope with the effects of a chronic illness.

EARLY STAGE

The early stage on the spectrum of HIV disease involves two groups: the "worried well" and those with initial HIV-positive infection. The worried well are individuals who fear having HIV infection because they have engaged in high-risk behaviors such as unprotected sexual activity or shared IV drug needles. The worried well also include health-care workers who fear exposure to HIV infection from caring for people living with HIV disease. The worried well may be individuals with no information or misinformation about HIV infection and HIV disease.

The worried well experience anxiety that interferes with their ability to function at home or work. Many require counseling to express their fears and gain correct information on the transmission of HIV. HIV counseling includes the choice of whether to have HIV testing.

Testing for HIV infection should be voluntary with informed consent obtained. Confidentiality and the avoidance of discrimination toward persons who test positive must be assured. Precede HIV testing with information and counseling about the testing procedure, the medical implications of the test, and assessment of risk, as well as an opportunity to ask questions and receive additional information.

Following testing, HIV-negative individuals should be informed that continued high-risk sexual and drug-use behaviors could result in HIV infection. HIV-negative individuals concerned about recent exposure should be advised to seek repeated testing at least 6 to 7 weeks after the suspected exposure.

The second group of individuals in the early stage of the spectrum of HIV disease are those with an initial HIV-positive infection. Tailor counseling to each individual and include an interpretation of the test results and a discussion of the medical, social, and psychological implications of a positive HIV test result. HIV-positive individuals should also be instructed about how to notify sex or needle-sharing partners and how to refer them for HIV counseling and testing. Confidentiality is important in protecting and not discouraging persons from seeking HIV testing. Individuals found to be HIV-positive require a medical assessment and evaluation, including immunologic monitoring, screening for other sexually transmitted diseases, prophylaxis against certain opportunistic illnesses, vaccinations, antiretroviral therapy, and other preventive and therapeutic services such as psychological and emotional support.[5]

Following initial HIV infection, the disease progression to full-blown AIDS varies greatly. Studies have shown that 5% of the total HIV-infected population will develop AIDS within 2 years of infection; without therapy, approximately 20 to 25% develop AIDS within 6 years after infection, and 50 percent within 10 years.[5] There are reports of individuals remaining asymptomatic after 5 to 10 years.

The initial reactions to a positive HIV test vary. According to Lego,[11] common psychological reactions include shock, anger, and panic; disappointment, loss, and sadness; fear; shame; denial; suicidal thoughts; and the "ego chill." Shock, anger, and panic are early reactions to a devastating disease. This reaction may be intensified because many individuals may have experienced HIV disease with their friends, family, or significant others. Those who have feared contracting the illness for years may have an initial reaction of relief now that the waiting is over that is quickly replaced with anger and panic.[11] The individual knows that AIDS is terminal, and a high percentage of those who are HIV-positive progress to an AIDS diagnosis. Panic sets in when the client realizes the potential devastation of the disease in social, psychological, and physical terms.[11]

Next, disappointment, loss, and sadness may occur. The person begins to internalize the meaning of an HIV-positive status. Disappointment occurs in the realization that life will be different. Losses for the HIV-positive individual and PLWAs are tremendous. The list of actual and potential losses is endless, including loss of independence, work, social connections, friends, self-image, physical abilities, and mental abilities. With these losses comes sadness and depression.

Some individuals may experience fleeting suicidal thoughts or actually formulate a plan. According to Lego,[11] the practitioner assesses suicidal risk for HIV-positive clients by determining whether they have a plan and means to carry out that plan, whether additional stressors and life-changing events have occurred in addition to the diagnosis, if the plan has been well thought out, if there are immediate and available means to carry out the plan, and whether a support system is available. Suicidal thoughts are not uncommon for individuals experiencing HIV disease. Usually the mention of suicide is an indication that people want assistance with coping; initiate interventions immediately.

Lego[11] points out that HIV-positive individuals may begin to feel the fear of incapacitation, physical and mental deterioration, deformity, and pain that leads to relying on others. The individual needs an opportunity to express these fears in an environment of acceptance. Loss of independence and the fear of dependence on others can be devastating, requiring supportive counseling. During this stage, the reality of certain death and Erikson's[12] ego chill may occur. According to Erikson, ego chill is "a shudder that comes from sudden awareness that our nonexistence . . . is entirely possible."

During the early stage, HIV-positive individuals are usually healthy. They are likely to be sexually active and may even continue to use drugs. They may cope with their illness and stress through continuing high-risk behaviors that place them at significant risk for transmitting the virus or becoming reinfected with different HIV strains. The nurse must continually provide support and prevention education.

Account of the HIV-Positive Result and Hope

I was afraid of knowing that which I didn't want to know. But beyond my then-incredible naiveté, I promised myself that if I ever found out I was infected with HIV, or, God forbid, found myself already sick and dying from "the plague," I would immediately overdose on Valium and peppermint schnapps, just peacefully end it all and not wait around to die in agony. Over the years, I'd witnessed far too many friends fade into ghostly shadows of their once-vital selves and die traumatic, slow, excruciating deaths from AIDS's myriad, multifaceted complications—at no time was it ever a pretty or pleasant sight. I didn't want it to happen to me. And if I didn't definitively know if I was HIV-positive or not, I could still believe that I wasn't, right?

Or so I thought back then—when then was "before" and I still lived in a once-upon-a-time, far, far away fairy-tale world. "After" was 2 years ago, when through no fault or design of my own, I was tested. The result: HIV antibody seropositive. My number came up and I became, at some point, the newest CDC statistic—another stricken, but not yet fallen, warrior in the savage battle against AIDS. I was catapulted from my enchanted never-never-land existence into the glaring, embittered reality of a life-and-death battlefield to join fellow comrades-in-arms living with and fighting AIDS.

Time, circumstances, and hopefully, people change. Fortunately, so did I. Now, I'm glad that I know I'm HIV positive. Why? For one thing, the worst part about not knowing is not knowing—at least, that foreboding cloud has been cleared. I have weathered its stormy turbulence and can now get on with the important matters at hand, which are taking better care of myself, educating myself on available treatment options, thereby enabling myself to make informed decisions in my treatment strategy, taking the necessary precautions against reinfections with HIV strains, educating others about AIDS—letting people know that if it can happen to a nice guy like me, it could happen to them or to someone they love, too—and, most important, protecting others from contracting the virus from me.

And now that I do know, how do I deal with that knowledge? Sometimes OK, sometimes not. I've finally stopped asking "why me?" and am working on not asking "why" anymore. I don't blame anyone, including myself, for my positive-antibody status: guilt and blame are negative energies that can be redirected and put to otherwise constructive use. And, I adamantly refuse to see myself or allow myself to be categorized as an "AIDS victim": I am still empowered to make decisions that affirm my being and positively affect the quality of my life. Nor am I ashamed anymore. I have found, fortunately, that some of the stigma once associated with HIV and AIDS has dissipated. I like to think that I have a pretty good handle on the situation as it is, but the truth of the matter is, I still freak out when I least expect to. It's hell living with the knowledge that you have a deadly virus coursing around in your body and that it isn't ever going to go away.

Yes, I walk through the valley of the shadow of death, and I'm afraid. But that's OK. It's OK because my being afraid has allowed me to truly and intimately experience hope, trust, faith, and love. These extraordinary encounters sustain me and provide a guiding beacon through the valley—a bright, iridescent beacon that ultimately outshines the valley's obscuring darkness.[9]

MIDDLE STAGE

During the middle stage, the HIV-positive individual first begins to experience symptoms of the HIV infection and declining health. It can be a difficult time for families and loved ones as well. Coping mechanisms are tested as health declines. The denial that was so strong in the early stage is no longer adequate to prevent distress. The central nervous system involvement may make the individual respond differently to internal and external stressors.

Although denial and other coping strategies may help all manage stress in the early stage, symptoms and the realization of impending illness may lead to increased anxiety and feelings of doom. At first, some individuals may have a short, flulike illness, whereas others have neuropathy that can lead to paralysis. The initial symptoms may overcome denial and result in fear, panic, feelings of confronting death, or loss of control. Regardless of the severity, the initial losses or fear of future losses can be extremely distressing for the client and family.

Alteration in appearance or loss of independence can cause the client with HIV-related illnesses to have changes in self-esteem or body image. Clients may isolate themselves and withdraw socially. HIV-infected persons may move between feeling mobilized to attend to their health and feeling overwhelmed and paralyzed.

The individual may experience a profound sense of loss of the illusion that he or she would be the "lucky one" who would never get sick and, instead, be forced to reject the myth that he or she had unlimited time to live. This can be an agonizing time for the client, yet a time when a positive outlook may be most important for sustaining health-promoting behaviors.

The individual's family and support system, too, have important psychosocial needs during this stage. With the onset of symptoms, the family, significant others, and friends can no longer deny the disease progression. Their own grief processes begin, and they may disagree about the HIV-positive client's decision to seek treatment, not to seek treatment, or to use alternative treatment modalities. The health-care practitioner provides the family with information about the individual's illness and, more important, may be the only person to whom the family members can express their grief, sense of burden, fears, and anger.

During this phase, it is appropriate for the individual, the family, and the health-care team to open a dialogue about loss and death. The clinician often has a key role in such dialogue, which should occur before life-threatening complications are likely. Death may be a frightening topic for all involved, including the practitioner, but one of the most important messages that the practitioner can convey is that death, no matter how tragic or premature, is an inevitable and natural part of life that can be faced with peace and dignity.

Clients who are still well may want to express exactly which measures they wish to be taken to sustain their lives. The clinician serves an important role in encouraging the verbalization of these thoughts and feelings and by explaining specific life-sustaining interventions such as emergency intubation, cardiopulmonary resuscitation, and indefinite mechanical ventilation. In most cases, these wishes can be translated into living wills, and the clinician should encourage such a declaration. Advance directives help to preserve autonomy and give clients a sense of control.

LATE STAGE

By the late stage, people living with HIV disease have, ideally, reached a realistic level of acceptance regarding their health status and uncertain future. They may have the capacity to enjoy life on a day-to-day basis but have several tasks left to accomplish. They are faced with physical or cognitive difficulties that hinder daily function and may need support in verbalizing a continued sense of loss as health declines or as memory or cognition decreases. They may also rely on the practitioner for continued acceptance despite increasing physical dependence or alteration in appearance.

By this stage, the client may be dealing with multiple losses such as health, job, physical and mental abilities, appearance, sexual intimacy, lifestyle, and autonomy. The multiple losses occur at different points in the course of the disease. These losses may reinforce feelings of powerlessness. The practitioner can assist the client in managing these losses and maintaining a realistic outlook through counseling and education.

Life review—looking at one's life and making peace with it—becomes one of the important tasks in the late stages of HIV disease as the individual makes final preparations for death. The goal of the life review is to achieve a sense of completion regarding one's life and come to terms with achievement or lack of achievement of life goals. The practitioner assists the client in identifying what has been accomplished, what has yet to be accomplished, and what will never be accomplished. A person may express joy about certain aspects of life and grief about those things not yet done. By creating a trusting and open atmosphere, the practitioner fosters an open discussion and expression of thoughts and feelings. The client's family also must do a life review as they recall past events and make peace with what has occurred. The clinician assists the family in understanding and experiencing their grief.

The client may want to make decisions to get his or her legal affairs in order, initiate the living will and power of attorney, and make funeral arrangements. The family may view these activities as giving up. The clinician should assist the family in understanding the importance of allowing the client to be as active as possible in his or her own care decisions.

During the late stage of HIV disease, the client confronts many fears as he or she progresses to acceptance. The client may experience the fears of death and dying, pain and suffering, developing dementia, and becoming a burden to others. The clinician can assist the client and family by allowing and encouraging the expression of these feelings.

NEUROPSYCHIATRIC TESTING

Psychiatric and psychological problems most common for those with HIV disease concern mood regulation. The alteration in mood is typically not caused by an underlying medical condition, but is presumed to be a response to psychological and social stressors. Neurological problems can cause cognitive or motor impairment, such as memory loss, confusion, headaches, and tingling or pain in the extremities, all of which are common hallmarks of neurological problems in HIV-infected individuals. Many times psychiatric or psychological and neurological problems coexist, causing difficulty in distinguishing between functional problems and organic disease.

A basic neuropsychological examination can be useful for evaluating the cognitive functioning of clients infected with HIV. Cognitive function can be assessed based on observable behaviors and responses to daily interactions with the nurse or other clients. Because the first indication of HIV-related cognitive impairment is often a change in mental status, it should be assessed often over time. With organic etiology, neuropsychological testing is effective in documenting subtle changes in cognition. It provides data on memory function, speed of information processing, reaction times, and ability to perform complex tasks.

Health-care providers working with clients with HIV disease should be familiar with screening for potential neurological involvement. A neurological history should include:

- Observing the client for appropriate emotional and behavioral responses. Does the client's affect match speech content? Is apathy more prominent than depression?
- Assessing for alteration in thought processes, such as concentration, memory, or organization skills.
- Noting any of the following signs or symptoms present that may be indicative of neurological disease requiring further workup:
  - Headache
  - Pain or numbness and tingling in the extremities
  - Loss of interest, drive, libido, and energy
  - Forgetfulness
  - Difficulty concentrating
  - Change in speech, with difficulty finding words or slurring
  - Visual problems
  - Changes in hearing
  - Loss of balance, frequent falls
  - Tremors or involuntary movements
  - Seizures
  - Unexplained injuries
- Considering the client's general appearance related to grooming and clothing.
- Determining if the client can organize thoughts in a logical manner.
- Assessing the client for the presence of hallucinations, delusions, suicidal thoughts, or obsessive thinking. What is the content of the client's thoughts?
- Noting intellectual function related to the client's orientation, memory function, and verbal skills and language.
- Assessing motor functions such as level of motor activity, gait, involuntary and purposeless movement, tremors, agitation, and inertia.

- Assessing mental status. Although the mental status assessment may not identify early cognitive changes related to HIV infection, it should become a routine part of a clinical encounter. It is useful for providing baseline evaluation information and is a simple clinical means for follow-up and evaluation.[13]

Neuropsychological tests are useful in the differential diagnosis of affective versus organic disorders. However, a conclusion or diagnosis of cognitive impairment or dysfunction is not made based upon the results of one measure or test. A diagnosis of neurological involvement is made on the combination of psychiatric symptoms, physical symptoms, and neuropsychological data.

NEUROPSYCHOLOGICAL COMPLICATIONS

Neurological complications are common in HIV disease with 10% of individuals presenting with neurological symptoms; between 60 and 70% of individuals with HIV disease eventually suffer some form of **AIDS-related dementia** (Figure 32–2). The neurobiological complications of HIV can be either primary or secondary: Primary complications are those that can be attributed directly to HIV infection of the central nervous system; secondary complications include infections and neoplasms facilitated by the immunodeficiency state, cerebrovascular complications, and toxic states produced either by HIV-associated medical illnesses or by toxic effects of various therapeutic agents.

The most important of the primary neurobiological complications are the HIV-associated neurocognitive disorders. The cardinal feature is impaired cognitive functioning, including slowed motor function and, sometimes, mood disturbances. "HIV encephalopathy" and "AIDS dementia complex (ADC)" are outdated terms that do not clearly outline the nature of the dysfunctions being described. **Mild neurocognitive disorder** and HIV-associated dementia are the more current terms used.[14]

An individual with mild neurocognitive disorder may experience some difficulty in concentrating, fatigue quickly when engaged in demanding mental tasks, feel subjectively slowed down, and have difficulty with short-term memory. Individuals may say that they are not as "sharp" or as "quick" as they once were. Neuropsychological testing may reveal difficulties with speed of information processing, sustained information processing, divided attention, and deficiencies in learning and recalling new information[13] Individuals may also experience difficulties with tasks involving problem solving and abstract reasoning, as well as slowing of simple motor tasks.

HIV-associated dementia is both more profound and more generalized than the mild neurocognitive disorder. Individuals report severe forgetfulness, difficulty in concentrating, problems with naming and word finding, marked mental slowness, and disorientation. Comprehensive neuropsychological testing usually reveals marked impairment in speed

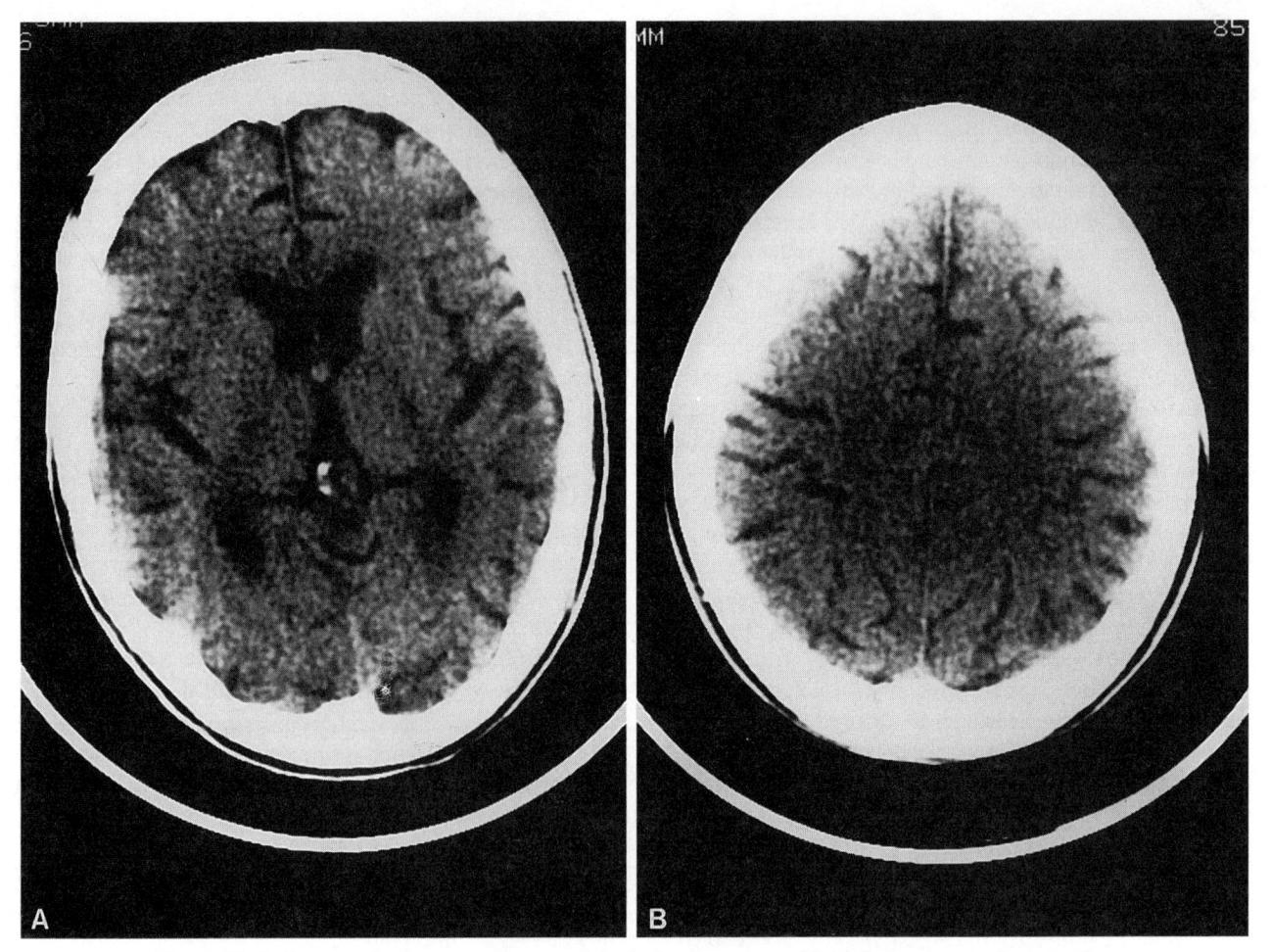

Figure 32-2. Computerized tomography scan of the brain of a patient with ADC showing cerebral atrophy.

of information processing, attention, abstracting ability, complex perceptual motor skills, learning new information, and recall.[14]

As the dementia progresses, the individual may become more apathetic, severely disoriented, and confused and have difficulty with independent living. Some individuals become markedly irritable or labile in mood. A small proportion of clients with dementia develop psychotic symptoms that have a paranoid theme and are accompanied by auditory and visual hallucinations.

There are three main areas to consider when intervening with neurological complications: cognitive, motor, and behavioral disturbance. When there is cognitive impairment, clinicians must make adjustments in the way care is provided, the nature of the interactions with the individual, the client's expectations, and the environment in which the person operates. Written or visual cues are more effective than verbal directions, which must be phrased in a way that the individual can understand and remember; for example, break lengthy directions into short, simple steps.

The practitioner will need to give clear, simple instructions, write out directions, and schedule repeated reminders. Information from the individual may need to be verified with significant others. Minimize abrupt changes in routine. The practitioner can involve the client in structured groups and activities to minimize isolation.

Assess the client's ability to think clearly and abstractly. Adjust teaching to give simple ideas or tasks. Ideas and tasks may need to broken down into smaller, simpler sections. Supplement teaching with written material, and include the input of caregivers in teaching to a greater degree. Decision-making options should be provided only to the individual's tolerance level. For an individual who has impaired abstract thinking or problem-solving ability, the clinician will need to provide extensive support in translating learning into new situations.

To maintain safety, the practitioner must adjust the environment for the individual with neurological complications. Stimuli should be kept to a minimum for the individual who has difficulty concentrating, especially during teaching and complex tasks. Assist the client in structuring her or his day. In an inpatient setting, more frequent checks on the confused and disoriented client may be required. Label the individual's room and bathroom.

When motor function is impaired, the individual requires additional safety measures and support. Attention to problems associated with immobility (such as skin breakdown and deep vein thrombosis) is essential, and the clinician may need to assist and encourage ambulation. Problems with bowel and bladder incontinence require the clinician to assess for other problems such as urinary tract infection, burning on urination, or skin breakdown. An individual with sensorimotor difficulties may need to be encouraged to speak slowly or point to what he or she wants.

There are no specific treatments for the cognitive disorders associated with HIV infection. Zidovudine (AZT) has been associated with subjective reports of improvement in mental functioning with early treatment. Another class of drugs used in treatment are calcium channel blockers; however, their efficacy is unknown. The remaining forms of treatment are principally supportive with behavior clues.

After diagnosis is clear, employ the usual supportive measures for neurocognitively impaired individuals. These include identifying areas of cognitive strength and weakness, reducing emphasis on those areas that are impaired, emphasizing efforts to maintain adequate orientation and reality testing, and avoiding medications that may further compromise cognitive functioning particularly benzodiazepine drugs. Antidepressants, benzodiazepines, and antipsychotics, if indicated, should be prescribed in low doses. Antidepressants and antipsychotics are ineffective in treating the underlying causes of symptoms.

Practitioners working with clients with HIV disease must be aware of the potential for meningitis; symptoms include photophobia, headaches, and neck stiffness as well as, in rare instances, confusion and clouding of consciousness. The course of the illness and treatment are typically self-limiting. Acute neuropathies, rapidly evolving symmetrical paralysis with variable sensory signs often beginning in the legs, can occasionally develop early in the course of HIV infection. Although these neuropathies tend to be self-limiting, more persistent types can occur during the middle and late stages, including a predominantly sensory neuropathy characterized by the onset of numbness, tingling, burning, or pain in the hands or feet. Symptoms are especially common in the feet and include both painful sensations and contact sensitivity without motor involvement. Zidovudine treatment is only sometimes effective. Treatment with low dosages of amitriptyline and carbamazepine is useful in managing symptoms.

OTHER PSYCHIATRIC DISORDERS

The emotional responses of shock, disbelief, grief, sadness, anger, and fear are normal and appropriate reactions to a disease as devasting as HIV.[13] Practitioners can facilitate the expression of these emotions while assessing for more severe or pathological responses.

Adjustment reactions are the most common emotional responses to HIV infection and often account for the "roller coaster" or "yo-yo" effect of hopeful highs and helpless lows.

It has been estimated that about two-thirds of HIV-positive clients experience adjustment disorders during the course of HIV disease. Adjustment reactions are most likely at times of significant medical events or transitional points in the illness, such as the manifestation of the first symptoms or the first time the CD4 cell count drops below 200. The clinical course of those HIV-related adjustment disorders is usually benign and responsive to education and supportive therapy. When emotional reactions have become so severe that individuals cannot meet their daily needs or are in danger of harming themselves or others, the practitioner must consider treatment: psychotherapy, relationship therapy, family therapy, environmental changes for safety, and medication.

Although anxiety is a common response to the stressors of any life-threatening illness, the diagnosis of anxiety disorders is less prevalent than that of depressive disorders. Anxiety disorders, such as major anxiety disorders, panic disorders, obsessive-compulsive disorders, and generalized anxiety disorders, occur in approximately 1 to 2% of HIV-infected individuals. The diagnosis and clinical features of the major anxiety disorders are usually straightforward, and, in many cases, a history of anxiety may precede the likely time of infection. The anxious HIV-positive client may experience diarrhea, nausea, sweating, tremors, visual disturbances, skin rashes, dizziness, or lethargy. Individuals with HIV disease have responded to medication, education, and support therapies. The HIV-positive individual may benefit from a referral to a community support group or cognitive-behavior therapy.

Depression is common in HIV-positive individuals and ranges from transient sadness to major depressive symptoms that require treatment. Grief is a natural response to an illness associated with so many losses, just as depression is a natural response to a chronic or fatal illness.

In individuals with more advanced HIV disease, some early estimates based on chart review suggest that 40% of hospitalized individuals with frank AIDS may meet the criteria for a major depressive disorder.[14] Whether HIV disease itself increases the likelihood of major depressive disorder beyond expected increases found in other chronic disease has not yet been determined. Although HIV disease's associated adverse physical and emotional impairments may potentiate the onset of a mood disorder, a history of previous mood disorders is the strongest predictor of a subsequent depressive illness with HIV disease.

The diagnosis of major depressive disorders is rather straightforward. As the HIV disease progresses, somatic symptoms such as fatigue, weight loss, and insomnia or neurocognitive impairment suggestive of depression may complicate diagnosis. In assessing thoughts of death, which might be expected in individuals with HIV disease, the practitioner must evaluate the client's level of preoccupation with death and determine whether it is a change in focus from usual thoughts about death and dying. Because the majority of HIV-positive individuals have considered suicide at some point during their illness, it is crucial to assess the lethality or seriousness of suicidal thoughts by asking whether the client has a plan and the means to carry out that plan. Treatment and prognosis are similar for that of the general psychiatric–mental health population. Individual depressive episodes are varied, with most individuals having infrequent episodes. The usual prognosis is remission, either spontaneously or with treatment. Most individuals with HIV disease and major depressive disorders respond well to antidepressant medications and supportive therapies.

Mood disorders with manic features, with or without hallucinations, delusions, or alterations in thought processes, occur rarely, but they can complicate the treatment of the HIV disease. Mania is characterized by excessive excitement, euphoria, irritability, paranoia, or agitation.

Some medications, such as steroids, zidovudine, and ganciclovir, as well as a wide variety of neurological conditions, such as cerebrovascular disorders and meningitis, can cause manic features. Typical case reports involve individuals previously described as stable, who, over a period of days or weeks, undergo changes in personality (for example, become pompous or belittling or act sexually inappropriately), and then progress into a fuller manic picture. The mood disturbance is generally elevated, with associated grandiosity. Diminished need for sleep, loquaciousness, racing thoughts, and unrealistic personal and financial plans may appear. Evaluation of medications, discontinuation of suspected medications, and a thorough assessment may reveal an underlying neurological source.

Psychotic symptoms, when they occur, are usually late-stage complications of HIV disease. They require immediate medical and neurological evaluation and often require antipsychotic management. Chart-review studies have found a frequency of psychotic disorders in HIV-infected populations ranging from 3 to 15 percent in individuals for whom obvious causes such as delirium have been excluded.[14] Some theories on the etiology of new-onset psychosis have been suggested: the direct effect of HIV on the brain; other CNS viruses, such as cytomegalovirus or herpes simplex virus; coinfection with two or more viruses; or brief psychotic disorders. The clinical presentation of psychosis in HIV-infected individuals is extremely variable. The most prevalent symptom seems to be delusions with persecutory, grandiose, or somatic components. Most individuals experience auditory hallucinations, with perhaps half of those also experiencing visual hallucinations. A majority of individuals also experience disorders of thought processes, including looseness of association or disorganized thinking. Disturbances in mood commonly coexist, with anxiety being the most prevalent symptom. Other symptoms may include depressed mood, euphoria, or irritability and mixed depressed and euphoric moods. Bizarre behavior is frequently present.

The treatment and prognosis are highly variable and depend partly on whether specific complicating conditions coexist. Psychosis and dementia due to HIV disease have a poor prognosis, whereas psychosis and other neurocognitive disorders may respond to effective treatment. Nevertheless, there is some evidence that death occurs earlier in psychotic than in nonpsychotic individuals who have similarly advanced HIV disease.[14] Psychotic symptoms can be managed with low doses of antipsychotic medications.

PATIENT CARE

Health-care interventions involve a holistic approach to care and treatment of the individual with HIV disease that takes into account the physical, emotional, and spiritual aspects of the individual and the family.

HIV Infection: One Man's Story

Where should I begin? Well, I'm 28 years old and I feel as if I died when I was 25; that's when I learned I had been infected. Two and a half years later, and I still find myself asking over and over again . . . what's happening inside of my body? What changes are going on? It's replicating with every breath I take; it makes me wonder, will I remain healthy for several more years or fall victim to the disease and die? Will I suffer, or will I die peacefully? Sometimes it's almost more than I can stand. I can try to maintain a positive attitude, and be optimistic; it's just so darn hard when your dearest friends are also HIV positive and slowly, one by one, they die. This may sound very grim but it's from my heart, and I feel as much pain. I hate the pain, I believe that it's the worst of our experience with the virus, seeing other people suffer and lose their dignity, and their pain is so obvious, I want to know how this could have happened. I feel no identity any longer; before I had it and now that it's gone, I can't remember what it feels like. I hate this virus and what it's doing to my friends, their families and friends, and my family and friends. This is a cruel virus and it's not going to go away any time soon, until a cure is found.

I will survive and exist. I strongly believe that a positive attitude will prolong my life and I really am for the most part "optimistic" that I may be one of the lucky ones spared the horrors this disease offers. I grieve the present, no longer feeling that I'm standing on solid ground, personally. That's vital to me—I don't believe that people realize just what HIV infection takes from us. In some ways this has taught me, I've grown—mentally—so quickly, it has made me realize that life can be over when you least expect it, and also that no matter how short life can be, it should be full of quality, happiness, love and dignity.

I grieve for the people we have already lost, I grieve for the people we are losing every day and I'm also grieving for the millions of people this virus will attack before it's stopped. People need to understand the pain each of us deals with every second of the day that we're awake. It's always there. We try to hide it, put it away; we pretend it isn't there; however, it's there and it's the most empty feeling I've ever felt personally. HIV-positive people have a lot of good to offer. The public (generally speaking) can be harmful to us (the ones HIV positive). Casually, we pose no threat to anyone. Ignorance must be converted into understanding and we need love and patience. I will not deny myself the right to feel the way I do; after all, I still walk in my own shoes. Let's pray for a cure; no one deserves the disease. Together, we can network support for each other, help each other get through this madness and be strong for each other. I know how weak I am at times.... Can we change things? What is real?[9]

ASSESSMENT

The individual experiencing HIV disease requires constant and consistent attention. In many cases, a timely and accurate assessment can mean the difference between independence and physical debilitation, or between life and death. However, the therapeutic relationship between the HIV-infected individual and the clinician can be complicated by factors beyond their control. Assessment of the HIV-infected client should address the individual's knowledge of HIV infection and HIV disease, his or her attitudes and behaviors related to HIV transmission and the course of HIV disease progression, understanding of treatment options for HIV disease, levels of coping and adjustment, and the neuropsychosocial involvement.

For example, a client's anger toward his or her disease or situation may often be directed at the practitioner, which can often hinder a therapeutic practitioner-client relationship. The clinician, by recognizing these signs of anger, can assist the client in recognizing and channeling anger in positive ways. An individual may be increasingly forgetful or apathetic and be identified as nonadherent when he or she misses appointments or inconsistently follows treatment regimens.

The Mini–Mental Status Examination (MMSE) is a global tool that provides a neurological status of individuals based on orientation and ability to perform simple tasks. The MMSE has not been demonstrated to be effective in detecting the subtle neurological changes in individuals with HIV disease. The MMSE used serially has been useful in providing data on neurological deterioration over time. One of the most important ways of detecting subtle neurological changes may be the therapeutic relationship and the clinician's understanding of baseline function for the individual. Through interaction and observation, the practitioner can discern something amiss in the individual's behavior. Through assessing for neurological changes the practitioner will be able to provide early intervention with behavioral and psychosocial support.

Clinicians can incorporate more structured assessments into regular assessments or even into the daily care routine. A simple structured assessment method is to have the individual recite a series of alternating patterns of numbers and letters as quickly possible. For example, have the client recite the alteration between consecutive numbers and letters such as A, 1; B, 2; C, 3; D, 4; and so forth for 15 seconds. The average person can achieve seven or eight without difficulty. An individual with HIV disease experiencing early onset of mild neurocognitive disorder or HIV-associated dementia may be able to achieve only two to four of a series. With severe cognitive impairment, the HIV-infected individual may be able to achieve only one, or possibly none.

Another structured assessment method to assess memory is to ask the client to recite a series of numbers. Most can recall a series of up to seven numbers. If the client cannot remember more than four numbers, memory deficit may be indicated. Sensory function might be assessed by asking the individual to identify sharp, dull, or soft objects touched to the arms, legs, or fingertips while his or her eyes are closed.

Assessment of motor function is concerned with speed, coordination, and mental manipulation. Practitioners assess speed in the individual's gait or the quantity and quality of spontaneous movements. Coordination is evaluated by using standard neurological assessment methods such as touching the nose with a finger with closed eyes, or by alternately pronating and supinating the hands on the thighs. Abstract thinking or problem solving can be assessed to determine an individual's motor function related to mental manipulation. An individual's response to a proverb such as "a stitch in time saves nine" might indicate concrete thinking, which impairs a person's ability to learn new behaviors or to apply past learning to new situations.

How an individual responds to a hypothetical situation might provide information about his or her ability to make important decisions and to solve problems. In a client with mild neurocognitive disorder or HIV-associated dementia, the clinician must assess the individual's functional ability to perform activities of daily living (ADLs). Assessment data may be obtained from the client, family, significant others, and caregivers.

NURSING DIAGNOSIS

Formulating nursing diagnoses for individuals with HIV disease involves considering how the neuropsychiatric effects of HIV may precipitate cognitive, affective, or behavioral symptoms. The nursing diagnoses must be considered within the context of clients' relevant age group and cultural environment. The clinician is usually called upon to provide care that focuses on both the physical and psychosocial aspects of the human experience. This is particularly true among individuals with severe or persistent mental illness who also have HIV disease. Nursing diagnoses that may be relevant in the psychiatric–mental health setting include:

- Thought Processes, altered
- Violence, risk for, directed at self/others
- Body Image Disturbance
- Injury, risk for
- Sensory/Perceptual Alterations
- Self Esteem disturbance
- Social Isolation
- Self Care Deficit, feeding, bathing/hygiene, dressing/grooming, toileting
- Role Performance, altered

- Spiritual Distress
- Anxiety
- Infection, risk for
- Hopelessness
- Grieving, dysfunctional
- Powerlessness
- Family Coping: ineffective, compromised

PLANNING AND THERAPEUTICS

Therapy for individuals with HIV disease is directed at supporting the individual to remain as independent as possible during each stage. The practitioner must attend to the psychosocial and medical aspects of the illness.

Emotions experienced upon being diagnosed as HIV-positive include fear, denial, guilt, anger, and anxiety. Feelings of powerlessness, hopelessness, depression, and social isolation are common. Practitioners must be prepared to provide crisis intervention and counseling to assist individuals in their coping. Normalize the overwhelming emotional responses by assuring the client that many people in this situation experience the same types of feelings and emotions.

Enhance the client's coping abilities by assisting the client to
- Identify internal strengths and abilities
- Identify family members who can serve as a source of support
- Connect with social services available in the community
- Use successful coping strategies used in past times of crisis
- Learn new coping strategies.

Support groups have benefited many individuals living with HIV disease by providing a chance for them to share their experiences and fears. Support groups also serve an important educational role; members can discuss their treatments and ways of solving day-to-day problems.

Individuals living with HIV disease and their families may benefit from family counseling or group support. The family may be defined as the family of procreation or the family of choice. It is the support structure within which the individual gives and receives nurturance, love, and care. Support groups help the family both during the illness and after the death of a loved one, and assist families to maintain a constructive involvement in the day-to-day activities of the person living with HIV disease. Support groups also assist the family with expression and resolution of anticipatory grief.[11]

HIV-infected clients, especially those with neurological complications in the acute care setting, may find it difficult to participate in the unit activities or groups. Some unit practices and program activities may need to be relaxed to accommodate the special needs of HIV-infected clients. A client's decision to reveal or not to reveal her or his HIV status should be respected and supported. The HIV-infected client should be offered the choice of whether to tell other clients within the therapeutic milieu. It is not imperative for other clients to be aware of the HIV-infected client's seropositive status. Universal precautions should be used for all clients regardless of known HIV status.

Intervene to preserve the self-esteem and self-respect of a client with behavioral disturbances. An individual's behavior is more easily redirected than controlled. The environment becomes a focus for therapeutic intervention as the clinician removes agitating stimuli while providing safety. The practitioner may need to teach stress-management techniques or limit contact with anxious family members or friends. Maintaining a therapeutic practitioner-client relationship may be the most important intervention of all. First and foremost, the clinician must retain the unconditional positive regard so commonly discussed in psychiatric settings.

HOPE FOR A FUTURE: PROTEASE INHIBITORS

Since the 1996 11th International AIDS Conference in Vancouver, Canada, **protease inhibitor drugs** have created a sense of optimism for the elimination of HIV. Like most viruses, HIV depends on the host cell it infects to make copies of itself. The new copies of HIV continue to infect other cells and duplicate rapidly. One step in making these new copies is to cut long chains of proteins and enzymes into shorter chains. Protease is an enzyme required in cutting these chains.

Protease inhibitors are drugs that slow the spread of HIV by interfering with the HIV-replication process. Protease inhibitors stop the protease enzyme from cutting the long chains into smaller chains for virus duplication. This interference comes toward the end of the HIV-replication process. At the end of the replication process, HIV has entered the infected cell's nucleus and has made the long chains of proteins and enzymes that will form new copies of HIV.

The new long-chain copies of HIV still push through the wall of the infected cell; however, these new copies are ineffective and are unable to infect other cells. Protease inhibitors can greatly reduce the number of new, infectious copies of HIV. When protease inhibitors are effective, the spread of HIV replication is slowed. Protease inhibitors do not rid an infected individual of HIV, but in clinical trials, these drugs have reduced the amount of virus by 99%. Researchers believe that some already-infected cells remain latent in the body and are not influenced by protease inhibitors.

Four protease inhibitors have been approved for use in the United States, and one is in the final stages of testing in people with HIV infection. Indinavir, ritonavir, saquinavir, and nelfinavir have been approved by the U.S. Food and Drug Administration (FDA) for use in combination with reverse transcriptase inhibitors. Most AIDS experts agree that protease inhibitors should be taken only in combination with the **antiretroviral drugs** called reverse transcriptase inhibitors. No one combination has been demonstrated most effective; the best combination for one person may not be the best for another.

Like other antiviral drugs, protease inhibitors become resistant. Resistance is the ability of HIV to change its chemical structure so that it resists the effects of drug therapies. All viruses can change themselves in this manner. Resistance to a drug may not necessarily mean that a person should stop taking that drug and will never be able to take it again. All of the virus in an HIV-infected person's body does not become resistant to a drug at the same rate. Therefore, the drug can continue to be effective against the many nonresistant viruses still in the body.

Protease inhibitors have created new questions: Has the AIDS epidemic become treatable? Will individuals participate in increased risk behaviors because of the belief in a "cure" for AIDS? Will HIV infection become more of a chronic, manageable disease? Will AIDS become a condition similar to diabetes or hypertension, that when correctly medicated, may allow individuals to live long and productive lives?

VULNERABLE POPULATIONS

THE SEVERELY AND PERSISTENTLY MENTALLY ILL

Many believe that the **severely and persistently mentally ill (SPMI)** are not at risk for HIV infection. However, because of their impairment in social skills and judgment and abuse of substances by some, the SPMI are at high risk for infection. Safe-sex practices are less likely with this population. HIV infection is higher among psychiatric inpatients than in the general population. Prevention and education strategies for the SPMI must be adapted to account for their impairment in concentration, cognitive functioning, and judgment.

In addition to the stigma associated with AIDS, the HIV-infected SPMI client faces the dual stigma of having a potentially fatal illness and a psychiatric disability. The challenges may be further complicated by the SPMI's cognitive impairment, poor judgment, affective instability, poor impulse control, or substance abuse. These challenges for the SPMI are likely to result in high-risk behaviors and practices such as unsafe sexual activity or drug use. An SPMI individual with a history of physical and sexual abuse is vulnerable to others' sexual exploitations and may have insufficient control over his or her sexual behaviors. Many have difficulty with interpersonal relationships, which may complicate their ability to negotiate safe sex practices.

The practitioner must assist the client who is SPMI to modify risk behaviors. The client who has mental illness has to perceive a need for changing risky behaviors and be motivated and committed to change. Social impairment associated with severe mental illness often leaves clients without the social skills and social routines to make needed behavioral changes. The caregiver who wants to assist the SPMI person to change behavior must understand why the SPMI client exhibits the behaviors. Reasons include:

- Most risk behaviors persist because they meet important unmet needs. The clinician must recognize and address these needs.
- Interventions focus on involving the SPMI person's peers and rewarding acquisition of positive attitudes toward safer behavior as a means of motivation.
- The SPMI individual must be an active decision maker. As with most populations, decisions that are based on compliance are less meaningful than those that are based on personal choice. An open examination of personal gains and losses related to changing behaviors is discussed and the clinician's willingness to recognize the client's priorities are acknowledged.
- All-or-nothing options set up the client for extremes of behavior in which rigid compliance can alternate with catastrophic relapse.
- Scare tactics are not useful for the SPMI because they only increase anxiety and escalate impulsive risk behaviors.[13]

The sexual risk of HIV infection for the SPMI population may be overlooked because of the widely held and false view that the SPMI are not sexual beings. Despite these stereotypical views, high-risk sexual activities appear to be common and in many cases may be the means by which the SPMI acquire or transmit HIV infection. Sexual activity for the SPMI may occur throughout the course of illness; it may be impulsive and take place during periods of impaired judgment.

The practitioner adapts prevention and educational interventions for the SPMI client with considerations for poor concentration, impaired cognitive functioning, and impaired judgment. Many SPMI clients have a limited ability to perceive the long-term consequences of high-risk behaviors. They lack cause-and-effect thinking skills and a future orientation. Interventions must focus on the here and now. The practitioner provides the client with relevant, usable, and understandable information. The educational experiences must be brief, simple, and relevant. Risk reduction requires access to condoms and clean needles, which may be difficult for clients who are isolated because of their impairment, are homeless, or live on a limited income.

WOMEN

HIV disease is affecting women at an alarming rate. Women in the United States account for almost 60,000 AIDS cases, and the proportion of women among AIDS cases has increased from 7% in 1985 to 18% in 1994. AIDS is the fourth leading cause of death for women ages 25 to 44. Conservatively, 11 million women worldwide had acquired HIV infection by January 1, 1996.[15] HIV disease follows the same course in men and women, with the exception of Kaposi's sarcoma, which is rare among HIV-infected women, and of women-specific illnesses such as gynecologic disease.[15]

One area the clinician is likely to encounter in managing women with HIV disease is the impact of childbearing and childrearing. Reproductive counseling and the opportunity to make informed choices regarding childbearing is a difficult and extremely sensitive issue of interaction between women living with HIV disease and the practitioner.[15] HIV disease is a long and protracted illness that makes child-rearing a frustrating and difficult job. The inability to fulfill the maternal role can lead to despair and depression.[11]

Women who are HIV infected and are pregnant or plan to become pregnant require HIV education, support, and counseling. Perinatal HIV transmission rates in the United States remain at or below 25%.[15] Opportunistic infections and other serious manifestations of HIV do occur in women with advanced HIV disease. Most women with HIV disease can experience a relatively normal pregnancy.

According to Williams,[15] the psychosocial factors on quality of life for women with HIV disease must be recognized and addressed. Correct information about the effects of HIV and the treatment options for women is imperative. The emotional and physical well-being of women with HIV disease is closely tied to that of significant support in their lives—children, partners, parents, and other family members. The nurse can assist women with HIV disease to use support networks and refer them to social services and support as needed.

SUBSTANCE ABUSERS

The issues of HIV disease and substance abuse are emotionally charged. Substance abusers are often unwilling to trust or believe warnings concerning HIV disease. Intravenous drug users (IVDU) are the second-largest transmission group for HIV disease in the United States. Substance abuse can influence the likelihood of HIV infection in at least two ways. First, sharing of used needles by IVDU can result in direct exposure of HIV into the bloodstream. Second, intoxication and decreased inhibitions can increase the likelihood of having unprotected sexual relations with one or multiple partners.

Individuals with HIV disease who are also substance abusers are doubly stigmatized within society. This group has two chronic, progressive, life-threatening conditions. Practitioners who treat one of the diseases and not the other sabotage the treatment and outcomes for both. Screening for substance abuse should be a part of the routine assessment for persons with HIV disease.

Most HIV-infected substance abusers are not well served by community groups providing services to people living with HIV disease. The major health issues for substance abusers include poor nutritional status, increased stress of the drug-use lifestyle, suppression of immune responses by most drugs that are abused, and histories of infectious diseases among abusers. These health issues make substance abusers a very high-risk population, vulnerable to opportunistic infections after they are infected with HIV.

Therapy for the substance abuser includes control of substance use and prevention of HIV infection. It is unrealistic to assume that simple education will make active substance abusers stop their risk behaviors out of fear of HIV infection. Open and frank discussions about methods to reduce risky behaviors are necessary. Scare tactics are counterproductive. Because many substance abusers use in an attempt to manage anxiety, fear may only elevate anxiety levels, leading to further risky behavior.[13]

The management of HIV disease has moved from acute episodic treatment to the treatment of a chronic illness. Psychiatric–mental health care providers for those with HIV disease will find their work challenging and rewarding. Clinicians must understand the neurobiological and psychosocial impact on the progression of HIV infection and disease. A general risk assessment as well as a sexual and substance-abuse risk assessment will assist them in providing prevention and education. The clinician is in an ideal position to provide encouragement, support, and education to the client and family.

AREAS FOR FUTURE RESEARCH

- What variables (such as hardiness, self-esteem, locus of control, and social support affect the HIV-positive population in maintaining wellness?
- What is the impact of a wellness program on length of survival and ability to manage psychosocial stressors?
- What is the impact of stress on the immune system in HIV-positive individuals? What stress-reduction techniques are most effective in maintaining or boosting immune functions?
- What are the best cognitive, motor, and behavioral interventions in managing mild neurocognitive disorders and AIDS-related dementia in HIV disease?
- What neuropsychological evaluations of the person with HIV disease are most predictive of psychiatric–mental health complications?
- How will new treatments such as protease inhibitors change the emotional well-being and expectations of HIV-infected individuals and families?
- How will life-prolonging treatments affect education and prevention of HIV infection?

KEY POINTS

◆ AIDS, more than any other chronic disease in recent history, is a multidimensional disease that challenges practitioners to use their physical, emotional, and social care skills.

◆ HIV is spread through exchange of body fluids that contain the virus; it cannot be spread through casual contact.

◆ The World Health Organization (WHO) conservatively estimates that 14 million people have been infected by HIV and that by the year 2000, between 30 and 40 million people will have been infected.

◆ HIV infection has become a pandemic affecting every region of the world. HIV is spread worldwide primarily

- through heterosexual contact, with women accounting for 5 of every 11 new HIV infections in adults.
- The counseling for HIV-positive individuals should be tailored for each individual and include an interpretation of the test results and a discussion of the medical, social, and psychological implications of a positive HIV test result.
- The spectrum of HIV disease ranges from an asymptomatic stage to severe immunodeficiency and associated serious secondary infections and neoplasms.
- Losses for the HIV-positive individual and persons living with AIDS are tremendous. AIDS is known as a disease of losses.
- Psychiatric and psychological problems most common for individuals with HIV disease concern mood regulation.
- A basic neuropsychological examination can be very useful for evaluating the cognitive functioning of clients infected with HIV.
- Neurological complications are common in HIV disease, with 10% of individuals presenting with neurological symptoms. Between 60 and 70% of individuals with HIV disease eventually suffer some form of dementia.
- The three main areas for neurological complications in the HIV-infected individual are cognitive, motor, and behavioral disturbance.
- Adjustment reactions are most likely to occur at times of significant medical events or transitional points in the illness, such as manifestation of the first symptoms or the first time the CD4 cell count drops below 200.
- Therapeutic interventions for individuals with HIV disease are directed at supporting the individual to remain as independent as possible during each stage of the HIV disease.
- Universal precautions are required during care of all clients, regardless of known HIV status.
- SPMI persons are at high risk for HIV infection.
- Individuals with HIV disease who are also substance abusers are doubly stigmatized within society.

REFERENCES

1. Bartlett, JG, and Finkbeiner, AK: The Guide to Living with HIV Infection. The Johns Hopkins University Press, Baltimore, MD, 1993.
2. American Health Consultants: Common sense about AIDS: The truth about AIDS. AIDS Alert 8(4):5, 1993.
3. Cassetta, R: The new faces of the epidemic. The American Nurse 25(3):16, 1993.
4. Merson, MH: The HIV pandemic: Global spread and global response. In Abstracts of the IX International Conference on AIDS/IV STD World Congress, vol. I. Berlin, Germany, 11:9, 1993.
5. Chamberland, ME, Ward, JW, and Curran, JW: Epidemiology and prevention of AIDS and HIV infection. In Mandell, GL, Bennett, JE, and Dolin, R (eds): Principles and Practice of Infectious Diseases. Churchill Livingstone Inc, New York, 1995.
6. Novello, A: HIV in adolescence. Report of the Surgeon General's Task Force on HIV in Children and Adolescents and Families. Department of Health and Human Services, Washington, DC, 1993.
7. Agency for Health Care Policy and Research: Clinical Practice Guideline: Evaluation and Management of Early HIV Infection. Publication No. 94-0572. Department of Health and Human Services, Washington, DC, 1994.
8. CDC Update: AIDS—United States. MMWR 44:64–67, 1994.
9. Regional HIV/AIDS Consortium. Speaking Heart to Heart: The Voice of AIDS. Foundation for the Carolinas, Charlotte, NC, 1991.
10. Farizo, KM, Buehler, JW, and Chamberland, ME: Spectrum of disease in persons with human immunodeficiency virus infection in the United States. JAMA 267:1798–1805, 1992.
11. Lego, S: Fear and AIDS/HIV: Empathy and Communication. Delmar Publisher, Inc, Albany, NY, 1994.
12. Erickson, EH: Young Man Luther: A Study in Psychoanalysis and History. WW Norton & Co Inc, New York, 1958.
13. Coalition of Psychiatric Nursing Organizations (COPNO): HIV/AIDS Education for Psychiatric–Mental Health Nurses. American Nurses Foundation, Washington, DC, 1995.
14. Grant, I, and Atkinson, JH: Psychiatric aspects of acquired immune deficiency syndrome. In Kaplan, HI, and Sadock, BJ (eds): Comprehensive Textbook of Psychiatry, VI. Williams & Wilkins, Baltimore, MD, 1995.
15. Williams, AB: Women and HIV/AIDS. Imprint September/October:62–64, 1995.

CHAPTER 33

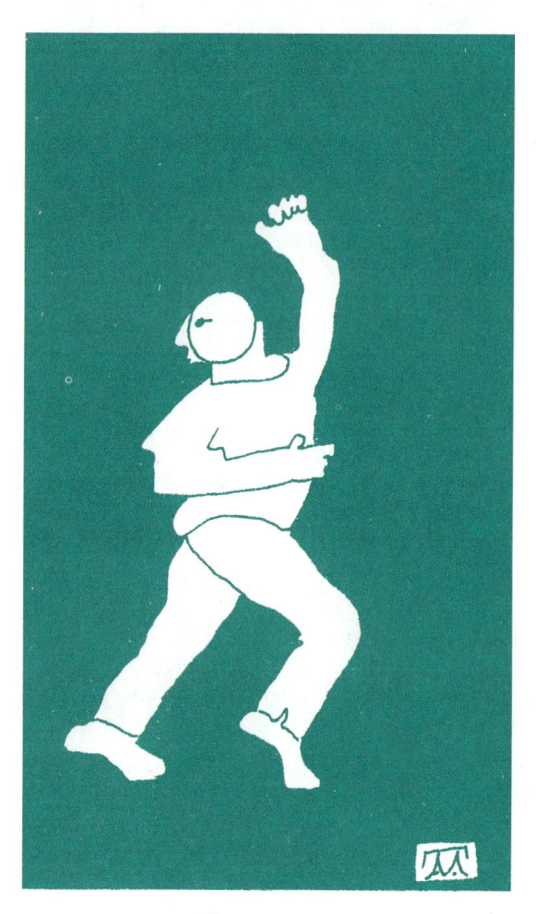

CHAPTER OUTLINE

Characteristics of the Client Population
  The Mentally Ill Offender
  Gender Issues
  Cultural Issues
Conflicting Convictions: Custody and Caring
The Context of Nursing Care in Correctional Facilities
  Nurse-Client Relationship
  Treatment Setting
  Professional Role Definition
  Societal Norms
Areas for Future Research

LEARNING OBJECTIVES

After completing this chapter, the reader should be able to:

- Describe general characteristics of clients in correctional facilities.
- Examine the clinical issues relevant to the development of therapeutic relationships with offenders.
- Identify the diversity in settings in which correctional nurses practice.
- Analyze the challenges of professional role development for correctional nurses.
- Describe the dilemmas embedded in the dual responsibility of providing both custody and caring.
- Evaluate the societal norms that affect the care and treatment of offenders.
- Identify questions for further research in correctional nursing.

KEY TERMS

contextual factors
correctional milieu
inmate
offender
therapeutic milieu

Cindy A. Peternelj-Taylor, RN, MSc

Care of Individuals in Correctional Facilities

The problems surrounding the care and control of the socially undesirable—the criminal, the dangerous, and the mentally ill—have historically plagued society. A milestone in the treatment of this group was reached when individuals were moved from jails to asylums and from asylums to hospitals. Unfortunately, people who are mentally ill and who are believed to have committed a crime, or those who have committed a crime and are believed to be mentally ill, continue to be enmeshed in a system that includes prisons, correctional facilities, jails, asylums, and the mental health–care delivery system.[1-3]

The deterioration of the mental health system following deinstitutionalization, coupled with a vigorous anticrime movement that is currently sweeping the nation, has resulted in an **offender** population that is spiraling upward. The mental health–care needs of this population are as complex and diverse as the nation as a whole (Fig. 33–1). Psychiatric–mental health nursing in corrections is emerging as a new and unique specialty, one of the most exciting and challenging developments in contemporary nursing practice. However, unlike many other specialties, there is little understanding of what correctional nursing represents.[1,4]

CHARACTERISTICS OF THE CLIENT POPULATION

It has been said that correctional facilities not only collect people with psychological problems but also create them.[5] In general, when studying offender populations, one quickly learns that the poor, ethnic minorities, the uneducated, and the mentally ill are overrepresented in correctional institutions. Often the lives of offenders have been marked by illiteracy, poverty, and homelessness. Many lack vocational skills, wander aimlessly, and get involved in the drug trade.[5,6] Furthermore, offenders demonstrate poor reasoning abilities and a history of not learning from past mistakes; many reveal a low tolerance for having requests denied and display uncontrolled, aggressive, and violent behaviors.[7] With **inmate** populations, mental health services must relate to the concerns experienced by the population. North American Nursing Diagnosis Association (NANDA) diagnoses common to the correctional population are listed in Box 33–1.

THE MENTALLY ILL OFFENDER

In comparison to the general population, mental disorders are two to three times more common in prison populations; 10 to 25% of incarcerated individuals require services usually associated with persistent mental illness.[7-9] Three distinct groups may be identified: (1) the mentally ill offender, (2) the offender who becomes mentally ill while incarcerated, and (3) those offenders who are classified as personality disordered[10]

As a psychiatric subpopulation, offenders fall into well-established diagnostic categories in the *Diagnostic and Statistical Manual of Mental Disorders, Fourth Edition (DSM-IV)*. In the correctional environment, most diagnoses are manifested by depression, self-harm, hallucinations, phobias, inability

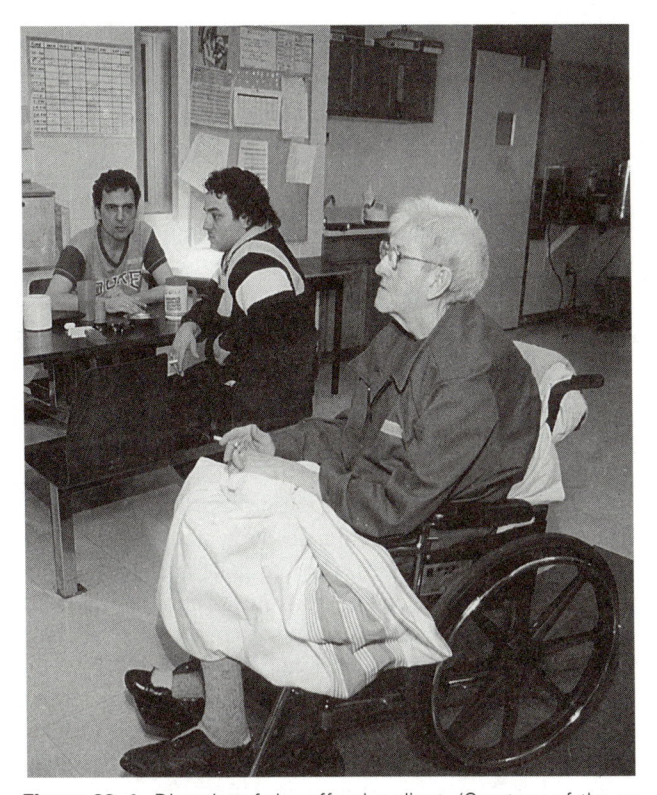

Figure 33–1. Diversity of the offender client. (Courtesy of the regional Psychiatric Centre-Prairies, Correctional Service of Canada. Photographer: David Mandeville, University of Saskatchewan.)

> **Box 33–1. Common NANDA Nursing Diagnoses**
>
> - Anxiety
> - Coping, defensive
> - Fear
> - Coping, individual, ineffective
> - Powerlessness
> - Self Esteem disturbance
> - Self-Mutilation, risk for
> - Sensory/Perceptual Alterations
> - Sexuality Patterns, altered
> - Social Interaction, impaired
> - Social Isolation
> - Thought Processes, altered
> - Communication, impaired verbal
> - Violence, risk for, directed at self/others

to relate to others, withdrawal, regressive behavior such as incontinence and thumb sucking, playing with food, poor hygiene, impulsive behavior, and sexually inappropriate conduct.[5,7,9,11]

A well-documented relationship exists between the rise in illegal drug use and criminality. Many offenders are substance abusers and continue to abuse illegal substances while incarcerated. Frequently, jails and prisons serve as detoxification centers; treatment programs are largely nonexistent, and many offenders who withdraw without medical or nursing care are at risk.[5–7] Many mentally ill offenders are substance abusers who have a tendency to self-medicate with drugs and alcohol because of their impaired mental state. Increasingly, dual disorder is recognized as a significant health-care problem in this population.[8,9]

The stress of the correctional environment can precipitate a psychiatric crisis, and psychotic presentations are often complicated by the coexistence of a personality disorder. Stressors associated with mental illness further compound the offender's ability to adapt to the realities of the correctional environment.[1,3,7]

Correctional facilities experience many challenges in caring for mentally ill inmates. Frequently, the mentally ill lack the social skills and physical strength for survival in the prison subculture, are victimized by other inmates, and endure torment, beatings, and sexual assault. Very often without timely treatment, their conditions deteriorate. Care for this group is inadequate in most situations, and often authorities find it necessary to confine inmates to segregation or protective custody units to keep them free from harm. This forced isolation can cause further decompensation of the illness and puts individual clients at risk for being labeled "crazy," thereby jeopardizing their safety and reintegration upon return to the general prison population.[3,5,9,12,13] The hierarchy assigns the mentally ill offender to the bottom of the pecking order of the prison subculture. In the words of one long-term offender, "It's okay to be labeled violent in the joint, but not crazy."[14]

GENDER ISSUES

In the past, women represented a very small portion of the prison population. Although the correctional population continues to be predominantly male, the last decade has seen a steady increase in the number and proportion of incarcerated females.[5,14]

Women's facilities are often inferior to male facilities, particularly for the female offender in need of psychiatric treatment. At times, female offenders who need treatment are housed in sections of male institutions.[3,5] As a consequence, it becomes necessary to supervise male and female interactions. Female offenders frequently report long histories of sexual violence at the hands of fathers, husbands, boyfriends, and strangers and are vulnerable to personal involvement with male clients (for all the wrong reasons) who are also in treatment.[7] The "jail house" relationships that can develop interfere with therapy, and animosity may build within the **correctional milieu**, as jealousies over intimate relationships develop. Acting out and volatile behaviors are common among women in prisons, and depression is often manifested by anger, fear, frustration, and loss.[3,5]

Adaptation to incarceration is complicated by the forced separation from family and children. Institutions for female offenders are often many miles from home, limiting contact with family members. Women are generally the primary caregivers, and many fear that they will lose custody of their children. Issues with female offenders often center around life inside prison and their families who await their return.[5,7,15]

Loneliness is an inevitable factor in prison settings that can affect and influence health. In a study on loneliness and social interaction, Desmond[14] found that, unlike male offenders, females form relationships with their peers upon entry into correctional facilities. The study concluded that women needed these relationships as a way of feeling accepted or of being in an accepting community and, ultimately, surviving incarceration. Correctional nurses who work with female offenders need to identify isolation as a clinical problem and assist clients in coping with their feelings of loneliness. Visits with children are often a stabilizing factor.[7,14]

CULTURAL ISSUES

In the United States, the inmate population is disproportionately ethnic minorities who are male and between the ages of 16 and 30. Offenders from ethnic minorities are also incarcerated at frequencies greater than expected in both Canada and the United Kingdom.[5,16,17] Depending on the geographic location of the institution, some specific ethnic groups may dominate. Nurses should be aware of the cultural components of illness, including relevant health beliefs, to provide competent nursing care to this diverse group.

Recognizing that traditional psychiatric approaches are often incompatible with Aboriginal or First Nations People, the Correctional Service of Canada has embarked on a partnership with the Aboriginal community to engage Native elders and healers to collaborate with correctional staff and to assist in healing the Aboriginal offender. Native Spiritual awareness, including traditional ceremonial activities—sweet grass ceremonies and sweat lodges—have become commonplace in many Canadian correctional facilities.[9,16]

Dvoskin[7] reports that African-Americans and Latinos who are incarcerated are typically less served by the mental health system. This may reflect an unwillingness to seek help from a predominantly white staff. Conversely, a subtle or even intentional racism may be found among some providers. Hiring staff who are more culturally and ethnically similar to the inmate population being served is recommended.

CONFLICTING CONVICTIONS: CUSTODY AND CARING

Providing mental health–nursing care in an environment in which health-care delivery is not the primary goal leads to many complex challenges for the nurse. Because the priorities of the correctional system are confinement and security, nurses will always face a basic conflict in values. Most often these conflicting philosophies are discussed as polar ends of a continuum—custody versus caring, treatment versus punishment, security versus therapy. Nurses charged with caring for offenders must find a balance between the security limitations of the milieu and the health-care needs of the inmate population. This contradiction, often referred to as *custody and caring*, can be immobilizing; as employees of correctional facilities, nurses frequently "walk the line" between the requirements of security, health care, and client advocacy.[3,4,18,19] Recognizing this dilemma, the American Nurses Association[20] published *Standards for Nursing Practice in Correctional Facilities* in 1985.

It's certainly a lot different than regular nursing, I guess more or less because of the security aspect. You are always taught that safety is a priority . . . so in this case, unless your environment is secure and you are feeling safe in your environment, you can't really go forward and provide the type of treatment that the client needs. Unfortunately, no matter what you do, you still have to be security conscious when you interact with the clients—everyone is a potential threat—yet at the same time, you have to develop a trusting relationship. . . . It's a bit of a conflict, but somehow we manage to squeak through it.[9]

RESEARCH NOTE

Caplan, CA: Nursing staff and patient perceptions on the ward atmosphere in a maximum security forensic hospital. Psychiatr Nurs 7(1), 23–29, 1993.

Findings: The Ward Atmosphere Scale (WAS), a 100-item true-false questionnaire originally designed to assess the social environment of psychiatric wards, was administered to a convenience sample of 70 nurses (69% response rate) and 39 patients (62% response rate). The findings indicate that structure and compliance with ward routine and behavioral standards are the most important factors influencing perceptions of the ward atmosphere.

Nursing staff perceived an above-average emphasis on the importance of planning activities and following schedules and routines, and they perceived that they communicated this emphasis clearly to the patients. The patients perceived emphasis on compliance with ward routine but felt that they did not clearly understand the ward rules or the staff expectations. At the same time, they perceived an above-average amount of staff control and perceived the staff as strict enforcers of behavioral standards and ward and hospital regulations. Nursing staff did not share this perception; instead, they perceived that they exerted minimal control over patient behavior.

Caplan refers to Goffman's work on total institutions to interpret these divergent positions. In correctional settings, nurses have two primary responsibilities: health care and security. In order to maintain this dual role, the emphasis on orderliness and strict behavioral standards in treatment programs represented a nursing intervention designed to maintain a safe, secure, therapeutic environment for treating dangerous patients.

Nursing staff and patients alike are so affected by the reality of violence in the forensic milieu that minimal environmental tolerance for open, unplanned expression of feelings, especially feelings of anger and aggression, was noted. However, despite the ongoing potential for violence, patients perceived above-average levels of concern, helpfulness, and comfort from both their fellow patients and staff. Based on these findings, Caplan concluded that relationships in the forensic setting can be characterized as caring, understanding, encouraging, and helpful.

Despite the ever-present conflict in providing caring within a secure environment, nursing staff in Caplan's study were able to maintain a therapeutic milieu by maintaining the delicate balance between the divergent goals of security and treatment.

Application to Practice: This study provides nurses practicing in correctional environments with an approach to the assessment of the ward atmosphere as perceived by both nursing staff and patients and could prove useful to the evaluation of treatment programs. Replication studies would not only contribute further to the evolving body of knowledge in this emerging specialty but also further assist nursing staff to establish levels of ward structure that enable effective provision of care in a safe manner.

In spite of this conflict, security and health care are not mutually exclusive and can coexist in the correctional environment. Security standards must be maintained to provide a safe environment for staff and clients alike.

THE CONTEXT OF NURSING CARE IN CORRECTIONAL FACILITIES

Caring is the essence of psychiatric–mental health nursing practice. The profession's obligation to this concept is not altered by the fact that the individuals being cared for are inmates and the practice setting the prison.[20,21] The impact of this distinctive environment on both nurses and offenders cannot be underestimated. Additionally, nursing practice in this domain is accountable to the public and reflects the social and political convictions of the society at large.[4,22] As such, the context of nursing care for clients in correctional facilities must be articulated in relation to the treatment setting, professional role definition, and societal values.[23] The profession's ability to adapt to and influence these **contextual factors** is critical in providing high-quality care to offender clients (Fig. 33–2).

NURSE-CLIENT RELATIONSHIP

The ability to establish a **therapeutic milieu** with an offender is important. The nurse-client relationship affects every aspect of the nursing process; it is the means by which nurses are able to assess clients, formulate nursing diagnoses, plan and implement nursing interventions, and evaluate their effectiveness. Four overlapping, yet distinct, phases of this relationship can be identified: preinteraction, orientation, working, and termination.

Preinteraction Phase

Correctional nurses care for a client population that is frequently stigmatized and stereotyped. The personal motivations, beliefs, and values of the nurse can greatly influence the nurse-client relationship. A "caregiver response" is more commonly expressed by nurses when the clients are perceived to be suffering from an illness; a more custodial, judgmental attitude prevails when they perceive that the client is not ill.[24] This attitude is a particular hazard in working with personality-disordered clients.

> *Sometimes it's a little more difficult, I find personally, when I have to deal with someone who has offended against young children, being a mother myself. But you really have to be professional about it and realize what your job is, and why you are here. If I bring those prejudices to my job, I'm not going to be effective with that person. And yet, like I said, being a mother, it is in my head and I think about it occasionally. I think if you don't, you aren't being honest with yourself.*[9]

Students—and nurses in general—have limited exposure to the distinctive attributes common to the offender population. Prior to entering into a helping role with offenders, it is important that nurses have opportunities to express and explore their preconceived ideas about offenders in general and the various alternate lifestyles and subcultures they may encounter.

> *You are going to feel apprehensive because you are dealing with a whole different field, per se. You are dealing with criminals, people who have taken lives and harmed people, physically, mentally, whatever. Don't judge the person, give the individual a chance at being exactly that—a person, an individual—help them to become aware of their behavior, their reasons for that behavior, and give them ideas how to change, help them gain some insight into themselves. I think if nurses can come in with that attitude of not judging, then in a snap, they will have no problem with anyone, period!*[9]

The following questions should be considered before entering a working relationship with offenders:
- What is motivating me to want to work with offenders?
- How do I feel about crimes of violence?
- What are my feelings about murderers, rapists, and pedophiles? Am I able to put my feelings aside and care for the individual who has committed these crimes?
- Can I balance the custodial and caring roles required to practice successfully in the correctional setting?

Orientation Phase

The orientation phase of the therapeutic relationship is frequently long and tense; the nurse's caring attributes are poorly understood by the offender and perceived as a weak-

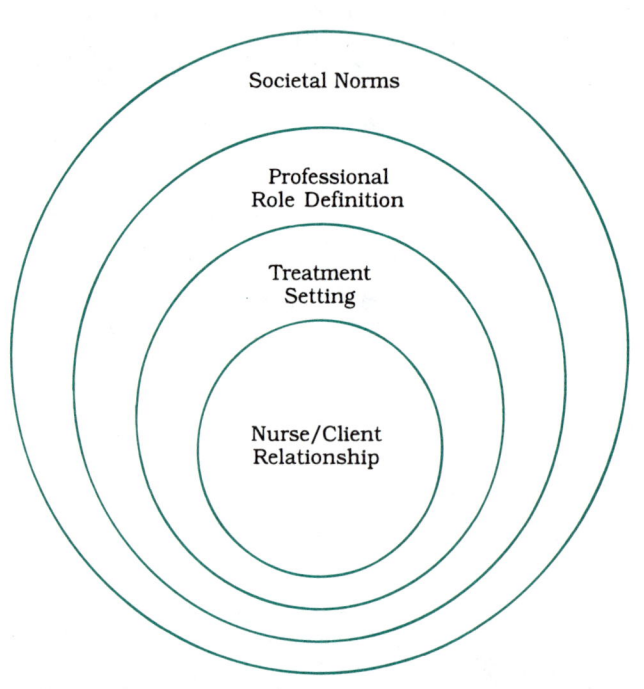

Figure 33–2. The context of nursing care for individuals in correctional facilities. (Adapted from Goering,[23] p 4, with permission.)

ness to be exploited.[1,4,25] Trust and rapport are critical to forming a helping therapeutic alliance; unfortunately, "the culture" of the inmate population does not lend itself to the whole notion of trust, or a trusting milieu. Instead, dishonesty, secretiveness, and paranoia are dominant. Inmates often view referrals for treatment with suspicion, and those who voluntarily seek treatment often have a hidden agenda of gaining "brownie points" for probation or parole.[6,25]

Because of the problems that most offenders have with the concepts of trust and rapport, absolute consistency in keeping scheduled appointments and congruence in verbal and nonverbal communication are recommended.[6] Clients will quickly learn how to relate to the nursing staff if they see the staff using the same approach from day to day and from client to client. Time, patience, and consistency are key.

I see nurses having to role model all the skills we are expecting these clients to incorporate into their behavior change. If I want someone to respect human beings, I believe I have to respect him and model that....[9]

Confidentiality of the nurse-client relationship is not absolute in corrections, and clients need to be informed of this. Those individuals who might be at risk following a therapy session need to be identified and discussed with the correctional personnel, particularly when suicidal, homicidal, or out-of-control behavior is of concern.[6] Furthermore, the disclosure of medical records is often a reality, and nurses may be subpoenaed to testify in court proceedings.

After their initial anxiety of being in a correctional setting, nurses are often shocked and surprised to see that the clients are young, often good looking, and like the "guy next door."[26]

I sat in the dayroom and immediately I had clients around me. It was really good. Sometimes it's hard to remember that these guys are criminals because some of them look really good to talk to. But, I keep reminding myself that they are here for a reason....

In the correctional setting, traditional approaches to therapeutic communication require modification. Major issues of concern relate to the use of touch and self-disclosure.

Touch. Touch is often described as a fundamental means of communication. However, in the correctional environment, the use of nonprocedural touch, other than a handshake, is generally frowned upon. In many cases it is prohibited, particularly between members of the opposite sex, because the touch may be misinterpreted by the client or by others who observe it. Likewise, procedural touch should be approached with caution in the correctional setting, particularly with a client experiencing psychosis and paranoia, who may incorrectly perceive the touch as a form of confrontation and strike the nurse. State the purpose of the touch in a matter-of-fact manner, for example, "I will need to touch your wrist to take your pulse." When intimate care is provided, it should, when possible, be provided by a staff member of the same gender.[3]

Therapeutic Self-Disclosure. In correctional settings, clients frequently ask nurses personal questions. On the surface, some of these questions may appear so insignificant that the nurse may feel awkward or uncomfortable in not disclosing the information requested. However, these requests are often a form of manipulation or a way that the client stays in control of information and the situation. Additionally, many offenders skillfully avoid talking about themselves by having the nurse do all the talking.

You always have in the back of your mind that you aren't supposed to reveal anything too personal about yourself. I find it easier to develop trust and rapport when I share something about myself with my client. In this setting, I find I have to think twice before I speak because I have a tendency to blurt things out. He asked me some direct questions about myself—"Where do you live?" "Boyfriend?" "Married?" I answered what I was comfortable answering, which was most of them. I tried to use humor, that is, "Who needs the hassle of having a boyfriend?" and it went over well....

The intent of therapeutic self-disclosure is to be empathetic and to let the clients know that their thoughts, feelings, and actions are understood by a nurse who is a normal human being.[27] Nurses in correctional environments can respond with caring and empathy by describing feelings without revealing extensive personal detail; self-disclosure should always be directed toward a therapeutic goal.

It was really important for the clients in the stress management group that I was teaching to know some of the things that were stressful for me. One of the exercises was to develop a list in response to the question, "What is stressful for you?" The clients always made sure that I also made a list. It was important for them to know that I had stress and to share that with them. It let them know that I was human too, and that stress is something that we all experience. Often at the end of the group, clients would stay and talk further about individual problems that they were experiencing.[28]

In corrections, good judgment must be exercised in all nurse-client situations. Nurses should reflect upon the following questions before self-disclosing: "Is what I am planning to reveal likely to demonstrate to my clients that I understand them?" "Do I feel comfortable (safe from repercussions and embarrassment, legally and morally secure) about revealing this information to my clients?"[27] If the nurse is unable to answer yes to both questions, then the self-disclosure should be avoided.

The nature of self-disclosure is important to acknowledge. Sometimes I could use it well if I used it generally. For example, in the self-awareness group, when we were talking about feelings and I could say sometimes I have problems too. There was one incident though, where I had gone too far, and it was too personal for me. I could tell there was a difference. It felt uncomfortable and I dropped it right then. It felt like it wasn't being helpful anymore.[28]

Regardless of the nature of the self-disclosure, it is critical to stay client focused and to redirect the interview back to the client, for example, "Is that how you felt?"

Working Phase

During the working phase of therapy, resistance, transference, and countertransference are common. Resistance to self-disclosure and expanding awareness are the greatest barriers to behavior change in this population. Most offenders are masters at denying and minimizing their problems and are reluctant to share their thoughts and feelings with peers or staff; to share is ego threatening and increases their vulnerability. As a result, they become experts at filtering out what they think is irrelevant and interacting on a superficial level.[6]

> Listening to what I have to say is important. It's hard to open up some of the things in my life, there is a lot of hurt there, and if I do open it up, I want the nurses to at least give me the benefit of listening to me and understand where I am coming from, before giving me an off-the-wall answer.[9]

When a therapeutic relationship is established, clients often incorrectly perceive the nurse's warmth and concern as love and caring in an intimate fashion, particularly if the nurse is female, young, and attractive, and the client is male.[9,25,26] Frequently misunderstood behaviors include flirtatious banter, ignoring sexual innuendos, allowing clients to minimize their problems, or relating in an over-friendly way.[26] Interestingly, until 1971, only male nurses were allowed to work with male offenders in Canadian correctional facilities.[29]

In some settings, nursing staff can spend up to 12 hours per day interacting with clients in individual and group activities. With this increased contact, many clients and nurses get to know each other very well. Unfortunately, this close association, coupled with the seductive pull of helping, can contribute to nurses' overinvolvement in their work and violation of the professional boundaries of the therapeutic relationship. The personal safety of nurses, coworkers, and other clients may be jeopardized.[4,30] Although all relationships have the potential for boundary violations, correctional institutions are "hotbeds" for potential problems, and transference and countertransference responses are generated more easily[4] (Box 33–2).

Issues that arise during this phase of the relationship need to be examined and processed within the context of the treatment team. Communication and information-sharing between nurses, other health-care professionals, and the correctional personnel are vital to safe and professional practice. The manipulative demeanor of many offenders makes it too easy to maneuver or "play" the nurse who tries to go it alone. It is not uncommon for offenders to try to pit one nurse against the other, or nurses against the guards, and vice versa.[25]

Nurses who are new to corrections (including students) often have difficulties with the subtleties of manipulation, particularly if their understanding of the role of the nurse in corrections is vague and ambiguous. Comments such as "You are not like the other nurses," "I have never told anyone this before," or "You really understand" can easily boost the fragile self-esteem of the novice, who genuinely and sincerely wants to be a good nurse. Although the clients may be sincere in their observations, these comments must be interpreted with caution.

Survival is dependent on the nurse's ability to question clients' sincerity and become wise to the ways that most offenders operate. Because most nurses are socialized to believe that trust and respect are inherent values of the nursing profession and that a basic goodness exists in all people,[31] adapting to the corrections milieu can be difficult. Self-awareness and recognition of feelings generated during therapy are critical; consultation, support, and mentoring are often required to cope with the magnitude of issues that arise in the correctional setting.

Termination Phase

The work of termination commonly begins during the orientation phase; nonetheless, this last stage is described as both the most difficult and the most important phase of the nurse-client relationship. Although agreement regarding termination between nurses and clients is desirable, it is not always possible in the correctional environment. At times clients may be transferred to other facilities without warning, for their own personal safety or for the safety of others, particularly if they are considered security risks. Violation of a

---

Box 33–2. Outsider

You arrive with a lot of new ideas
Saying that you understand our fears.
But you don't understand a damned thing
Because you don't live here.

You may sincerely want to help
And may try in every way,
But you can never know us—
You don't live here 24 hours a day.

You may be able to see the tensions
And may wish it wasn't so.
But what can you do about it?
You don't live here, so you don't really know.

You may try to make our time easier
And get rid of some of the hate.
But how can you understand;
You're not locked behind this gate.

It may hurt to see hope is gone.
It may pain you to hear us cuss.
But you can never know or understand
Cause you're not one of us.

Anonymous

treatment contract—for instance, drug or alcohol usage or possession of contraband or a weapon—may result in immediate discharge from treatment facilities and return to the parent institutions. Some treatment programs are of fixed duration (for example, 6 months), and many clients may leave the treatment setting prior to feeling a sense of accomplishment or true closure to the therapeutic relationship. Treatment settings are often much pleasanter than parent institutions, and it is not uncommon for clients to regress or create new problems as termination approaches. Assessment for malingering is then required.

Termination is also a time to mutually explore the progress that was made during treatment and the continued work that needs to take place. Frequently, nurses are responsible for the timely completion of discharge summaries and referrals. Transition to the community can be extraordinarily difficult, and most offenders require a higher degree of support and follow-up than other client groups, particularly offenders who have served very long sentences and know no life other than incarceration. Unfortunately, continuity of care is virtually nonexistent for offenders once they leave the correctional system, and many mentally ill offenders experience high rates of recidivism, high symptom levels, and a poor quality of life.[23]

Collaboration with community-based agencies and services is required to assist with the long-term community management of offenders and ultimately to decrease the rate of recidivism. Services required to prevent this group from returning to prison include the early identification of problems, crisis intervention, case management, and housing assistance. Diverting mentally ill clients from the criminal justice system to the mental health–care system must be a priority for all community partners.[1,11]

Termination can also be a difficult time for student nurses, particularly if they feel as if they are leaving their clinical practicum too soon. Often, students are just beginning to gain some confidence with roles in corrections, and their practicum is completed.

I was quite emotional leaving my clinical placement in corrections. Just before I left, all the guys came up to me, shook my hand, and then we exchanged farewells. I was quite choked up by this. I never knew I was so attached to them. Even though they have committed crimes, they are people, too. I think that is one of the most important things I have learned during this placement.

TREATMENT SETTING

The health-care services implemented in the criminal justice system are largely dependent on the jurisdiction, mission of the facility, and the security classification of the offenders. The setting can be jails, prisons, forensic hospitals, locked wards, and correctional facilities; the most common practice site for the correctional nurse is the health-care center operated within the prison system. Such a facility varies in security classification from a community correctional center to a maximum security facility.[3,7,9,11,20] International consensus regarding the best approach to caring for those in custody is largely nonexistent.[12]

Although management of the therapeutic milieu has always been, and will continue to be, a powerful intervention strategy for psychiatric–mental health nurses,[32,33] creating a healing therapeutic milieu in a correctional facility is complicated by societal values, the uniqueness of the environment, the physical setting, the clientele, and the authoritarian interpersonal climate.[1,3,34] The context of care (treatment setting), and institutional protocol, can challenge the nurse's ability to provide the necessary services for the mentally disordered offender.

Security Awareness

Safety and security are major concerns in controlled environments. Security-awareness training prepares nurses to function within the static and dynamic security systems of the facility. *Static* refers to the cameras, bars, fences, and locks; *dynamic* refers to policies, staffing patterns, and methods of operation. Orientation for nurses includes such topics as radio procedures, key control, personal portable alarms, and contraband (Box 33–3). Burrow[34] concludes that these technological artifacts serve to enhance nurses' security

---

Box 33–3. Security Awareness Tips

- Always let staff know where you are at all times, who you will be seeing, and the anticipated length of the interview. Always talk to offenders in designated interview rooms, or in places visible to staff members. Be aware of blind spots and avoid them; maintain good lighting.
- Be aware of the location of offenders in relation to staff members. Use a "buddy system" (e.g., another staff member) any time you are uncomfortable entering an area inhabited by offenders.
- Familiarize yourself with policies and procedures relating to the security of the institution. Observe institutional policies regarding personal protection alarms (body alarms). Ask questions to understand the rationale behind the policies that are in place.
- Dress as per institutional policy. In some settings, nurses wear uniforms or lab coats in order to be easily identified. A professional appearance and decorum are desired. Offenders respect this even though they may not demonstrate it.
- Never take anything out of, or bring anything into, the correctional institution for an offender, no matter how insignificant the request. Administrative approval is always required.
- Report any suspicious behavior as soon as possible. Information sharing is vital to safe and competent nursing practice.
- If a client touches you, even if on the surface it appears accidental, discuss it with the client, and report it to staff members.

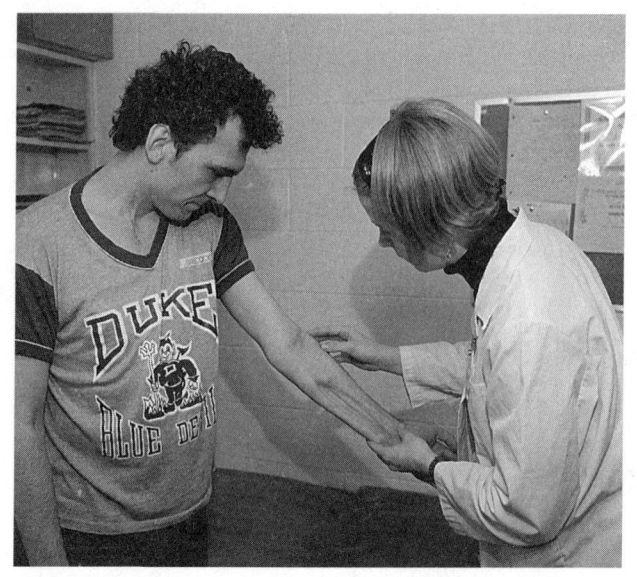

Figure 33–3. Assessment following an attempted suicide. (Courtesy of the regional Psychiatric Centre-Prairies, Correctional Service of Canada. Photographer: David Mandeville, University of Saskatchewan.)

awareness and are essential to the creation of a mental health milieu.

Nurses may eventually become accustomed to the clanging bars, the constant searches, and the casual brutality, but they must never become desensitized to the adversities of correctional environments by adopting a casual attitude toward the activities that go on within the prison walls.[18] A high incidence of sexual assault occurs in both male and female institutions, and young offenders are particularly at risk. These assaults are generally not sexually motivated but carried out to gain power, control, or revenge; offenders may be prostituted by pimps for drugs, smokes, or gambling debts. This degradation may result in a lost sense of safety for the victim.[5,9,18] Inmate violence, deteriorating environmental conditions, and overcrowding exacerbate the stress of institutional life.

Suicide in Prisons

A correlation exists between increases in prison populations and increases in rates of suicide.[18] A retrospective study of inmate suicide found that offenders commit suicide three and one-half times more often than do their nonincarcerated counterparts in the general population.[35] These findings have direct implications for nurses working in correctional environments. Cooperation and collaboration between the health-care staff and the corrections personnel are critical to the successful implementation of a suicide-prevention protocol. Otherwise, offenders in need of treatment may be overlooked, identified as troublemakers, or simply dismissed as manipulative individuals unworthy of attention. Suicide attempts and self-mutilation need to be addressed as a serious breakdown in coping resources for the individual client. Nurses can assist in keeping high-risk inmates safe through accurate assessments, observations, appropriate hospitalizations, and follow-up counseling (Fig. 33–3).

(Following a client's attempted suicide) . . . I'm not sure where to begin. I guess I need to look at myself. I can't imagine being at a point so low that death is the only answer. For the most part, I am surrounded by healthy, happy individuals, people with strong support systems and reasons to get through the day—people with someone to turn to with their problems. Then I look at Jack E and think that this guy is so screwed up. How do I convince him that life is worthwhile? He has nothing. He has extensive neurological damage from repeated substance and solvent abuse, and he is in a maximum security psychiatric hospital . . . his attempt forced me to look at something that I'd always thought was a selfish and cowardly act. However, it made me see the world through his eyes a little better than

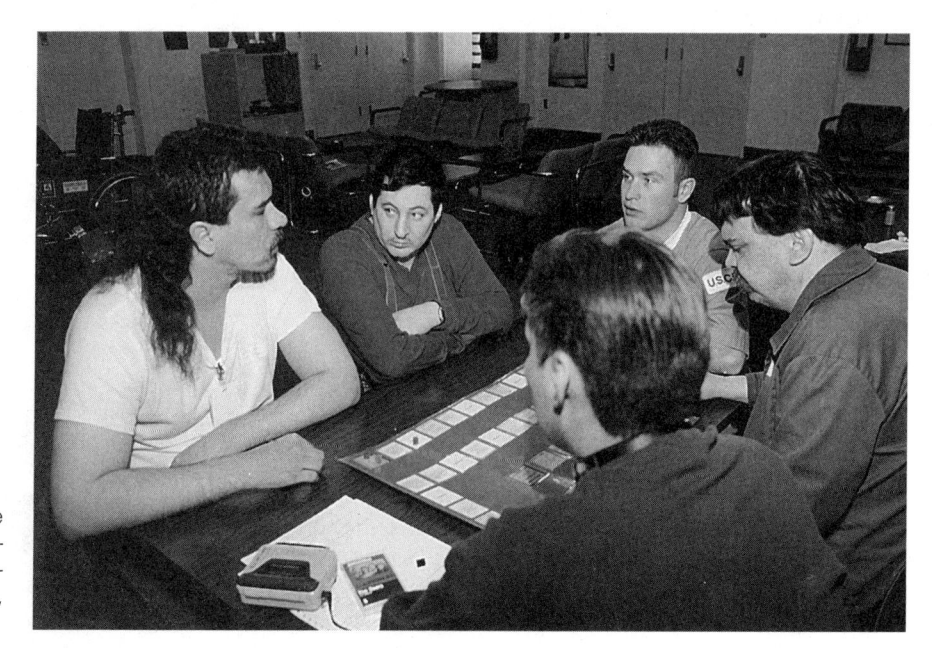

Figure 33–4. Social skills board game (Courtesy of the regional Psychiatric Centre-Prairies, Correctional Service of Canada. Photographer: David Mandeville, University of Saskatchewan.)

I may have before. After talking with him, I realized that he is a man consumed with guilt about his life.

PROFESSIONAL ROLE DEFINITION

Psychiatric–mental health nursing has evolved in response to the social, political, and economic ideologies of society.[2,22] Historically, role development for correctional nurses has been particularly difficult because of the myth that correctional nurses are "second class" and unable to seek employment in more traditional settings. Contrary to this stereotype, psychiatric–mental health nurses need to be highly skilled and able to provide the offender with a level of care comparable to the community standard.[1,9,20] The role of the nurse in correctional settings includes but is not limited to assessing, planning, implementing, evaluating, and coordinating nursing care consistent with the needs of the inmate population. In some settings, long-term access to offenders facilitates a trusting relationship necessary for state-of-the-art mental health treatment programming and case management; elsewhere, the length of stay is so short, and the role of the nurse so minimal, that the nurse may provide only ambulatory and emergency services.[20] Innovation and creativity in adapting nursing care to the correctional environment is the key to success (Fig. 33–4). Roles and responsibilities of the nurse in correctional settings are outlined in Box 33–4.

How the role of the nurse is defined may restrict or enlarge the nurse's image and potential influence within the correctional setting and the community at large. Nurses have a pivotal role in caring for mentally disordered offenders and assisting them to become law abiding citizens (see Research Note). Professional identity, professional isolation, and territoriality are factors impacting on professional role development for correctional nurses.[4]

Professional Identity

One of the greatest challenges facing nurses working in corrections is to remain true to nursing and avoid the seduction of institutionalization and the pull toward the role of the correctional officer, whose functions and responsibilities are more clearly defined.[4,18,19] Nurses working in corrections need to be cooperative with the corrections personnel and collaborate with them, but they must not be coopted into forgoing caring and empathy,[1,36] which leads to failure to individualize client care, limited positive client outcomes, and difficulty establishing trust.[1]

Professional Isolation

Because correctional environments can be lonely and frightening workplaces, to succeed, nurses must adapt to the demands associated with professional isolation and conflicting goal expectations.[1] Depending on the setting and nature of the institution, nurses may work alone or as members of a large nursing team. Nurses may be isolated from other nurses within their institution of employment or, more commonly, isolated from noncorrectional nurse colleagues, who have little understanding of what correctional nursing rep-

---

Box 33–4. Roles and Responsibilities of the Correctional Nurse

Administrative-Research-Clinical Practice-Teaching-Community Service

Psychosocial Evaluation
- Mental status examination
- Mental health screening
- Suicide risk assessment
- Assessment of criminogenic factors
- Identifying individual risk factors

Individual Therapy
- Crisis intervention
- Conflict resolution
- Short-term supportive therapy
- Episodic counseling
- Psychotherapy

Group Therapy
- Therapeutic community
- Anger management
- Empathy training
- Cognitive behavior therapy for relapse prevention
- Substance-abuse treatment
- Sex-offender treatment

Psychoeducation
- Social skills training
- Life skills training
- Health promotion counseling
- Leisure and vocational skills
- Illness management

Psychopharmacological
- Medication administration and management
- Monitoring and evaluating therapeutic efficacy
- Educating clients in mechanism of action, compliance, side effects, and self-care strategies

Milieu Management
- Role modeling socially appropriate behavior and communication skills
- Adapting the nursing process to the correctional client
- Case management

Consultation
- Advocacy for the offender
- Community involvement
- Hostage negotiation (requires specialized training)

Education
- Political advocacy
- Teaching correctional staff signs and symptoms of illness, medication side effects
- Teaching offenders self-care
- Teaching nursing and other health-care students

Research
- Classification of stressors
- Data collection
- Interpretation of research to corrections personnel
- Identification of questions for further research

> **RESEARCH NOTE**
>
> Scheela, RA: Remodeling as metaphor: Sex offenders perceptions of the treatment process. Issues in Mental Health Nursing 16, 493–504, 1995.
>
> **Findings:** The perceptions of 43 adult male sex offenders were examined to generate a grounded theory of the sexual abuse treatment process. Through the use of interviews, direct observations, and record analysis, the "Remodeling as Metaphor" framework emerged to describe the process offenders experience while in treatment.
>
> Participants in Scheela's study described the treatment process as one that involved remodeling themselves, their relationships, and their environments. Six components were identified: "falling apart" both physically and emotionally; "taking on" responsibility for the abuse and deciding to work; "tearing out" the damaged parts; "rebuilding" to make the necessary changes in their lives; doing the "upkeep" to prevent recidivism; and "moving on" to new remodeling projects and life after treatment.
>
> Remodeling as a metaphor offers offenders a concrete, visual, individualized, and safe way to approach the treatment process. Offenders in treatment may experience "falling apart," "taking on," or "tearing out" more than once in treatment and need to see this as part of the remodeling process and not a sign of failure. Furthermore, remodeling indicates that although certain parts of the old structure remain (histories, memories, personality disorders, the abuse), the foundation is strengthened. This concept is critical to sex offenders who need to constantly guard against reoffending and use the remodeling tools to cope with their personal struggles in a healthy and constructive manner.
>
> **Application to Practice:** The remodeling metaphor provides nurses with a conceptual framework to use when working with adult male sex offenders. Identifying and understanding the process helps nurses to provide timely interventions most appropriate to the individual offender. This metaphor may also be applicable to other offenders in treatment and provides a mechanism whereby the treatment process and expectations may be discussed with offenders in a meaningful way. Correctional nurses are in an excellent position to adapt and apply the principles of remodeling in their treatment of offenders in general, to assist them to become safe productive members of society.

resents. Correctional facilities are essentially closed systems, which adds to nurses' isolation.[4,5,19]

Territoriality

Although territoriality is not unique to correctional settings, the concepts of boundary overlap and role blurring are noteworthy in corrections because of the addition of the correctional officer to the treatment team. The priorities of the correctional system center on confinement and security, and these principles always come before nursing care. In terms of professional authority, matters of security often override sound nursing care plans, and decisions related to health care may be taken away from the nurse for the greater good of the institution.[1,9]

Hall[32] concludes that the lack of power and control over nursing practice conditions have thwarted the profession's efforts to study and implement care within the therapeutic milieu.

I don't know if you ever work through it. I think there is always some kind of conflict there between the two obligations, because what is necessarily best for your client, the institution may not approve of, or it may even be contradictory to policy.[9]

SOCIETAL NORMS

Correctional facilities are particularly controversial; various sectors debate their proper function and place in society. The need to provide a humane level of care is defined by society and subject to changing convictions regarding offenders' worthiness.[1,3,4,22] Unfortunately, the current attitude of public animosity toward offenders in general precludes the allotment of more than the absolute minimum to correctional settings.

The "three strikes and you're out" legislation that was passed in California in March 1994 is gaining momentum in other jurisdictions, leading to a general warehousing of offenders in existing correctional facilities. This draconian legislation concerns advocates of the mentally ill.[37] Although these measures were designed as a deterrent to crime, many nonviolent and mentally ill offenders are indiscriminately given 30-year sentences without consideration for the seriousness of the crime or, more important, their mental status. Many believe this legislation will further perpetuate the criminalization of the mentally ill.[13,37,38] Lego[39] concludes, "As state hospitals empty, forcing people into the streets, and as policies such as mandatory drug sentencing and 'three strikes and you're out' continue, prisons are becoming the 1990's state psychiatric hospital."

Working in correctional environments forces nurses to contemplate the broader health issues that face society—interpersonal and family violence, substance abuse, housing, education, and poverty. How might a nurse approach these issues? Who is responsible for primary crime prevention, justice, or health? How might nurses collaborate with community agencies and bridge the gap between the justice system and the mental–health care system? The following story may inspire the reader to ponder this critical contemporary problem.

> Confucius was hired to run the jails in his home province in China. The legend says that within 2 years he had managed to empty the jails. When asked how he did it, he explained that those in jail were the poor, or

the children of the poor; or the ignorant, or the children of the ignorant. He went on to explain that he took the next logical step and educated the ignorant and provided the poor with the skills to earn a living.[40]

Certainly it would be a gross oversimplification to suggest that any one factor such as poverty, lack of education, or illiteracy is the sole cause of criminal behavior and ultimately crime. However, it would be irresponsible to ignore the combined impact of these factors. Osborne[41] challenges all nurses to "examine the moral dilemma of supporting a society that incarcerates increasing numbers of its citizens in both correctional and mental institutions—often carelessly failing to make distinctions between these institutions."

AREAS FOR FUTURE RESEARCH

Peplau[2] observes that changes are made by nurses who observe new challenges in the field of psychiatric nursing care. Correctional nurses, as members of a dynamic and evolving specialty, often have the most intensive contact with offender clients, and therefore issues influencing crime, violence, victimization, and criminalization of the mentally ill are relevant to nursing curricula.[42] Correctional nursing represents a gold mine of learning opportunities for student nurses and is a challenging and rewarding nursing experience. There is a great need for nurses with basic and advanced preparation to embrace correctional nursing and address offenders' complex problems. Scales and associates[43] invite correctional nurses to "come out of the closet" and educate the public and the profession about the exciting and rewarding work done by nurses in correctional facilities.

Continuing education and professional development relevant to and grounded in the practice setting are essential to the advancement of correctional nursing as a specialty. Since 1989, the College of Nursing, University of Saskatchewan, in collaboration with the Regional Psychiatric Center—Prairies, Correctional Service of Canada, have sponsored a biennial nursing conference that focuses on the unique clinical and work-life issues that affect nurses working within the criminal justice system. The ongoing evolution of correctional nursing as a specialty is further dependent on the establishment of a research culture that supports and nurtures the development of nursing research.[4]

Although nurses have been writing about correctional nursing for more than a decade, the literature remains largely anecdotal and requires nurses to further explore relevant problems from a qualitative and quantitative research perspective. Similarly, evaluation and outcome studies are required to demonstrate program efficacy, with recommendations geared specifically to research-based practice.

- How do nurses carry out a therapeutic role in corrections? How long does the orientation phase last?
- Caring for many offender clients challenges the empathic skills of the nurse. How do nurses care for an offender who has committed a repugnant and heinous crime?
- What are the common countertransference responses experienced by correctional nurses? What is the best approach to dealing with these responses?
- What coping strategies do correctional nurses adopt in caring for the mentally disordered element of society?
- How do the behaviors of staff and clients affect the potential for aggression within the correctional milieu?
- What is the role of the nurse in primary prevention? How might success be evaluated?

This chapter has focused on the unique role of the psychiatric–mental health nurse in providing care to individuals in custody. The correctional nurse can have a significant impact on the health and well-being of offender clients by attending to the contextual factors affecting psychiatric–mental health nursing in the correctional milieu.

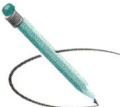

Key Points

- Correctional nurses are members of a dynamic specialty, changing to meet the needs of the mentally disordered offender and the public at large. Nursing practice in most correctional settings is characterized by a high degree of autonomy.

- Deinstitutionalization, homelessness, criminalization of drug abuse, and dwindling community mental health services have all served to accelerate the movement of individuals from the streets to the correctional system.

- Offenders present with complex and multifaceted issues compounded by environmental and social factors unique to the correctional milieu. Common NANDA nursing diagnoses are identified.

- The opposing philosophies of custody and caring result in direct implications for nurses working in correctional environments. Nurses constantly "walk the line" between the requirements of security, health care, and client advocacy.

- Therapy issues with the inmate population are complicated. The ability to establish a therapeutic nurse-client relationship is the most important competency required by nurses in correctional settings. Modification of therapeutic communication strategies may be required.

- Historically, role development for nurses working in corrections has been difficult. Correctional nurses must grapple with issues surrounding professional identity, professional isolation, and territoriality.

- Correctional nurses are actively involved in a continuum of care that includes crisis intervention, early identification of problems, acute inpatient psychiatry, and rehabilitation of offenders with long-term mental illness.

- Specialized programming often includes suicide prevention, management of self-mutilation, aggressive-behavior

control, sex-offender treatment, and substance-abuse management.
- Attending to the contextual factors—nurse-client relationship, treatment setting, professional role definition, and societal norms—allows nurses to provide care to inmate populations.

CASE STUDY

George T was a 32-year-old man serving time in a federal prison. He had a long psychiatric history and had been transient and homeless most of his adult life. He was a self-proclaimed "street person" who had spent time in foster homes, psychiatric units, shelters, low-rate inner city hotels, jails, and prisons. Many of his criminal charges stemmed from experiencing symptoms of illness in public places, and he was charged twice with assaulting a police officer. He was serving a 5-year sentence for aggravated assault in a maximum security institution.

He grew up in a rural community, the eldest of three boys, and generally did well in school until grade 8. In high school he was described as "odd" and began having problems with his friends and his teachers. He seemed to be frightened all the time and had difficulty concentrating on his school work. He began to experiment with alcohol and drugs and smoked pot regularly. His mother was very concerned about her son's odd behavior and understood his drug use as a symptom of a much greater problem. His father, however, thought all he needed was "a good swift kick in the pants" and believed that his problems could easily be cured by hard physical work around the farm.

At age 16, George quite school and left home, believing that his brothers and parents were part of an intricate conspiracy to harm him. He cut off all communication with his family and only once tried to contact them. He had no job, no money, and quickly found himself involved in criminal activities—shoplifting, vandalism, and drug trafficking.

His first winter away from home, he was identified by an outreach worker as an individual in need of mental health services, and arrangements were made for his placement in a shelter for the homeless. His stay in the shelter was short-lived; he assaulted a staff member with a hammer, believing that the worker was poisoning his food. Charges were laid, and he was ordered to spend time at the local psychiatric facility for a psychiatric assessment. He stayed only a few days before he assaulted a psychiatrist and the nurse who was attempting to give him his medication. He ran away from the hospital and believed that if he moved west everything would be okay.

In his early 20s he found himself certified and treated against his will in a state psychiatric facility. He responded favorably to medication and participated in individual and group therapy. He was subsequently discharged and lived in a one-room apartment in the community. Although he had done well in the program, he had difficulty maintaining his treatment regimen, and without sufficient professional support, he quickly relapsed. When he was well, he said he had schizophrenia and stated, "I could use someone to take care of me."

George had recently been transferred to the psychiatric unit from the general population of the prison. Correctional staff observed that he had not attended his job in the laundry for 3 days, was frequently absent at meal times, and was withdrawing from the other inmates with whom he usually associated. Their report stated that he looked "spooked" and they were concerned about his safety because the other inmates were referring to him as a "goof" (crazy). He refused all offers of help, stating he was not ill and that the medication was poison. He was certified based on the knowledge that he was too ill to make a rational decision regarding treatment.

While in the psychiatric unit, he purposefully avoided staff and other clients and stated, "The more I interact with others, the more I lose focus on the conspiracy at hand." He isolated himself in his room and spoke only when striking out at individuals who he believed were part of the conspiracy. At times he participated in off-ward activities, "to avoid the poisonous gas that was being released through the vents in his room." He attended exercise time regularly, as he believed he was "training for the end."

Although George was a small man, the nurses and correctional officers were intimidated by him; he had a long history of assaults against staff. As a result, a pattern of staff avoidance ensued with this client. The staff related "stories" of previous attempts at treating this client and feared for their personal safety.

CRITICAL THINKING QUESTIONS

1. Discuss the stressors that George may have experienced during his incarceration.
2. What additional information does the nurse need to assess at this time? Identify the potential sources of data collection.
3. What assumptions might the staff be making about George? How are these assumptions directing their behavior? What approach should be used to gain George's confidence?
4. What short-term goals might be established with this client?
5. What concerns might the nurse have regarding George's prognosis upon his release from prison? What additional factors will the nurse consider in planning for his long-term case management?

REFERENCES

1. Hufft, AG, and Fawkes, LS: Federal inmates: A unique psychiatric nursing challenge. Nurs Clin North Am 29(1):35, 1994.
2. Peplau, HE: Psychiatric mental health nursing: Challenge and change. J Psychiatric and Mental Health Nursing 1(1):3, 1994.
3. Phillips, RTM, and Caplan, C: Administrative and staffing problems for psychiatric services in correctional and forensic settings. In Rosner, R (ed): Principles and Practice of Forensic Psychiatry. Chapman and Hall, New York, 1994.
4. Peternelj-Taylor, CA, and Johnson, RL: Serving time: Psychiatric mental health nursing in corrections. J Psychosoc Nurs Ment Health Serv 33(8):12, 1995.
5. Bernier, SL: Mental health issues and nursing in corrections. In McFarland, GK, and Thomas, MD (eds): Psychiatric Mental Health Nursing. JB Lippincott Co, Philadelphia, 1991.
6. Rynerson, BC: Cops and counselors. J Psychosoc Nurs Ment Health Serv 27(2):12, 1989.
7. Dvoskin, JA: The structure of correctional mental health services. In Rosner, R (ed): Principles and Practice of Forensic Psychiatry. Chapman and Hall, New York, 1994.
8. Jemelka, R, Trupin, E, and Chiles, JA: The mentally ill in prisons: A review. Hospital and Community Psychiatry 40:481, 1989.

9. Peternelj-Taylor, CA, Johnson, RL (producers), and Bulk, F (director): Custody and Caring: A Challenge for Nursing [video]. (Available from Division of Audiovisual Services, University of Saskatchewan, 28 Campus Drive, Saskatoon, SK S7N OX1), 1993.
10. Canadian Nurses Association: Mental Health Care Reform: A Priority for Nurses. Canadian Nurses Association, Ottawa, 1991.
11. Burrow, S: An outline of the forensic nursing role. Br J Nurs 2(18):899, 1993.
12. Conacher, GN: Issues in psychiatric care within a prison service. Canada's Mental Health 41(1):11, 1993.
13. Torrey, EF, et al: Criminalizing the seriously mentally ill: The abuse of jails as mental hospitals. Innovations and Research 2(1):11, 1993.
14. Desmond, AM: The relationship between loneliness and social interaction in women prisoners. J Psychosoc Nurs Ment Health Serv 29(3):5, 1991.
15. Umlauf, MG: Women in white. Nursing Forum 27(1):12, 1992.
16. Correctional Service of Canada: Annual Report of the Regional Psychiatric Centre (Prairies). Correctional Service of Canada, Saskatoon, 1992.
17. Faulk, M: Basic Forensic Psychiatry, ed 2. Blackwell Scientific Publications, London, 1994.
18. Alexander-Rodriguez, T: Prison health: A role for professional nursing. Nurs Outlook 31(2):115, 1983.
19. Gulotta, KC: Factors affecting nursing practice in a correctional health care setting. Journal of Prison and Health Care 6(1):3, 1987.
20. American Nurses Association: Standards of Nursing Practice in Correctional Facilities. ANA, Kansas City, 1985.
21. Kent-Wilkinson, A: After the crime, before the trial. The Canadian Nurse 89(11):23, 1993.
22. Osborne, O, and Thomas, MD: On public sector psychosocial nursing: A conceptual framework. J Psychosoc Ment Health Serv 29(8):13, 1991.
23. Goering, P: Psychiatric nursing and the context of care. In Lamb, HR (series ed) and Chafetz, L (vol ed): New Directions for Mental Health Services: No 58, A. Nursing Perspective on Severe Mental Illness. Jossey-Bass Publishers, San Francisco, 1993.
24. Nussbaum, D, Lang, M, and Repaci, R: How forensic mental health staff cope: Results of a preliminary study. Forum on Corrections Research 5(1):19, 1993.
25. Dighton, S: Tough minded nursing . . . correctional nursing. AJN 86(1):48, 1986.
26. Petryshen, P: Nusing the mentally ill offender. The Canadian Nurse 77(6):26, 1981.
27. Balzer-Riley, JW: Communications in Nursing, ed 3. Mosby, St. Louis, 1996.
28. Peternelj-Taylor, CA (producer), and Bulk, F (director): Psychiatric Nursing Practicum in Corrections [video]. (Available from Division of Audiovisual Services, University of Saskatchewan, 28 Campus Drive, Saskatoon, SK S7N OX1), 1994.
29. Smale, SL: Nursing behind bars: A decade of change. The Canadian Nurse 78(7):31, 1983.
30. Gallop, R: Sexual contact between nurses and patients. The Canadian Nurse 89(2):28, 1993.
31. Stevens, R: When your clients are in jail. Nursing Forum 28(4):5, 1993.
32. Hall, BA: Use of milieu therapy: The context of environment as therapeutic practice for psychiatric mental health nurses. In Anderson, CA (ed): Psychiatric Nursing 1974 to 1994: A Report on the State of the Art. Mosby, St. Louis, 1995.
33. Walker, M: Principles of a therapeutic milieu: An overview. Perspectives in Psychiatric Care 30(3):5, 1994.
34. Burrow, S: Inside the walls. Nursing Times 89(37):38, 1993.
35. Suicide prevention: Working toward a better approach. Let's Talk 19(3):6, 1994.
36. Standing Bear, ZG: Forensic nursing and death investigation: Will the vision be co-opted? J Psychosoc Nurs Ment Health Serv 33(9):59, 1995.
37. Jacobs, C: "Three strikes" = 30 years for mentally ill man. NAMI Advocate 16(5):3, 1995.
38. Honberg, R: Harsh crime measures could be trouble for offenders with mental illness. NAMI Advocate 16(5):3, 1995.
39. Lego, SF: Review of the book Live from Death Row. Journal of the American Psychiatric Nurses Association 1(5):174, 1995.
40. Strauss, JM: Public ignorance: Whose problem is it? Let's Talk 19(3):14, 1994.
41. Osborne, OH: Editorial: Public sector psychosocial nursing. J Psychosoc Nurs Ment Health Serv 33(8):4, 1995.
42. Lynch, VA: Editorial: Forensic nursing: What's new? J Psychosoc Nurs Ment Health Serv 33(9):6, 1995.
43. Scales, CJ, Mitchell, JL, and Smith, RD: Survey report on forensic nursing. J Psychosoc Nurs Ment Health Serv 31(11):39, 1993.

CHAPTER 34

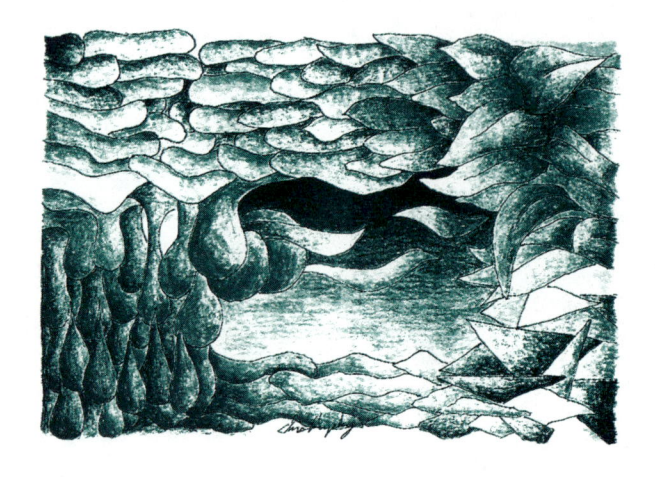

CHAPTER OUTLINE

Characteristics of the Grieving Process
Types of Grieving Experienced by Clients
The Context of Nursing Care in the Grieving Process
  The Nurse-Client Relationship
  Assisting Clients in the Grieving Process

LEARNING OBJECTIVES

After completing this chapter, the reader should be able to:

- Describe general characteristics of clients experiencing grief.
- Understand the grieving process and pinpoint where clients are in that process.
- Understand the differences among grief reactions and differentially diagnose grief reactions versus other conditions such as major depression.
- Identify questions for further research in the area of grief reactions.

KEY TERMS

anticipatory grieving
grief
healthy grieving

Shari Petronis-Gibson, MSW, LSW

Grieving

Every death represents a person with family members and friends who experience their loss and grieve. As common as this experience is, professionals often have great difficulty reaching out to those who are grieving. This chapter provides general guidelines for understanding the stages of the normal grieving process, which all who are experiencing grief go through. Professionals have to be able to define and distinguish this normal process from bona fide mental health problems such as depression.

In her seminal work, *On Death and Dying*, Elisabeth Kubler-Ross[1] outlined five stages that each individual passes through in a normal grieving process:

- Denial and isolation
- Anger
- Bargaining
- Depression
- Acceptance.

These stages constitute the traditional framework within which the grieving process has been viewed.[1,2] More recently, researchers and authors have reframed the stages of the grieving process to reflect the basic, universal parts of the process experienced by those who grieve. These stages place more emphasis on the tasks that grieving individuals must undertake and accomplish to effectively grieve a loss.

CHARACTERISTICS OF THE GRIEVING PROCESS

> Sara A is a 68-year-old woman who was recently widowed. Her husband experienced a long battle with cancer, during which Sara was emotionally supportive. At the end of his illness, Sara provided care for her husband at home with the help of a hospice home care program; care included visiting nurses, social workers, and volunteers who provided help with cooking and cleaning. Now that her husband is gone, Sara has gone back to some of her former hobbies, such as playing bridge and traveling. Her friends are surprised that she has taken his death so well. Sara has periods when she breaks down and cries while remembering her husband, but these periods are less frequent than they were 6 months ago, when he died.

Sara A went through a great deal in the 6 months since her husband died and in the period during his illness. Although Sara knew that her husband's death was impending, her initial response to his death was overwhelming shock, followed by a period of emotional numbness. It is not uncommon for family members or friends to cry out when they first learn of the death of a loved one. This initial period may also be marked by disbelief that the loved one is actually dead, especially if the death was not anticipated or was due to an accident.

Denial of the death of a loved one may play an important psychological function in preventing the family member from becoming completely overwhelmed and overwrought upon hearing the news. This period may allow the bereaved individual to slowly come to the full realization that his or her loved one has died. Denial may persist beyond the early stages of the grieving process. The best recent societal example of this denial is the never-ending series of "sightings" of Elvis Presley. Bereaved individuals have the sensation of catching a glimpse of their deceased loved ones or may inadvertently set a place at the table for them days, months, or even years after the death.

Bereaved individuals, either during or after a period of denial, often experience feelings of numbness, during which they feel little, if anything at all. This numbed state may have an important function for the psyche, enabling the bereaved person to attend to the details surrounding the death, including planning and attending a wake and funeral, receiving guests and condolence calls, and dealing with the finances and the insurance matters necessary to close an estate.

The second stage is marked by fully experiencing the many emotions involved in the grieving process. After numbness, shock, and disbelief subside, the death becomes a reality, and the bereaved person begins to fully experience the loss of the loved one. This period, which may last from a few months to a period of years, may be marked by confusion, unstable moods, sadness, anxiety, guilt, and anger.

Recently bereaved individuals may appear to be confused and disorganized. They may have difficulty coping with the tasks of daily living and forget to do the grocery shopping, pay bills, or return telephone calls. Those close to the bereaved may comment on how they seem to be "not themselves" since the loss.

Periods of emotional instability are common. One moment the bereaved individual may appear calm and well-adjusted and may the next moment experience overwhelming feelings of sadness and begin to cry. Those experiencing grief have described this period as an emotional roller coaster of ups and downs and unpredictable behavior. One grieving man stated, "If I don't like the mood I'm in at a given point, I never worry about it very much because my mood will change to something else pretty quickly."

The sadness experienced by grieving individuals may seem overwhelming and disabling at times. One bereaved man described periods of uncontrollable crying during the work day, as he waited for the traffic light to turn green when driving in his car, and during his daughter's ballet recital. Some of these experiences reminded him of his wife; some of the crying episodes were unexplainable. Although the frequency and intensity of these periods generally decreases with the passage of time, they may increase during stressful times and near the anniversary of the loss. Others who are grieving may experience periods of great anxiety, during which the grieving person may become restless, unable to concentrate, and panicked at the thought of performing even the smallest, most routine tasks of daily living. At times, anxious bereaved persons may fear that they are dying. Periods of anxiety, similar to periods of sadness, appear to lessen in frequency and intensity with time but may reappear during difficult times and at the anniversary of the death of the loved one.

Those who are grieving often experience and express feelings of guilt.

> One older woman whose husband had complained of stomach discomfort for a few hours before he died of a massive heart attack expressed her guilt at not recognizing his symptoms and taking them more seriously. "I told him to take an antacid and encouraged him to take a nap," she said. "If only I had taken him to the doctor or the emergency room, he might still be alive today. I think about this all the time. I can't sleep at night sometimes because I feel so guilty."

Others who grieve express guilt about the quality of their relationships with those deceased. A daughter may feel guilty that she did not visit her mother more often before she died. A husband may express guilt that he did not take his wife on the trip to Florida that she had been asking for before she died. The degree of emotional closeness between the deceased person and the grieving family member or friend may not be determinative of the amount of guilt experienced or expressed.

Many grieving people are angry: angry that those they loved died and left them alone, angry at the illness or physicians or hospitals who treated the loved one. Some grieving people are justifiably angry at the criminals who murdered their loved ones or the drunk drivers who killed them. Others who grieve are angry at themselves for their behavior towards the deceased. Some grieving people feel overwhelming periods of anger and rage, during which they vent this anger at other family members or friends. Still others whose faith is important to them may be angry at God for taking their loved ones away from them.

The final stage of the grieving process is acceptance, during which the grieving person can assimilate the loss into his or her life, accept the loss, and begin the task of rebuilding life without the loved one. Although many expect those who are grieving to recover quickly and to reach this stage in weeks or months, realistically, some who grieve need a much longer period to experience the loss before reaching this last stage. One older man's family knew that he had reached the final stage of his grieving process when, 4 years after his wife had died unexpectedly, he was finally able to store her clothing in the attic and honor her dying request to give a few items of her jewelry to her daughter. Others are finally able to talk openly about their loved ones, remembering both their good qualities and idiosyncrasies and honoring the fullness of their relationships. During this final stage of the grieving process, the survivors may have found some source of hope that allows them to carry on their lives. They may once again feel in control of their lives. Most important, in the final stage people can select and incorporate into their lives memories of the deceased that are both positive and reflective of the person's true character.

TYPES OF GRIEVING EXPERIENCED BY CLIENTS

Most often, grieving is associated with feelings of sadness. **Healthy grieving** may also include feelings of anger, frustration, guilt, and sorrow. Everyone experiences losses differently, so the way that one client grieves may be very different from the way another experiences a similar loss.[3]

Different types of losses may lead to different grieving processes. A family member who loses a loved one unexpectedly as a result of a traumatic injury (such as a motor vehicle accident or a violent murder) may experience a strong initial feeling of denial. Feelings of extreme anger may follow. Family members and friends of suicide victims may experience overwhelming feelings of guilt or anger that persist for months or even years.

In the previous example, Sara A and her husband knew for 6 months of his impending death and had a chance to process their feelings about his illness. Sara A went through a period of **anticipatory grieving**, during which she saw her husband lose his health and many of his abilities, including his ability to work and, eventually, his ability to care for himself. Sara A experienced, in a sense, her husband's death slowly over several months. As a result, when her husband finally died, Sara had already begun her grieving work with the help of his hospice nurse and chaplain.

Men and women may grieve differently. Stereotypically, men are expected to grieve and mourn quietly and privately, whereas women are expected to be more emotionally expressive. These stereotypes may create expectations that are very difficult for grieving individuals to fulfill. As a result, some older men, socialized to suppress their emotions, are so effective at denying their feelings that they fail to recognize them. Emotions that are not dealt with may lead to dangerous or inappropriate expressions in the form of *externalization* (ventilation of anger toward undeserving family members or friends) or *internalization* (including self-abusive behaviors like abuse of alcohol or drugs, self-neglect that leads to personal-care deficits, or the development of medical problems).

Similarly, older women who may be expected to grieve in a more emotionally demonstrative way may be tempted to label their grief as depression. They may readily accept this diagnosis from mental health professionals and numb the pain of their grief with antidepressants, antianxiety medications, or other psychotropics.

Both men and women may experience prolonged periods of sadness that may result in unresolved grief. The symptoms of unresolved grief may parallel those of depression: changes in weight, eating, and sleeping patterns and loss of interest in formerly pleasurable activities. Social withdrawal and feelings of hopelessness and worthlessness may also be present.

As a result of advances in medical treatment, people are living longer lives than ever before and experiencing more losses throughout their lives. Older adults may, as a result, experience *cumulative grief*, as a result of multiple losses within a few years, including spouses, several close friends, beloved pets, and their own physical health. Added to these may be job loss as a result of planned or forced retirement, loss of caregiver roles for ill relatives who died, and the loss of financial and emotional security that these relationships provided.

THE CONTEXT OF NURSING CARE IN THE GRIEVING PROCESS

THE NURSE-CLIENT RELATIONSHIP

Grieving is a universal experience that may occur at any point in life. Although it is more anticipated and expected in later life, younger adults and children also grieve. The nature of the nurse-client relationship and the role of the professional nurse may change, depending on the age and ethnicity of the client and the type of grief the client is experiencing.

ASSISTING CLIENTS IN THE GRIEVING PROCESS

No two clients grieve in the same way. The task of the nurse is to assess the expressed needs and unmet needs, strengths, and existing support systems of the grieving client, taking into consideration that everyone's grief experience is unique. The nurse has to reassess and anticipate needs and issues frequently as the client passes through the stages of the grieving process.

As seen in Table 34–1, the needs of grieving children require special attention.[4] Young children are limited in their abilities to understand and deal with the loss of a friend or family member. It is often helpful to explain death to very young children by using terms and phrases that are simple and familiar. For example, very young children may not fully understand the details of a grandparent's death, but affirming their understanding that their grandfather had been ill

TABLE 34–1. Children's Understanding of Death

Age	Understanding of Death	Common Behaviors in Response to Death
Infant/toddler	• Unable to comprehend death • Fears separation and abandonment	• Frightened, difficulty separating
3–5 years	• Views illness as punishment for real or imagined wrongdoings • May view death as sleep; cannot comprehend death • Magical thinking; may think they caused the event by their thoughts or actions	• Sadness • Clinging to parent • Nightmares, sleep disruption • Regression in toilet habits • Complaints of stomachache and headaches • Temper tantrums
School age	• Associates death with punishment, mutilation, violence • May feel responsible for event • By age 9, understands that death is final	• School phobia, diminished school performance • Aggressive behavior • Preoccupation with parent's health • Loss of appetite • Change in relationship with friends
Adolescence	• Understands own mortality • May seem to have adult view of death but not emotional view	• Acting out; substance abuse • Increased time with peers • Withdrawal from family • Depression

Source: With permission, Gorman, LM, Sultan, DF, and Raines, ML. Davis's Manual of Psychological Nursing. FA Davis, Philadelphia, 1996.

for a long time may be helpful. Explaining that the grandfather will not be able to take them to the park as he did before may help to make the grandfather's death more real.

Older children have a better understanding of the finality of death. They know that death is not a temporary or reversible condition. They also may have a great degree of intellectual curiosity about death and the rituals that surround it. Children over the age of 5 or 6 have a basic understanding of the human body's functioning and may be able to connect their knowledge to an explanation of the causes of the death of their loved ones. The nurse can explain, in general terms, that a grandparent died of cancer and go into some detail in describing the effects of cancer. Older children may fear that they, too, will fall victim to the same medical problems and need further explanations to be reassured. During their grieving process, they may regress to behavior more characteristic of younger children.

Adolescents may possess an adultlike understanding of the circumstances surrounding death. For this reason, it may be tempting to treat them like adults and to expect them to grieve as adults would. Grieving adolescents may regress to earlier forms of behavior or struggle to behave more maturely than normal in an attempt to take on an adult persona as a result of the death, particularly in the case of the death of a same-sex parent whose role the adolescent may feel pressure to fill. It is important to acknowledge the differences between adolescents and adults in their abilities to cope with loss and, perhaps more important, in their abilities to provide support to family members in the grieving process.

Children and adolescents may assist adults in the grieving process. Although children and adolescents should not be expected to provide emotional support for grieving adults, they can actively listen to adults as they reminisce about the life of the deceased.

The nurse should be prepared to help grieving individuals in all of the different tasks necessary to move through the grieving process.[5] First, the nurse will need to assist clients in acknowledging the loss and its meaning and effects on their lives. This process may take place over several weeks or months. Honoring the religious and cultural background and preferences of grieving people is also important. For example, some cultural and religious traditions place greater importance on the idea of an afterlife, whereas others emphasize the actions and accomplishments of the deceased during life. Some cultures encourage a full expression of emotions at wakes and funerals; others emphasize a more restrained, emotionally contained approach to death.

Throughout the grieving process, the nurse needs to help clients identify their needs within that stage, as well as current and potential support systems. Some clients have extended families and close friends who can provide emotional help. Others may benefit from grief counseling or support groups in which they are able to connect with others who have experienced similar losses. Some clients may require more intensive psychological, psychosocial, or psychiatric intervention in order to grieve. Clients with preexisting mental health problems or those with few or no supports are particularly at risk.

As part of the therapeutic relationship, the nurse may need to assist clients in redefining their role in the family or in society following the death of a loved one.[6] For example, the surviving spouse may have assumed the role of caregiver to the exclusion of other roles and activities; the death of the care receiver marks the end of this all-consuming role. Often, the caregiver has difficulty rediscovering former interests and redefining a role within the family, separate from caregiving. Through the therapeutic alliance with the client, the professional nurse may be instrumental in assisting the client to identify and set new goals and to explore new or former interests.

TABLE 34–2. Differentiating Symptoms of Grief from Major Depression

Normal Grief	versus	Major Depression
The client experiences sadness but can switch to more normal moods in the same day.		The client feels sadness mixed with anger, sometimes directed toward himself or herself.
The client has changeable moods, activity levels, appetite, and sleep patterns.		The client may consistently feel tired, lose appetite, or have trouble sleeping.
The client expresses anger at appropriate times even if not in appropriate ways.		The client expresses anger in the form of rage or denies being angry altogether.
The client dreams and fantasizes, particularly about the loss.		The client may not recall dreams and fantasizes infrequently.
The client may blame himself or herself for somehow not preventing the loss.		The client may see himself or herself as bad and worthless and is preoccupied with himself or herself and feelings.
The client may be able to respond to warmth and reassurance.		The client may be unresponsive to others, or only responsive to much pressure or urging on the part of family members or friends.
The client is able to experience happiness and pleasure, at times, with varying success.		The client is rarely able to express pleasure or happiness.

Source: From The Seasons of Grief by Donna Aman Gaffney. Copyright © 1988. Used by permission of Dutton Signet, a division of Penguin Book USA Inc.

Reconnecting to friends, family, and community supports is an important task in the grieving process for many clients. Colleagues, close friends, and family may facilitate the process of healthy grieving and help clients rebuild a life without the deceased person.

Clients may experience anniversary reactions to loss or death. As part of the initial psychosocial assessment performed by the professional nurse, request historical information including the dates of major losses or other traumatic incidents. Keep in mind that clients may grieve over a variety of situations, which may or may not be an immediate death. These situations include, but are not limited to:

- Miscarriage (early or late in pregnancy)
- Abortion
- Kidnapping
- Having a loved one missing in action in the armed forces
- Giving a child up for adoption
- Having a child run away from home
- Loss of a marriage or significant love relationship
- Loss of role, including loss of a job
- Loss of a beloved pet
- Loss of physical health
- Loss of familiar neighborhood surroundings and friendships as a result of a move.

The nurse may provide crucial support to a client who grieves over these and other losses.[7] Crisis intervention may be the first task of the nurse, who should assess the client's need for intervention and arrange for immediate support, if necessary. As the client moves out of the denial phase and more fully experiences the reality of the loss, the nurse's primary role becomes active listening and emotional support. The nurse may also provide a safe environment for venting feelings (especially those that the client may be unable to express or may be uncomfortable expressing to family and friends). Later in the grieving process, the nurse's ability to help the client process the thoughts, feelings, and behaviors associated with the grieving process may greatly help the client heal and begin to plan for life after the loss. Encouraging healthy memories and assisting the client in recognizing and coping with anniversary reactions to the loss are also important tasks for the psychiatric nurse.

At times, grief persists longer than expected. When grief is prolonged or accompanied by serious emotional health problems, the client is likely to be suffering from major depression (see Table 34–2).

Most clients experience a range of normal, healthy thoughts, feelings, and behaviors associated with the grieving process. Those clients with unresolved grief that leads to depression may benefit from intensive group or individual psychotherapy, antidepressants, or antianxiety medications. Any of these may improve mood and functioning and lessen the risk of self-injurious behaviors. Table 34–3 lists behaviors that indicate a need for professional consultation.

TABLE 34–3. When to Call for Help

Professional consultation is important if the patient exhibits:
- Disturbing behavior including hallucinations, delusions, obsessions
- Evidence of intense prolonged preoccupation with lost person
- Long periods of depression possibly including suicidal thoughts or gestures
- Living in the past many months or years after loss occurred
- No emotional reaction to loss for a prolonged period of time

Or, if the staff exhibits:
- Intense emotional reaction to death of patient
- Difficulty in dealing with personal grief to the extent that it impacts on patient care

Source: With permission, Gorman, LM, Sultan, DF, and Raines, ML: Davis's Manual of Psychosocial Nursing, FA Davis Co, Philadelphia, 1996.

CASE STUDY

Ed A is a 64-year-old man whose wife recently died after a bout with breast cancer. Approximately 6 months passed between her initial diagnosis and her death, during which time Ed's family described him as becoming angry and very self-isolating. When his wife died, Ed at first appeared relieved but quickly began to express escalating feelings of anger, regret, and remorse toward his wife, his adult children, and his wife's caregivers. From his children's accounts, Ed has always been a private man who shared few of his emotions with his family members. His only close personal friend was recently placed in a nursing home as a result of a debilitating, dementing illness. Ed formerly shared his thoughts and feelings with this friend.

Ed's adult children have expressed concern for his mental health. They have also noticed that his ability to care for himself has deteriorated, and when they visited recently they noticed several unpaid bills and late-payment notices on his desk.

CRITICAL THINKING QUESTIONS

1. What losses has Ed experienced? What losses will he likely experience in the next year?
2. In what stage of grieving does Ed appear to be? What stages does he appear to have passed through successfully?
3. Is Ed experiencing healthy grieving, or might he be depressed? What symptoms suggest a normal grieving response, and what symptoms suggest a depressed mood?
4. From what interventions and supports might Ed benefit? What might be done to provide support to his adult children?

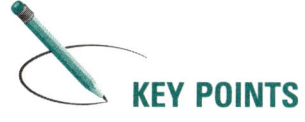

KEY POINTS

◆ One of the most important roles of the professional nurse is to prepare clients and their families for the experience of grieving.

- Normalize clients' grief, anger, anxiety, and sadness by explaining that these feelings are an expected part of the grieving process.
- Adults who experience grief may need assistance in dealing with the loss of their caregiving roles as well as the loss of the individuals from their lives.
- Children and adolescents need to be assessed, keeping in mind their relative abilities to understand death and that their own grieving processes will differ based on their previous experience (or lack of experience) with death.
- Clients who have experienced multiple or cumulative losses are especially at risk for developing symptoms of depression.

REFERENCES

1. Kubler-Ross, E: On Death and Dying. Macmillan, 1991.
2. Ahronheim, J, and Weber, D: Final Passages. Simon and Schuster, New York, 1992.
3. Buckman, R: I Don't Know What to Say. . . . Little, Brown & Co, Boston, 1989.
4. Gaffney, DA: The Seasons of Grief: Helping Children Grow through Loss. New American Library: New York, 1988.
5. Hughes, J: Cancer and Emotion: Psychological Preludes and Reactions to Cancer, John Wiley & Sons, Chichester, England, 1987.
6. Sanders, CM: How to Survive the Loss of a Child: Filling the Emptiness and Rebuilding Your Life. Prima Publishing, Rocklin, CA, 1992.
7. Zunin, LM, and Zunin, HS: The Art of Condolence. HarperCollins Publishers, New York, 1991.

UNIT Six

Future Challenges to Delivering Care to the Mentally Ill

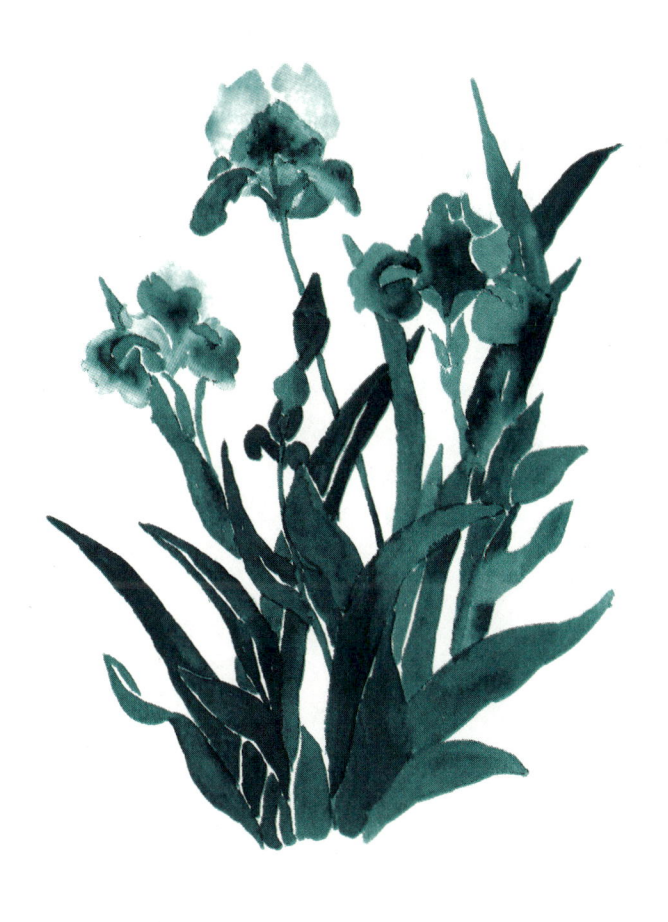

CHAPTER 35
Future Trends

APPENDIX 1
DSM-IV Classification

APPENDIX 2
A Patient's Bill of Rights

APPENDIX 3
Tips for Psychiatric Home Visits

APPENDIX 4
Psychopharmacology Guidelines

APPENDIX 5
Comparison of the Major Features of Alzheimer's Disease, Parkinson's Disease, Acquired Immunodeficiency Syndrome—Dementia Complex

APPENDIX 6
Selected Resources

GLOSSARY

INDEX

CHAPTER 35

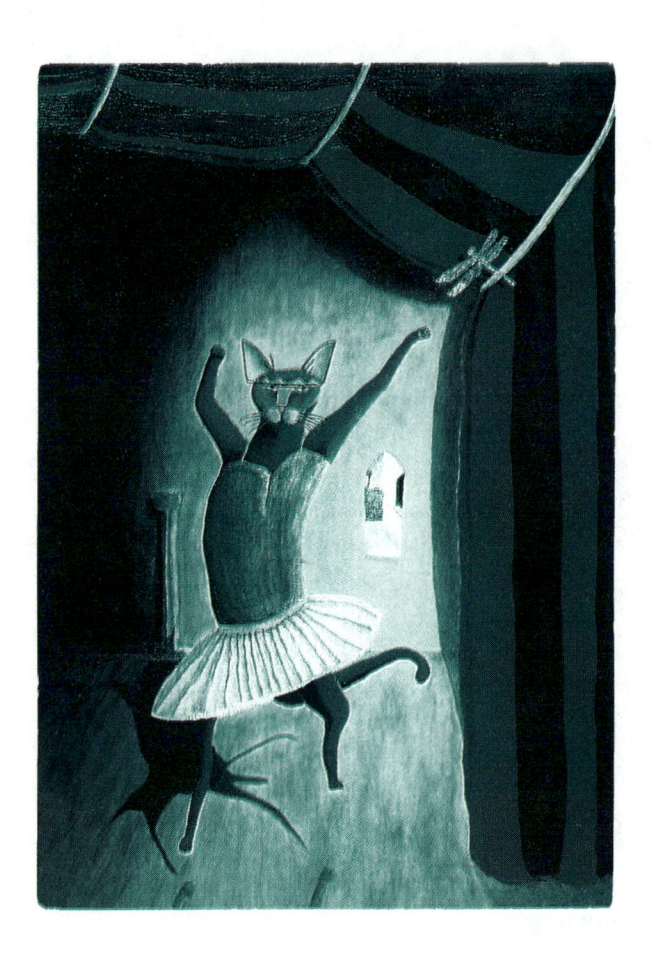

CHAPTER OUTLINE

The Present and Future of Psychiatric–Mental Health Care: Managed Care
The Fee-for-Service Delivery System
The Managed Care Delivery System
The Effects of Managed Care on Psychiatric–Mental Health Care Delivery
Opportunities for Psychiatric Nurses
Roles for the Psychiatric-Generalist Nurse
Roles for the Psychiatric Clinical Nurse Specialist (CNS)
Challenges for Future Psychiatric Nurses

KEY TERMS

capitation
carve out
fee-for-service
managed care
organized systems of care (OSCs)
retrospective payment

Nancy Valentine, RN, MPH, PhD, FAAN
Carol A. Glod, RN, CS, PhD

Future Trends

"Before the beginning of great brilliance, there must be chaos." This statement from the I Ching sets the theme for consideration of the future trends in psychiatric nursing. Over the past decade, the process of change has gained increased momentum and now has reached a point of recognized chaos for all users and providers of services. Terms such as *change*, *reform*, and *reengineering* have become part of every nurse's experience and language. These are challenging times for those who have devoted their professional energies to the specialty of psychiatric–mental health nursing, as well as for those just starting. Administrators in policy, financial, and clinical arenas are questioning nursing traditions, present contributions, and perceptions of "value-added" that will ultimately determine the future of psychiatric nursing. Major changes are refocusing fragmented delivery systems. Nurses are faced with balancing and integrating competing forces, such as the development of a primary care model, incentive-based payment mechanisms for doctors and hospitals, aggressive growth in competition among providers and institutions for clients, a potential surplus of health-care providers, and mounting problems in financing the care of the poor and the very sick, including the long-term needs of the chronically mentally ill.[1] According to the Pew Health Professions Commission Report,[2]

> In five brief years the organizational, financial, and legal framework of much of health care in the U.S. have been transformed to emerging systems of integrated care that combine primary and specialty hospital services. These systems attempt to manage the care delivered to enrolled populations in such a manner as to achieve some combination of cost reduction, enhanced patient and consumer satisfaction, and improvement of health care outcomes. Within another decade 80–90% of the insured population of the U.S. will receive its care through one of these systems.

Given these predictions, one of the greatest challenges for psychiatric nurses is to determine the best response and how to adapt to these fundamental redirections. Professional associations such as the American Nurses Association warn of the replacement of professional nurses with unlicensed assistive personnel and suggest that high-quality care remain the primary goal.[3,4] Other groups such as the TriCouncil for Nursing suggest that nurses reengineer professional care to be truly client centered.[5] Different perspectives, opinions, and political positions translate into confusing times fraught with uncertainty as well as opportunity. As in any dramatic period of change, psychiatric nurses face the pressure for change. Many systems are in need of a complete overhaul. These realities spell opportunities for both the demise of some systems and growth of others. Psychiatric nurses must retain their "internal gyroscopes" and seize one of the few opportunities to position nurses as leaders—capable of articulating new priorities—and architects of improved methods of service. This is nursing's chance to shine with "great brilliance." Along with the daily focus on the present, psychiatric nurses must simultaneously plan for the future. As the poet Rainer Maria Rilke mused, "The future enters into us in order to transform itself within us long before it ever happens."[7] The future of psychiatric nursing and its value to mental health delivery in this country depend on nurses' collective abilities to embrace, harness, and redirect these changes.

Psychiatric nursing is also charged with mental health advocacy and staying close to the customer.[8] The goal is to achieve excellence in education, research, and practice patterns in a consumer-driven, high-quality, and cost-conscious environment.

THE PRESENT AND FUTURE OF PSYCHIATRIC MENTAL–HEALTH CARE: MANAGED CARE

THE FEE-FOR-SERVICE DELIVERY SYSTEM

Managed care signals a major shift from the traditional fee-for-service delivery of care in both medical and psychiatric settings. **Fee-for-service** was a cost-based delivery system; the insurer paid for whatever the hospital billed or the private practitioner charged, so-called **retrospective payment.** These arrangements contained no specific cost controls. For instance, an insurance company might receive a bill for $1 million for one client's intensive hospitalization of several years. To cap these costs, some insurance companies placed limits on the amount of coverage for an individual's lifetime. The insurance paid for a set amount; once that was reached, no further mental health benefits were paid. Under the current managed care system, these high levels of coverage are unlikely. New approaches instead focus on "predicting" how much will be spent on psychiatric care in the coming year for each insured individual.

THE MANAGED CARE DELIVERY SYSTEM

Managed care is the financing and delivery of systems of health care that are held clinically and fiscally accountable for the health outcomes of the insured population. Ideally, managed care fosters the development of **organized systems of care** (OSCs). The key concepts that differentiate OSCs from other existing systems are accountability, integration, client-centered care, and continuous improvement. As these systems develop, several shifts occur simultaneously: (1) a purposeful move away from fragmentation to integration, (2) passive participation to active participation, (3) paying for services to buying real value, (4) shifting responsibility to taking responsibility, and (5) focusing on health as opposed to sickness. The ideal system includes true partnerships between insurers and providers who focus on their unique strengths and use integrated systems to manage large client populations.

Managed Care Using the Carve-Out System

Two different mechanisms restructure how mental health services are reimbursed: carve out and capitation. **Carve out** refers to separating mental health services from the overall medical benefits package. In this arrangement, the insurance company independently contracts with mental health providers to provide care for their participants. Characteristics of a "carved out" plan include a coordinated, managed approach to providing mental health and substance-abuse care that is totally separate from the medical plan. A specialty managed behavioral health-care plan oversees and provides the care. For the client, the plan features easy access to providers around the clock, 7 days per week. In this system, the client pays little or nothing out-of-pocket such as a deductible. No insurance claim forms are necessary to access services. The incentive is to care for the client in a system with mental health providers who supply a range of services, but only within that health plan. These plans have proliferated over the past 5 years; approximately half of all insured Americans are enrolled in some type of carve-out managed behavioral health care plan.[9]

Managed Care Using Capitation

Capitation is the other form of financing mental health care under managed care. In this arrangement, payment is based upon the entire population enrolled in a plan. The provider (hospital, agency, clinic) agrees to provide all care for a fixed amount of money. The contract pays the provider in advance to cover all its members, usually for 1 year. The contracts are renegotiated annually, depending on the cost and quality of services delivered. These arrangements can be risky if the number of clients requiring care is underestimated.[10] Capitation differs in several ways from traditional approaches such as fee-for-service.[11,12] Because practitioners usually have greater financial incentives to minimize services, clients do not always receive certain services or expensive testing such as magnetic resonance imaging (MRI) scans to detect psychiatric problems. In a capitated system, a primary provider usually must approve access to specific services. More creative options for treatment also exist.

TABLE 35–1. Stages of Managed Care Evolution

Stage	Major Feature	Characteristics and Consequences
I Unstructured	Consists of little managed care	Overuse of hospital care, oversupply of hospital beds, providers maintain control over fees
II Loose Framework	"Discounted" fee-for-service	Limits on amounts of payments (capitation), money saved through competition, hospitals consolidate, insurer partnerships with providers and groups of physicians, oversupply of hospital beds, lower rates for hospital beds
III Managed Care	Heavy managed care penetration	Managed care–dominated payment including government insurance plans such as Medicare, capitation for primary care clinicians, hospital mergers, groups of specialty physicians; physicians and hospitals dropped from health plans; development of alternative care-delivery systems
IV Managed Competition	Employer groups purchase health care	Managed care–dominated payment system, little fee-for-service billing, strong alignment of providers and insurer, elimination of hospital beds, decreased use of specialists, full continuum of health-care delivery
V End Game	Partnerships between provider and insurers	Health-care delivery is an integrated system that manages large groups of clients

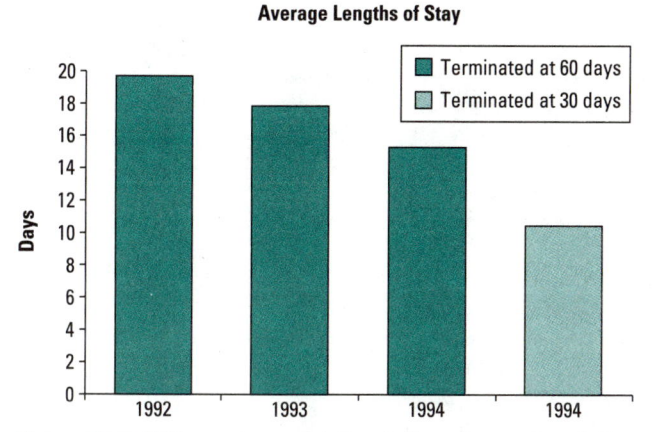

Figure 35–1. With greater availability of alternatives to hospitalization and with improvements in medication management, the length of stay continues to decrease. (The impact of managed care is evidenced in the 1995 Annual Survey, "Trends in Psychiatric Health Systems," published by the National Association of Psychiatric Health Systems.)

THE EFFECTS OF MANAGED CARE ON PSYCHIATRIC–MENTAL HEALTH CARE DELIVERY

Over the past several years, the effects of managed care have evolved incrementally in five stages.[13] As seen in Table 35–1, the stages range from little managed care to an integrated system of managed care with a network of providers. The stages progress from placing limits on the amount of money supplied to insure individuals, so-called capitation, to a system that includes only groups of organized providers whose goals are consistent with the managed care plan. As a result, psychiatric hospitals close, health plans begin to drop doctors and hospitals, and alternative continua of care such as crisis and urgent care systems develop. Primary care practitioners see more clients, and visits to specialists and the resultant fees decrease dramatically.

Two major themes have grown out of managed care: (1) the fundamental shift in focus from inpatient to outpatient care and (2) client management by a primary care provider working to "manage" the client through the system, often with the assistance of a case manager. State psychiatric hospitals and clinics have shifted to privatizing care, consolidating costly service-delivery programs, and closing state hospitals. As seen in Figure 35–1, private psychiatric hospitals have responded to this fiscal pressure by admitting fewer clients to the hospital. Hospital stays have decreased from an average length of 20 days in 1992 to 10 days in 1994. Specialty hospitals have evolved into behavioral health delivery systems offering a spectrum of treatment services[14] (Figure 35–2). Successful mental health plans devise a full continuum of care. Clients are carefully managed for only as long as necessary for stabilization. Acute care may begin with brief treatment in the hospital, a day program, or a crisis center, with follow-up care in the community.[15]

OPPORTUNITIES FOR PSYCHIATRIC NURSES

These are complex times for every health-care provider, and psychiatric nurses are no exception. With reforms occurring so rapidly, there are many views and opinions on every treatment, finance, and change issue.[16,17] For example, with this amount of change, many individuals have difficulty shifting from fundamental beliefs about long-term hospitalization to a private, entrepreneurial focus for mental health care.[18] Anger, frustration, and apprehension can cloud the picture. With all of the changes in financing and service delivery, every discipline, including nursing, has been forced to ask the difficult questions: Who will buy psychiatric nursing services? Under what circumstances? How much will be paid? Psychiatric nurses have to find the best matches between the marketplace, needs of clients, and their skills and even actively design alternatives.[19] Nurses need to think flexibly and take risks; some new roles may work and others may not.

Although traditional roles such as staff nurse and nurse manager are diminishing because of the introduction of assistive personnel, a reduction in inpatient beds, and the trend toward self-managed teams, psychiatric nursing opportunities are expanding for generalists and specialists. Aiken and Salmon[20] note that the educational levels of the nursing workforce may not be compatible with the growing demand for nurses educated at the bachelor's and master's

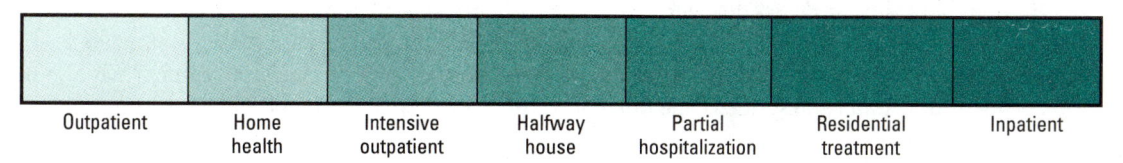

Figure 35–2. Specialty hospitals have continued to evolve into behavioral health delivery systems offering a range of treatment services. (The impact of managed care is evidenced in the 1995 Annual Survey, "Trends in Psychiatric Health Systems," published by the National Association of Psychiatric Health Systems.)

levels with independent decision-making and practice skills. Because psychiatric nurses have effectively lobbied for prescriptive privileges and have broken down many of the barriers to independent practice, they are now working more in direct primary care and case management.[21,22]

These changes have particular implications for the current nurse workforce. In some cases, nurse generalists are being cross-trained for home care, whereas psychiatric clinical nurse specialists are returning to school for post-master's certificates as nurse practitioners; both are expanding their roles into areas of physical as well as psychosocial assessment.[23] The goals of cross-training are to assist nurses in fine-tuning their basic nursing skills and adapting these skills to new and challenging environments.

ROLES FOR THE PSYCHIATRIC-GENERALIST NURSE

Because the health-care arena is changing so rapidly, psychiatric nurses play an increasing role in treating psychiatric disorders and in promoting mental health. Psychiatric nurses, traditionally found on an inpatient unit, are expanding into nontraditional settings and developing new roles. The primary settings include community-based mental health treatment and home care. Psychiatric symptoms take time to remit, and long-term care is necessary for individuals with severe and recurrent illnesses. As a result, the client may initially receive care in nonhospital treatment centers, such as a day program or emergency evaluation center that provides an alternative to hospitalization. The majority of psychiatric treatment occurs in the community.

Underserved populations such as abused children, homeless individuals, criminals, and the elderly commonly need mental health services. Child and elder abuse, domestic violence, substance abuse, acquired immunodeficiency syndrome (AIDS), immigration, and homelessness are pervasive sociocultural problems that lead to a complex array of psychiatric difficulties. Psychiatric nurses are desperately needed to provide mental health care to these groups.

As members of the health-care team, psychiatric nurses are in a prime position to identify the psychiatric needs of high-risk individuals in the community, advocate for them, and coordinate service delivery. As seen in Table 35–2, psychiatric nurses work in a variety of treatment settings: home care of individuals with dementia, day treatment and residential programs for persistently mentally ill clients, and nursing clinics in homeless shelters. The nursing roles can include case manager, client educator and client advocate, triage nurse, utilization and resource or risk manager, provider liaison, and benefits interpreter.[24]

For instance, a 60-year-old woman living at home is diagnosed with diabetes, and insulin is prescribed. The nurse makes a home visit and realizes that the woman has not been caring for herself or her home. According to the client's neighbors, her functioning has gradually declined over the past few months. The psychiatric nurse uses a variety of skills to treat the client; she teaches about diet and insulin administration, while simultaneously assessing mental status and social support available. She discovers that the woman is somewhat confused and refers her for further assessment of her physical condition and for potential psychiatric problems such as depression and dementia. In this case, the specialized skills of the psychiatric nurse help to identify the confusion and determine whether it is related to a medical condition such as diabetes or to beginning dementia or depression.

This example illustrates the complexity of mental health–care delivery. The psychiatric nurse is actively involved in applying an integrated knowledge of physical and psychiatric conditions, while making a care plan that blends medical and psychosocial interventions. Inherent in these interventions is a shift to understanding the interplay between conditions: Medical illness can produce psychiatric symptoms, and psychiatric disorders can masquerade as physical symptoms. An in-depth knowledge of pharmacology and psychopharmacology is necessary for the psychiatric nurse to determine the difference between uncomfortable side effects due to medication and the exacerbation of an underlying illness. For instance, some medications may cause sleep disruption, but sleeplessness may also be a symptom of an underlying mood or sleep disorder. A careful holistic assessment is crucial for identifying whether psychiatric symptoms have an organic basis: An individual with dementia may show worsening memory problems and agitation when an undetected urinary tract infection is present. After the physical condition is treated, the symptoms may abate.

TABLE 35–2. Opportunities for the Psychiatric Nurse Generalist in the Community

- Programs for women with postpartum depression
- Utilization review for insurance companies
- Day treatment programs for persistently mentally ill
- Risk management
- Day care for children who have been physically or sexually abused
- Day treatment program for elders with dementia
- Prisons
- Home-based programs for clients with HIV and AIDS
- Elderly housing and retirement centers
- Court advocacy programs for battered women
- Home-based programs for children with developmental disabilities
- Home-based detoxification programs for clients with alcohol and substance abuse
- Headstart programs for children at risk
- Day treatment programs for mothers with dual diagnosis
- Medication clinics at an outpatient mental health center
- Clozapine management group treatment
- Residential treatment centers, such as halfway houses
- Nursing clinics in homeless shelters
- Projects testing new psychopharmacologic agents
- Alzheimer's disease residential treatment centers

As care continues to shift from hospital settings to the community, creative thinking is required to redesign every component of care from the use of privileges to treatment care plans.[25] For example, in home care settings, part of the care plan may be to review medication administration, discuss family relationships, and assist the client and family in socializing or preparing for an upcoming job interview. In lieu of customary nursing routines in the hospital setting, home-based treatment plans need to be fluid and customized to the clients to meet their needs or the designated goals of treatment. With these desired outcomes in mind, the nurse prioritizes the amount of time spent on each activity.

For some individuals, the lack of institutional boundaries can be threatening and unsettling, especially when personal safety is felt to be at risk. To thrive amid change, the new psychiatric nurse must be culturally competent and able to negotiate complex systems, able to deal with and manage change, and comfortable with involving consumers every step of the way.[26]

ROLES FOR THE PSYCHIATRIC CLINICAL NURSE SPECIALIST (CNS)

The role of the psychiatric specialist is being expanded in general hospital acute care settings, nursing homes, and psychiatric residential treatment centers. Psychiatric nurse practitioners and psychiatric CNSs are in great demand as high-quality, cost-effective providers of care in urban and rural settings. Some clinical specialists are developing subspecialization within their psychiatric consultation-liaison roles. In these cases, the nurse has extensive experience or formal certification in a defined medical-surgical area of expertise.[27]

In community-based settings, the psychiatric CNS may function as psychiatric triage nurse in a primary health-care center. By making the judgment for referring or conducting a psychiatric assessment, the psychiatric CNS can contribute to improved outcomes. Another role is medication assessment and management for persistently mentally ill clients. Psychiatric CNSs are effective in helping clients manage their medications by offering support, diet counseling, and education. Because of their training in both physical and mental illnesses, psychiatric nurses are good managers of dual-diagnosis programs and of geriatric populations across all care settings.

At the Veterans' Administration Medical Center in Salem, Virginia, a physician and nurse, both with dual preparation, colead the primary care team. Together with a panel of other providers, they care for both the psychosocial and physical needs of a large population of veteran clients. Their outcomes have been very encouraging. The morale of the team and client satisfaction are high. Their team has less need for consultations, decreased fragmentation, and the freedom to provide timely, integrated, holistic care. Their ability to integrate and manage the total range of care needs, case manage, and consistently evaluate their results has dramatically reduced recidivism, leading to significantly fewer days of hospitalization than a year earlier. Reorganized teams such as this one can meet client needs in settings such as homes, clinics, nursing homes, and other community settings. A team can become portable and go to the client rather than require that the client to travel to a specific location.

CHALLENGES FOR FUTURE PSYCHIATRIC NURSES

At first glance, nurses may think that the technicalities of financing and service-delivery redesign and reengineering are not a major concern for them or an area they influence, but financing and developing programs are very much the business of nursing. As psychiatric units and hospitals close, large numbers of clients continue to need psychiatric nursing services in the community. Changes in Medicare and Medicaid legislation also affect psychiatric nurses. Medicare does not currently reimburse advanced practice psychiatric nurses for services to the mentally ill or to the elderly with psychiatric symptoms, except in federally designated rural areas. Medicare does pay primary care nurse practitioners (NPs) for services provided in a nursing facility, regardless of geographic area. However, Medicare reimbursement rates for NPs are 85% of what a physician is paid for the same service, and 75% for services furnished in rural areas. Such reimbursement restrictions limit access to cost-effective physical and mental health services and represent a significant barrier to nursing practice.

Groups of psychiatric nurses have organized and crafted legislative amendments to continue community treatment and to expand reimbursement to psychiatric nurses.[28] Nurses can work together to break through these barriers and form new programs that integrate psychiatric nurse generalists and specialists. They can develop cost-effective, high-quality alternatives such as nurse-managed clinics and nurse-managed home care programs.[29,30] These are dreams that deserve to become realities.

As nurses enter this revolutionary time in service delivery, psychiatric nursing needs to identify its strengths, the areas that need to be developed, and the sources of support available. Although anxiety is natural in uncertain environments, individual health-care organizations have responded by instituting educational programs for supporting staff to transition into network assignments, new roles, and expanded scopes of responsibility. Psychiatric nurses must take responsibility for seeking out growth experiences.

In addition to workplace support systems, psychiatric nurses need to join and participate in professional organizations, which play a significant role in introducing new information, political lobbying, collegial sharing, patient advocacy, and the change process. Specialty psychiatric nursing organizations typically offer continuing education, periodic updates on issues relevant to practice, and a network of committees (Table 35–3). These activities help

TABLE 35-3. Psychiatric Nursing Organizations

American Psychiatric Nurses Association
Timothy Gordon
Executive Director
1200 19th St., NW, Suite 300
Washington, DC 20036-2401
Ph: 202-857-1133
Number of Members: 3000

Association of Child & Adolescent Psychiatric Nursing
Joseph Braden
Executive Director
1211 Locust St.
Philadelphia, PA 19107
Ph: 800-826-2950
Number of Members: 500

International Society of Psychiatric Consultation Liaison Nurses
Ann Robinette, MS, RN, CS, ARNP
Chairperson
437 Twin Bay Dr.
Pensacola, FL 32534-1350
Ph: 904-474-4147
Number of members: 200

Society for Education and Research in Psychiatric–Mental Health Nursing
Dr. Melva Jo Hendrix, RN, CS
437 Twin Bay Dr.
Pensacola, FL 32534
Ph: 904-474-9024
Number of Members: 400

---

nurses stay abreast of trends and changes and keep the "bigger picture" in focus. Most important, these organizations bring psychiatric nurses together for mutual sharing and problem solving. They provide a healthy counterbalance to work settings where an atmosphere of fear and uncertainty may demoralize even the most seasoned optimist.

Psychiatric nursing organizations have been woefully undersubscribed, especially compared to other specialty nursing groups; only about 6% of all psychiatric nurses are members. However, the trend may be changing because of the many shifts in the workplace. Psychiatric nurses are increasingly searching for ways to expand colleagueship, gain new knowledge, and take an active role in policy issues. As we know from our clinical practice, it is important to seek out others for support and communication during times of stress. A sense of helplessness can quickly be replaced with a sense of a broader mission and the recognition that strength lies in numbers, knowledge, and attitudes.

As new thinking is applied and new systems created, we will be living through the single greatest health-care transformation in history. Each psychiatric nurse has the opportunity to be a part of this journey. We can and will influence the process of change every step of the way. All nurses have to choose their missions to make a difference. As the demand in the marketplace changes, nurse educators must prepare graduates for the complexity of practice and new role development. As the demand for outcome data increases, nurse researchers must design studies that serve to improve care. As consumers clamor for client-centered care, psychiatric nurses can take a leadership role to revise treatment regimens with the client and family as the first and most important determinant of priorities. And as organizations search for leaders and managers who can inspire employees to do their creative best, let nurse administrators be role models for transformational leadership.

REFERENCES

1. Fagin, C: Poised for the 21st Century: Interview. Nurs Health Care 14(1):14–17, 1993.
2. Pew Health Professions Commission: Critical challenges: Revitalizing the health professions for the twenty-first century. Philadelphia. Place
3. American Nurses Association (Sept 16, 1994). Written testimony of the ANA before the Institute of Medicine. Commission on the agency of nurse staffing. Washington, DC.
4. Lewin-VHI, Inc: Nursing Report Card for Acute Care. American Nurses Association, Washington, DC, 1995.
5. TriCouncil for Nursing: Statement on assistive personnel to the registered nurse. American Nurses Association, Washington, DC, 1995.
6. Rilke, RM: Letters to a Young Poet. Norton, New York, 1954, pp 11–123.
7. Goering, P: Psychiatric nursing and the context of care. New Dir Ment Health Serv 58:3–12, 1993.
8. Frank, RG, McQuire, TG, and Newhouse, JP: Risk contracts in managed mental health care. Health Affairs 14(3):50–64, 1995.
9. Holloway, D: Implications for Capitation for Stanford Hospital. University Hospital Consortium, Chicago, 1995.
10. McFarland, BH, George, RA, Pollack, DA, and Angell, RH: Managed mental health in the Oregon health plan. In Goldman, W, and Feldman, S (eds): Managed Mental Health Care. Jossey-Bass, San Francisco, 1993, pp 41–54.
11. Shern, DL, Donahue, SA, Felton, C, Joseph, GR, and Brier, N: Partial capitation versus fee-for-service in mental health care. Health Affairs 14(3):208–219, 1995.
12. Yang, T: Managed Care: Paradox of the 90s. Presentation at Georgetown University Medical Center Grand Rounds, Washington, DC, October 1995.
13. National Association of Psychiatric Health Systems: Trends in Psychiatric Health Systems: 1995 Annual Survey. National Association of Psychiatric Health Systems, Washington, DC, 1995.
14. Valentine, NM: Policy partners: Nursing and psychiatry in the capital: An interview with Dr. Mary Jane England. J Am Psychiatr Nurses Association 1(3):76–82, 1995.
15. Harper, M (Interview): Meet Mary Harper, co-chair, health care reform, mental health task force. J Psychosoc nurs Ment Health Serv 31(8):34–36, 1993.
16. Osborne, OH, Hagerott, RJ, Hilliard, I, and Thomas, MD: The rise of public sector psychosocial nursing. Arch Psychiatr Nurs 7(3):133–138, 1993.
17. Kane, CF: Deinstitutionalization and managed care: Deja vu? Psychiatric Services 46(9):883–889.
18. Peplau, HE: Some unresolved issues in the era of biopsychosocial nursing. J Am Psychiatr Nurses Association 1(3):92–96, 1995.
19. Aiken, LH, and Salmon, ME: Health care workforce priorities: What nursing should do now. Inquiry 31:318–319, 1994.
20. Talley, S, and Brooke, PS: Prescriptive authority for psychiatric clinical specialists: Framing the issues. Arch Psychiatr Nurs 6(2):71–82, 1992.

21. Talley, S, and Caverly, S: Advanced-practice psychiatric nursing and health care reform. Hosp Community Psychiatry 45(6):545–547, 1994.
22. Malone, JA: What's happening to clinical nurse specialists in psychiatric mental health nursing? J Psychosoc nurs Ment Health Serv 31(7):37–39, 1993.
23. Betts, VT: Management perspectives. The Nursing Spectrum 5(23), 1995.
24. Delaney, K, Ulsafer-Van Lanen, J, Pitula, C, and Johnson, M: Seven days and counting: How inpatient nurses might adjust their practice to brief hospitalization. J Psychosoc nurs Ment Health Serv 33(8):36–39, 1995.
25. Shea, CA: Moving into the mainstream. J Psychosoc nurs Ment Health Serv 31(3):5–6, 1993.
26. Moschler, LB, and Finacannon, J: Subspecialization within psychiatric consultation-liaison nursing. Arch Psychiatr Nurs 6(4):234–238, 1992.
27. Haber, J: Legislative priorities for 1995: Medicare and Medicaid reimbursement. Clin Nurse Spec 9(3):143, 148, 1995.
28. Murphy, B (ed): Nursing Centers: The Time Is Now. National League for Nursing, New York, 1995.

APPENDIX 1

DSM-IV Classification

NOS = Not Otherwise Specified.

An *x* appearing in a diagnostic code indicates that a specific code number is required.

An ellipsis (. . .) is used in the names of certain disorders to indicate that the name of a specific mental disorder or general medical condition should be inserted when recording the name (e.g., 293.0 Delirium Due to Hypothyroidism).

If criteria are currently met, one of the following severity specifiers may be noted after the diagnosis:
  Mild
  Moderate
  Severe

If criteria are no longer met, one of the following specifiers may be noted:
  In Partial Remission
  In Full Remission
  Prior History

DISORDERS USUALLY FIRST DIAGNOSED IN INFANCY, CHILDHOOD, OR ADOLESCENCE

MENTAL RETARDATION

Note: These are coded on Axis II.
317	Mild Mental Retardation
318.0	Moderate Mental Retardation
318.1	Severe Mental Retardation
318.2	Profound Mental Retardation
319	Mental Retardation, Severity Unspecified

LEARNING DISORDERS

315.00	Reading Disorder
315.1	Mathematics Disorder
315.2	Disorder of Written Expression
315.9	Learning Disorder NOS

MOTOR SKILLS DISORDER

315.4	Developmental Coordination Disorder

COMMUNICATION DISORDERS

315.31	Expressive Language Disorder
315.31	Mixed Receptive-Expressive Language Disorder
315.39	Phonological Disorder
307.0	Stuttering
307.9	Communication Disorder NOS

PERVASIVE DEVELOPMENTAL DISORDERS

299.00	Autistic Disorder
299.80	Rett's Disorder
299.10	Childhood Disintegrative Disorder
299.80	Asperger's Disorder
299.80	Pervasive Developmental Disorder NOS

ATTENTION-DEFICIT AND DISRUPTIVE BEHAVIOR DISORDERS

314.xx	Attention-Deficit/Hyperactivity Disorder
.01	Combined Type
.00	Predominantly Inattentive Type
.01	Predominantly Hyperactive-Impulsive Type
314.9	Attention-Deficit/Hyperactivity Disorder NOS
312.8	Conduct Disorder
	Specify Type: Childhood-Onset Type
	Adolescent-Onset Type
313.81	Oppositional Defiant Disorder
312.9	Disruptive Behavior Disorder NOS

FEEDING AND EATING DISORDERS OF INFANCY OR EARLY CHILDHOOD

307.52	Pica
307.53	Rumination Disorder
307.59	Feeding Disorder of Infancy or Early Childhood

TIC DISORDERS

307.23	Tourette's Disorder
307.22	Chronic Motor or Vocal Tic Disorder
307.21	Transient Tic Disorder
	Specify if: Single Episode/Recurrent
307.20	Tic Disorder NOS

ELIMINATION DISORDERS

—.—	Encopresis
787.6	With Constipation and Overflow Incontinence
307.7	Without Constipation and Overflow Incontinence
307.6	Enuresis (Not Due to a General Medical Condition)

Specify type: Nocturnal Only/Diurnal Only/Nocturnal and Diurnal

OTHER DISORDERS OF INFANCY, CHILDHOOD, OR ADOLESCENCE

309.21	Separation Anxiety Disorder

Specify if: Early Onset

313.23	Selective Mutism
313.89	Reactive Attachment Disorder of Infancy or Early Childhood

Specify type: Inhibited Type/Disinhibited Type

307.3	Stereotypic Movement Disorder

Specify if: With Self-Injurious Behavior

313.9	Disorder of Infancy, Childhood, or Adolescence NOS

DELIRIUM, DEMENTIA, AND AMNESTIC AND OTHER COGNITIVE DISORDERS

DELIRIUM

293.0	Delirium Due to . . . *[Indicate the General Medical Condition]*
—.—	Substance Intoxication Delirium (*refer to Substance-Related Disorders for substance-specific codes*)
—.—	Substance Withdrawal Delirium (*refer to Substance-Related Disorders for substance-specific codes*)
—.—	Delirium Due to Multiple Etiologies (*code each of the specific etiologies*)
780.09	Delirium NOS

DEMENTIA

290.xx	Dementia of the Alzheimer's Type, With Early Onset (*also code 331.0 Alzheimer's disease on Axis III*)
.10	Uncomplicated
.11	With Delirium
.12	With Delusions
.13	With Depressed Mood

Specify if: With Behavioral Disturbance

290.xx	Dementia of the Alzheimer's Type, With Late Onset (*also code 331.0 Alzheimer's disease on Axis III*)
.0	Uncomplicated
.3	With Delirium
.20	With Delusions
.21	With Depressed Mood

Specify if: With Behavioral Disturbance

290.xx	Vascular Dementia
.40	Uncomplicated
.41	With Delirium
.42	With Delusions
.43	With Depressed Mood

Specify if: With Behavioral Disturbance

294.9	Dementia Due to HIV Disease (*also code 043.1 HIV infection affecting central nervous system on Axis III*)
294.1	Dementia Due to Head Trauma (*also code 854.00 head injury on Axis III*)
294.1	Dementia Due to Parkinson's Disease (*also code 332.0 Parkinson's disease on Axis III*)
294.1	Dementia Due to Huntington's Disease (*also code 333.4 Huntington's disease on Axis III*)
290.10	Dementia Due to Pick's Disease (*also code 331.1 Pick's disease on Axis III*)
290.10	Dementia Due to Creutzfeldt-Jakob Disease (*also code 046.1 Creutzfeldt-Jakob disease on Axis III*)
294.1	Dementia Due to . . . *[Indicate the General Medical Condition not listed above]* (*also code the general medical condition on Axis III*)
—.—	Substance-Induced Persisting Dementia (*refer to Substance-Related Disorders for substance-specific codes*)
—.—	Dementia Due to Multiple Etiologies (*code each of the specific etiologies*)
294.8	Dementia NOS

AMNESTIC DISORDERS

294.0	Amnestic Disorder Due to . . . *[Indicate the General Medical Condition]*

Specify if: Transient/Chronic

—.—	Substance-Induced Persisting Amnestic Disorder (*refer to Substance-Related Disorders for substance-specific codes*)
294.8	Amnestic Disorder NOS

OTHER COGNITIVE DISORDERS

294.9	Cognitive Disorder NOS

MENTAL DISORDERS DUE TO A GENERAL MEDICAL CONDITION NOT ELSEWHERE CLASSIFIED

293.89	Catatonic Disorder Due to . . . *[Indicate the General Medical Condition]*
310.1	Personality Change Due to . . . *[Indicate the General Medical Condition]*

Specify type: Labile Type/Disinhibited Type/Aggressive Type/Apathetic Type/Paranoid Type/Other Type/Combined Type/Unspecified Type

293.9	Mental Disorder NOS Due to . . . *[Indicate the General Medical Condition]*

SUBSTANCE-RELATED DISORDERS

[a]The following specifiers may be applied to Substance Dependence:

    With Physiological Dependence/Without Physiological Dependence

    Early Full Remission/Early Partial Remission
    Sustained Full Remission/Sustained Partial Remission
    On Agonist Therapy/In a Controlled Environment

The following specifiers apply to Substance-Induced Disorders as noted:

    [I]With Onset During Intoxication/[W]With Onset During Withdrawal

ALCOHOL-RELATED DISORDERS

Alcohol Use Disorders

303.90   Alcohol Dependence[a]
305.00   Alcohol Abuse

Alcohol-Induced Disorders

303.00   Alcohol Intoxication
291.8   Alcohol Withdrawal
            Specify if: With Perceptual Disturbances
291.0   Alcohol Intoxication Delirium
291.0   Alcohol Withdrawal Delirium
291.2   Alcohol-Induced Persisting Dementia
291.1   Alcohol-Induced Persisting Amnestic Disorder
291.x   Alcohol-Induced Psychotic Disorder
   .5   With Delusion[I,W]
   .3   With Hallucinations[I,W]
291.8   Alcohol-Induced Mood Disorder[I,W]
291.8   Alcohol-Induced Anxiety Disorder[I,W]
291.8   Alcohol-Induced Sexual Dysfunction[I]
291.8   Alcohol-Induced Sleep Disorder[I,W]
291.9   Alcohol-Related Disorder NOS

AMPHETAMINE (OR AMPHETAMINE-LIKE)– RELATED DISORDERS

Amphetamine Use Disorders

304.40   Amphetamine Dependence[a]
305.70   Amphetamine Abuse

Amphetamine-Induced Disorders

292.89   Amphetamine Intoxication
            Specify if: With Perceptual Disturbances
292.0   Amphetamine Withdrawal
292.81   Amphetamine Intoxication Delirium
292.xx Amphetamine-Induced Psychotic Disorder
   .11   With Delusions[I]
   .12   With Hallucinations[I]
292.84   Amphetamine-Induced Mood Disorder[I,W]
292.89   Amphetamine-Induced Anxiety Disorder[I]
292.89   Amphetamine-Induced Sexual Dysfunction[I]
292.89   Amphetamine-Induced Sleep Disorder[I,W]
292.9   Amphetamine-Related Disorder NOS

CAFFEINE-RELATED DISORDERS

Caffeine-Induced Disorders

305.90   Caffeine Intoxication
292.89   Caffeine-Induced Anxiety Disorder[I]
292.89   Caffeine-Induced Sleep Disorder[I]
292.9   Caffeine-Related Disorder NOS

CANNABIS-RELATED DISORDERS

Cannabis Use Disorders

304.30   Cannabis Dependence[a]
305.20   Cannabis Abuse

Cannabis-Induced Disorders

292.89   Cannabis Intoxication
            Specify if: With Perceptual Disturbances
292.81   Cannabis Intoxication Delirium
292.xx Cannabis-Induced Psychotic Disorder
   .11   With Delusions[I]
   .12   With Hallucinations[I]
292.89   Cannabis-Induced Anxiety Disorder[I]
292.9   Cannabis-Related Disorder NOS

COCAINE-RELATED DISORDERS

Cocaine Use Disorders

304.20   Cocaine Dependence[a]
305.60   Cocaine Abuse

Cocaine-Induced Disorders

292.89   Cocaine Intoxication
            Specify if: With Perceptual Disturbances
292.0   Cocaine Withdrawal
292.81   Cocaine Intoxication Delirium
292.xx Cocaine-Induced Psychotic Disorder
   .11   With Delusions[I]
   .12   With Hallucinations[I]
292.84   Cocaine-Induced Mood Disorder[I,W]
292.89   Cocaine-Induced Anxiety Disorder[I,W]
292.89   Cocaine-Induced Sexual Dysfunction[I]
292.89   Cocaine-Induced Sleep Disorder[I,W]
292.9   Cocaine-Related Disorder NOS

HALLUCINOGEN-RELATED DISORDERS

Hallucinogen Use Disorders

304.50   Hallucinogen Dependence[a]
305.30   Hallucinogen Abuse

Hallucinogen-Induced Disorders

292.89	Hallucinogen Intoxication
292.89	Hallucinogen Persisting Perception Disorder (Flashbacks)
292.81	Hallucinogen Intoxication Delirium
292.xx	Hallucinogen-Induced Psychotic Disorder
.11	With Delusions[I]
.12	With Hallucinations[I]
292.84	Hallucinogen-Induced Mood Disorder[I]
292.89	Hallucinogen-Induced Anxiety Disorder[I]
292.9	Hallucinogen-Related Disorder NOS

INHALANT-RELATED DISORDERS

Inhalant Use Disorders

304.60	Inhalant Dependence[a]
305.90	Inhalant Abuse

Inhalant-Induced Disorders

292.89	Inhalant Intoxication
292.81	Inhalant Intoxication Delirium
292.82	Inhalant-Induced Persisting Dementia
292.xx	Inhalant-Induced Psychotic Disorder
.11	With Delusions[I]
.12	With Hallucinations[I]
292.84	Inhalant-Induced Mood Disorder[I]
292.89	Inhalant-Induced Anxiety Disorder[I]
292.9	Inhalant-Related Disorder NOS

NICOTINE-RELATED DISORDERS

Nicotine Use Disorder

305.10	Nicotine Dependence[a]

Nicotine-Induced Disorder

292.0	Nicotine Withdrawal
292.9	Nicotine-Related Disorder NOS

OPIOID-RELATED DISORDERS

Opioid Use Disorders

304.00	Opioid Dependence[a]
305.50	Opioid Abuse

Opioid-Induced Disorders

292.89	Opioid Intoxication
	Specify if: With Perceptual Disturbances
292.0	Opioid Withdrawal
292.81	Opioid Intoxication Delirium
292.xx	Opioid-Induced Psychotic Disorder
.11	With Delusions[I]
.12	With Hallucinations[I]
292.84	Opioid-Induced Mood Disorder[I]
292.89	Opioid-Induced Sexual Dysfunction[I]
292.89	Opioid-Induced Sleep Disorder[I,W]
292.9	Opioid-Related Disorder NOS

PHENCYCLIDINE (OR PHENCYCLIDINE-LIKE)–RELATED DISORDERS

Phencyclidine Use Disorders

304.90	Phencyclidine Dependence[a]
305.90	Phencyclidine Abuse

Phencyclidine-Induced Disorders

292.89	Phencyclidine Intoxication
	Specify if: With Perceptual Disturbances
292.81	Phencyclidine Intoxication Delirium
292.xx	Phencyclidine-Induced Psychotic Disorder
.11	With Delusions[I]
.12	With Hallucinations[I]
292.84	Phencyclidine-Induced Mood Disorder[I]
292.89	Phencyclidine-Induced Anxiety Disorder[I]
292.9	Phencyclidine-Related Disorder NOS

SEDATIVE-, HYPNOTIC-, OR ANXIOLYTIC-RELATED DISORDERS

Sedative, Hypnotic, or Anxiolytic Use Disorders

304.10	Sedative, Hypnotic, or Anxiolytic Dependence[a]
305.40	Sedative, Hypnotic, or Anxiolytic Abuse

Sedative-, Hypnotic-, or Anxiolytic-Induced Disorders

292.89	Sedative, Hypnotic, or Anxiolytic Intoxication
292.0	Sedative, Hypnotic, or Anxiolytic Withdrawal
	Specify if: With Perceptual Disturbances
292.81	Sedative, Hypnotic, or Anxiolytic Intoxication Delirium
292.81	Sedative, Hypnotic, or Anxiolytic Withdrawal Delirium
292.82	Sedative-, Hypnotic-, or Anxiolytic-Induced Persisting Dementia
292.83	Sedative-, Hypnotic-, or Anxiolytic-Induced Persisting Amnestic Disorder
292.xx	Sedative-, Hypnotic-, or Anxiolytic-Induced Psychotic Disorder
.11	With Delusions[I,W]
.12	With Hallucinations[I,W]
292.84	Sedative-, Hypnotic-, or Anxiolytic-Induced Mood Disorder[I,W]
292.89	Sedative-, Hypnotic-, or Anxiolytic-Induced Anxiety Disorder[W]
292.89	Sedative-, Hypnotic-, or Anxiolytic-Induced Sexual Dysfunction[I]
292.89	Sedative-, Hypnotic-, or Anxiolytic-Induced Sleep Disorder[I,W]
292.9	Sedative-, Hypnotic-, or Anxiolytic-Related Disorder NOS

POLYSUBSTANCE-RELATED DISORDER

304.80 Polysubstance Dependence[a]

OTHER (OR UNKNOWN) SUBSTANCE-RELATED DISORDERS

Other (or Unknown) Substance Use Disorders

304.90 Other (or Unknown) Substance Dependence[a]
305.90 Other (or Unknown) Substance Abuse

Other (or Unknown) Substance–Induced Disorders

292.89 Other (or Unknown) Substance Intoxication
Specify if: With Perceptual Disturbances
292.0 Other (or Unknown) Substance Withdrawal
Specify if: With Perceptual Disturbances
292.81 Other (or Unknown) Substance–Induced Delirium
292.82 Other (or Unknown) Substance–Induced Persisting Dementia
292.83 Other (or Unknown) Substance–Induced Persisting Amnestic Disorder
292.xx Other (or Unknown) Substance–Induced Psychotic Disorder
   .11 With Delusions[I,W]
   .12 With Hallucinations[I,W]
292.84 Other (or Unknown) Substance–Induced Mood Disorder[I,W]
292.89 Other (or Unknown) Substance–Induced Anxiety Disorder[I,W]
292.89 Other (or Unknown) Substance–Induced Sexual Dysfunction[I]
292.89 Other (or Unknown) Substance–Induced Sleep Disorder[I,W]
292.9 Other (or Unknown) Substance–Related Disorder NOS

SCHIZOPHRENIA AND OTHER PSYCHOTIC DISORDERS

295.xx Schizophrenia

The following Classification of Longitudinal Course applies to all subtypes of Schizophrenia:
  Episodic With Interepisode Residual Symptoms (*specify if:* With Prominent Negative Symptoms)/Episodic With No Interepisode Residual Symptoms/Continuous (*specify if:* With Prominent Negative Symptoms)
  Single Episode In Partial Remission (*specify if:* With Prominent Negative Symptoms)/Single Episode In Full Remission
  Other or Unspecified Pattern

   .30 Paranoid Type
   .10 Disorganized Type
   .20 Catatonic Type
   .90 Undifferentiated Type
   .60 Residual Type

295.40 Schizophreniform Disorder
Specify if: Without Good Prognostic Features/With Good Prognostic Features
295.70 Schizoaffective Disorder
Specify type: Bipolar Type/Depressive Type
297.1 Delusional Disorder
Specify type: Erotomanic Type/Grandiose Type/Jealous Type/Persecutory Type/Somatic Type/Mixed Type/Unspecified Type
298.8 Brief Psychotic Disorder
Specify if: With Marked Stressor(s)/Without Marked Stressor(s)/With Postpartum Onset
297.3 Shared Psychotic Disorder
293.xx Psychotic Disorder Due to . . . [Indicate the General Medical Condition]
   .81 With Delusions
   .82 With Hallucinations
—.— Substance-Induced Psychotic Disorder (*refer to Substance-Related Disorders for substance-specific codes*)
Specify if: With Onset During Intoxication/With Onset During Withdrawal
298.9 Psychotic Disorder NOS

MOOD DISORDERS

Code current state of Major Depressive Disorder or Bipolar I Disorder in fifth digit:
  1 = Mild
  2 = Moderate
  3 = Severe Without Psychotic Features
  4 = Severe With Psychotic Features
    Specify: Mood-Congruent Psychotic Features/Mood-Incongruent Psychotic Features
  5 = In Partial Remission
  6 = In Full Remission
  0 = Unspecified

The following specifiers apply (for current or most recent episode) to Mood Disorders as noted:
[a]Severity/Psychotic/Remission Specifiers/[b]Chronic/[c]With Catatonic Features/[d]With Melancholic Features/[e]With Atypical Features/[f]With Postpartum Onset

The following specifiers apply to Mood Disorders as noted:
[g]With or Without Full Interepisode Recovery/[h]With Seasonal Pattern/[i]With Rapid Cycling

DEPRESSIVE DISORDERS

296.xx Major Depressive Disorder
   .2x Single Episode[a,b,c,d,e,f]
   .3x Recurrent[a,b,c,d,e,f,g,h]
300.4 Dysthymic Disorder
Specify if: Early Onset/Late Onset
Specify: With Atypical Features
311 Depressive Disorder NOS

BIPOLAR DISORDERS

296.xx	Bipolar I Disorder
.0x	Single Manic Episode[a,c,f]
	Specify if: Mixed
.40	Most Recent Episode Hypomanic[g,h,i]
.4x	Most Recent Episode Manic[a,c,f,g,h,i]
.6x	Most Recent Episode Mixed[a,c,f,g,h,i]
.5x	Most Recent Episode Depressed[a,b,c,d,e,f,g,h,i]
.7	Most Recent Episode Unspecified[g,h,i]
296.89	Bipolar II Disorder[a,b,c,d,e,f,g,h,i]
	Specify (current or most recent episode): Hypomanic/Depressed
301.13	Cyclothymic Disorder
296.80	Bipolar Disorder NOS
293.83	Mood Disorder Due to . . . [Indicate the General Medical Condition]
	Specify type: With Depressive Features/With Major Depressive-Like Episode/With Manic Features/With Mixed Features
—.—	Substance-Induced Mood Disorder *(refer to Substance-Related Disorders for substance-specific codes)*
	Specify type: With Depressive Features/With Manic Features/With Mixed Features
	Specify if: With Onset During Intoxication/With Onset During Withdrawal
296.90	Mood Disorder NOS

ANXIETY DISORDERS

300.01	Panic Disorder Without Agoraphobia
300.21	Panic Disorder With Agoraphobia
300.22	Agoraphobia Without History of Panic Disorder
300.29	Specific Phobia
	Specify type: Animal Type/Natural Environment Type/Blood-Injection-Injury Type/Situational Type/Other Type
300.23	Social Phobia
	Specify if: Generalized
300.3	Obsessive-Compulsive Disorder
	Specify if: With Poor Insight
309.81	Posttraumatic Stress Disorder
	Specify if: Acute/Chronic
	Specify if: With Delayed Onset
308.3	Acute Stress Disorder
300.02	Generalized Anxiety Disorder
293.89	Anxiety Disorder Due to . . . [Indicate the General Medical Condition]
	Specify if: With Generalized Anxiety/With Panic Attacks/With Obsessive-Compulsive Symptoms
—.—	Substance-Induced Anxiety Disorder *(refer to Substance-Related Disorders for substance-specific codes)*
	Specify if: With Generalized Anxiety/With Panic Attacks/With Obsessive-Compulsive Symptoms/With Phobic Symptoms
	Specify if: With Onset During Intoxication/With Onset During Withdrawal
300.00	Anxiety Disorder NOS

SOMATOFORM DISORDERS

300.81	Somatization Disorder
300.81	Undifferentiated Somatoform Disorder
300.11	Conversion Disorder
	Specify type: With Motor Symptom or Deficit/With Sensory Symptom or Deficit/With Seizures or Convulsions/With Mixed Presentation
307.xx	Pain Disorder
.80	Associated With Psychological Factors
.89	Associated With Both Psychological Factors and a General Medical Condition
	Specify if: Acute/Chronic
300.7	Hypochondriasis
	Specify if: With Poor Insight
300.7	Body Dysmorphic Disorder
300.81	Somatoform Disorder NOS

FACTITIOUS DISORDERS

300.xx	Factitious Disorder
.16	With Predominantly Psychological Signs and Symptoms
.19	With Predominantly Physical Signs and Symptoms
.19	With Combined Psychological and Physical Signs and Symptoms
300.19	Factitious Disorder NOS

DISSOCIATIVE DISORDERS

300.12	Dissociative Amnesia
300.13	Dissociative Fugue
300.14	Dissociative Identity Disorder
300.6	Depersonalization Disorder
300.15	Dissociative Disorder NOS

SEXUAL AND GENDER IDENTITY DISORDERS

SEXUAL DYSFUNCTIONS

The following specifiers apply to all primary Sexual Dysfunctions:
Lifelong Type/Acquired Type
Generalized Type/Situational Type
Due to Psychological Factors/Due to Combined Factors

Sexual Desire Disorders

302.71	Hypoactive Sexual Desire Disorder
302.79	Sexual Aversion Disorder

Sexual Arousal Disorders

302.72 Female Sexual Arousal Disorder
302.72 Male Erectile Disorder

Orgasmic Disorders

302.73 Female Orgasmic Disorder
302.74 Male Orgasmic Disorder
302.75 Premature Ejaculation

Sexual Pain Disorders

302.76 Dyspareunia (Not Due to a General Medical Condition)
306.51 Vaginismus (Not Due to a General Medical Condition)

Sexual Dysfunction Due to a General Medical Condition

625.8 Female Hypoactive Sexual Desire Disorder Due to . . . [Indicate the General Medical Condition]
608.89 Male Hypoactive Sexual Desire Disorder Due to . . . [Indicate the General Medical Condition]
607.84 Male Erectile Disorder Due to . . . [Indicate the General Medical Condition]
625.0 Female Dyspareunia Due to . . . [Indicate the General Medical Condition]
608.89 Male Dyspareunia Due to . . . [Indicate the General Medical Condition]
625.8 Other Female Sexual Dysfunction Due to . . . [Indicate the General Medical Condition]
608.89 Other Male Sexual Dysfunction Due to . . . [Indicate the General Medical Condition]
—.— Substance-Induced Sexual Dysfunction (refer to Substance-Related Disorders for substance-specific codes)
Specify if: With Impaired Desire/With Impaired Arousal/With Impaired Orgasm/With Sexual Pain
Specify if: With Onset During Intoxication
302.70 Sexual Dysfunction NOS

PARAPHILIAS

302.4 Exhibitionism
302.81 Fetishism
302.89 Frotteurism
302.2 Pedophilia
Specify if: Sexually Attracted to Males/Sexually Attracted to Females/Sexually Attracted to Both
Specify if: Limited to Incest
Specify type: Exclusive Type/Nonexclusive Type
302.83 Sexual Masochism
302.84 Sexual Sadism

302.3 Transvestic Fetishism
Specify if: With Gender Dysphoria
302.82 Voyeurism
302.9 Paraphilia NOS

GENDER IDENTITY DISORDERS

302.xx Gender Identity Disorder
 .6 in Children
 .85 in Adolescents or Adults
Specify if: Sexually Attracted to Males/Sexually Attracted to Females/Sexually Attracted to Both/Sexually Attracted to Neither
302.6 Gender Identity Disorder NOS
302.9 Sexual Disorder NOS

EATING DISORDERS

307.1 Anorexia Nervosa
Specify type: Restricting Type; Binge-Eating/Purging Type
307.51 Bulimia Nervosa
Specify type: Purging Type/Nonpurging Type
307.50 Eating Disorder NOS

SLEEP DISORDERS

PRIMARY SLEEP DISORDERS

Dyssomnias

307.42 Primary Insomnia
307.44 Primary Hypersomnia
Specify if: Recurrent
347 Narcolepsy
780.59 Breathing-Related Sleep Disorder
307.45 Circadian Rhythm Sleep Disorder
Specify type: Delayed Sleep Phase Type/Jet Lag Type/Shift Work Type/Unspecified Type
307.47 Dyssomnia NOS

Parasomnias

307.47 Nightmare Disorder
307.46 Sleep Terror Disorder
307.46 Sleepwalking Disorder
307.47 Parasomnia NOS

SLEEP DISORDERS RELATED TO ANOTHER MENTAL DISORDER

307.42 Insomnia Related to . . . [Indicate the Axis I or Axis II Disorder]
307.44 Hypersomnia Related to . . . [Indicate the Axis I or Axis II Disorder]

OTHER SLEEP DISORDERS

780.xx Sleep Disorder Due to ... *[Indicate the General Medical Condition]*
 .52 Insomnia Type
 .54 Hypersomnia Type
 .59 Parasomnia Type
 .59 Mixed Type
—.— Substance-Induced Sleep Disorder *(refer to Substance-Related Disorders for substance-specific codes)*
Specify type: Insomnia Type/Hypersomnia Type/Parasomnia Type/Mixed Type
Specify if: With Onset During Intoxication/With Onset During Withdrawal

IMPULSE-CONTROL DISORDERS NOT ELSEWHERE CLASSIFIED

312.34 Intermittent Explosive Disorder
312.32 Kleptomania
312.33 Pyromania
312.31 Pathological Gambling
312.39 Trichotillomania
312.30 Impulse-Control Disorder NOS

ADJUSTMENT DISORDERS

309.xx Adjustment Disorder
 .0 With Depressed Mood
 .24 With Anxiety
 .28 With Mixed Anxiety and Depressed Mood
 .3 With Disturbance of Conduct
 .4 With Mixed Disturbance of Emotions and Conduct
 .9 Unspecified
Specify if: Acute/Chronic

PERSONALITY DISORDERS

Note: These are coded on Axis II.
301.0 Paranoid Personality Disorder
301.20 Schizoid Personality Disorder
301.22 Schizotypal Personality Disorder
301.7 Antisocial Personality Disorder
301.83 Borderline Personality Disorder
301.50 Histrionic Personality Disorder
301.81 Narcissistic Personality Disorder
301.82 Avoidant Personality Disorder
301.6 Dependent Personality Disorder
301.4 Obsessive-Compulsive Personality Disorder
301.9 Personality Disorder NOS

OTHER CONDITIONS THAT MAY BE A FOCUS OF CLINICAL ATTENTION

PSYCHOLOGICAL FACTORS AFFECTING MEDICAL CONDITION

316 ... *[Specified Psychological Factor]* Affecting ... *[Indicate the General Medical Condition]* Choose name based on nature of factors:
Mental Disorder Affecting Medical Condition
Psychological Symptoms Affecting Medical Condition
Personality Traits or Coping Style Affecting Medical Condition
Maladaptive Health Behaviors Affecting Medical Condition
Stress-Related Physiological Response Affecting Medical Condition
Other or Unspecified Psychological Factors Affecting Medical Condition

MEDICATION-INDUCED MOVEMENT DISORDERS

332.1 Neuroleptic-Induced Parkinsonism
333.92 Neuroleptic Malignant Syndrome
333.7 Neuroleptic-Induced Acute Dystonia
333.99 Neuroleptic-Induced Acute Akathisia
333.82 Neuroleptic-Induced Tardive Dyskinesia
333.1 Medication-Induced Postural Tremor
333.90 Medication-Induced Movement Disorder NOS

OTHER MEDICATION-INDUCED DISORDER

995.2 Adverse Effects of Medication NOS

RELATIONAL PROBLEMS

V61.9 Relational Problem Related to a Mental Disorder or General Medical Condition
V61.20 Parent-Child Relational Problem
V61.1 Partner Relational Problem
V61.8 Sibling Relational Problem
V62.81 Relational Problem NOS

PROBLEMS RELATED TO ABUSE OR NEGLECT

V61.21 Physical Abuse of Child *(code 995.5 if focus of attention is on victim)*
V61.21 Sexual Abuse of Child *(code 995.5 if focus of attention is on victim)*
V61.21 Neglect of Child *(code 995.5 if focus of attention is on victim)*
V61.1 Physical Abuse of Adult *(code 995.81 if focus of attention is on victim)*

V61.1 Sexual Abuse of Adult (*code 995.81 if focus of attention is on victim*)

ADDITIONAL CONDITIONS THAT MAY BE A FOCUS OF CLINICAL ATTENTION

V15.81	Noncompliance With Treatment
V65.2	Malingering
V71.01	Adult Antisocial Behavior
V71.02	Child or Adolescent Antisocial Behavior
V62.89	Borderline Intellectual Functioning
	Note: This is coded on Axis II
780.9	Age-Related Cognitive Decline
V62.82	Bereavement
V62.3	Academic Problem
V62.2	Occupational Problem
313.82	Identity Problem
V62.89	Religious or Spiritual Problem
V62.4	Acculturation Problem
V62.89	Phase of Life Problem

ADDITIONAL CODES

300.9	Unspecified Mental Disorder (nonpsychotic)
V71.09	No Diagnosis or Condition on Axis I
799.9	Diagnosis or Condition Deferred on Axis I
V71.09	No Diagnosis on Axis II
799.9	Diagnosis Deferred on Axis II

MULTIAXIAL SYSTEM

Axis I	Clinical Disorders
	Other Conditions That May Be a Focus of Clinical Attention
Axis II	Personality Disorders
	Mental Retardation
Axis III	General Medical Conditions
Axis IV	Psychosocial and Environmental Problems
Axis V	Global Assessment of Functioning

APPENDIX 2

A Patient's Bill of Rights*

1. The patient has the right to considerate and respectful care.
2. The patient has the right to and is encouraged to obtain from physicians and other direct caregivers relevant, current, and understandable information concerning diagnosis, treatment, and prognosis.

   Except in emergencies when the patient lacks decision-making capacity and the need for treatment is urgent, the patient is entitled to the opportunity to discuss and request information related to the specific procedures and/or treatments, the risks involved, the possible length of recuperation, and the medically reasonable alternatives and their accompanying risks and benefits.

   Patients have the right to know the identity of physicians, nurses, and others involved in their care, as well as when those involved are students, residents, or other trainees. The patient also has the right to know the immediate and long-term financial implications of treatment choices, insofar as they are known.
3. The patient has the right to make decisions about the plan of care prior to and during the course of treatment and to refuse a recommended treatment or plan of care to the extent permitted by law and hospital policy and to be informed of the medical consequences of this action. In case of such refusal, the patient is entitled to other appropriate care and services that the hospital provides or transfer to another hospital. The hospital should notify patients of any policy that might affect patient choice within the institution.
4. The patient has the right to have an advance directive (such as a living will, health care proxy, or durable power of attorney for health care) concerning treatment or designating a surrogate decision maker with the expectation that the hospital will honor the intent of that directive to the extent permitted by law and hospital policy.

   Health care institutions must advise patients of their rights under state law and hospital policy to make informed medical choices, ask if the patient has an advance directive, and include that information in patient records. The patient has the right to timely information about hospital policy that may limit its ability to implement fully a legally valid advance directive.
5. The patient has the right to every consideration of privacy. Case discussion, consultation, examination, and treatment should be conducted so as to protect each patient's privacy.
6. The patient has the right to expect that all communications and records pertaining to his/her care will be treated as confidential by the hospital, except in cases such as suspected abuse and public health hazards when reporting is permitted or required by law. The patient has the right to expect that the hospital will emphasize the confidentiality of this information when it releases it to any other parties entitled to review information in these records.
7. The patient has the right to review the records pertaining to his/her medical care and to have the information explained or interpreted as necessary, except when restricted by law.
8. The patient has the right to expect that, within its capacity and policies, a hospital will make reasonable response to the request of a patient for appropriate and medically indicated care and services. The hospital must provide evaluation, service, and/or referral as indicated by the urgency of the case. When medically appropriate and legally permissible, or when a patient has so requested, a patient may be transferred to another facility. The institution to which the patient is to be transferred must first have accepted the patient for transfer. The patient must also have the benefit of complete information and explanation concerning the need for, risks, benefits, and alternatives to such a transfer.
9. The patient has the right to ask and be informed of the existence of business relationships among the

---

*These rights can be exercised on the patient's behalf by a designated surrogate or proxy decision maker if the patient lacks decision-making capacity, is legally incompetent, or is a minor.

hospital, educational institutions, other health care providers, or payers that may influence the patient's treatment and care.
10. The patient has the right to consent to or decline to participate in proposed research studies or human experimentation affecting care and treatment or requiring direct patient involvement, and to have those studies fully explained prior to consent. A patient who declines to participate in research or experimentation is entitled to the most effective care that the hospital can otherwise provide.
11. The patient has the right to expect reasonable continuity of care when appropriate and to be informed by physicians and other caregivers of available and realistic patient care options when hospital care is no longer appropriate.
12. The patient has the right to be informed of hospital policies and practices that relate to patient care, treatment, and responsibilities. The patient has the right to be informed of available resources for resolving disputes, grievances, and conflicts, such as ethics committees, patient representatives, or other mechanisms available in the institution. The patient has the right to be informed of the hospital's charges for services and available payment methods.

The collaborative nature of health care requires that patients, or their families/surrogates, participate in their care. The effectiveness of care and patient satisfaction with the course of treatment depend, in part, on the patient fulfilling certain responsibilities. Patients are responsible for providing information about past illnesses, hospitalizations, medications, and other matters related to health status. To participate effectively in decision making, patients must be encouraged to take responsibility for requesting additional information or clarification about their health status or treatment when they do not fully understand information and instructions. Patients are also responsible for ensuring that the health care institution has a copy of their written advance directive if they have one. Patients are responsible for informing their physicians and other caregivers if they anticipate problems in following prescribed treatment.

Patients should also be aware of the hospital's obligation to be reasonably efficient and equitable in providing care to other patients and the community. The hospital's rules and regulations are designed to help the hospital meet this obligation. Patients and their families are responsible for making reasonable accommodations to the needs of the hospital, other patients, medical staff, and hospital employees. Patients are responsible for providing necessary information for insurance claims and for working with the hospital to make payment arrangements, when necessary.

A person's health depends on much more than health care services. Patients are responsible for recognizing the impact of their life-style on their personal health.

Hospitals have many functions to perform, including the enhancement of health status, health promotion, and the prevention and treatment of injury and disease; the immediate and ongoing care and rehabilitation of patients; the education of health professionals, patients, and the community; and research. All these activities must be conducted with an overriding concern for the values and dignity of patients.

APPENDIX 3

Tips for Psychiatric Home Visits

Preparation		Rationale/Clarification
Call client	Introduce self	• Clarify what agency you represent. Some clients receive services from many resources.
	Specify goals of visit	• Clients do not always understand the roles of all of the health-care providers who visit them.
	Set up time of visit	• Always give a half-hour range to plan for the unexpected.[†]
	Confirm address	• The record may be hard to read, may not specify apartment number, etc.
Review record	Review diagnoses	• Usually multiple. Refer to the "Physicians Plan of Care" and/or the admission orders for all pertinent diagnoses.
	Review biographical information	• Age, sex, culture, language, etc.
	Read Mental Status Examination	• Structure visit: Teaching potential, need for safety assessment, discharge potential.
	Find out who lives with the client	• Clients who live alone may need more community resources to remain safely at home.
	Note insurance source	• Nurses may need to document on specific forms for various insurance companies. Supplies and medications are not covered by all insurance companies.
Gather supplies	BP cuff Stethoscope Other	• Most supplies are delivered to the home. Always check with the client before visit regarding supplies needed.

Home Visit*	Rationale/Clarification
Subjective	
Focus on chief complaint	• Nurses must adapt to the client's immediate concerns. The nurse's goals of a home visit may be changed if the client has other priorities.
Collect data specific to diagnoses	• Most insurance providers mandate that nursing assessments are specific to the client's problems, as listed on the physian's orders. If the assessment/documentation does not address these diagnoses, a bill may be denied and the client may become responsible for payment.
Collect data specific to functional/safety needs	• A good deal of nursing care at home is justified based on a client's functional status and personal safety. Documentation must reflect the client's current functional and safety status.
Objective	
Focus on chief complaint	• A skilled nursing assessment of new client problems must be documented. A psychiatric home care nurse may be the first health-care provider to assess a new problem. Document all conversations with the interdisciplinary team and teaching provided to the client.

Continued on following page

Home Visit*	Rationale/Clarification
Collect data specific to diagnoses on Form 485	• All diagnoses must correlate with the medication list and the problem list. All home nursing visits must address each diagnosis/problem and reflect the status of the problem. Discharge planning begins when problems are resolving.
Assessment	• The home care nurse must document the assessment of the client based on subjective and objective data collection. Every client has specific goals of care that have been set during the first client visit. The nursing assessment specifies the status of the client's condition in terms of these goals. New goals may be added to the plan of care as needed. A client is discharged when all goals have been met.
Plan	• Document plans for the next nursing visit. This ensures that the care provided to the client is consistent, focused, and meeting the documented goals. Include plans for teaching, discharge, and interdisciplinary coordination.

*A psychiatric home care nurse must be particularly sensitive to a client's right to privacy and to autonomy. When entering someone's home, remember that the environment is controlled by the client. Any rules and regulations set by the client should be respected and maintained by all health-care providers.

†Always let a client know how long you anticipate your visit to last. This allows the client to plan for personal comfort.

Courtesy of Carolyn O'Brien, Northeastern University College of Nursing, Boston, MA.

APPENDIX 4

Psychopharmacology Guidelines

This document describes the knowledge base psychiatric–mental health nurses need in relation to one aspect of practice—psychopharmacology. It is intended only to inform and guide psychiatric–mental health nursing education, practice, and research in this area. Thus, this document should not be considered part of any state's nurse practice act, or viewed as a requirement for licensure, or construed as a legal standard by which to judge psychiatric nursing practice.

These guidelines will be evaluated and updated regularly. Psychiatric–mental health nurses will demonstrate expanding expertise in psychopharmacology based on the state of the science, education, experience, practice setting, patient needs, and professional goals.

NEUROSCIENCES

Commensurate with level of practice, the psychiatric–mental health nurse integrates current knowledge from the neurosciences to understand etiologic models, diagnostic issues, and treatment strategies for psychiatric illness.

OBJECTIVES

The psychiatric–mental health nurse can:
- Describe basic central nervous system structures and functions implicated in mental illness, such as the cerebrum, diencephalon, brain stem, basal ganglia, limbic system, and extrapyramidal motor system.
- Describe basic mechanisms of neurotransmission at the synapse, such as neurochemical metabolism, role(s) of the presynaptic and postsynaptic membranes, reuptake, receptor binding, and autoregulation.
- Describe the general functions of the major neurochemicals implicated in mental illness, such as serotonin, norepinephrine, dopamine, acetylcholine, GABA, and the peptides.
- Describe the basic structure and function of the endocrine system, particularly as it is affected by the various hypothalamic-pituitary endocrine axes.
- Identify the neurotransmitter system implicated in side-effect profiles of psychopharmacologic agents, such as blockade of cholinergic receptors (blurred vision, dry mouth, memory dysfunction), histaminic receptors (sedation, weight gain, hypotension), and adrenergic receptors (dizziness, postural hypotension, tachycardia).
- Discuss the relevance of current biological hypotheses underlying major mental illnesses and the use of psychopharmacologic agents.
- Demonstrate a familiarity with the increased lifetime risk of mental illness—for people who have a mentally ill first-degree (biological) relative—compared to the general population, based on genetic, epidemiologic, family, adoption, and twin research.
- Describe normal sleep stages and identify circadian rhythm disturbances, such as decreased REM latency and phase-shift disturbances as evidenced in psychiatric disorders.
- Demonstrate familiarity with recent research findings from neuroimaging techniques such as computerized tomography (CT), magnetic resonance imaging (MRI), positron-emission tomography (PET), and single photon emission computerized tomography (SPECT) as well as the psychiatric uses of these techniques.
- Discuss the purposes and limitations of current biological tests used in the diagnosis and monitoring of mental illness.

PSYCHOPHARMACOLOGY

The psychiatric–mental health nurse involved in the care of patients who have been prescribed psychopharmacologic agents demonstrates knowledge of psychopharmacologic

Source: With permission. American Nurses Association: Psychopharmacology guidelines for psychiatric mental health nurses. In Psychiatric Mental Health Nursing Psychopharmacology Project. ANA: Washington, DC, 1994, pp 41–45.

principles—including pharmacokinetics, pharmacodynamics, drug classification, intended and unintended effects, and related nursing implications.

OBJECTIVES

The psychiatric–mental health nurse can:
- Describe psychopharmacologic agents based on the similarities and differences among drugs of the same and different classes.
- Discuss the actions of psychopharmacologic agents that range from global human behavioral responses to those at a cellular level, such as the actions of lithium from mood stabilization to glomerular effects.
- Differentiate the psychiatric symptoms targeted for psychopharmacologic intervention from medication side effects and toxicities, and the appropriate interventions to minimize each.
- Apply basic principles of pharmacokinetics and pharmacodynamics, such as half-life, steady state, absorption, and metabolism, in general and as they relate to age, gender, race/ethnicity, and organ system function.
- Identify the appropriate use of psychotherapeutic agents related to the psychiatric needs of special populations.
- Involve patients and their families and significant others in the design and implementation of the medication treatment plan, taking into account patient readiness, knowledge, environment, beliefs and preferences, and lifestyle.
- Identify factors that may prevent the active collaboration of patients with medication regimens and strategies to minimize these risks.
- Describe nonpsychopharmacologic interventions for target symptoms that are not responsive to psychopharmacologic interventions, psychiatric symptoms unlikely to respond to drug treatments, and drug side effects that are not treated with drugs.
- Discuss the use of standardized rating scales for measuring symptom severity and clinical response to psychopharmacologic treatment, such as changes in target symptoms of illness and medication side effects.
- Demonstrate the knowledge necessary to develop psychopharmacologic education and treatment plans based on current neurobiological concepts and the patient's lifestyle and recovery environment.

CLINICAL MANAGEMENT

The psychiatric–mental health nurse applies principles from the neurosciences and psychopharmacology to provide safe and effective management of patients being treated with psychopharmacologic agents. Clinical management includes assessment, diagnosis, and treatment considerations.

ASSESSMENT

The psychiatric–mental health nurse has the knowledge, skills, and ability to conduct and interpret patient assessments in relation to psychopharmacologic agents. Assessments include physical, neuropsychiatric, psychosocial, and psychopharmacologic parameters.

Physical Assessment

Objectives. The psychiatric–mental health nurse can:
- Collect health data related to past and present health problems and concurrent treatments for other psychiatric or medical problems the patient may have.
- Collect health data related to current and past drug use (prescribed, over-the-counter, and illicit), current and past substance use (caffeine, nicotine, alcohol), and related health practices.
- Conduct and/or interpret findings from a physical examination and laboratory studies to obtain information about pertinent organ system functioning.
- Evaluate laboratory results that reflect drug effects on organ systems, drug blood levels and toxicities, and concurrent medical problems that may mimic or exacerbate psychiatric symptoms or drug effects.
- Assess baseline and ongoing status of motor activity and sleep patterns, appetite, dietary practices and preferences, and functional status.

Neuropsychiatric Assessment

Objectives. The psychiatric–mental health nurse can:
- Conduct and/or interpret findings from a basic neuropsychiatric examination including gross cranial and peripheral nerve function; gait; muscle strength, function, and range of motion; and mental status.
- Identify chief neuropsychiatric complaints, presenting symptoms, and goals for psychopharmacologic interventions.
- Make appropriate use of available informants and records to augment self-reports of neuropsychiatric assessment and premorbid patterns.
- Demonstrate appropriate use of standardized rating scales to document mental status, drug effects on the core psychiatric symptomatology, and side effects such as those occurring in the extrapyramidal system.

Psychosocial Assessment

Objectives. The psychiatric–mental health nurse can:
- Use demographic and personal information for the development of a patient-centered medication treatment plan, considering the patient's ethnic/cultural background, developmental stage, cognitive ability, educational level, reading level and comprehension, socioeconomic status, and capacity to ask questions and seek answers.

- Assess the effects of psychopharmacologic interventions on the patient's quality of life, including the impact on interpersonal relationships, appearance, work and leisure functioning, diet, sleep, sexual performance, family planning, functional status, financial status, self-esteem, and perception of stigma associated with medication intervention.
- Identify actual and potential sources of support for the patient such as significant others; household and family members; friendships and informal relationships; work relationships; and affiliations with community, social, and religious organizations.
- Identify actual and potential barriers to treatment within the patient and the environment, such as impaired functional status, cultural/ethnic/religious beliefs and practices, absence of a support system, limited cognitive abilities, stressors, financial hardships, deficient coping skills, impaired capacity to collaborate with treatment, limited transportation, and patient and family perceptions of illness and medication treatment.

Psychopharmacologic Assessment

Objectives. The psychiatric–mental health nurse can:
- Identify patient-related variables pertinent to the risk/benefit assessment of psychopharmacologic treatment such as demographic (age, gender, ethnicity/race); physical (organ system function, concurrent illnesses); treatment (concurrent treatments); and personal (past history, self-care practices, goals for treatment, ability to pay, and quality of life) characteristics.
- Identify drug-related variables important in the risk/benefit assessment of psychopharmacologic agents, such as safety and efficacy, advantages and disadvantages compared to other drugs in the same class, therapeutic range, side-effect profile, toxicities, contraindications, potential interactions with other drugs or diet, polypharmacy considerations, safety in overdose, availability of information on long-term side effects, and cost.
- Evaluate the appropriateness and least restrictive nature of psychopharmacologic interventions for each patient.
- Assess the ability and willingness of the patient and significant others to give informed consent for treatment with psychopharmacologic agents.
- Use standardized behavioral rating scales to assess and monitor drug effects and changes in target symptoms.

DIAGNOSIS

The psychiatric–mental health nurse has the knowledge, skills, and ability to utilize appropriate nursing, psychiatric, and medical diagnostic classification systems to guide psychopharmacologic management of patients with mental illness.

Objectives. The psychiatric–mental health nurse can:
- Use standardized diagnostic systems as appropriate for making nursing (North American Nursing Diagnostic Association—NANDA or other nursing systems) and psychiatric diagnoses (*Diagnostic and Statistical Manual—DSM*), and interpreting medical diagnoses (*International Classification of Diseases—ICD*).
- Elicit information—from the patient and other appropriate informants or records—that is relevant to the diagnostic process.
- Make nursing diagnostic judgments that include information about but are not limited to the psychiatric diagnosis, symptoms targeted for psychopharmacologic intervention, clinical diagnoses, physical symptoms, coping responses, functional status, developmental level, learning capabilities, and the patient's quality of life and preferences.
- Use these diagnostic judgments as the basis for setting treatment priorities and selecting and assessing nursing interventions, including management of psychopharmacologic agents.
- Communicate and integrate diagnostic impressions with other members of the health-care team. This can include representatives of managed care enterprises.

TREATMENT

The psychiatric–mental health nurse takes an active role in the treatment of patients with mental illness and integrates prescribed psychopharmacologic interventions into a cohesive, multidimensional plan of care.

Initiation

Objectives. The psychiatric–mental health nurse can:
- Use information obtained during the nursing assessment to develop a medication treatment plan that considers target symptoms, side effects, concurrent treatments and health status, requirements of specific drugs, dietary and activity considerations, and patient-related variables.
- Demonstrate an understanding of pharmacokinetic and pharmacodynamic principles that underlie safe and effective psychopharmacologic management, such as how dosing and tapering schedules are adjusted, and how patient-related variables are integrated.
- Relate the length of time it may take a drug to have a therapeutic effect, the time it takes for expected side effects to occur and remit, early signs of unexpected or adverse events, and nursing interventions to reduce side effects and facilitate therapeutic response.
- Apply principles of health education and nursing ethics and legal parameters in informing patients about medication treatments, risks/benefits, concurrent and alternative treatments, and informed consent.

- Apply least restrictive principles and advance directives to avoid the overuse or underuse of medications as chemical restraints, and to anticipate safety needs, such as potential for harm to self or others, suicidality, aggression, assaultiveness, and violence.

Stabilization

Objectives. The psychiatric–mental health nurse can:
- Monitor target symptoms, acute medication effects, and functional status throughout the course of treatment.
- Use information obtained from therapeutic drug monitoring, laboratory values, standardized rating scales, and patient and family reports to monitor progress.
- Recognize indications for modifying dosing schedules and describe alternative medication strategies as needed.

Maintenance

Objectives. The psychiatric–mental health nurse can:
- Develop a plan of care—in collaboration with the patient, family, and other care providers as appropriate—that includes monitoring outcomes such as efficacy of treatment, changes in target symptoms, emergence of long-term side effects, laboratory values and physical findings relevant to specific medications, and occurrence of destabilizing stressors.
- Identify possible barriers to maintenance care, such as issues regarding transportation, finances, birth control, child care, support system, relocation, cultural/ethnic differences, therapeutic relationship, and psychosocial stressors, and the patient's understanding of symptom reduction, symptom exacerbation, and side effects.
- Facilitate the patient's transition from one treatment setting to another, such as from the hospital to the community, from one care provider to another, and from one treatment to another.
- Develop a patient-education program for relapse prevention that can include self-monitoring techniques and teaching tools such as medication cards, handouts, diaries, bibliographies, and other materials to enhance ongoing education of patients, families, and significant others.
- Enhance health promotion with restoration techniques that can be individualized for the patient and integrated with medication treatments, such as diet; exercise; leisure activities; and community, social, and religious affiliations.
- Assist the patient, family, and significant others to establish advance directives regarding emergency interventions, including the use of psychopharmacologic agents.

Discontinuation and Follow-Up

Objectives. The psychiatric–mental health nurse can:
- Relate current recommended practices regarding psychopharmacologic maintenance requirements and duration of treatment for specific psychiatric disorders.
- Discuss issues related to discontinuation of medication, including tapering schedules, and potential sequelae, such as withdrawal, dependence, rebound effects, and return of symptoms of illness.
- Develop with the patient, family, and significant others a plan for self-care in a postmedication phase that considers assessments of quality of life, predisposing stressors, reemergence of symptoms, appropriate use of support systems, and contact sources for potential reevaluation of treatment status.
- Assess the patient before, during, and after the course of treatment, clearly differentiating between changes in the patient as a result of illness effects, drug effects, premorbid personality characteristics, effects of aging, and effects of the environment.

RECOMMENDATIONS

These *Guidelines* are designed to be used as a tool for psychiatric–mental health nurses to determine their knowledge and skill in psychopharmacology and to design a plan for their continued growth in this field. The *Guidelines* can also be used as the basis for the development of curricula and continuing education programs for psychiatric–mental health nurses in psychopharmacology. New information in this field should be added to the *Guidelines* on a regular basis.

As a set of guidelines, this document should not be used in legal proceedings or as an evaluation of nurses' competence in this field by institutions or state or federal agencies.

APPENDIX 5

Comparison of the Major Features of Alzheimer's Disease, Parkinson's Disease & Acquired Immunodeficiency Syndrome–Dementia Complex

	Alzheimer's Dementia	**Parkinson's Disease**	**Acquired Immunodeficiency Syndrome–Dementia Complex**
Etiology/Cause	Unknown	Unknown	Human immunodeficiency virus (HIV)
	Postulated Abnormal protein theory Genetic predisposition Slow virus theory Aluminum toxicity theory	*Postulated* **Primary:** Genetic theory Viral theory Environmental toxin theory **Secondary** (drug induced): Neuroleptics Antiemetics Antihypertensives	Transmitted through sexual contact or contact with bodily fluids of infected individuals Blood transfusions or organs from HIV donors Children born to HIV-positive mothers
Occurrence	Primarily middle or late in life	Primarily middle or late in life	Generally infects adults both male and female in the prime of life **Subgroups most affected:** Homosexual/bisexual males IV drug users Dementia occurs in up to 75% of people living with AIDS
Neuroanatomy/Pathology	Cerebral cortex Hippocampus **Alterations include:** Neurofibrillary tangles and neuritic plaques interfering with transmission of	Basal ganglia Substantia nigra Subthalamic nucleus Extrapyramidal system **Alterations include:** Degeneration of pigmented cells in the substantia nigra	HIV invades the brain shortly after infection, mechanism of viral invasion of CNS tissue unknown Free virus theory Infected macrophage theory

Continued on following page

Comparison of Alzheimer's Disease, Parkinson's Disease & Acquired Immunodeficiency Syndrome–Dementia Complex

	Alzheimer's Dementia	**Parkinson's Disease**	**Acquired Immunodeficiency Syndrome–Dementia Complex**
	neurochemicals at the synaptic cleft	Depleting dopamine stores and unique deposits of pigmented inclusion bodies called "Lewy bodies"	**Alterations include:** Subcortical areas Central white matter Thalamus Brain stem Basal ganglia
Neurotransmitter	**Reduction in:** Acetylcholine Choline acetyl transferase Serotonin γ-aminobutyric acid (GABA) Norepinephrine Somatostatin	Imbalance between dopamine inhibitory and acetylcholine excitatory control of movement	Unknown: Researchers have proposed that infected cells release toxins that lead to neuron damage and abnormal neurotransmission
Neuropsychiatric Manifestation: Cognitive/Thought/ Mood/Behavior/ Motorsensory	Impaired ability to learn new information or recall previously learned information Inability to express or understand written or spoken language (aphasia) Impaired ability to carry out learned motor activities (apraxia) Failure to recognize or identify objects (agnosia) Disturbance in executive functioning disorganized thinking Predominantly depressive mood, lability Impulsivity, aggression, loss of social skills, frustration, personality deterioration Eventually incapable of independent function	Generally intellect is intact, but may have some cognitive impairment, such as visual spatial loss, language difficulties, executive dysfunction No thought disorder—psychosis secondary to drug therapy Depression common—younger clients are at risk for suicide Decreasing abilities to perform ADLs, bradykinesia, tremor, rigidity, and postural instability Increasing apathy manifested by ungratefulness or lack of recognition for family's caring responses	Characterized by progressive dementia, global cognitive impairment with severe intellectual dysfunction Later in disease, delusion and visual hallucinations have been described Reactive depression with suicide a serious risk Social withdrawal, isolation Increasing difficulty with ADLs Eventually incapable of independent function—bedridden Progressive motor deterioration and sensory dysfunction Autonomic dysfunction

Table from: Judy Matana and Jinx Tull, Somerville Hospital School of Nursing, Somerville, MA.

APPENDIX 6

Selected Resources

General Resources

Referral to private practitioners
National Mental Health Association
1021 Prince St.
Alexandria, VA 22314-2971
(800) 969-6642
www.nmha.org

National Alliance for the Mentally Ill
200 N. Glebe Rd.
Suite 1015
Arlington, VA 22203
(800) 950-6264
www.nami.org

Depression

Centers specializing in the treatment of depressive disorders
National Foundation for Depressive Illness
Box 2257
New York City 11016
(212) 268-4260
www.depression.org

National Depressive and Manic Depressive Assn.
730 N. Franklin, Suite 501
Chicago, IL 60610
(312) 642-0049

Depression/Awareness, Recognition and Treatment (D/ART)
National Institute of Mental Health
Room 7C-02
5600 Fisher Ln.
Rockville, MD 20857
(301) 443-4513
www.nimh.nih.gov

Research funding for depression and schizophrenia
National Alliance for Research of Schizophrenia and Depression (NARSAD)
60 Cutter Mill Rd.
Great Neck, NY 11021

Obsessive-Compulsive Disorder

Anxiety Disorders Association of America (ADAA)
6000 Executive Blvd., Suite 513
Rockville, MD 20852
(301) 231-9350

Obsessive Compulsive Foundation (OCF)
P.O. Box 70
Milford, CT 06460
(203) 878-5669
(203) 874-3483 (information line with national referral list)

Obsessive Compulsive Information Center
Dean Foundation
2711 Allen Blvd.
Middleton, Wisconsin 53562
(608) 827-2390

Abuse

National Coalition against Domestic Violence
1500 Massachusetts Ave.
Washington, DC 20005

Resources

Excerpts from National Committee to Prevent Child Abuse (NCPCA)
Working Paper #867332
S. Michigan Ave., Suite 1600
Chicago, IL
(312) 663-3520

Hotlines

National Directory of Hotlines and Crisis Intervention Centers
(800) 999-9999

Childhelp USA/IOF National Child Abuse Hotline
(800) 422-4453 (4-A-CHILD)

Directories

Public Welfare Directory, American Public Welfare Association
(202) 682-0100

NCPCA publishes a variety of educational materials that deal with parenting, child abuse, and prevention (800) 835-2671

ADHD

Support Groups. The largest organization network for those with ADHD is a group called CHADD (Children and Adults with ADD). They have local groups and publish a newsletter. They can be reached by calling (800) 233-4050, or writing CHADD, 499 N.W. 70th Ave, Suite 308, Plantation, FL 33317.

Self-Help Books. A number of self-help books are available for parents of children and adults with the symptoms. For practical help and information for parents with ADHD children, the following books are recommended:

Garber, S, Garber, M, and Spizman, RF: Is Your Child Hyperactive? Inattentive? Impulsive? Distractible? Villard Books, New York, 1995.

Barkley, R: Taking Charge of ADHD: The Complete Authoritative Guide for Parents. The Guilford Press, New York, 1995.

Ingersoll, B and Goldstein, S: Attention Deficit Disorder and Learning Disabilities: Realities, Myths, and Controversial Treatments. Doubleday, New York, 1993.

Recommended reading for adults with ADHD is the following:

Hartmann, T: ADD Success Stories: A Guide to Fulfillment for Families with Attention Deficit Disorder. Underwood Books, Grass Valley, California, 1995.

Recommended educational video for adults is the following:

Phelan TW: Adults with Attention Deficit Disorder: Essential Information for ADD Adults. Child Management Inc, Glen Ellyn, Illinois, 1994.

Homelessness

The National Coalition for the Homeless
1612 K St. NW, Suite 1004
Washington, DC 20006
(202) 775-1322

Interagency Council on the Homeless
451 Seventh St. SW, Suite 7274
Washington, DC 20410
(202) 708-1480

National Law Center on Homelessness and Poverty
918 F St. NW, Suite 412
Washington, DC 20004
(202) 638-2535

National Alliance to End Homelessness
1518 K St. NW
Washington, DC 20005
(202) 638-1526

Institute for Children and Poverty
Homes for the Homeless
36 Cooper Sq.
New York, NY 10003
(212) 529-5252

Health Care for the Homeless Resource Center
210 Lincoln St.
Boston, MA 02111
(617) 482-9485

National Association of State Coordinators for the Education of Homeless Children and Youth
c/o Louisiana Department of Education
645 Main St., 3rd Floor
Baton Rouge, LA 70801
(504) 342-3431

Glossary

A-B-C model: a behavioral analysis model that attempts to identify antecedents to certain consequences and promote adaptive behaviors.

Abuse: physical, sexual, or psychological maltreatment.

Acquired immunodeficiency syndrome (AIDS): a manifestation of infection with the human immunodeficiency virus (HIV) characterized by the presence of one or more diseases as defined by the Centers for Disease Control and Prevention (CDC). These diseases occur following a depression of an individual's immune system function. The affected person becomes susceptible to unusual infections and malignancies.

Acting out: expressing oneself in an overt manner without self-understanding; usually instead of expressing feelings directly. Often the term used to describe negative behaviors of children, such as acting out anger toward a parent by being defiant. Can be confused with the term *act up*, which means to misbehave.

Active listening: a therapeutic skill that requires more than listening: hearing the client, interpreting the language, noticing nonverbal and paraverbal enhancements, and identifying underlying feelings.

Addiction: repetitive behavior, generally reserved to indicate dependence on narcotics, drugs of abuse, alcohol, or tobacco.

Adjustment: the process of adapting to emotions and psychological distress.

Affect: the emotional reactions associated with an experience.

Agonist: a drug or agent that mimics the action or effects of another drug or agent.

Agoraphobia: literally "fear of the marketplace." Fears and anxieties that lead to avoidance of places or situations such as stores, movie theaters, or crowded places.

AIDS-defining illness: a disease marker in which an HIV-positive individual experiences one of the opportunistic infections as well as a CD4 cell count below 200.

AIDS-related dementia: an HIV-associated neurocognitive disorder that causes memory impairment and mental slowness.

Akathisia: a persistent and uncomfortable state of motor restlessness, experienced as the need to pace or move. Clients pace, shift position frequently, jiggle their legs, or are unable to sit still. Akathisia is an extrapyramidal symptom. It commonly arises from antipsychotic medications, particularly high-potency agents, and less frequently with some of the newer antidepressants.

Alzheimer's disease: a progressive disorder that significantly impacts short- and long-term memory, functional and cognitive abilities; it terminates in dementia and death.

Ambivalence: the experience of having opposite feelings or behaviors for a situation, triggering indecision.

Amenorrhea: a physical sign of anorexia nervosa in females, characterized by the absence or loss of menstruation usually related to weight loss and malnutrition.

Amnesia: loss of memory caused by emotional trauma or brain damage.

Amnestic disorder: a persistent disorder that severely disturbs memory to cause noticeable impairment in social or occupational functioning.

Anhedonia: an inability to experience pleasure.

Anorexia nervosa: an eating disorder characterized by a pursuit for thinness, driven by the fear of gaining weight and distorted body image, resulting in abnormally low body weight.

Anorgasmia: difficulty achieving orgasm in women.

Antagonists: drugs or agents that block or reverse the action or effects of another drug or agent.

Anterograde amnesia: loss of the ability to retain newly learned information. This type of memory loss results frequently from electroconvulsive therapy (ECT).

Anticipatory grieving: the process by which a person anticipates the loss of a loved one by experiencing a grief reaction in response to an upcoming loss.

Anticipatory intervention: intervention in anticipation of stressors to prepare an individual, family, or group for such experiences as birth, death, separation, stress, and loss.

Antiretroviral drug: a drug that reduces the replication rate of HIV and is used to treat HIV-infected persons. The most common are zidovudine, didanosine, and zalcitabine.

Antisocial: a personality disorder characterized by lying, deceit, irresponsibility, disregard for the welfare of others, and possibly criminal behavior.

Anxiety: a normal human emotion experienced in varying degrees. In moderate to severe forms it is a state of nervousness, worry, or fear sometimes associated with physical symptoms such as muscle tension and tachycardia.

Anxiolytics: medications that reduce or alleviate anxiety; also called *antianxiety agents*.

Apraxia: an impairment in the ability to use objects or to perform deliberate activities.

Attention-Deficit/Hyperactivity Disorder (ADHD): diagnosed when children are distractible, impulsive, hyperactive, and unable to sustain attention. Their behavioral and attention difficulties affect school performance and home and social interactions.

Avoidant: a personality disorder characterized by extreme social inhibition. Individuals typically shun social and close relationships because of fear of rejection, criticism, and humiliation.

Behavioral analysis: analysis focusing on problems in behavior, as opposed to focusing on early childhood experiences or biological factors.

Benign homelessness: homelessness of short duration, with minimal effects and a long-lasting resolution.

Binge eating disorder: a proposed diagnostic eating disorder category in *DSM-IV* characterized by recurrent binge eating episodes in the absence of inappropriate compensatory behaviors to prevent weight gain.

Biofeedback: a behavior therapy technique used to help clients control physical responses to emotions such as heart rate. A mechanical device provides immediate feedback about physiological responses through reinforcement and punishment.

Bipolar: indicating the two extremes of manic-depressive illness: mania and depression.

Blunted: showing less emotional response than expected.

Borderline: a personality disorder characterized by intense and inappropriate anger, emptiness, mood shifts, suicidal feelings or actions, impulsivity, and frantic efforts to avoid abandonment.

Boundary: the limits an individual uses to separate himself or herself from an event or another person. Also the line of demarcation between a therapeutic and a nontherapeutic relationship.

Bulimia nervosa: an eating disorder characterized by recurring binge episodes and inappropriate compensatory behaviors, such as self-induced vomiting, to prevent weight gain.

Capitation: a managed care plan in which payment is based on the whole population enrolled in the plan. The provider agrees to provide all care for a set amount of money.

Capsulotomy: a psychosurgical procedure that involves either lesioning the brain by gamma irradiation, or targets the anterior limb of the internal capsule under local anesthesia.

Carve out: the separation of mental health services from a larger medical benefits package.

Catastrophic reaction: an outburst of rage that is a result of a client's unchecked frustration over less-than-maximum independence. Often followed by a period of withdrawal and depression.

Catecholamines: the monoaminergic neurotransmitters dopamine, norepinephrine, and epinephrine that contain a catechol ring in their chemical structure. These "brain chemicals" are implicated in many psychiatric disorders, including schizophrenia, mood disorders, and anxiety disorders.

CCU-psychosis: delirium that is found in critical care environments and is most likely related to environmental factors such as sensory deprivation or overload or medication.

Central sleep apnea: a breathing-related sleep disorder characterized by periods of 20–90 seconds of breathing cessation due to cardiac or neurological problems.

Changes: the inevitable experiences of moving from one state to another. Change can be planned or unexpected and results in varying degrees of stress.

Chronic homelessness: homelessness for more than 1 year and sometimes for many years. People in this state accept their life experiences on the streets as normative, are usually identifiable as homeless, and are suspicious of mainstream society.

Chronic sorrow: a normal grief process occurring throughout an individual's life as a reaction to the experience of either living with a prolonged illness or disability or being a caregiver to an individual with a life-long disability.

Cingulotomy: a psychosurgical procedure that involves inserting heated electrodes into two adjacent bilateral holes into the cingulate bundle, creating lesions. Commonly used to treat severe obsessive-compulsive disorder, intractable pain, and major depression unresponsive to conventional treatment.

Client advocacy: a role of the nurse that emphasizes protection of the client's rights, protection from exploitation, and interventions to promote health.

Clients' rights: privileges accorded to the client of a psychiatric facility that must be honored by nurses. Included are basic client rights as well as special rights of the mentally ill specified in state laws.

Cognition: the mental process by which knowledge is acquired. Having perception and memory.

Cognitive restructuring: the basis of cognitive therapy. The process of changing distorted negative thinking and substituting more adaptive thoughts.

Cognitive-behavior intervention: a method of helping individuals change their behavior and conduct as they become aware of self-perceptions, thoughts, and consequences.

Cognitive-behavior therapy: specific techniques, based on learning theories, that help individuals directly confront distorted negative thoughts, thereby changing their behavior.

Commitment: the legal process through which a client may be admitted to a psychiatric agency.

Communication roadblocks: anything that impedes communication, including language barriers, age and developmental level, level of health, knowledge level, time constraints, or faulty communication techniques.

Community support programs: resources in the community that provide an array of rehabilitative and treatment services for clients experiencing severe and prolonged mental illness.

Compulsions: repetitive behaviors or mental acts that often attempt to neutralize obsessional thoughts and anxious feelings. These behaviors usually make little sense and include excessive checking, handwashing, or ordering.

Conduct disorder: a diagnosis that identifies a pattern of asocial behaviors characterized by disregard for the basic rights of others and social rules. It is associated with ADHD in children and adolescents.

Confabulation: a coping mechanism that involves the fabrication of events or experiences as a way of supplying information for gaps in memory.

Confidentiality: protecting the identity of individuals receiving psychiatric care.

Conscious: refers to thoughts and feelings that are accessible to the individual.

Consensual validation: the mutual agreement by two or more individuals regarding a particular meaning that is attributed to verbal and nonverbal behavior.

Containment: an essential function of the therapeutic milieu that provides safety for the milieu by maintaining appropriate physical and social boundaries.

Contextual factors: the individual, interpersonal, and environmental variables that make up an individual's unique life experience.

Conversion: the unconscious use of a somatic symptom to reduce or repress a psychological conflict that creates anxiety.

Coping: those behaviors and psychological reactions that occur in response to a threat or stressor. Coping can be adaptive and promote functioning, or maladaptive and lead to work and school problems.

Coping mechanisms: the behaviors of an individual used in an attempt to reduce stress and improve an immediate situation. Coping mechanisms are directly associated with the individual's level of psychodynamic functioning and can be effectively adaptive or maladaptive.

Corpus callosum: the major myelinated pathway connecting the left and right brain hemispheres.

Correctional milieu: secure or controlled settings, commonly jails, prisons, correctional facilities, or penitentiaries, including those for women, juveniles, and the mentally ill.

Countertransference: the mental process by which a person transfers feelings from important figures in his or her life onto clients. Sometimes defined as the nurse's feelings about the client, regardless of origin.

CPAP: continuous positive-airway pressure used to keep the upper airway open for clients with sleep apnea. An effective and noninvasive procedure used nightly.

Creutzfeldt-Jakob disease: a transmissible progressive neurological disease caused by spongiform encephalopathies that are slow-acting viruses.

Crisis: an unstable period in a person's life, characterized by an inability to adapt quickly to a change resulting from a precipitating event.

Crisis intervention: a conceptual framework that provides brief, short-term, action-oriented intervention focused on problem solving with the goal of restoring those involved to the maximum level of functioning in the precrisis state.

Critical incident stress debriefing: the method of reviewing an event that provides the individuals involved with a process for education and psychological or emotional catharsis.

Critical social thinking: a framework intended to provide the reconceptualization of the understanding of the individual's lived experience as it related to social, cultural, economic, and political influences.

Culture: an abstract concept that describes the way of life of a particular group of people who live together. The patterns of lifestyle of a group, often identifiable by speech, dress, and behavior. Recognized to exert considerable influence on the individuals in the group.

Defense mechanisms: unconscious ways of protecting the self (ego) from unwanted or unpleasant feelings, impulses, and anxiety.

Deindustrialization: the ongoing shift in the job market in this country from relatively well-paid manufacturing jobs to lower-paid employment in service industries.

Deinstitutionalization: the movement of the chronically mentally ill from long-term facilities to the community, beginning in the 1950s with the introduction of neuroleptic medications, and again now, with renewed interest in psychosocial rehabilitation.

Delayed sleep phase disorder: a circadian rhythm sleep disorder characterized by going to bed very late and arising late in the morning or afternoon. Common in adolescence.

Delirium: an acute-onset disturbance of consciousness that affects the client's ability to attend to stimuli in the environment. It fluctuates over the course of the day and is the direct result of an underlying medical condition, exposure to a toxin, drug withdrawal, or a combination of these problems.

Delusions: false beliefs and disturbances in thinking; firm convictions and thoughts about the world that are not based in reality. When challenged about the unlikelihood of their beliefs, clients persevere relentlessly.

Dementia: a constellation of symptoms resulting in impairment of both short- and long-term memory, associated with deterioration in judgment and abstract reasoning.

Dendrite: the receiving end of a neuron.

Dependent: a personality disorder characterized by the need to rely on others to an extreme degree for support, love, decision making, and advice.

Depersonalization: a specific form of dissociation characterized by detachment from feelings or the body.

Development: the formulation of an autonomous, self-sufficient "separate self," usually attained though mastery of sequential crises or stages.

Developmental plasticity: the capacity for experience to alter the brain's structure and function, particularly during the first decade or so of life. Also called *neural* or *brain plasticity*.

Disclosure: the process of the abuse victim revealing the occurrence of abuse.

Disinhibitions: behavior demonstrating poor impulse control such as inappropriate offensive language or inappropriate sexual behavior.

Dissociation: feeling detached or disconnected from reality. It refers to a severe disruption in consciousness, memory, identity, or perception of the environment.

DSM-IV: (*Diagnostic and Statistical Manual of Mental Disorders, Fourth Edition*) a classification system used by all disciplines for the diagnosis of psychiatric illness.

Dura mater: the leatherlike covering that protects the brain.

Dysfunctional family: a family that cannot cope or accommodate stresses that arise from changes in its life cycle. Family members tend to be unresponsive to the developmental needs of the members, role expectations go unfulfilled, communication becomes distorted or indirect, and cooperation and support cannot occur.

Dyspareunia: genital pain during sexual intercourse.

Dysphoria: an irritable and angry mood that frequently occurs during extreme states of mania.

Dysphoric: a sad, tearful feeling.

Dyssomnia: a group of primary sleep disorders characterized by difficulty initiating or maintaining sleep or by sleeping excessively.

Dysthymia: a milder, chronic form of depression that is different from major depression, characterized by 2 or more years of depressed mood on most days.

Dystonias: acute muscle spasms that mainly affect muscles of the head and neck. Less commonly, dystonic reactions of the trunk and legs lead to gait disturbances. They often appear as spasms of the neck (head turned to one side) or tongue protrusion. Dystonias emerge during acute antipsychotic therapy and are treated effectively with anticholinergic agents (often administered intramuscularly).

Economic abuse: the control or withholding of financial resources from the abused person by the dominant person.
Empathy: the ability to place oneself into the feelings and experiences of another and imagine what it's like.
Environment: the physical circumstances that surround the client including temperature, air, and setting, for example.
Euphoria: a state of excessive happiness and elevated mood.
Euphoric: overly buoyant for the circumstances.
Euthymia: normal mood and behavior states.
Extinction: removing a desired event when an unwanted behavioral response occurs to decrease the frequency of that behavior.
Extrapyramidal syndrome (EPS): a triad of three side effects induced by antipsychotic therapy: akathisia, dystonias, and drug-induced parkinsonian side effects.
False memories: confabulations of abuse; so-called recovered traumatic memories that describe events that never occurred.
Family: a group of interdependent persons with identified members who relate to one another. Individuals in the unit are emotionally dependent on each other and may be responsible for financial and material support, meeting growth and developmental needs, and providing stability, care, and protection.
Family boundary: a psychological barrier that serves to protect and enhance (1) the integrity of the family as a whole unit, (2) the separateness of individual family members, and (3) the subsystems of parents, siblings, and generations.
Family of origin: the family into which an individual is born or adopted; an individual's first and original family.
Family of procreation: the family formed by two individuals entering a relationship into which children are born and the individuals become parents.
Family process: the totality of the transactions occurring in the family during interaction sequences.
Family structure: the organization of the family and its functioning. This organization or structure determines the manner in which members interact, communicate, and fulfill roles.
Family system: a network of transactions by members that contributes to maintaining the stability (homeostasis) of the group and also facilitates changes. This network of transactions is determined by the behavior of individuals and in turn influences the behavior of individual members.
Fee-for-service: a cost-based system in which an insurer pays what a hospital or practitioner charges.
Fight or flight: the generalized response to an emergency situation, characterized by stimulation of the sympathetic nervous system, as the body prepares to either flee or fight.
Flashbacks: the spontaneous memory, feeling, or perceptual reexperiencing of traumatic events. One of the persistent reexperiencing symptoms of PTSD.
Flat: showing no emotional response.
Flat affect: the absence of emotion or changes in feeling normally evident in facial expressions or tone of voice. Commonly, facial expressions do not change, and the tone of voice is monotonous. No emotions are evident in response to sad, angry, or happy events.
Formal thought disorder: disordered thinking or use of language.
Fugue: a dissociative disorder characterized by unexpected abrupt travel associated with loss of identity or assuming a new identity.

General adaptation syndrome: a three-stage process of response to stress. It includes the alarm reaction (the fight-or-flight response), in which the sympathetic nervous system is stimulated; the stage of resistance, in which there is some resistance to the stressor and the individual functions at a level lower than optimal and requires greater energy consumption to survive; and the stage of exhaustion, in which all energy has been expended and the ability to adapt fails.
Gentrification: the redevelopment of urban areas with a consequence of losing many low-cost housing units; it occurs when the more affluent members of society move into and rehabilitate areas once inhabited by the poor.
Grief: the emotional state wherein an individual experiences the loss of a loved one.
Group-as-a-whole: the overall themes that emerge in a group that affect the whole group, such as anxiety about competition, anger, and confrontation.
Group content: the topic or issue discussed within the group, and the leader's ability to present the topic in a language that can be understood by all group members.
Group dynamics: the way in which each group develops a unique set of norms, values, and roles.
Group process: the way in which group members interact with each other. Interruptions, silences, glares, and scapegoating are all examples of group processes.
Group therapy: a treatment modality for two or more individuals who meet on a regular, predetermined basis, with one or more therapists, for the purpose of achieving health-related goals.
Hallucinations: problems with sensory perception that seem to reflect reality. The individual is convinced that he or she can hear, see, smell, and so forth, something that is not perceived by others.
Healthy grieving: grieving that is appropriate in scope, severity, and time for a given situation, without being indicative of a larger psychological problem.
Healthy sexual functioning: the ability to engage and perform in three primary stages of sexual activity to achieve satisfaction as a result of the sexual activity.
Helpful communication techniques: those nondirective comments made by a nurse that encourage self-expression by the client. Basic skills for therapeutic interaction.
Hemispheres: the major division of the brain into left and right parts.
Histrionic: a personality disorder characterized by the need to draw attention and by extremely dramatic and emotional speech, dress, and behaviors.
HIV disease: the period from initial infection with the human immunodeficiency virus through the symptomatic stage of acquired immunodeficiency syndrome (AIDS).
Homelessness: (1) a situation in which individuals or families do not have a stable residence or a place where they can sleep and receive mail; also includes those who are forced to move in with family members or friends because they lack housing alternatives. (2) A human condition of disaffiliation and detachment (sociological definition). (3) More than the lack of a home, it is a profound disconnection from other people and social institutions (intrapsychic definition). (4) A situation that occurs when one lacks adequate shelter, resources, and community ties (ADAMHA definition).
Human immunodeficiency virus (HIV): the organism isolated and recognized as the etiologic agent of AIDS. HIV is

classified as a lentivirus in a subgroup of the retroviruses. It infects and destroys a class of lymphocyte, CD4 cells, thereby causing progressive damage to the immune system.

Huntington's disease: a chronic, progressive, hereditary condition that results in involuntary, purposeless, rapid motions, called chorea, and mental deterioration that progresses to dementia.

Hyperactivity: excessive or constant overactivity.

Hyperarousal: a state of excitement experienced as one of the core symptoms of posttraumatic stress disorder (PTSD). It may include increased pulse or blood pressure, difficulty concentrating, sleep disruption, angry outbursts, being easily startled, or hypervigilance.

Hypersomnia: increased sleep duration, evidenced by prolonged sleep during the day and night.

Hypervigilance: a state of extreme alertness and being "on guard."

Hypochondriasis: preoccupation for at least six months with the fear or belief that one has a serious disease, based on individual misinterpretation of physical symptoms.

Hypomania: periods of elated mood and behaviors similar to mania, but not sufficient to cause social or occupational impairment; it lasts at least 4 days.

Impulsivity: acting on impulse rather than thought.

Inappropriate: behavior that does not match the circumstances, such as glee after a death in the family.

Inattention: the lack of notice or regard for environmental stimuli.

Indolamines: the monoaminergic neurotransmitters serotonin and melatonin that contain an indole ring in their chemical structure.

Informative reminiscence: storytelling and oral history through which an elder passes knowledge on to younger generations.

Inmate: a male or female of any age who is incarcerated in a jail, prison, juvenile detention facility, or similar setting, where freedom and movement are restricted and controlled.

Insight: the ability to understand one's own character and the inner meaning of one's behavior.

Insomnia: difficulty falling asleep, multiple nighttime wakenings, or waking early in the morning and being unable to resume sleep. Insomnia can be transient (lasting a few days), short-term (lasting 3 or 4 weeks), or long-term (lasting more than 4 weeks).

Institutionalization: a process in which an individual has remained in a hospital or institution for an extended period and becomes dependent on caregivers for basic needs as well as decision making.

Intoxication: an abnormal psychological state, essentially a poisoning by a substance.

Involvement: an essential function of the therapeutic milieu that addresses clients' active participation in treatment and in other interactions within the milieu.

Kindling: a leading theory of bipolar disorder, borrowed from neurology, that refers to the process that shifts normal mood and behaviors to depression and mania. Mild episodes of depression (dysthymia) or mania repeat, build on the previous episode, and finally culminate in a full-blown manic or depressive state.

La belle indifference: an attitude suggesting a lack of concern about the manifestation of physical symptoms during somatization.

Lability: rapid change in emotions.

Lanugo: a physical sign of anorexia nervosa characterized by fine hair growth on the facial area or trunk of the body.

Libido: sexual desire or sex drive.

Life review: evaluative reminiscence covering the lifespan to integrate the individual's life experiences into a whole and discern its meaning.

Lux: a measure of the intensity of light.

Malignant homelessness: long-term or recurrent episodes of homelessness that create significant hardships for the homeless individual or family.

Managed care: a system for the financing and delivery of health care in which costs are contained by controlling the provision of services.

Mania: a period of increased euphoric mood, energy, thoughts, and activity, along with decreased need for sleep.

Marginal homelessness: homeless individuals or families living just below or slightly above the poverty line. They are not often recognized or counted as homeless, but frequently use the services offered for the homeless community. This group includes many women.

Mental health: a state of well-being in which individuals function well in society and are generally satisfied with their lives.

Mental illness: clinically significant behaviors or psychological syndromes associated with present distress or impairment in one or more important areas of functioning, or with a significantly increased risk of suffering death, pain, disability, or an important loss of freedom.

Mental Status Examination: a series of interactions designed to elicit information on the mental functioning of the client.

Mild neurocognitive disorder: an HIV-associated neurocognitive disorder in which individuals experience poor concentration, fatigue, and difficulty with short-term memory.

Milieu therapy: based on the French word for environment, a setting consciously sculpted to promote structured interactions and communications. Also called *therapeutic milieu*. Staff retains authority and responsibility for the milieu's functioning.

Misuse: the nonmedical use of a psychoactive drug in greater amounts than prescribed, more frequently than prescribed, or without a prescription.

Mood: temporary state of mind evidenced by one's thoughts or actions.

Mood stabilizers: medications used to treat the depressive and manic cycles of bipolar disorder. This class is comprised of lithium carbonate, carbamazepine, and valproic acid.

Myelin: a fatty substance that wraps around neurons to increase the speed of information exchange.

Narcissistic: a personality disorder characterized by extreme "self-love"; a sense of arrogance, self-importance, and entitlement. These individuals tend to lack empathy for others and exploit them for their own needs.

Narcolepsy: short periods of irresistible sleepiness ("sleep attacks") that occur several times each day. Hallucinations and muscle paralysis and weakness also occur.

Negative reinforcement: the process by which undesirable events increase the likelihood that a behavior will recur in the future.

Negative symptoms: refers to the functional deficits observed in schizophrenia. They include flat affect, lack of motivation, social withdrawal, poor attention, and alogia (poverty of speech, using few words).

Neuroleptic malignant syndrome (NMS): muscle rigidity, altered levels of consciousness, autonomic instability (hyperthermia, tachycardia, increased blood pressure, diaphoresis), and possible elevations in creatinine kinase, which is an uncommon result from antipsychotic medications. This life-threatening condition requires immediate drug discontinuation and treatment to correct fluid and electrolyte imbalances and reduce fever; it demands careful observation. Bromocriptine or dantrolene may be instituted in severe conditions.

Neurotransmitters: chemical messengers in the brain, including dopamine, norepinephrine, epinephrine, serotonin, melatonin, histamine, acetylcholine, neuropeptides, and amino acids.

"New" homeless: those who became homeless beginning in the 1980s; this group is increasing rapidly now. They are shelterless as well as homeless, quite young, disproportionately from minority groups, and die at an average age of 50. They are much poorer than the "old" homeless, and there are substantial numbers of women and children among them.

Norms: standards of behavior that are expected within a particular group.

Nonverbal communication: the unspoken messages people give. Often more reliable than verbal content.

Nuclear family: a marital or ongoing relationship between two individuals and their child or children.

Numbing: a condition of being detached, indifferent, and devoid of feeling, particularly for traumatic events.

Object relations: the psychological and emotional connection with others; may be described as the capacity to love and react appropriately to others.

Obsessions: uncomfortable thoughts or impulses that are repetitive, intrusive, and lead to extreme anxiety.

Obsessive-compulsive personality disorder: a personality disorder characterized by extreme orderliness, need to control, lack of emotion, and perfectionism.

Obstructive sleep apnea: a breathing-related sleep disorder characterized by periods of 20–90 seconds of breathing cessation due to an obstructed airway.

Offender: an individual who has broken the law. See also *inmate*.

"Old" homeless: individuals who were homeless during the 1930s to 1950s; they were mostly men, average age of 50 years, white, unmarried, and intermittently employed, with about 25% on Social Security. They did not have permanent residences but were seldom without shelter.

Operant conditioning: the investigation of how the events that follow a particular behavior affect the occurrence of that behavior in the future.

Opioids: chemicals produced by the body that act like natural narcotics. Under extremely stressful conditions, the body releases opioids to decrease the emotional responses and fear.

Organized systems of care (OCSs): an outgrowth of managed care with an emphasis on developing accountability, integration, client-centered care, and continuous improvement. The ideal system strives for a genuine partnership between insurers and providers.

Orgasm: the peaking of sexual pleasure with a subsequent release of sexual tension accompanied by rhythmic contractions of the perineal muscles and, in men, the emission of semen.

Orientation: ability to comprehend and adjust oneself to one's environment with regard to time, location, and the identity of persons.

Orientation phase: a beginning phase of the nurse-client relationship that is characterized by assessment, bonding, identification of problems, and designation of a plan of care.

Outcomes: measurable, attainable changes in the client's condition.

Panic attack: a brief unexpected period of extreme anxiety, usually lasting for several minutes. Characteristic symptoms include shortness of breath, heart palpitations, chest pain, spaciness, and fears of having a heart attack or of going crazy.

Panic disorder: a condition with recurrent unexpected panic attacks about which there is persistent concern or worry.

Paranoia: a pervasive sense of suspiciousness or sense that one is being watched or followed. Paranoia may be a symptom of a psychotic disorder or other psychiatric conditions. Paranoid delusions are those false beliefs involving mistrust and suspiciousness or threat of harm.

Paranoid: a personality disorder characterized by suspiciousness, mistrust, and belief that others are "plotting" harm or talking about the client behind his or her back.

Paraphilia: ongoing sexually arousing feelings or fantasies involving nonhuman objects, suffering or humiliation, or children or nonconsenting individuals, lasting at least 6 months. They include exhibitionism, frotteurism, pedophilia, sexual masochism and sadism, and transvestic fetishism.

Parasomnia: a group of primary sleep disorders characterized by abnormal behaviors or physiological events linked to sleep, certain sleep stages, or sleep-wake transitions.

Perpetrator: an individual responsible for inflicting abuse or violence on another.

Pharmacodynamics: the process of how medications affect the individual.

Pharmacokinetics: the principles of drug movement within the body, including absorption, distribution, metabolism, and half-life.

Phase advanced sleep pattern: a circadian rhythm sleep disorder characterized by going to bed very early and arising early in the morning. Common in the elderly.

Phobia: extreme and excessive fears leading to significant anxiety and avoidance of the feared object or situation. Examples include fear of heights, animals, blood, germs, or social situations.

Phototherapy: the direct administration of artificial light treatment, commonly used to treat seasonal affective disorder (SAD), jet lag, and some sleep disorders. Phototherapy devices include the light box, light visor, and dawn simulator.

Physical abuse: physical injury resulting from punching, beating, kicking, biting, burning, or otherwise harming a person. The injury is not an accident; however, the perpetrator may not have intended to hurt the victim. The injury may be the result of a single episode or of repeated episodes ranging in severity from bruising to death.

Physiological dependence: an altered physiological state resulting from prolonged substance use; regular use is necessary to prevent withdrawal.

Play therapy: therapeutic medium through which a child can communicate with the therapist through action play, fantasy play, or artistic expression such as drawings, instead of words alone.

Positive reinforcement: the process in which environmental events that are desirable increase the likelihood that a behavior will recur in the future.

Positive symptoms: the psychotic processes most evident in schizophrenia: delusions, hallucinations, formal thought disorder, and odd, bizarre, or disorganized behaviors.

Precipitating factor: the critical event, as perceived by the individual, that results in the experience of unresolved stress and eventual disequilibrium and crisis.

Precrisis state: the level of functioning for an individual, family, or group preceding the experience of a crisis or critical event.

Premature ejaculation: ejaculation occurs before, during, or shortly after sexual intercourse and prior to when the individual desires it. Occurs with minimal sexual stimulation.

Primary gain: responsibilities that are avoided as a result of somatization.

Primary mental health care: a model for practice that incorporates both physical and mental health care.

Primary prevention: reducing the incidence of an illness in a community. Also referred to as *health maintenance*.

Primary sexual dysfunction: a dysfunction in which there has never been a time of adequate functioning; the dysfunction has always been present and is lifelong.

Progressive muscle relaxation: a behavioral technique in which individuals alternatively tense and relax different major muscle groups in sequence. By systematically contrasting tension and relaxation, clients learn to control anxiety and substitute relaxation for tension. Also called *deep muscle relaxation*.

Prolonged mental illness: an illness that is serious and lasts the duration of an individual's life. It can include periods of remission and exacerbation.

Protease inhibitor drug: a drug that slows down the spread of HIV by inhibiting protease, which is one of the HIV enzymes needed to continue the process of HIV infection. The most commonly used are indinavir, ritonavir, and saquinavir.

Psychiatric disability: a disability resulting from a severe and prolonged mental illness in which the affected individual needs to participate in rehabilitative programs.

Psychiatric–clinical nurse specialist (CNS): a psychiatric nurse with a master's degree in psychiatric nursing, who has successfully passed a national certification exam, demonstrating advanced knowledge of treating clients with psychiatric conditions.

Psychiatric–mental health generalist nurse: a licensed RN with aptitude for and demonstrated expertise in psychiatric–mental health practice.

Psychiatric–mental health nursing: a subspecialty of nursing that emphasizes the use of the nursing process with clients who have unmet psychiatric or psychosocial needs. It involves applying theories of human behavior, purposeful use of self, and a focus on human aspects and responses to psychiatric illness.

Psychoactive substances: drugs or chemicals that may alter perception, awareness, consciousness, thinking, judgment, decision making, insight, mood, and/or behavior.

Psychobiology: the study of structure and function of the brain and the relationship between cellular and molecular processes and behavior.

Psychological abuse: includes acts or omissions by the parents or other persons responsible for the child's care that have caused or could cause serious behavioral, cognitive, emotional, or mental disorders. Emotional abuse is the most difficult form of maltreatment to identify.

Psychological dependence: a compulsive need to experience pleasurable responses from a substance.

Psychomotor retardation: excessively slowed movements and behaviors.

Psychopharmacotherapy: the process of using psychotropic medications to treat psychiatric disorders. Also called *pharmacotherapy*.

Psychosis: misperceptions of reality, false beliefs, disordered thoughts, and lack of insight or awareness into the discrepancy between reality and something that is actually false or unreal.

Psychosocial rehabilitation: special type of treatment and supportive services for assisting an individual experiencing a prolonged mental illness.

Psychosocial stages: Erikson's eight stages of human development. Each stage is characterized by a critical developmental issue that can be resolved either positively or negatively.

Psychostimulants: methylphenidate, d-amphetamine, and pemoline are the most widely used medications to treat ADHD. Stimulants calm overactivity and improve attention in ADHD children.

Psychosurgery: surgical manipulation of normal brain tissue, similar to neurosurgery for intractable pain or uncontrollable seizures. Used to treat severe psychiatric disorders unresponsive to conventional methods.

Punishers: effects that decrease the likelihood that a behavior will be repeated in the future.

Punishment: the addition of an unpleasant event to decrease the frequency or likelihood that a problematic behavior will occur.

Racing thoughts: a rapid series of ideas or thoughts that occur during manic episodes.

Rapid cycling: a subtype of bipolar disorder characterized by at least four episodes of depression, mania, or mixed states each year.

Reality orientation: an intervention intended to orient clients in the early stages of delirium or dementia, using frequent reminders of date, time, names, and whereabouts.

Recent homelessness: homelessness within the past 9 months. People still identify with the mainstream communities and have hope of regaining a lost home, job, and social standing; they avoid living on the streets. This group encounters many problems with depression, substance abuse, low self-esteem, and shame. They use episodic or emergency health-care services.

Receptor: a binding site for a neurotransmitter.

Reinforcers: events that increase the likelihood that a behavior will recur in the future at an increased frequency.

REM (Rapid Eye Movement) sleep: the final part of the nighttime sleep cycle characterized by actual eye movements, decrease in muscle tone (atonia), and dreaming.
Reminiscence: the act or process of recalling the past.
Reminiscence therapy: the use of reminiscence as a nursing intervention for treatment of specific psychosocial nursing diagnoses.
Remotivation therapy: an approach used with cognitively impaired elders, designed to interrupt self-absorption and isolation. Consisting of five stages, it focuses on experiencing the world and becoming a part of a group; learning about the theme of the group, having some experience that relates to the group's theme, reminiscing in relation to the group's theme, and then establishing a climate of appreciation for being a member of the group.
Response prevention: a cognitive behavior technique used to treat obsessive compulsive disorder (OCD), in which the client is prevented from engaging in ritual behaviors, beginning with less feared situations.
Retrograde amnesia: loss of the ability to recall information learned prior to electroconvulsive therapy (ECT).
Retrospective payment: payment in a fee-for-service system.
Reuptake: the process of neurotransmitter inactivation in which the neurotransmitter reenters the presynaptic neuron from which it had been released.
Revolving door syndrome: when an individual with a mental illness continues experiencing recurrent hospitalizations and discharges from treatment settings.
Russell's sign: a physical sign of an eating disorder characterized by calluses and abrasions on the knuckles caused by the client's teeth during self-induced vomiting.
Schizoid: a personality disorder characterized by lack of emotion and pleasure, extreme isolation, and little to no desire to engage in social or close relationships.
Schizotypal: a personality disorder characterized by odd and peculiar speech, thoughts, and behaviors, ideas of reference, suspiciousness, and inappropriate affect.
Seasonal affective disorder (SAD): a subtype of major depression. It commonly involves a fall-winter pattern of symptoms that occur each fall and remit spontaneously in the spring. The cycle tends to repeat each year without treatment.
Secondary gain: the caring responses from others that result from somatization.
Secondary prevention: reducing the deviance of an illness after it has developed. Comparable to care and curative aspects of an illness. Also referred to as *health restoration*.
Secondary sexual dysfunction: the dysfunction follows a period of normal functioning; an acquired problem in functioning.
Selective serotonin reuptake inhibitors (SSRIs): a class of antidepressants that specifically block the reentry of serotonin into the presynaptic neuron. The net result is that more serotonin is available for transmission, inducing antidepressant effects.
Self-disclosure: the ability to express feelings. A concept that is encouraged in the client during therapeutic interaction, but used with discretion and supervision by the nurse.
Self-in-relation theory: proposes that women's development emphasizes connection and relationship to others, rather than separation and independence, as the primary goal.
Severely and persistently mentally ill (SPMI): persons who are chronically mentally ill.
Sexual abuse: behaviors that include fondling a child's genitals, intercourse, rape, sodomy, exhibitionism, and commercial exploitation through prostitution or the production of pornographic materials. Sexual abuse includes acts committed by a person responsible for the care of the child.
Sexual arousal: affective, cognitive, and physiological changes that serve to prepare persons for sexual activity.
Sexual assault: acts committed by a person who is not responsible for the care of the child.
Sexual desire: a natural drive to behave sexually that is influenced by biological, psychological, social, and cultural factors.
Sexual dysfunction: a change in sexual health or function, usually characterized by disruption in the sexual response cycle or pain during intercourse.
Sexual response cycle: normal healthy sexual functioning characterized by four stages: desire, excitement, orgasm, and resolution.
Shaping: a method of conditioning behavior that incrementally reinforces small behavioral steps until the target behavior is reached.
Signs: observable, objective evidence of an illness in a client.
Simple reminiscence: the recollection of past experiences without analysis or evaluation that occurs spontaneously or is triggered in response to a stimulus.
Sleep deprivation: a form of therapy that does not allow the individual to sleep. Used to treat depression.
Sleep diary: detailed subjective reports of 24-hour sleeping and waking times that clients complete for at least several days.
Sleep hygiene: techniques used to promote sleep. They include environmental manipulation, adjustments to facilitate sleep, and avoidance of behaviors that disrupt sleep.
Sleep restriction: a type of sleep deprivation therapy that allows sleep in the early part of the night, usually from 9:00 pm to 1:00 am. Used to treat depression.
Social distress theory: a theory that provides a structure for understanding the phenomenon of homelessness in terms of conflicting societal issues and values.
Sociocultural crisis: a crisis resulting from the inability of the individual to manage the stressors associated with the social or cultural influences of the situation.
Somatization: the process or an instance of expressing emotional problems and psychosocial stress as a disturbed bodily function, with physical symptoms.
Somatosensory amplification: somatic sensations experienced as intense, noxious, and disturbing. An individual first has heightened attention to bodily sensations, then a focus on relatively mild and infrequent sensations, then a tendency to react with thoughts and feelings that make the sensations more disturbing and frightening.
Spectrum of HIV disease: the continuum of HIV disease or AIDS that ranges from asymptomatic stage of illness to severe immunodeficiency and associated serious secondary infection and neoplasms.
Startle response: exaggerated alarm and fear in response to usual stimuli.

Stigma: a negative perception about an individual who experiences a psychiatric disability, mental illness, or deviation in some way from what the society values.

Stressor: an event leading to marked distress and impairment.

Structure: an essential function of the therapeutic milieu that defines the milieu in terms of time and orientation, providing a sense of organization and concreteness.

Subcaudate trachotomy: a form of psychosurgery that targets an area beneath the caudate nucleus, the substantia innominata. Used for treatment-resistant affective disorders.

Substance abuse: a pattern of maladaptive substance use outside the limits acceptable by society that negatively affects the psychological, physiological, and social functioning of an individual.

Substance dependence: a reliance on a substance or chemical to a degree that its absence will cause impairment in psychological or physiological function.

Substantiation: after the process of investigating allegations of abuse, sufficient evidence is found to indicate that abuse occurred.

Support: an essential function of the therapeutic milieu that maintains a sense of connection, worth, and hope.

Survivor: an individual who has been subjected to abuse; indicates strength and the ability to overcome victimization.

Symptoms: subjective statement by client of conditions of illness.

Synapse: the point where two neurons meet and communicate.

Systematic desensitization: a series of behavioral techniques used to help clients manage feared or anxious situations. After learning progressive relaxation, the client applies these techniques to increasingly feared situations, first through visualizing them and then by actual exposure.

Tardive dyskinesia (TD): tardive (late onset) dyskinesia (abnormal movements) refers to abnormal involuntary movements usually in the face, mouth, or tongue that result from prolonged antipsychotic therapy. Examples include lip smacking, sucking, and puckering, grimacing, and snakelike movements of the tongue, fingers, or toes. This effect may be sustained and lifelong; however, some individuals will experience remission after medication is discontinued.

Termination phase: the ending phase of the therapeutic relationship.

Tertiary prevention: reducing the impairment resulting from having had an illness. Also referred to as *rehabilitation*.

Therapeutic community: specific social setting, emphasizing health and rehabilitation, with characteristics including democracy, egalitarianism, focus on group processes, permissiveness, and community self-regulation. Differs from therapeutic milieu by deemphasizing differences between staff and "clients" in roles or power structures.

Therapeutic milieu: the physical and interpersonal environment manipulated in a systematic manner for therapeutic purposes, such as for the promotion of optimal functioning in activities of daily living or for the improvement of interpersonal skills.

Therapeutic relationship: the systematic interaction of a nurse and a client for the purpose of providing assistance or care to the client.

Tolerance: the decreased psychoactive effect of a drug resulting from repeated exposure. It is also possible to develop cross-tolerance to other drugs in the same category.

Transference: the mental process by which a person transfers feelings from important figures in his or her life onto the nurse or other practitioners.

Trauma response: responses to abuse, immediate or long-lasting, that affect an individual's functioning.

Unconscious: unwanted and uncomfortable thoughts and feelings hidden from awareness.

Unipolar depression: states of depressed mood, loss of interest, sleep and appetite disturbance, lack of energy, and suicidal thoughts, lasting 2 weeks or longer. Also called *major depression*.

Vaginismus: ongoing involuntary contraction of the lower vaginal muscles.

Validation: an essential function of the therapeutic milieu that affirms a client's individuality within the milieu through the nurse-client relationship.

Validation therapy: an approach for treating the demented client, in which nursing staff attempt to enter the client's world rather than force him or her to relate to an external world that he or she can no longer comprehend.

Vascular dementia: dementia that is a result of multiple cerebral infarctions.

Ventricles: hollow cavities in the brain filled with cerebrospinal fluid.

Violence: behaviors by individuals that intentionally threaten, attempt, or inflict physical harm on others.

Withdrawal: a period after the discontinuance of an addictive substance, frequently characterized by painful physical and/or psychological symptoms.

Working phase: that phase of the nurse-client relationship in which progress occurs, largely because the client knows the nurse better and trusts more.

Index

An "f" following a page number indicates a figure; a "t" following a page number indicates a table.

AA. *See* Alcoholics Anonymous
Abbreviated Connors Rating Scale (ACRS), 538
A-B-C model, 133–134
Abnormal Involuntary Movement Scale (AIMS), 118, 119–120t
Abuse, 591–602. *See also* specific types of abuse
   abuse-related symptoms, 596–598
   assessment of, 595–598
   case study of, 602
   client's perception of shame or vulnerability, 600
   cognitive distortions in, 600
   components of, 593–594
   confidentiality issues in, 599
   disclosure and substantiation of, 593
   empowering abused individual, 598
   false memories of, 597–598
   identifying symptom clusters in, 599–600
   indicators of, 595–596, 595–596t
   mandated reporting laws, 596, 598, 598f
   minimizing intrusiveness, 599
   perpetrator of, 593
   prevalence of, 591–592
   principles of treatment of, 598–600
   reassuring client that symptoms are normal, 600
   resources about, 670–671
   safety of client, 598
   survivor of, 594
   trauma responses in, 594–595
   treatment of survivor of, 600–602
     family, couples, and sex therapy, 601
     group psychotherapy, 601
     individual psychotherapy, 601
     pharmacologic treatment, 601–602
     potential countertransference, 602
   types of, 592–593
   violence in environment, 594
   violence in home, 593–594
Acceptance stage, of grieving, 636
Acetylcholine, 80t, 83, 84t, 248
Acetylcholine receptor, 80t, 83
Acetylcholinesterase, 83
Acidosis, 266t
Acquired immunodeficiency syndrome. *See* AIDS
ACRS. *See* Abbreviated Connors Rating Scale
ACTH, 87
Actigraphy, 490t, 492f
Acting out, 544
Action potential, 79–80, 79f
Active listening, 54

Activity group, 163–165
Acute intoxication, 292
Acute retroviral syndrome, 605
Acute stress disorder, 440, 506
Acute withdrawal, 292–295, 295–296t
Acyclovir (Zovirax), 267t
Adaptation theory, of somatization disorder, 404
Addiction, 297
Addiction Research Foundation Clinical Institute Withdrawal Assessment for Alcohol (CIWA-Ar), 294t
Addison's disease, 264t
Addressing client, 50
Adenosine hypothesis, of panic disorder, 386
ADHD. *See* Attention-deficit/hyperactivity disorder
Adinazolam, 127t
Adjustment, 501
Adjustment disorder(s), 501–508
   care plan for, 503–504
   case study of, 507–508
   characteristic behaviors in, 501–503
   chronic, interventions for, 505
   client and family education in, 506
   clinical management of, 504
   cognitive-behavior therapy for, 505–506
   culture and age and, 503
   current research on, 507
   diagnostic criteria for, 502
   differential diagnosis of, 440, 506–507
   DSM-IV classification of, 12t, 658
   etiology of
     neuropharmacologic theories, 503
     stress-adaptation theories, 503
   expected outcomes in, 506
   future research on, 507
   in HIV-positive client, 613
   interventions for clients in community, 504–506
   nursing diagnoses in, 507
   pharmacologic interventions in, 506
   prevalence of, 503t
   prognosis of, 503
   psychosocial and environmental problems causing, 502t
   subtypes of, 501–502
Adolescence, 70–71
Adolescent
   abused, 599
     warning signs of abuse, 595t

   attention-deficit/hyperactivity disorder in, 533–534, 542
   bipolar disorder in, 365
   body dysmorphic disorder in, 421
   communication training, 190
   dating violence among, 538
   depression in, 134, 348–349
   generalized anxiety disorder in, 381
   grieving process in, 638
   HIV-infected, 607
   homeless, 580
   obsessive-compulsive disorder in, 392–393
   panic disorder in, 384
   rating scales for, 41
   runaway teens, 599
   suicide among, 352f
Adolescent and Adult Brown Attention-Deficit Disorder Scale, 539t
Adoption study(ies), 86
Adrenal gland, 87–88, 88f
Adulthood
   attention-deficit/hyperactivity disorder in, 533–534, 533t
   developmental problems of, 71
Adventitious crisis, 147–148
Advice to client, 60t
Affect
   assessment of, 34
   instability in borderline personality disorder, 522
   types of, 34
Affective disorder, rating scales for, 41
Affective factor(s), in family, 185
African(s), culture-bound syndromes among, 38t
African-American(s), culture-bound syndromes among, 38t
Age
   adjustment disorders and, 503
   amnesia and, 256
   attention-deficit/hyperactivity disorder and, 534
   bipolar disorder and, 365
   body dysmorphic disorder and, 421
   as communication barrier, 59
   critical care unit psychosis and, 272
   delirium and, 235
   dementia and, 245–246
   depression and, 348–349
   eating disorders and, 463
   gender identity disorder and, 453
   generalized anxiety disorder and, 381

683

Age—Continued
  mental illness due to general medical condition and, 264–265
  obsessive-compulsive disorder and, 392–393
  panic disorder and, 384
  personality disorders and, 514, 518–519
  phobias and, 389
  posttraumatic stress and dissociative disorders and, 433
  schizophrenia and, 313
  sleep disorders and, 481–485
  substance-related disorders and, 284f, 285
Ageism, 33t
Aggression, pharmacologic treatment of, 253–254
Aging
  development and, 71–72
  normative, 233–234
Agitation, pharmacologic treatment of, 253–254
Agonist (drug), 299
Agoraphobia, 379, 383–384, 386–387
Agranulocytosis, 106t
Agreeing with client, 60t
AIDS, 496t, 605. *See also* HIV disease
  definition of, 605
  epidemiology of, 606–608
  pediatric, 607
AIDS-defining illness, 605, 606t
AIDS-related dementia, 611–613, 612f
  comparison to Alzheimer's and Parkinson's diseases, 668–669
AIMS. *See* Abnormal Involuntary Movement Scale
Akathisia, 103, 116, 325, 332, 333t
Akinesia, 332, 333t
Akineton. *See* Biperiden
Alanine aminotransferase, 291t
Al-Anon, 298–299
Alarm reaction, 143
Albuterol, 268t
Alcohol abstainer, 285
Alcohol abuse, 281–282, 283t. *See also* Substance-related disorder(s)
  acute intoxication, 292
  adverse reactions to, 197t
  alcohol-related car crashes, 277, 278f
  binge drinking, 281, 284–285, 284f
  blood alcohol level, 290, 291t
  CIWA-Ar, 294t
  costs of, 11f
  denial of, 287
  dual diagnosis, 318
  pharmacologic treatment of, 299t, 300
  prevalence of, 281
  safe drinking guidelines, 295–296
  screening tests for, 289, 289t
  short alcohol and drug history, 289
  stages of alcoholism, 281–282
  type I alcoholism, 281
  type II alcoholism, 281
  withdrawal symptoms and nursing actions, 293t, 295
Alcoholics Anonymous (AA), 166, 296, 296–297t
Aldehyde dehydrogenase, 286
Aldomet. *See* Methyldopa

Alexithymia, 404, 469
Alkalosis, 266t
Almshouse, 6
Alogia, 309
Alprazolam (Xanax), 102t, 121t, 122–124, 382t, 387
"Alters," 431
Altruism, 161, 209t
Alzheimer's disease, 78, 83, 239–246, 397t, 496t. *See also* Dementia
  biological theories of, 246–248
  caring for patient with, 245, 254, 257
  compared to Parkinson's disease and AIDS-related dementia, 668–669
  genetics of, 257
  Global Deterioration Scale, 243–244t
  neurotransmitters in, 80t, 84t
  stages of, 241–242, 242t
  treatment of, 80t
  writing deficits and, 249
Amantadine, 99, 102, 234, 237t
Ambien. *See* Zolpidem
Ambivalence, 36, 71
Amenorrhea, 461
American Nurses' Association (ANA)
  Code of Ethics for Nurses, 19, 20t
  Psychopharmacology Guidelines for Psychiatric Mental Health Nurses, 8, 9t
  standards of care, 15, 15t
  Statement on Psychiatric-Mental Health Clinical Nursing Practice, 3
Amino acid(s)
  excitatory, 84–85
  inhibitory, 84–85
Amitriptyline (Elavil), 96t, 97–98, 234
Amnesia/amnestic disorder(s), 255–256
  age and, 256
  anterograde, 223, 256
  care plan for, 256
  characteristic behaviors in, 255–256
  definition of, 255
  diagnostic aids in, 256
  dissociative. *See* Dissociative amnesia
  DSM-IV classification of, 12t, 652
  etiology of
    biological theories, 256
    neuropharmacologic theories, 256
  expected outcomes in, 256
  interventions for clients in community, 256
  prevalence of, 248
  prognosis of, 256
  retrograde, 223
Amnestic disorder due to general medical condition, 255
Amoxapine (Ascendin), 96t, 234
Ampalex, 257
Amphetamine(s), 100t, 542
  abuse of, 283t
  adverse reactions to, 268t
  withdrawal symptoms and nursing actions, 293t
Amplification, 408
Amulet, 12
Amygdala, 76f, 78
Amyloid cascade hypothesis, of Alzheimer's disease, 246–248, 248f

ANA. *See* American Nurses' Association
Anafranil. *See* Clomipramine
Analgesic(s), psychiatric effects of, 234
Anger stage, of grieving, 636
Angina, 397t
Angry client, clinical management of, 520
Anhedonia, 345
Anniversary reaction, 639
Anorexia, 38t
Anorexia nervosa, 461. *See also* Eating disorder(s)
  age and gender features of, 463
  care plan for, 473
  characteristics of, 467, 468f
  cognitive-behavior therapy for, 139t
  critical pathway for, 475–476
  diagnostic criteria for, 461
  differential diagnosis of, 472
  medical complications of, 467t
  neurobiological factors in, 464
  neurotransmitters in, 84t
  nursing diagnoses for, 473
  pharmacologic treatment for, 471
Anorgasmia, 447
Antabuse. *See* Disulfiram
Antagonist (drug), 299
Anterograde amnesia, 223, 256
Anticholinergic(s), 237t, 268t
Anticipatory grieving, 636
Anticipatory intervention, in crisis, 151
Anticonvulsant(s)
  adverse reactions to, 267–268t
  for bipolar disorder, 370–371, 371t
Antidepressant medication(s), 95–107, 359–361, 359–370f
  adverse reactions to, 106, 197t, 268t, 451
  for attention-deficit/hyperactivity disorder, 543–544, 545t
  during breastfeeding, 105
  case study of, 106–107
  current research on, 126, 127t
  for dementia, 254
  for eating disorders, 471
  general information on, 95–96
  mechanism of action of, 111, 350, 350f, 375
  novel. *See* Novel antidepressant(s)
  nursing considerations for, 105–106
  for obsessive-compulsive disorder, 395
  for panic disorder, 387
  for parasomnias, 494
  for posttraumatic stress disorder, 439
  psychiatric effects of, 234
  tricyclic. *See* Tricyclic antidepressant(s)
Antidiuretic hormone, 286
Antigen, 88
Antihistamine(s), 268t
  adverse reactions to, 197t
  psychiatric effects of, 237t
Antihypertensive(s)
  adverse reactions to, 197t, 451
  for attention-deficit/hyperactivity disorder, 544, 545t
  for posttraumatic stress disorder, 440
  psychiatric effects of, 237t
Anti-inflammatory(ies), psychiatric effects of, 234
Antimicrobial(s), psychiatric effects of, 237t
Antiobesity medication, 126

Antiparkinsonism drug(s), 234, 237t
Antipsychotic medication(s), 331–334, 331t
   for acute vs. chronic schizophrenia, 338
   adverse reactions to, 112–113t, 116–117, 332, 451
   atypical, 94, 112–118, 113t, 115f, 331, 331t, 333–334, 337
   for bipolar disorder, 371
   case study of, 120
   clinically significant interactions of, 118, 118t
   contraindications and precautions, 115–116
   current research on, 126, 127t, 337
   extrapyramidal symptoms, 333, 333t
   general information about, 112–118
   indications for, 113
   mechanism of action of, 94, 113–114, 114–115f
   nursing considerations for, 118, 119–120t
   patient's perspective on, 332
   pharmacokinetics of, 113
   potency of, 112, 112t
   typical, 112–113, 112t, 114f, 116–117, 331
Antiretroviral drug(s), 616–617
Antisocial personality disorder, 512t
   characteristic behaviors in, 517
   diagnostic criteria for, 516
   prevalence of, 512t
Antispasmodic(s), 197t
Anxiety, 379
   level of, 379
   therapeutic relationship to assist, 52
Anxiety continuum, 379, 379t
Anxiety disorder(s), 379–400
   attention-deficit/hyperactivity disorder and, 537t, 547
   care plan in, 385
   case study of, 398–399
   clinical management of, 396
   cognitive-behavior therapy for, 139t
   critical pathway for, 390–391
   current research on, 398
   differential diagnosis of, 301, 374, 396–397, 496, 526
   DSM-IV classification of, 12t, 656
   expected outcomes in, 397
   future research on, 398
   generalized. See Generalized anxiety disorder
   in HIV-positive client, 613
   medical conditions causing anxiety, 397t
   neurotransmitters in, 80t, 82
   nursing diagnoses in, 385, 397
   prevalence of, 380t
   rating scales for, 41
   treatment of, 80t
Anxiety disorder due to general medical condition, 263
Anxiolytic(s), 121t
   case study of, 124
   current research on, 126, 127t
   for delirium, 237
   general introduction to, 120–121
   nursing considerations for, 123–124
   for posttraumatic stress and dissociative disorders, 440
   withdrawal symptoms and nursing actions, 293t

Apo E, 248, 257
Appearance, assessment of, 32–33
Appetite suppressant, 125–126
Apraxia, 245
Arachnoid mater, 76
Arctic native(s), culture-bound syndromes among, 38t
Aricept. See Donepezil
Aromatic amino acid decarboxylase, 82
Artane. See Trihexyphenidyl
Arts and crafts group, 163
Ascendin. See Amoxapine
Asian(s), culture-bound syndromes among, 38t
Asian flush reaction, 284
Aspartate, 249
Aspartate aminotransferase, 291t
Aspirin, 234
Assertiveness training, 138, 139t
Assessment, 25–41
   of abuse, 595–598
   of attention-deficit/hyperactivity disorder, 537–539
   behavioral, 133–134
   of body dysmorphic disorder, 422
   case study of, 44
   of conversion disorder, 412
   in crisis intervention, 149–151
   of delirium, 235
   of dementia, 249, 252
   of depression, 353, 357
   determination of strengths, 37
   of eating disorders, 465, 466–467t
   in emergency room, 36
   of family. See Family assessment
   of HIV-positive client, 615
   of hypochondriasis, 418–419
   identifying information, 29
   of life cycle developments, 29
   making nursing diagnosis, 40
   of medication side effects, 35
   Mental Status Examination. See Mental Status Examination
   of pain disorder, 415
   physical, 29
   prelude to, 25–26
   problem statement, 29
   of prolonged mental illness, 556–560
   psychiatric rating scales, 41
   of psychotic disorders, 319–325
   for reminiscence therapy, 206
   responding to interview, 40
   of sexual functioning, 195, 196t, 198t, 446
   of sexual identity disorder, 446
   of sleep disorders, 488, 490t, 491f
   of sociological variables, 37
   of somatization disorders, 408–409
   of substance-related disorders, 288–289
   of suicidal potential, 35–37, 37t, 353
   testing beyond initial assessment, 40–41, 40–41t
   of violence potential, 37, 37t
Assessment interview, 54–55
Association area(s), 78
Astemizole, 102t
Asymmetrical relationship, 185
Ataque de nervios, 38t

Ataxia, 106t
Atenolol (Tenormin), 299t
Ativan. See Lorazepam
Atonia, 479
Atropine, 237t
Attention, assessment of, 33
Attention-deficit/hyperactivity disorder (ADHD), 531–548
   antidepressants for, 543–544, 545t
   antihypertensives for, 544, 545t
   anxiety disorders and, 547
   assessment of, 537–539
      assessment instruments, 538–539, 539t
      clinical assessment interview, 537–538, 537t
   care plan for, 539–541
   case study of, 125–126, 547–548
   characteristic behaviors in, 531–533
   clinical management of, 535
   cognitive-behavior therapy for, 139t, 542
   conduct disorder and, 546
   consequences of, 533t
   culture, age, and gender features of, 533–535
   current research on, 547
   diagnostic criteria for, 532
   differential diagnosis of, 302, 374, 544–546
   etiology of, 535–537
      disinhibitory psychopathology hypothesis, 536
      genetic theory, 535
      impaired brain development, 536
      motivational deficit hypothesis, 536
      neurotransmitter abnormalities, 536–537
   expected outcomes in, 544
   future research on, 547
   home-based interventions for, 542–543
   interventions in
      for clients in community, 541–544
      for hospitalized clients, 541
   learning deficit and, 545
   magnetic resonance imaging in, 536–537
   mental retardation and, 546
   mood disorders and, 544–545
   neurotransmitters in, 80t, 82
   oppositional behaviors and, 546
   pervasive developmental disorders and, 546
   pharmacologic interventions for, 542–544, 545t
   with psychiatric disorders, 537t
   psychostimulants for, 124, 542–543, 545t
   resources about, 671
   school-based interventions for, 542
   subtypes of, 537
   tic disorders and, 547
   time-management strategies for, 542, 544t
   trauma and, 545–546
   treatment of, 80t
Attitude of client, assessment of, 32–33
Auditory channel, 53
Auditory hallucination, 311, 431
Autism, 66, 84t
Autobiography, 204
Autocratic leadership, 175
Autoimmune disease, 88–89
Aversive conditioning, 456

Avoidant personality disorder, 512t
  characteristic behaviors in, 523
  diagnostic criteria for, 524
  pharmacologic treatment of, 525
  prevalence of, 512t
Avolition, 309
AZT. See Zidovudine

Bactrim. See Trimethoprim/sulfamethoxazole
Bahamian(s), culture-bound syndromes among, 38t
BAL. See Blood alcohol level
Balancing factor(s), in assessment of crisis, 149–150, 150f
Barbiturate(s), 237t, 267t
Basal ganglia, 76f, 78–79
  abnormalities in obsessive-compulsive disorder, 393
BDI. See Beck Depression Inventory
BEAM. See Brain electrical activity map
Beck Depression Inventory (BDI), 348
Behavior program, clinical management for implementing, 542
Behavior rehearsal, 138
Behavior therapy
  for eating disorders, 470–471
  for sleep disorders, 492
Behavior therapy procedure(s), 135–138, 139t
Behavioral assessment, 32–33, 133–134
Behavioral theory(ies), 132–133, 133t
  of development, 68
  of substance-related disorders, 286–287
Behaviorism, 132–133, 132t
Belittling client's feeling(s), 60t
Benadryl. See Diphenhydramine
Benign homelessness, 576
Benzodiazepine(s), 94
  adverse reactions to, 122, 237t, 267–268t
  for bipolar disorder, 371
  characteristics of, 121t
  clinically significant interactions of, 122–123
  contraindications and precautions, 122
  for delirium, 237
  for generalized anxiety disorder, 382, 382t
  indications for, 121
  mechanism of action of, 122, 381
  for panic disorder, 386–387
  pharmacokinetics of, 121–122, 121t
  pharmacologic treatment of dependence, 300
  psychiatric effects of, 234
  withdrawal symptoms, 295
Benztropine (Cogentin), 116t
Bereavement, 507. See also Grieving
Beta-alanine, 84
Beta-blocker(s), 267–268t
Bethanechol, 457
Bias, in assessment, 33t
Bilis and colera, 38t
Bill of rights, patient's, 660–661
Binge drinking, 281, 284–285, 284f
Binge eating, 462
Binge eating disorder, 461–463
Biofeedback, 135–136, 382
Biogenic amine(s), 81–83
Biological rhythm(s), 86, 226–227, 348

Biological rhythm theory
  of bipolar disorder, 367
  of depression, 351
Biological theory
  of amnesia, 256
  of bipolar disorder, 366–367, 367f
  of dementia, 246–248
  of depression, 350, 350f
  of gender identity disorder, 453
  of generalized anxiety disorder, 381, 381f
  of hypochondriasis, 417
  of obsessive-compulsive disorder, 393
  of pain disorder, 413–414
  of panic disorder, 384t, 385
  of paraphilia, 456
  of personality disorders, 514, 519
  of sexual dysfunctions, 450
  of substance-related disorders, 285–286
Biological therapy(ies), 221–229
  current research on, 228–229
  future research on, 229
  types of, 221–228
Biperiden (Akineton), 116t
Bipolar disorder, 343, 363–373, 363f
  anticonvulsants for, 370–371, 371t
  antipsychotics for, 371
  benzodiazepines for, 371
  calcium channel blockers for, 371
  care plan for, 368
  case study of, 111, 372–373, 572
  characteristic behaviors in, 363–365, 366t
  client and family education in, 371–372
  culture, age, and gender features of, 365–366
  current research on, 374–375
  differential diagnosis of, 373–374
  etiology of
    biological theories, 366–367, 367f
    circadian and other rhythm theories, 367
    genetic theory, 367, 369–370
  expected outcomes in, 372
  family and, 369
  future research on, 375
  interventions in
    for clients in community, 368–371
    for hospitalized clients, 368
  monitoring compliance, 369
  mood stabilizers for, 370, 370t
  nursing diagnoses in, 374
  pharmacologic treatment in, 370–371
  prevalence of, 343t, 554t
  prognosis for, 368
  rapid cycling, 364, 370
  resources about, 371–372
  self-management in, 369
  subtypes of, 364–365, 365t
  in women, 366
Bipolar I disorder, 363–364, 365t
Bipolar II disorder, 364, 365t
Bipolar III disorder. See Cyclothymia
Bipolar IV disorder, 365t
Blacking out, 38t
Blocking of speech, 311
Blood alcohol level (BAL), 290, 291t
Blood-brain barrier, 76, 89
Blunted affect, 34
Board and care, 568

Body dysmorphic disorder, 319, 421–422, 472
  age and, 421
  assessment of, 422
  care plan for, 422
  characteristic behaviors in, 421
  cultural and gender features of, 406t
  diagnostic criteria for, 405t, 421
  etiology of
    neurobiological theory, 421
    psychological theory, 421
  expected outcomes in, 422
  interventions for clients in community, 422
  prevalence of, 405t
Body fluid(s), chemical analysis of, 85
Borderline personality disorder, 512t
  affect instability in, 522
  characteristic behaviors in, 517–518
  cognitive-behavior therapy for, 139t
  developmental problems and, 71
  diagnostic criteria for, 516
  pharmacologic treatment of, 522–523, 523t
  prevalence of, 512t
Boston University Center for Psychiatric Rehabilitation, 571
Boundary(ies), of therapeutic relationship, 48–50
Boundary crossing, 48
Boundary violation. See Boundary crossing
Bowen's family emotional system therapy, 186, 187t
BPRS. See Brief Psychiatric Rating Scale
Brain
  abnormalities in schizophrenia, 316–317f, 317
  anatomy of, 75–79, 76–77f
  developmental plasticity of, 5
  impaired development and ADHD, 536
Brain electrical activity map (BEAM), 41t
Brain fag, 38t
Brain stem, 76f
Brain tumor, 266
Breastfeeding
  antidepressant use during, 105
  pharmacotherapy during, 94–95
Breathing-related sleep disorder(s), 480, 486
  characteristic behaviors in, 481t, 486
  diagnostic criteria for, 482
  etiology of
    genetic theories, 486
    physiological theories, 486
Brief hospitalization, 215
Brief intervention, in substance-related disorders, 295
Brief Psychiatric Rating Scale (BPRS), 313, 314t
Brief psychotherapy, 19
Brief psychotic disorder, 319
  course of, 324t
  diagnostic criteria for, 320–321
  pharmacologic treatment of, 334
  symptoms of, 324t
Briquet's syndrome. See Somatization disorder
Bromocriptine, 117, 234, 237t
Brujeria, 38t
Bulimia, 38t
Bulimia nervosa, 461–462. See also Eating disorder(s)
  age and gender features of, 463
  care plan for, 474

case study of, 473–476
characteristics of, 467–468, 468f
cognitive-behavior therapy for, 139t
diagnostic criteria for, 462
differential diagnosis of, 472
medical complications of, 467t
neurobiological factors in, 464–465
nursing diagnoses for, 474
pharmacologic treatment for, 471
Buprenex. *See* Buprenorphine
Buprenorphine (Buprenex), 299t, 300–301
Bupropion (Wellbutrin), 96t, 104–105, 359, 360t, 544, 545t
sustained-release, 126
BuSpar. *See* Buspirone
Buspirone (BuSpar), 100t, 101, 121t, 123, 237, 382
adverse reactions to, 123
clinically significant interactions of, 123
contraindications and precautions, 123
indications for, 123
mechanism of action of, 123
pharmacokinetics of, 123

Caffeine, 283t
CAGE screening test, 289, 289t
Calcium channel blocker(s), for bipolar disorder, 371
Calculation ability, 34
Cancer, mental status changes due to, 265, 267, 271
Candidiasis syndrome, chronic, 408
Cannabis, 283t
Capitation, 644–645
Capsulotomy, 224
Carbamazepine (Tegretol), 107, 234, 299t, 370–371, 370t, 522
adverse reactions to, 109–110
clinically significant interactions of, 99, 108t, 110
contraindications and precautions, 109
indications for, 109
mechanism of action of, 109
pharmacokinetics of, 109
Carbidopa, 237t
Cardiac drug(s), 237t
psychiatric effects of, 234
Cardizem. *See* Diltiazem
Care plan, 42
for adjustment disorders, 503–504
for amnesia, 256
for anorexia nervosa, 473
for anxiety disorders, 385
for attention-deficit/hyperactivity disorder, 539–541
for bipolar disorder, 368
for body dysmorphic disorder, 422
for bulimia nervosa, 474
collaborative, 25, 44
for conversion disorder, 412
for dementia, 247, 249
for depression, 353–357
designing interventions, 42
for dissociative disorders, 435–436
for eating disorders, 468–469
establishing priority, 42

for hypochondriasis, 419
for mental illness due to general medical condition, 268, 270
for pain disorder, 415
for personality disorders, 515
for posttraumatic stress disorder, 435–436
for prolonged mental illness, 562
for psychotic disorders, 327
for schizophrenia, 326–327
setting goals, 42
for sexual dysfunctions, 451
for sleep disorders, 488
for somatization disorder, 409
for substance-related disorders, 291–292
Caregiver, for Alzheimer's patient, 245, 254, 257
Caribbean society, culture-bound syndromes among, 38t
Caring, in therapeutic relationship, 47, 48t
Caring touch, 53
Carve out, 644
CASE. *See* Cognitive Adaptation to Stressful Events Scale
Case management, in prolonged mental illness, 567–568
Case manager, 17, 17t
Cataplexy, 312, 486
Catapres. *See* Clonidine
Catastrophic reaction, 250–251
Catatonia, 222
Catecholamine(s), 81
Catecholamine theory, of depression, 361
Catharsis, 161, 204, 209t
Caudate, 76f, 79
glucose metabolism in, 393
CCK. *See* Cholecystokinin
CCU-psychosis. *See* Critical care unit psychosis
Center for Community Health Education, Research, and Service, 8–9
Central sleep apnea, 481t, 486
Centrax. *See* Prazepam
Cerebellum, 76–77f
Cerebrospinal fluid, 76
Cerebrum, 76f
Chakore, 38t
Challenging, 60t
Change(s), 146
Channel (element of communication), 53
"Checking" behavior, 391
Chibih, 38t
Child
attention-deficit/hyperactivity disorder in, 531–532, 534
treatment of, 541, 541f
boundaries of therapeutic relationship with, 50
depression in, 348–349
developmental problems of, 70–71
generalized anxiety disorder in, 381
grieving process in, 637–638, 637t
HIV-infected, 607
homeless, 579–580
obsessive-compulsive disorder in, 392–393, 395
panic disorder in, 384
rating scales for, 41
understanding of death, 637–638, 637t

Child abuse, 591–593f, 592, 595–598
false memories of, 597–598
among psychiatric outpatients, 433
recall in adulthood, 69
warning signs of abuse, 595t
Child Behavior Checklist, 538, 539t
Child development, assessment of family, 183
Childhood abuse theory, of personality disorders, 520
Chloral hydrate, 237t
Chlordiazepoxide (Librium), 121t, 299t, 382t
Chlorpromazine (Thorazine), 112t, 115–118, 237t
Chlorprothixene (Taractan), 112t
Cholecystokinin (CCK), 83, 84t, 464, 464t
Choline, 83
Choline acetyltransferase, 248
Cholinergic(s), 83
Cholinergic theory, of Alzheimer's disease, 248, 248f
Cholinesterase inhibitor, 253
Choreathetoid movement(s), 333t
Chronic fatigue syndrome, 496t
Chronic homelessness, 583
Chronic mental illness. *See* Prolonged mental illness
Chronic sorrow, 554, 565
Cimetidine, 99, 102t, 103–105, 234, 237t
Cingulotomy, 224
Cipro. *See* Ciprofloxacin
Ciprofloxacin (Cipro), 268t
Circadian rhythm, 79, 86–87, 348, 351
light effects on, 87, 87f
Circadian rhythm sleep disorder, 480–481, 487
characteristic behaviors in, 481t, 487, 489t
diagnostic criteria for, 482
etiology of, 487
treatment of, 493
Circular questioning, 180
Circumstantial thought process, 34t
Cirrhosis, 373t
Citalopram, 127t
CIWA-Ar. *See* Addiction Research Foundation Clinical Institute Withdrawal Assessment for Alcohol
Clanging, 312
Classic conditioning, 68, 132–133, 132t
Client advocacy, 21–22
for homeless individuals, 584
Client education
in adjustment disorders, 506
in bipolar disorder, 371–372
job training in prolonged mental illness, 566–567, 567t
in personality disorders, 526
in posttraumatic stress and dissociative disorders, 440
in psychotic disorder, 335
in sleep disorders, 494
Client-centered therapy, 67–68
Clients' rights, 20–21
patient's bill of rights, 660–661
Clinical Assessment of Confusion, 235
Clinical depression. *See* Depression, major
Clinical management, 9t
Clinical nurse specialist, psychiatric, 16, 16t, 18, 647

Clomipramine (Anafranil), 96t, 97–98, 101, 395, 419–420
Clonazepam (Klonopin), 121t, 122–123, 370t, 371, 382t, 387, 395
Clonidine (Catapres), 80t, 116t, 237t, 267t, 299t, 545t, 602
Clorazepate (Tranxene), 121t, 382t
Closed group, 166
Clozapine (Clozaril), 80t, 81, 112–117, 113t, 315, 331t, 332–334, 554
Clozaril. See Clozapine
Coalition, 185
Cocaine, 100t, 283t, 286
 pharmacologic treatment of dependence, 299t
 withdrawal symptoms and nursing actions, 293t
Code of Ethics for Nurses (ANA), 19, 20t
Codeine, 237t
Cogentin. See Benztropine
Cognition, 34, 233–234
Cognitive Adaptation to Stressful Events Scale (CASE), 507
Cognitive disorder(s), 233–257
 current research on, 256–257
 future research on, 257
 HIV-associated, 611–613
 medication-related, 234
 prevalence of, 248
Cognitive distortion, 134–135, 146
Cognitive function, assessment of, 34
Cognitive restructuring, 134, 139t, 387
Cognitive theory, of development, 67
Cognitive therapy, for schizophrenia, 327
Cognitive-behavior group therapy, 165
Cognitive-behavior theory
 of depression, 352–353, 352t
 of phobias, 389
Cognitive-behavior therapy, 131–140
 for adjustment disorders, 505–506
 applications of, 131–132, 135, 139t
 for attention-deficit/hyperactivity disorder, 542
 behavior therapy procedures, 135–138, 139t
 behavioral assessment in, 133–134
 behavioral theories, 132–133, 132t
 case study of, 140
 components of, 134
 current research on, 139
 for depression, 134, 358–359
 for dissociative disorders, 438
 for eating disorders, 470–471
 expected outcomes for, 138–139, 139t
 future research on, 139–140
 for hypochondriasis, 418
 nurse's role in, 131–132
 for obsessive-compulsive disorder, 395
 for panic disorder, 387
 for paraphilias, 456–457
 for personality disorders, 521–522
 for phobias, 389
 for posttraumatic stress disorder, 438
 purpose of, 131
 for sexual dysfunctions, 451
 for substance-related disorders, 295–296
Cognitive-behavioral model, of sexual therapy, 197, 199t

Cognitive-perceptual theory, of somatization disorder, 407–408
Coherence, 33
Cohesiveness, 209t
Collaboration, 16–17
Collaborative plan of care, 25, 44
Co-localization, 83, 84t
Communication
 elements of, 53–54
 levels of, 52–53
 nonverbal, 53, 53t, 55
 therapeutic. See Therapeutic communication
 with treatment team, 55
 within family, 184
Communication pattern, 47, 48t
Communication process, 52–54
Communication roadblock(s), 55–60
Communication style
 closed patterns, 184
 congruent, 184
 open patterns, 184
Communication technique, in eating disorders, 469–470
Communication training, for families, 190
Community mental health movement, historical aspects of, 6–9
Community support group, 553
Community support system, 37
Comorbid disorder(s), in pain disorder, 414
Competency, 21
Compliance, 332, 369
Compulsion, 35t, 391
Computed tomography (CT), 41t, 85, 85t
Computerized patient record, 42
Concept formation, 34
Conceptual models of nursing, 4–9, 4t
Concordance rate, 86
Conditioning, 286–287
 classic, 68, 132–133, 132t
 operant, 132–133
Conduct disorder, 534, 546
 with attention-deficit/hyperactivity disorder, 537t
 cognitive-behavior therapy for, 139t
Confabulation, 34, 241
Confidentiality, 19–20, 49–50, 168, 599, 625
Confusion Assessment Method, 235
Congestive heart failure, 397t
Connors Rating Scale, 538, 539t
Conscious mind, 65
Consensual validation, 161
Constipation, side effect of medication, 106t
Constrictive response, 596
Consultation-liaison nurse, 18
Consumerism, 555
Containment, as function of milieu, 213–214, 214t
Contextual factor(s), 624, 624f
Contextual family therapy, 186–188, 187t
Continuous performance test, 538–539
Continuous positive airway pressure (CPAP), for sleep apnea, 493, 493f
Continuous treatment team, in prolonged mental illness, 568
Continuum of care, 645f
Contract, group, 168–169
Conversion, 411

Conversion disorder, 411–413
 assessment of, 412
 care plan for, 412
 case study of, 413
 characteristic behaviors in, 411
 cultural and gender features of, 406t
 diagnostic criteria for, 405t, 412
 etiology of, 411–412
 expected outcomes in, 413
 familial patterns of, 406t
 gender features of, 411
 interventions in
  for clients in community, 413
  for hospitalized clients, 412
 prevalence of, 405t
Coping, 503
Coping mechanism(s), 146, 150, 507
 assessment of, 29
 of homeless individuals, 582
Coprophilia, 456
Coronary artery bypass surgery, 267
Corpus callosum, 76
Correctional facility. See Offender population
Correctional milieu, 622
Correctional nurse. See also Offender population
 professional identity for, 629
 professional isolation of, 629–630
 professional role definition, 629–630
 roles and responsibilities of, 629
 territoriality issues, 630
Corrective recapitulation, of family group, 161
Cortex, 76–78, 77–78f
Cortical function, assessment of, 34
Corticosteroid(s), 87
 mental status changes due to, 267–268, 267–268t
Corticotropin-releasing factor (CRF), 84t, 87
Cortisol, 87, 346, 367, 434, 466
Cost(s)
 of homelessness, 577
 of mental illness, 11f
 of prolonged mental illness, 554–555
 of substance abuse, 11f
Cotherapist, 175
Counseling, 43, 55
 in bipolar disorder, 371–372
 crisis, 153
Counterconditioning, 68, 136
Countertransference, 40, 50, 436, 602
Couple development, 183–184
Couples therapy
 for abuse survivor, 601
 for sexual dysfunctions, 451–453
Covert sensitization, 456
CPAP. See Continuous positive airway pressure
Creutzfeldt-Jakob disease, 89, 238, 245
CRF. See Corticotropin-releasing factor
Criminalization, of mentally ill, 630–631
Crisis
 adventitious, 147–148
 characteristics of, 144–145
 Chinese symbol for, 144–145, 144f
 definition of, 143–149
 developmental phases in crisis situation, 145–146
 dysfunctional responses to, 145–146

Index

maturational, 146–147
situational, 146
sociocultural, 148–149
types of, 146–149
Crisis counseling, 153
Crisis intervention, 143–155
  assessment phase of, 149–151
    analysis of balancing factors, 149–150, 150f
    sociocultural assessment, 150–151
  case study of, 155
  coping with crisis work, 154
  education and research on, 154–155
  evaluation of nursing process, 154
  expected outcomes in, 154
  future research on, 155
  generic approach in, 151
  historical evolution of, 143
  individual approach in, 151–152
    pharmacologic intervention, 152
    therapeutic techniques, 152
  nurse's role in, 143
  nursing diagnoses in, 151
  nursing process and, 149–154
  planning and implementation phase of, 151–154
  purpose of, 143
  types of intervention programs, 152–154
Crisis theory, 143
  Baldwin's corollaries to, 144
Critical care unit psychosis (CCU-psychosis), 235
  age and, 272
  case study of, 273
  characteristic behaviors in, 272
  differential diagnosis of, 273
  etiology of
    prolonged immobilization, 272
    sensory overload and deprivation, 272
    sleep deprivation, 272
  expected outcomes in, 273
  interventions for hospitalized clients, 272–273
  prognosis of, 272
Critical incident stress debriefing, 153
Critical social thinking, 144
Cross-cultural diagnosis, 43
Cross-dressing, 453, 456
Crucifix, 13
CT. See Computed tomography
Cultural bias, in assessment, 33t
Cultural factor(s), in selecting group members, 166
Culture
  adjustment disorders and, 503
  attention-deficit/hyperactivity disorder and, 533–534
  as communication barrier, 59
  cross-cultural diagnosis, 43
  definition of, 11
  delirium and, 235
  dementia and, 245
  depression and, 348
  eating disorders and, 463
  family assessment and, 182
  gender identity disorder and, 453
  generalized anxiety disorder and, 381

group, 172–173
mental illness and, 10–13
obsessive-compulsive disorder and, 392
offender population and, 622–623
personality disorders and, 514, 524–525
pharmacokinetics and, 94
posttraumatic stress and dissociative disorders and, 433
schizophrenia and, 313
sleep disorders and, 481
somatoform disorders and, 406t
substance-related disorders and, 284
Culture-bound syndrome(s), 37, 38t
Cumulative grief, 637
Current events group, 163
Cushing's disease, 397t
Cushing's syndrome, 264t
"Cycle of violence," 435
Cyclosporine, 268t
Cyclothymia, 364, 365t
Cylert. See Pemoline
Cyproheptadine, 99–100, 102, 457
Cystic fibrosis, 496t
Cytochrome P-450, 101, 102t, 105

D8/17 antibody, 395
Dalmane. See Flurazepam
Dantrolene, 117
DAST-10. See Drug Abuse Screening Test
Dating violence, among adolescents, 538
Dawn simulator, 226–227
Daydreaming, as communication barrier, 59
DBT. See Dialectic behavior therapy
Defending, 60t
Defense mechanism(s), 65, 66t
  in group therapy, 169
Deindustrialization, 581
Deinstitutionalization, 7, 576, 581
Delayed sleep phase disorder, 481, 481t, 485f
Delirium, 233
  assessment of, 235
  characteristic behaviors in, 234–235
  course of, 251t
  culture, age, and gender factors in, 235
  definition of, 234
  diagnostic criteria for, 236
  differential diagnosis of, 255
  DSM-IV classification of, 12t, 652
  etiology of, 235
  expected outcomes in, 237
  in hospitalized elderly, 269
  interventions for hospitalized clients, 235–237
  medications causing, 237t
  pharmacologic interventions for, 237
  precipitating factors during hospitalization, 262
  prevalence of, 248
  prognosis of, 235
  risk factors for, 235t
Delirium due to general medical condition, 236, 261–262
Delirium due to multiple etiologies, 236
Delusion, 35, 35t
  characteristics of, 308, 308t
  clinical management of client, 329

Delusion of alien control, 35t
Delusion of grandeur, 35t
Delusion of a paranoid nature, 35t
Delusion of reference or persecution, 35t
Delusion of thought broadcasting, 35t
Delusion of thought insertion, 35t
Delusional disorder, 319
  course of, 324t
  diagnostic criteria for, 320
  pharmacologic treatment of, 334
  prevalence of, 324t
  symptoms of, 324t
Dementia. See also Alzheimer's disease
  AIDS-related, 611–613, 612f
  assessment of, 249, 252
  care plan for, 247, 249
  case study of, 257
  characteristic behaviors in, 241–245
  client and family education in, 254
  clinical management of, 251
  course of, 251t
  critical pathway, 240–241
  culture, age, and gender features of, 245–246
  definition of, 239–241
  depression vs., 249, 251
  diagnostic aids in, 245
  diagnostic criteria for, 238–239
  differential diagnosis of, 254–255
  diseases presenting as, 250t
  DSM-IV classification of, 12t, 652
  etiology of
    biological theories, 246–248
    genetic theory, 249
    neuroanatomical changes, 246
  expected outcomes in, 254, 257
  frontal, 78
  Global Deterioration Scale, 243–244t
  interventions for clients in community, 250–253, 251t
  medications causing, 237t
  multiple, 245
  nursing diagnoses in, 247
  in nursing home residents, 252
  pharmacologic interventions in, 253–254
  prevalence of, 248
  prognosis of, 249
  remotivation therapy for, 252–253
  reversible causes of, 250t
  treatable, 250t
  validation therapy for, 252
  writing deficits and, 249
Dementia due to Creutzfeldt-Jakob disease, 238
Dementia due to general medical condition, 238
Dementia due to head trauma, 238
Dementia due to HIV disease, 238–239, 611–613, 612f
Dementia due to Huntington's disease, 238–239
Dementia due to medical condition, 245
Dementia due to multiple etiologies, 239
Dementia due to Parkinson's disease, 238–239
Dementia due to Pick's disease, 238–239
Dementia of the Alzheimer's type, 241–244. See also Alzheimer's disease
  diagnostic criteria for, 246
Dementia praecox. See Schizophrenia

Demerol. *See* Meperidine
Democratic leadership, 175
Demographic factor(s), assessment of family, 182
Dendrite, 80
Denial, 66t
  alcoholic, 287
Denial stage, of grieving, 635
Depakote. *See* Valproic acid
Dependent client, clinical management of, 519
Dependent personality disorder, 512t
  characteristic behaviors in, 523
  diagnostic criteria for, 524
  prevalence of, 512t
Depersonalization disorder, 427, 431–432
Depolarization, 80
Depressant, withdrawal symptoms and nursing actions, 293t, 295
Depression
  in adolescent, 134
  course of, 251t
  definition of, 343
  dementia vs., 249, 251
  marital therapy for, 184
  medications that cause, 267t
  neurotransmitters in, 80t, 82, 84t
  therapeutic relationship to assist, 52
  treatment of, 80t
Depression, major, 345–362. *See also* Bipolar disorder
  assessment of, 353, 357
  with atypical features, 347t
  care plan for, 353–357
  case study of, 22, 106–107, 216–217, 229, 362
  characteristic behaviors in, 345–346
  cognitive-behavior therapy for, 134, 139t, 358–359
  critical pathway for, 354–355
  culture and age features of, 348–349
  current research on, 374–375
  definition of, 345
  dexamethasone suppression test in, 88, 346–347, 347t
  diagnostic aids for, 346–347
  diagnostic criteria for, 347
  differential diagnosis of, 373–374, 396
  electroconvulsive therapy for, 221–224, 361–362
  etiology of
    biological theories, 350, 350f
    catecholamine theory, 361
    circadian and other rhythm theories, 351
    cognitive-behavior theories, 352–353, 352t
    genetic theories, 350–351
    psychoanalytic theory, 351–352
  expected outcomes in, 362
  future research on, 375
  grieving vs., 638t, 639
  in HIV-positive client, 613–614
  interventions in
    for clients in community, 357–362
    for hospitalized clients, 357
  nursing diagnoses in, 356, 374
  organic conditions that present as, 373t
  pattern integration in, 346

  pharmacologic treatment for, 359–361, 359–370f
  phototherapy for, 361
  physical and social functioning in, 345, 345f
  postpartum, 346, 347t, 351
  prevalence of, 343t, 554t
  prognosis of, 353
  with psychotic features, 347t, 361
  rating scales for, 348
  recurrent, 347t
  resources about, 670
  with seasonal pattern, 347t
  severity of, 346
  single episode, 347t
  sleep deprivation therapy for, 228
  subtypes of, 346, 347t
  thought patterns in, 352t
  treatment-resistant, 357, 361
  unipolar, 350
Depressive disorder not otherwise specified, 374
Derogatis Sexual Functioning Index, 195
DES. *See* Dissociative Experience Scale
Desensitization, 197, 199t
Desipramine (Norpramin), 96t, 97, 99, 102t, 299t, 543
Desyrel. *See* Trazodone
Development, 65
  aging and, 71–72
  behavioral theories of, 68
  effects of trauma on, 71
  ego psychology, 65–66
  Erikson's life cycle theory of, 66–67, 67–68t
  Freud's psychosexual theory of, 65, 68t
  interpersonal theories of, 67–68, 68t
  object relations theory of, 66
  Piaget's cognitive theory of, 67
  psychoanalytic theories of, 65–66
  women's, 68–70
Development level, as communication barrier, 59
Developmental delay, 70
Developmental plasticity, 5
Developmental problem(s)
  of adulthood, 71
  of childhood, 70–71
Developmental stage, 29
Dexamethasone suppression test, 88
  in depression, 346–347, 347t
  in posttraumatic stress disorder, 346, 347t, 434
Dexedrine. *See* Dextroamphetamine
Dexfenfluramine (Redux), 126
Dextroamphetamine (Dexedrine), 124, 124t, 545t
Diagnostic and Statistical Manual of Mental Disorders, Fourth Edition (DSM-IV)
  axis I, 13
  axis II, 13
  axis III, 13
  axis IV, 13, 13t
  axis V, 13, 14t
  classification of mental illness, 12t, 13, 651–659
Diagnostic Survey for Eating Disorders (DSED), 467

Dialectic behavior therapy (DBT), 137, 521–522
Diarrhea, side effect of medication, 106t
Diazepam (Valium), 80t, 102t, 121t, 234, 299t, 382, 382t
Diencephalon, 76f, 79
Diet pill(s), 126
Dietary log, 470, 470f
Digit Span Test, 235
Digitalis, 237t, 267–268t
Digitoxin, 234
Digoxin, 234
Dihydroxyphenylacetic acid, 82
Diltiazem (Cardizem), 370t
Diphenhydramine (Benadryl), 116t, 237t
Direct questioning, 54–55
Direct victimization, 593–594
Directed masturbation, 451
Disability, psychiatric, 567
Disagreeing with client, 60t
Disempowerment, 598
Disenfranchisement, in prolonged mental illness, 562–565
Disillusionment, in prolonged mental illness, 565–566
Disinhibition, 262, 522, 536
Disinhibitory psychopathology hypothesis, for attention-deficit/hyperactivity disorder, 536
Disopyramide, 234
Disorders usually first diagnosed in infancy, childhood, or adolescence (*DSM-IV*), 12t, 651–652
Dissociation, 71, 427, 582
Dissociative amnesia, 427, 429, 432
Dissociative disorder(s), 427–442
  care plan for, 435–436
  characteristic behaviors in, 428–431
  client and family education in, 440
  clinical management of, 437
  cognitive-behavior therapy for, 438
  culture, age, and gender features of, 433
  current research on, 441
  differential diagnosis of, 440–441
  DSM-IV classification of, 656
  etiology of
    endogenous opioid theory, 434
    neurodevelopmental and neurobiological theories, 434–435
    neuroendocrine theory, 434
    neuropharmacologic theories, 434
    repetition and family influences theory, 435
  expected outcomes in, 440
  future research on, 441
  hypnosis in, 439
  interventions in
    for clients in community, 436–440
    for hospitalized clients, 436
  nursing diagnoses in, 441
  pharmacologic treatment of, 439–440
  prevalence of, 433
  prognosis of, 435
  risk factors for, 431–433
  therapeutic exposure in, 438–439
  traumatic events leading to, 428t
Dissociative disorder not otherwise specified, 427

Dissociative Experience Scale (DES), 428–429, 430–431t
Dissociative fugue, 427, 429–432
Dissociative identity disorder, 427, 431, 436, 438
 diagnostic criteria for, 432
 trauma and, 71
Disulfiram (Antabuse), 267–268t, 299t, 300
Diuretic(s), 197t, 237t
Divalproex. See Valproic acid
Dizziness, side effect of medication, 106t
DNA, 85–86, 86f
"Do you" question, 60t
Domestic violence, 593–595
Donepezil (Aricept), 253
Dopamine, 80t, 81–82, 84t, 313, 361, 464–465, 464t, 514, 536
Dopamine beta-hydroxylase, 82
Dopamine receptor, 80t, 82, 313, 315, 315f, 332f
Dopaminergic reward pathway, 286
Doral. See Quazepam
Down syndrome, 86
Doxepin (Sinequan), 96t, 98
Draw-A-Person, 40t
Dreaming, 479
Drug abuse. See Substance-related disorder(s)
Drug Abuse Screening Test (DAST-10), 290, 290t
Drug holiday, 101–102, 125
Drug screen(s), 290–291, 291t
Dry mouth, 106t
DSED. See Diagnostic Survey for Eating Disorders
DSM-IV. See Diagnostic and Statistical Manual of Mental Disorders, Fourth Edition
Dual diagnosis, 318, 622
Dura mater, 76
Duty to warn, 20
Dynamic security system, 627
Dyskinesia, 333t
Dyslexia, 86
Dysmorphophobia, 421
Dyspareunia, 446, 449
Dysphoria, 364
Dysphoric affect, 34
Dysphoric mania, 364
Dyssomnia(s), 480, 481t
Dyssomnia not otherwise specified, 480, 481t, 487
Dysthymia, 345–346, 357, 365t
 diagnostic criteria for, 358
 differential diagnosis of, 373
 prevalence of, 343t
Dystonia, 116, 118

EAT. See Eating Attitudes Test
Eating Attitudes Test (EAT), 467
Eating disorder(s), 461–476
 assessment of, 465, 466–467t
 behavior therapy for, 470–471
 care plan for, 468–469
 case study of, 473–476
 characteristic behaviors in, 463
 cognitive-behavior therapy for, 139t, 470–471
 communication strategies in, 469–470
 critical pathway for, 475–476
 culture, age, and gender features of, 463
 differential diagnosis of, 472
 DSM-IV classification of, 12t, 657
 etiology of, 463–464
  genetic factors, 465
  neurobiological factors, 464–465, 464t
 expected outcomes in, 471–472
 future research on, 473
 interpersonal therapy for, 470–471
 interventions in
  for clients in community, 471
  for hospitalized clients, 469–471
 medical complications of, 467t
 milieu therapy for, 470
 nursing diagnoses in, 472–473, 472t
 pharmacologic treatment for, 471
 prognosis of, 465
 psychiatric comorbidity in, 472, 472t
 rating scales for, 41
 referral in, 469
Eating disorder not otherwise specified, 462–463
Eating Disorders Inventory (EDI), 467
Echolalia, 312
Echopraxia, 312
Economic abuse, 593
ECT. See Electroconvulsive therapy
Edema, side effect of medication, 106t
EDI. See Eating Disorders Inventory
Education, of homeless children, 580
EEG. See Electroencephalogram
Effexor. See Venlafaxine
Ego, 65
Ego chill, 608–609
Ego dystonic thought, 389
Ego psychology, 65–66
Ego syntonic thought, 389
Elavil. See Amitriptyline
Eldepryl. See Selegiline
Elderly
 abuse of, 595
 bipolar disorder in, 365–366
 delirium in hospitalized clients, 269
 depression in, 349
 development and, 71–72
 generalized anxiety disorder in, 381
 homeless, 580–581
 normative aging and cognition, 233–234
 panic disorder in, 384
 suicide among, 72
Elective abstraction, 135
Electroconvulsive therapy (ECT), 221–224, 222f
 adverse reactions to, 223
 bilateral, 221
 case study of, 229
 contraindications to, 222–223, 222t
 for depression, 361–362
 expected outcomes in, 224
 indications for, 222, 222t
 nursing considerations in, 223
 for obsessive-compulsive disorder, 395–396
 patient selection for, 221–222
 for psychotic disorders, 334
 theory of action of, 221
 unilateral, 221

Electroencephalogram (EEG), 41t
Electrolyte imbalance(s), mental status changes due to, 265, 266t
Emergency room, assessment in, 36
Emotional constriction, 594, 596
Emotional neglect, 593
Empathy, 47, 48t, 52, 170
Employment
 prolonged mental illness and, 566–567, 567t
 transitional employment position, 570
Encephalitis, 397t
Endocrine disorder(s), 397t
 mental status changes due to, 264t, 265
Endogenous depression. See Depression, major
Endogenous opioid theory, of posttraumatic stress and dissociative disorders, 434
Endorphin, 83
Enkephalin, 83
Environment
 definition of, 13
 in hypochondriasis, 417–418
 in mental illness, 10–13
 in schizophrenia, 316–317
Environmental manipulation, in crisis, 151
Environmental support, in crisis, 150
Environmental violence, 594
Epinephrine, 82, 84t, 434
Erikson's life cycle theory, 66–67, 67–68t
Erythromycin, 102t
Espanto, 38t
Ethical issue(s), 19–22
Ethnocentrism, 33t
Euphoria, 363
Euphoric affect, 34
Euthymia, 107, 363, 365t
Evaluation phase, of nursing process, 43–44
Evil eye, 38t
Excitotoxic hypothesis, 249
Exercise, 357, 490
Exhaustion, effect of stress, 143
Exhibitionism, 454–456
Existential factor(s), in group therapy, 161–162
Experience(s), assessment of, 34–35
Exposure therapy, 138, 139t, 387, 389
Expressed emotion, 190
Externalization, 637
Extinction (behavioral therapy), 137, 139t
Extrapyramidal symptom(s), 79, 116t, 333, 333t
Extrapyramidal system, 79
Eye movement desensitization and reprocessing, 438

Facial expression, 53t
Factitious disorder(s), DSM-IV classification of, 12t, 656
Falling out, 38t
False memory, 597–598
Family, 179
 bipolar disorder and, 369
 of client with prolonged mental illness, 558–559, 563–564
 homeless, 578, 585

Family—Continued
  involvement in substance-related disorders, 290, 298–299
  nuclear, 182
Family assessment, 37, 179–185, 181t
  affective factors, 185
  boundaries, 185
  communication patterns, 184
  couple development, 183–184
  demographic information, 182
  development of children, 183
  developmental factors, 183
  genogram, 181, 182f
  historical factors, 182–183
  life cycle development, 184
  meanings, 185
  mood and tone, 185
  power structure, 185
  preassessment questions, 179, 180t
  problem solving, 185
  relational integrity, 185
  roles of family members, 184
  sociocultural factors, 182
  structural mapping, 181–182, 183f
  transactional factors, 184
  trust within family, 185
Family boundary(ies), 185
Family education
  in adjustment disorders, 506
  in bipolar disorder, 371–372
  in dementia, 254
  in personality disorders, 526
  in posttraumatic stress and dissociative disorders, 440
  in psychotic disorders, 335–336
  in sleep disorders, 494
Family emotional system therapy, 186, 187t
Family of origin, 183
Family process, 181
Family reenactment, 209t
Family structure, 189
Family study (genetics), 86
Family system, 189
Family therapy, 179–192
  for abuse survivor, 601
  approaches in, 185–190
  case study of, 191–192
  communication training, 190
  compared to individual and group therapy, 179, 180t
  contextual, 186–188, 187t
  current research on, 191
  expected outcomes in, 190–191
  family emotional system therapy, 186, 187t
  future research on, 191
  indications for, 179
  multigenerational theories and therapies, 186–189
  nurse's role in, 179–180
  nursing diagnoses in, 185–186
  object relations theory, 187t, 188–189
  preassessment questions in, 179, 180t
  psychiatric diagnoses in, 185–186
  psychoeducational approach to, 190
  purpose of, 179
  structural, 187t, 189
  systematic and strategic, 187t, 189–190

Fananserin, 127t
Fatigue, side effect of medication, 106t
Feedback (element of communication), 54
Fee-for-service system, 643–644
"Feeling talk," 138
Female orgasmic disorder, 447–448
Female sexual arousal disorder, 446–448
Fenfluramine (Pondimin), 126
Fetishism, 454–456
Fibromyalgia, 496t
Fight-or-flight response, 82, 143, 386
Flashback, 428
Flat affect, 34, 308
Flesinoxan, 127t
Flight of ideas, 34t, 364
Flooding, 387
Florida Obsessive-Compulsive Inventory, 392
Fluency, 33
Fluoxetine (Prozac), 80t, 81, 96t, 101–104, 102t, 359, 360t, 395, 419–420, 439, 456, 522
Fluphenazine (Prolixin), 112t
Flurazepam (Dalmane), 121t, 234, 494t
Fluvoxamine (Luvox), 96t, 101, 102t, 126, 395
Focused phase, of group development, 172–173
Forensic evidence, 16
Formal thought disorder, 308, 309t
Fornix, 76f, 78
Fountain House, 569
Frenzy witchcraft, 38t
Freud's psychosexual theory, 65, 68t
Frontal cortex, 78
  abnormalities in obsessive-compulsive disorder, 393
Frontal dementia, 78
Frontal lobe, 76, 76–77f, 78
Frotteurism, 454–456
Fugue, dissociative. See Dissociative fugue
Future trends in nursing, 643–648

GABA, 80t, 84, 84t, 249, 313
GABA receptor, 80t, 84–85, 381, 381f
GABA transaminase, 84
GABA-benzodiazepine hypothesis, of panic disorder, 386
GAD. See Generalized anxiety disorder
GAF. See Global Assessment of Functioning
Galactorrhea, 332f
Gamma-glutamyltransferase, 291t
Gamma-hydroxybutyrate, 84
Gastrointestinal disturbance, side effect of medication, 106t
GDS. See Global Deterioration Scale
Gender
  attention-deficit/hyperactivity disorder and, 534–535
  bipolar disorder and, 366
  conversion disorder and, 411
  delirium and, 235
  dementia and, 246
  eating disorders and, 463
  gender identity disorder and, 453
  generalized anxiety disorder and, 381
  obsessive-compulsive disorder and, 392

  offender population, 622
  paraphilias and, 456
  personality disorders and, 514, 519, 525
  pharmacokinetics and, 94
  posttraumatic stress and dissociative disorders and, 433
  schizophrenia and, 313
  sleep disorders and, 485
  somatization disorder and, 404
  somatoform disorders and, 406t
  substance-related disorders and, 285
Gender identity disorder, 445–458
  assessment of, 446
  characteristic behaviors in, 453
  client and family education in, 457
  culture, age, and gender features of, 453
  current research on, 457
  diagnostic criteria for, 454
  DSM-IV classification of, 12t, 656–657
  etiology of
    biological theories, 453
    learning theories, 453–454
  expected outcomes in, 457
  further research on, 457–458
  interventions for clients in community, 454
  nursing diagnoses in, 457
  prevalence of, 450
  prognosis of, 454
Gene, 85–86
General adaptation syndrome, 143
General recall, 34
Generalist nurse, 15–16, 15t, 646–647, 646t
Generalized anxiety disorder (GAD), 379–382
  benzodiazepines for, 382, 382t
  buspirone for, 382
  characteristic behaviors in, 380
  culture, age, and gender features of, 381
  diagnostic criteria for, 380
  etiology of
    biological theories, 381, 381f
    genetic theories, 381
  interventions in
    for clients in community, 382
    for hospitalized clients, 381–382
  pharmacologic treatment of, 382
  prevalence of, 380t
  prognosis of, 381
Generativity, 66
Genetic testing, 41t
Genetic theory
  of attention-deficit/hyperactivity disorder, 535
  of bipolar disorder, 367, 369–370
  of breathing-related sleep disorders, 486
  of dementia, 249
  of depression, 350–351
  of eating disorders, 465
  of generalized anxiety disorder, 381
  of narcolepsy, 487
  of obsessive-compulsive disorder, 393
  of panic disorder, 384–385
  of personality disorders, 514–515, 514t, 519
  of phobias, 389
  of schizophrenia, 315–316, 337
  of substance-related disorders, 286
Genetics, 85–86, 86f
  of Alzheimer's disease, 257

Genogram, 181, 182f
Gentamicin, 237t
Gentrification, 581
Gestalt, 203
Ghost sickness, 38t
Gift giving, between nurse and client, 49–50
Global Assessment of Functioning (GAF), 13, 14t
Global Deterioration Scale (GDS), 243–244t
Global statement(s), 60t
Globus pallidus, 76f, 79
Glucocorticoid, 88
Glucocorticoid receptor, 87
Glucose metabolism, in caudate nucleus, 393
Glutamate, 84, 249, 313
Glutamate receptor, 84
Glutamine, 315
Glycine, 84
Goal(s)
　long-term, 42
　short-term, 42
"Good-enough mother," 66
Gray matter, 80
Grief
　cumulative, 637
　unresolved, 637, 639
Grieving, 635–640
　in adolescents, 638
　anticipatory, 636
　case study of, 639
　characteristics of grieving process, 635–636
　in children, 637–638, 637t
　depression vs., 638t, 639
　healthy, 636
　indications for professional consultation, 639, 639t
　life events leading to, 639
　nurse-client relationship in, 637
　nursing care in grieving process, 637–639
　types of, 636–637
Grisi siknis, 38t
Grounded theory, 369
Group cohesiveness, 161, 171
Group communication, 55, 555t
Group content, 168
Group contract, 168–169
Group culture, 172–173
Group development
　focused phase of, 172–173
　initial phase of, 170–171
　responsive phase of, 171–172
　termination phase of, 173
Group dynamics, 53, 174
Group norm(s), 171
Group process, 162
Group proposal, 168
Group size, 167
Group therapy, 159–175
　case study of, 163–164
　client preparation for group, 168–169
　compared to individual and family therapy, 179, 180t
　cotherapists, 175
　creation of group, 162
　definition of, 159–160
　expected outcomes in, 173–174
　frequency of meetings, 167

group environment, 166–167
group purpose and goals, 162–169
implications for research, 175
inpatient, 167
intervention strategies in
　balancing group-as-whole and individual interpretations, 170
　being curious about group behavior, 170
　being empathetic and supportive, 170
　fostering connections to other members, 169
　observing defensive maneuvers, 169
membership selection, 166, 172
nurse's role in, 163–166, 174–175
　educational preparation, 174
　group leadership, 174–175
　leadership style, 175
　supervision, 174
purpose of, 160–162
reminiscence, 205–208
single therapist, 174–175
stages of group development, 170–173
therapeutic factors in, 160–162
Growth hormone, 480
Guanfacine (Tenex), 545t
Guidance, 209t
Guilt stage, of grieving, 636
Gyrus, 76

Haitian(s), culture-bound syndromes among, 38t
Halazepam (Paxipam), 121t
Halcion. See Triazolam
Haldol. See Haloperidol
Half-life, 94
Halfway house, 568, 645f
Hallucination, 35, 35t
　assessment of, 324–325
　auditory, 311, 431
　characteristics of, 308, 308t
　clinical management of client, 329
　in narcolepsy, 486
　visual, 311
Hallucinogen(s), 283t
Haloperidol (Haldol), 80t, 102t, 112–113t, 237t, 253, 331t, 332, 371, 515
Hamilton Depression Rating Scale (HDRS), 348
HDRS. See Hamilton Depression Rating Scale
Head trauma, 238, 265, 496t
Headache, side effect of medication, 106t
Health, level of, as communication barrier, 59
Health insurance. See Insurance coverage
Health risk factor(s), in prolonged mental illness, 558
Healthy grieving, 636
Healthy sexual functioning, 195
Hearing impairment, 206
Heart disease, 397t
Helpful communication technique(s), 55, 58
Hemisphere, 76
　sex differences in, 89
Hemispheric laterality, 76, 89
Hepatitis, 373t
Heredity, 85–86, 86f
Heterogenous group, 166
Heterosexism, 33t

Hippocampus, 76f, 78
　volume in posttraumatic stress disorder, 435, 441
Histamine, 83
Histamine antagonist(s), 268t
Histamine receptor, 83
Histrionic personality disorder, 512t
　characteristic behaviors in, 518
　diagnostic criteria for, 516
　prevalence of, 512t
HIV disease, 238–239, 605
　assessment of client with, 615
　clinical manifestations of, 608–610
　coping in infected mothers, 505
　early stage of, 608–609
　epidemiology of, 606–608
　future research on, 618
　HIV-associated dementia, 611–613. See also AIDS-related dementia
　late stage of, 610
　middle stage of, 609–610
　mode of HIV transmission, 606
　neuropsychiatric testing in, 610–611
　neuropsychological complications of, 611–613, 612f
　nurse's knowledge and attitudes about, 608
　nursing diagnoses in, 615–616
　patient care in, 614–617
　planning and therapeutics in, 616
　protease inhibitors for, 616–617
　psychiatric disorders in, 613–614
　in severely and persistently mentally ill, 617
　spectrum of, 608–610
　substance-related disorders and, 618
　vulnerable populations, 617–618
　in women, 617–618
HIV testing, 608
Home visit, psychiatric, 662–663
Homeless individual(s), 575–586
　adolescents, 580
　case study of, 585–586
　children, 579–580
　coping mechanisms of, 582
　elderly, 580–581
　families, 578, 585
　needs, resources, and services for, 147
　new homeless, 576
　old homeless, 576
　with physical illness, 581
　prolonged mental illness among, 554, 566–567, 578
　psychiatric-mental health concerns about, 577–581
　psychiatric-mental health nursing and advocacy, 584
　　historical background, 583
　　intervention strategies, 584
　　theoretical basis, 583–584
　schizophrenia in, 575
　subgroups of, 577–581
　substance-related disorders in, 7, 580
　women, 578–579, 585–586
Homelessness
　benign, 576
　chronic, 583
　definition of, 575–576
　deinstitutionalization and, 576

Homelessness—Continued
  economic and public policy factors in, 577
  historical perspective and related issues, 576–577
  malignant, 576
  marginal, 582
  McKinney Act, 577
  model of homelessness process, 582–583
  process of becoming homeless, 581–583
  as psychological trauma, 578
  recent, 582–583
  resources about, 671
  social distress theory of, 581–582
Homeostasis, 286–287
Homogenous group, 166
Homophobia, 33t
Homovanillic acid, 82, 465, 514
Homunculus, 78, 78f
Hope, instillation of, 160, 209t
Hospitalization. See also Inpatient care
  brief, 215
  partial, 645f
Hotline, 153
Housing, low-income, 577–578, 581
Human Genome Project, 85
Human immunodeficiency virus. See HIV disease
Huntington's disease, 79, 86, 238–239, 245, 397t, 496t
Hurricane Andrew, 148
Hydralazine, 237t
5-Hydroxyindoleacetic acid, 83, 465
Hydroxyzine, 237t
Hyperactivity-impulsivity, 533
Hyperarousal, 427–428
Hypercalcemia, 266t, 271, 373t
Hyperinsulinism, 264t
Hyperkalemia, 266t
Hypernatremia, 266t
Hyperparathyroidism, 264t
Hypersomnia, 346, 480
  primary. See Primary hypersomnia
Hypersomnia related to Axis I or Axis II disorder, 483
Hyperthyroidism, 264t, 397t, 496t
Hypervigilance, 428
Hypnosis, in posttraumatic stress and dissociative disorders, 439
Hypoactive sexual desire disorder, 446–447
Hypocalcemia, 266t
Hypochondriasis, 35t, 416–420
  assessment of, 418–419
  care plan for, 419
  case study of, 420
  characteristic behaviors in, 416–417
  cognitive-behavior therapy for, 418
  culture, age, and gender features of, 406t, 417
  diagnostic criteria for, 405t, 417
  etiology of
    biological theory, 417
    perceptual-cognitive theory, 417
    psychological theory, 417
    sociocultural and environmental factors, 417–418
  expected outcomes in, 420
  familial patterns of, 406t

  interventions for clients in community, 419–420
  obsessive-compulsive disorder and, 417
  prevalence of, 405t
  prognosis of, 418
Hypoglycemia, 397t
Hypoglycemic(s), 237t
Hypokalemia, 266t, 373t
Hypomania, 363–364, 365t
Hyponatremia, 266t
Hypoparathyroidism, 264t, 397t
Hypophosphatemia, 266t
Hypopnea, 486
Hypothalamic-pituitary-adrenal axis, 87–88, 88f
Hypothalamus, 76f, 79
Hypothyroidism, 264t, 373t
Hysteria. See Somatization disorder

"I statements," 138
Id, 65
Identification (defense mechanism), 66t
Identification (positive feeling), 209t
Identifying information, 29
Illness management group, 165
Image habituation training, 439
Imipramine (Tofranil), 96t, 97, 99, 102t, 543, 545t
Imitative behavior, 161
Immobilization, in critical care unit psychosis, 272
Immune function, mental illness and, 88–89, 89t
Implementation of care plan, 42–43
Implosive therapy, 387
Inappropriate affect, 34, 311
Inattention, 309, 531–533
Incarcerated population. See Offender population
Income, of poor and near poor, 577
Independence, in client with dementia, 250–251
Inderal. See Propranolol
Indinavir, 616
Indirect victimization, 594
Indolamine(s), 81
Indomethacin, 234, 237t
Infectious mononucleosis, 373t
Informative reminiscence, 203
Informed consent, 21, 540
  exceptions to, 21
Infradian rhythm, 87, 351
Infrared motion-analysis system, 539, 539–540f
Inhalant abuse, 283t
Inmate population. See Offender population
Inpatient care, 645f
  admission to, 20, 25–26
  decision to hospitalize emergency room client, 36
  discharge from, 20
  historical aspects of, 6
  insurance coverage for, 22
  length of hospital stay, 645, 645f
  short-stay units, 215
Inpatient group, 167

Insight, 35
  assessment of, 29
  poor, 312
Insight-oriented therapy, 165
Insomnia, 357, 480
  primary. See Primary insomnia
Insomnia related to Axis I or Axis II disorder, 483
Institutionalization, 554
Insulin, 237t
Insurance coverage
  for inpatient vs. outpatient care, 22
  trends in, 643–645
Intellectual function, assessment of, 34
Interferon, 268t
Internal locus of control, 379–380
Internalization, 637
International Pilot Study of Schizophrenia (IPSS), 43
Interpersonal communication, 53, 55, 55t
Interpersonal learning, 161, 209t
Interpersonal skill(s), 51–52
Interpersonal theory, of development, 67–68, 68t
Interpersonal therapy, for eating disorders, 470–471
Intoxication. See Substance intoxication
Intrapersonal communication, 53
Intravenous drug user, 618. See also Substance-related disorder(s)
Intrusion, 599
Intrusive recollection(s), 428
Intrusive trauma, 596
Involvement, as function of milieu, 213–214, 214t
Ionamin. See Phentermine
IPSS. See International Pilot Study of Schizophrenia
Isoniazid, 237t, 267t
Isoptin. See Verapamil
Isordil. See Isosorbide dinitrate
Isosorbide dinitrate (Isordil), 267t

Jail. See Offender population
Jet lag, 227, 480, 481t, 487, 493
Judgment, assessment of, 34
Justice, within family, 188

Kindling, 93–94, 109, 366–367, 367f
Kinesthetic channel, 53
Klonopin. See Clonazepam
Knowledge level, as communication barrier, 59
Korsakoff's syndrome, 78
K-SADS, 539t

La belle indifference, 411
Lability, 34
Laboratory testing, 41t
Lactate hypothesis, in panic disorder, 384t, 385
Lactation. See Breastfeeding
Laissez-faire leadership, 175
Lamictal. See Lamotrigine
Lamotrigine (Lamictal), 127t, 370t

Language
  assessment of language function, 33–34, 34t
  as communication barrier, 58–59
Lanugo, 466
Latent content, 171
Latin American(s), culture-bound syndromes among, 38t
L-dopa, 82, 100t, 234, 237t, 267t
Leadership style
  autocratic, 175
  democratic, 175
  laissez-faire, 175
Learning, in group therapy, 161
Learning deficit, attention-deficit/hyperactivity disorder and, 545
Learning disorder, 537t
Learning theory
  of gender identity disorder, 453–454
  of paraphilia, 456
Legal issue(s), 19–22
Leisure skills group, 163
Leptin, 126
Lethargy, side effect of medication, 106t
Levodopa. See l-dopa
Lexical retrieval, 249
Libido, 445
Librium. See Chlordiazepoxide
Lidocaine, 237t
Life cycle development(s)
  assessment of, 29
  family, 184
Life cycle theory, 66–67, 67–68t
Life review, 203–204, 206, 610
Life review therapy, 204, 208–209
Light, circadian rhythms and, 87, 87f
Light box therapy, 225–227, 225f
Light sleeper, 480
Light therapy. See Phototherapy
Light visor, 225–226
Limbic system, 76f, 78
  dysfunction, 386, 433, 435, 441
"Listening attitude," 311
Listening to Prozac, 104
Lithium
  adverse reactions to, 108–109, 237t
  for bipolar disorder, 370, 370t
  blood levels of, 107, 370
  case study of, 111
  clinically significant interactions of, 108t, 109
  contraindications and precautions, 107–108
  for depression, 361
  indications for, 107
  mechanism of action of, 107, 370
  pharmacokinetics of, 107, 107–108t
  toxicity of, 109
Locus caeruleus, 82
Long-term memory, 34
Loose association(s), 34t, 311
Lorazepam (Ativan), 116t, 121t, 237, 253, 371, 382t
Lower functioning group, 167
Loxapine (Loxitane), 112t, 117
Loxitane. See Loxapine
Loyalty, within family, 188
LSD, 83

Luteinizing hormone, 480
Luvox. See Fluvoxamine
Lux, 225

"Mad cow disease," 89
"Madhouse," 6
Magical knowing, 60t
Magical thinking, 35t
Magnetic resonance imaging (MRI), 41t, 85, 85t
  in attention-deficit/hyperactivity disorder, 536–537
Major depression. See Depression, major
Mal de ojo, 38t
Mal puestro, 38t
Male erectile disorder, 446–448, 453
Male orgasmic disorder, 447–448
Malignant homelessness, 576
Managed care delivery system, 643–645
  capitation, 644–645
  carve-out system, 644
  effects on psychiatric-mental health care, 645
  stages of managed care evolution, 644t, 645
Mania, 343, 363. See also Bipolar disorder
  diagnostic criteria for manic episode, 365
  differential diagnosis of, 373–374, 373t
  dysphoric, 364
Manic-depressive illness. See Bipolar disorder
Manifest content, 171
Manipulative patient, clinical management of, 518
MAOI. See Monoamine oxidase inhibitor(s)
Marginal homelessness, 582
Marital Satisfaction Inventory, 195
Marital therapy, as treatment for depression, 184
Masturbation, directed, 451
Maturational crisis, 146–147
Mature group, 173
Mazapertine, 127t
McKinney Homeless Assistance Act, 577
Mean corpuscular volume, 291t
Medial forebrain bundle, 82
Medication
  assessment of side effects of, 35
  as cause of dementia or delirium, 237t
  as cause of depression, 267t
  as cause of psychotic symptoms, 268t
  misuse of, 277, 285
  psychiatric effects of, 234
  treatment of common side effects of, 106t
Medication management group, 165
Medicine bag, 13
Mediterranean(s), culture-bound syndromes among, 38t
Medulla oblongata, 76f
Melatonin, 79, 82–83, 87, 351, 480–481
  for insomnia, 493–494
Melatonin hypothesis, of seasonal effective disorder, 348
Mellaril. See Thioridazine
Memory. See also Reminiscence therapy
  assessment of, 34
  of childhood sexual abuse, 69
  false, 597–598

  impaired, 72. See also Amnesia/amnestic disorder(s)
  long-term, 34
  repressed, 69, 597–598
  short-term, 34
Memory enhancer(s), for dementia, 253, 253f
Meninges, 76
Meningitis, 76
Mental health, definition of, 9
Mental health promotion, 17
Mental health team, 16–17
  assessment by, 40–41, 40–41t
  communication with, 55
Mental illness
  biological basis of, 75–89
  "cause" of, 5
  costs of, 11f
  culture and, 10–13
  definition of, 9–10
  developmental theories of, 65–72
  DSM-IV classification of, 12t, 13, 651–659
  environmental factors in, 10–13
  historical aspects of, 6
  percentages of Americans with, 10f
  prevention of, 17
  prolonged. See Prolonged mental illness
  psychological theories of, 65–72
  spirituality and, 10–13
Mental illness due to general medical condition, 261–274, 262t
  age and, 264–265
  care plan for, 268, 270
  case study of, 271
  characteristic behaviors in, 261–264
  current research on, 273
  differential diagnosis of, 271
  DSM-IV classification of, 12t, 652
  etiology of
    cancer, 265, 267, 271
    drug side effects and interactions, 267–268, 267–268t
    metabolic, 265
    neurological, 265–266
    vascular, 265
  expected outcomes in, 271
  future research on, 273–274
  interventions in
    for clients in community, 271
    for hospitalized clients, 268–271
  nursing diagnoses for, 270
  prognosis of, 268
Mental retardation, 537t
  attention-deficit/hyperactivity disorder and, 546
Mental Status Examination (MSE), 25, 29, 30f
  appearance, behavior, and attitude, 32–33
  attention, 33
  components of, 32
  cortical and cognitive functions, 34
  cultural and common biases, 33t
  intellectual evaluation and memory, 34
  language function and characteristics of speech, 33–34, 34t
  mood and affect, 34
  orientation, 33
  performance of, 29–35

Mental Status Examination (MSE)—Continued
  in prolonged mental illness, 558
  in psychotic disorders, 323–324
  in substance-related disorders, 290
  thought content, 34–35
Meperidine (Demerol), 100–101, 100t, 237t, 268t
Meridia. See Sibutramine
Mesocortical system, 81–82, 332f
Mesolimbic system, 81, 332f
Mesoridazine (Serentil), 112t, 117
Message (element of communication), 53
Metabolic disorder(s), 265, 397t
Metabolism, 94
  brain, 89
Methadone, 299t, 300–301
3-Methoxy-4-hydroxymandelic acid, 82
3-Methoxy-4-hydroxyphenylglycol, 82, 465
Methyldopa (Aldomet), 234, 237t, 267t
Methylphenidate (Ritalin), 80t, 124–126, 124t, 268t, 286, 361, 542, 545t
Metoclopramide (Reglan), 267t
Midazolam (Versed), 382t, 494t
Midbrain, 76f
Migraine, 496t
Mild neurocognitive disorder, HIV-associated, 611–613
Milieu therapy, 213–217
  case study of, 216–217
  definition of, 213
  for eating disorders, 470
  expected outcomes in, 215–216
  functions of milieu, 213–214
  future research on, 216
  historical aspects of, 6
  nurse's role as manager, 214–215
  purpose of, 213, 214t
  for schizophrenia, 329
Mindfulness, 139t
Mini-Mental State Examination (MMSE), 29, 31–32f, 235, 615
Mirtazapine (Remeron), 96t, 102t, 104–105, 359, 360t
Mixed state, 364
MMSE. See Mini–Mental State Examination
Moban. See Molindone
Mobile crisis team, 153
Moclobomide, 127t
Modeling, 138, 139t
Molindone (Moban), 112t
Monoamine deficiency hypothesis, of depression, 361
Monoamine oxidase (MAO), 367
Monoamine oxidase inhibitor(s) (MAOI), 96, 96t, 359–360
  adverse reactions to, 96t, 100–101, 100t
  clinically significant interactions of, 99, 100t, 101, 105, 125
  contraindications and precautions, 100
  indications for, 99
  mechanism of action of, 81, 100, 360f
  pharmacokinetics of, 99–100
Monopolizing, 169
Monosodium glutamate (MSG), 84
Monosymptomatic phobia, 140
Mood, assessment of, 34

Mood disorder(s), 343–375
  attention-deficit/hyperactivity disorder and, 537t, 544–545
  clinical management of, 344
  cognitive-behavior therapy for, 139t
  current research on, 374–375
  differential diagnosis of, 301, 336, 373–374, 496, 506, 526
  DSM-IV classification of, 12t, 655–656
  future research on, 375
  in HIV-positive client, 614
  nursing diagnoses in, 374
  prevalence of, 343t
Mood disorder due to general medical condition, 263
Mood enhancer(s), 104
Mood stabilizer(s), 93–94, 107–112
  for bipolar depression, 370, 370t
  case study of, 111
  current research on, 127t
  general information about, 107
  nursing considerations for, 110–111
  for posttraumatic stress disorder, 439
Mood swings, 364
Moodswing (book), 364
Moral treatment, 19
Morphine, 237t
Motivation of client, assessment of, 29
Motivational deficit hypothesis, for attention-deficit/hyperactivity disorder, 536
MRI. See Magnetic resonance imaging
MSE. See Mental Status Examination
MSG. See Monosodium glutamate
Muina, 38t
Multicausal theory, of sexual dysfunctions, 450–451
Multidirectional partiality, 188
Multigenerational therapy, 186
Multiple dementia(s), 245
Multiple personality disorder. See Dissociative identity disorder
Multiple sclerosis, 89, 265
Multiple sleep latency test, 490t
Muscarinic receptor, 83
Music therapy, 257
Mutism, 34t
Myelin, 80
Myocardial infarction, 397t
Myxedema. See Hypothyroidism

NA. See Narcotics Anonymous
Nadolol, 234
Naloxone (Narcan), 299t, 300
Naltrexone (ReVia), 299t, 300
Naming, 33
NANDA (North American Nursing Diagnosis Association)
  nursing diagnoses, 39–40t, 40
  steps in nursing process, 25, 25f
Narcan. See Naloxone
Narcissistic personality disorder, 512t
  characteristic behaviors in, 518
  developmental problems and, 71
  diagnostic criteria for, 516
  prevalence of, 512t

Narcolepsy, 480, 486–487
  characteristic behaviors in, 481t, 486, 489t
  diagnostic criteria for, 482
  etiology of
    genetic theories, 487
    physiological theories, 487
  prevalence of, 481t
  psychostimulants for, 494
Narcotic(s). See also Substance-related disorder(s)
  psychiatric effects of, 237t
Narcotics Anonymous (NA), 166, 296, 296–297t
Nardil. See Phenelzine
National Alliance for the Mentally Ill, 166
Native American(s), culture-bound syndromes among, 38t
Natural disaster, 147–148
  disaster response, 153
Nature versus nurture controversy, 86
Nausea, side effect of medication, 106t
Navane. See Thiothixene
Necrophilia, 456
Nefazodone (Serzone), 96t, 102t, 104–105, 359, 360t, 362
Negative reinforcer, 133
Neighborhood health center, 8–9
Nelfinavir, 616
Neologism, 33, 34t, 311–312
Nervios, 38t
Neural plasticity, 5
Neuroanatomy, 75–79, 76–77f
  changes in dementia, 246
Neurobiological theory
  of body dysmorphic disorder, 421
  of eating disorders, 464–465, 464t
  of posttraumatic stress and dissociative disorders, 434–435
  of somatization disorder, 404
Neurocognitive disorder(s), HIV-associated, 611–613
Neurodevelopmental factor(s), in schizophrenia, 316–317, 316f
Neurodevelopmental theory, of posttraumatic stress and dissociative disorders, 434–435
Neuroendocrine theory, of posttraumatic stress and dissociative disorders, 434
Neuroimaging, 85, 85t
  in dementia, 245
  in substance-related disorders, 286, 286f
Neuroleptic(s). See Antipsychotic medication(s)
Neuroleptic malignant syndrome, 116–117
Neuroleptic-induced deficit syndrome, 332f
Neurological condition(s), mental status changes due to, 265–266
Neuron
  activity of, 79–80
  structure of, 79–80
Neuropeptide(s), 83–84, 84t
Neuropeptide Y, 84t, 464, 464t
Neuropharmacologic theory
  of adjustment disorders, 503
  of amnesia, 256
  of posttraumatic stress and dissociative disorders, 434
  of schizophrenia, 313–315, 315f

Neuropharmacology, 93–94
Neurophysiologic theory, of schizophrenia, 313–315, 315f
Neuropsychiatric testing, in HIV disease, 610–611
Neuropsychologic testing, 41t
Neuroscience, 5–6, 9t, 664
Neurotensin, 83, 84t
Neurotransmission, 79–81
Neurotransmitter(s), 80–85
　amino acids, 84–85
　in attention-deficit/hyperactivity disorder, 536–537
　biogenic amines, 81–83
　cholinergics, 83
　inactivation of, 81
　neuropeptides, 83–84, 84t
　neuropharmacologic effects on, 93–94, 94t
　in psychiatric disorders, 80, 80t
　receptors for, 80–81, 80t
　release of, 80
　response to, 80–81
　reuptake of, 81, 93, 95f, 111
　storage of, 80
　synthesis of, 80
New homeless, 576
Nicorette. *See* Nicotine gum
Nicotine, 283t
Nicotine gum (Nicorette), 299t
Nicotine withdrawal
　pharmacologic treatment of, 299t, 301
　symptoms and nursing actions, 293t
Nicotinic receptor, 83
Nicotrol. *See* Transdermal nicotine
Nifedipine (Procardia), 102t, 267t, 370t, 371
Night owl, 487
Nightmare disorder, 480, 487–488, 489t
　characteristic behaviors in, 481t
　diagnostic criteria for, 483
Nigrostriatal system, 81–82, 332f
Nihilistic delusion, 35t
Nocturnal myoclonus, 487
Nolvadex. *See* Tamoxifen
Nonverbal message, 53, 53t, 55
Nootropic(s), 257
Norepinephrine, 80t, 82, 84t, 88, 93–94, 94t, 111, 313, 350–351, 359, 361, 367, 375, 434, 464, 464t, 536
Norepinephrine receptor, 80t, 82
Norepinephrine theory
　of Alzheimer's disease, 248–249
　of panic disorder, 384t, 386
Norfluoxetine, 81
Norpramin. *See* Desipramine
North American(s), culture-bound syndromes among, 38t
North American Nursing Diagnosis Association. *See* NANDA
Nortriptyline (Pamelor), 96t, 97, 99, 234
Novel antidepressant(s), 96t
　adverse reactions to, 104–105, 360t
　clinically significant interactions of, 105
　contraindications and precautions, 104
　dosages of, 360t
　indications for, 104
　mechanism of action of, 104
　pharmacokinetics of, 104
Nuclear family, 182
Numbed state, 635
Numbing, 428, 582, 594, 596
Nurse. *See* Psychiatric–mental health nurse
Nurse case manager, 17, 17t
Nurse practitioner, psychiatric, 16
Nurse psychopharmacologist, 19
Nurse psychotherapist, 18–19
Nursing diagnosis, 40. *See also* specific disorders
　in family therapy, 185–186
　NANDA, 39–40t, 40
Nursing history form, 26, 26–28f
Nursing home, dementia in residents of, 252
Nursing process. *See also* specific steps
　assessment phase of, 25–41
　care plan, 42
　definition of, 25
　evaluation phase of, 43–44
　implementation phase of, 42–43
　steps in, 25, 25f
Nursing theorist(s), 4t
Nutritional deficiency, 255, 265, 397t

OA. *See* Overeaters Anonymous
Obesity, treatment of, 126
Object constancy, 66, 71
Object relations theory, 66
　in family, 187t, 188–189
Objectivity, 54
Obsession, 35, 35t, 389
Obsessive-compulsive disorder (OCD), 79, 379, 389–395
　antidepressants for, 395
　case study of, 398–399
　characteristic behaviors in, 389–392, 472
　cognitive-behavior therapy for, 139t, 395
　culture, age, and gender features of, 392–393
　current research on, 398
　diagnostic aids for, 392, 394–395t
　diagnostic criteria for, 392
　differential diagnosis of, 336, 441
　electroconvulsive therapy for, 395–396
　etiology of
　　biological theories, 393
　　genetic theories, 393
　hypochondriasis and, 417
　immune system and, 89
　interventions in
　　for clients in community, 393–396
　　for hospitalized clients, 393
　prevalence of, 380t
　prognosis of, 393
　psychosurgery for, 395–396
　resources about, 670
　screening test for, 394–395t
　strep-induced, 395
Obsessive-compulsive personality disorder, 512t
　characteristic behaviors in, 523–524
　diagnostic criteria for, 524
　prevalence of, 512t
Obstructive sleep apnea, 486
　case study of, 497–498
　characteristic behaviors in, 481t
　prevalence of, 481t
　treatment of, 492–493, 493f
Occipital lobe, 76, 76–77f, 78
OCD. *See* Obsessive-compulsive disorder
Offender population, 621–632, 621f. *See also* Correctional nurse
　case study of, 632
　characteristics of clients in, 621–623
　cultural issues in, 622–623
　drug use and, 622
　future research on, 631
　gender issues in, 622
　nurse-client relationship in, 624–627
　　custody and caring, 623–624
　　orientation phase, 624–626
　　preinteraction phase, 624
　　restrictions on touch, 625
　　termination phase, 626–627
　　therapeutic self-disclosure, 625–626
　　working phase, 626
　nursing diagnoses for, 622
　personality disorders in, 622
　prolonged mental illness in, 554, 566–567, 621–622
　public animosity toward, 630–631
　sex offenders, 630
　suicide among, 628–629, 628f
　treatment setting, 627–629
　　security issues, 627–628
　　ward atmosphere, 623
Oklahoma City bombing, 147–148, 439
Olanzapine (Zyprexa), 112, 113t, 117, 126, 253, 331t, 332–333, 337
Old homeless, 576
Open group, 166
Operant conditioning, 132–133
Opioid(s), 84t, 197t
　abuse of, 283t
　adverse reactions to, 267–268t
　endogenous, 434
　pharmacologic treatment of dependence, 299t, 300–301
　withdrawal symptoms and nursing actions, 293t, 295
Opportunistic infection(s), 605–606, 606t
Oppositional defiant disorder, 544, 546
Oral contraceptive(s), 197t, 267t
Oral history, 203–204
Orap. *See* Pimozide
Orem, Dorothea, 4t
Organic brain syndrome(s), 373t
Organic mental disorder
　rating scales for, 41
　substance-induced, 279t
Organizational communication, 53
Organized systems of care, 644
Orgasm, 196
Orgasmic disorder(s), 446–447, 451
Orientation, assessment of, 33
Orientation phase, of therapeutic relationship, 50
Orlistat (Xenical), 126
Orthostatic hypotension, 99, 106t

Outcome, 42
Outcome criteria, 42
Outpatient care, insurance coverage for, 22
Overeaters Anonymous (OA), 166
Overgeneralization, 135
Oxazepam (Serax), 121t, 237, 382t, 494t

Pain disorder, 413–416
  assessment of, 415
  care plan for, 415
  case study of, 416
  characteristic behaviors in, 413
  cultural and gender features of, 406t
  diagnostic criteria for, 405t, 414
  etiology of
    biological theories, 413–414
    comorbid disorders, 414
    sociocultural theories, 414–415
  expected outcomes in, 415
  familial patterns of, 406t
  interventions in
    for clients in community, 415
    for hospitalized clients, 415
  prevalence of, 405t
Pamelor. *See* Nortriptyline
Pamipexole, 127t
Pancreatic cancer, 373t
PANDAS. *See* Pediatric autoimmune neuropsychiatric disorder
Panic attack, 383
  diagnostic criteria for, 382–383
Panic disorder, 379, 383
  age and, 384
  agoraphobia and, 382–387
  antidepressant medication for, 387
  benzodiazepines for, 386–387
  case study of, 124, 398
  characteristic behaviors in, 382–384
  cognitive-behavior therapy for, 139t, 387
  current research on, 398
  etiology of
    biological theories, 384t, 385
    genetic theories, 384–385
  interventions for clients in community, 386–387
  neurotransmitters in, 82
  pharmacologic treatment for, 387
  prevalence of, 380t
  prognosis of, 386
  selective serotonin reuptake inhibitors for, 386
Papaverine, 453
Paradoxical intention, 387
Paralysis
  conversion, 411
  sleep, 486
Paranoia, 311
Paranoid personality disorder, 512t
  characteristic behaviors in, 512
  diagnostic criteria for, 513
  prevalence of, 512t
Paraphilia(s), 445, 454–457
  characteristic behaviors in, 454–456
  cognitive-behavior therapy for, 456–457

etiology of
  biological theories, 456
  learning theories, 456
  gender features of, 456
  interventions for clients in community, 456–457
  pharmacologic treatment of, 456–457
  prevalence of, 450
  prognosis of, 456
Paraphilia not otherwise specified, 456
Paraphrasing, 153
Parasomnia(s), 480, 487–488
  characteristic behaviors in, 481t, 487–488
  etiology of, 488
  prevalence of, 481t
  treatment of, 493–494
Parasomnia not otherwise specified, 480, 481t
Paraverbal cue, 53
Parietal lobe, 76, 76–77f, 78
Parkinson's disease, 79, 84t, 238–239, 245, 257, 265, 397t
  compared to Alzheimer's disease and AIDS-related dementia, 668–669
Parkinsonian symptom(s), 116, 332, 333t
Parkinsonism, drug-induced, 332f
Parnate. *See* Tranylcypromine
Paroxetine (Paxil), 101, 102t, 103, 126, 359, 360t, 395
Partial hospitalization, 645f
Pasmo, 38t
Patient record, computerized, 42
Pattern integration, in depression, 346
Pavlov, Ivan, 132, 132t
Paxil. *See* Paroxetine
Paxipam. *See* Halazepam
PDD. *See* Pervasive developmental disorder(s)
Pediatric autoimmune neuropsychiatric disorder (PANDAS), 395
Pedophilia, 454–456
Peer support group, 165–166
Pemoline (Cylert), 124, 124t, 361, 542, 545t
Pentazocine, 237t
Peplau, Hildegard, 4, 4t
Perception, 53
Perceptual-cognitive theory, of hypochondriasis, 417
Perdida del alma, 38t
Performance anxiety, 451
Perpetrator, 593
Perphenazine (Trilafon), 112t
Perseveration, 34t
Personality change(s)
  due to general medical condition, 263
  medication-related, 104
Personality disorder(s), 511–527
  case study of, 527
  client and family education in, 526
  cluster A (odd, eccentric), 512t
    care plan for, 515
    characteristic behaviors in, 511–514
    culture, age, and gender features of, 514
    diagnostic criteria for, 513
    etiology of, 514–515
    interventions for clients in community, 515–517
    interventions for hospitalized clients, 515

    pharmacologic treatment, 515–517
    prognosis of, 515
  cluster B (dramatic, emotional, erratic), 512t
    age and gender features of, 518–519
    characteristic behaviors in, 517–518
    cognitive-behavior therapy for, 521–522
    diagnostic criteria for, 516
    etiology of, 519–520
    interventions for clients in community, 521–523
    interventions for hospitalized clients, 520–521
    pharmacologic treatment of, 522–523, 523t
    prognosis of, 520
  cluster C (anxious, fearful), 512t
    characteristic behaviors in, 523–524
    culture and gender features of, 524–525
    diagnostic criteria for, 524
    etiology of, 525
    expected outcomes in, 525
    interventions for clients in community, 525
    pharmacologic treatment of, 525
    prognosis of, 525
  cognitive-behavior therapy for, 139t
  current research on, 526–527
  differential diagnosis of, 301–302, 336, 374, 396, 441, 525–526
  DSM-IV classification of, 12t, 658
  future research on, 527
  nursing diagnoses in, 526
  in offender population, 622
  prevalence of, 512t
Personality testing, 40–41t
Personality trait(s), with genetic contribution, 514, 514t
Personalization, 135
Pervasive developmental disorder(s) (PDD)
  attention-deficit/hyperactivity disorder and, 546
  differential diagnosis of, 336–337
PET. *See* Positron emission tomography
Pharmacodynamics, 94
Pharmacokinetics, 94. *See also* specific drugs
Pharmacologic challenge testing, 41t
Pharmacotherapy. *See* Psychopharmacology
Phase-advance theory, of depression, 351
Phase-advanced sleep pattern, 485, 485f
Phase-delay theory, of depression, 351
Phase-shift hypothesis, of phototherapy, 226
Phenelzine (Nardil), 96t
Phenergan. *See* Promethazine
Phentermine (Ionamin), 126
Phentolamine, 453
Phenylethanolamine-N-methyl transferase, 82
Phenytoin, 102t, 234
Pheochromocytoma, 397t
Phobia(s), 35, 35t, 68, 379, 387–389
  age and gender features of, 389
  case study of, 140
  characteristic behaviors in, 387–389
  cognitive-behavior therapy for, 389
  diagnostic criteria for, 388
  etiology of
    cognitive-behavior theories, 389
    genetic theories, 389

interventions for clients in community, 389
monosymptomatic, 140
pharmacologic therapy for, 389
simple, prevalence of, 380t
social. *See* Social phobia
Photoperiod effect, 226, 348
Photosensitivity, 116
Phototherapy, 87, 225–228, 225f
   adverse reactions to, 227
   for circadian rhythm sleep disorder, 493
   contraindications to, 227
   for depression, 361
   expected outcomes in, 228
   nursing considerations in, 227–228
   patient selection for, 227
   for seasonal affective disorder, 361
   theory of action of, 226–227
Physical abuse, 592, 595–596
Physical assessment, 29
Physical contact, between nurse and client, 49
Physical setting, for group therapy, 166–167
Physiological dependence, 282
Physiological theory
   of breathing-related sleep disorders, 486
   of narcolepsy, 487
Pia mater, 76
Piaget's cognitive theory, 67
Pibloktoq, 38t
Pick's disease, 238–239
Pimozide (Orap), 112t, 117
Pineal gland, 76f, 79, 83, 87, 87f
Pituitary disorder(s), 264t
Pituitary gland, 87–88, 88f
Plan of care. *See* Care plan
Plaque, in Alzheimer's disease, 246
Play therapy, 541, 541f
Polarized thinking, 135
Polysomnography, 41t, 488, 490t, 491f
Pondimin. *See* Fenfluramine
Pons, 76f
Porphyria, 397t
Positive reinforcer, 133
Positron emission tomography (PET), 41t, 85, 85t, 89
Postoperative client, 267
Postpartum depression, 346, 347t, 351
Posttraumatic stress disorder (PTSD), 379, 427–442, 520. *See also* Abuse
   attention-deficit/hyperactivity disorder and, 545–546
   care plan for, 435–436
   case study of, 442
   characteristic behaviors in, 428
   client and family education in, 440
   clinical management of, 437
   cognitive-behavior therapy for, 438
   culture, age, and gender features of, 434
   current research on, 441, 526
   dexamethasone suppression test in, 346, 347t, 434
   diagnostic criteria for, 429
   differential diagnosis of, 397, 440–441, 506
   etiology of
      endogenous opioid theory, 434
      neurodevelopmental and neurobiological theories, 434–435

      neuroendocrine theory, 434
      neuropharmacologic theories, 434
      repetition and family influences theory, 435
   expected outcomes in, 440
   future research on, 441
   hippocampal volume in, 435, 441
   hypnosis in, 439
   interventions in
      for clients in community, 436–440
      for hospitalized clients, 436
   neurotransmitters in, 80t, 82
   nursing diagnoses in, 441
   pharmacologic treatment of, 439–440
   prevalence of, 433
   prognosis of, 435
   risk factors for, 431–433
   therapeutic exposure in, 438–439
   traumatic events leading to, 428t
   treatment of, 80t
   veterans' reaction to Oklahoma City bombing, 439
Postviral infection syndrome, 373t
Potter Place, 569–570
Prazepam (Centrax), 121t
Precipitating event, in crisis, 149
Precontemplation, 285, 297
Precrisis state, 144
Prednisolone, 234
Prednisone, 234
Prefrontal leukotomy. *See* Psychosurgery
Pregnancy, pharmacotherapy during, 94–95
Pregroup meeting, 168
Preinteraction phase, of therapeutic relationship, 50
Premature discussion, 60t
Premature ejaculation, 446–447
   case study of, 458
   cognitive-behavior therapy for, 451
   diagnostic criteria for, 449
Preoccupation(s), assessment of, 34–35
Prescription drug(s). *See* Medication
Prescriptive authority, 19
Prescriptive practice, 19
Priapism, 105, 106t
Primary care nurse, 16
Primary gain, 404, 411
Primary hypersomnia, 480, 481t
   characteristic behaviors in, 486, 489t
   diagnostic criteria for, 482
   etiology of, 486
Primary insomnia, 480–481, 485–486
   characteristic behaviors in, 481t, 485, 489t
   diagnostic criteria for, 482
   etiology of, 485–486
   prevalence of, 481t
Primary mental health care, 15–16
Primary prevention, 17
Primidone, 234
Prison. *See* Offender population
Proband, 465
Problem solving, in family, 185
Problem statement, 29
Procainamide, 234
Procaine derivative, 268t
Procardia. *See* Nifedipine

Procedural touch, 53
Process recording, 55, 56–57t
Professional nursing organization(s), 647–648, 648t
Program director, 17–18
Progressive relaxation, 135, 136t, 382
Projection, 66t
Projective identification, 66, 66t
Prolactin, 480
Prolixin. *See* Fluphenazine
Prolonged mental illness, 533–572
   assessment of, 556–560
      access to health care, 559, 559t
      family system and social supports, 558–559
      health risk factors, 558
      history of illness, 558
      mental status examination, 558
      physical health, 557
      review of medication, 558
      subjective and objective data, 560
   care plan for, 562
   case management in, 567–568
   case study of, 572
   characteristics of, 553
   concept of recovery, 553–554
   continuous treatment teams in, 568
   costs of, 554–555
   decreased sense of control in, 560–561
   dilemmas experienced by clients, 560–561
   disenfranchisement and stigma in, 562–565
      anticipation and recreation, 564–565
      need to belong, 564
      strategies relevant to family, 563–564
   disillusionment with self and life in, 565–566
   disorganization of time and tasks in, 562
   educational opportunities and, 566–567, 567t
   employment and, 566–567, 567t
   environments in, 561–567
   evaluation of outcomes in, 571
   expected outcomes in, 560–561
   future research on, 571–572
   historical perspectives of, 554–556, 556t
   HIV disease in, 617
   among homeless, 554, 566–567, 578
   impact of, 554
   intervention strategies in, 560–561
   managed costs and rationed care, 554–556
   nursing considerations for, 553–554
   nursing diagnoses in, 560–561
   nursing process within systems concept, 556, 557f
   in offender population, 554, 566–567, 621–622
   open systems model within community, 556–557
   prevalence of, 554t
   prognosis of, 554, 555f
   psychiatric social club in, 569–571
   psychopharmacologic therapy for, 555–556
   psychosocial rehabilitation program in, 569–571, 570t
   residential care in, 568
   safety nets in, 561

Prolonged mental illness—Continued
  stressors and target symptoms in, 560–561
  support systems in, 558–559, 561–567
  treatment and rehabilitation in, 567–571
Promethazine (Phenergan), 268t
Pronoun(s), troublesome, 60t
Propranolol (Inderal), 102t, 108, 116t, 234, 237t
Protease inhibitor(s), 616–617
Protriptyline (Vivactil), 96t
Prozac. See Fluoxetine
Pseudocyesis, 422–423
Pseudodementia, 254
Pseudoephedrine, 268t
Psychiatric clinical nurse specialist, 16, 16t, 18, 647
Psychiatric consultation–liaison nurse, 18
Psychiatric disability, 567
Psychiatric home visit, 662–663
Psychiatric nurse practitioner, 16
Psychiatric social club, 569–571
Psychiatric-mental health nurse
  challenges for future, 647–648
  community-based education, 8–9
  consultation-liaison nurse, 18
  as counselor, 43
  definition of, 3
  director of therapeutic milieu, 17–18
  feelings which interfere with communication, 59
  future trends in nursing, 643–648
  generalist, 15–16, 15t, 646–647, 646t
  among homeless, 583–584
  influence of conceptual models of nursing on, 4–9, 4t
  leadership role of, 43
  as member of mental health team, 16–17
  in mental health promotion, 17
  nurse case manager, 17, 17t
  opportunities for, 645–647
  primary care nurse, 16
  professional organizations for, 647–648, 648t
  psychopharmacologist, 19
  psychotherapist, 18–19
  role in mental health care, 15–19
  specialist, 16, 16t, 18, 647
  teaching role of, 43
Psychoactive substance, 277
Psychoanalytic theory
  of depression, 351–352
  of development, 65–66
Psychoanalytic-developmental theory, of personality disorders, 515, 519–520, 525
Psychobiology, 5
Psychodynamic group therapy, 165
Psychodynamic-psychosexual model, of sexual therapy, 197
Psychoeducation, 526
Psychoeducational approach, to family therapy, 190
Psychological abuse, 593, 595
Psychological dependence, 285
Psychological testing, 40t
Psychological theory
  of body dysmorphic disorder, 421
  of hypochondriasis, 417
  of somatization disorder, 404

Psychology
  of men, 70
  of women, 68–70
Psychomotor retardation, 346
Psychoneuroimmunology, 87–89
  hypothalamic-pituitary-adrenal axis and, 87–88, 88f
  immune function and mental illness, 88–89, 89t
Psychopharmacologic agent(s), clinical management and, 665–667
Psychopharmacologist, nurse, 19
Psychopharmacology, 6, 9t, 93–127
  current research on, 126–127, 127t
  definition of, 93
  future research on, 127
Psychopharmacology guidelines, 664–667
Psychopharmacology Guidelines for Psychiatric Mental Health Nurses (ANA), 8, 9t
Psychosexual development, 65
Psychosis, 313
Psychosocial rehabilitation program
  in prolonged mental illness, 569–571, 570t
  in psychotic disorders, 334–335
Psychosocial stage(s), 66–67, 67t
Psychosocial theory, of somatization disorder, 404
Psychostimulant(s), 124–125
  adverse reactions to, 125
  for attention-deficit/hyperactivity disorder, 124, 542–543, 545t
  case study of, 125–126
  clinically significant interactions of, 125
  contraindications and precautions, 125
  current research on, 126
  for depression, 361
  drug holiday from, 125
  general information about, 124, 124t
  indications for, 124
  mechanism of action of, 125
  for narcolepsy, 494
  overprescription of, 124
  pharmacokinetics of, 124–125, 124t
Psychosurgery, 224–225
  adverse reactions to, 224–225
  contraindications to, 224
  expected outcomes in, 225
  nursing considerations in, 225
  for obsessive-compulsive disorder, 395–396
  patient selection for, 224, 224t
  theory of action of, 224
Psychotherapist, nurse, 18–19
Psychotherapy
  for abuse survivor, 601
  brief, 19
  historical aspects of, 6
Psychotherapy group, 165
  case study of, 163–164
Psychotic disorder(s), 307–338. See also Schizophrenia
  altered thought processes in, 324–325
  assessment of acute episodes, 319–325
  care plan in, 327
  case study of, 338
  client education in, 335
  current research on, 337
  diagnostic criteria for, 320–321

differential diagnosis of, 301, 336–337, 336t, 374, 440, 526, 547
DSM-IV classification of, 12t, 655
electroconvulsive therapy for, 334
expected outcomes in, 337
family education in, 335–336
future research on, 337–338
in HIV-positive client, 614
interventions in
  for clients in community, 330–336
  for hospitalized clients, 327–329, 329t
mental status examination in, 323–324
nursing diagnoses in, 337
nursing interventions in, 330–331
pharmacologic treatment of, 331–334
prevalence of, 324t
prognosis of, 319
providing structure for client, 329
psychosocial rehabilitation in, 334–335
rating scales for, 41
safety of client, 325t, 329, 329t
self-care deficits in, 325t
therapeutic communication in, 327–329, 329t
Psychotic disorder due to general medical condition, 262, 321
Psychotic symptom(s), medications that cause, 268t
Psychotropic medication(s)
  mechanism of action of, 111
  psychiatric effects of, 237t
PTSD. See Posttraumatic stress disorder
Public opinion/policy
  attitudes toward offender population, 630–631
  homelessness and, 577
Pulmonary hypertension, primary, 126
Punisher, 133
Punishment (behavioral therapy), 137
Putamen, 76f, 79
Pyridoxine, 100–101

Quazepam (Doral), 121t, 494t
Quetiapine (Seroquel), 112, 113t, 117, 126, 127t

Race, pharmacokinetics and, 94
Racing thoughts, 364
Racism, 33t
Radical behaviorism, 132–133, 132t
Ranitidine, 234
Rape, 16, 593
Rapid cycling bipolar disorder, 364, 370
Rapid eye movement sleep. See REM sleep
Rapprochement, 66
Rash, side effect of medication, 106t
Reaction formation, 66t
Reality orientation, 205, 251
Reality testing, 327
Reassurance, 60t
Rebound symptom(s), after discontinuing benzodiazepines, 122
Recall, general, 34
Receiver (element of communication), 53
Recent homelessness, 582–583

Receptor, 80–81, 80t
Recovery, concept of, 553–554
Recreational activity(ies), in prolonged mental illness, 564–565
Redux. See Dexfenfluramine
Reflective delay, 522
Refusal of treatment, 21
Reglan. See Metoclopramide
Regression, 65, 66t
Reinforcer, 132–133
  negative, 133
  positive, 133
Relational integrity, 185
Relaxation exercise(s), 135, 136t
Religion, 13, 37, 313
REM sleep, 228, 479–480, 479t, 496
Remeron. See Mirtazapine
Reminiscence, 203
  autobiography, 204
  informative, 203
  life review, 203–204
  oral history, 204
  reparative, 209
  retentive, 208–209
  simple, 203–204
  as social activity, 206
  types of, 203–204
  universality of, 206
Reminiscence therapy, 203–210
  assessment of client for, 206
  case study of, 210
  definition of, 204
  evaluating quality of reminiscences, 208, 208t
  expected outcomes in, 208–209, 209t
  future research on, 209
  group, 205–208
  increased self-esteem from, 209
  indications for, 205, 205f
  intervention strategies for, 207–208
  nurse's role in, 205–207, 205f
  purpose of, 204–205
  topics for, 206, 207t
Remotivation therapy, 205
  for dementia, 252–253
Remotivation therapy group, 163
Reparative reminiscence, 209
Repetition and family influences theory, of posttraumatic stress and dissociative disorders, 435
Repressed memory, 69, 597–598
Repression, 66t
Reserpine (Serpasil), 80, 237t, 267t, 373t
Residential care, 568, 645f
Resiliency, 432
Resistance to stressor, 143
Respiratory and carbon dioxide hypothesis, in panic disorder, 384t, 385–386
Respiratory disease, 397t
Response prevention, 138, 139t
Responsive phase, of group development, 171–172
Restless legs syndrome, 487
Restoril. See Temazepam
Restraint, 21
  guidelines for use of, 21, 22t
  indications for, 21, 21t

Restriction fragment length polymorphism(s) (RFLP), 41t
Retentive reminiscence, 208–209
Reticular formation, 76f
Retrograde amnesia, 223
Retrospective payment, 643
Reuptake of neurotransmitter, 81, 93, 95f, 111
Reversal (defense mechanism), 66t
ReVia. See Naltrexone
Revictimization, 435
Revolving door syndrome, 554
RFLP. See Restriction fragment length polymorphism(s)
Rhythm theory. See Biological rhythm theory
Risk-taking behavior, 241
Risperdal. See Risperidone
Risperidone (Risperdal), 80t, 102t, 112, 113t, 117, 253, 331t, 333, 337
Ritalin. See Methylphenidate
Ritonavir, 616
RNA, 86
Rogers, Martha, 4t
Role playing, 138
Rootwork, 38t
Rorschach, 41t
Roy, Calista, 4t
Runaway teen(s), 599

SAD. See Seasonal affective disorder
Safe drinking guideline(s), 295–296
Safety
  of abused client, 598
  of client with dementia, 251, 251t
SANE. See Sexual Assault Nurse Examiner
Saquinavir, 616
Schizoaffective disorder, 319
  course of, 324t
  diagnostic criteria for, 320
  pharmacologic treatment of, 334
  prevalence of, 324t
  symptoms of, 324t
Schizoid personality disorder, 512t
  characteristic behaviors in, 512
  diagnostic criteria for, 513
  prevalence of, 512t
Schizophrenia, 307–317. See also Psychotic disorder(s)
  active phase of, 311–312
  care plan in, 326–327
  case study of, 75, 120, 585
  catatonic type, 310, 312, 312t
  characteristic behaviors in, 308–313, 324t
  chronic, 338
  cognitive therapy for, 327
  concordance rates of, 86
  course of, 324t
  critical pathway for, 322–323
  cross-cultural diagnosis of, 43
  culture, age, and gender features of, 313
  diagnostic aids in, 313, 314t
  diagnostic criteria for, 310–311
  disorganized type, 310, 312, 312t
  dopamine receptors in, 82
  DSM-IV classification of, 12t, 655
  dual diagnosis, 318

  etiology of
    abnormalities in brain, 316–317f, 317
    environmental factors, 316–317
    genetic theory, 315–316, 337
    neurodevelopmental factors, 316–317, 316f
    neurophysiologic and neuropharmacologic theories, 313–315, 315f
    two-hit model, 315
  first-episode, 337–338
  formal thought disorder in, 308, 309t
  among homeless, 575
  milieu therapy for, 329
  negative symptoms in, 309, 309t
  neurotransmitters in, 80t, 82, 84t
  nursing diagnoses in, 326–327
  paranoid type, 310, 312, 312t
  pharmacologic treatment of, 331–334
  positive symptoms in, 308–309, 309t
  prevalence of, 324t, 554t
  prodromal phase of, 309, 325–327
  prognosis of, 317, 317t
  residual type, 311–312, 312t
  subtypes of, 312
  thalamus in, 79
  treatment of, 80t
  undifferentiated type, 310, 312, 312t
Schizophreniform disorder, 319
  course of, 324t
  diagnostic criteria for, 320
  pharmacologic treatment of, 334
  prevalence of, 324t
  symptoms of, 324t
Schizotypal personality disorder, 512t
  characteristic behaviors in, 514
  diagnostic criteria for, 513
  pharmacologic treatment of, 515–517
  prevalence of, 512t
Seasonal affective disorder (SAD), 87, 346, 348
  phototherapy for, 225–228, 361
Seclusion, 21
  guidelines for use of, 21, 22t
  indications for, 21, 21t
Secondary gain, 404
Secondary prevention, 17
Second-messenger system, 81
Security issue(s), in prison setting, 627–628
Sedative-hypnotic(s)
  abuse of, 283t
  adverse reactions to, 106t, 197t, 267–268t
  characteristics of, 121t
  current research on, 126
  general introduction to, 120–121
  nursing considerations for, 123–124
  for parasomnias, 493–494, 494t
  pharmacologic treatment of dependence on, 300
  psychiatric effects of, 237t
  withdrawal symptoms and nursing actions, 293t, 295
Seizure disorder, 265–266
Selective serotonin reuptake inhibitor(s) (SSRI), 96, 96t, 359, 360t
  adverse reactions to, 96t, 102–103
  case study of, 106–107
  clinically significant interactions of, 103–104, 122–123

Selective serotonin reuptake inhibitor(s) (SSRI)—Continued
  contraindications and precautions, 102
  indications for, 101
  mechanism of action of, 81, 101–102, 103f, 350, 350f, 360f
  for panic disorder, 386
  pharmacokinetics of, 101
  sexual dysfunction related to, 101–102
Selegiline (Eldepryl), 96t, 99, 257
Self-control training, in substance-related disorders, 295
Self-determination, 21
Self-disclosure, 47
  by nurse, 49
  therapeutic, 625–626
Self-esteem
  decrease in depression, 358
  effect of reminiscence therapy on, 209
Self-evaluation, in reminiscence therapy, 205
Self-help group(s), 165–166
  for client with dual diagnosis, 318
  in substance-related disorders, 296, 296–297t
Self-in-relation theory, 68–70
Self-statement training, 382
Self-talk, 53, 59, 134
Self-understanding, 209t
Sender (element of communication), 53
Sensate focus, 197, 199t, 451
Sensory deprivation, in critical care unit psychosis, 272
Sensory impairment, 254
Sensory overload, in critical care unit psychosis, 272
Separation-individuation, 65–66
Sequencing of normal activities, 34
Serax. *See* Oxazepam
Serentil. *See* Mesoridazine
Serlect. *See* Sertindole
Seroquel. *See* Quetiapine
Serotonin, 80, 80t, 82–83, 84t, 87, 93–94, 94t, 111, 313, 350–351, 359, 361, 374–375, 398, 434, 457, 464–465, 464t, 536
  in obsessive-compulsive disorder, 393
Serotonin receptor, 80t, 83, 315, 315f
Serotonin syndrome, 101, 105
Serotonin theory
  of Alzheimer's disease, 248–249
  of panic disorder, 386
Serpasil. *See* Reserpine
Sertindole (Serlect), 112, 113t, 117, 126, 331t, 333, 337
Sertraline (Zoloft), 80t, 96t, 101, 102t, 254, 359, 360t, 395
Serzone. *See* Nefazodone
Severely and persistently mentally ill, HIV disease in, 617
Sex offender, 456–457, 630
Sexism, 33t
Sexual abuse, 592–593, 595
  adult recall of childhood abuse, 69
  in prisons, 628
Sexual addiction, 456
Sexual arousal, 196

Sexual arousal disorder(s), 447
  cognitive-behavior therapy for, 451
  pharmacologic interventions in, 453
Sexual assault, 593
Sexual Assault Nurse Examiner (SANE), 16
Sexual aversion disorder(s), 446–447
Sexual desire, 196
Sexual desire disorder(s), 446–447
Sexual disorder(s), 445–458
Sexual disorder not otherwise specified, 445
Sexual dysfunction(s), 196, 445–453
  assessment of, 446
  beginning symptoms of, 446
  care plan for, 451
  case study of, 458
  characteristic behaviors in, 446–449
  client and family education in, 457
  clinical management of, 445
  cognitive-behavior therapy for, 451
  couples therapy for, 451–453
  culture, age, and gender features of, 449–450
  current research on, 457
  DSM-IV classification of, 12t, 656–657
  etiology of
    biological theories, 450
    multicausal theories, 450–451
  expected outcomes in, 457
  further research on, 457–458
  interventions for clients in community, 451–453
  medical conditions associated with, 450
  medications that lead to, 106t, 197t, 451, 457
  nursing diagnoses in, 457
  pharmacologic interventions in, 453
  prevalence of, 450
  prognosis of, 451
  sexual therapy for, 451–453
  SSRI-related, 101–102
Sexual dysfunction due to medical condition, 452
Sexual functioning
  assessment of, 195, 196t, 198t
  healthy, 195
  normal, 445–446
  nurse's reactions to, 195
Sexual harassment, 593
Sexual Interaction Inventory, 195
Sexual interview, 195, 196t
Sexual masochism, 454–456
Sexual Opinion Survey, 195
Sexual pain disorder(s), 449, 451
Sexual response cycle, 445–446
Sexual sadism, 454–456
Sexual task(s), 197, 200
Sexual therapy, 195–200
  for abuse survivor, 601
  case study of, 199–200
  cognitive-behavioral model of, 197, 199t
  current research on, 199
  expected outcomes in, 198–199
  future research on, 199
  nurse's role in, 195–196
  psychodynamic and psychosexual model of, 197
  purpose of, 195

  referral for, 196
  for sexual dysfunction, 451–453
  systems model of, 197–198
Shaping, 137, 139t
Shared psychotic disorder, 321
Shenjing, 38t
Shift work, 481t, 487
Shin-byung, 38t
Short Michigan Alcoholism Screening Test (SMAST), 289, 289t
Short sleeper, 480
Short-term memory, 34
Shuairuo, 38t
Sibutramine (Meridia), 126
Sign, 43
Simple phobia, cognitive-behavior therapy for, 139t
Simple reminiscence, 203–204
Sinequan. *See* Doxepin
Single photon emission computed tomography (SPECT), 41t, 85, 85t
Situational crisis, 146
Skinner, B.F., 132, 132t
Sleep apnea, 486, 492–493, 493f, 497–498
"Sleep attack." *See* Narcolepsy
Sleep deprivation, 228
  in critical care unit psychosis, 272
Sleep deprivation therapy, 228
  contraindications to, 228
  expected outcomes in, 228
  nursing considerations in, 228
  patient selection for, 228
  theory of action of, 228
Sleep diary, 490t, 494, 495t
Sleep disorder(s), 479–498
  assessment of, 488, 490t, 491f
  behavioral therapy for, 492
  care plan for, 488
  case study of, 497–498
  characteristic behaviors in, 481t
  client and family education in, 494
  clinical management of, 497
  culture, age, and gender features of, 481–485
  current research on, 496–497
  differential diagnosis of, 495–496
  distinguishing among, 488, 489t
  DSM-IV classification of, 12t, 657–658
  expected outcomes in, 494–495
  future research on, 497
  interventions in
    for clients in community, 490–494
    for hospitalized clients, 488–489
  normal sleep-wake patterns, 479–481, 479t, 480f
  nursing diagnoses in, 496
  overlap with psychiatric disorders, 496
  prevalence of, 481t
  primary, 480, 481t
  prognosis of, 488
  secondary, 480
Sleep disorder due to general medical condition, 484, 495–496, 496t
Sleep disorder due to medical and psychiatric disorders, 488
"Sleep drunkenness," 486
Sleep hygiene, 490, 494, 495t

Sleep paralysis, 486
Sleep restriction, 228
Sleep terror disorder, 480, 487–488, 489t
　characteristic behaviors in, 481t
　diagnostic criteria for, 483
Sleep-wake pattern, normal, 479–481, 479t, 480f
Sleepwalking disorder, 480, 487–488, 489t
　characteristic behaviors in, 481t
　diagnostic criteria for, 483
　prevalence of, 481t
Small group communication, 53
SMAST. *See* Short Michigan Alcoholism Screening Test
Snoring, 486
Snow phobia, 140
Social distress theory, of homelessness, 581–582
Social encounter, between nurse and client, 50
Social factor(s), in family assessment, 182
Social learning, 161
Social phobia, 387–389, 472
　cognitive-behavior therapy for, 139t
　diagnostic criteria for, 388
　prevalence of, 380t
Social relationship, 47–48
　between nurse and client, 50
Social skills training, 138, 139t, 165
　board game, 628f
　in substance-abuse disorders, 295
Social support, in prolonged mental illness, 558–559
Socialization, in psychotic disorders, 330
Socializing technique, development of, 161
Sociocultural assessment, in crisis, 150–151
Sociocultural crisis, 148–149
Sociocultural factor(s), in hypochondriasis, 417–418
Sociocultural theory, of pain disorder, 414–415
Sociological variable(s), assessment of, 37
"Soft signs," 313
Somatic delusion, 35t
Somatization
　definition of, 403–404
　as trauma response, 595
Somatization disorder, 403–411
　assessment of, 408–409
　care plan for, 409
　case study of, 411
　characteristic behaviors in, 404
　cultural and gender features of, 406t
　diagnostic criteria for, 405t, 407
　differential diagnosis of, 410–411
　etiology of
　　adaptation theory, 404
　　cognitive-perceptual theory, 407–408
　　multifactorial theory, 408
　　neurobiological theories, 404
　　psychological and psychosocial theories, 404
　expected outcomes in, 410
　familial patterns of, 406t
　gender features of, 404
　interventions in
　　for clients in community, 409
　　for hospitalized clients, 409, 410t
　prevalence of, 405t
　prognosis of, 408
Somatoform, definition of, 403
Somatoform disorder(s), 403–424
　clinical management of, 424
　cultural and gender features of, 406t
　current research on, 423–424
　diagnostic criteria for, 405t
　DSM-IV classification of, 12t, 656
　familial patterns of, 406t
　future research on, 424
　nursing diagnoses in, 423
　prevalence of, 405t
Somatoform disorder not otherwise specified, 422–423
　cultural and gender features of, 406t
　diagnostic criteria for, 405t, 423
　expected outcomes in, 423
　prevalence of, 405t
Somatosensory amplification, 407
Somatostatin, 84t
Sorrow, chronic, 554, 565
South American(s), culture-bound syndromes among, 38t
Space, effect on communication, 54
Spanish culture, culture-bound syndromes in, 38t
Specific phobia, 388
SPECT. *See* Single photon emission computed tomography
Speech, assessment of, 33–34, 34t
Spirit possession, 38t
Spiritual need, 37
Spirituality, 10–13
Splitting, 66t, 71, 517
Squeeze technique, 199t
SSRI. *See* Selective serotonin reuptake inhibitor(s)
Standards of care (ANA), 15, 15t
Startle response, 428
State amplification, 408
Statement on Psychiatric–Mental Health Clinical Nursing Practice (ANA), 3
Static security system, 627
Stelazine. *See* Trifluoperazine
Steroid(s), psychiatric effects of, 234, 237t
Steroid psychosis, 373t
Stigma, in prolonged mental illness, 562–565
Stimulant(s)
　pharmacologic treatment of withdrawal, 301
　withdrawal symptoms and nursing actions, 293t, 295
Storytelling, 203
Storytelling group therapy, 163
Strengths of client, assessment of, 37
Streptococcal infection, obsessive-compulsive disorder and, 395
Stress, 427–428
　general adaptation syndrome, 143
Stress management, in substance-related disorders, 296
Stress management group, 165
Stress response
　hypothalamic-pituitary-adrenal axis in, 87–88
　immune function and, 88–89, 89t
Stress-adaptation theory, of adjustment disorders, 503
Stroke, 244
Structural family therapy, 187t, 189
Structural mapping, 181–182, 183f
Structure, as function of milieu, 213–214, 214t
Structured lifestyle, for client with dementia, 251–252
Subcaudate tractotomy, 224
Sublimation, 66t
Substance abuse, 277–282. *See also* Substance-related disorder(s)
　diagnostic criteria for, 280
　percentages of Americans with, 10f
　prevalence of, 281
　among women in homeless shelter, 7
Substance dependence, 282
　diagnostic criteria for, 280
　long-term, 297–298, 297t
Substance intoxication, 278, 282, 283t. *See also* Substance-related disorder(s)
　acute intoxication, 292
　diagnostic criteria for, 282
Substance intoxication delirium, 236
Substance P, 83, 84t
Substance withdrawal, 278, 282. *See also* Substance-related disorder(s)
　acute, 292–295, 295–296t
　diagnostic criteria for, 282
　symptoms and nursing actions, 293t
Substance withdrawal delirium, 236
Substance-induced organic mental disorder, 279t
Substance-induced persisting amnestic disorder, 255
Substance-induced persisting dementia, 239
Substance-induced psychotic disorder, 321
Substance-induced sexual dysfunction, 452
Substance-induced sleep disorder, 484, 496
Substance-related disorder(s), 277–303
　alcohol abuse. *See* Alcohol abuse
　assessment of, 288–289
　brief interventions in, 295
　care plan in, 291–292
　case study of, 302–303
　characteristic behaviors in, 278
　cognitive-behavior therapy for, 295–296
　common drugs of abuse, 283t
　conditions causing anxiety, 397t
　costs of, 11f, 277, 278f
　culture, age, and gender features of, 284–285
　definition of, 277–278
　diagnostic criteria for, 280
　differential diagnosis of, 254–255, 301–302, 336, 374, 396, 441, 526
　DSM-IV classification of, 12t, 653–655
　dual diagnosis, 318
　etiology of
　　behavioral theories, 286–287
　　biological theories, 285–286
　　genetic theories, 286
　　imaging studies, 286, 286f
　expected outcomes in, 301
　family and significant others and, 290
　family interventions in, 298–299
　future research on, 302
　HIV disease and, 618
　in homeless population, 580

Substance-related disorder(s)—Continued
  interventions in
    for clients in community, 295–297
    for hospitalized clients, 292–295
  intoxication and withdrawal, 282
  laboratory findings in, 290–291, 291t
  long-term substance dependence, 297–298, 297t
  mental status examination in, 290
  nursing diagnoses in, 302
  in offender population, 622
  with other mental disorders, 288, 288f
  pharmacologic treatment of, 299–301, 299t
  physical findings in, 290
  prevalence of, 281
  prognosis of, 287–288
  rating scales for, 41
  screening tools for, 289–290, 289–290t
  self-help groups in, 296, 296–297t
  short alcohol and drug history, 289
  stages of behavior change and interventions, 297–298, 298t
  stress management in, 296
  substances with potential for abuse, 278–279
Substantia nigra, 79
Suicidal ideation, 36, 216, 353
  medication-related, 102–103, 106
Suicidal potential
  assessment of, 35–37, 37t, 353
  case study of, 44
  for HIV-positive clients, 609
Suicide
  death rates due to, 352f
  in elderly, 72
  in offender population, 628–629, 628f
  risk factors for, 349–350
Suicide plan, 36, 353
Suicide prevention, 153
Sulcus, 76
Sulfonamide(s), 267–268t
Sulfonylurea, 237t
Sulindac, 234
Sundowning, 241, 242t
Superego, 65
Support
  as function of milieu, 213–214, 214t
  in prolonged mental illness, 558–559, 561–567
Supported apartment program, 568
Suprachiasmatic nucleus, 87, 87f
Surmontil. See Trimipramine
Survivorship, 594
Susto, 38t
Symbiosis, 66
Symmetrical relationship, 185
Symptom, 43
Synapse, 80
Systematic desensitization, 136–140, 136t, 139t, 387, 451
Systemic and strategic family therapy, 187t, 189–190
Systems model, of sexual therapy, 197–198

Tacrine, 80t, 248, 253
Talisman, 12

Tamoxifen (Nolvadex), 267–268t
Tangential thought process, 34t
Tangentiality of speech, 311
Tangle(s), 246
Taractan. See Chlorprothixene
Tarasoff case, 20
Tardive dyskinesia, 117–118, 333t
TAT. See Thematic Apperception Test
Tau protein, 257
Taurine, 84
Teaching and behavioral change group, 165
Tegretol. See Carbamazepine
Telephone counseling, 153
Temazepam (Restoril), 121t, 494t
Temporal lobe, 76, 76–77f, 78
Tenderness, 52
Tenex. See Guanfacine
Tenormin. See Atenolol
Termination phase
  of group development, 173
  of therapeutic relationship, 51
Tertiary prevention, 17
TGIF. See Therapeutic Group Interaction Factors Scale
Thalamus, 76f, 79
Thematic Apperception Test (TAT), 41t
Theophylline, 102t
Therapeutic communication
  active listening, 54
  barriers to, 55–60
  case study of, 59–60
  objectivity in, 54
  in psychotic disorders, 327–329, 329t
  techniques of, 55, 56–57t, 58
    allowing client to begin conversation, 58
    conveying recognition to client, 58
    focusing on client's feelings, 58
    promoting thinking, 58
    with prompting quality, 58
    responding to leads from client, 58
    unhelpful techniques, 59, 60t
  types of, 54–55
Therapeutic community, 213, 214t
Therapeutic community residence, 568
Therapeutic exposure
  in dissociative disorders, 438–439
  in posttraumatic stress disorder, 438–439
Therapeutic Group Interaction Factors Scale (TGIF), 162
Therapeutic milieu, 624
  director or manager of, 17–18
Therapeutic privilege, 21
Therapeutic relationship, 47–52
  boundaries of, 48–50
    with children, 50
    decision making about, 50
    establishment of, 49–50
  defining parameters of, 49
  definition of, 47
  elements of, 47, 48t
  guidelines for conducting, 51–52
  nurse's reaction to clients' behavior, 48, 49t
  phases of
    orientation phase, 50
    preinteraction phase, 50

    termination phase, 51
    working phase, 50–51
  social relationship vs., 47–48
Therapeutic window, 97
Thiazide diuretic(s), 234
Thiorazine. See Chlorpromazine
Thioridazine (Mellaril), 112t, 116–117, 237t
Thiothixene (Navane), 112t, 237t, 515
Thought blocking, 34t
Thought content, assessment of, 34–35
Thought disorder, 308
Thought pattern(s), impaired, 35t
Three-quarter way house, 568
Thyroid hormone(s), 267–268t
Thyroiditis, 397t
Thyroid-stimulating hormone, 351
Thyrotoxicosis, 397t
Tic disorder, 81, 547
Time, effect on communication, 54, 59
Time-management strategy(ies), for attention-deficit/hyperactivity disorder, 542, 544t
Tofranil. See Imipramine
Token economy program, 137, 139t
Tolerance, 282
Touch, 53
  in therapeutic relationship, 625
Tourette's syndrome, 496t, 537t
Toxicology testing, 290–291, 291t
Trait amplification, 408
Transaction(s), among family members, 184
Transdermal nicotine (Nicotrol), 299t
Transference, 40
Transitional employment position, 570
Transitional object, 66
Transsexual, 453
Transsexualism. See Gender identity disorder
Transvestic fetishism, 453–456
Tranxene. See Clorazepate
Tranylcypromine (Parnate), 96t
Trauma, 428
  attention-deficit/hyperactivity disorder and, 545–546
  effect on development, 71
  intrusive, 596
  repetition of, 71
Trauma response(s), 594–595
Trauma theory, of personality disorders, 520
Trazodone (Desyrel), 96t, 100, 104–105, 234, 254, 360t
Tremor, side effect of medication, 106t
Triangulation, 185
Triazolam (Halcion), 102t, 121t, 122, 234, 256, 494t
Tricyclic antidepressant(s), 359
  adverse reactions to, 96t, 97–99, 237t
  clinically significant interactions of, 99
  contraindications and precautions, 97
  indications for, 96
  mechanism of action of, 81, 97, 98f
  pharmacokinetics of, 96–97, 96t
  therapeutic blood levels and monitoring of, 97
Trifluoperazine (Stelazine), 112t
Trihexyphenidyl (Artane), 116t
Trilafon. See Perphenazine

Trimethoprim/sulfamethoxazole (Bactrim), 267–268t
Trimipramine (Surmontil), 96t, 98
Tripa ida, 38t
Trisomy 21, 86
Trust
  within family, 185
  in therapeutic relationship, 47, 48t, 50–51
Tryptophan, 80, 375, 464
Tuberoinfundibular pathway, 332f
Twelve-step program(s), 296
Twin study(ies), 86
Tyramine, 100
Tyrosine hydroxylase, 82

Ultraradian rhythm, 87
Unconditional positive regard, 47, 48t
Unconscious mind, 65
Undifferentiated somatoform disorder, 411
  cultural and gender features of, 406t
  diagnostic criteria for, 405t, 407
  prevalence of, 405t
Undoing, 66t
Uninhibited behavior, 241
Unipolar depression, 350
Universality, 161, 209t
Unresolved grief, 637, 639

Vaginismus, 446, 449
Validation, as function of milieu, 213–214, 214t
Validation therapy, for dementia, 252
Valium. *See* Diazepam
Valproic acid (Depakote), 107, 370–371, 370t
  adverse reactions to, 110
  clinically significant interactions of, 99, 108t, 110
  indications for, 110
  mechanism of action of, 110
  pharmacokinetics of, 110
Vanlafaxine, 100t
Vascular dementia, 238, 244

Vascular disease, mental status changes due to, 265
Vasoactive intestinal peptide (VIP), 83
Vasopressin, 84t
Venlafaxine (Effexor), 96t, 104–105, 126, 359, 360t
Ventricle, 76
Verapamil (Isoptin), 370t, 371
Verbal message, 53
Versed. *See* Midazolam
Vesicle, 80
Victim-blaming, 582
Victimization
  direct, 593–594
  indirect, 594
Vigilance "A" Test, 235
Violence, 591. *See also* Abuse
  assessment of violence potential, 37, 37t
  dating, 538
  in environment, 594
  in home, 593–594
  in prisons, 628
VIP. *See* Vasoactive intestinal peptide
Viral load, 606
Vision disturbance, side effect of medication, 106t
Visual channel, 53
Visual hallucination, 311
Vivactil. *See* Protriptyline
Vomiting, side effect of medication, 106t
Voodoo, 38t
Voyeurism, 454–456

WAIS-R. *See* Wechsler Adult Intelligence Scale-Revised
Warfarin, 102t
Watson, J.B., 132, 132t
Wechsler Adult Intelligence Scale-Revised (WAIS-R), 40t
Wechsler Intelligence Scale for Children (WISC), 40t
Wechsler Preschool and Primary Scale of Intelligence (WPPSI), 40t

Weight gain, side effect of medication, 106t
Wellbutrin. *See* Bupropion
White matter, 80
"Why" question, 60t
WISC. *See* Wechsler Intelligence Scale for Children
Witchcraft, 38t
Withdrawal. *See* Substance withdrawal
Woman
  HIV disease and, 617–618
  homeless, 578–579, 585–586
  memories of childhood sexual abuse, 69
  psychology of women, 68–70
Word finding, 33
Word salad, 33, 34t, 312
Work group, 173
Working phase, of therapeutic relationship, 50–51
Worried well, 608
WPPSI. *See* Wechsler Preschool and Primary Scale of Intelligence

Xanax. *See* Alprazolam
Xenical. *See* Orlistat
Xenophobia, 33t

Yale-Brown Obsession Compulsion Scale (YBOCS), 392
YBOCS. *See* Yale-Brown Obsession Compulsion Scale
Yohimbine, 99, 102, 457

Zidovudine (AZT), 268t, 613
Ziprasidone, 127t
Zoloft. *See* Sertraline
Zolpidem (Ambien), 121–122, 121t, 254, 494t
Zovirax. *See* Acyclovir
Zung Rating Scale, 348, 349t
Zyprexa. *See* Olanzapine